PRIMARY CARE OF THE

CHILD *with a*
CHRONIC CONDITION

PRIMARY CARE OF THE

CHILD *with a*

CHRONIC CONDITION

THIRD EDITION

Patricia Ludder Jackson, RN, MS, PNP, FAAN

Clinical Professor,
Director, Advanced Practice Pediatric Nursing Program
Department of Family Health Care Nursing
University of California, San Francisco
San Francisco, California

Judith A. Vessey, PhD, RN, DPNP, FAAN

Professor
Johns Hopkins University
School of Nursing
Baltimore, Maryland

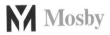 Mosby

A *Harcourt Health Sciences Company*
St. Louis   Philadelphia   London   Sydney   Toronto

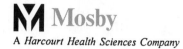

A *Harcourt Health Sciences Company*

Editor-in-Chief: Sally Schrefer
Executive Editor: Barbara Nelson Cullen
Senior Developmental Editor: Sandra Clark Brown
Project Manager: Dana Peick
Production Editor: Jodi Everding
Designer: Amy Buxton

THIRD EDITION
Copyright © 2000 by Mosby, Inc.

Previous editions copyrighted 1992, 1996

NOTICE
Pharmacology is an ever-changing field. Standard safety precautions must be followed, but as new research and clinical experience broaden our knowledge, changes in treatment and drug therapy may become necessary or appropriate. Readers are advised to check the most current product information provided by the manufacturer of each drug to be administered to verify the recommended dose, the method and duration of administration, and contraindications. It is the responsibility of the appropriately licensed health care provider, relying on experience and knowledge of the patient, to determine dosages and the best treatment for each individual patient. Neither the publisher nor the editor assumes any liability for any injury and/or damage to persons or property arising from this publication.

Mosby, Inc.
A Harcourt Health Sciences Company
11830 Westline Industrial Drive
St. Louis, Missouri 63146

Printed in the United States of America

ISBN 0-323-00883-6

00 01 02 03 CL/FF 9 8 7 6 5 4 3 2

To Heather, may she soar with eagles

To Robert, may his recent triumphs make him reach for the stars

To Scott, may his adolescent years be safe and full of wonder

And to Bruce and Dad, may their memory continue to warm my heart and guide my way

P.L.J.

To my parents, with love and affection

J.A.V.

Contributors

Elizabeth A. Boland, MSN, APRN, PNP, CDE
Pediatric Nurse Practitioner,
Yale New Haven Children's Hospital,
New Haven, Connecticut
Chapter 19 **Diabetes Mellitus (Type I)**

Elena Bosque, RNC, NNP, PhD
formerly Neonatal Research Practitioner/Research
  Associate,
Newborn Services,
California Pacific Medical Center,
San Francisco, California
Chapter 32 **Prematurity**

Barbara A. Carroll, MN, RN, CPNP
Clinical Nurse Specialist-Pediatric Hematology,
Palmetto Richland Memorial Hospital,
Columbia, South Carolina
Chapter 35 **Sickle Cell Disease**

Elizabeth H. Cook, MS, RN, CS, PNP
Assistant Clinical Professor,
Department of Family Health Care Nursing,
University of California, San Francisco,
San Francisco, California
Chapter 17 **Congenital Heart Disease**

Beverly Corbo-Richert, PhD, RN, CRNP
Lecturer,
West Virginia University School of Nursing,
Morgantown, West Virginia;
Adjunct Assistant Professor,
University of Pittsburgh School of Nursing,
Pittsburgh, Pennsylvania
Chapter 30 **Organ Transplants**

Ann W. Cox, PhD, MN
Director of Preservice Training,
Virginia Institute for Developmental Disabilities;
Assistant Professor of Education and Nursing,
Virginia Commonwealth University,
Richmond, Virginia
Chapter 8 **Transition to Adulthood**

Ginny Curtin, MS, RNC, PNP
Clinical Nurse Specialist,
Craniofacial Center,
Children's Hospital Oakland,
Oakland, California
Chapter 15 **Cleft Lip and Palate**

Mary Alice Dragone, MS, RN, CS, PNP
Pediatric Oncology Clinical Consultant,
The Degge Group, Ltd.,
Arlington, Virginia
Chapter 13 **Cancer**

Mary Jo Dunleavy, BSN, RN
Coordinator, Myelodysplasia Program,
Children's Hospital,
Boston, Massachusetts
Chapter 29 **Myelodysplasia**

Rita Fahrner, RN, MS, PNP
Assistant Clinical Professor, Department
  of Physiological Nursing,
University of California, San Francisco;
Coordinator, Occupational Infectious Diseases
  Program,
San Francisco General Hospital,
San Francisco, California
Chapter 24 **HIV Infection and AIDS**

Judith A. Farley, MSN, RN, CNRN
Director of Nursing and Patient Services,
Neuroscience Program,
Children's Hospital,
Boston, Massachusetts
Chapter 21 **Epilepsy**
Chapter 29 **Myelodysplasia**

Betty M. Flores, RN, MS, PNP, CDE
Pediatric Nurse Practitioner,
Department of Endocrinology,
Children's Hospital Oakland,
Oakland, California
Chapter 16 **Congenital Adrenal Hyperplasia**

Margaret Grey, DrPH, FAAN, CPNP
Independence Foundation Professor of Nursing,
Associate Dean for Research Affairs,
Yale University School of Nursing,
New Haven, Connecticut
Chapter 19 **Diabetes Mellitus (Type I)**

Randi J. Hagerman, MD
Professor of Pediatrics,
Section Head of Developmental and Behavioral
  Pediatrics,
University of Colorado Health Sciences Center
and Child Development Unit,
The Childrens Hospital,
Denver, Colorado
Chapter 22 **Fragile X Syndrome**

Joyce Harvey, RNC, PNP
Nurse Practitioner,
Pediatric Rehabilitation,
Oakland Children's Hospital,
Oakland, California
Chapter 25 **Hydrocephalus**

Kayla Harvey, RN, MS, PNP
Pediatric Pulmonary and Cystic Fibrosis Center,
Children's Hospital Oakland,
Oakland, California;
California Pacific Medical Center,
San Francisco, California
Chapter 12 **Bronchopulmonary Dysplasia**

Sarah S. Higgins, PhD, RN, FAAN
Associate Professor,
University of California, San Francisco,
San Francisco, California
Chapter 17 **Congenital Heart Disease**

Toshiko Hirata, BS, MD
Clinical Professor of Pediatrics and Medical
  Director,
University of California, San Francisco,
Whitney High Risk Infant Follow-Up Clinic,
California Pacific Medical Center,
San Francisco, California
Chapter 32 **Prematurity**

Patricia Ludder Jackson, RN, MS, PNP
Clinical Professor,
Director, Advanced Practice Pediatric Nursing
  Program,
Department of Family Health Care Nursing,
University of California, San Francisco,
San Francisco, California
Chapter 1 **The Primary Care Provider and
  Children with Chronic Conditions**
Chapter 5 **School and the Child with a Chronic
  Condition**
Chapter 25 **Hydrocephalus**

Susan Karp, RN, MS
Nurse Coordinator, Hemophilia Program,
University of California, San Francisco,
San Francisco, California
Chapter 11 **Bleeding Disorders**

Gail Kieckhefer, PhD, ARNP
Associate Professor,
University of Washington,
Seattle, Washington
Chapter 9 **Asthma**

Elizabeth A. Kuehne, PNP, MSN
Pediatric Nurse Practitioner,
Children's Aid and Family Services, Inc.,
Paramus, New Jersey
Chapter 33 **Prenatal Cocaine Exposure**

Carole Low, RN, MS, CPNP†
Clinical Neurology Clinical Nurse Specialist,
Nurse Practitioner,
University of California, Davis,
Medical Center,
Sacramento, California
Chapter 23 **Head Injury**

Margaret M. Mahon, PhD, RN, CPNP
Advanced Practice Nurse,
Hospital of the University of Pennsylvania,
Philadelphia, Pennsylvania
Chapter 3 **Chronic Conditions and the Family**

Estrella B. Manio, MS, PNP, RN
Pediatric Nurse Practitioner,
University of California, San Francisco,
San Francisco, California
Chapter 24 **HIV Infection and AIDS**

Marion McEwan, BSN, MS
Staff Nurse III,
Children's Hospital,
Boston, Massachusetts
Chapter 21 **Epilepsy**

Gail McIlvain-Simpson, MSN, RN, CS
Advanced Practice Nurse-Pediatric Rheumatology,
Alfred I. DuPont Hospital for Children,
Wilmington, Delaware
Chapter 27 **Juvenile Rheumatoid Arthritis**

Ann Hix McMullen, MS, CPNP
Senior Advanced Practice Nurse,
University of Rochester Medical Center,
Rochester, New York
Chapter 18 **Cystic Fibrosis**

Dionne J. Mebane, BSN, RN, MSN
Johns Hopkins University,
Baltimore, Maryland
Chapter 2 **Chronic Conditions and Child
Development**

Stephanie G. Metzger, MS, RN, CS, PNP
Advanced Practice Nurse,
Children's Hospital,
Clinical Faculty, School of Nursing,
Virginia Commonwealth University,
Richmond, Virginia
Chapter 8 **Transition to Adulthood**

Patricia A. Murphy RN, MS, PNP
Pediatric Neurosurgery Nurse Practitioner,
Department of Neurosurgery,
UCSF Stanford Health Care,
Palo Alto, California
Chapter 23 **Head Injury**

Wendy M. Nehring, RN, PhD
Associate Professor,
Southern Illinois University Edwardsville,
School of Nursing,
Edwardsville, Illinois
Chapter 14 **Cerebral Palsy**
Chapter 20 **Down Syndrome**

Beverly Kosmach Park, MSN, CRNP
Clinical Nurse Specialist,
Starzl Transplantation Institute,
Children's Hospital of Pittsburgh,
Pittsburgh, Pennsylvania
Chapter 30 **Organ Transplants**

Nancy Pike, RN, MN, FNP, CCRN
Nurse Practitioner,
Lucile Salter Packard Children's Hospital at
  Stanford,
Stanford University Medical Center,
Stanford, California
Chapter 30 **Organ Transplants**

Veronica Perrone Pollack, MSN, RN
Doctoral Student,
University of Michigan,
Ann Arbor, Michigan
Chapter 26 **Inflammatory Bowel Disease**

†Deceased.

Marijo Ratcliffe, RN, MN, PNP
Pediatric Pulmonary CNS,
Children's Hospital and Regional Medical Center,
Seattle, Washington
Chapter 9 Asthma

Anne DelSanto Ravenscroft, MSN, PNP
Pediatric Nurse Practitioner,
Division of Pediatric Gastroenterology
    and Nutrition,
Rhode Island Hospital,
Providence, Rhode Island
Chapter 26 Inflammatory Bowel Disease

Roberta S. Rehm, RN, PhD
Assistant Professor,
College of Nursing,
University of New Mexico,
Albuquerque, New Mexico
Chapter 4 Family Culture and Chronic Conditions

Marianne Warguska Reilly, BSN, MSN
PNP Pediatric OPD,
Holy Name Hospital,
Teaneck, New Jersey
Chapter 33 Prenatal Cocaine Exposure

Judith A. Ruble, MS, RN, CPNP
Medical Analyst,
Crosby, Heafey, Roach and May,
Oakland, California
Chapter 16 Congenital Adrenal Hyperplasia

Cindy Hylton Rushton, DNSc, RN, FAAN
Clinical Nurse Specialist in Ethics,
The Johns Hopkins Children's Center,
Baltimore, Maryland;
Assistant Professor of Nursing,
Johns Hopkins University,
School of Nursing;
Core Faculty,
Bioethics Institute,
Baltimore, Maryland
Chapter 6 Ethics and the Child with a Chronic
    Condition

Teresa A. Savage, BSN, MS, PhD
Research Assistant Professor,
Maternal-Child Nursing,
University of Illinois at Chicago,
College of Nursing,
Chicago, Illinois
Chapter 6 Ethics and the Child with a Chronic
    Condition

Kathleen J. Sawin, DNS, RN, CS, FAAN
Postdoctoral Fellow,
Indiana University School of Nursing,
Indianapolis, Indiana;
Associate Professor,
Virginia Commonwealth University,
Richmond, Virginia
Chapter 8 Transition to Adulthood

Janice Selekman, DNSc, RN
Professor and Chair,
Department of Nursing,
University of Delaware,
Newark, Delaware
Chapter 28 Learning Disabilities and/or Attention
    Deficit Hyperactivity Disorder

Maureen Sheehan, RN, MS, CPNP
Pediatric Nurse Practitioner,
Pediatric Neurology,
Packard Children's Hospital at Stanford,
Palo Alto, California
Chapter 10 Autism

Margaret P. Shepard, PhD, RN
Assistant Professor,
Director of Graduate Studies,
Temple University College of Allied Health,
Philadelphia, Pennsylvania
Chapter 3 Chronic Conditions and the Family

Marybeth Snyder, RN, BSN, MS
Instructor,
Department of Nursing,
University of Delaware College of Health and
    Nursing Sciences,
Newark, Delaware
Chapter 28 Learning Disabilities and/or Attention
    Deficit Hyperactivity Disorder

Judy H. Taylor, MPH, BSN, RN, CNN
Pediatric Nephrology Nurse Coordinator,
University of South Florida,
Tampa, Florida
Chapter 34 **Renal Failure, Chronic**

Judith A. Vessey, PhD, RN, DPNP, FAAN
Professor,
Johns Hopkins University,
School of Nursing,
Baltimore, Maryland
Chapter 2 **Chronic Conditions and Child Development**
Chapter 5 **School and the Child with a Chronic Condition**
Chapter 7 **Financing Health Care for Children with Chronic Conditions**
Chapter 20 **Down Syndrome**

Kathleen Schmidt Yule, RN, MS
Coordinator,
California Newborn Screening Program,
Department of Pediatrics, Division of Medical Genetics,
University of California, San Francisco,
San Francisco, California
Chapter 31 **Phenylketonuria**

Reviewers

Tonya M. Andrade, PhDc, CRNP
Pediatric Critical Care Nurse Practitioner,
Doctoral Candidate,
Johns Hopkins School of Nursing,
Sinai Hospital of Baltimore,
Baltimore, Maryland

Michelle A. Beuchesne, DNSc, RN, PNP
Associate Professor and Coordinator of Primary
    Care Specialization,
Northeastern University,
Graduate School of Nursing,
Boston, Massachusetts

Karen G. Duderstadt, RN, MS, PNP
Associate Clincal Professor,
Department of Family Health Care Nursing,
University of California San Francisco,
School of Nursing,
San Francisco, California

Ardis Hanson, RN, MS, PNP
Assistant Clinical Professor,
Director of School Nurse Practitioner
    Subspeciality,
Department of Family Health Care Nursing,
University of California San Francisco,
San Francisco, California

Veronica Kane, RN, MSN, CPNP
Assistant Clinical Professor,
Massachusetts General Hospital,
Institute of Health Professions,
Boston, Massachusetts

Monica Hubbard, RN, MS, PNP
Assistant Clinical Professor,
Department of Family Health Care Nursing,
University of California San Francisco,
School of Nursing,
San Francisco, California

Judith Robinson, PhD, RN
Executive Director,
National Association of School Nurses,
Scarborough, Maine

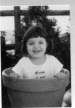

Preface

Growing up is not easy. Seemingly limitless potential is juxtaposed with devastating possibilities. Medical advances over the past 50 years have dramatically decreased the mortality and morbidity rates in children, especially from infectious diseases that annually killed thousands in previous decades. With many devastating illnesses controlled, pediatric health care providers shifted their focus of care from illness management to prevention, with the goal of maximizing each child's potential through health promotion, disease and injury prevention, and growth and development counseling.

During this same period, however, a new childhood morbidity profile emerged. Children with chronic conditions and special health care needs who would have died decades ago as a result of their condition are now surviving. Their medical care is often complex, frequently requiring multiple treatment modalities. In addition, treatments that were previously only provided by professionals in acute care hospitals are now being provided by family members at home, shifting medical responsibilities from hospital professionals to community providers.

In an attempt to keep pace with the rapid developments in medical and surgical treatment for children with chronic conditions, care has often become specialized, focused on the disease process instead of on holistic care for the child. In part, this shift has happened because primary care providers have been hesitant to care for a child with a serious chronic condition for fear of not knowing how to manage the chronic condition well, and specialists have not thought it their role to provide care beyond that needed for management of the chronic condition. Managed care plans now expect primary care providers to assume more comprehensive care responsibilities for children with chronic conditions, including managing their chronic condition and acting as "gate keepers" for specialty services to reduce health care costs. These changes, along with the increasing complexity of treatment protocols for children with special health care needs, require primary care providers to be dedicated lifelong learners.

Growing up with a chronic condition or disability is inherently more difficult. A child's growth and development may be compromised by the stress of the illness and treatments; a child's susceptibility to common childhood illnesses, behavioral dysfunctions, and injuries may be increased as a result of the chronic condition; and many children with chronic conditions also come from impoverished families with little or no access to preventive health care, increasing the potential morbidity from the chronic condition, as well as the general health risks. This book provides pediatric health care professionals with the knowledge necessary to provide comprehensive primary care to children with special health care needs.

Part I addresses the major issues common to care of all children with chronic conditions: the role of the primary care provider, effect of a chronic condition on a child's development and on a family, school issues, transition to adulthood, ethical and cultural concerns, and the financial resources—or lack thereof—available and necessary to support the care of a child with a chronic condition. This knowledge is not condition-specific but forms the framework for delivery of care to all children with chronic conditions.

Part II identifies 27 chronic conditions found in children that necessitate alterations in standard primary care practices. Each condition-specific chapter was written and reviewed by health care professionals with extensive experience in caring for the complex needs of children with the condition. The information provided briefly covers causes and clinical manifestations of the chronic condition but mainly focuses on how these affect the primary care needs of the child. The emphasis is on the need for and provision of primary care. Each chapter follows the same format for ease of reading, and the primary care needs are summarized at the end of each chapter for quick reference.

Decisions about which chronic conditions were included in this text were based on two criteria. First, the prevalence of the condition needed to be at least 1 in 10,000 or would likely reach this level if underreporting were not a problem. For a few other conditions, the decision of inclusion was based on how rapidly the incidence was increasing. The second criterion for inclusion was that the condition requires significant adaptations in primary care.

Whenever possible, inclusive language regarding health care providers has been used throughout the text. We have extended this terminology to include nurse practitioners, physicians, and other health care providers because individuals with a variety of professional preparations provide primary care to children with chronic conditions. Readers will also note that the terms *patient* and *chronic illness* are rarely used and, whenever possible, we have used the wording "the child with (condition name)" rather than the "(condition name) child." Although we recognize that this sometimes makes for awkward grammar, it reflects our philosophy that children are children first instead of being defined by their condition and that wellness and illness are relative.

It would be presumptuous to edit such a text without acknowledging its scope and limitations. First, we assume that readers have a basic knowledge of growth and development and of common pediatric conditions and their management. Second, it is impossible to provide detailed information on treatment options for all secondary problems that may occur in conjunction with those highlighted. Wherever possible, readers are re-ferred to another chapter of the text. If referral was not feasible, readers should consult the general pediatric literature for management protocols. Third, we also decided to exclude most pediatric mental health conditions despite the fact that over 40% of these are treated in the primary care arena. In part, this decision was due to the broad range of conditions and the current disparity in treatment regimens.

The preparation of this text has been a professionally challenging and personally rewarding endeavor for us. As with any text, its successful completion depended on the help of numerous others. We wish to extend our gratitude to the contributors and reviewers for their excellent careful and timely work. Our sincere thanks is also extended to Kelly Wilson for secretarial support. The contributions of the University of California, San Francisco, Department of Family Health Care Nursing, and the Johns Hopkins University School of Nursing are recognized. The assistance and support of the Mosby staff editors, Barbara Nelson Cullen, Sandra Brown, and Jodi Everding, are also greatly acknowledged.

In summary, we hope the information provided in this book will help ensure that children with chronic conditions receive more holistic primary care that will promote their growth and development and maximize their potential in all areas. This care can only be provided if health care professionals are willing to assume the challenge of helping these children to reach their maximum potential—and beyond.

Patricia Ludder Jackson
Judith A. Vessey

Contents

1

CONCEPTS IN PEDIATRIC PRIMARY CARE

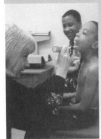

CHAPTER 1

The Primary Care Provider and Children with Chronic Conditions

Patricia Ludder Jackson

Chronic Conditions in Children

A chronic health condition is defined as one that at the time of diagnosis or during its expected course will produce one or more of the following current or future long-term sequelae: limitation of functions appropriate for age and development; disfigurement; dependency on medication or special diet for normal functioning or control of condition; dependency on medical technology for functioning; need for more medical care or related services than usual for the child's age; or special ongoing treatments at home or in school (Stein, 1992).

There are basic differences in the type and profile of chronic conditions in children and adults. Children are affected by a large number of rare diseases and genetic or prenatal conditions, and adults are affected by a relatively small number of common diseases (e.g., heart disease, emphysema, hypertension, diabetes) that increase in morbidity with age (Halfon and Hochstein, 1997). Children with chronic conditions have unique health and social needs. Chronic illness in children is often not stable but subject to acute exacerbations and remissions that are superimposed on the child's growth and development. If the effects of the chronic condition or disability are to be minimized and the children allowed to develop to their maximum potential, then comprehensive, family-centered, community-based, coordinated care must be provided (Committee on Children with Disabilities, 1993, 1998).

The exact number of children who have a chronic condition and the relative severity of the conditions are unknown. The National Health Interview Survey on Child Health (NHIS-CH), which was conducted by the National Center for Health Statistics in 1988, estimated that 31% of children under 18 years of age, or almost 20 million children nationwide, had one or more chronic conditions—not including mental health conditions—based on parent reports (Aday, 1992; Newacheck, McManus, and Fox, 1991; Newacheck and Taylor, 1992). The majority of the children (66%) in the NHIS-CH study reportedly had only mild conditions that resulted in little or no "bother" or limitation of activity. The high incidence of reported respiratory, skin, and digestive allergies probably accounts for the significant number of mild chronic conditions.

Although 31% of children have chronic physical conditions, only a portion of these children require additional health, education, or social services. In 1995, the federal Maternal and Child Health Bureau's Division of Services for Children With Special Health Care Needs (DSCSHCN) established a group to develop a definition of children with special health-care needs (McPherson et al, 1998). Health, education, social policy changes, as well as changes in child health and disability patterns warranted a definition that was easily understood and used by federal and state programs for planning and developing comprehensive community-based, family-centered services for children with special health-care needs. While this new definition was created, eligibility criteria for existing state and federal Title V programs, special education, and Supplemental Security Income (SSI) programs were reviewed. The following definition was developed:

> Children with special health care needs are those who have or are at risk for a chronic physical, developmental, behavioral, or emotional condi-

tion and who also require health and related services of a type or amount beyond that required by children generally. (McPherson, Arango, Fox et al, 1998)

This definition of children with special health care needs focuses on the criteria of need for additional services instead of an identified medical condition or functional impairment, recognizing the variability in disease severity, degree of impairment, and service needs among children with the same or differing diagnosis. This definition also recognizes that children "at risk" for developing chronic physical, developmental, behavioral, or emotional conditions because of biological or environmental characteristics also require health and related services beyond those generally required by children (McPherson, Arango, Fox et al, 1998).

Applying the new definition of children with special health care needs developed by the federal Maternal and Child Health Bureau to the 1994 National Health Interview Survey on Disability in children, it is estimated that 18% of U.S. children under 18 years of age (i.e., 12.6 million children) have a chronic physical, developmental, behavioral, or emotional condition and require health and related services beyond those generally required by children (Newacheck, Strickland, Shonkoff et al, 1998). This estimate does not include children "at risk" for special health care needs because this was not measured by the National Health Interview Survey. Adding "at risk" children would significantly increase the number of children in this category. The new Maternal and Child Health Bureau definition for children with special health care needs helps to delineate those children needing additional services to maintain health and allow them to function at their full potential.

Children with chronic conditions at the highest need for services can be determined by identifying those children with disabilities or limitations in age-appropriate activities as a result of their chronic condition or secondary complications. The National Health Interview Survey for the years 1992 to 1994 indicates that 6.5% of children under 18 years of age (i.e., 4.4 million children) had some disability, with 0.7% of this group having a severe disability that made them unable to participate in a major, age-appropriate activity (e.g., playing for

younger children; attending school for older children). The survey results can be further delineated: 4% of the children were limited in their ability to perform expected activities, and 1.8% were able to perform major activities but were restricted in other activities (Newacheck and Halfon, 1998). The three major condition categories resulting in disability are respiratory conditions (i.e., principally asthma), impairment of speech or intelligence (i.e., principally mental retardation), and mental and nervous system disorders. Black males, children from families with incomes below the poverty level, and children in single-parent families increased the prevalence of disability in children with chronic conditions and exerted an independent effect on the probability of disability (Newacheck and Halfon, 1998).

Figure 1-1 compares the percentage of U.S. children with a chronic physical condition with those children identified as having special health care needs under the new Maternal and Child

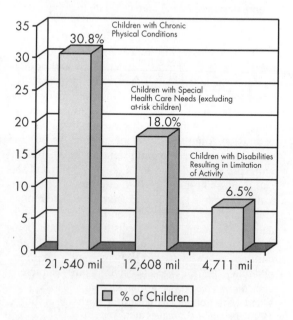

Figure 1-1 Chronic conditions, special needs, and disabilities for children under the age of 18 years in the United States. (Adapted from Newcheck PW and Halfon N: Prevalence and impact of disabling chronic conditions in children, Am J Pub Health 88(4):610-617, 1998.)

Health Bureau definition, as well as with children with disabilities or limitations in activities as a result of their condition.

The survey also found that children with existing special health care needs, including but not limited to those with disabilities, spent three times as many days ill in bed and three times as many days absent from school as other children (Newacheck, Strickland, Shonkoff et al, 1998). In addition, the survey found that children with existing special health care needs had more than two times the number of physician contacts and five times as many days in the hospital as other children in 1994 (Newacheck, Strickland, Shonkoff et al, 1998).

These numbers increased dramatically when only children with identified disabilities were evaluated; these children had physician contact three times as often as other children and spent eight times as many days in the hospital (Newacheck and Halfon, 1998). Table 1-1 shows the prevalence of chronic conditions found in the National Health Interview Survey that result in disability, the propor-

Table 1-1
Prevalence of Chronic Conditions Causing Disability with Limitations of Activity Appropriate for Age in Children Under 18 Years: United States, 1992 to 1994

	Main or Secondary Cause of Disability: # of Cases per 100,000	% of Children Unable to Conduct Major Age-Appropriate Activity	% of Children Limited in School Attendance	% of Children Hospitalized in Past Year
Impairments				
Impairment of vision	108	3.6	6.5	14.7
Impairment of hearing	247	4.1	4.7	6.2
Impairment of speech, intelligence	1942	3.7	2.5	4.6
Absence or loss of extremity	26	9.5	19.9	20.7
Paralysis—complete or partial	190	29.2	18.0	20.4
Deformity of limb, trunk, back	198	12.2	19.9	20.5
Nonparalytic orthopedic problem	239	4.0	13.7	12.9
Abnormality, special impairment	103	30.0	35.8	22.0
Disease and Injuries				
Infectious and/or parasitic	64	19.4	62.0	22.7
Neoplasms	62	21.2	41.8	40.2
Endocrine, metabolic, nutritional, blood	177	16.2	53.9	36.3
Mental, nervous system	1262	9.4	15.8	8.4
Diseases of eye, ear	236	4.9	18.7	5.4
Diseases of circulatory system	143	13.5	18.4	13.2
Diseases of respiratory system	1952	12.5	46.8	12.4
Diseases of digestive system	105	20.4	72.2	16.0
Genitourinary and/or reproductive	55	24.8	54.8	25.6
Diseases of skin	108	13.4	42.5	9.3
Diseases of musculoskeletal system	110	10.8	27.3	8.9
Congenital anomalies and/or perinatal morbidity	211	21.2	22.0	25.7
Ill-defined condition	295	13.3	25.0	15.5
Injuries	51	20.3	38.9	45.8

Data from 1992-1994 National Health Interview Survey.
Adapted from Newacheck PW and Halfon N: Prevalence and impact of disabling chronic conditions in childhood, Am J Pub Health 88(4):610-617, 1998.

Table 1-2
Leading Causes of Death for Infants, Children, and Adolescents in the United States, 1979 and 1997

Infant Mortality Rates for Selected Conditions: Rate per 100,000 Live Births

	1979	1997
All Causes	1306.8	711.0
Congenital Anomalies	255.4	155.7
Disorders Related to Short Gestation	100.0	95.7
Sudden Infant Death	151.1	69.4
Respiratory Distress Syndrome	156.2	32.4
Unintentional Injuries	30.9	19.3
Complications of Pregnancy	37.1	27.9

Mortality Rates for Children 1 to 4 Years: Rate Per 100,000 Population in Specified Group

	1979	1997
All Causes	64.2	35.6
Unintentional Injuries	26.5	12.8
Congenital Anomalies	8.1	3.9
Malignant Neoplasms	4.6	3.0
Homicide	2.5	2.3
Diseases of the Heart	2.1	1.3

Mortality Rates for Children 5 to 9 Years: Rate Per 100,000 Population in Specified Group

	1979	1997
All Causes	31.1	18.5
Unintentional Injuries	16.0	7.7
Malignant Neoplasms	4.7	2.6
Congenital Anomalies	1.7	1.1
Homicide	1.0	0.8
Diseases of the Heart	2.3	0.7

tion of children in each category who were limited in their school attendance because of their condition, and the proportion of children in each category hospitalized in the past year. Although some chronic conditions and disabilities have minimal effect on a child's daily activities, 1.5 million children and adolescents under the age of 22 years are deemed severely disabled and require daily assistive care (McNeil, 1997). There is clearly a hierarchy of health and social risk among children with chronic conditions, as well as a hierarchy of those with increased service needs.

Incidence and Prevalence of Chronic Conditions

The percentage of the pediatric population with a chronic condition is increasing because the patterns of childhood morbidity and mortality have changed due to advances in technology, improved treatment of infectious diseases that were previously fatal, improved diagnoses and case findings of children with previously unrecognized illnesses, and implementation of public and preventive health measures that have saved the lives of infants and chil-

Table 1-2
Leading Causes of Death for Infants, Children, and Adolescents in the United States, 1979 and 1997—cont'd

Mortality Rates for Children 10 to 14 Years: Rate Per 100,000 Population in Specified Group

	1979	1997
All Causes	31.8	23.1
Unintentional Injuries	16.2	9.5
Malignant Neoplasms	4.1	2.5
Homicide	1.2	1.5
Suicide	0.8	1.6
Diseases of the Heart	0.9	1.1

Mortality Rates for Adolescents 15 to 19 Years: Rate Per 100,000 Population in Specified Group

	1979	1997
All Causes	98.8	73.3
Unintentional Injuries	59.4	33.6
Homicide	10.3	12.8
Suicide	8.4	9.5
Malignant Neoplasms	5.3	3.5
Diseases of the Heart	1.9	2.0

Adapted from Guyer, MacDorman, Martin, Peters, and Strobino: Annual summary of vital statistics—1997, Pediatrics, 102(6): 1333-1349, 1998.

dren who would have previously died (Kleiman and Perloff, 1997). Mortality rates have fallen from 870 per 100,000 children aged 1 to 14 years in 1900 to 27.5 per 100,000 in 1997 (Guyer et al, 1998; Newacheck and Taylor, 1992).

During the past 20 years, mortality rates have dropped significantly in all categories except homicide and suicide. See Table 1-2 for mortality rates for the leading causes of death in infants, children, and adolescents for 1979 and 1997. The dramatic drop in mortality rates is not mirrored in the prevalence rate of chronic conditions. Infants, children, and adolescents are surviving requiring additional health care and social services. Each year an estimated 50,000 children acquire a permanent disability as a result of serious injury or acute illness (Guyer and Ellers, 1990). Children with disabilities are more likely to have behavioral problems, be a victim of emotional or sexual abuse, drop out of school, and be involved in the juvenile justice system than their unaffected peers—all situations requiring "health and related services of a type or amount beyond that required by children generally" (Center for the Future of Children, 1997; Gortmaker et al, 1990).

The overall incidence of most childhood chronic conditions has not changed significantly over the past 20 years. In contrast to these relatively stable incidence rates, however, the estimates of survival of children with a variety of chronic conditions have shown considerable change during the same time. Today most children survive requiring continued, often complex, care. For example, children with cystic fibrosis now frequently survive into adulthood (see Chapter 18). Improved surgical intervention and control of urinary tract infections have prolonged the life expectancy of children with spina bifida (see Chapter 29). Newborn screening programs and early dietary intervention have dramatically improved the quality of life and reproductive capability of children with phenylketonuria (see Chapter 31). Advanced trauma care has enabled children to survive brain injury, which often results in a chronic disability (see Chapter 23).

New categories of childhood chronic conditions are also emerging. Infants surviving extreme prematurity or very low birth weight are posing new medical and management problems (see Chapter 32). A large population of infants and children with prenatal drug exposure present new challenges to the health care and educational systems (see Chapter 33). Children with acquired immunodeficiency syndrome (AIDS) are living longer due to advances in treatment (see Chapter 24). The health care system with its advanced technology has created a spectrum of children with chronic iatrogenic conditions (e.g., infants with bronchopulmonary dysplasia [see Chapter 12], children with immune suppression as a result of drug therapy following organ transplantation [see Chapter 30], and survivors of childhood cancer who later suffer the residual effects of treatment [see Chapter 13].

Barriers to Optimal Health Care

Not all children in the United States are equally affected by chronic conditions. Poverty and ethnicity play important roles in the incidence and severity of chronic conditions (Starfield, 1997). National health indicators for children and adolescents show appreciable movement toward meeting the Healthy People 2000 Objectives (Annie E. Casey Foundation, 1997; Maternal and Child Health Bureau, 1997). The goals of reducing health disparities among groups of children and providing preventive services for all children, however, are far from being accomplished and may actually be farther from being attained because of rapidly changing population demographics and changes in federal and state health care and welfare policies affecting low income and immigrant families (Children's Defense Fund, 1997; Department of Health and Human Services, 1997; Montgomery, Kiely, and Pappas, 1996). The Federal Interagency Forum on Child and Family Statistics (1997) has identified poverty, access to health care, and difficulty speaking English as key indicators of a child's well-being.

Financial Barriers

Nationally, a disproportionate number of children (21% vs. 11% of adults) live in poverty and poverty continues to be associated with minority/immigrant status, higher rates of mortality, morbidity, chronic illness, and disability (McNeil, 1997; Newacheck and Jameson, 1994; Center for the Future of Children, 1997; Newacheck and Halfon, 1998) (Table 1-3). Children with disabilities caused by chronic conditions who are in low-income families without Medicaid coverage received only half the number of health care visits as children with similar disabilities who are in higher-income families or have Medicaid coverage (Newacheck et al, 1995). Although health status is an important predictor of children's use of services (e.g., the sicker the child, the more frequent the use of health services), poor, minority, and uninsured children, as well as those

Table 1-3
Relative Frequency and Severity of Health Problems in Low-Income Children Compared with Other Children

Frequency	
Low birth weight	Double
Delayed immunization	Double
Asthma	Double
Bacterial meningitis	Double
Rheumatic fever	Double-triple
Lead poisoning	Triple
Mild retardation	Double

Severity	
Neonatal mortality	1.5 times
Postnatal mortality	Double-triple
Child deaths due to:	
Accidents	Double-triple
Disease-related	Triple-quadruple
Diabetic ketoacidosis	Double
Complications of bacterial	
meningitis	Double-triple
% with conditions limiting	
school activity	Double-triple
Missed school days	Double
Severely impaired vision	Double-triple
Severe iron-deficiency anemia	Double

Adapted from Starfield B: Childhood morbidity: comparisons, clusters, and trends, Pediatrics 88(3):519-526, 1991.
Crain EF et al: An estimate of the prevalence of asthma and wheezing among inner-city children, Pediatrics 94(3):356-362, 1994.
Yeargin-Allsopp M et al: Mild mental retardation in black and white children in metropolitan Atlanta: A case-control study, Am J Pub Health 85(3):324-328, 1995.

living with only their mother, were most likely to experience barriers to access or less apt to seek care than other children with comparable needs (Aday et al, 1993; Cunningham and Hahn, 1994; Starfield, 1997; Wood et al, 1990).

If a child is covered by insurance, access to care is usually improved, but out-of-pocket medical expenses for the family can be significant. Many services required to prevent or ameliorate the effects of the child's condition, to aid in the child's overall physical and mental development, or to assist the child in achieving or maintaining functional capacity may not be covered by the family's insurance. On average, families with children with special health-care needs have three times the level of expenditures per child (Sherry, Gentry, and Restuccia, 1997). Insurance may not cover services such as physical therapy, speech therapy, or mental health services, or may place a cap on the amount of these services covered. Insurance plans usually limit home health care and respite care services and rarely cover the additional costs of transportation, special diets and clothing, or necessary home remodeling, placing a heavy financial and emotional burden on families.

Insurance Barriers

According to the Census Bureau, the largest number ever of children age 18 years and under—11.3 million children—are uninsured (Dorn, Teitelbaum, and Cortez, 1998). The National Health Interview Survey found that 11.2% of children with special health care needs had no health insurance (Newacheck et al, 1998a). Children from low-income families and minorities are more likely to be uninsured, receive fewer health care services than insured children, and be hospitalized more often than children who are not poor (Center for The Future of Children, 1997; McConnochie, Roghmann, and Liptak, 1997; Newacheck, Hughes, and Stoddard, 1996; Newacheck et al, 1997). Minority children with chronic conditions were found to use emergency rooms as their primary source of illness care two to three times as often as white children (Newacheck, Stoddard, and McManus, 1993). Hispanic children are the least likely to have health insurance, with only 73% insured in 1996 as compared with 85% of black children and 87% of white

children (Department of Health and Human Services, 1997).

Lack of insurance coverage is the most important barrier to health care, and the number of children without insurance for all or part of a year continues to grow because of the decline in employment-related health benefits and the changes brought about by the Welfare Reform Act of 1996 (Children's Defense Fund, 1997; Newacheck et al, 1997). In 1996, 14% of children (i.e., 11.3 million) age 18 years and under were without health insurance; 13% of white children, 17% of black children, and 28% of Hispanic children were affected (Department of Health and Human Services, 1997; Children's Defense Fund, 1997). The percentage of children covered by private insurance declined from 74% in 1989 to 66% in 1996. Medicaid was preserved for most children and families who would have qualified for Aid to Families with Dependent Children, but Medicaid eligibility (except for medical emergencies) was lost for hundreds of thousands of legal and illegal immigrants residing in the United States. In addition, one fifth of the children losing Supplemental Security Income (SSI) assistance because of a more narrow definition of disability will have lost their Medicaid coverage (Children's Defense Fund, 1997).

Uninsured children are less likely to have a "medical home" and more likely to receive their care in community clinics than their insured peers (Newacheck et al, 1997). Continuity care in community clinics is often limited, which may result in poor identification of chronic health conditions, inconsistency in management, and lack of appropriate referrals. Access to health care—even for those children with chronic or disabling conditions—is more likely to be sporadic and delayed if a family does not have adequate insurance.

Minority and/or Immigrant Status Barrier

Minority children are at greater risk for disabilities, as well. Based on information from the Survey of Income and Program Participation, the incidence of disability in white children was 5.6% as compared with 11.8% in black children and 6.7% in Hispanic children (McNeil, 1997). One in every five children under age 18 years (i.e., 14 million children in the United States) are immigrants or have parents who are immigrants (National Research Council, Institute of Medicine, 1998). The Welfare Reform Act of 1996 curtails eligibility of children of immigrant parents—even those residing in the United States legally—from income assistance, including SSI, food stamps, Women, Infants, and Children (WIC) programs, and general health care through Medicaid, dramatically increasing the number of children without health insurance and at risk for complications of health conditions associated with inconsistent health care and poverty (Children's Defense Fund, 1997; Geltman et al, 1996; Mihaly, 1997; National Research Council, Institute of Medicine, 1998).

Barriers Created by Fragmentation of Care

Many children with chronic conditions receive the majority of their medical care in specialty clinics that do not provide routine health-care management (Stein, 1997). Shuffled from specialist to specialist, children often miss the screenings, developmental assessments, anticipatory guidance, and immunizations that healthy children of the same age receive. This lack of routine health care appears to cross disease categories. Jessop and Stein (1994) interviewed mothers of children with a variety of chronic conditions and found that although 56% could identify a usual source of care, few could identify a provider who would listen to their concerns (27%), provide them with general advice about the child's condition (24%), or facilitate case-management services with other agencies (22%) (Table 1-4). Newacheck and associates (1998a) found that nearly one in five children with a special health care need were dissatisfied with at least one dimension of their health care and that more than one in ten children with an existing special health care need reported having an unmet health care need, such as a need for dental, vision, medications, or mental health services that was unmet in the past year.

The development of medical specialization, which has improved the disease control and life ex-

pectancy of children with special health care needs, has also resulted in fragmentation of health-care delivery and increased medical costs (Ireys et al, 1997; Stein, 1997). The families of these children—far more than other families—have to interact with multiple institutions providing some aspect of care for their child (e.g., early intervention programs; equipment vendors; social services; special education programs; and federal, state, or private financial providers of care). In addition, there are often medical subspecialists whose expectations may or may not be realistic for the family or child. Demands are sometimes conflicting, uncoordinated, and incomprehensible to the family.

Knowledge Barriers

Knowledge barriers to optimal health care can be present for both the family and the practitioner. A recent study of caretakers' knowledge about their children's medical problems found that only half of the caretakers interviewed in specialty clinics could provide a lay diagnosis of the condition, 29% could not provide an accurate list of current medications, and 25% could not identify the subspecialist providing care to the child (Carraccio et al, 1998). This lack of knowledge jeopardizes the child's health care if continuity providers are not available for care. Not knowing the need for or value of early intervention may delay the initiation of care. Not knowing how to access services with proper referrals and eligibility identification may prevent a family from obtaining the care they are entitled to receive. Parents may not appreciate the need for health maintenance care in addition to specialty care.

Because of the explosive growth of medical knowledge and technology, it is difficult for practitioners to stay abreast of the current management techniques for children with chronic conditions. The specific condition and its severity, the availability of specialists in the community, and the parental requests all affect a primary-care provider's perceived ability and role in caring for children with chronic conditions (Blancquaert et al, 1992; Young, Shyr, and Schork, 1994). This recognition of knowledge limitations, possibly coupled with concern over potential legal consequences if

Table 1-4
Health Services Provided to Families with Children with Chronic Conditions and the Questions
Used to Elicit Them

Area	Question	% Indicating Services Currently Provided
1. Usual source of care	Is there a place you usually go for care and a particular person you usually see there?	56%
2. Coordination with specialists	Does this provider make arrangements if the child needs to see a specialist?	50%
3. Coordination with other agencies	Does this provider talk to other agencies (e.g., school, daycare center, Medicaid)?	22%
4. General advice	Does anyone give general advice about your child and things such as special schooling, handicaps, behavior problems, and what to expect later in childhood or adulthood?	24%
5. Family risk	Does anyone discuss with you whether the child's illness runs in the family or could occur in other family members?	38%
6. Listen to concerns	Does anyone listen to your concerns about your child and understand the problems of raising a child with an illness?	27%
7. Explanation of illness	Has the child's illness been explained to you?	62%
8. Intercurrent illness	Is there someone you go to when the child has a fever or an ear infection or something similar?	72%
9. Health care maintenance	Does anyone measure the child's height and weight, talk about development and eating, etc.?	80%

Adapted from Jessop DJ and Stein REK: Providing comprehensive health care to children with chronic illness, Pediatrics 93(4):602-607, 1994.

subtle but important changes in a chronic condition are not recognized early, may be the reason some primary care practitioners do not want to assume medical or health care responsibilities for children with chronic conditions. Lack of specialist support of primary-care providers was also identified as a barrier to care (Young, Shyr, and Schork, 1994).

Need for Universal Access to Health Care

Concern over the large number of children without adequate health care caused the American Academy of Pediatrics Committee on Child Health Financing to release a new policy statement on access to health care for infants, children, adolescents, and pregnant women (Committee on Child Health Financing, 1998). The American Academy of Pedi-

atrics advocates universal access to quality health care, which includes preventive care services, acute and chronic care services, emergency care services, and all necessary services that: (1) are appropriate for the child's age and health status; (2) will prevent or ameliorate the effects of a condition, illness, injury, or disorder; (3) will aid in the overall physical and mental development of the individual; and/or (4) will assist in achieving or maintaining functional capacity (Committee on Child Health Financing, 1998).

Managed Care and Children with Chronic Conditions

Managed care health plans are quickly becoming the dominant form of health care coverage. From their inception, managed care plans were designed to provide services for adults, whose care consumed 86% of health care dollars, so the needs of children received little attention (Deal, Shiono, and Berman 1998). With the rapid expansion of managed care—especially for Medicaid-eligible clients, the roles and responsibilities of state Title V Programs for children with special health care needs are also changing (McManus et al, 1996). Across the United States, the direct services provided by specialty clinics funded through Title V have decreased while managed care systems attempt to provide services to children within the managed care organization (Newacheck et al,1995). The consequences of these changes are unknown (Newacheck et al, 1996). Managed care plans have the potential to establish a medical home for care and offer increased and coordinated services (e.g., preventive health care and specialty care at a fixed price for enrolled families) to children with special health care needs (Committee on Children with Disabilities, 1998). The provision of coordinated services within one system of care can increase access to services and reduce the number of bureaucracies with which families need to negotiate.

Managed care plans are constructed to be cost-efficient, however, and focus on providing services to relatively healthy populations. Health care plans can discourage the enrollment of high-risk individuals by excluding enrollment of individuals with certain preexisting conditions, having higher rates of cost sharing for out-of-plan referrals, restricting the use of specialists or choice of hospitals, and having a narrow interpretation of what is medically necessary (Berman, 1997; Fowler and Anderson, 1996). Many managed care plans have a built-in economic disincentive for enrolling children with special health care needs and, when they are enrolled, for offering them additional services or referrals to specialists—especially specialists outside of their care plan (Newacheck et al, 1996). For families used to receiving care in specialty centers supported by Title V Children's Services where their child's condition and service needs are well-understood, moving into managed-care plans requiring them to use only providers in the organization can disrupt long-standing relationships and bonds of trust (Ireys, Grason, and Guyer, 1996). Many of the conditions of children with special health care needs are fairly rare, so providers as-

signed to care for them who were not trained in pediatric specialty centers will not be as knowledgeable in caring for the child, prioritizing services that could prevent or ameliorate the effects of the condition, aiding the overall physical and mental growth and development of the child, or using the available community resources to support the child and family. Therefore the quality of care may be decreased (Committee on Child Health Financing, 1998; Ireys, Grason, and Guyer, 1996; Newacheck et al, 1996). In some instances, internal medicine subspecialists are being required to see children as young as 10 years of age to save the additional cost of a pediatric specialist (Walker, 1998).

Providing care to children with chronic or disabling conditions is expensive, but clear standards of care or clinical guidelines have not been established to mandate a higher expenditure for services (Committee on Children with Disabilities, 1998; Fowler and Anderson, 1996; Ireys et al, 1997; Neff and Anderson, 1995). Changing technology and limited outcomes data, especially regarding mental health and rehabilitation services to promote normal growth and development, often result in arbitrary caps on services provided by managed care organizations (Committee on Children With Disabilities, 1998). Increased capitation fees for providers willing to care for children with special health-care needs and continued fee-for-service "carveouts" for these children are two of the risk-adjustment methods that have been tried. Any risk-adjustment method must recognize the increased time and frequency of health care visits, service referrals and coordination, and family counseling necessary for quality care (Committee on Children With Disabilities, 1998).

Primary care providers have a central role in managed care systems. All clients are assigned a primary care provider who is a "gatekeeper" to health services. This central role increases the responsibility of primary care providers to care for children with chronic or disabling conditions and requires that providers be more knowledgeable about the direct care of these children and the availability and effectiveness of potential referrals. In conjunction with the family, primary care providers are now more responsible for accessing services through a system of care predicated on cost savings and profit margins.

Role of the Primary Care Provider in Caring for Children with Chronic Conditions

Few professionals would argue that the pediatric specialists with advanced training and skills gained from caring for many children with similar conditions are not the best professionals to deal with the medical complexities of many chronic conditions. On the other hand, if the broader needs of the child and family (i.e., education, support, advocacy, and health promotion—needs that families have regardless of the specific chronic condition) are seen as the major focus of care, there is an obvious role for a primary care provider.

The primary care provider should be an integral part—if not the leading force—in the care of children with chronic conditions for the following reasons. (1) Holistic health care of children requires that they be viewed first and primarily as children with the health care and developmental needs of any child. (2) The family must be seen as an integral part of the child's growth and development and recognized for its individual strengths and weaknesses (Allmond, Tanner, and Gofman, 1999; Briskin and Liptak, 1995). (3) Health promotion, disease prevention, and anticipatory guidance have even greater significance when children already have a condition putting them at increased risk. Subspecialists are experts in their area of disease management but often have limited knowledge of normal growth and development and standard health care practices for health maintenance. (4) Primary care providers most likely know a family's community resources better than subspecialists, who may have practices many miles from the family's home. This knowledge of community resources is extremely important in helping families receive optimal care and support for their child.

In our rapidly changing health care system, financing of care, access to care, provision of care, and place of care are all in flux. To control health care costs, it is apparent that more families will be insured under health maintenance organizations (HMOs) and capitated managed-care systems than in previous years (see Chapter 7). The role of the primary-care provider as the "gatekeeper" to specialist services will be expanded, and primary care providers will be expected to provide higher levels of care to children with a variety of chronic conditions to decrease costs of specialist care.

Caring for children with chronic conditions is a challenging, rewarding, and time-consuming proposition. It requires a commitment to service beyond that required for routine ambulatory pediatric care, increased knowledge about children with chronic conditions, and additional interpersonal communication and organizational skills necessary to provide optimal child and family care.

Levels of intervention in the primary care of children, as well as the knowledge base and skills primary-care providers need at each level of intervention, are outlined in Box 1-1. These levels of intervention are cumulative (i.e., level 3 intervention cannot be attained until the knowledge base and skills of levels 1 and 2 are mastered). As the levels increase, so do the commitment of the provider and the comprehensiveness of care for the child and family. This model of care was inspired by work done in the area of family-centered care by Doherty and Baird (1987).

Level 1 care is the provision of routine health care maintenance and common illness management to healthy children and their families. Some health care providers may elect not to care for children with chronic conditions because of practice restrictions, a knowledge base limited to the care of normal children, or a lack of skills necessary to adequately manage more complex medical and psychosocial problems. Optimal care can be provided at level 1 but only to children and families without complex health care needs.

Level 2 care is task-oriented care requiring minimal interaction with the child or family and no commitment to continuity care. Level 2 care is not primary care but may be used to supplement primary care when a certain task must be accomplished. The knowledge base and skill level needed for task-oriented care are limited to those necessary to complete the task efficiently, effectively, and safely. Examples of this level of care include the primary care provider administering immunizations, ordering laboratory tests, or performing a prehospitalization physical examination at the request of the managing subspecialist.

Level 3 care is provided when the health care professionals offer routine primary care to children

Box 1-1

Hierarchical Intervention Framework for Practitioners Caring for Children with Chronic Conditions

Level 1

Ongoing health care and illness management for children without chronic conditions

Knowledge base needed

Routine health care maintenance and common illness management for children without chronic conditions and their families

Skills needed

1. The ability to collect subjective and objective data related to child health maintenance and common pediatric illnesses
2. The ability to elicit relevant family data related to family structure, medical history, and current health problems and concerns
3. The ability to listen effectively
4. The ability to assess the information obtained
5. The ability to identify a treatment plan for an individual child without a chronic condition and family
6. The ability to effectively communicate the treatment plan to the child and family
7. The ability to identify children with more complex needs requiring additional services
8. The ability to provide culturally sensitive care to the child and family.

Level 2

Task-oriented care for children with chronic conditions; primary care needs and specialty care needs managed by other professionals

Additional knowledge base needed

Task-related knowledge

Additional skills needed

Performance of task in efficient, correct manner

Level 3

Management of routine health care needs for children with chronic conditions; collaboration or referral for care related to the chronic condition

Additional knowledge base needed

1. Basic pathophysiology of chronic conditions

2. Child and family reactions to the stress of chronic conditions
3. Noncategorical effect of chronic conditions on child development
4. Collaborative role function
5. Specialists, community agencies, tertiary care centers, and other professionals to assume responsibility for care of child's chronic condition

Additional skills needed

1. The ability to educate the child and family about health care maintenance needs, management plans, and accessing services
2. The ability to work with family members in their efforts to manage the child's normal growth and development
3. The ability to assess the child with a chronic condition identifying change requiring consultation or referral to specialist
4. The ability to identify family dysfunction requiring referral
5. The ability to communicate physical or psychosocial changes in the child or family to the appropriate professional
6. The ability to provide culturally sensitive care to the child and family experiencing a chronic health condition

Level 4

Comprehensive primary care of children with chronic conditions and their families

Additional knowledge base needed

1. In-depth pathophysiology of chronic conditions
2. Unique primary care needs of children with chronic conditions
3. Common associated problems found in chronic conditions and effective management
4. Differential diagnosis for common pediatric illnesses occurring in children with chronic conditions
5. Specific stressors for child and family with chronic condition
6. Effect of chronic condition on child's growth, development, and activities of daily living

Hierarchical Intervention Framework
for Practitioners Caring for Children
with Chronic Conditions—cont'd

Additional knowledge base needed—cont'd

7. Health care system resources and consultants available to assist child and family
8. Resource needs associated with chronic condition and means of accessing services
9. Basic cost of services provided to family and health system
10. Community resources, including educational resources, available to assist child and family and means of accessing these services

Additional skills needed

1. The ability to systematically assess the medical condition and health care needs of the child with a chronic condition
2. The ability to plan and implement primary health care, including common illness management that is individualized for the child, the family, and the chronic condition
3. The ability to identify complications of the chronic condition requiring more complex care and to make appropriate referrals
4. The ability to educate the family on the special health care needs of the child with a chronic condition, management plans, and accessing of services
5. The ability to access services within the health care system and community, including educational system, to meet child's health care needs
6. The ability to work with families to plan short- and long-term care consistent with medical needs and family function
7. The ability to assist parents and child in problem solving both medical and family concerns
8. The ability to help families recognize the needs of individual members and balance these needs.
9. The ability to assist families in planning services and activities to reduce stress.
10. The ability to make interdisciplinary referrals communicating child and family needs and expectations
11. The ability to provide consistent, available, long-term care

Level 5

Case management of families and children with chronic conditions

Additional knowledge base needed

1. Service network available to child and family
2. Information systems available to collect and evaluate outcome data
3. Cost of resources
4. Quality outcome measures
5. Service planning and systems coordination
6. Team building and coordination
7. Eligibility requirements, referral process, and utilization measures for agencies or services that might benefit the family and child

Additional skills needed

1. The ability to identify outcome measures of quality care for children with chronic conditions
2. The ability to develop an alliance with family and child to work together to plan and provide optimum care
3. The ability to make a comprehensive needs assessment for child and family
4. The ability to plan and initiate appropriate and successful referrals for services within the health care system and community
5. The ability to analyze cost/benefit ratio for services provided
6. The ability to coordinate services and personnel working with the family and child
7. The ability to utilize information systems to collect and evaluate outcome data
8. The ability to measure and monitor child and family progress
9. The ability to make changes in management and service plan as necessary
10. The ability to communicate findings from multiple interdisciplinary sources to family, child, and other involved personnel or agencies
11. The willingness to function as child and family advocate

Level 6

Advocate for children with chronic conditions and their families

Additional knowledge base needed

1. Institutional structure governing practice priorities
2. Community leadership network
3. Legislative process

continued

---

with chronic conditions, recognizing the unique health-care needs of the child and family. Providers are able to assess the child's chronic condition but refer this care to other individuals or agencies. Because of the complexity of some conditions, the provider's personal interest and/or knowledge base, or practice restriction, primary care providers may elect to manage some children with chronic conditions at this level while managing children with other conditions at a higher level.

Level 4 care is comprehensive primary health care that incorporates the unique complexities of the chronic condition, the child, and the family. At this level the practitioner assumes the primary health care responsibilities of the child and family and uses consultations or referrals for complex situations. This is the level of care often expected of primary care providers serving as "gatekeepers" in managed care systems. Practitioners do not abdicate care to specialists but work with them and the family to provide optimal care. As the health professional with the greatest knowledge of the family, the child, the health care system, and the community, the primary care provider assumes a leadership role in providing comprehensive continuity care.

Level 5 care takes the role of the primary provider one step further to that of case manager. A case manager assesses, plans, implements, coordinates, monitors, and evaluates the options and services needed by a child and family, using available resources to assure quality, cost-effective outcomes

of care (Mullahy, 1995). Case management of children with complex health care needs has become more critical as managed care and capitation require coordinated, efficient, team-based approaches to care (May, Schraeder, and Britt, 1996). Information systems will enable providers to evaluate outcome data to measure the effectiveness of specific interventions, resource utilization, and revenue expenditures.

It is the responsibility of the case manager to enhance the coordination, continuity, integration, and communication of services, as well as to actively engage the family and child in this process. The case manager must be able to perform a needs assessment of the child and family; plan, negotiate, and arrange for medical and nonmedical services; facilitate and coordinate services, including the education and training of community providers; assume responsibility for follow-ups to monitor services and client progress; and empower children and families through counseling, education, training, and advocacy (Liptak, 1995; Kaufman, 1992).

As the complexity of medical management increases with knowledge and technology and the health care financial system becomes overtaxed with health care costs, service efficiency and cost-effectiveness will be central concerns. In the past, practitioners have been more likely to emphasize the quality of services and intensive care needs of clients, while administrators and funding sources often viewed service efficiency and cost-effectiveness as more important (Weil and Karls, 1985). With the advent of new federal health care programs and managed-care organizations based on a cost-containment model, providers will have to be effective child and family advocates to obtain necessary services. Primary care providers must function as case managers and learn to assess and document the effectiveness of the treatment programs used by their clients to support the continuation of these programs in this era of shrinking health care dollars and rising incidences of chronic conditions in children.

Level 6 care goes beyond direct health care services and management of services to the policies and political activism of child advocacy. Provision of quality health care services to individual children with special health care needs is critical and requires knowledgeable and skilled providers willing to take on the additional care requirements of these children. The barriers to optimal health for children with chronic conditions will not be altered, however, without significant changes in health care delivery systems, community awareness and acceptance of the special needs of such children, and legislative mandates for improved health care for all children.

Pediatric primary care providers must become leaders in child advocacy at the institutional, community, state, and federal level—especially during this period of financial competition for service priorities (Berman, 1998). The barriers to optimal health care identified earlier (i.e., poverty, lack of insurance, minority/immigrant status, and fragmentation of care) will not be reduced without fundamental changes in society's awareness and recognition of the health care needs of children. Pediatric health care providers can become effective child advocates by getting involved in the governing structure of health care organizations to ensure that the needs of children are addressed, by conducting or participating in research to determine outcome measures of quality care, by performing community service as a professional and community leader, by getting involved in the legislative process to change laws or regulations affecting children's health care, and by becoming a pediatric health care expert in development of policies governing pediatric health care (Berman, 1998).

Summary

Primary care providers working with children with complex needs must identify their role and the roles of other health care professionals working with the child and family and communicate this role to all concerned, including the family. If primary care providers plan to only intervene at levels 1 to 3, the family must be informed of this decision and an appropriate professional identified to provide level 4 and 5 care. Leaders in the care of children with special health care needs should aspire to level 6 care in order to have the greatest effect on these children.

If the chronic condition is medically complicated, uses complex technology, or requires prolonged use of resources housed in a tertiary care center, the primary specialist (i.e., often more than one specialist is working with a child) may be the appropriate professional to assume the leadership role in total health care management of the child. In this situation the specialist is required to consult with or refer to a primary practitioner for normal health care maintenance appropriate for the child. Many specialty clinics are now using advanced nurse practitioners knowledgeable in both the specialty area and primary care to help facilitate communication and care among the specialty clinic, the primary provider, and the family.

Most chronic conditions of childhood are not so complex that the primary care practitioner with additional knowledge about the chronic condition and its implications for primary care, as well as a commitment to effective communication, cannot assume a leadership role in health care management. In many managed care plans, this is a requirement of the primary care provider as a "gatekeeper" to additional services. Providers of pediatric health care have long embraced the philosophy that it encompasses much more than disease management (Green, 1994). Regionalized systems of care that link high-quality specialized health services with community-based primary care services are needed to coordinate the special needs of children with chronic conditions (Perrin et al, 1994). The primary care provider must play a key role in establishing, organizing, and participating in these systems if they are to exist and provide

the holistic, family-centered, health care maintenance needed to ensure the maximum health and
potential of each child (Committee on Children
with Disabilities, 1993, 1998). Care—rather than
cure—assumes greater meaning when working
with children with chronic conditions, but there is
much care in common with that needed by all children and their families.

The goal of health care maintenance for these
children is to promote normal growth and development; to maximize the child's potential in all areas;
to prevent or diminish the behavioral, social, and
family dysfunction frequently accompanying a
chronic condition; and to confine or minimize the
biological disorder and its sequelae (Stein, 1997;
Committee on Children with Disabilities, 1993,
1998). The primary care provider who knows the
child and family well, knows the resources of the
community, and specializes in health care maintenance is most often the appropriate health care professional to assume leadership in the often complex
care and case management of these children.

References

Aday LA: Health insurance and utilization of medical care for
  chronically ill children with special needs: health of our nation's children, United States, 1988, Advanced Data from
  the Centers for Disease Control/National Center for Health
  Statistics 215:1-8, August 18, 1992.

Aday LA et al: Health insurance and utilization of medical care
  for children with special health care needs, Medical Care
  31(11):1013-1026, 1993.

Allmond BW, Tanner JL, and Gofman HF: The family is the patient, Baltimore, 1999, Williams & Wilkins.

Annie E. Casey Foundation: Kids count data book: State profiles of child well-being, Baltimore, 1997, The Foundation.

Berman S: A pediatric perspective on medical necessity, Arch
  Pediatr Adolesc Medicine 51:858-859, 1997.

Berman S: Training pediatricians to become child advocates,
  Pediatrics 102(3):632-636, 1998.

Blancquaert IR et al: Referral patterns for children with chronic
  diseases, Pediatrics 94(3):284-290, 1994.

Briskin K and Liptak GS: Helping families with children with
  developmental disabilities, Pediatr Ann 24(5):262-266,
  1995.

Carraccio CL et al: Family member knowledge of children's
  medical problems: the need for universal application of an
  emergency data set, Pediatrics 102(2):367-370, 1998.

Center for the Future of Children, The David and Lucile
  Packard Foundation: Children and poverty, Future Child
  7(2), 1997.

Children's Defense Fund: The state of America's children,
  Washington, DC, 1997.

Committee on Child Health Financing, American Academy of
  Pediatrics: Principles of child health financing, Pediatrics 102(4):994-995, 1998.

Committee on Children with Disabilities, American Academy of
  Pediatrics: Pediatric services for infants and children with
  special health care needs, Pediatrics 92(1):163-165, 1993.

Committee on Children with Disabilities, American Academy of
  Pediatrics: Managed care and children with special health care
  needs: A subject review, Pediatrics 102(3):657-659, 1998.

Crain EF et al.: An estimate of the prevalence of asthma and
  wheezing among inner-city children, Pediatrics 94(3):356-
  362, 1994.

Cunningham PJ and Hahn BA: The changing American family:
  implications for children's health insurance coverage and
  use of ambulatory care services—in the future of children:
  critical health issues for children and youth, Future Child
  4(3):24-42, 1994.

Deal LW, Shiono PH, and Behrman RE: Children and managed
  health care: analysis and recommendations, Future Child
  8(2), 1998.

Department of Health and Human Services: Trends in the well-
  being of America's children and youth, 1997, Website:
  aspe.os.dhhs.gov.

Doherty W and Baird MA: Family centered medical care: a clinical casework, New York, 1987, Guilford Press.

Dorn S, Teitelbaum M, and Cortez C: An advocate's tool kit for
  the State Children's Health Insurance Program, Washington
  DC, 1998, Children's Defense Fund.

Federal Interagency, Forum on child and family statistics:
  America's children: key national indicators of well being,
  Washington DC, 1997, US Government Printing Office.

Fowler EJ and Anderson GF: Capitation adjustment for pediatric populations, Pediatrics 98(1):10-17, 1996.

Freys HT, Grason HA, and Guyer B: Assuring quality of care for
  children with special needs in managed care organizations:
  roles for pediatricians, Pediatrics 98(2):178-185, 1996.

Geltman P et al.: Welfare reform and children's health, Arch Pediatr Adolesc Medicine 150:384-389, 1996.

Gortmaker SL et al.: Chronic conditions, socioeconomic risks
  and behavioral problems in children and adolescents, Pediatrics 85(3):267-276, 1990.

Green M (editor): 1994 Bright futures: national guidelines for
  health supervision of infants, children, and adolescent, Arlington, Va., 1994, National Center for Education in Maternal and Child Health.

Guyer B and Ellers B: Childhood injuries in the United States:
  mortality, morbidity, and cost, J Dis Child 144(6):649-652,
  1990.

Guyer B et al: Annual summary of vital statistics 1997, Pediatrics 102(6):1333-1349, 1998.

Halfon N and Hochstein M: Developing a system of care for all:
  what the needs of vulnerable children tell us. In Stein R (editor): Health care for children: what's right, what's wrong,
  what's next, New York, 1997, United Hospital Fund.

Ireys HT et al: Expenditures for care of children with chronic
  illnesses enrolled in the Washington state Medicaid program
  fiscal year 1993, Pediatrics 100(2):197-204, 1997.

Ireys HT, Grason H, and Gwyer B: Assuring quality of care for
  children with special needs in managed care organization:
  roles for pediatricians, Pediatrics 98:178-185, 1996.

Jessop DJ and Stein REK: Providing comprehensive health care to children with chronic illness, Pediatrics 93(4):602-607, 1994.

Kaufman J: Case management services for children with special health care needs: a family centered approach, J Case Management 2:53-56, Summer 1992.

Kleiman L and Perloff JD: Recent trends in the health of U.S. children. In Stein R (editor): Health care for children: what's right, what's wrong, what's next, New York, 1997, United Hospital Fund.

Liptak GS: The role of the pediatrician in caring for children with developmental disabilities: overview, Pediatr Ann 24(5):232237, 1995.

Maternal and Child Health Bureau: Child Health USA '96-97, Rockville, Md., 1997, US Department of Health and Human Services.

May CA, Schraeder C, and Britt T: Managed care and case management: roles for professional nursing, Washington, DC, 1996, American Nurses Publishing.

McConnochie KM, Roghmann KJ, and Liptak GS: Socioeconomic variation in discretionary and mandatory hospitalization of infants: an ecological analysis, Pediatrics 99(6):774-784, 1997.

McManus P et al: Strengthening partnerships between state programs for children with special health needs and managed care organizations, Washington, DC, March 1996, US Department of Health and Human Services, Public Health Service, Health Resources & Services Administration, Maternal and Child Health Bureau.

McNeil JM: Current population reports: Americans with disabilities: 1994-1995, Maryland, 1997, US Census Bureau.

McPherson M et al: A new definition of children with special health care needs, Pediatrics 102(1):137-140, 1998.

Mihaly LK: Impact of federal welfare reform on children in San Francisco, San Francisco, 1997, Mayor's Office of Children, Youth and Their Families.

Montgomery LE, Kiely JL, and Pappas G: The effects of poverty, race, and family structure on US children's health: Data from the NHIS, 1978-1980 and 1989-1991, Am J Pub Health 86(10):1401-1405, 1996.

Mullahy C: The case manager's handbook, Gaithersburg, Md., 1995, Aspen Publishers, Inc.

National Research Council, Institute of Medicine: From generation to generation, Washington, DC, 1998, National Academy Press.

Neff JM and Anderson G: Protecting children with chronic illness in a competitive market place, JAMA 274(23):1866-1869, 1995.

Newacheck PW et al: Children's access to health care: the role of social and economic factors. In Stein R (editor): Health care for children: what's right, what's wrong, what's next, New York, 1997, United Hospital Fund.

Newacheck PW et al: The effect on children of curtailing Medicaid spending, JAMA 274:1468-1471, 1995.

Newacheck PW et al: An epidemiologic profile of children with special health care needs, Pediatrics 102(1):117-121, 1998.

Newacheck PW et al: Monitoring and evaluating managed care for children with chronic illness and disabilities, Pediatrics 98(5):952-958, 1996.

Newacheck PW and Halfon N: Prevalence and impact of disabling chronic conditions in childhood, Am J Pub Health 88(4):610-617, 1998.

Newacheck PW, Hughes DC, and Stoddard JJ: Children's access to primary care: differences by race, income, and insurance status, Pediatrics 97(1):26-32, 1996.

Newacheck PW and Jameson WJ: Health status and income: the impact of poverty on child health, J Sch Health 64(6):229-233, 1994.

Newacheck PW, McManus MA, and Fox HB: Prevalence and impact of chronic illness among adolescents, Am J Dis Child 145:1367-1373, 1991.

Newacheck PW, Stoddard JJ, and McManus M: Ethnocultural variations in the prevalence and impact of childhood chronic conditions, Pediatrics 91(5):1031-1039, 1993.

Newacheck PW and Taylor WR: Childhood chronic illness: prevalence, severity, and impact, Am Public Health 82(3):364-371, 1992.

Perrin JM et al: Health care reform and the special needs of children, Pediatrics 93(3):504-506, 1994.

Rappo PD: Capitation and chronic illness, Contemp Pediatrics 14(4):155-156, 1997.

Sherry S, Gentry C, and Restuccia R: The changing role of consumer advocates. In Stein R (editor): Health care for children: what's right, what's wrong, what's next, New York, 1997, United Hospital Fund.

Starfield B: Childhood morbidity: comparisons, clusters, and trends, Pediatrics 88(3):519-526, 1991.

Starfield B: Social, economic, and medical care determinants of children's health. In Stein R (editor): Health care for children: what's right, what's wrong, what's next, New York, 1997, United Hospital Fund.

Stein R: Health care for children: what's right, what's wrong, what's next, New York, 1997, United Hospital Fund.

Stein REK: Chronic physical disorders, Pediatr Review 13(6):224229, 1992.

Walker WA: A subspecialist's view of training and pediatric practice in the next millennium, Part I, Pediatrics 102(3): 636644, 1998.

Weil M and Karls J: Case management in human service practice, San Francisco, 1985, Jossey-Bass.

Wood DL et al: Access to medical care for children and adolescents in the United States, Pediatrics 86:666-673, 1990.

Yeargin-Allsopp M et al: Mild mental retardation in black and white children in metropolitan Atlanta: a case-control study, Am J Pub Health 85(3):324-328, 1995.

Young PC, Shyr Y, and Schork MA: The role of the primary care physician in the care of children with serious heart disease, Pediatrics 94(3):284-290, 1994.

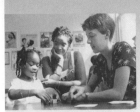

CHAPTER *2*

Chronic Conditions and Child Development

Judith A. Vessey and Dionne J. Mebane

Development does not exist in a vacuum; the developmental domains of children are significantly influenced by their physiologic state, psychologic competence, and external environment (Hertzman, 1998). The presence of a chronic condition adds a dimension of developmental and behavioral risk (Patterson and Blum, 1996). Because children with chronic conditions are more similar than different, a noncategorical approach focusing on the commonalties of these children instead of on just the disease process is useful (Stein, 1996). This approach is the foundation for this chapter.

Children with chronic conditions may experience developmental lags in acquiring cognitive, communicative, motor, adaptive, and social skills compared with their unaffected peers. These maturational alterations may range from minor to all-encompassing and transient to permanent. The presence of a chronic condition, while complicating the attainment of developmental tasks, does not necessarily connote the presence of a developmental disturbance or permanent disability. The development of many children with chronic conditions progresses without interruption.

The maturational alterations that accompany chronic conditions may be characterized in several ways. Some alterations are manifested within a single area of development (e.g., motor difficulty in a child with mild cerebral palsy). Other developmental alterations (e.g., those seen in a child with Down syndrome) are more global in nature. Alterations may also be classified as delayed or deviant. Children with delayed development will advance through the normal sequence of milestones but at a rate slower than that of their peers of the same chronologic age. Such is the case of a child with an uncorrected congenital heart defect. Deviant development, which occurs from unevenly developed or damaged neurologic processes, involves a disruption in the normal developmental sequences (e.g., a child with autism).

Variables that contribute to the occurrence and severity of maturational alterations associated with chronic conditions include the natural history of the condition, personal characteristics of the child, and larger social networks, with the latter two categories appearing to play more significant roles (Clay et al, 1995).

The Condition's Natural History

The severity, pathophysiology, and prognosis of the condition, as well as any iatrogenic insults that may have occurred, influence a child's developmental outcome (Patterson and Blum, 1996).

Severity and Pathophysiology

The severity of the condition and numerous specific pathophysiologic mechanisms (i.e., including chronic hypoxemia in serum glucose levels and malabsorption) are known to alter development, although the correlation between severity and developmental attainment is not very robust (Wallander and Thompson, 1995). It appears that children in the least and most disabled groups are at greater risk than those at intermediate levels of severity (Northam, 1997). The pathophysiologic changes that children with mild conditions experience lack sufficient severity or are ameliorated by treatment so that such children readily adapt to them, and the potential for developmental insult is minimized. When conditions are marked by only occasional exacerbations, limited visibility, or appear to cause only marginal problems, they may be ignored or denied by children and their families (Patterson and Blum, 1996). This denial is often motivated by an effort to normalize the child's condition. Unfortunately, these children may have poorer developmental outcomes if denial interferes with symptom recognition or ongoing management regimens. Children experiencing significant disability related to neurologic impairment or multisystem involvement are also at significantly greater developmental risk. The interaction of pathophysiologic changes, availability for learning, and contact with the environment often compromise developmental attainment.

Developmental sequelae secondary to prolonged disease states are also emerging. As research continues to advance health care technology, the mortality previously associated with many chronic conditions has been reduced. Often reductions in mortality, however, initially result in escalating morbidity. The survival of very low birth weight infants is one example (Chapieski and Evankovich, 1997; McCarton et al, 1996). (See Chapter 32).

Other developmental limitations are secondarily imposed by the condition's pathophysiology and management. Conditions that are painful, embarrassing, or energy-depleting place a child at greater developmental risk (Patterson and Blum, 1996). Tremendous exertion may be necessary to cope with intensive treatment protocols or the time-consuming activities of daily life. For example, children with cystic fibrosis may spend more than 3 hours each day receiving pulmonary care. Additional energy is also required in adjusting to new or exacerbated symptoms (e.g., persistent pain, malaise, and/or fatigue). The activities of children who are dependent on technology are limited by physical constraints and the time needed to care for such things as ventilators and infusion pumps. Such expenditures of time and energy may limit children's opportunities to engage in recreational activities or predispose them to significant fatigue because participation requires too much effort.

Prognosis

Maturational progression is superimposed on the natural course of the condition. In conditions associated with ongoing pathophysiological deterioration, children may initially achieve milestones but lose them as the condition worsens. It is always noted when there is progressive degeneration of the neurologic system (e.g., as with Tay-Sachs disease), but this is also a problem with any seriously compromised physiologic state. Even in nonprogressive conditions, developmental lags become noticeable as children mature and developmental expectations are higher. In part, the ability to sustain development is dependent on effectively managing the effects of the disease and promoting the child's functional status and psychosocial adjustment.

Another area of concern is for children who have limited or uncertain futures or whose significant others (i.e., family, teachers, etc.) consider them to have a poor prognosis for reaching adulthood. These children may be deprived of a past-present-future perspective of learning about one's cultural heritage or forming goals and personal aspirations. This longitudinal perspective plays an integral role in shaping cognitive processes. If individuals are misguided into thinking that such information is not worth transmitting or would be unduly upsetting—especially for children who recognize their potentially diminished longevity, this lack of information limits children's ability to learn. Predicting prognoses is a risky business in light of rapid advances in medical science (Van Dyke and Lin-Dyken, 1993); the life expectancies for children with cystic fibrosis, organ transplantation, cancer, and many other conditions continue to increase at dramatic rates. If a poor prognosis is communicated to the family without a broader perspective of the child's future, it may become a self-fulfilling prophecy.

Iatrogenic Insults

Selected treatment protocols impose their own risks (Northam, 1997). *Developmental iatrogeny* refers to health care interventions that hinder children from progressing through their normal developmental milestones. Therapeutic interventions commonly associated with developmental iatrogeny are the associations between amino-glycosides and hearing loss (Borradori et al, 1997; Fischel-Ghodsian et al, 1997); cancer therapies, transplantation, and late effects (Fochtman, 1995; Kramer et al, 1997); and oxygen administration and retinopathy of prematurity (Gaynon et al, 1997). Numerous other interventions, however, directly or indirectly influence development. Many classes of drugs (e.g., anticonvulsants and steroid therapy) have been shown to alter cognition, perceptual abilities, and/or behavior and make children less available for learning (Lehne, 1998).

Characteristics of the Child

Each age group gives rise to different sets of challenges for children with chronic conditions. The child's age at onset of a condition, however, affects progression from one stage of development to the next. Achieving a developmental task that has never been acquired is very different from regaining a skill mastered and then lost. Overall, children with congenital conditions have greater developmental plasticity; they more readily adjust to condition-imposed limitations as greater adaptive mechanisms come into play (Weiss and Wagner, 1998). Yet evidence suggests that the risk of behavioral difficulty is inversely correlated with age (Frank et al, 1998), with younger children being at higher risk.

Infancy

The major developmental tasks of infancy include establishing trust and learning about the environment through sensorimotor exploration. For infants with congenital chronic conditions, these tasks may be difficult to accomplish. Parents who are mourning the loss of their perfect child may have little energy, but their infants may be very tiring to care for. Parents may find little gratification in trying to meet their child's basic needs despite their best efforts. They may begin to view their child as vulnerable because of the extensive care required, and this attitude can affect future development (Goldberg, 1990). A poor prognosis may lead some par-

ents to emotionally divorce themselves from their infants in an effort to insulate themselves from further emotional hurt. Infants subjected to prolonged or frequent hospitalizations may encounter repeated separations, the unpredictability associated with numerous caregivers, potentially unreliable or inadequate care, and painful experiences. All of these factors can inhibit attachment and the subsequent development of a trusting relationship. For infants whose conditions are physically limiting or painful, exploration and interaction with their environment is limited, further curtailing development.

Toddlerhood

The major developmental tasks of toddlerhood include acquiring a sense of autonomy, developing self-control, and forming symbolic representation through the acquisition of language. If a child's chronic condition requires careful limit setting and control of activities of daily living, independence in tasks such as toileting, feeding, or acquiring larger social networks may not be encouraged. For example, toddlers who are immunosuppressed need to be restricted in their social contacts and play arenas. Mandatory prolonged dependency can make separation difficult and contribute to a fragile self-image. Developmental tasks that have just been mastered are often easily lost in toddlers experiencing acute exacerbations of disease—with or without hospitalization. This behavioral regression is a means of social and emotional adaptation whereby children revert to earlier, previously abandoned stages when they do not have the necessary psychic energy to maintain functioning at developmental levels already achieved (Freud, 1966). Behavioral regression is exacerbated by stress, including that associated with separation and pain. Although regression can happen at any point along the developmental continuum, it is most commonly noted in this age group.

Preschool Children

The primary developmental task for preschoolers is acquiring a sense of initiative to successfully meet the challenges of their ever-expanding world. Preschoolers with chronic conditions may not have the physical energy or resources to design and perform such activities; therefore opportunities for learning about the environment, developing social relationships, and cultivating self-confidence and a sense of purpose are diminished. They may have difficulty forming a healthy body image and sexual identity, particularly if most of their body awareness is associated with disability and discomfort. The egocentricity and naive reasoning processes of preschoolers directly influence their understanding and interpretation of their condition, although recent research suggests that their understanding of illness and its relationship to morality is less enmeshed than previously thought (Kato, Lyon, and Rasco, 1998). Regardless, preschoolers' developing self-esteem and motivation to undertake new tasks may be compromised by their condition.

School-aged Children

For school-aged children, increasing independence and mastery over their environment are important developmental landmarks. A lack of physical stamina may prevent children with chronic conditions from participating in school and extracurricular activities. Such activities contribute to gaining social skills, developing a sense of accomplishment, learning to effectively cope with stress, and acquiring the skills that result in self-sufficiency. Children with a condition that is not highly visible may try to hide its existence until forced by circumstances to admit otherwise when they recognize that it distinguishes them from their peers. If not provided with the necessary skills to communicate information about their condition to peers, these children may withdraw with a diminished self-concept. Moreover, enforced dependency—whether required by the treatment regimen or instituted by overprotective parents—creates additional social and emotional barriers between these children and their unaffected peers.

Adolescence

Adolescents, in the transitional period from childhood to adulthood, should become increasingly independent of their parents. Many want to assume total responsibility for their care despite their relative inexperience, but extensive care needs may preclude this from happening (Vessey and Miola,

1997). Adolescents need to begin to make decisions about future career and personal goals. For an adolescent who requires complex care or has a limited life expectancy, these developmental tasks may go unmet. Adolescents are prone to the following two dangers in planning for the future: they may (1) overemphasize the potential barriers that accompany their condition and succumb to a sense of futility or despair, or (2) deny realistic limitations and set themselves up for failure by holding unrealistic expectations. Puberty, which is always a time of rapid change and uncertainty for adolescents, makes this already complex period more confusing for teens with chronic conditions. Integrating limitations into a changing body image and self-concept is difficult. Delayed puberty accompanies many conditions, emphasizing the differences between affected and unaffected adolescents. Adolescence is a particularly difficult time to be viewed as different by one's peers, and some adolescents may withdraw from social activities and relationships that promote healthy psychosexual development. Others may choose to engage in risky behaviors (e.g., smoking and unprotected sex) despite the potentially damaging effects to be accepted by peers (Britto et al, 1998).

Gender

Although the information on the influence of gender on the developmental outcomes of children with chronic conditions is meager, it does appear that boys may demonstrate more problems than girls (Pless, Power, and Peckham, 1993). This may be because boys experiencing behavioral problems tend toward externalizing disorders (e.g., conduct or oppositional disorders), and girls tend toward internalizing disorders (e.g., depression). Externalized disorders are more readily detected and diagnosed. Girls, however, tend to report more symptoms of distress (Wallander and Thompson, 1995).

Individualism

Despite great odds, many children have intrapsychic and interpersonal resources that allow them to conquer virtually any disability and excel in life. A child's individualism, or the rubric of those relatively stable behavioral attributes that underlie a child's behavior (i.e., temperament, motivation, hardiness, intellect, attitudinal qualities, and interpersonal skills), influence developmental attainment and adaptation to their condition (Frank et al, 1998; Zeanah, Boris, and Larrieu, 1997).

Children with chronic conditions display the same scope of individual differences as children without chronic conditions. Some behavioral traits, such as temperament, are present at birth, and others, such as self-concept, develop over time. A child's individualism is influenced by environmental factors, although there is little correlation between familial attitudes and practices and a child's psychologic development.

A child's self-concept is linked to fully mastering a variety of physical, intellectual, social, and emotional tasks. Failing such tasks at critical developmental periods does not bode well for physical or socioemotional health. Although children with chronic conditions are at a somewhat higher risk for developing a vulnerable personality, many are remarkably resilient and approach life's challenges with aplomb (Committee on Children with Disabilities, 1993). They learn to rapidly identify threats to their integrity, respond with justifiable anger to those who are prejudiced against them, and reject biased individuals as inferior. These children often work to simultaneously educate those around them, dispelling myths and inaccuracies that might interfere with their own developmental competence.

Children with multiple chronic conditions are at increased risk (Lavigne and Faire-Routman, 1992; Newacheck and Stoddard, 1994), although the severity of a single condition does not appear to affect a child's psychologic outcome. Factors known to place children at greater risk for psychologic co-morbidity are as follows: (1) a poor self-concept, (2) dependence on others, (3) a dysfunctional family, (4) residence in an isolated area, and/or (5) poverty (Committee on Children with Disabilities, 1993; Dadds, Stein, and Silver, 1995; Newacheck et al, 1998). Moreover, selected therapeutic interventions can affect psychologic wellbeing. Psychologic co-morbidity can be reduced when comprehensive preventive care is provided for the child and family (Stein and Jessop, 1991).

The interrelationships of a child's positive self-esteem, perceived autonomy, easy temperament, internal locus of control, at least normal intelligence, adequate perceptual and communication skills, and accurate cognitive appraisal of the condition in conjunction with environmental and family support all purport better adaptation (Northam, 1997). Development is dynamic, however, and these traits are subject to change. When children are provided with the protective factors needed to balance out risk exposure, positive behavioral attributes and adaptability are fostered in concordance with positive development (Patterson and Blum, 1996).

Role of Family and Social Networks

Healthy development depends on repeated, varied positive interactions between the growing child and the environment. Such reciprocity results in a spiral of mutually effective interactions. A child's family is the most important influence on development during early childhood (Wallander and Thompson, 1995). Most parents are tremendously resilient despite the demands of the child's condition and effectively balance their role in normative parenting with meeting specific demands of the condition (Reiss, Steinglass, and Howe, 1993). For a minority of parents, the converse is also true. Parental guilt, despair, or unfinished grief over the loss of the fantasied child may negatively affect a child's development. Other factors include maternal depression, "nerves," poor self-esteem, and a chronically stressful environment (Dadds, Stein, and Silver, 1995; Thompson and Gustafson, 1996). Well-functioning families enhance their child's development, whereas those with discordant functioning curtail it (Patterson and Blum, 1996). Differences between children and families who successfully adapt are related to their coping abilities and access to needed resources (see Chapter 3).

Differing cultural orientation, social class, and economic status of the family influence development in children with chronic conditions (Sterling, Peterson, and Weekes, 1997). As these orientations vary, so do the symbolic and semantic significance of the events, perceived origins, and potential consequences (Brookins, 1993; Geber and Latts, 1993; Groce and Zola, 1993). Practitioners working with children from varied circumstances need to recognize the variations in intrafamily communication patterns, temporal orientation, religiousness, and the value placed on childhood because these are known to influence development (see Chapters 3) and 4).

As children mature, their environments and social networks naturally expand, and extended family members, teachers, friends, and acquaintances influence their developmental attainment. Informal and voluntary support appears to be the most critical. Individuals who offer practical, tangible support, provide intellectual stimulation, plan activities that help the child excel, and take pride in the child's accomplishments truly serve as the child's advocates. Unfortunately, some individuals have had few experiences with children with special needs and may overcompensate for or reject a child's limitations. For children whose conditions are associated with disfigurement, their development may be unwittingly at risk because of the reactions of others. Many uninformed individuals automatically assume that a physical handicap is associated with cognitive impairment. Children may be spoken of as if they are not present, or questions may be addressed to nearby family members or peers. The damage that can be done to a child's sense of self-worth is inestimable. The family can be helped to educate significant others about the child's strengths and limitations, mainstream their child into community activities, and use effective methods for working with insensitive individuals.

Developmental Perspectives of the Body, Illness, Medical Procedures, and Death

Children's perspectives about their bodies, illness, medical procedures, and death differ depending on age and experience. Early research investigating how children conceptualized topics used a developmental approach (Bibace and Walsh, 1981) and was influenced by cognitive stage theory. Another paradigm explaining how children learn about these subjects is now showing credence. In this framework, learning about such topics is not as dependent on cognitive level as on previous experience (Crisp, Ungerer, and Goodnow, 1996; Yoos, 1994). Children with chronic conditions may develop expertise about selected topics within the range of their experiences and beyond that expected at their cognitive levels, but they may hold less sophisticated views about general concepts of anatomy, physiology, illness, procedures, and treatments. Children may use advanced terminology that could confuse others into thinking that their comprehension exceeds what is normally expected. For example, a 4-year-old stated that he was receiving "methotrexate intravenously," but thought his blood filled an empty body cavity because blood vessels were an unknown entity.

Children's self-concepts, interpersonal abilities, and therapeutic adherence to treatment regimens are related to the beliefs they hold. For those who perceive their chronic condition as totally negative and restricting, functional status, school performance, and psychosocial competence are more likely to be compromised. These perspectives need to be taken into account when children are taught about their condition and their help is enlisted in therapeutic adherence.

Understanding of the Body

Toddlers can point to various body parts, but by the preschool period, children have well-defined concepts of their external bodies and the relationships of its parts. Their understanding of anatomy and physiology, however, is primitive in keeping with experience, cognitive level, and perceptual abilities. By the early school years, children can name several body parts, with the heart, brain, bones, and blood being the most common. Children's descriptions of the parts and how they function tend to be global, undifferentiated, and laced with fantasy, although there is a great deal of variation among children about their specific ideas. Knowledge of the interrelationships of the parts and their functions are equally hazy. Physiologic processes are seen as a series of static states, with each organ having a singular, autonomous function. By middle to late grade school age, when children's causal reasoning and ability to differentiate matures, they begin to understand the complexities of anatomy and physiology. Levels of the body's organization are differentiated and hierarchically integrated with each other. Progressively more complex information about bodily functions, much of it from required academic classes, is incorporated throughout adolescence. Children with chronic conditions hold a slightly different—though not more sophisticated—view of their internal bodies than that of their unaffected peers. They may focus on the affected part of the body but do not identify fewer organs or organ systems. Evidence indicates that these children do develop the increasing differentiation seen in children without chronic conditions, although some may remain fixated on their defective part (Vessey, in press; Vessey and O'Sullivan, in review).

Understanding of Illness

If children are considered by their parents to be sick, their developing views and personalization of illness will significantly influence how they interpret their condition. As children mature and their view of illness evolves, primary care practitioners and significant others can assist children in developing positive images of their condition.

Infants are concerned about illness only as it directly interferes with their comfort and attachment to their parents. By toddlerhood, children begin to understand the concept of illness. For children with chronic conditions, this is usually interpreted by how the condition interferes with desired activities. Many condition-specific tasks (e.g., injections of insulin or wearing a seizure helmet) are particularly onerous for this age group. As children mature, they form ideas and articulate their feelings about illness. Preschoolers' understanding of illness—although naïve—is more sophisticated than once thought. It appears that a child's understanding of illness is related to the difficulty of comprehending why things are happening to them (Kato, Lyon, and Rasco, 1998). Relying on phenomenism (i.e., attributing illness to any external concrete phenomenon) or ascribing the causes of illness to other temporally occurring events is common. As children reach school age, their view of illness begins to reflect their evolving causal reasoning. Illness is initially perceived as occurring

from contamination of or physical contact with the causal agent. Over time their understanding matures, and the cause of illness is believed to be external (e.g., germs that enter the body). With the development of formal operations in adolescents, illness causation is seen as a complex, multifaceted process. Biologic and physiologic explanations initially emerge as the basis for illness and later evolve into psychophysiologic explanations. The relationship of behavior and emotion to illness is usually acknowledged during adolescence.

Understanding of Medical Procedures and Treatments

Children's understanding of medical procedures and treatments is intrinsically linked to their knowledge about their body and illness. Infants and young children have no specific initial understanding of procedures, which are only interpreted in light of how they intrude on personal comfort. By preschool age, children's comprehension of medical procedures is marked by magical thinking, transductive reasoning, and overgeneralization. The purpose of a procedure is independent of a child's health status, and little discrimination about its diagnostic or therapeutic purpose is made except by children who have undergone repetitive procedures. All procedures are designed to make them "better" or "sicker." Many associate treatment with punishment (Kato, Lyon, and Rasco, 1998); and because preschoolers' understanding of body boundaries are not well-developed, virtually all invasive procedures are perceived as threats to their body integrity.

As children mature, their view of medical procedures evolves from overgeneralization to overdiscrimination and then to correct identification of their functions. Multistep procedures and their purposes can be understood by school-age children, who can classify and order variables. Information may be interpreted quite literally, however, and misunderstandings can occur if the content taught is not validated. Children of grade school age respect health care personnel and their hierarchical position, but expressions of affection are often ambivalent. Often intrigued with understanding medical procedures, children are usually pleased when asked to participate in their own care.

Adolescents can understand the efficacy of specific medical procedures and the relationships between procedures and their health status, although their sense of invincibility and desire for experimentation affect their decision-making. Informed decisions about alternative treatments are possible. Adolescents view the health care provider's authority as extending only as far as their willingness to adhere to the therapeutic regimen. Although the need for therapeutic adherence is understood, treatments are not automatically affectively and behaviorally assimilated into an adolescent's daily activities.

Understanding of Death

Death is the ultimate experience of separation and loss for children and their families. Children's understanding of death is formed along a developmental progression and reflects their cognitive maturation (Mahon, 1993). Infants do not comprehend death per se but react to phenomena (e.g., pain and separation) associated with death. By late toddlerhood and preschool age, children may talk freely about death but may describe its occurrence and attributes with magical thinking and an egocentric viewpoint. They may perceive their impending death as punishment yet do not view death as permanent but rather as "sleep" or departure from the family. The permanence of death is not realized until the grade school-age period, when the concepts of reversibility and irreversibility are learned. Children in this age group tend to personify death as the bogeyman or some kind of monster. For children who are dying, this newly found knowledge can enhance their fears of the unknown. Adolescents, with their new metacognitive abilities, conceptualize death as a process of the life cycle, readily comprehending the emotional, social, and financial implications of the loss occurring from death for themselves and their families. Of all age groups, adolescents have the most difficulty in dealing with death.

Children with chronic conditions are often subjected to many intrusive and painful experiences and may have experienced the death of friends in the hospital. These experiences often exacerbate their anxieties about death. Depending on individual experience, a child's understanding of death may not follow the projected trajectory. Although information about how affected children's views of death differ from their nonaffected peers is limited, it appears that the fears associated with death are remarkably similar to the fears of hospitalization and intrusive procedures. Even preschool-aged children may express fear of separation, despite the fact that death may not yet be conceptualized as irreversible.

For the dying child, how issues such as separation, mutilation, and loss of control are handled plays an important role in their personal conceptualization of death. Care must be taken to prevent unnecessary separation and help these children maintain their autonomy, sense of mastery, and other developmental skills whenever possible. (See Chapter 4 for additional information.)

The Primary Care Provider's Role in Promoting Development

Because a cure is not possible for many chronic conditions, practitioners must focus on care. The goal of care is to minimize the manifestations of the disease and maximize the child's physical, cognitive, and psychosocial potential. Realization of this goal is facilitated by adopting a family-centered approach to care. Family-centered care recognizes that the family is the constant in the child's life and as such is vital to children successfully meeting their potential. Practicing family-centered care requires professionals to do the following: (1) recognize and respect a family's strengths and individuality, (2) promote a family's confidence and competence in caring for the child, and (3) empower a family to advocate for their child when working with the health care system. A noncategorical approach, incorporated with specific disease management strategies, provides a nexus on which to base assessments and develop holistic management plans. A good maxim to follow is to generalize developmental information across diagnostic groups and then individualize it for each child and family (Stein and Jessop, 1989).

Assessment and Management

In today's climate of cost constraint, children are being discharged earlier—and often sicker—than before. This places increased care demands on family members who may feel unprepared to handle these increased responsibilities. The primary care provider is in an ideal position to provide assistance during this transition.

Maturational alterations are rarely immutable and should not be thought of as such. Children with chronic conditions require comprehensive care to achieve their optimal level of functioning (Curry and Duby, 1994). Therefore a developmental surveillance program must be established. Developmental surveillance is a broader approach than detection; it is comprehensive, continuous, and contains the following components: (1) general and condition specific screening, (2) child and parental observation, (3) identification of concerns, and (4) general primary care guidance (Gilbride, 1995). Although developmental surveillance falls under the primary care provider's purview, it can involve input from an interdisciplinary group of professionals. The composition of the group is dynamic and varies depending on the child's age, disability, level of impairment, familial involvement, and environmental resources. Coordination is critical to preventing omissions and duplications of services (Smith, Layne, and Garell, 1994). Involvement of the primary care provider helps ensure consistency across the disciplines.

Ideally, children at risk for developmental lags and/or behavioral problems should be identified as soon as possible and followed closely. Primary care providers should anticipate and, whenever possible, vigorously intervene before significant aberrations occur. This is best accomplished by identifying and initiating treatment in the preclinical period when slight indications of developmental impairment may be detected, but gross manifestations are not yet evident. A "wait and see" attitude is not warranted because these children are at developmental risk. Early intervention may prevent or ameliorate many secondary problems or those resulting from neglect or mistreatment of the original condition. Although a child may suffer hearing loss from aminoglycosides, for example, subsequent language and cognitive delays may be prevented with aggressive intervention. Because a chronic condition generally persists throughout a child's life, ongoing surveillance of physical development and psychosocial adjustment is helpful.

Assessment of the child's physical development normally consists of evaluating basic indicators of health—including growth measures and vital signs, performing a comprehensive physical examination, and noting any changes in the status of the chronic condition. Additional dimensions, which include screening specific developmental domains and rating the child's functional status, should also be an integral part of the assessment. An evaluation of functional status provides information about the child's ability to engage in the activities of daily living that heavily influence developmental outcomes.

Although the tendency may be to focus attention on the child's physical status, assessing the child's psychosocial adjustment is of critical importance. Not all of the psychosocial stresses experienced by children with chronic conditions are caused by their condition, nor do only affected children experience stress. These children, however, are at increased risk of psychologic difficulties, much of which can be attributed to the child's condition (Wallander and Thompson, 1995). It is estimated that two to three times as many children with chronic conditions have behavioral problems as their nonaffected peers. Moreover, 30% to 40% of these children also have school-related problems, only one half of which are directly related to their condition (Andrews, 1991).

Assessment has traditionally focused on identifying how children with chronic conditions differ from their nonaffected peers. This information is useful in developing an explanatory theory about the effects of chronic conditions but does little to help an individual child. Evaluating if a child is effectively coping with the condition and adjusting to school, peer groups, and the like provides guidelines on which interventions can be based.

Standardized assessment instruments are useful, necessary adjuncts to a complete history and physical examination for a comprehensive developmental evaluation. When used at regular intervals, these instruments provide objective data so that small developmental changes can be detected. Considering the ever-growing number of children with special needs being cared for in the community, primary care practitioners need to have a compendium of readily administered standardized instruments from which to draw (Table 2-1). They

Text continued on page 43

Table 2-1
Instruments Used in Developmental Assessment

Types of Screening Tools	Test/Score	Age Level	Method	Comments
General development	Alberta Infant Motor Scale *Authors:* M Piper , J Darrah, L Pinnell, T Maguire, and P Byrne *Source:* Piper MC, Darrah J: Motor assessment of the developing infant, Philadelphia, 1993, W.B. Saunders.	Birth to 18 months	Observation	*General Information:* • Measures gross motor developmental milestones • Assesses postural control in supine, prone, and sitting positions *Time Required:* varies*
	Battelle Developmental Inventory (BDI) (1984) *Authors:* J Newborg, J Stock, L Wnek, J Guidubaldi, and J Svinicki *Source:* Riverside Publishing Co, 8420 Bryn Mawr Avenue, Chicago, IL 60631	Birth to 8 years	• Structured test format • Parent and teacher interview • Observation	*General Information:* • Includes a screening test that can be used to identify areas of development in need of a complete comprehensive BDI • Full BDI consists of 341 test items in five domains: personal-social, adaptive, motor, communication, and cognitive • Screening test consists of 96 items taking 20 to 35 minutes to administer *Time Required:* 1-1½ hours to administer*
	Bayley Scales of Infant Development, ed 2 (1993) *Author:* N. Bayley *Source:* The Psychological Corporation Harcourt, Brace, Jovanovich, Inc. 6277 Sea Harbor Drive Orlando, Fla. 32887 *Phone:* 1-800-211-8378 *Website:* www.psychcorp.com	1 to 42 months	Observation/ demonstration	*General Information:* • Evaluates motor, mental, and social behavior of infants and toddlers • Diagnoses normal vs. delayed development • New scoring procedures allow examiners to determine a child's developmental age equivalent for each ability domain

*Can be administered by a professional or paraprofessional. Some special training required. Must understand testing procedures and develop rapport with children.

Continued

Table 2-1
Instruments Used in Developmental Assessment—cont'd

Types of Screening Tools	Test/Score	Age Level	Method	Comments
General development —cont'd				• Requires a qualified practitioner to examine and evaluate an infant *Time Required:* <15 months, 25 to 35 minutes; >15 months, 60 minutes
	Bender Visual Motor Gestalt Test *Author:* L Bender *Source:* American Orthopsychiatric Association, Inc., Seventh Avenue, 18th Floor, New York, NY 10001 *Phone:* 212-564-5930 *Website:* www.amerortho. org	≥3 years	Demonstration	*General Information:* • A drawing test for evaluating developmental problems, learning disabilities, retardation, psychosis, organic brain disorders in children • Requires a qualified practitioner *Time Required:* 10 minutes to administer
	Brigance Diagnostic Inventory of Early Development (Revised) (1991) *Author:* A Brigance *Source:* Curriculum Associates, Inc, 5 Esquire Road North Billerica, Mass. 01862-2589 *Phone:* 978-667-8000 *Website:* www. curriculumassociates. com	Birth to 7 years	Performance task by child	• Assesses skills in all areas required for PL 101-476 eligibility • Criterion and normative referenced, curriculum based • May be administered by a paraprofessional with supervision *Time Required:* varies
	Developmental Profile II *Author:* G Alpern, T Boll, and M Shearer *Source:* Western Psychological Services, 12031 Wilshire Blvd, Los Angeles, Calif. 90025-1251	Birth to 9½ years	Parent or teacher report	*General Information:* • Screens children for delays in five domains: physical (motor and muscle development), self-help, social, academic, and communication.

Table 2-1
Instruments Used in Developmental Assessment—cont'd

Types of Screening Tools	Test/Score	Age Level	Method	Comments
General development —cont'd				• Can be computer-scored *Time Required:* 186 items takes 20 to 30 minutes to administer
	The Early Screening Inventory (Revised) (1997) *Authors:* S Meisels, D Marsden, M Wiske, and L Henderson *Source:* Rebus, Inc., P.O. Box 479, Ann Arbor, Mich. 48106 *Phone:* 1-800-435-3085 *Website:* mail@ rebusinc.com	3 to 6 years	Observation	*General Information:* • Two separate tests: one for age 3 to 4½ years, and one for 4½ to 6 years • Assesses visual-motor/adaptive skills; language; gross motor and cognition • Also includes a parental checklist • Must be administered by a trained professional *Time Required:* varies
	Hawaii Early Learning Profile (HELP) (1979) *Authors:* SF Furuno, KA O'Reilly, CM Hosaka, TT Inatsuka, TL Allman, B Zeisloft, and S Parks *Source:* Vort Corporation, P.O. Box 60880, Palo Alto, Calif. 94306	Birth to 36 months	Observation and parent interview	*General Information:* • 685 developmental tasks used to assess six domains: cognition, language, gross motor, fine motor, social-emotional, and self-help • Criterion-referenced, curriculum-based *Time Required:* Each domain takes 15 to 30 minutes to administer. Domains may be selected for individual use
	• Minnesota Infant Development Inventory (1988) • Minnesota Early Child Development Inventory (1988) • Minnesota Preschool Development Inventory (1984) *Authors:* H Ireton and E Thwing	• Birth to 15 months • 1 to 3 years • 3 to 6 years	• Observation/interview • Parent report • True/False	*General Information:* • A first-level screening tool • Measures the infant's development in five domains: gross motor, fine motor, language, comprehension, and personal-social

Continued

Table 2-1
Instruments Used in Developmental Assessment—cont'd

Types of Screening Tools	Test/Score	Age Level	Method	Comments
General development —cont'd	*Source:* Behavior Science Systems, P.O. Box 1108 Minneapolis, Minn. 55458			• Provides a profile of the child's strengths and weaknesses • 60 to 80 items on each inventory *Time Required:* varies
	Movement Assessment of Infants *Authors:* LS Chandler, MW Swanson, and MS Andrews *Source:* Infant Movement Research, P.O. Box 4631 Rolling Bay, Wis. 18060	Birth to 12 months	Observation	*General Information:* • Provides uniform approach to the evaluation of high-risk infants • Assesses muscle tone, reflexes, automatic reactions, volitional movement • Must be administered by a trained professional *Time Required:* varies
	Peabody Developmental Motor Scales *Authors:* M Folio and R Fewell *Source:* DLM Teaching Resources, One DLM Park, Allen, Tex. 75002	Birth to 7 years	Observation	*General Information:* • Assesses reflexes, gross motor, and fine motor skills to assess developmental level • Must be administered by a trained professional *Time Required:* varies
	Rapid Developmental Screening Checklist *Authors:* Committee on Children with Handicaps, American Academy of Pediatrics *Source:* MJ Giannini, MD Director, Mental Retardation Institute, New York Medical College, Valhalla, NY 10595 *Phone:* 914-493-8215	1 month to 5 5 years	Checklist	*General Information:* Tests general developmental milestones and tasks *Time Required:* minimal time allotment
	Riley Motor Problems Inventory (RMPI) *Author:* GD Riley	≥4 years	Performance tasks by the child	*General Information:* • Provides a quantified system for observation and

Table 2-1
Instruments Used in Developmental Assessment—cont'd

Types of Screening Tools	Test/Score	Age Level	Method	Comments
General development —cont'd	*Source:* Western Psychological, 12031 Wilshire Blvd, Los Angeles, Calif. 90025			measurement of neurologic signs that lead to problems in speech, language, learning, and behavior • Needs to be administered by a qualified practitioner *Time Required:* varies
	Wheel Guide to Normal Milestones of Development *Author:* U Hayes *Source:* A Developmental Approach to Case Findings, ed 2, U.S. Dept of Health and Human Services, Superintendent of Documents, Washington, DC 20402 *Phone:* 202-690-6782 *Website:* www.acf.dhhs.gov	1 to 3 years	Observation	*General Information:* • Assesses basic reflexes and developmental milestones • Reinforces the normal growth and development patterns of children *Time Required:* varies
Adaptive Behavior	AAMR Adaptive Behavior Scale-School, ed 2 ABS-S:2 (1981-1993) *Authors:* N Lambert, K Nihira, and H Leland *Source:* PRO-ED, Inc, 8700 Shoal Creek Blvd, Austin, Tex. 76758-6897 *Phone:* 512-451-3246 *Website:* www.Proedinc.com	3 to 21 years	Performance tasks, observation, and parent report	*General Information:* • Used as a screening tool and for instructional planning • Can be an indicator in assessing children whose adaptive behavior indicates possible mental retardation, learning difficulties, or emotional disturbances; provides 16 domain scores • Previously called AAMD Adaptive Behavior Scale • Software for scoring available *Time Required:* 15 to 30 minutes

Continued

Table 2-1
Instruments Used in Developmental Assessment—cont'd

Types of Screening Tools	Test/Score	Age Level	Method	Comments
Adaptive Behavior —cont'd	AAMR Adaptive Behavior Scale Residential and Community, ed 2, ABS-RC:2 (1969-1993) *Authors:* N Lambert, K Nihira, and H Leland *Source:* PRO-ED, Inc, 8700 Shoal Creek Blvd, Austin, Tex. 76758-6897 *Phone:* 512-451-3246 *Website:* www.Proedinc.com	3 to 21 years	Performance tasks, observation, and parent report	*General Information:* • Similar to AAMR-School • Provides scores in 18 domains including: independent functioning, language development, social behavior, and physical development • Software for scoring available *Time Required:* 15 to 30 minutes
	Vineland Adaptive Behavior Scales *Authors:* SS Sparrow, DA Balla, and DV Cicchetti *Source:* American Guidance Services Inc., 4201 Woodland Road, Circle Pines, Minn. 55014-1796 *Phone:* 612-786-4343 *Website:* www.agsnet.com	Birth to 19 years	Semistructured interview with caregiver observation	*General Information:* • Assesses adaptive behavior in four sectors: communication, daily living skills, socialization, and motor skills • Can be used with mentally retarded and disabled individuals *Time Required:* 20 to 40 minutes to administer
Temperament	Temperament Assessment Battery for Children (TABC) (1988) *Author:* RP Martin *Source:* Clinical Psychology Publishing Co, Inc., #4 Conant Square, Brandon, Vt 05733	3 to 7 years	Structured test format	*General Information:* Measures basic personality-behavioral dimensions in the areas of: activity, adaptability, approach/withdrawal, intensity, distractibility, persistence *Time Required:* 10 to 20 minutes to administer
	Carey and McDevitt Revised Temperament Questionnaire: Toddler Temperament Scale	1 to 3 years	Interview	*General Information:* • Provides an objective measure of the child's temperament profile

Table 2-1
Instruments Used in Developmental Assessment—cont'd

Types of Screening Tools	Test/Score	Age Level	Method	Comments
Temperament —cont'd	*Authors:* W Fullard, SC McDevitt, and WB Carey *Source:* W Fullard, PhD Dept. of Educational Psychology, Temple University, Philadelphia, Pa. 19122 *Phone:* 215-204-8087			• Fosters more effective interaction between parent and child • 95 items, 6-point frequency scale *Time Required:* varies
	Carey and McDevitt Revised Temperament Questionnaire: Behavior Style Questionnaire *Authors:* SC McDevitt and WB Carey *Source:* SC McDevitt, PhD Dev Profile II, Devereaux Center, 6436 E Sweetwater Scottsdale, Az. 85254 *Phone:* 602-922-5440	3 to 7 years	Interview	*General Information:* • Provides an objective measure of the child's temperament profile • Fosters more effective interactions between parent and child *Time Required:* varies
	Infant Temperament Questionnaire (ITQ) *Authors:* WB Carey and SC McDevitt *Source:* WB Carey, MD 319 West Front Street Media, Pa. 19063 *Phone:* 610-543-0818	4 to 8 months	Interview and parent report	*General Information:* • Provides an objective measure of the infant's temperament profile • Fosters more effective interaction between parent and infant *Time Required:* varies
Vision	Allen Picture Card Test of Visual Acuity *Author:* HF Allen *Source:* LADOCA Project and Publishing Foundation, E 51st Avenue and Lincoln Street, Denver, Co. 80216 *Phone:* 303-295-6379	2½ to 6 years	Observation	*General Information:* • Preschooler screening test for visual acuity • Must teach child names of pictures before testing *Time Required:* varies
	Denver Eye Screening Test (DEST) (1973) *Authors:* WK Frankenberg, AD Goldstein, and J Barker	6 months to 6 years	Observation	*General Information:* • Includes three different tests according to age

Continued

Table 2-1
Instruments Used in Developmental Assessment—cont'd

Types of Screening Tools	Test/Score	Age Level	Method	Comments
Vision—cont'd	*Source:* LADOCA Project and Publishing Foundation E 51st Avenue and Lincoln Street, Denver, Co. 80216 *Phone:* 303-295-6379			• Identifies children with acuity problems • 6 months to 2½ years—fixation test • 2½ to 3 years (preschool-age children unable to respond to the Snellen Illiterate E Test) Do a picture card test—takes 5 minutes • 3 to 6 years—Snellen Illiterate E Test *Time Required:* 6 months to 3 years—5 minutes; 3 to 6 years—10 minutes
	HOTV (matching symbol test) *Author:* O Lippmann *Source:* Wilson Ophthalmic Corp, P.O. Box 49 Mustang, Ok. 73064 *Phone:* 405-376-9114	≥2½ or when the child can identify shapes	Flashcards	*General Information:* • Good for young children or those who do not like to verbalize • Children name the four letters *H, O, T,* and *V* on a chart for testing at 10 to 20 feet and match them to a demonstration card • Avoids the problem with image reversal and eye-hand coordination that can occur with the letter E *Time Required:* varies
	Picture Card Test (adaptation of the Preschool Vision Test) *Author:* HF Allen	≥ 2½ years	Interview—"name the picture"	*General Information:* Identifies children with acuity problems *Time Required:* 10 minutes

Table 2-1

Instruments Used in Developmental Assessment—cont'd

Types of Screening Tools	Test/Score	Age Level	Method	Comments
Vision—cont'd	*Source:* LADOCA Project and Publishing Foundation E 51st Avenue and Lincoln Street, Denver, Co. 80216 *Phone:* 303-295-6379			
	Snellen Illiterate E Test *Author:* H Snellen *Source:* National Society for Blindness; American Association of Ophthalmology, 1100 17th Street NW, Washington, DC 20036	≥3 years	Observation using two persons as a team in screening	*General Information:* Intended as a screening measure for central acuity of preschool-aged children and other children who have not learned to read *Time Required:* varies
Speech and Language	The Bzoch-League Receptive Expressive Emergent Language Scale (REEL) *Authors:* KR Bzoch and R League *Source:* University Park Press, 360 N. Charles Street, Baltimore, Md. 21201	Birth to 3 years	Paper-pencil inventory; parent interview	*General Information:* Identifies children needing further follow-up in language *Time Required:* 15 to 20 minutes to administer
	Denver Articulation Screening Exam (DASE) (1971-1973) *Authors:* AF Drumwright and WK Frankenberg *Source:* Denver Developmental Materials, Inc. P.O. Box 6919, Denver, Co. 80206-0919 *Phone:* 303-355-4777	2½ to 7 years	Observation	*General Information:* • Designed to identify significant developmental delay in the acquisition of speech sounds • Good for screening children who may be economically disadvantaged and have a potential speech problem with articulation or pronunciation • Administered by a qualified professional or a nonprofessional with special training *Time Required:* 10 to 15 minutes to administer

Continued

Table 2-1
Instruments Used in Developmental Assessment—cont'd

Types of Screening Tools	Test/Score	Age Level	Method	Comments
Speech and Language —cont'd	Emergent Language Milestone Scale (ELM) (1984) *Source:* Education Corporation P.O. Box 721 Tulsa, Ok. 74101	Birth to 36 months	Interview/ observation	*General Information:* Screening instrument for auditory expressive, auditory receptive, and visual components of language *Time Required:* varies
	McCarthur Communicative Development Inventory *Authors:* L Fenson, PS Dale, D Thal, E Bates, JP Harding, S Pethick, and JS Reily *Source:* Singular Publishing Group Inc., San Diego, Calif.	8 to 30 months and older developmentally delayed children	Parent report measuring vocabulary development	*General Information:* • Measures vocabulary development (words and sentences) in children with and without developmental delays • Includes an extensive vocabulary checklist containing words that children typically produce in the second and third years of life; parents are asked to review and check all words that their child can spontaneously produce • Must be administered by a speech therapist or pathologist, physician, or nurse *Time Required:* varies
	Peabody Picture Vocabulary Test, Revised (PPVT-R) (1981) *Authors:* LM Dunn and LM Dunn *Source:* American Guidance Service, 4201 Woodland Road, Circle Pine, Minn. 55014-1796 *Phone:* 612-786-4343 *Website:* www.agsnet.com	2½ to 40 years	Individual "point to" response test	*General Information:* • IQ used to assess receptive vocabulary; not a measure of speech and language skills • Measures hearing vocabulary for standard American English

Table 2-1

Instruments Used in Developmental Assessment—cont'd

Types of Screening Tools	Test/Score	Age Level	Method	Comments
Speech and Language —cont'd				• Used with non-English-speaking students to screen for mental retardation or giftedness • Requires a qualified practitioner to administer *Time Required:* 10 to 20 minutes to administer
	Riley Articulation and Language Test, Revised (RALT-R) *Author:* GD Riley *Source:* Western Psychological, 12031 Wilshire Blvd Los Angeles, Calif. 90025	≥4 years	Performance tasks by the child	*General Information:* • 2 to 3 minute screening test that identifies children in need of speech therapy • Provides a quantified system for observing and measuring neurologic signs leading to problems in speech, language, learning, and behavior • Must be administered by a qualified clinician *Time Required:* varies
Hearing	Noise Stik *Author:* LH Eckstein *Source:* Eckstein Bros, Inc. 4807 W 118th Place Hawthorne, Calif. 90250 *Phone:* 310-772-6113	Birth to 3 years	Behavioral response to auditory stimulation	*General Information:* Handheld free-field screener for early detection of infant hearing loss *Time Required:* varies
Child Behavior and Cognition	Kaufman Brief Intelligence Test (K-BIT) (1990) *Authors:* AS Kaufman and NL Kaufman *Source:* American Guidance Service, 4201 Woodlawn Road, Circle Pines, Minn. 55014-1796 *Phone:* 612-786-4343 *Website:* www.agsnet.com	4 to 90 years	Structured test format	*General Information:* • Quick measure of intelligence, may not be substituted for comprehensive measure of intelligence • Assesses expressive vocabulary, definitions, matrices *Time Required:* 15 to 30 minutes to administer

Continued

Table 2-1
Instruments Used in Developmental Assessment—cont'd

Types of Screening Tools	Test/Score	Age Level	Method	Comments
Child Behavior and Cognition —cont'd	Brazelton Neonatal Behavioral Assessment Scale *Author:* TB Brazelton *Source:* JB Lippincott, 227 Washington Square Philadelphia, Pa. 19106-3780 *Phone:* 215-238-4200 *Website:* www.lww.com	3 days to 4 weeks		*General Information:* • Used as a predictive tool in clinical practice and research for behavioral and neurologic assessment • Tests 27 behavioral items in the areas of habitation, orientation, motor maturity, variation, self-quieting, and social • Requires a trained examiner *Time Required:* 20 to 30 minutes
	Child Behavior Checklist *Author:* TM Achenbach *Source:* Center for Children, Youth, and Families University of Vermont 1 S. Prospect Street Burlington, Vt. 05401	2 to 30 years	Observation/ interview	*General Information:* • Provides an overview of the child's behavior • Parent and teacher forms available *Time Required:* administrative form—15 minutes scoring—3 minutes via computer, 20 minutes by hand
	Pediatric Symptom Checklist *Authors:* M Murphy and M Jellinek *Source:* Dr. Mike Jellinek Child Psychology Service Massachusetts General Hospital in Boston ACC725 Boston, Mass. 02114 *Phone:* 617-726-2724	6 to 18 years	Completed by parent	*General Information:* • Used to screen for areas of weakness requiring more detailed diagnostic testing in scholastic achievement • Parent completed form • A child self-report version • Version for children 2 to 5 years of age also available *Time Required:* 5 minutes to administer

Table 2-1
Instruments Used in Developmental Assessment—cont'd

Types of Screening Tools	Test/Score	Age Level	Method	Comments
Child Behavior and Cognition —cont'd	Peabody Individual Achievement Test: Revised (PIAT-R) (1970-1989) *Authors:* LM Dunn and FC Markwardt, Jr *Source:* American Guidance Service, 4201 Woodland Road, Circle Pines, Minn. 55014-1796 *Phone:* 612-786-4343 *Website:* www.agsnet.com	Kindergarten to 12th grade	Interview and written test	*General Information:* • Used to screen for areas of weakness requiring more detailed diagnostic testing in scholastic achievement • Assesses reading recognition comprehension, total reading, mathematics, spelling, written expression • Must be administered by a psychologist *Time Required:* 50 to 70 minutes to administer
	Riley Preschool Development Screening Inventory (RPDSI) *Author:* CMD Riley *Source:* Western Psychological, 12031 Wilshire Blvd Los Angeles, Calif. 90025	3 to 5 years	Observation	*General Information:* • For children who tend to have academic problems • Used to screen for emotional, learning, and behavioral problems • Requires a qualified clinician to administer *Time Required:* varies
	Wide Range Achievement Test (WRAT) 3(1940-1993) *Author:* GS Wilkinson *Source:* Jastak Associates, Wide Range Inc, P.O. Box 3410, Wilmington, DE 19804-0250 *Phone:* 302-652-4990	5 to 75 years	Paper-pencil subtests	*General Information:* • Used for education placement, vocational assessment, and job placement training • Large print edition is available • Measures the skills needed to learn reading, spelling, and arithmetic *Time Required:* 15 to 30 minutes to administer

Continued

Table 2-1
Instruments Used in Developmental Assessment—cont'd

Types of Screening Tools	Test/Score	Age Level	Method	Comments
Stress anxiety	State-Trait Anxiety Inventory for Children (STAIC) (1970-1973) *Authors:* CD Spielberg, CD Edwards, RE Lushene, J Montuori, and D Platzek *Source:* Mind Garden, 1690 Woodside Road Redwood, Calif. 94061 *Phone:* 650-261-3500 *Website:* www.mindgarden.com	Grades 4 to 6	Self-administered in groups or individually	*General Information:* • Measures anxiety in elementary school children • Title on test is "How I Feel Questionnaire" *Time Required:* 20 minutes to administer
	State-Trait Anxiety Inventory (STAI) (1968-1984) *Authors:* CD Spielberg, RL Gorsuch, RE Lushene, PR Vagg, and D Platzek *Source:* Mind Garden, 1690 Woodside Road Redwood, Calif. 94061 *Phone:* 650-261-3500 *Website:* www.mindgarden.com	9 to 16 years and adults	Group administration; test booklet available in Spanish and English	*General Information:* Designed to assess anxiety as an emotional state (S-Anxiety) and individual differences in anxiety proneness as a personality trait (T-Anxiety) *Time Required:* 10 to 20 minutes to administer
Self-concept	Piers-Harris Children's Self-Concept Scale (The Way I Feel About Myself) (PHCSCS) (1969-1984) *Authors:* EV Piers and DB Harris *Source:* Western Psychological Services, 12031 Wilshire Blvd, Los Angeles, Calif. 90025	8 to 18 years	Descriptive statements used by groups or individual	*General Information:* • 80 questions requiring yes-no response • Assesses a raw self-concept score plus cluster scores for behavior, intellectual and school status, physical appearance and attributes, anxiety, popularity, happiness, and satisfaction *Time Required:* 15 to 20 minutes to administer
Family function	Feetham Family Functioning Survey (FFFS) (1982)	Family	Self-reporting instrument	*General Information:* • 25 questions evaluating six areas of

Table 2-1
Instruments Used in Developmental Assessment—cont'd

Types of Screening Tools	Test/Score	Age Level	Method	Comments
Family function —cont'd	*Authors:* S Feetham and S Humenick *Source:* Nursing Systems and Research Children's National Medical Center 111 Michigan Avenue NW Washington, DC 20010 *Phone:* 312-996-8008			functioning: household tasks, child care, sexual and moral relations, interaction with family and friends, community involvement, and sources of support • Used for identifying specific areas of dysfunction in a stressed family *Time Required:* 10 minutes to administer
	Home Observation for Measurement of the Environment (HOME) (1984) *Authors:* R Bradley and B Caldwell *Source:* Center for Research on Teaching & Learning, University of Arkansas at Little Rock, 2801 S. University Avenue, Little Rock, Ark. 72204-1099 *Phone:* 501-569-8542	Birth to 3 years; 3 to 6 years	Interview and direct observation of the interaction between the caretaker and the child	*General Information:* • Two separate instruments designed to assess the quantity and quality of social, emotional, and cognitive support available to a child within his home • The inventory for children at birth to 3 years contains 45 items; the inventory for 3- to 6-year-olds contains 55 items *Time Required:* each inventory takes about 1 hour

also should not rely only on basic developmental screening instruments (e.g., DDST II), which are designed to identify global delay rather than provide in-depth information on the type and severity of developmental problems (Bennett and Nickel, 1995). Focused instruments provide specific information that is useful as part of in-depth evaluation.

Instruments should be carefully chosen and results thoroughly interpreted because most of each are norm-referenced instead of criterion-referenced.

Other instruments and/or results are invalid if they measure one developmental construct based on performance in a different arena of development (e.g., the cognitive development of a child with a tracheostomy should not be assessed by an instrument requiring verbal responses). Timed tests may also bias results, particularly if a child has a motor or learning deficit. If a child tires easily, it is best to perform developmental assessments in short intervals so as not to obscure the child's true capabilities.

In general, children with chronic conditions who are at risk for developmental deviations but have no indications of problems should participate in developmental surveillance programs similar to those of their unaffected peers. For those children exhibiting warning signs of developmental problems, more frequent assessments are appropriate. If at-risk but nonsymptomatic children are assessed too frequently, parents' perceptions may be altered so that they believe their child is unduly vulnerable, creating a self-fulfilling prophecy. Practitioners need to walk the fine line between errors of commission and those of omission when determining the frequency and intensity of assessment. The best defense is to place efforts on prevention rather than detection.

When untoward developmental manifestations are detected, the primary care provider can either provide treatment or, more likely, refer the child to specialists with expertise in the area of concern. Referrals should ideally be made to individuals who are a part of the specialty team or within the child's school setting, but additional local referrals may be necessary if the specialty team is far away or school services are inadequate. Adding another layer of care providers requires exquisite coordination of services if the child is to receive appropriate care without overlaps, gaps, or too many demands to cause fatigue.

Obtaining services may require that the child's condition and associated problems be diagnostically labeled, although recent legislation has made this less common. Providing a label may help validate the concerns of children and families and direct future interventions and activities but must be done judiciously. Labeling often sets children apart from their peers and may result in different treatment by family members, teachers, and significant others. Diagnostic labels assigned in childhood follow children into adulthood and might prevent them from pursuing selected careers, joining the military, or being eligible for insurance. Although it is usually feasible to label specific disease entities, labeling associated with developmental manifestations should be done carefully. The ultimate long-term goal of care is for a child to reach and sustain optimal levels of functioning. Developing precise, measurable, short-term goals helps ensure that optimal functioning is obtained.

Education

In addition to providing health maintenance, primary care helps prepare children in self-care behaviors and development of self-advocacy skills for dealing with the health care community. This is important for children and adolescents with chronic conditions because they are likely to use the health care system often throughout their lives. The transition between pediatric and adult care is never easy, especially for those with conditions that used to be fatal in early childhood. Providers of adult care often have little experience with these conditions and their management. Educating children and adolescents will help empower them to negotiate with the health care system effectively.

To accomplish the objectives of primary care, children must initially have a basic understanding of the workings of their body, characteristics of their condition, and the intricacies of the health care system. It is often assumed that children are well-versed about these topics because they know the jargon, appear comfortable with the health care environment, and have been diagnosed "for years," but developmentally appropriate teaching guides need to be incorporated into the primary care of all children with chronic conditions. Learning is more likely to occur in a nonthreatening environment where children are in a comparatively good state of health than when they are sick and/or hospitalized. A comprehensive plan managed by the primary care provider in conjunction with parents and specialty providers will help ensure that this learning occurs. Teaching methods must be altered to fit the child's developmental age. Children will learn best when the material presented to them remains within one level above their current cognitive functioning.

A multisensory approach (i.e., one that brings all of the child's senses to bear on the learning task at hand) is more likely to be effective with preschool and school-aged children than more traditional methods. For example, using anatomic rag dolls to explain anatomy and physiology (Vessey, 1988) or doll hospitals to explain various procedures has been highly effective. A variety of options (e.g., books, discussion, videos, and interactive computer programs) are appropriate for use with older children without cognitive deficits.

Many commercially available materials are excellent and useful adjuncts to individualized teaching plans. Practitioners should examine all materials in advance to determine if the information presented will correspond to the child's experiences. The language of all materials must be accurate and age-appropriate. There is little sense in providing cute but inaccurate information to a child, because these myths will just need to be dispelled when the child matures. This is of particular significance for younger children who have not developed causal reasoning, engage in fantasy, and tend to interpret their environment from a singular perspective.

Therapeutic Adherence

Promoting therapeutic adherence is a critical role of the primary care provider, especially in light of current health care trends shifting the onus of treatment responsibilities to the client. Therapeutic adherence is enhanced when a child actively participates in health care decisions. Practitioners who gradually involve children and adolescents in decisions about their care improve their therapeutic adherence and self-care abilities (Brady, 1994). Considering a child's individualism when determining treatment regimens can improve adherence. For example, a child who has a low activity level, is given appropriate autonomy, and adapts easily to new situations is more likely to comply with a regimen of bedrest and nutritional restrictions than a very active child who has difficulty adapting to new situations. Therapeutic adherence can be encouraged through open discussion and adoption of activities such as those listed in Box 2-1.

When a child does not adhere to the treatment regimen, determining why is critical before taking any action. Nonadherence is usually not deliberate but due to poor time management, forgetfulness, or other related behaviors. Smaller groups of children (and their parents) deliberately do not adhere to a treatment regimen because they do not believe in its efficacy or want to deal with the side effects, it is too costly, or similar reasons. Regardless, family reports of adherence frequently are exaggerated.

Advocacy

Many professionals are called on to care for the complex needs of children with chronic conditions. Although all have the same goal—to help the child

Box 2-1
Promoting Therapeutic Adherence

Teach Children in a Developmentally Appropriate Manner About:
Anatomy and physiology.
The pathophysiology of their condition.
Medication and treatment effectiveness.

Explore the Thoughts and Feelings of Children and Parents about the Treatment Plan.

Adjust the Treatment Plan to Fit Within the Child's and Family's Lifestyle.

Suggest the Use of "Props" to Serve as Reminders:
Use wristwatch alarms for medication reminders.
Coordinate medications with mealtimes.
Use sticker charts or tokens with younger children.

reach maximum potential—conflicts may arise over the best approach for realizing it. Moreover, recent scientific advances in genetics have significant implications for children and families (Fanos, 1997). Primary care providers are in the unique position to advocate for a child by identifying the range of treatment options and their implications, informing the child and family of available resources, and helping coordinate these interdisciplinary services. This support is critically important in light of the changing service delivery and reimbursement patterns for chronic conditions (see Chapter 7)

Hospitalization

Hospitalization is not uncommon with this population of children, and so care is usually transferred to the specialty team during this time. Primary care providers can assist in a smooth transition. In addition to giving information about the child's physical condition, parents must be encouraged to inform the specialty team of developmental stimulation programs or schooling that the child is receiving. If the hospitalization is planned, every effort should be made for hospital-based educators or tutors to confer with school officials before the child's admission so that schooling is not interrupted. Properly preparing the child and family—especially for new situations—also smooths the adjustment to hospitalization. Preparation must include procedural information about situations the child and family will encounter, definitions of medical jargon specific to the condition, and opportunities to process (i.e., through play, role playing, or discussion) new situations they may experience. For families who are nonassertive or overly aggressive, primary care providers can help to appropriately empower the child and family members for self-advocacy by working through these tasks.

Monitoring the child's adjustment to hospitalization and how it affects the child's future development is also an important part of advocacy. The individualism of the child and the severity of the condition affect the adaptation to hospitalization. Hospitalization is an intrusion into the lives of many children with chronic conditions, but other children have positive memories of previous hospitalizations and may see the hospital as a safe environment. These children may perceive the staff as friends and are often relieved to have a temporary respite from the stress of school, the harassment of other children, or the demands of daily activities. Primary care providers need to recognize that children will occasionally try to become hospitalized to remove themselves from home or school situations that are particularly onerous, although this is uncommon.

Schooling

The role of the educational arena should not be undervalued. Participating in school provides a measure of independence and opportunities for self-mastery and self-esteem building that are not readily achieved at home (Sylva, 1994). Primary care providers can promote the benefits of schooling in numerous ways. Suggestions for altering treatment protocols and medications that interfere with school activities may be offered. Attempts to schedule appointments around the school day should be made to avoid unnecessary absenteeism. A careful history of absenteeism needs to be collected; if it seems excessive for the child's condition, an interdisciplinary conference should be called.

After hospitalization, primary care providers can facilitate a child's transition to school by helping parents provide information about the condition and its ramifications for school participation to school authorities (Andrews, 1991; Committee on Children with Disabilities and Committee on School Health, 1990). Although they may be reluctant to do so, parents should be encouraged to interact with their child's teacher and school nurse unless there is a good reason not to do so. Suggesting methods for preparing classmates for the return of the child is equally important, especially for children with noticeable physical changes (Sexson and Madan-Swain, 1993). "Sanctioned staring," or encouraging classmates to preview the new appearance of the child without fear of recrimination or causing embarrassment, is conducive to a child's acceptance on returning to school. For example, a child can share hospital experiences with classmates by writing a letter and including a picture or making a videotape to send to school. Because many teachers have little knowledge of chronic conditions, offering the address and telephone number of specialty agencies (e.g., the American Cancer Society) initially provides an important source of useful information.

Counseling

Because children with chronic conditions have a higher percentage of psychosocial problems, careful attention must be paid to the child's mental and emotional health (Pless, Power, Peckham, 1993). Growing up is difficult, and the incidence of violence, substance abuse, depression, suicide, and other risks continues to climb among all children. Children with chronic conditions—especially those with diminished self-esteem—may be particularly vulnerable, although research findings on this point remain controversial and unclear (Vessey, 1999). Proactive efforts to prevent mental health problems from occurring include the following: (1) encouraging normal life experiences, (2) improving coping and adaptive abilities, (3) helping children empower themselves, (4) expanding social support networks, and (5) coordinating care (Committee on Children with Disabilities and Committee on Psychosocial Aspects of Child and Family Health, 1993).

Despite the prevalence of mental health concerns among children, only 2% receive services from a mental health professional in a given year. The burden of identifying psychosocial problems falls on primary care providers. The longitudinal relationship that such individuals have with children and families is critical in helping to recognize that mental health problems might develop or may already exist. Unfortunately, the mental health problems of many children are overshadowed by the symptomatology associated with their chronic condition and may go unrecognized and undiagnosed.

The first step for all pediatric providers is to recognize and appreciate the scope of psychologic comorbidity in children with chronic conditions. Mental health problems may present as global behavioral or achievement problems or aberrant behaviors (e.g., psychosomatic complaints, extreme apprehension, deliberate therapeutic nonadherence, or dysfunctional communication) to family members and others. Adopting a healthy suspicion, conducting a careful health history, and providing an atmosphere for discussion will help identify children at risk. Research has shown that mental health concerns are missed if only the parents or the child is interviewed (Canning et al, 1992). Moreover, less than one half of parents will initiate discussions about psychosocial concerns, so it is important to explore this possibility in discussions with all family members. Standardized behavioral screening instruments also have low sensitivity with populations of children with chronic conditions (Canning and Kelleher, 1994).

If no problems are apparent, the focus is on primary prevention with a community-centered approach (Committee on Children with Disabilities et al, 1993). Primary prevention programs are directed toward high risk children without psychiatric diagnoses for whom measures can be undertaken to avoid onset of emotional disturbance or enhance mental health. Programs may be based on counseling, skills training, health education, discussion groups, or combinations of these and are designed to develop resilience and coping skills. Most of these approaches have been shown to be effective (Bauman et al, 1997). Referral may also be appropriate to help a child adapt to a new diagnosis or deteriorating prognosis; deal with school,

family, and peer group issues; or clarify interpersonal and career goals, which are usually very private concerns for older children and adolescents.

Secondary prevention seeks to treat symptoms of emotional distress early to prevent long-term sequelae of mental illness. When problems exist, an accurate diagnosis in accordance with the Diagnostic and Statistical Manual of Mental Disorders IV (American Psychiatric Association, 1994) or the Diagnostic and Statistical Manual: Primary Care Version (American Psychiatric Association, 1995) is important. After the diagnosis is made, appropriate interventions must begin without delay. Individual or group counseling, judicious use of psychotropic medications, and/or referral to a mental health provider are all appropriate measures. Unfortunately, the current insurance and health care delivery infrastructure, accompanied by family resistance to mental health intervention, are significant barriers to the referral process. Moreover, seeking help while maintaining privacy may be difficult for children and families if their mobility around the community is limited. Primary care providers can facilitate such help.

Dying

Despite everyone's best efforts, some children will die. Primary care providers can assist in planning for and providing psychologic care during this difficult time. One of the key roles is to encourage and facilitate the family's ability to provide this care. The emotional needs and fears of children need to be addressed from their perspective. Primary care providers can help family members with this by modeling ways to communicate these sensitive issues and offering insights on how children's developmental levels affect their ability to conceptualize death. Children's questions are often upsetting to parents, such as when a 6-year-old requests detailed information about death rituals or a preschooler asks, "Who will read me stories after I die?". Helping family members and other significant individuals communicate effectively with the child and each other makes death easier to bear.

Many children want to die at home, where they are in familiar surroundings, separation is minimized, care is individualized, and they are in greater control of their situation. Other children may feel insecure at home and prefer to be hospitalized, surrounded by professionals they trust. Home care and hospitalization both have advantages and disadvantages, and the decision of which to pursue must be made in concert with the child's wishes and the family's capabilities. Primary care providers can be instrumental in facilitating either option in conjunction with local hospice services.

Summary

Children with chronic conditions are at a higher risk for negative developmental sequelae than their nonaffected peers. The severity of the condition, the individualism of the child, and the available network of social supports all influence the child's developmental outcomes. Comprehensive prospective care, however, can eliminate or significantly ameliorate negative outcomes. Careful assessment with an interdisciplinary approach helps identify potential or emerging problems associated with the child's disease progression, functional status, social interactions, or global development. Individualized intervention strategies—including therapeutic management, education, counseling, and advocacy—can then be designed and implemented to help children with chronic conditions reach their developmental potential.

References

American Psychiatric Association: Diagnostic and statistical manual of mental disorders, DSM-IV, Washington, 1994, The Association.

American Psychiatric Association: Diagnostic and statistical manual of mental disorders, DSM-PC, Washington, 1995, American Psychiatric Association.

Andrews SG: Informing schools about children's chronic illness: parents' opinions, Pediatrics 88:306-311, 1991.

Bauman LJ et al: A review of psychosocial interventions for children with chronic health conditions, Pediatrics 100(2): 244251, 1997.

Bennett FC and Nickel RE: Developmental screening surveillance. Paper presented at The Child with Special Needs, San Francisco, April 1995.

Bibace R and Walsh M. (editors): New directions for child development: children's conceptions of health, illness, and bodily functions, San Francisco, 1981, Jossey-Bass.

Borradori C et al: Risk factors of sensorineural hearing loss in preterm infants, Biol Neonate 71:1-10, 1997.

Brady TJ: Patient control of treatment is essential, Arthritis Care and Research 38(2):195-202, 1994.

Britto MT et al: Risky behavior in teens with cystic fibrosis or sickle cell disease: a multicenter study, Pediatrics 101:250-256, 1998.

Brookins GK: Culture, ethnicity, and bicultural competence: implications for children with chronic illness and disability, Pediatrics 91:1056-1062, 1993.

Canning EH and Kelleher K: Performance of screening tools for mental health problems in chronically ill children, Arch Pediatr Adolesc Med 148:272-278, 1994.

Canning EH et al: Mental disorders in chronically ill children: parent-child discrepancy and physician identification, Pediatrics 90:692-696, 1992.

Chapieski ML and Evankovich KD: Behavioral effects of prematurity, Semin Perinatol 21:221-239, 1997.

Clay DL et al: Examining systematic differences in adaptation to chronic illness: a growth modeling approach, Rehabilitation Psychol 40:85-98, 1995.

Committee on Children with Disabilities and Committee on Psychosocial Aspects of Child and Family Health: Psychosocial risks of chronic health conditions in childhood and adolescence, Pediatrics 92:876-877, 1993.

Committee on Children with Disabilities and Committee on School Health: Children with health impairments in schools, Pediatrics 86:636-638, 1990.

Crisp J, Ungerer JA, Goodnow JJ: The impact of experience on children's understanding of illness, J Pediatr Psychol, 21(1):57-72, 1996.

Curry DM and Duby JC: Developmental surveillance by pediatric nurses, Ped Nurs 20:40-44, 1994.

Dadds MR, Stein REK, Silver EJ: The role of maternal psychological adjustment in the measurement of children's functional status, J Pediatr Psychol 20:527-544, 1995.

Fanos JH: Developmental tasks of childhood and adolescence: implications for genetic testing. Am J Med Genet 71:22-28, 1997.

Fischel-Ghodsian N et al: Mitochondrial gene mutation is a significant predisposing factor in aminoglycoside ototoxicity, Am J Otolaryngol 18:173-178, 1997.

Fochtman D: Follow-up care for survivors of childhood cancer, Nurse Pract 6:194-200, 1995.

Frank RG et al: Trajectories of adaptation in pediatric chronic illness: the importance of the individual, J Consult Clin Psychol 66:521-532, 1998.

Freud A: The ego mechanism of defense, New York, 1966, International Universities Press.

Gaynon MW et al: Supplemental oxygen may decrease progression of prethreshold disease to threshold retinopathy of prematurity, J Perinatol 17:434-438, 1997.

Geber G and Latts E: Race and ethnicity: issues for adolescents with chronic illness and disabilities, an annotated bibliography, Pediatrics 91:1071-1081, 1993.

Gilbride KE: Developmental testing, Pediatr Rev, 16:338-345, 1995.

Goldberg S: Chronic illness and early development: parent-child relationships, Pediatr Ann 19:35, 39-41, 1990.

Groce NE and Zola IK: Multiculturalism, chronic illness and disability, Pediatrics 91:1048-1055, 1993.

Hertzman C: The case for child development as a determinant of health, Can J Pub Health 89:S14-S19, 1998.

Kato PM, Lyon TD, and Rasco C: Reasoning about moral aspects of illness and treatment by preschoolers who are healthy or who have a chronic illness, J Dev Behav Pediatr 19(2):68-76, 1998.

Kramer JH et al: Cognitive and adaptive behavior 1 and 3 years following bone marrow transplantation, Bone Marrow Transplant 19:607-613, 1997.

Lavigne JV and Faire-Routman J: Psychological adjustment to pediatric physical disorders: A meta-analytic review, J Pediatr Psychol 17:133-157, 1992.

Lehne RA: Pharmacology for nursing care, ed 3, Philadelphia, 1998, W.B. Saunders.

Mahon MM: Children's concept of death and sibling death from trauma, J Pediatr Nurs 8:335-344, 1993.

McCarton CM et al: Cognitive and neurologic development of the premature, small for gestational age infant through age 6: comparison by birth weight and gestational age, Pediatrics 98:1167-1178, 1996.

Newacheck PW and Stoddard JJ: Prevalence and impact of multiple childhood chronic illnesses, J Pediatr 124:40-48, 1994.

Newacheck PW et al: An epidemiologic profile of children with special health care needs, Pediatrics 102:117-121, 1998.

Northam E: Psychosocial impact of chronic illness in children, J Paediatr Child Health 33:369-372, 1997.

Patterson J and Blum RW: Risk and resilience among children and youth with disabilities, Arch Pediatr Adolesc Med 150:692-698, 1996.

Pless IB, Power C, and Peckham CS: Long-term psychosocial sequelae of chronic physical disorders in childhood, Pediatrics 91(6):1131-1136, 1993.

Reiss D, Steinglass P, and Howe G: The family's organization around the illness. In Cole R, Reiss D (editors): How do families cope with chronic illness?, Hillsdale, 1993, Lawrence Erlbaum Associates Inc.

Sexson SB and Madan-Swain A: School re-entry for the child with chronic illness, J Learning Disabilities 26:115-125, 1993.

Smith K, Layne M, and Garell D: The impact of care coordination on children with special health care needs, Child Health Care 23:251-266, 1994.

Stein REK: To be or no to be . . . noncategorical, J Dev Behav Pediatr 17:36-37, 1996.

Stein REK and Jessop DJ: What diagnosis does not tell: the case for a noncategorical approach to chronic illness in children, Soc Sci Med 29:769-778, 1989.

Sterling YV, Peterson J, and Weekes DP: African-American families with chronically ill children: oversights and insights, J Pediatr Nursing 12:292-300, 1997.

Sylva K: School influences on children's development, J Child Psychol Psychiatry 35:135-170, 1994.

Thompson RJ and Gustafson KE: Models of adaptation, adaptation to chronic childhood illness, Washington DC, 1996, American Psychological Association.

Van Dyke DC and Lin-Dyken DC: The new genetics, developmental disabilities, and early intervention, Infants and Young Children 5:8-19, 1993.

Vessey JA: Psychologic comorbidity and chronic conditions, J Pediatr Nursing, 25:211-214, 1999.

Vessey JA and O'Sullivan P: A study of children's concepts of their internal bodies: a comparison of children with and without congenital heart disease, J Pediatr Nurs, in review.

Vessey JA: Comparison of two teaching methods on children's knowledge of their internal bodies, Nurs Res 37:262-267, 1988.

Vessey JA and Miola ES: Teaching adolescents self-advocacy skills, J Pediatr Nurs, 23:53-56, 1997.

Wallander JL and Thompson RJ: Psychosocial adjustment of children with chronic physical conditions. In Roberts MC, editor: Handbook of pediatric psychology, ed 2, New York, 1995, Guilford Press.

Weiss MJS and Wagner SH: What explains the negative consequences of adverse childhood experiences on adult health?, Am J Prev Med 14(4):356-360, 1998.

Yoos HL: Children's illness concepts: old and new paradigms, J Pediatr Nurs 20:134-140, 145, 1994.

Zeanah CH, Boris NW, and Larrieu JA: Infant development and developmental risk: a review of the past 10 years, J Am Acad Child Adolesc Psychiatry 36:165-178, 1997.

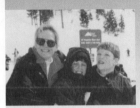

CHAPTER 3

Chronic Conditions and the Family

Margaret P. Shepard and Margaret M. Mahon

The Family

Caring for a child with a chronic condition also involves caring for the child's family. Defining the family is not as easy as it once seemed. The family can be represented by many different configurations of its members. Although there are still nuclear families, a variety of family structures exist, including single-parent families by choice or as a result of death or divorce; blended families; multigenerational families; children raised by gay or lesbian parents; children living in foster or adoptive homes; and children living with grandparents, aunts or uncles, older siblings, or nonrelatives.

The definitions and expectations of family members vary from culture to culture. Regardless, families generally create an environment in which the basic necessities to sustain life and growth are met. When a family functions in a manner supportive or enabling the growth of its members, it is functioning well (Thomas, 1987). Unfortunately, the bonds that tie family members together may be those of obligation or ambivalence instead of affection (Yost, Hochstadt, and Charles, 1988). Regardless, the family influences individual members' expressions of illness and health through socialization and transmission of basic values, beliefs, attitudes, hopes, and aspirations, although these vary among families. When working with a child and family, practitioners must determine who is defined as the family and work within those parameters. This information must be updated over time because of the high rate of flux within families today.

The literature on families who have children with chronic conditions is prolific, but relatively few articles provide comprehensive, organized ways to think about caring for the whole family. This is profoundly important as families and communities increasingly assume day-to-day responsibility for children with chronic conditions in this changing health care climate (Hayes, 1997). The clearest guidance a practitioner can gain comes from the families themselves. In the process of caring for a child with a chronic condition, it is essential to know and understand the family, as well.

Family Crisis and the Child with a Chronic Condition

All families experience crises, which can generally be categorized into two types: developmental and situational. Developmental crises are an expected part of the maturational process of all individuals and families (e.g., marriage, birth of a child, toilet training, starting school, or leaving home). Situational crises, however, are not universal but are determined by circumstances the family encounters. Although all families experience situational crises, they do not necessarily experience the same crises (e.g., having a child with a chronic condition is a situational crisis).

Regardless of the type of crisis, family coping is challenged and adaptation is required. How a family perceives a situation, their problem-solving strategies and coping repertoire, as well as their usual patterns of functioning, will influence their ability to adapt to the new situation (McCubbin, 1993). Adaptation, or the attempt to adapt, leaves the family stronger, weaker, or dissolved. Any crisis—whether developmental or situational—changes the family in some way.

When assessing the effect of a child's chronic condition on the family, practitioners must consider the situational crisis in the context of any concomitant or proximal developmental crisis. For example, the family whose newborn has a condition necessitating surgery or other treatment is also dealing with the birth of a newborn and the accompanying role change. It is important when working with individual families to identify the stresses they are experiencing regarding the burden of caring for a child with a chronic condition and other life stresses.

Family Responses to Diagnosis of a Chronic Condition

Factors that affect the family's response to their child's diagnosis include usual coping patterns, concurrent stressors, and culturally determined values about health and illness. A child previously thought of as "healthy" may now be thought of as "ill." Such labeling may change perceived abilities, values, responsibilities, and other factors that affect all members of the family system. Other factors that affect the responses of parents and others are as follows: (1) the visibility of the condition, (2) the potential for functional limitations (Silver, Westbrook, and Stein, 1998), (3) the presence or absence of mental retardation, (4) the expectation of suffering for the child, (5) the uncertainty about change in the course of condition, (6) family members' experience with others who have chronic conditions, and (7) family members' preconceived ideas about the condition.

Awareness and Initial Diagnosis

Parents have described the time between their initial awareness of the child's symptoms and the diagnosis as overwhelming and characterized by uncertainty and a sense of "groping in the dark" (Horner, 1997). Parents often experience great relief when the diagnosis is made because it relieves some of the uncertainty. New areas of uncertainty, however, are created. Parents may wonder how the condition will effect the whole family, as well as each of the individual members. The diagnosis of a chronic condition often causes disequilibrium for families as some find that their "taken-for-granted world" has been replaced with less predictable conditions (Cohen, 1993).

When a newborn or older child is diagnosed with what will become a chronic condition, the initial reaction is often similar to the reaction to an acute illness. In each of these situations, the parents are likely to grieve the loss of the healthy infant or child they envisioned (Meyers and Weitzman, 1991; Solnit and Stark, 1962). Initial reactions may include shock, disbelief, denial (Holaday, 1984), disgust, guilt, despair, rage, or confusion. Some parents question if there has been some kind of mix-up or mistake or whether the diagnosis is incorrect. If the condition is inherited, many parents feel guilty that they are the cause of their child's condition, and some will search for reasons to fault the other parent. For some parents, their initial reactions interfere with their abilities to respond to their child, or they may distance themselves from the situation.

The magnitude of the crisis that is perceived by the family is an important area for assessment. As with all families in crisis, it is important to determine family member's perceptions of the event, their previous patterns of coping, and the available support systems and resources. In addition, primary care providers must consider the facts, condition, management requirements, and nuances of each condition. Primary care providers should not attempt to change the family's perceptions with statements such as, "It really isn't as bad as you think," but should give objective information that the family can use. Providers also should be aware that it is not inappropriate for parents to temporarily distance themselves from the situation so this behavior should not be treated as maladaptive. It is equally important to ensure that appropriate support from providers, family, and friends is available. These individuals will help the family to cope and reappraise their situation over time.

Search for Information

Having a diagnosis sets some parents on a search for information about causes, treatments, and effects of their child's condition. This quest is usually appropriate and is the first step in having some control over the situation (Hobbs, Perrin, and Ireys, 1985). As such, it should be supported as part of the family's efforts to cope. For other parents, however, the search for information is a denial of the reality of their child's situation. Some parents will read medical books, talk with specialists and subspecialists, and access information on the internet. Such self-education allows families to make informed choices or can start a search exclusively for a cure, possibly delaying the immediate medical care the child needs. Primary care providers must evaluate this information—some of which will be inaccurate, some of which might be dangerous, and some of which may be very helpful.

Some parents search for religious or philosophic reasons for their child's condition (Holaday, 1984). Family functioning can be enhanced if parents have a more positive than negative interpretation (i.e., the child is a "gift from God" not a punishment for prior sins). Being able to define the chronic condition and resultant situations within a previously existing personal, medical-scientific, and/or religious philosophy of life is helpful (Coyne, 1997; Venters, 1981). Primary care providers need to explore the role religious beliefs play in the understanding and decision-making of families.

Fear of Death

The prognosis of the condition affects a family's response to their child. If the condition is, or might be life-threatening, terror about the child's possible or impending death is likely to pervade the initial reactions of family members. Although many health care providers do not discuss death while there is possibility of a cure, this is not helpful. Fear of a child's death is likely to be in the forefront of the parents' thinking. Other information that is conveyed will only be heard through this veil of fear. It is only after dealing with this fear that information about the condition and the available interventions can be readily processed.

Guidelines for Working with Families

Primary care providers should consider the following several important guidelines when working with families and their newly diagnosed children.

1. **Be concrete.** Families should be given as much information as is immediately necessary but not much more. Parents should fully participate in the decision-making process and receive information in enough time to make informed decisions, which is especially difficult because parents are juggling this information with the shock of the diagnosis. Encourage families to ask questions, and then take the time to answer them. Collaboration with a subspecialist is essential because divergent information increases potential anxiety. Provide information in writing. Encourage families to tape record discussions with providers about the condition so that parents and children can review the explanations repeatedly. Family members may not assimilate even the best explanations because of their need for appropriate distraction from the nature of the news they are receiving. Give children developmentally appropriate information, and periodically assess how the parents and child are responding to and using the information provided. Cultural considerations (see Chapter 4) of providing information (e.g., needing to speak to the senior male family member or recognizing the hesitancy of family members to question the provider) must also be considered.

2. **Provide resources.** Personnel may include the primary care provider, other key members of the health care team, and community resource personnel. Previously evaluated websites, books, pamphlets, and referrals to support groups, can also be very helpful for families. Supply them with information about "what comes next," and if possible do this in writing or on tape. Consider the cultural background of the family and the community when recommending supportive and other resources (Garwick et al, 1998).

3. **Help the family put the diagnosis and treatment plan in perspective.** Ascertain what expectations and knowledge the family already has and clarify any misconceptions. Help parents identify the child's strengths (e.g., comment on the alertness of an infant born with myelomeningocele)—

not in an attempt to minimize the seriousness of the situation but to focus on the child as an individual who demonstrates the same needs as other children. Primary care providers can provide a reality check for what children can do and how they will and will not be different.

There are no right or wrong responses for family members at the time of diagnosis. The coping strategies of families are rich and diverse and may reflect ethnic or other cultural values unfamiliar to the primary care provider. Different cultural and religious belief systems should be explored, understood, and accepted by primary care providers (Hostler, 1991), who should look for cues from family members about their readiness to learn, their obstacles to accepting the diagnosis, or their unique fears and stressors. Primary care providers should supportively respond to these cues, but family strengths and prior coping patterns must be considered when intervening. Families will not adopt new patterns of communication in times of crisis. Every interaction at this critical juncture should end with a statement on what to expect next and when the family will be seen again.

When the diagnosis of a chronic condition is made by someone other than the primary care provider, the family often turn to the primary care provider for information, help, or advice. It is important for the primary care provider to consult with the specialist to help the family to understand the diagnosis and treatment options. The primary care provider can act as an advocate or intermediary with the subspecialist, as well as an advisor to the family on how to interact with other providers (e.g., by rehearsing questions or suggesting important areas on which to focus) (Stainton, 1994). Because the child's care ultimately lies with the family, the family must be a part of—and not merely the recipient of—interventions.

Responses to Treatment and Chronicity

Families perceive the chronic condition, as well as its effects and implications, in a variety of ways. Some families can integrate the condition as just another part of the daily routine; whereas to others, it is a feared and loathsome intrusion into their lives. Knafl and associates (1993) categorized families' views of chronic illness as either a "manageable condition," an "ominous situation," a "hateful restriction," or else stated that the family had a "limited understanding of the condition." Each family may define the roles and responsibilities of caring for a child with a chronic condition in different—yet equally effective—ways. Moreover, how roles and responsibilities are assigned is likely to change over time because of the changing developmental and environmental demands on the family.

Parent Response and Responsibilities

Psychologic Effect

Early studies suggested that parents of a child with a chronic condition were likely to experience significant negative psychologic sequelae. Although caring for a child with a chronic condition is associated with unique stressors and hardships, recent studies have uncovered fewer negative sequelae than were previously supposed, as well as considerable variation in outcomes (Drotar, 1997; Wallander and Varni, 1998). The interplay of family functioning and the inherent qualities of the child help determine outcomes. When chronic conditions included functional limitations, parents often experienced greater distress and mothers were at greater risk for depression (Jessop, Reissman, and Stein, 1988; Silver, Westbrook, and Stein, 1998). Other studies demonstrated a relationship between a child's chronic condition and maternal depression, parental care burdens, and passive familial coping (Frank et al, 1998; Ievers and Drotar, 1996). An array of protective factors associated with family functioning have been identified. Higher family competence is associated with better adjustment in the children; and these relations were particularly true for younger adolescents and girls (Kell et al, 1998).

The parenting stress associated with the chronic condition or resultant treatments may bring about behavioral changes that affect the relationship between parents and child (Sheeran, Marvin, and Pianta, 1997). Some parents view certain aspects of the treatment of chronic conditions as disruptive to their relationship with their child (Goldberg and Simmons, 1988) (e.g., parents of children with cystic fibrosis who must perform postural drainage, or the decreased physical contact that might be required if a child has osteogenesis imperfecta, or the blood testing and insulin injections required by children too young to care for their diabetes). The gender of the child also may affect how parents perceive the burden of caring for the child.

Caregiving

Although managing a chronic condition is a family affair, it rarely falls equally on family caregivers. It is well-documented that the mother is usually primarily responsible for the day-to-day care and management of the child (Gallo and Knafl, 1998). Some mothers leave outside employment in order to care for their child and meet the demands of medical treatment (Mastroyannopoulou et al, 1997; Stein et al, 1989). Limited day care availability for children with chronic conditions requires other mothers who might have been employed to stay at home.

Many mothers evaluate their caregiving experience very positively but say it is helpful to have someone with whom they can talk (Jessop, Reissman, and Stein, 1988). This person does not have to be a family member (Kazak, Reber, and Carter, 1988), and support groups may meet this need (Hostler, 1991). These groups are most often helpful around the time of diagnosis, probably because of the need for concrete information that is shared among the relatively small number of people in similar situations. Primary care providers may consider engaging the assistance of one or several parents to plan a parent support group. Parent-led groups may be more effective than ones led by professionals.

Marital Relations

Many health professionals assume that the rate of family dissolution is greater because of increased familial stress from the presence of a chronic condition in a family. On the contrary, carefully controlled studies have indicated differences neither in marital functioning nor in the rates of divorced or single-parent families of children with chronic conditions (Cadman et al, 1991; Kazak, 1989; Spaulding and Morgan, 1986). Although divorce is not more prevalent, tension and stress are more common in families of a child with a chronic condition (Hobbs, Perrin, and Ireys, 1985). These families may experience more strain and conflict over the roles of their members, as well as fewer exchanges of affection. Parents of children with chronic conditions, however, are not more likely to experience higher levels of depression or marital dissatisfaction than families of healthy children (Quittner et al, 1998).

Finances

Finances are an issue for many parents because there are many additional expenses beyond those directly for care of the child with a chronic condition. Additional costs for families include foods for special diets; transportation; baby-sitters for siblings while a child receives treatment or other care; time lost from work or school; cosmetics, wigs, or clothing to hide the effects of the disease or treatment; and incidentals such as bandages, test kits, diapers, and bed pads (Hobbs, Perrin, and Ireys, 1985). Other expenses are the need for structural modifications to the home, counseling and mental health services, and respite homemaker services. Not many of these expenses are covered by most third-party payers. If these costs are covered, the amount of reimbursement is likely to be limited (see Chapter 7).

Privacy

The trend toward shorter hospital stays has resulted in children being discharged when they are sick and with more complex care demands. Sometimes children return home with nurses or other caregivers; and having "outsiders" in the home regularly can be very stressful for families. The increase in the acuity and number of care providers requires more vigilant efforts in communication between care providers.

Response of Siblings

The effect of a chronic condition on siblings varies. Many children neither perceive having a sibling with a chronic condition as a significant stressor nor experience greater problems in behavior and social competence (Gallo et al, 1992). Others experience a variety of stressors—including their brother or sister (Barbarian et al, 1995), but most siblings of children with chronic conditions feel stress and sadness during the hospitalization of their brother or sister (Morrison, 1997).

Parents may have difficulty accurately perceiving how their children are coping. Furthermore, if problems do exist, it may be difficult to distinguish if they are related to the sibling's chronic condition (Gallo et al, 1993) or to other developmental or environmental issues. It is often helpful for the primary care provider to ask how siblings are doing and what they understand about the recent changes in the family.

A lack of accurate and understandable information about the chronic condition is stressful. Siblings may hear things from friends who received information from their parents. Adolescents and even younger siblings increasingly use the Internet to obtain information. What siblings overhear or piece together is often much worse than the reality; they often imagine gruesome things about the experiences associated with illness, hospitalization, and treatment. If possible, siblings should be allowed to visit the hospital, treatment rooms, and perhaps witness treatments (i.e., if acceptable to the affected child). Psychologic preparation is necessary for siblings, just as it is for children being admitted to hospitals.

Throughout the course of the chronic condition, information for the siblings needs to be updated for two primary reasons. First, what is known about the condition changes, both as the affected child and parents learn more about the condition and as the manifestations of the condition in this particular child evolve. Second, the developmental level of the siblings changes, improving their ability to understand and integrate information.

Among siblings of hospitalized children, children older than 7 years of age and those with more than one visit to the hospital had more behavioral changes (Morrison, 1997). Williams, Lorenzo, and Borja (1993) found that siblings of children with chronic conditions had significantly more responsibilities at home, involving both housework and child care. Gender-biased expectations of siblings occurs with older sisters, who might be called on more often than younger sisters to perform caregiving tasks, and should be avoided if at all possible. Siblings' perceptions of the home environment are

likely to differ from the impressions of their parents (Feeman and Hagen, 1990).

There is some disagreement about the degree to which siblings should be involved in the care of a child with a chronic condition. Two areas should be considered: the developmental abilities of the siblings and their desire to be involved. The most important consideration is consistency; for example, are demands being made regardless of whether a chronic condition is present or absent in any particular child? Siblings who want to be involved in care should be allowed to be involved, just as one would involve a helpful child in other areas of family life. Siblings' abilities to contribute to family life should be recognized (Kiburz, 1994).

Primary care providers are often in an ideal position to educate and counsel siblings throughout the course of their brother or sister's illness. Within the context of the preexisting relationship, sibling responses, patterns of communication, and reactions to stress are helpful in guiding these dialogs. If the parents are unable to talk to the siblings, it is important to find someone else (e.g., the primary care provider) who can speak with the siblings in a developmentally appropriate way. It also is important for health care providers to monitor for depression.

Some siblings complain, and often not incorrectly, that the child with the chronic condition is treated more leniently. Parents may be unaware that they are treating their children with different standards, or may think that the child's condition warrants leniency. For example, Quittner and Opipari (1994) concluded that there were both qualitative and quantitative differences in parenting when a child with cystic fibrosis was in the family, despite the parents' lack of awareness. It is appropriate for primary care providers to question families about methods and consistency of discipline. The need for consistent discipline is crucial. Discipline supplies limits and structure and should be consistent within families and between siblings.

The effects of a condition or treatment (e.g., hair loss, flatulence, or copious secretions) may be embarrassing for siblings. At the same time, however, children want to protect their affected sibling from the derisive statements or stares of others. Any feelings of shame and embarrassment are usually not severe, although they can engender simultaneous or subsequent feelings of guilt or depression.

The developmental level of siblings (i.e., both physical and psychosocial) further influences their reaction to the child with a chronic condition. If a child is to be cared for at home and needs to use equipment and medications, planning for sibling safety is required. Cases of children injuring or potentially injuring themselves or their siblings by changing intravenous flow rates or by not understanding the danger of electric equipment have been reported (Andrews and Nielson, 1988).

Siblings are usually very aware of their negative feelings, which may include anger; neglect; fear of causality, contagion, or responsibility; as well as other founded and unfounded feelings. As a result of their negative feelings, siblings may experience guilt. Children need to be told that their emotions are acceptable, but misconceptions must simultaneously be clarified. This may be a time-consuming process calling for self-realization, which is a difficult task for some families. For example, a sibling's perception of receiving less attention can be confirmed. Children should also be told that it is okay to feel angry about receiving less attention. This process can be very difficult if a family does not usually share emotions.

Siblings have also described many positive effects of having a brother or sister with a chronic condition, including greater maturity, supportiveness, and independence (Barbarian et al, 1995). Siblings of children with myelomeningocele were found to have a high degree of empathy and concern for the affected child (Kiburz, 1994). Siblings of children with chronic conditions have been reported to be cooperative and able to cognitively master situations earlier than their peers (Lynn, 1989). Positive responses were even more likely to occur among adolescents and first-born siblings, as well as when the sibling's prognosis was less positive (Barbarian et al, 1995). Parental attitudes about the child and efforts at normalization are very important in developing positive responses in siblings.

Family Management Styles

Family management style has been conceptualized as the configuration formed by individual family members' definitions of their situations, the man-

agement behaviors they engage in with respect to the chronic conditions, and the sociocultural context in which these definitions and behaviors occur. The definition of a situation is its subjective meaning for a person. Management behaviors are the discrete behavioral accommodations that family members use to manage a chronic condition on a daily basis. Five distinct family management styles have been described: thriving, accommodating, enduring, struggling, and floundering (Deatrick and Knafl, 1990; Knafl et al, 1996).

Thriving and accommodative families view the condition and the child as "normal." Parents have confidence in and a proactive stance toward their ability to manage the illness. Children view themselves as "healthy." Accommodative families differ from thriving families by viewing their situation as essentially normal, although somewhat more negatively. Accommodative parents may also take a more compliant approach to illness management. Enduring families tend to perceive more difficulty in raising a child with a chronic condition and associate greater negative consequences to their situation. Although they may view the child as normal, some enduring families describe their child with a chronic condition as a "tragic figure" and tend to be more protective of the child. Struggling families are characterized by conflict over how to best manage their child's condition. Struggling parents perceive less support and mutuality from one another—particularly mothers who feel they receive insufficient support from their spouses. Children in struggling families perceive the illness as a greater intrusion in their lives and an ongoing source of worry. The hallmark of floundering families is their sense of confusion. Parents define themselves and their situation negatively. They are uncertain about the best management approaches, and condition management is perceived as difficult and burdensome. They also view the child as a tragic figure.

Children with chronic conditions are superimposed on families with preexisting management styles. As such, most parents continue to parent as they have been doing, and most families function how they have been. Management styles are not immutable, however, and over one half of the participating families described using a different management styles 1 year apart (Knafl et al, 1996).

Primary care providers must recognize family management style as a dynamic process that changes as a result of not only the changes in the child's condition but also other developmental and situational stressors or supports. Ongoing assessments of family management styles contribute to targeted interventions based on information about whether challenges to adaptation are due to problems in the family definition of the situation, management approaches, or differences between the parents.

Normalization

Normalization is the overriding theme that characterizes the successful management process used by many families of children with chronic conditions. Normalization is an ongoing process of actively accommodating the child's evolving physical, emotional, and social needs (Deatrick, Knafl, and Walsh, 1988). Acknowledging the condition is essential as the foundation of normalization. There is no denial involved; instead the family is making a statement that this child is a part of their family, and their family is just like every other family. Normalization also involves viewing the social effects of having a child with a chronic condition as minimal and engaging in behaviors that show others that this is a normal family (Knafl and Deatrick, 1986).The child is integrated into the mainstream to the greatest extent possible (Holaday, 1984). The child's age and the condition's severity, however, affect the ability of the family to use the process of normalization (Knafl and Deatrick, 1986).

Krulik (1980) described several antecedent principles necessary for the normalization process, as follows: (1) Those involved in the care of the child, including the child, are prepared for the effects of the condition and treatment. (2) The child is involved in self-care and decisions made about care. (3) The child is not treated differently from others in the family. (4) The child's condition is not kept secret but shared with others when appropriate. (5) The parents' role in managing care is recognized.

Normalization is important because it focuses on the child—not the condition. Although most parents who have used normalization have discovered these techniques on their own, the process involves some concrete steps that can be taught. Par-

ents may go through a series of stages while learning to care for their child day-to-day. In this process, family tasks and activities may be reorganized so the condition regimen becomes a routine part of family life (Jerret, 1994). Primary care providers can demonstrate some of these steps by recognizing the normalcy, strengths, and weaknesses of the family system; by being open and supportive about the child's condition and treatment; and by actively involving the family in all aspects of care. Reinforcing the family's successful use of these tactics can improve self-esteem and motivate further development.

Therapeutic Adherence

Families have successfully demonstrated a variety of approaches to managing the condition with their lifestyle. The following are three predominant approaches: (1) strict adherence, (2) flexible adherence, and (3) selective adherence (Gallo and Knafl, 1998). Families that take a strict-adherence approach work closely with health professionals and strictly comply with the prescribed treatment plan. The primary goal of this approach is to control the condition and related symptoms. Families that take a flexible approach to adherence focus on streamlining treatment and making life more "livable" while controlling the illness. Flexible parents work closely with health professionals to achieve their goals. Families that follow a selective approach to adherence share the goal of controlling the condition and its symptoms but may develop alternative treatment plans and work independently of professionals.

When the family's management approach veers from the prescribed treatment plan, health care providers tend to view such families as noncompliant without considering that their underlying goals may be the same. Awareness of differing approaches to managing a child's condition provide important information for health care professionals and parents as they mutually strive to address the needs of the child's condition (Gallo and Knafl, 1998). Encouraging families to articulate their goals and management approaches may provide key information on how to intervene more thoughtfully with families based on their treatment approach; after all, they manage their child's condition on a daily basis.

Social Support

The amount and type of social support received by families is an essential factor in their adjustment to the chronic condition (Frankel and Wamboldt, 1998). In general, families receive adequate support from a variety of sources including other family members, friends, and health care providers (Garwick et al, 1998), but parents may differentiate the types of support received from these sources. Mothers may be more critical of and more dissatisfied with the quality of help received—especially from extended family members and health professionals (Patterson et al, 1997). Offers of support from uninformed neighbors and community members may be perceived as unhelp.ful. Well-intentioned neighbors and friends who lack adequate knowledge and understanding of the child's condition or treatment may make insensitive remarks suggesting that the parents are to blame for their child's condition (Garwick et al, 1998).

Race and ethnicity may influence how families perceive and use social supports (Garwick et al, 1998). In a comparison study of black and white families, white families were more likely to identify affective support (i.e., support conveying empathy and understanding) as the primary type of support, whereas black families identified instrumental assistance (i.e., help with other children or transportation) as the primary means of support from friends and families (Williams, 1993).

At the time of diagnosis there is often an influx of concerned people. After the initial crisis period and during periods of acute hospitalizations, parents may find they are without support from friends and family, which often results in social isolation (Andrews and Nielson, 1988). Tangible types of support that families have found helpful include transportation for siblings, arranging for siblings to stay with friends during hospitalizations, providing meals, doing laundry, running errands, or baby-sitting in the home so that the parents can have some time for personal needs. This latter form of assistance may entail learning skills such as cardiopulmonary resuscitation (CPR), use of monitors, or emergency care. It is extremely important that someone besides the mother be able and willing to do this. Families usually rely on other family members and close friends to assist them at this time.

There are a number of factors related to both the chronic condition and to the familial context that may influence a family's ability to seek and use supportive resources. If the condition is relatively common or well-understood, the child is less likely to face societal prejudice. The issue of familiarity with the condition is one reason some parents turn to support groups; they do not have to explain and re-explain the condition because the support group members are experiencing similar situations.

Practitioners should assess the type of support needed before planning supportive interventions. Practitioners may help families early in the diagnostic and treatment process by encouraging them to plan for and use helpful resources. Parents may also benefit from the notion that it is okay to refuse certain types of "well-intended" support from family and friends. Families often express that they need help finding community resources and/or recreational activities for their children with chronic conditions (Williams, 1993), and primary care providers can facilitate family support by identifying the types of support that may be most helpful for a family and by being knowledgeable and culturally sensitive about community resources and parents' groups.

Health professionals have been perceived as most helpful when they provide expert informational support to address specific stressors identified by the family. Research by Burke and associates (1997) found that responding to specific stress points identified by the family members improved family coping and functioning and eliminated hospitalization-induced developmental regression in the children. It may be helpful to encourage families to outline practical planning steps for the next phases of treatment and the caring process (Dokken and Sydnor-Greenberg, 1998). Families perceived it as unhelpful when primary care providers were unable to furnish complete information about the child's condition or care, or when they lacked adequate knowledge of services and referral options (Garwick et al, 1998). Primary care providers who have established long-term relationships with the child and the family may be relied on for emotional and informational support, but the principal supportive role for the primary care provider should be to provide expert knowledge and facilitate seamless transitions throughout the increasingly complex health care system.

Chronic Sorrow

Olshansky (1962) first described the phenomenon of "chronic sorrow" as a pattern of sadness in response to a child's differences that is an ongoing process differing from grief. Chronic sorrow is not static (Gravelle, 1997) but includes elements of permanence with episodic surges in the presence of situational or developmental crisis (Hainsworth, 1996).

Although complex and multifaceted, chronic sorrow is not pathologic. For some parents, chronic sorrow includes feelings of anger, guilt, and failure, which does not mean that the parents are always sad or wish this was not their child. They may have a tremendous appreciation of small victories and are proud of their children. Chronic sorrow occurs while parents redefine parental expectations and the parameters for judging the child's accomplishments. There is the recognition, often daily, that their child is not normal. External events, such as the passage of a child's expected date of graduation or internal awareness (e.g., an awareness that a child will need these treatments every day for the rest of his or her life), trigger resurgences of chronic sorrow (Lindgren et al, 1992). Chronic sorrow does not necessarily occur uniformly within families. There may be clear-cut differences in maternal and paternal patterns of overall adjustment (Damrosch and Perry 1989), with most fathers depicting their adjustment as steady, gradual, and bound to time, and most mothers perceiving their own adjustment as chronic, periodic crises.

Developing Family Expertise

Parenting a child with a chronic condition "involve[s] qualitatively different work than parenting a child" without a chronic condition (Deatrick, Knafl, and Walsh, 1988). Family members and providers must differentiate between assuming that having a child with a chronic condition is inherently negative and specifying which aspects of the situation are problematic (Knafl and Deatrick, 1987). Many parental concerns for their children are the same as those of parents whose child does not have a chronic condition. All parents worry; the extent to which the parent of a child with a chronic condition worries cannot be predicted from the severity of symptoms (Stein et al, 1989).

Many parents are concerned about what implications their child's diagnosis may have for future children. A major factor is whether or not the chronic condition has a genetic component. Potential of inheritance, availability of prenatal diagnosis, conditions, symptomatology, and trajectory of a condition are all known to influence the decision-making of parents about conceiving other children. Parents who feel guilty about having a child with a genetically transmitted chronic condition revisit this each time they consider having another child, as well as later in life when their children reach child-bearing age (Goldberg and Simmons, 1988). As children with chronic conditions get older, concerns about the ability to have children become their own. For example, with the increased survival time of people with cystic fibrosis, more women are surviving to childbearing age, which has implications not only for these women but also for families and primary-care providers. Another common concern for parents is that of the parental (usually maternal) workload (i.e., can they physically and fiscally care for another child?). Again, these concerns are often the same as for those families with no children with chronic conditions.

Family and child adaptation are mutually interrelated. Children tend to adapt most successfully to living with a chronic condition when family functioning remains strong (Grey et al, 1996; Hamlett, Pelligrini and Katz, 1992; Ievers et al, 1998; Kell et al, 1998). When families are not functioning optimally, however, they tend to experience greater severity in effects related to the chronic condition. The negative effects experienced by the child are not likely to be related to the chronic condition (Drotar, 1997; Frank et al, 1998; Holden et al, 1997).

The relationship of the family with the primary care provider often, and appropriately, changes over time as the locus of expertise shifts to the family. Primary care providers must recognize the family's increasing acquisition of knowledge, as well as its management behaviors and styles (Deatrick, Knafl, and Guyer, 1993). Some parents have reported that they and their children are not respected, especially for their expertise in managing the child's condition (Faux and Seidemann, 1996). Families who do not follow the care plan precisely as given to them may be judged negatively (Gallo and Knafl, 1998). Respecting and using knowledge the family has acquired—not only about the condition but also about the child and his or her individual responses—is important. Empowerment of the family by providers can enhance the family's quality of life (Hartley and Fuller, 1997).

Foster Care

Because some families are unable to provide care, some children with chronic conditions need medical foster care. The need for families capable of providing this service has dramatically increased in recent years. When foster care is not available, these children sometimes become boarder infants in hospitals at great cost to the hospital and the public and at significant personal risk to the child. Placing children in medical foster care results in a 40% to 98% monetary savings and provides a home environment for the children (Yost, Hochstadt, and Charles, 1988).

Over time, foster care has developed two major problems—inequitable placements and decreased access to care—that became increasingly apparent. In addition, it was recognized that for many children foster care was not to be a temporary arrangement. As a result, the Adoption Assistance and Child Welfare Act of 1980 (PL96-272) was enacted to limit the number of children in foster care, in part by limiting the time that children can spend in foster care (Alexander and Alexander, 1995). By 1982, the number of children in foster care had decreased by one-half to less than 250,000 (Rosenfeld et al, 1997). Many social problems have developed since then, however, and the number of children in foster care currently exceeds 500,000 (Gitlitz and Kuehne, 1997; Rosenfeld et al, 1997).

There are several types of foster care placements: group homes, kinship family foster care, and nonrelated family foster care (Gitlitz and Kuehne, 1997). Group homes are often for children whose emotional and/or behavioral problems or severe medical problems make family placement impossible. In kinship family foster care, the child is placed with family, usually on the mother's side of the family.

Foster care parents often have difficulty obtaining services for the children in their care (Barton, 1998). Primary care providers can improve access, as well as direct health of the child (Blatt and Simms, 1997; Brodie, Berridge, and Beckett, 1997; Carlson, 1996; Cohen et al, 1995) through efforts focused on the following three areas: (1) gathering as much data as possible regarding past health and risk factors; (2) compiling a broad and thorough database for the present (recognizing that it is likely to travel with the child); and (3) being aware of the risk factors for children in foster care and the implications of these factors on a child's chronic condition.

The Dying Child and the Family

Caring for a child who dies at home is a positive experience for most families (Collins, Stevens, and Cousens, 1998). Once a child's condition has reached the terminal phase, the focus of care should switch from cure to palliation. Although palliative care for children is not widely available, emphasis should be on complete symptom management in the context of the child and family. Discussions with families must include the child whenever possible. Decision-making must take into consideration the child's quality of life, family values, and other personal and ethical dimensions (Fleischman et al, 1994). Having this broader focus before death provides a foundation for continuing support for the family after the death. Receiving quality family-focused care during the terminal phase of a child's illness makes a positive difference in the long-term bereavement and adaptation of the family. Families do recognize and value the concept of a "good death," even given the fact that they would do almost anything to prevent the death from happening.

The Dying Child

Children who have been sick for a long time often have an understanding of sickness and death well beyond their chronologic age. These children can judge who is comfortable dealing with their impending death and who is not. Dying children may use the way care givers have handled other deaths as a test. For example, if children and families get to know other children and families (i.e., in the clinical setting or during hospitalization) who later die, they are likely to use the response of staff and others to gauge how their own death will be handled and to measure how helpful others are likely to be when preparing for death.

Maintaining Normalcy

Families of children who are dying want to sustain normalcy (James and Johnson, 1997). It is important to maintain the usual activities of childhood, such as playing and reading. Play is important because it enhances the child's feelings of control (Vessey and Mahon, 1990). Although dying children may be less able to participate in familiar and favorite activities, modifications can usually be made if this is something the child really wants to do (e.g., someone else can roll dice and move a game piece). If children are no longer able to read their own books, many love having books read to them. Music is also a favorite distraction for children; even children of 1 or 2 years of age have favorite tapes. Older children may want to be involved in planning their own funeral. This is often difficult for the family, but it is the last act of control for some children. In the past, children have chosen particular readings or music for their funerals. One child asked that balloons be released outside of the church "to go up in the same way his spirit would go." Others might want to leave a videotaped message for siblings or classmates.

Dying children often seem ambivalent about the role of those around them. They may be adamant about not being left alone, but they are also likely to be selective about who they want with them. It may seem that their world is becoming progressively smaller. They are likely to become less verbal because of decreased energy or possibly a physical inability to talk. These children might also be in a coma, depending on the condition. If this is the case, parents can be encouraged to continue physical and verbal contact with them. When possible, the presence of a few people and physical contact are very important to a child.

Parents often turn to the practitioner for advice on communicating with the ill child or the siblings about death. A good guideline is to answer the question the child asks while understanding why the child is asking the question. Often the subtext is "Who will take care of me?", or "Does it hurt to die?". The inclination may be to either avoid answering the questions altogether or inundate children with information. If primary care providers take the time to listen and are clearly willing to respond, children will most often ask what they are ready to hear.

Pain Control

Pain control is an extremely important issue when a child is dying, so it must not go underrecognized and undertreated. Pain is a subjective experience. A child's developmental level affects not only perceptions of pain but also descriptions of pain (Vessey and Carlson, 1996). The pain experienced by the dying child is often a focus for both the child and the parents. Children's pain contributes to parental feelings of impotence. Not only can the parents not provide a cure for the child, but they are also unable to protect the child from pain. Because a child can play with a video game for 30 minutes without complaining does not mean the child is not in pain. It is more likely that the child has excellent self-distraction abilities. Fears about addiction and tolerance should not preclude adequate treatment of pain.

Providers sometimes believe that pain is an inevitable part of dying or that they would be hastening death by managing pain adequately. Community-based providers are ideal to manage dying children (Dawson, 1995; Margolius, Hudson, and Michel, 1995), however, the provider who cares for the dying child must be aware of personal attitudes about dying, pain management, and using what is necessary to completely alleviate pain. Assessment of pain also must be geared to children and can include instruments like the FACES or Oucher scale. Cultural differences also need to be considered (Abu-Saad and Hamers, 1997). Pain management should include optimal use of pharmacologic and nonpharmacologic methods in treating acute and chronic pain (Schanberg et al, 1997). Appropriate use of opiates and other methods (e.g. nerve blocks) must be considered (Liben, 1996; Staats and Kost-Byerly, 1995; Stevens et al, 1994). In addition, pain management must include pain from procedures, which is often undertreated (Ashburn, 1995; Stevens et al, 1994).

Parents

Parents are often experts in providing complete care for their child. At the same time, however, families need specific interventions related to the child's impending death. Caring for a dying child can be physically and emotionally exhausting (Davies et al, 1996).

The death of a child is the most painful loss an individual can experience. Bereavement is a complex and long-term adaptation process. Families will never be as they were before and should not be urged to "get over it." Bereavement involves putting the child who died in a new place in the survivors' lives. There is not one specific right thing to say to support parents, but there are wrong responses. Parents should never be told "at least you have other children," "at least he was young enough so you didn't have time to know him well," "You're young. You can have more children," or worst, "I know how you feel." Even those who have experienced the death of a child will not experience the same responses.

Within families there will be variation in response to the death of a child. Mothers are more likely to receive social support and recognition of the depth of their loss. Fathers are expected to support the mothers. This may help to explain why fathers' grief is different from that of mothers (Hogan, 1988). Whether the death was sudden or followed a long illness, many families have found it helpful to have contact with the primary care provider about 1 month after the death. By this time, friends and relatives may be expecting the family members to manage their grief, but family members' pain is still fresh. Not uncommonly, many parents want to learn more about their child's death.

Siblings

Siblings often feel isolated while the child is dying, especially if the child is hospitalized. If the child is dying at home, siblings can have a more active role in the dying process. This does not necessarily mean a task orientation, although doing tasks can help siblings feel less isolated. Regardless of where the child is dying, it is very important that siblings be kept informed of the child's condition. The lack of sureness about when death will occur is difficult for siblings, so when the child does die, they are often surprised. If siblings had been told many times that death was imminent, but it did not occur, they were sure that again, death would be thwarted. Siblings (and parents) should be prepared for what is likely to happen at the time of death.

After the child dies, siblings' reactions are based on their own feelings in conjunction with their parents' grief reactions. Children who depend on their parents now see them in such pain that it exposes a vulnerability not previously evident. This is difficult and potentially frightening for the child. As a result, siblings might act cheerful in an effort to spare the parents pain, while parents may misinterpret this response and believe siblings are not grieving. This can increase tension at an already difficult time (Hogan, 1988).

Parents are often so overwhelmed with grief that it is difficult for them to understand and support the bereavement of their surviving children. Children are often reluctant to talk to their parents about the deceased sibling or matters related to the death for fear of causing their parents more pain. Bereavement is a healthy process, though painful and difficult. Those who interact regularly with the bereaved child (e.g., teachers) may not feel qualified or otherwise able to provide support for the child (Mahon, Goldberg, and Washington, in press). Some families benefit from counseling or support groups or referrals to tertiary centers with appropriate services.

The Primary Care Provider's Role

A death at home gives the family greater freedom, privacy, and fewer disruptions in family life (Collins, Stevens, and Cousens, 1998). Most pediatric primary care providers do not often deal with the death of a child; however, dying children are increasingly becoming their purview as chronic care management shifts to community clinicians. Primary care providers should consult with a palliative care team early in the disease course (Frager, 1996). To be honest with the child and family does not mean to take away hope; hope should be interwoven with the course of the illness. As the inevitability of death becomes clearer, the focus of the hope changes (i.e., perhaps from cure to minimal pain and control in the process of dying).

The death of a child can be a painful and awkward situation for primary care providers. The greatest difficulty for some may be a perception that the death of a child is a failure (Charlton, 1996). At the same time, because of the long-term involvement of primary care providers with the family, they can be a valuable resource and advocate. Unfortunately, siblings of all ages often inappropriately assume some responsibility for the death or feel guilty about their responses to the death (Mahon, Goldberg, and Washington, 1999; Mahon and Page, 1995). Siblings should be told that they had no responsibility for the death. As is true with all crucial developmental issues, this information will probably have to be repeated several times.

Primary care providers are likely to have more experience with survivors (e.g., parents and siblings) than with a terminally ill child. Primary care providers may be best able to answer any questions the parents have about the death, any last words, or if the child was in pain—particularly if it was a sudden death or the parents were not present at the time of death. Meeting with parents also shows the family that someone remembers how recent the death was and how acute the pain is.

Practitioners can offer support and guidance for parents and provide concrete information and reassurance for surviving children. If a referral is made for counseling, the primary care provider must ensure that the facilitator is comfortable with and qualified to address death-related issues. A "loss" group, in which bereaved children are clustered with those of children whose parents have divorced, is not appropriate.

Summary

The family unit, which varies in structure and composition, is the primary unit of care and support for the child. A child's chronic condition alters the roles and expectations of all family members by creating stressors to which the family must learn to adapt. Primary care providers can be instrumental in assisting the child and family to cope with a chronic condition by supporting coping strategies, by providing accurate and understandable information on the condition and all aspects of the child's care, by implementing preventive health measures to minimize complications of the condition and promote optimal well-being, by accessing services needed by the family, and by offering support for the long-term emotional needs of each family member.

References

Abu-Saad HH and Hammers JP: Decision making and pediatric pain: a review, J Adv Nurs 26:946-952, 1997.

Alexander R and Alexander CL: The impact of Suter v. Artist M. on foster care policy, Social Work: J Natl Assoc Soc Workers 40:543-8, 1995.

Andrews MM and Nielson DW: Technology dependent children in the home, Pediatr Nurs 14:111-114, 1988.

Ashburn MA: Burn pain: the management of procedure related pain, J Nurs Care Rehab 16:365-71, 1995.

Barbarian et al: Sibling adaptation to childhood cancer collaborative study: parental views of pre- and postdiagnosis adjustment of siblings of children with cancer, J Psychosoc Oncol 13(3): 1-20, 1995.

Barton SJ: Foster parents of cocaine exposed infants, J Pediatr Nurs 13:104-112, 1998.

Blatt SD and Simms M: Foster care: special children, special needs, Contemp Pediatrics 14:109-10, 112-113, 117-118, 1997.

Brodie I, Berridge D, and Beckett W: Children's nursing: the health of children looked after by local authorities, British Nursing 6:386-90, 1997.

Burke SO et al: Stress-point intervention of parents of repeatedly hospitalized children with chronic conditions, Res Nurs Health 20:475-485, 1997.

Cadman D et al: Children with chronic illness: family and parent demographic characteristics and psychological adjustment, Pediatrics 87:884-889, 1991.

Carlson KL: Providing health care for children in foster care: a role for advanced practice nurses, Pediatr Nurs 22:418-422, 1996.

Charlton R: Medical education—addressing the needs of the dying child, Palliat Med 10:240-246, 1996.

Cohen FL et al: Family experiences when a child is HIV positive, Pediatr Nurs 21:248-253, 1995.

Cohen MH: Diagnostic closure and the spread of uncertainty, Issues Compr Pediatr Nurs 16:135-146, 1993.

Collins JJ, Stevens MM, and Cousens P: Home care for the dying child: a parent's perception, Aust Fam Physician 27:610-614, 1998.

Coyne IT: Chronic illness: the importance of support for families caring for a child with cystic fibrosis, J Clin Nurs 6:121-129, 1997.

Damrosch SP and Perry LA: Self-reported adjustment, chronic sorrow, and coping of parents of children with Down syndrome, Nurs Res 38:25-30, 1989.

Davies B et al: Canuck place: a hospice for dying children, Can Nurs 92:22-25, 1996.

Dawson SA: A dying child, Can Fam Physician 41:534-540, 1995.

Deatrick JA, Knafl KA, and Guyer K: The meaning of care-giver behaviors: inductive approaches to family theory development. In the nursing of families: theories, research, education, practice, 1993, Newbury Park, Calif., Sage.

Deatrick J and Knafl K: Management behaviors: day to day adjustments to childhood chronic conditions, J Pediatr Nurs 5:15-22, 1990.

Deatrick JA, Knafl KA, and Walsh M: The process of parenting a child with a disability: normalization through accommodations, J Adv Nurs 13:15-21, 1988.

Dokken DL and Sydnor-Greenberg N: Helping families mobilize their personal resources, Pediatr Nurs 24:66-69, 1998.

Drotar D: Relating parent and family functioning to the psychological adjustment of children with chronic conditions: what have we learned? what do we need to know?, J Pediatr Psychol 22:149-165, 1997.

Faux SA and Seidemann RY: Health care professionals and their relationships with families who have members with developmental disabilities, J Fam Nurs 2:217-238, 1996.

Feeman DJ and Hagen JW: Effects of childhood chronic illness in families, Soc Work Health Care 14(3):37-53, 1990.

Fleischman AR et al: Caring for gravely ill children, Pediatrics 94:433-439, 1994.

Frager G: Pediatric palliative care: building the model, bridging the gaps, J Palliat Care 12:9-12, 1996.

Frank RG et al: Disease and family contributors to adaptation in juvenile rheumatoid arthritis and juvenile diabetes, Arthritis Care Res 11:166-176, 1998.

Frankel K and Wamboldt MZ: Chronic childhood illness and maternal mental health—why should we care? J Asthma 35:621-630, 1998.

Gallo A and Knafl K: Parents' reports of "tricks of the trade" for managing childhood chronic illness, J Pediatr Nurs 3:93-102, 1998.

Gallo AM et al: Well siblings of children with chronic illness: parents' reports of their psychological adjustment, Pediatr Nurs 18:23-27, 1992.

Gallo AM et al: Mothers' perceptions of sibling adjustment and family life in childhood chronic illness, J Pediatr Nurs 8:318-324, 1993.

Garwick AW et al: Families' recommendations for improving services for children with chronic conditions, Arch Pediatr Adolesc Med 152:440-448, 1998.

Garwick AW et al: Parents perceptions of helpful vs. unhelpful types of support in managing the care or preadolescents with chronic conditions, Arch Pediatr Adolesc Med 152:665-671, 1998.

Gitlitz B and Kuehne E: Caring for children in foster care, J Pediatr Health Care 11:127-129, 1997.

Goldberg S and Simmons RJ: Chronic illness and early development, Pediatrician 15:13-20, 1988.

Gravelle AM: Caring for a child with a progressive illness during the complex chronic phase: parents' experience of facing adversity, J Adv Nurs 25:738-745, 1997.

Grey et al: Personal and family factors associated with quality of life in children with diabetes, Diabetes Care 21(6):909-914, 1998.

Hainsworth MA: Helping children with chronic sorrow related to multiple sclerosis, J Psychosoc Nurs Mental Health Serv 34(6):36-42, 1996.

Hamlett KW, Pellegrini DS, and Katz KS: Childhood chronic illness as a family stressor, J Pediatr Psychol 17:33-47, 1992.

Hartley B and Fuller CC: Juvenile arthritis: a nursing perspective, J Pediatr Nurs 12:100-109, 1997.

Hayes V: Families and children's chronic conditions: knowledge development and methodological considerations, Sch Inq Nurs Pract 11:259-290, 1997.

Hobbs N, Perrin JM, and Ireys HT: Chronically ill children and their families, San Francisco, 1985, Jossey-Bass.

Hogan NS: The effects of time on the adolescent sibling bereavement process, Pediatr Nurs 14:333-335, 1988.

Holaday B: Challenges of rearing a chronically ill child, Nurs Clin North Am 19:361-368, 1984.

Holden EW et al: Controlling for general and disease-specific effects in child and family adjustment to chronic childhood illness, J Pediatr Psychol 22:15-27, 1997.

Horner SD: Uncertainty in mothers' care for their ill children, J Adv Nurs 26:658-663, 1997.

Hostler SL: Family-centered care, Pediatr Clin North Am 38:1545-1560, 1991.

Ievers CE et al: Family functioning and social support in the adaptation of caregivers of children with sickle cell syndromes, J Pediatr Psychol 23:377-388, 1998.

Ievers CE and Drotar D: Family and parental functioning in cystic fibrosis, J Dev Behav Pediatr 17:48-55, 1996.

James L and Johnson B: The needs of parents of pediatric oncology patients during the palliative care phase, J Pediatr Oncol Nurs 14:83-95, 1997.

Jerret M: Parents' experience of coming to know the care of a chronically ill child, J Adv Nurs 19:1050-1056, 1994.

Jessop DJ, Reissman CK, and Stein REK: Chronic childhood illness and maternal mental health, J Dev Behav Pediatr 9:147-156, 1988.

Kazak AE: Families of chronically ill children: a systems and social-ecological model of adaptation and challenge, J Consult Clin Psychol 57:25-30, 1989.

Kazak AE, Reber M, and Carter A: Structural and qualitative aspects of social networks in families with young chronically ill children, J Pediatr Psychol 13:171-182, 1988.

Kell RS et al: Psychological adjustment of adolescents with sickle cell disease: relations with demographic, medical, and family competence variables, J Pediatr Psychol 23:301-312, 1998.

Kiburz JA: Perceptions and concerns of the school-age siblings of children with myelomeningocele, Issues Comp Pediatr Nurs 17:223-231, 1994.

Knafl K et al: Family responses to childhood chronic illness: description of management styles, J Pediatr Nurs 11:315-326, 1996.

Knafl KA and Deatrick JA: How families manage chronic conditions: an analysis of the concept of normalization, Res Nurs Health 9:215-222, 1986.

Knafl KA and Deatrick JA: Conceptualizing family response to a child's chronic illness or disability, Fam Relat 36:300-304, 1987.

Knafl KA et al: Family response to a child's chronic illness: a description of major defining themes. In Funk S and Tornquist E, editors: Key aspects of caring for the chronically ill: home and hospital, New York, 1993, Springer.

Krulik T: Successful "normalization" tactics of parents of chronically ill children, J Adv Nurs 5:573-578, 1980.

Liben S: Pediatric palliative care: obstacles to overcome, J Palliat Care 12:24-28, 1996.

Lindgren CL et al: Chronic sorrow: a lifespan concept, Sch Inq Nurs Pract 6:27-40, 1992.

Lynn MR: Siblings' response in illness situations, J Pediatr Nurs 4:127-129, 1989.

Mahon MM and Page ML: Childhood bereavement after the death of a sibling, Holistic Nurs Pract 9(3):15-26, 1995.

Mahon MM, Goldberg EZ, and Washington S: Concept of death in a sample of Israeli children, Death Studies 23:43-59, 1999.

Mahon MM, Goldberg R, and Washington S: Discussing death in the classroom: beliefs and experiences of educators and education students, Omega, in press.

Margolius FR, Hudson KA, and Michel Y: Beliefs and perceptions about children in pain: a survey, Pediatr Nurs 21:111-115, 1995.

Mastroyannopoulou K et al: The impact of childhood nonmalignant life threatening illness on parents: gender differences and predictors of parental adjustment, J Child Psychol Psychiatry 38:823-829, 1997.

McCubbin MA: Family stress theory and the development of nursing knowledge about family adaptation. In Feetham SL et al, editors: The nursing of families: theory/research/education/practice, Newbury Park, Calif., 1993, Sage Publications.

Meyers A and Weitzman M: Pediatric HIV disease: the newest chronic illness of childhood, Pediatr Clin North Am 38:169-191, 1991.

Morrison L: Stress and siblings, Paediatr Nurs 9:26-27, 1997.

Olshansky S: Chronic sorrow: a response to having a mentally defective child, Soc Casework 43:190-193, 1962.

Patterson JM et al: Social support in families of children with chronic conditions: supportive and nonsupportive behaviors, J Dev Behav Pediatr 18:383-391, 1997.

Quittner AL et al: Role strain in couples with and without a child with a chronic illness: associations with marital satisfaction, intimacy, and daily mood, Health Psychol 17(2):112-124, 1998.

Quittner AL and Opipari LC: Differential treatment of siblings: interview and diary analysis comparing two family contexts, Child Dev 65:800-814, 1994.

Rosenfeld AA et al: Foster care: an update, J Am Acad Child Adolesc Psychiatry 36:448-457, 1997.

Schanberg LE et al: Pain coping and the pain experience in children with juvenile chronic arthritis, Pain 73:181-189, 1997.

Sheeran T, Marvin RS, and Pianta RC: Mother's resolution of their child's diagnosis and self-reported measures of parenting stress, marital relations, and social support, J Pediatr Psychol 22:197-212, 1997.

Silver EF, Westbrook LE, and Stein RE: Relationship of parental psychological distress to consequences of chronic health conditions in children, J Pediatr Psychol 23:5-15, 1998.

Solnit A and Stark M: Mourning the birth of a defective child, Psychoanal Study Child 16:523-536, 1962.

Spaulding BR and Morgan SB: Spina bifida children and their parents: a population prone to family dysfunction?, J Pediatr Psychol 11:359-374, 1986.

Staats PS and Kost-Byerly S: Celiac plexus blockade in a 7 year-old child with neuroblastoma, J Pain Symptom Manage 10:321-324, 1995.

Stainton MC: Supporting family functioning during a high risk pregnancy, MCN Am J Matern Child Nurs 19:24-28, 1994.

Stein A et al: Life threatening illness and hospice care, Arch Dis Child 64:697-702, 1989.

Stevens MM et al: Pain and symptom control in paediatric palliative care, Cancer Surv 21:211-231, 1994.

Thomas RB: Family adaptation to a child with a chronic condition. In Rose MH and Thomas RB, editors: Children with chronic conditions: nursing in a family and community context, Orlando, Fla., 1987, Grune & Stratton.

Venters M: Family coping with chronic and severe childhood illness: the case of cystic fibrosis, Soc Sci Med 15a:289-297, 1981.

Vessey JA and Carlson KL: Nonpharmacological interventions to use with children in pain, Issues Comp Pediatr Nurs 19:169-182, 1996.

Vessey JA and Mahon NM: Therapeutic play and the hospitalized child, J Pediatr Nurs 5:328-333, 1990.

Wallander JL and Varni JW: Effects of pediatric chronic physical disorders on child and family adjustment, J Child Psychol Psychiatry 39:29-46, 1998.

Williams HA: A comparison of social support and social networks of black parents and white parents with chronically ill children, Soc Sci Med 37:1509-1520, 1993.

Williams PD, Lorenzo FD, and Borja M: Pediatric chronic illness: effects on siblings and mothers, Matern Child Nurs 21:111-121, 1993.

Yost DM, Hochstadt NJ, and Charles P: Medical foster care: achieving permanency for seriously ill children, Child Today 17(5):22-26, 1988.

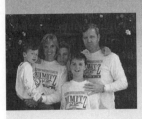

CHAPTER 4

Family Culture and Chronic Conditions

Roberta S. Rehm

Historical Roots of Diversity

Americans have long recognized—though not always valued—their multicultural heritage. It is important for health care providers to understand the roles that culture plays in modern U.S. society in order to provide sensitive and appropriate care for children and families from diverse cultural backgrounds. The components of cultural identity are complex and vary even between people of the same ethnic, racial, or religious group. This chapter explores the interaction of culture and health care and discusses the cultural implications for providing care to children with chronic conditions and their families.

The North American Multicultural Heritage

The early seventeenth century English Pilgrims are the best known of the early permanent immigrants to the United States, but explorers, refugees, and immigrants seeking a better life began arriving on North American lands long before the Pilgrims. Scientists believe that humans began migrating to North America from Asia across the Bering Land Bridge perhaps 12,000 years ago and may be ancestors of some of the peoples now called Native Americans or American Indians (Bogucka and Boyd, 1996). Although the exact history of the earliest settlers varies according to each tribe's origination myths, it is certain that migration has always been an important factor in U.S. history. Spanish conquistadors began exploring what would become the American Southwest in the early sixteenth century. They led the first permanent colonial era settlers, who arrived in New Mexico in 1598. This group of 800 colonists were mostly natives of Spain or Iberia but also included Mexican-Indians and Africans who were servants to the soldiers and settlers (Preston, 1998).

The foreign-born proportion of the U.S. population reached its peak at 14.7% in 1910. In 1996, foreign-born U.S. residents constituted 9.3% of the total population, or 24.6 million people (U.S. Department of Commerce, 1996). Europeans made up the largest percentage of immigrants to the United States from 1820 (when formal immigration records began) until 1970. Since then the proportion of Latino and Asian immigrants has grown significantly (U.S. Department of Commerce, 1993). In 1996, 16.9% of immigrants came from Europe; 25% from Asia; and over 50% from the Western hemisphere, including 25% from Mexico, 10.5% from the Caribbean, 7% from Central America, 4.9% from South America, and 2.7% from Canada (U.S. Department of Commerce, 1996). Besides these legal entrants, about 275,000 immigrants illegally enter the United States each year. Although this number has dropped since the early 1990s, about 5 million undocumented immigrants still reside in the United States (U.S. Immigration and Naturalization Service, 1998).

The Dynamic Nature of Culture

These trends in immigration reflect the changing face of our society and the dynamic nature of American culture. It was once presumed that most immigrants would give up traditional values, languages, and ways of life to join the "melting pot" of U.S. society, but scholars now recognize that the "melting pot" is an American myth. In reality the United States is a multicultural nation with an immensely heterogeneous population (Boyle, 1995; Groce and Zola, 1993). There are many—not one—American cultures, and no one set of values and practices clearly defines the United States. Increasing migration around the world in the last decade has contributed to the heterogeneity of many nations. Women and children now constitute the largest portion of transnational migrants around the world (McGuire, 1998).

Culture can simply be characterized as "the informal practices of everyday life" (Rosaldo, 1993) or can be defined in complex terms that account for tradition, history, recurrent patterns, and common values (Leininger, 1995). Important definitions of cultural terms are found in Table 4-1. Definitions of culture must be fluid enough to recognize that although all cultural groups have commonalties, there is a great deal of intracultural variation. Racial and ethnic identity form strong components of culture, but many people may identify more with cultural subgroups based on less obvious factors than ethnic or racial identity.

Among the shared understandings that constitute cultural subgroups are those based on factors such as religious belief or affiliation (e.g., fundamentalist Christian, Sunni Moslem), physical ability (e.g., mobility impairment, athletic nature), sexual preference or identity (e.g., heterosexual, lesbian), occupation (e.g., plumber, college professor), educational attainment (e.g., illiterate, college student), socioeconomic status (e.g., inherited wealth, homeless) women's issues (e.g., feminism, maternal status), and many others (Lipson, 1996b; Purnell and Paulanka, 1998).

Religious and Spiritual Influences

Religious and spiritual beliefs are among the most powerful forces that shape human experience. Although specific belief systems vary widely and are even sometimes directly contradictory, religious faith and spiritual beliefs usually provide a sense of comfort, strength, and direction for families coping with concerns about health and illness (Andrews and Hanson, 1995; Rehm, 1999; Wright, 1998).

Table 4-1
Definitions of Cultural Terms

Culture	A dynamic and negotiated social construction arising from interaction and resulting in shared understandings among people in contact with one another.
Race	Originally, it was human biological variation, but racial mixing has given the term little biological significance. Race retains social and political significance and may reflect individual or group identity factors.
Ethnicity	A socially, culturally, and/or politically constructed group of individuals that holds a set of characteristics in common; often based on language, national origin, and/or religion.
Racism	An oppressive system of racial relations justified by an ideology in which one racial group benefits from dominating another and defines itself and others through this domination.
Institutional Racism	Intentional or unintentional manipulation or toleration of institutional policies that unfairly restrict the opportunities of particular groups.
Ethnocentrism	The belief that one's own ways are the best or preferred way to think, believe, or behave.
Prejudice	Preconceived ideas or opinions about an individual or group based solely on factors such as race, sex, or physical ability.
Discrimination	Different treatment, including restricted opportunities or choices, of people because of factors such as race, class, or physical ability.

Spirituality is a concept that includes practices and beliefs that give meaning to life and help an individual to cultivate inner strength to meet the challenges of daily life (Purnell and Paulanka, 1998). Spirituality may be expressed in an organized religious setting with formal rituals of prayer and worship or more independently with individual practices. Both organized religious belief systems and spirituality that arises from life experiences may provide a set of values by which life can be lived (Andrews and Hanson, 1995; Wright, 1998).

Chronic conditions of childhood may present particular challenges for families, especially in the face of children's suffering, the need for ongoing care, and the possibility of disability or death. Many families seek an explanation for these difficulties in religious beliefs; others use their beliefs to find solace or strength to face the future. A recent study found that Mexican-American parents recognized three key factors in determining the outcome of their child's chronic condition: God, family, and health care providers. Although these parents gave the ultimate authority to God, they felt that it was important to take excellent care of the child themselves and to seek the best possible professional care in order to ensure the greatest chance for survival and healing (Rehm, 1999).

Families' religious tenets rarely bring them into conflict with health care providers (e.g., when beliefs preclude certain forms of medical care, such as blood transfusion, or lead to preferences for prayer or other healing rituals over biomedical treatment); but in such cases, an open dialog must be maintained with families and legal and ethical concerns must be formally balanced. When negotiation does not reach a solution acceptable to both the family and the care provider, the courts may be consulted. Because the dominant value in the United States usually includes preservation of a child's life, families are sometimes forced to accept care that is against their wishes and belief systems (Furrow et al, 1997). Health care providers must recognize the profound effect of such a situation and work to preserve respectful relationships with the family to ensure ongoing care for the child and to try to avoid future legal conflicts if possible.

Socioeconomic Status and Health

Many studies have found that socioeconomic status exerts a profound influence—sometimes even more than ethnic or racial characteristics—on the health and well-being of many people. Although the majority of poor Americans are white, people of color are disproportionately burdened by poverty and health problems (Kinsman, Sally, and Fox,

1996). American children are profoundly affected by poverty. One in four American children are born poor, and one in three will be poor at some point during childhood (Children's Defense Fund, 1998). Morbidity and mortality rates in the United States rise as income and educational levels decrease and are higher for the unemployed and those in working-class occupations when compared with professionals, managers, and executives (Krieger and Fee, 1994). Moreover, higher morbidity and mortality rates persist as socioeconomic status increases in nonwhite ethnic groups, particularly among African Americans and at lower socioeconomic levels (Anderson and Armistead, 1995). Poverty and ethnicity alone, however, are not sufficient to explain excess mortality in all locations. Research has shown that poor blacks in Alabama had lower rates of excess mortality than those in Harlem, despite being poorer, which provides evidence that additional sociocultural factors are important to health (Geronimus et al, 1996).

Several mechanisms have been suggested for this link between socioeconomic factors and health, including interactions of socioeconomic variables (e.g., income, education, and occupation) and social and environmental factors (e.g., residential characteristics, occupational environment, social support, discrimination, and access to health care) (Anderson and Armistead, 1995). Little is known about how other factors (e.g., psychologic and behavioral characteristics) that interact with physiologic mechanisms are linked to socioeconomic status and ethnicity. Because nonwhite ethnic groups are disproportionately represented in lower socioeconomic groups, it is important to ask how ethnicity interacts with socioeconomic status to influence health outcomes, and what factors may be protective in some populations and locations.

Cultural Power Struggles

Perhaps because of the nation's long association with European immigrants and their descendants, political and decision-making power has traditionally been held by white European-Americans. This tendency is evidently changing in cities and states where other immigrant groups have gathered in large numbers over a long time, such as San Francisco, which has many Asian politicians, and

New Mexico, where Latinos and Hispanics play a large role in municipal and legislative activities. Of immigrants, 32% have become naturalized U.S. citizens—a percentage that tends to increase with length of residence (U.S. Department of Commerce, 1996). Over time, most residents of the United States adopt English for official and public transactions, although many people continue to speak other languages in their homes and communities.

Ethnocentrism and Racism

Ethnocentrism and racism (see definitions in Table 4-1) arise when those in privileged or powerful positions fail to recognize nondominant viewpoints as legitimate or are prejudiced against those from other racial and ethnic groups. These forms of discrimination can be enacted by individuals or become institutionalized and reflective of wider societal attitudes (Barbee, 1993). Health care providers are sometimes ethnocentric in expecting children and families to accept advice or treatment based on their own values instead of on those of the family. For example, children and parents are sometimes given diagnostic information and asked to make critical decisions without being able to first consult members of the extended family. This is an untenable position for families from cultures in which decision-making is not necessarily centered in the nuclear family (Brink, 1993). Institutional racism also affects children and families. For example, black women who had recently given birth were reported to authorities 10 times more frequently than white women, despite similar rates of positive toxicology screenings at the time of birth (Neuspiel, 1996). Another example is the targeted marketing of tobacco and alcohol products to children and youths (e.g., billboards near schools, sponsorship of sporting and music events), especially in areas and venues frequented by young people from ethnic minorities (Moore, Williams, and Qualls, 1996).

Barbee (1993) describes three forms of racism that are common among nurses in the United States: denial, color-blind perspectives, and aversive racism. Barbee posits that denial arises from attributes of the profession of nursing (i.e., a preference for homogeneity and a need to avoid conflict), as well as the idealistic mission of nursing to serve all persons, which has allowed nurses to avoid acknowledging and examining racism within the profession. Idealism may also lead nurses to adopt a color-blind perspective, which occurs when nurses assert that they treat all people the same regardless of race or ethnicity and can lead to a lack of recognition and respect for cultural differences, which may then be labeled as deviance. Aversive racism occurs when clinicians do not acknowledge the conflict between an egalitarian value system and negative feelings and beliefs toward other cultural groups. Because aversive racists may believe they are not prejudiced, discrimination becomes subtle and nurses experience great ambivalence. Health care providers can and must learn to recognize ethnocentrism and racism and enhance their sensitivity to all clients by working to establish personal and institutional cultural competence.

Intracultural Variation and Diversity

Although it is helpful to learn about the common history, values, and practices of particular cultural groups, it can never be presumed that any particular individual or family is fully represented by these descriptions (Lipson, 1996a). Written descriptions of broad cultural groups are offered by authors in order to facilitate the acquisition of knowledge of other cultures; but these depictions often present the most conservative cultural viewpoint, which stands in greatest contrast to that presumed to be "typically" American. These general descriptions rarely account for the dynamic nature of culture, in which traditional values and ways of life are incorporated into modern circumstances and familial needs (Rosaldo, 1993). There is great diversity within particular ethnic, racial, and religious populations; and many people belong to several subcultures while identifying themselves with one major cultural group.

Acculturation and Biculturalism

Acculturation is the process whereby one group of people adapts to living with another, which often includes learning the dominant group's language, as well as adopting certain behaviors and practices (Herberg, 1995). Acculturation can be bidirectional (i.e., both groups influence each other), although the most established culture is likely to remain dominant and to wield greater influence than less-powerful subgroups (e.g., ethnic foods, rituals, and holidays have become popular and are widely enjoyed in America without changing the political dominance of powerful groups in most locales). In individuals exposed to two cultures or languages over long periods, it is common to see biculturalism and bilingualism enabling them to function well in both cultures (Brookins, 1993). Biculturalism can be helpful to children and families, allowing them to meet the demands of the dominant culture while retaining aspects of their cultural heritage (e.g., language, rituals, and family relationships). Biculturalism may cause strain, however, when family members have different levels of acculturation and varying expectations about family roles and obligations.

Despite acculturation or biculturalism, people often retain significant preferences for language, relating to others, and values from their culture of origin. This principle was confirmed in part by Rueschenberg and Buriel (1989), who studied Mexican-American families at three levels of acculturation, which they evaluated using language preference and proficiency, generational status, and when migration took place. Using the Family Environment Scale (FES), they determined that external family system variables (e.g., independence of family members, achievement orientation, intellectual-cultural orientation, and active recreational orientation) all grew with increasing acculturation. There was no change, however, in internal family system variables such as cohesion, expressiveness, conflict, organization, or control. "Patterns of intrafamilial relationships and interactions do not appear to differ substantially from one generation to the next despite the fact that English becomes the primary language and family members become active participants in U.S. society" (Rueschenberg and Buriel, 1989, p. 241).

Potential Differences in the Values of Health Care Providers and Families

Throughout the world the family is the basic unit of society; however, different societies use family members in various ways to fulfill their basic functions of protecting, nurturing, and educating chil-

dren (Brink, 1993). In the United States—unlike many parts of the world, it is common for the nuclear family (i.e., parents and their children) to live apart from other family members; therefore presumptions of nuclear family autonomy are widespread among health care providers. It is necessary to recognize the wide variety of existing family constellations and the interdependence of extended family members that are common throughout the world, as well as in many subcultures in the United States. Hospital policies here have traditionally epitomized this potential conflict, and many health care providers are harried and distressed when large family groups arrive to visit in small hospital rooms, or when family members besides parents seek information about hospitalized children.

When extended family interdependence is customary, decisions about a child's health and well being are often reach far beyond the parents. Parents may wish to consult with, or even rely on, a variety of important people (e.g., grandparents, family or community elders, religious leaders or counselors, or native healers) when making critical decisions. When possible, parents should be given time and opportunities for these important consultations; and when the situation is critical or immediate decisions are crucial, families should be encouraged to keep vigil with important members present or nearby (Kinsman et al, 1996).

Although there is no one "American" value system in the multicultural United States, there are many values held widely among particular groups of people—including health care providers, who often share many common traits (e.g., most are white, middle-class, and relatively well-educated). Some values commonly held by providers (e.g., gender equality) may contrast with those of certain families. When providing care for people who live by contrasting values of male superiority or family protection, professionals may find themselves in conflict with those they seek to serve. One way to deal with such potential conflicts is to use cultural relativism, in which values and behaviors are judged only from the context of the client's cultural system (Baker, 1997). Many caregivers are comfortable with a large degree of cultural relativism and can use this principle to avoid ethnocentrism in most clinical encounters; however, providers rarely find that there are problematic situations or behaviors that cross their "bottom line" belief systems so that they cannot espouse tolerance and understanding. Examples might include spousal dominance that becomes physical abuse or certain rituals that cause pain or physical complications (e.g., female genital excision or infibulation).

Underlying the principles of cultural competence is the goal of achieving a level of cultural relativism that allows care to be both congruent with a client's cultural beliefs and understanding of familial viewpoints and decisions from the family's perspective. Nevertheless, Baker (1997) points out that nurses are not required to abandon their own principles in such conflictual encounters. Rather, they have an obligation to dialog with families, to try to understand the clients' viewpoints and prejudices, and to critically examine their own biases. In such a dialog, neither the caregiver nor the client may change stances, but each may understand the other better. Where good communication and constructive relationships continue, change may eventually result.

Cultural Competence

Culturally competent health care is sensitive to the needs, backgrounds, and wishes of children with chronic conditions and their families. To be truly culturally competent requires care providers to acquire knowledge about themselves and others; to adopt attitudes of tolerance, curiosity, patience, and appreciation of difference; and to practice interpersonal skills that foster good communication and trust (Lipson, 1996a, Lynch, 1992).

Hallmarks of culturally competent care giving and care-giving systems are described in Boxes 4-1 and 4-2. The information given there reiterates that

---

Box 4-1

Hallmarks of Culturally Sensitive Caregiving

An asset model based on recognizing cultural differences in child rearing, family strengths, and culturally based coping methods should be used:

- Information gathering: health records, cultural reading, family interviews
- Family strengths serve as the basis for planning care for child

Families are directly involved in the family treatment and service plan:

- Family decision makers are consulted.
- Family helps to prioritize goals of care.
- Family's orientation to care providers as authority figures or joint decision makers is determined before care is planned.

Family goals permit intracultural variation on a case-by-case basis:

- Standard care plans are altered as needed or desired.
- Alternative modes of care are incorporated as possible.

Self-sufficiency of the family is encouraged by promotion of self-esteem, cultural identification, and skill-building to negotiate complicated medical systems:

- Importance of family decision makers and caregivers is acknowledged.
- Family strengths are recognized and praised.
- Community resources are used.

Individual family/cultural values are respected:

- Parent-child interaction patterns are taught in a culturally appropriate manner.
- Differences between family and care giver goals are negotiated with goodwill, patience, and a willingness to compromise.

Modified from Adams EV: Policy-planning for culturally comprehensive special services: bureau of maternal and child health, Washington DC, 1990, US Department of Health and Human Services.

Bernstein HK and Stettner-Eaton B: Cultural inclusion in part H: system development, Infant-Toddler Intervention 4(1):43-50, 1994.

Leininger M: Culture, care, diversity, and universality: a theory of nursing, New York, 1991, National League of Nursing.

Box 4-2

Hallmarks of Culturally Sensitive Caregiving Systems

1. *Primary care providers and care-giving systems seek community participation in all stages of program design, development, implementation, and evaluation, including outreach, policy making, and problem solving.*
   - Formal and informal community leaders (e.g., church leaders, traditional healers, elders) are involved in defining culturally appropriate care.
   - Community outreach to families is ongoing and culturally appropriate, involving bilingual, bicultural providers, and/or community members when possible.

2. *Intake systems are sensitive to family and cultural values:*
   - Family privacy and previous experiences leading to mistrust must be respected.

3. *Team members must have ongoing, culturally appropriate training.*

4. *Educational materials, media, evaluation, and monitoring instruments are field-tested for cultural appropriateness and congruency in language content and emotional meaning.*

5. *Programs are continuously evaluated to ensure cultural appropriateness and program effectiveness:*
   - The child's progress is monitored by the family, the program, and external evaluators.
   - Family perceptions of interventions are sought and used in program revisions.

Modified from Adams EV: Policy-planning for culturally comprehensive special services: bureau of maternal and child health, Washington DC, 1990, US Department of Health and Human Services.

Bernstein HK and Stettner-Eaton B: Cultural inclusion in part H: system development, Infant-Toddler Intervention 4(1):43-50, 1994.

Leininger M: Culture, care, diversity, and universality: a theory of nursing, New York, 1991, National League of Nursing.

---

culturally competent care is only achieved when care givers and institutions form individual relationships with families. In a study of African-American, Hispanic, and European-American families interviewed about improving services for children with chronic conditions, the authors stated, "Surprisingly, there were no distinctive differences in families' recommendations based on ethnicity alone. Participants stressed the importance of individualizing care rather than providing culturally specific care for particular ethnic groups" (Garwick et al, 1998, p. 446).

Lipson (1996a) describes three interacting viewpoints that constitute a cultural perspective: objective, subjective, and the context of the cross-cultural encounter. The objective viewpoint focuses providers on the client, family, and community, including communication, world view, and other cultural patterns and social characteristics. The subjective viewpoint scrutinizes the personal and cultural characteristics of the primary care providers themselves. Providers seeking cultural

competence must explore their own contribution to enhancing or impeding cross-cultural interactions (i.e., their own values, beliefs, and communication patterns). Unconscious prejudices or ethnocentrism may be reflected in strained cross-cultural interactions and require thoughtful self-reflection to identify and rectify. The cross-cultural context of encounters between individuals, providers, and the health care system includes both societal factors (e.g., economic, political, and policy influences) and the immediate environment of the clinical setting (e.g., language congruency, privacy, and the acuity of the client's health needs).

Cultural competence is a complex phenomenon that requires knowledge of self and others; an open-minded and tolerant attitude toward human differences; and skills in critical thinking, communication, and assessment of the outcomes of cross-cultural interactions. An ongoing effort is generally required to develop cultural competence over time. Orlandi (1992) has expressed this idea as a continuum in which cognitive, affective, and skill dimensions may be at different levels. Care providers can progress from incompetence to sensitivity and then to competence as growth occurs in each dimension. Culturally incompetent individuals might be oblivious to cross-cultural differences, apathetic to the need for change, and unskilled in personal interactions. Culturally sensitive individuals, however, are aware of differences and sympathetic to necessary changes but lack some skills to enhance interactions. Culturally competent care providers are knowledgeable about themselves and others, committed to making necessary changes, and highly skilled in fostering communication and creating productive environments for both clients and professionals. Progress along this continuum changes the overall effect of cross-cultural encounters from destructive to constructive as competence is developed.

Culturally Competent Care of Children with Chronic Conditions

Cultural Variations in the Impact of Childhood Chronic Conditions

A variety of chronic conditions have been reported to occur more frequently in certain ethnic or racial groups, and a summary is presented in Table 4-2. Recent immigrants must be assessed for conditions that are prevalent in their region of origin, and all children with chronic conditions need comprehensive family and developmental assessment, as well as well-child care in addition to care for their chronic condition (Niederhauser, 1989).

Children who have or are at increased risk for chronic physical, developmental, behavioral, or emotional conditions and also require health and related services beyond those generally required for children are estimated to make up 18% of U.S. children less than 18 years of age (i.e., about 12.6 million children). Newacheck et al (1998) created an epidemiological profile of these children and found that 18.6% are white, 19.8% are black, 15% are Hispanic, and 13% fall into other categories. Boys were about one-third more likely to have a special health need than girls; and children whose family incomes were at or below the federal poverty level were also about one-third more likely to have special needs than those with

higher income levels. Children from single-parent families are about 40% more likely to have special health care needs than those from two-parent families.

It is important to recognize that definitions of chronic conditions may vary and some cultures may consider minor differences in health or ability as acceptable variants of normal (Groce and Zola, 1993). This point is apparent in data collected from The National Health Interview Survey on Child Health (Newacheck, Stoddard, and McManus, 1993), which revealed that clinically minor conditions that caused little or no bother or limitation in activities were more commonly reported by parents of white children than those of blacks or Hispanics. Whites were somewhat more likely to report conditions causing some bother or limitation, but all groups were equally likely to report severe conditions that were frequently bothersome and caused activity limitations.

Newacheck and associates (1993) found that most of the children with chronic conditions had a usual source of care for routine needs, but black and Hispanic children were more likely to receive sick care in hospital emergency departments than white children. In addition, minority children used fewer ambulatory care services on average and received fewer medications for their chronic conditions. These findings indicate that access to health care—particularly ambulatory care—varies by race and ethnicity and is diminished for children of color with chronic conditions. As increasing numbers of children with chronic conditions are enrolled in managed-care programs (i.e., through Medicaid, Supplemental Security Income, SSI/Disability, or private insurance plans), it will be important to monitor access and use of care to ensure appropriate services are available for both well-child and sick care (Kuhlthau et al, 1998).

Communications

At the heart of all successful relationships is good communication, although the parameters of "good" may vary among different cultural groups. For example, cultural factors (e.g., respect for authority or differences in social class) between fam-

Table 4-2
Conditions Found More Frequently in Minority or Immigrant Populations

Ethnic Groups	Condition	Screening Tests	Age of Child
All adolescents	HIV infection	Culture, antibody, or antigen	13 to 21
All immigrants	Tuberculosis	PPD	Newborn to adult
	PKU	Guthrie	Newborn to adult
	Iron deficiency anemia	Hgb/Hct	>6 months
All immigrants and high-risk teens	STDs	Examination/laboratory serology	High-risk
All immigrants	Vitamin A deficiency	Serum test for Vitamin A deficiency	All children
Asian	Anencephaly	Imaging studies,	Newborn
	VSD, PDA	Examination, ECG, echocardiogram,	Newborn, child
	Down syndrome	amniocentesis, MSAFP, chromosome analysis	Fetus, newborn
	Cleft lip	Examination	Newborn
	Congenital hip	Examination, radiograph	Newborn
African-Americans	Sickle Cell disease	Hgb electrophoresis	All ages
African-Americans Mediterranean, Jewish, Thai Filipino/Chinese	G6PD	Assay for enzyme	Newborn
African-Americans	Prematurity	Early prenatal care	Fetus, newborn
	perinatal drugs	Toxicology screen	Newborn
	alcohol/drugs	Toxicology screen	Adolescent
	microcephaly	Examination, imaging	Newborn
	PDA and pulmonary artery stenosis	Examination, radiograph, ECG	Child
	Low birth weight	Growth chart	Fetus, newborn
	High infant mortality	Prenatal care	Fetus, newborn
French Canadian	Tyrosinemia (1)	Serum tyrosine	High-risk newborn
Filipino	Gout	Serum uric acid	Symptomatic
Hispanic/ Puerto Rican	Prematurity/LBW Obesity, low SES	Growth chart	Preschoolers/teens
Jewish	Tay-Sachs disease	Amniocentesis chromosome analysis	Fetus, newborn child
Mediterranean	Thalassemia	Hemoglobin electrophoresis	All children
Native American (including Eskimos)	Low birth weight	Prenatal care	Fetus Neonate
	SIDS	Apnea monitor	Infant
	Persistant otitis	Otoscopy, tympanometry	Infant/school age

Modified from Alexander MA et al: Obesity in Mexican-American preschool children—a population group at risk, Ped Health Nurs 8(1):53-58, 1991.
Behrman et al: Nelson textbook of pediatrics, Philadelphia, 1996, W.B. Saunders.
Centers for Disease Control and Prevention: Trends in HIV/AIDS infections, Website: http://www.cecapin.org/geneval1998/trends/trends_4htm
Groce NE et al: Multiculturalism, chronic illness, and disability, Pediatrics Suppl 5 1(15):1048-1055, 1993.
Heruada GA et al: Weaning: historical perspectives, practical recommendations, and current controversies, Curr Probl Pediatr 22(5):223-240, 1992.
Hoekelman RA et al: Primary pediatric care, ed 3, St Louis, 1997, Mosby.
Newacheck PW et al: Ethnocultural variations in the prevalence and impact of childhood chronic conditions, Pediatrics 91:1031-1039, 1993.
Newacheck PW et al: An epidemiological profile of children with special health needs, Pediatrics 102:117-123, 1998.
Palafox N et al: A cross-cultural caring: a handbook for health care professionals, Honolulu, 1980, University of Hawaii Press.
Ramer L: Culturally sensitive caregiving and child bearing families, White Plains, NY, 1992, March of Dimes Birth Defects Foundation.
Wuest J: Harmonizing: a North American Indian approach to management of middle ear disease with transcultural nursing implications, J Transcultural Nurs 3:5-14, 1991.

Table 4-2
Conditions Found More Frequently in Minority or Immigrant Populations—cont'd

Ethnic Groups	Condition	Screening Tests	Age of Child
Native American (including Eskimos) —cont'd	Juvenile diabetes	Blood glucose	School age/teenager
	Fetal alcohol syndrome	Toxicology, examination	All ages
	Alcohol/inhalants	Drug screens,	Adolescent
	PDA, valve stenosis/artesia	Examination, radiograph, ECG	Neonate/child
	Cleft lip	Examination, amniocentesis	Newborn
	Hydrocephalus	Amniocentesis, examination	Newborn
	Congenital hip	Examination	Infant
Southeast Asian Pacific Islander and Haitian	Parasites/diarrhea	Corneal scars, stool for O & P, peripheral eosinophilia	All children
	Malaria	Blood smear/parasitemia	All ages
	Hepatitis	Hepatitis surface antigen	All ages
	Hemoglobinopathy	CBC with RBC indices	Any child
Caucasian	Cystic fibrosis	Sweat test	School age
	Club foot	Examination	Newborn
	Congenital hip	Examination, radiograph	Newborn
	Hypospadias	Examination	Newborn
	Asthma	Examination, radiograph	Postnewborn
	Allergic phenomena	Examination, CBC/Diff	Infant,
	Otitis media		Toddler,
			School age
British	Neutral tube defect	MSAFP amniocentesis	Fetus, Newborn

ilies and providers may influence a family's attitude about accepting advice from health care providers or willingness to share reservations or objections to treatment plans. Some families may consider care providers to be consultants whose advice can be considered and either accepted or discarded, but others may consider caregivers to be authority figures whose advice—accepted or not—should never be openly questioned. Therefore follow-ups and ongoing dialog are necessary to ensure that mutually acceptable care and outcomes are established.

Besides words, communication is established through body language, touch, eye contact, and other nonverbal indicators (Lipson, 1996a). To convey respect and establish comfort, health care providers must be good observers and responsive to cues from children and families. Many care providers use direct, to-the-point communication; full eye contact; and firm handshakes, which are common courtesies for many people but may be aggressive or rude gestures to individuals used to indirect approaches and a lack of physical contact between strangers (McCubbin et al, 1993).

The subtleties of effective communication are particularly complicated when interpreters are necessary. Children or friends of the family should not be used as interpreters because their presence may inhibit parents from a frank discussion of sensitive issues (Faust, 1996; Lipson, 1996a). Family members who can usually communicate adequately in English may find themselves tongue-tied or unable to understand complex medical concepts and vocabulary during times of crisis or stress (Rehm, 1996). Moreover, parents may desire interpretation of their native language to fully understand explanations related to a child's chronic condition. It is important that interpreters be highly skilled communicators in both languages and cultures, and that they convey more than simple, word-for-word translations of dialog in clinical settings so that the actual meaning of the message is accurately portrayed (Purnell and Paulanka, 1998). When an interpreter is used, it is important to speak in short units of speech; to use simple, nontechnical language; to speak to family members directly—not just to the interpreter; and to listen to the client and family and check their understanding often by asking them to restate the message in their own words (Lipson, 1996a).

Variations in Perceptions of Causality and Meaning of Chronic Conditions

Perceptions about the cause and meaning of disability and chronic conditions of childhood vary widely among families. Some of these variations are associated with cultural or religious beliefs or may be related to parental educational levels and past experiences. Groce and Zola (1993) point out three important issues that influence interactions of children with chronic conditions, their families, and health care providers: culturally perceived causes of disability or illness, expectations for survival, and expectations of social roles for children and adults with chronic conditions. These issues are all influenced by multiple social factors, including traditional community- and family-belief systems, educational levels, financial and social support networks, exposure and access to modern health care and community support services, and levels of acculturation to dominant values within the medical and social service sector of the United States.

Families with belief systems that consider social factors and spiritual influences, as well as pathophysiological associations, may attribute a child's condition to multiple factors, including environmental, interpersonal, and genetic influences. Chronic conditions may be stigmatizing if thought to result from unacceptable behavior, inherent weaknesses, or external threats that could endanger the rest of the family or community (e.g., hexes or spirit possession). Children with such conditions may be kept at home and out of view to protect either the family from shame or the child from potentially disapproving or threatening community restrictions (Scheper-Hughes, 1990).

In many communities, however, families caring for children with chronic conditions are admired and offered ongoing support. Belief in causative factors beyond those generally recognized by biomedicine does not often interfere with acceptance and use of modern medical diagnosis and treatment. For example, Mardiros (1989) found that Mexican-American parents recognized both biomedical and sociocultural causes for their children's disabilities. Within the biomedical domain, parents described pregnancy problems, iatrogenic causes, substance abuse, genetic factors, and toxic exposures. Sociocultural causation included both familial and personal domains (e.g., difficulties within the marriage, spousal abuse, prior attitudes, and past transgressions). Parents in this study placed responsibility for naming the illness with physicians and—regardless of their own predominant view of causation—recognized the necessity of a formal medical label in order to access desired services for their child.

Expectations for the survival of infants and children influence the kinds of familial and community resources that parents seek and provide for their children with chronic conditions. Residents or recent immigrants from parts of the world that are less technologically oriented than the U.S. medical system may be unaware of recent advances in medical care that facilitate survival for many children who would ordinarily die or be profoundly disabled without the surgical, pharmacologic, and mechanical supports routinely available here. Moreover, there may be philosophic and ethical traditions that do not necessarily value survival in the face of stigmatizing factors such as altered appearance or disability (Scheper-Hughes, 1990). Societies that condone infanticide or neglect of children with physical or developmental impairments are increasingly rare throughout the world because of improved access to sophisticated services and governmental policies that disapprove of such practices. Nevertheless, expectations for children with chronic conditions vary widely and require ongoing education in the face of changing life circumstances, available support services, and official policies.

Family- and community-sanctioned roles for children and adults with chronic conditions help to determine the kinds of educational, health, and other resources that are expended on such individuals. The official U.S. policy (i.e., in the form of laws such as the Americans with Disabilities Act

[ADA] and the Individuals with Disabilities Education Act [IDEA]) explicitly entitles children and adults with disabling conditions to the same educational, occupational, and social opportunities as those without such conditions (see Chapter 5). These laws reflect the widely held American beliefs that most people should be independent and self-supporting and therefore are entitled to education and opportunities to ensure such measures of success. These expectations are often modified depending on individual circumstances, but the belief that each person should strive for the highest possible level of independence remains and may be seen, for example, in the widespread practice of group-home living for individuals who cannot live alone. This value is not universally held, however, and notions of independence may not be the highest priority of families who value interdependence of family members and do not perceive ongoing home care as excessively burdensome. Throughout the world, however, most people are expected to contribute their labor to their families as their abilities allow (Groce and Zola, 1993).

Alternative Therapies

Much of the literature on health care of children from non-U.S. cultures describes exotic folk-healing practices and rituals. Many systems of health care and beliefs other than those of Western biomedicine exist throughout the world. Two of the best known are Chinese medicine, which uses herbs, acupuncture, and religious rituals (e.g., prayer and healing touch) that are common to many spiritual systems. In most cases, there is little conflict between biomedical care and traditional practices, and provider support of the alternative therapies favored by a family may foster the growth of trust (Kinsman et al, 1996). Even if the suggestions of primary care providers are found to be acceptable, a family's current practices must be determined, and planned treatments besides those proposed by primary care providers must be recognized. It may be important to determine the effects of herbs or other pharmacologic agents to assess drug interactions and safety, but folk healers are often willing to cooperate with health care providers;

and a blending of rituals and healing techniques can be both medically effective and helpful to the family (Chin, 1996). Pediatric care providers may facilitate joint practices when blessing ceremonies are conducted before an invasive procedure (e.g., Mormons) or amulets (e.g., some American Indians) are worn by children for protection.

Cultural Assessment

Cultural competence requires that children with chronic conditions and their families are assessed to determine their cultural identities and any particular beliefs or needs that should be incorporated into care plans. There are many excellent, in-depth cultural assessment tools (Andrews and Boyle, 1995; Leininger, 1995; Lipson, 1996a). "Cross-cultural assessment of a family with a child with a chronic condition" is reprinted in Table 4-3. These tools are particularly helpful when care providers see families repeatedly over time because the many questions can be incorporated into several interviews. Many times, however, care providers are uncertain if they will see families repeatedly or the nature of the contact is time-limited and problem-focused. In such cases, it is helpful to distill a few key questions from these larger tools and focus attention on the aspects of assessment that are most relevant to the current encounter.

Key Questions for Brief Encounters in the Primary Care Setting

In the primary care setting, it is helpful to supplement the general client and family history with key questions, such as the following: (1) Would you be more comfortable with a translator present? (2) Who are your child's primary care givers at home? (3) Is there anyone else who needs to know the treatment plan and have the opportunity to ask questions? (4) What kinds of home remedies have you been using for your child, and what others might you use for this situation? (5) Are you satisfied with the care plan made at this visit, and is there anything that you anticipate might interfere with your ability to carry it out? In an acute situa-

---

Table 4-3
Cross-Cultural Assessment of a Family with a Child with a Chronic Condition

---

Family Demographics	Who lives in your family (i.e., members, ages, sexes)?
	What kind of work do members of the household do?
	What is your family's socioeconomic status?
	What kind of health insurance coverage do you have?
	Which family members are covered?
	Which child are you seeking care for today?
	What chronic conditions or symptoms does the child have?
	How would you describe the problems that have brought you here today?
	Who is the primary care taker in your family?
Orientation	Where were the members of the family born?
	What is the ethnic background of the family members?
	How many years have family members lived in the United States? (NOTE: Only ask if appropriate.)
	In your family is it important to be on time for an appointment or to get to an appointment based on everyone's schedule for that day?
	Why do you think your child has (the above-named) chronic condition (e.g., punishment for a parent's past behavior such as conceiving a child out of wedlock, the result of a genetic problem, or a gift given because of the family's patience and love)?
Communication	What language(s) and dialect(s) are spoken at home?
	Who reads English in the family? If no one reads English, in what language would you prefer printed materials?
	Do parents and children make eye contact when spoken to or do they look down?
	To whom should questions be addressed?
	What can be asked of the child directly? (NOTE: Avoid using the child as a translator because of the strain this imposes.)
Family Relationships	Besides the immediate household, who else makes up the members of this family?
	Who makes the decisions in this family (e.g., mother-in-law, father, both partners, other family or friends, group decision)?
	Who cares for the child and the child's medical needs?

Modified from Davis B and Voegtle K: Culturally competent health care for adolescents, Chicago, 1994, American Medical Association.
Fong CM: Ethnicity and nursing practices, Top Dlin Nurs 7(3):4, 1985.
Jackson SF: Native American Health, Ann Rev Nurs Res 12:193-213, 1994.
Lynch EW and Hanson MJ: Developing cross-cultural competence: a guide for working with young children and their families, Baltimore, Md., 1992, Paul Brookes.
Ramer L: Culturally sensitive caregiving and childbearing families, White Plains, NY, 1992, March of Dimes Birth Defects Foundation.

---

tion or when it is necessary to make major decisions or changes in the care plan, it is important to add the following questions about the family's decision-making procedures: (1) Who are the appropriate people to make this decision for your child? (2) Do you need to bring in other family members or authority figures to receive information and help you make this decision?

It may be useful to get to know the family with these key questions and incorporate the answers into a larger assessment that can be left in the chart and completed over time. Primary care providers can bring in additional questions relating to the reason for the visit (e.g., questions about medication acceptability and use, dietary preferences and restrictions, or developmental goals). Many questions asked by clinicians as part of the routine history and physical clearly have cultural relevance, and once practitioners are sensitive to that fact, cultural assessment can be incorporated into all en-

Table 4-3
Cross-Cultural Assessment of a Family with a Child with a Chronic Condition—cont'd

Family Relationships —cont'd	What are the housing arrangements (e.g., space, number of rooms, members living in the home)?
	What is the child's or family's usual daily routine like?
	To whom do you turn when you need help with or have questions about your child?
Beliefs about Health	What is the present health status of family members?
	What illnesses or conditions are present in the current family members?
	What illnesses or conditions were present in deceased family members?
	How often and for what reasons have family members used western medicine in the past?
	What complimentary therapies are used by your family routinely and specifically for the child (e.g., acupuncture, healers, prayer, massage)?
	What do you do when your child is in pain?
	Who takes care of the child if the child is hospitalized?
	Is it important to keep the child at home or to use institutional placement?
	What do you think will help clear up the problem?
	Are there things that help your child get better that the doctors should know?
	What problems has your child's illness caused your family?
Education	How much schooling have members of the family completed?
	What ways are the best for you to learn about your child's condition (e.g., pamphlets, videos, direct patient teaching, home visits, return demonstrations)?
	From whom are you most comfortable learning about your child's condition (e.g., doctor, nurse, social worker, home health aide, other family members)?
Religion	What religion(s) are practiced in your family?
	What religious things do you do to help your child (e.g., pray, meditate, attend a support group, practice the laying on of hands)?
	What things does your religion say you should *not* do for this child (e.g., have blood transfusions, allow strangers or dangerous circumstances to affect child)?
Nutrition	When are usual mealtimes for your family?
	With whom does the child eat?
	What foods does the child usually eat?
	What special foods does the child eat when the child is sick?
	What foods do you *not* give the child and when?

counters and does not have to take up large blocks of time. A clinician's respect, nonjudgmental attitude, and sincere interest and curiosity about clients is likely to foster trust and open communication. It is important to assure clients that their input is valuable and to verify that the plan of care is acceptable to them.

Research and Culture

Investigators have extensively described the effect of chronic conditions on children and their family members in both qualitative and quantitative studies (see Chapters 2 and 3). Despite this extensive research foundation, it is often difficult to find databased information on the experiences of chronic childhood conditions for particular cultural groups. Sterling, Peterson, and Weeks (1997) reviewed the literature of African-American families with children with chronic illnesses and concluded that although these children are often included in research studies, their numbers are often small, so the information related to African-Americans is subsumed into the findings of the larger study. Sterling, Peterson, and Weeks (1997) also found that African-Americans are not studied within the context of their own culture. It is likely that these two factors also apply to other cultural groups and contribute to the false impression that common symptoms lead to similar family reactions regardless of cultural affiliations (McCubbin et al, 1993).

Despite current regulations that require the inclusion of across-the-lifespan and ethnically diverse samples in government-funded studies, children, women, and nondominant ethnic groups continue to be underrepresented in many forms of research studies, particularly clinical trials (King, 1996). Although these regulations help to ensure that all U.S. residents are represented in research, few studies focusing on particular cultural groups, which could help to overcome oft-repeated stereotypes, are conducted. Perhaps these studies are rare because there is an assumption that such research is best conducted by members of a particular culture (Jackson, 1993). If this assumption is accepted, then important questions about particular cultural groups may never be answered because cultural minority groups are vastly underrepresented among the ranks of scholars. Therefore cross-cultural research is necessary—but inherently difficult—because of the potential for ethnocentrism and cultural misunderstandings.

Ethnocentrism may arise in research studies when investigators assume that findings in one group of people are necessarily applicable across the board, especially if the context or other relevant variables are not considered. Starns (1996) describes two such examples: care of Native American infants on cradleboards and use of marijuana by Jamaican mothers, both of which might be thought to restrict infant development and lead to poor childhood outcomes. Researchers have found, however, that Native American newborns have traits that are well-suited to cradleboards, low activity, little crying, and well-modulated infant states. Hanging a cradleboard near the mother as she works increases upright stimulation and therefore facilitates development (Chisholm, 1989). For a sample of Jamaican infants, higher levels of maternal education and a more nurturing home environment were found to overcome the potentially harmful effects of heavy marijuana use. These infants were more alert, self-regulating, and less irri-

table when compared with a nondrug-using but poorer peer group (Dreher, Nugent, and Hudgins, 1994).

Studies of disadvantaged cultural populations must also recognize the effects of racial, class, and other forms of discrimination, as well as seek solutions to health problems through interventions beyond those aimed at individuals who do not conform to generally accepted healthy behaviors (Jackson, 1993). Researchers have demonstrated the effects of poverty and social class on health (Adler et al, 1994; Anderson and Armstead, 1995) but seldom acknowledge other societal factors, such as repeated discrimination, exposure to high levels of pollutants and violence, and lack of opportunity for educational or occupational advancement. Interventions that address these factors, as well as those most commonly aimed at individual behavior changes, are necessary.

Prejudice against children with chronic conditions has received relatively little attention among researchers. In a recent study, however, 35% of 365 parents of school-age children with chronic illnesses reported discrimination, particularly in school settings and from peers (Turner-Henson et al, 1994). These results, coupled with previous findings that children of ethnic minorities with chronic conditions have fewer ambulatory care visits and are more likely than white children to use emergency rooms as a usual source of care (Newacheck, Stoddard, and McManus, 1993), suggest that social factors and poverty are important areas for future investigation in this population as well.

Summary

As the United States becomes more culturally diverse, health care providers must develop cultural competence to ensure that sensitive and effective care is delivered. Cultural competence will help to prevent racism and ethnocentrism in practice and research by helping providers to assess their own cultural viewpoints and biases while learning about the issues and needs of children and their families. Care should be congruent with the cultural beliefs and practices of clients whenever possible, and increasing cultural competence will enhance effective communication and facilitate respect and appreciation for the range of human diversity. Researchers must investigate culturally relevant questions and test interventions in a wide variety of populations in order to develop the baseline knowledge that will provide clinicians with a sound foundation upon which to develop primary care practices that are culturally competent.

References

Adler NE et al: Socioeconomic status and health, the challenge of the gradient, Am Psychol 49(1):15-24, 1994.

Anderson NB and Armistead CA: Toward understanding the association of socioeconomic status and health: a new challenge for the biopsychosocial approach, Psychosom Med 57:213-225, 1995.

Andrews MM and Boyle JS: Transcultural concepts in nursing care, Philadelphia:, 1995, J.P. Lippincott.

Andrews MM and Hanson PA: Religion, culture, and nursing. In Andrews MM and Boyle JS, editors: Transcultural concepts in nursing care, Philadelphia, 1995, J.P. Lippincott.

Baker C: Cultural relativism and cultural diversity: implications for nursing practice, ANS Adv Nurs Sci 20:3-11, 1997.

Barbee EL: Racism in U.S. nursing, Med Anthropol Q 7:346-362, 1993.

Bogucka R and Boyd D: The Bering Land Bridge, website: http://www.earthsky/com/1996/es960110.html.

Boyle JS: Culture and the community. In Andrews MM and Boyle JS: Transcultural concepts in nursing care, Philadelphia, 1995, J.P. Lippincott.

Brink PJ: Culture and the family ethic, J Child Psychiatr Mental Health Nurs 6(4):3-5, 1993.

Brookins GK: Culture, ethnicity, and bicultural competence: implications for children with chronic illness and disability, Pediatrics Suppl 91:1056-1062, 1993.

Children's Defense Fund: The state of America's children yearbook 1998, Washington DC, 1998, Website: www.childrensdefense.org/keyfacts.html.

Chin P: Chinese americans. In Lipson JG, Dibble SL, and Minarek PA, editors: Culture and nursing care: a pocket guide, San Francisco, 1996, UCSF Nursing Press.

Chisholm J: Biology, culture, and the development of temperament. In Nugent JK, Lester BM, and Brazelton TB, editors: The cultural context of infancy, vol 1, Norwood, NJ, 1989, Ablex.

Dreher M, Nugent JK, and Hudgins R: Prenatal marijuana exposure and neonatal outcomes in Jamaica: an ethnographic study, Pediatrics 93:254-260, 1994.

Furrow BR et al: Bioethics: Health care law and ethics, ed 3, St. Paul, Minn., 1997, West Publishing Co.

Garwick AW et al: Families' recommendations for improving services for children with chronic conditions, Arch Pediatr Adolesc Med 152:440-448, 1998.

Geronimus AT et al: Excess mortality among blacks and whites in the United States, N Engl J Med 335:1552-1558, 1996.

Groce NE and Zola IK: Multiculturalism, chronic illness, and disability, Pediatrics Suppl 91: 1048-1055, 1993.

Herberg P: Theoretical foundations of transcultural nursing. In Andrews MM and Boyle JS, editors: Transcultural concepts in nursing care, Philadelphia, 1995, J.P. Lippincott.

Jackson EM: Whiting-out difference: why U.S. nursing research fails black families, Med Anthropol Q 7:363-385, 1993.

King G: Institutional racism and the medical/health complex: a conceptual analysis, Ethnicity and Disease 6:30-46, 1996.

Kinsman SB, Sally M, and Fox K: Pediatr Rev 17:349-354, 1996.

Krieger N and Fee E: Social class: the missing link in U.S. health data, Int J Health Serv 24(1):25-44, 1994.

Kuhlthau K et al: Assessing managed care for children with chronic conditions, Health Aff 17(4):42-52, 1998.

Leininger M: Transcultural nursing: concepts, theories, research, and practices, New York, 1995, McGraw-Hill.

Lipson JG: Culturally competent nursing care. In Lipson JG, Dibble SL, and Minarek PA, editors: Culture and nursing care: a pocket guide, San Francisco, 1996a, UCSF Nursing Press.

Lipson JG: Diversity issues. In Lipson JG, Dibble SL, and Minarek PA, editors: Culture and nursing care: a pocket guide, San Francisco, 1996b, UCSF Nursing Press.

Lynch EW: Developing cross-cultural competence. In Lynch EW and Hanson MJ, editors: Developing cross-cultural competence: a guide for working with young children and their families, Baltimore, 1992, Paul H. Brookings Publishing Co.

Mardiros M: Conceptions of childhood disability among Mexican-American parents, Medical Anthropology 12:55-68, 1989.

McCubbin HI et al: Culture, ethnicity, and the family: critical factors in childhood chronic illnesses and disabilities: Pediatrics Suppl 91:1063-70, 1993.

McGuire S: Global migration and health: ecofeminist perspectives, ANS, Adv Nurs Sci 21(2):1-16, 1998.

Moore DJ, Williams JD, and Qualls WJ: Target marketing of tobacco and alcohol and related products to ethnic minority groups in the U.S., Ethnicity and Disease 6:83-98, 1996.

Newacheck PW et al: An epidemiologic profile of children with special health care needs, Pediatrics 102:117-123, 1998.

Newacheck PW, Stoddard JJ, and McManus M: Ethnocultural variations in the prevalence and impact of childhood chronic conditions, Pediatrics 91, 1031-1039, 1993.

Niederhauser VP: Health care of immigrant children: incorporating culture into practice, Pediatr Nurs 15:569-74, 1989.

Orlandi MA: Defining cultural competence: an organizing framework. In Orlandi MA, Weston R and Epstein LG, editors: Cultural competence for evaluators: a guide for alcohol and other drug abuse prevention practitioners working with ethnic/racial communities (DHHS Publication No. [ADM] 92-1884), Washington, D.C., 1992, Department of Health and Human Services.

Preston C: The royal road: El Camino Real from Mexico City to Santa Fe, Albuquerque, 1998, University of New Mexico Press.

Purnell LD and Paulanka BJ: Purnell's model for cultural competence. In Purnell LD and Paulanka BJ editors: Trancultural health care: a culturally competent approach, Philadelphia, 1998, F.A. Davis Co.

Rehm RS: Religious faith in Mexican American families living with chronic childhood illness, Image J Nurs Sch 31:33-38, 1999.

Rehm RS: Mexican American family experiences with chronic childhood illness, unpublished doctoral dissertation, 1996.

Rosaldo R: Culture and truth: the remaking of social analysis, Boston, 1993, Beacon Press.

Rueschenberg E and Buriel R: Mexican American family functioning and acculturation: a family systems perspective, Hispanic Journal of Behavioral Sciences 11:232-244, 1989.

Scheper-Hughes N: Difference and danger: the cultural dynamics of childhood stigma, rejection, and rescue, Cleft Palate J 27:301-310, 1990.

Starns JR: Family culture and chronic conditions. In Jackson PL and Vessey JA, editors: Primary care of the child with a chronic condition, ed 2, St Louis, Mosby, 1996.

Sterling YM, Peterson J, and Weekes D: African-American families with chronically ill children: oversights and insights, J Pediatr Nurs12:292-300, 1997.

Turner-Henson A et al: The experiences of discrimination: challenges for chronically ill children., Pediatr Nurs 20:571-577, 1994.

US Department of Commerce: Current population reports: the foreign-born population: 1996, (Economics and Statistics Administration Publication P 20-494), Washington DC, 1996, Bureau of the Census.

US Department of Commerce: We the American . . . foreign born, 1993, Bureau of the Census Website: http://www.census.gov/apsdwww/wepeople.html.

US Immigration and Naturalization Service: Illegal alien resident population, 1998, INS Website: http://www.ins.usdoj.gov/stats/illegalalien/index.html.

Wright KB: Professional, ethical, and legal implications for spiritual care in nursing, Image J Nurs Sch 30:81-83, 1998.

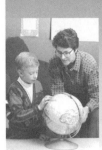

CHAPTER 5

School and the Child with a Chronic Condition

Judith Vessey and Patricia Jackson

The Role of School in a Child's Life

The role of school should not be underestimated in a child's life. School provides opportunities for social, emotional, and cognitive development. In addition to the family, school is the major context in which children develop their sense of self and understanding of their place in relation to peers. More importantly, most children genuinely enjoy school, despite their protestations. This enjoyment of school may be particularly true for children with chronic conditions because they may have fewer opportunities to socialize outside of the school setting. Another positive benefit of including children with chronic conditions in school activities is that nondisabled children can develop attitudes of acceptance and respect for their peers with special needs.

Integrating children with chronic needs into the school setting, however, is not without problems. These children and their families may experience community resistance and resentment. Moreover, many schools have inadequate resources to educate these children, despite the fact that educational services are mandated by law. Parents' fears, guilt, and values need to be carefully assessed because these play critical roles in their children's school success. This chapter will initially examine the legislative underpinnings of special education and then explore ways primary care providers can facilitate a child's school experience.

Laws on the Education of Children with Chronic Conditions

Legislative and judicial rulings over the past 25 years have dramatically changed the role of public educational institutions in providing services to children with chronic conditions (Box 5-1). The change in public policy actually started with the civil rights movement when the landmark decision of *Brown v. Board of Education* (1954) banned segregated schools and affirmed education as a right of all Americans. The principle of "separate is not equal" was used almost 20 years later in *Pennsylvania Association for Retarded Citizens v. Pennsylvania* (1972) to challenge the state's right to exclude children with mental retardation from public education (Burns and Thornan, 1993). That same year the Supreme Court ruled that a free, public education must be provided to all school-age children regardless of disability or degree of impairment (*Mills v. Board of Education of the District of Columbia,* 1972). This landmark Supreme Court decision paved the way for the federal government to enact legislation supporting public education for all children regardless of health or ability.

In 1975 Congress passed Public Law 94-142, the Education for All Handicapped Children Act, as an educational bill of rights for children 5 to 18 years of age (Box 5-2). Public Law 94-142 entitles

<table>
<tr><td>

Box 5-1

Major Legislative Rulings on Education for Children with Disabilities or Chronic Conditions

- Brown v. Board of Education, 1954
- Public Law 93-112, 1973, The Civil Rights Act, Rehabilitation Act, Section 504
- Public Law 94-142, 1975, The Education for All Handicapped Children Act; amended by Public Law 99-457, 1986, The Education of Handicapped Amendments, became Public Law 102-119
- Public Law 100-407, 1988, The Technology Related Assistance for Individuals With Disabilities Act.
- Public Law 101-476, 1990, Individuals With Disabilities Education Act (IDEA); amended by Public Law 102-119, 1991, IDEA Revisions of 1991
- Public Law 101-336, 1992, Americans With Disabilities Act
- Public Law 103-239, 1994, The School to Work Transition Act
- Public Law 105-17, 1997, Individuals with Disabilities Education Act Amendments of 1997
- *Cedar Rapids v. Garret F.,* No. 96-1793, 1999

</td><td>

Box 5-2

Goals of Public Law 94-142

Public Law 94-142, The Education of All Handicapped Children Act of 1975, is to provide:
1. A free and appropriate education for all children.
2. An education in the least restrictive environment based on individual needs.
3. An assessment of needs that is racially and culturally unbiased and given in the individual's native language or mode of communication.
4. An individualized education program (IEP) prepared by a team of professionals that includes parents.
5. Due process and a procedure for complaints to ensure the rights of the individual.

</td></tr>
</table>

children to a "free and appropriate public education" including "special education and related services provided at public expense, under public supervision and direction, without charge, which meet the standards of the state educational agency, and are provided in uniformity with the Individualized Educational Program (IEP)" (PL 94-142, 1975a).

The term *related services* includes "transportation and other developmental, corrective, and supportive services, including speech pathology and audiology, psychologic devices, physical and occupational therapy, recreation, early identification and assessment of disabilities in children, counseling services, and medical services for diagnostic or evaluative purposes. The term also includes school health services, extended school year and school day services, social work services in schools, and

parent counseling and training" (PL 94-142, 1975b).

Public Law 94-142 was amended in 1986 by Public Law 99-457, which included The Handicapped Infants and Toddlers Program, Part H of the amended law. Public Law 99-457 extended services to children from birth to 21 years of age and required interagency and interdisciplinary collaboration, development of a child identification system, a care manager designated for the family, and the implementation of an Individualized Family Service Plan (IFSP) for children from birth through 2 years, analogous to the IEP for children (PL 99-457, 1986). This amendment dramatically increased the school systems' role in providing services to infants and young children. In 1990 and 1991, these laws were further amended under the Individuals with Disabilities Education Act (IDEA), Public Law 101-476 (PL 101-476, 1990), and Public Law 102-119, the IDEA Revisions (PL 102-119, 1991) (Table 5-1).

In May, 1997 after 2 years of intense analysis and hearings, Congress passed legislation reauthorizing and amending IDEA again. Public law 105-17 reaffirms and strengthens the language about the importance of educating children in the least restrictive environment, including participation in the curriculum of general education, the rights of

Table 5-1
Number of Students Ages 6 to 21 Served* During the 1990-1991 to 1994-1995 School Years

Disability Condition	School Year					Change from 1990-1991 to 1994-1995	
	1990-1991	1991-1992	1992-1993	1993-1994	1994-1995	Number	Percent
Specific learning disabilities	2,144,017	2,247,004	2,366,487	2,428,112	2,513,977	369,960	17.3
Speech or language impairments	987,778	998,904	998,049	1,018,208	1,023,665	35,887	3.6
Mental retardation	551,457	553,262	532,362	553,869	570,855	19,398	3.5
Serious emotional disturbance	390,764	400,211	401,652	415,071	428,168	37,404	9.6
Multiple disabilities	97,629	98,408	103,279	109,730	89,646	−7,983	−8.2
Hearing impairments	59,211	60,727	60,616	64,667	65,568	6,357	10.7
Orthopedic impairments	49,340	51,389	52,588	56,842	60,604	11,264	22.8
Other health impairments	56,349	58,749	66,063	83,080	106,509	50,160	89.0
Visual impairments	23,682	24,083	23,544	24,813	24,877	1,195	5.0
Autism	NA	5,415	15,580	19,058	22,780	22,780	—
Deaf-blindness	1,524	1,427	1,394	1,367	1,331	−193	−12.7
Traumatic brain injury	NA	245	3,960	5,395	7,188	7,188	—
All disabilities	4,361,751	4,499,824	4,625,574	4,780,212	4,915,168	553,417	12.7

From the U.S. Department of Education, Office of Special Education Programs, Data Analysis System (DANS)
*The data for 1990-1991 through 1993-1994 include children 6 to 21 years of age served under IDEA, Part B, and Chapter 1 Handicapped Program. For 1994-1995 all children ages 6 to 21 were served under Part B, which includes children previously counted under the Chapter 1 Handicapped Program. Autism and traumatic brain injury were introduced as separate reporting categories in the 1991-1992 school year as a result of PL 101-476, the 1990 Amendments to IDEA.

parents to be involved in educational decisions affecting their children, the importance of functional behavioral assessments and strategies to promote positive behavior, and the requirement that states develop performance goals and outcome measurements for children with disabilities as part of school reform issues and district-wide assessments (Lipton, 1997). This legislation clarifies that states are required to identify, locate, and evaluate all children with disabilities residing in the state, including children in private schools. This directive is referred to as "child find." Directives for services provided to infants and toddlers with disabilities are now Part C of PL 105-17. In addition, the 1997 amendment to IDEA expanded related services to include orientation and mobility services, transition services, and supplemental aids and supports

needed to enable children with disabilities to be educated with nondisabled children to the most appropriate extent (Public law 105-17, 1997). In 1999 in *Cedar Rapids v. Garret F.,* the Supreme Court reaffirmed the requirement of schools to provide special education and related services to all children with disabilites, even if this requires one-on-one, full-time registered nursing services for a child with complex medical needs (Supreme Court Decision No. 96-1793).

Today, one in ten students receives some level of special education services. This number continues to increase because of state funding incentives for schools to label children as disabled, ongoing pressures of schools to improve academic performance, and parental recognition that without appropriate educational intervention minor disabling conditions

Box 5-3

Conditions Identified as Disabilities in Children under the Individuals with Disabilities Education Act (1990)

A. *Disabilities as Defined for Children 5 to 21 Years of Age:*

1. *Autism:* A developmental disability significantly affecting verbal and nonverbal communication and social interaction.
2. *Deaf-blindness:* Children with both deafness and blindness; communication with others is severely impaired.
3. *Deafness:* Children with a hearing deficiency that impairs process of linguistic information through hearing with or without amplification.
4. *Hearing Impairment:* Permanent or fluctuating hearing loss that adversely affects the child's educational process.
5. *Mental Retardation:* Significant subaverage general intelligence existing with deficits in adaptive behavior.
6. *Multiple Disabilities:* Concomitant impairments other than deaf-blindness resulting in severe educational problems that cannot be addressed in a special education program solely for one impairment.
7. *Orthopedic Impairments:* Severe orthopedic impairments that adversely affect the child's educational performance.
8. *Other Health Impairments:* Limited strength, vitality, or alertness due to chronic or acute health problems that affect the child's educational performance.
9. *Serious Emotional Disturbance:* A child who exhibits over a prolonged period of time one or more of the following characteristics: an inability to learn that cannot be explained by intellectual, sensory, or health factors; an inability to build or maintain satisfactory interpersonal relationships; inappropriate behavior or feelings; depression or unhappiness; and a tendency to develop physical symptoms or fears associated with personal or school problems.

10. *Specific Learning Disability:* A disorder in one or more of the psychologic processes involved in understanding or using spoken or written language. This term does not apply to children who have learning problems primarily due to other disabilities listed here or environmental, cultural, or economic disadvantages.
11. *Speech or Language Impairment:* A communication disorder due to impaired articulation, problems with language development, or voice impairment that adversely affects a child's educational performance.
12. *Traumatic Brain Injury:* Acquired injury to the brain resulting in total or partial functional and/or psychosocial impairment.
13. *Visual Impairments (including blindness):* Visual impairments, including ones that can be corrected, that adversely affect a child's educational performance.

B. *Disabilities as Defined for Children 3 to 5 Years of Age:*

Children experiencing developmental delays, as defined by the state, in one or more of the following developmental areas: physical, cognitive, communication, social, emotional, or adaptive.
Children meeting these requirements are eligible for services from their school district at age 3 years.

C. *Disabilities as Defined for Infants and Toddlers:*

Infants and toddlers from birth to age 2 years who: (1) experience delay in cognitive, physical, communicative, social/emotional, or adaptive development; (2) are diagnosed with a physical or mental condition that has a high probability or resulting in developmental delay; or (3) are at risk of having developmental delays if early intervention services are not provided.

Adapted from Publication 99-457, Individuals with Disabilities Education Act (IDEA), Part B.

can have a profound effect on a child's academic success (Terman et al, 1996) (see Table 5-1). In addition, the number of children and youths served through special education is expected to continue to grow as a result of changing laws and interpretations of laws, the legal recognition of new disability categories (e.g., autism and traumatic brain injury, which were added in 1990), and the rising numbers of children in society with sociodemographic and personal characteristics (e.g., poverty, minority/immigrant status, and chronic health conditions) that increase their risk for disabilities and failure in school (Parrish and Chambers, 1996).

The number of people requesting services and special accommodations due to disabilities—especially learning disabilities—has recently led to a backlash by some educators, particularly at the college level, who think that some individuals requesting services are not truly disabled but seeking public-supported assistance with academic work (Shalit, 1997).

Problems with the Implementation of Laws

Identification of Eligible Children

The intent of these legislative acts is honorable and an improvement over previous inequities and lack of services for children with disabilities. Problems exist, however, with interpretation, funding, responsibility for services, and the actual provision of services to the targeted child. Public Law 94-142 (the Education for All Handicapped Children Act) and 99-457 (IDEA) identified only certain chronic health conditions as handicapping and as making a child eligible for special education and related services (Box 5-3). To be eligible for special education, a child must have an identified condition and test at or below a designated level of performance (i.e., often 1.5 to 2.0 standard deviations below the norm in specific or multiple areas of function). Children with milder handicaps or chronic conditions that do not result in significant disability in a given functional area (e.g., speech, learning, motor function, or cognition) are not eligible for special education. The 1990 IDEA Part B, restricted "related services" to only children eligible for special education, thereby limiting services to many chil-

dren with milder disabilities or chronic conditions who would also benefit from services to support their learning (Committee on Children with Disabilities, 1993).

Section 504 of the Rehabilitation Act of 1973 (PL 93-112) protects individuals with physical or mental impairment from discrimination in education or employment. This federal law has been used in the courts to extend "related services" to children with milder disabilities not eligible for special education designation (Ballard, 1977). Children protected under Section 504 of the Rehabilitation Act must receive services required for them to participate in the educational system, but these services must be paid for with general education funds—not special education funds. The Americans with Disabilities Act (ADA) in 1990 further strengthened Section 504 of the Rehabilitation Act by giving civil rights protection to individuals with disabilities by guaranteeing equal opportunity to public accommodations, employment, transportation, state and local government services, and telecommunications (ADA, 1990). This act has been extremely helpful in facilitating the transition of youths with disabilities into employment positions and independent housing.

The Lack of Sufficient Funding

Lack of adequate funding to support public education and services for children with special needs is the basis for most controversies. Federal programs mandate services but do not adequately provide the financial resources to supply these services to all children who would benefit from them. For example, federal aid only funds an estimated 8% of special education costs (Terman et al, 1996). Although the range varies widely, on average the states pay 56% of the costs, and local school districts are responsible for the remainder. This results in poor communities having fewer financial resources to commit to special education services even though there may be more children needing services due to the risks associated with sociodemographic characteristics. States are mandated to provide the services to "eligible" children—not to all children who would benefit, setting up a complex mechanism for establishing eligibility. This often results in an adversarial relationship between the parents seeking services for their children and the educational departments of school systems functioning under severe budgetary constraints. States that actively embrace the call for early case findings and intervention may increase their financial obligations without receiving additional money from the federal government. School districts that identify therapeutic interventions for children with special needs in the IEP process are generally required to pay for these services, although Medicaid fee-for-service or other public funding can often be billed. For children covered by Medicaid managed care, coverage varies substantially among plans (Fox and McManus, 1998). Private insurance will not usually cover services provided in the school setting. The inability of school systems to collect revenue for services provided often results in minimal services. As a result, parents often feel they have to fight for each service provided.

Provision of "Related Services"

Because educational systems are responsible for the "related services" or therapies provided to children in the school setting, they have become overseers of medical care, often quite independent of the child's primary or specialty care providers. The medical role, as determined under Public Law 94-142, is to determine a child's medically related handicapping condition that results in the need for special education and related services (PL 94-142, 1975c). This limited role may further fragment delivery of health care, resulting in duplicated or omitted services, and puts the responsibility of health care on an institution designed to provide education—not health care (Committee on Children with Disabilities, 1993; Palfrey et al, 1990).

As children with chronic conditions live longer and medical technology enables them to participate in school, concern has surfaced about the qualifications of school personnel to provide services to children with special needs (Krier, 1993; McCarthy, Williams, and Eidahl, 1996). School systems must provide services that are essential for the child to have access to school. All services that can be provided by someone with less training than a physician are the responsibility of the school district (Martin, Martin, and Terman, 1996). Public

Law 94-142 identified "a qualified school nurse or other qualified person" as the appropriate person to provide school health services (PL 94-142, 1975d). As the complexity of health conditions increases, the number of school nurses has increased only slightly. Over 90,000 public schools currently exist, but the number of school nurses is around 40,000 (Igoe, 1999). The number of school-based clinics operating in elementary, middle, and high schools is approximately 300, with an additional 20 school-linked clinics (Passarelli, 1994).

When school nurses are available, they can be instrumental in identifying children needing services, initiating assessments, and participating in the development of an individualized health plan (IHP) and the IEP. The nurse can also train and supervise unlicensed personnel in performing health-related services. Primary care providers are not adequately represented in the school setting to directly provide services to children with special health care needs. Therefore whenever possible, they should work collaboratively with school nurses to identify children who would benefit from services, as well as provide staff education and training on medical procedures necessary to perform during school to enable children with special health care needs to safely and effectively participate in school. Procedures such as tracheotomy care, ileostomy care, gavage feedings, and intermittent clean catheterization are all procedures done routinely in school settings, often by unlicensed health care personnel (Harrison, Faircloth, and Yaryan, 1995; Krier, 1993). Krier (1993) found that educators were performing medical procedures, such as medication administration (35%), tube feeding (12%), ostomy care (5%), catheter care (2%), and tracheostomy care (1%). Of the educational staff, 68% felt unprepared to care for medically fragile children, and only 30% had any training in health care procedures including first aid or CPR (Krier, 1993).

Public Law 100-407, the Technology-Related Assistance for Individuals with Disabilities Act, defines technology assistance as any item or equipment used to increase, maintain, or improve a disabled person's functional capabilities (PL 100-407, 1988). Under IDEA Public Law 101-476, schools must provide "assistive technology services" to eligible students if these services are identified as necessary to help a child benefit from the special education program (Parette and Parette, 1992). Assistive technology may be as simple as a spoon designed to support independent feeding or as complex as a laser-operated computer to establish communication with a severely physically disabled but cognitively intact child. School systems are financially responsible for providing the necessary equipment to support the child's educational program but can attempt to obtain reimbursement or funding from other resources such as Crippled Children Services, Medicaid, the State Children's Insurance Plans (SCHIP), or other private health insurance plans. Cooperative funding arrangements may be negotiated to pay for equipment used across environments (Parette and Parette, 1992). The high cost of many modern technological assistive devices has put a major financial strain on the already underfunded special education programs.

Special Education Services

Special education services can be provided in a regular classroom, special classroom or facility, home, private nonprofit preschool, college, hospital, and even state prison. Children eligible for services who attend private schools are still eligible through the public school system, but parents will need to bring them to public schools for services.

Inclusion is the term used when a child receiving special education services is in a regular daycare, preschool, or school program (Hocutt, 1996). This environment is seen as the least restrictive, providing the child the fullest educational potential (Figure 5-1). Most children in special education are in regular classes. They receive special education services (e.g., speech, physical or occupational therapy) in the classroom or are removed briefly for services and then return to the classroom when the intervention is completed.

Children with severe disabilities or who are medically fragile will require services in special classrooms often found within regular school settings or in special schools, institutions, hospitals, or at home (if the individual is unable to attend other facilities). Special day classes usually fall into four categories and serve children with various

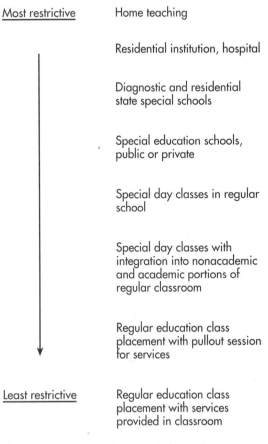

Figure 5-1 Most to least restrictive environments for educational services.

severe disabilities (Table 5-2). Even the profoundly handicapped are required by law to receive educational services for a designated period of time each week. Depending on the size of the school district and the population served, these special classes may be available in the child's actual school district or in adjoining school districts that contract out services. In some situations, school districts contract special education services to private institutions or programs.

Although the momentum has been toward full inclusion of children with special needs, additional research is needed to determine the degree of benefit or detriment to the child with special needs and the other children in the classroom. In general,

Table 5-2
Categories of Special Day Classes

Special Day Classes	Diagnostic Category
Learning Handicapped (LH)	Severely learning disabled
	Educably mentally handicapped
	Mildly mentally handicapped
Communicatively Handicapped (CH)	Severe disorder of language
	Hearing handicapped
	Language delayed
	Severely learning disabled
Physically Handicapped (PH)	Orthopedically handicapped
	Physically handicapped/ disabled
	Multihandicapped
	Visually impaired/handicapped or disabled
Severely Handicapped (SH)	Profoundly mentally handicapped
	Severely mentally handicapped
	Moderately mentally handicapped
	Severely emotionally disturbed
	Autistic
	Multihandicapped

there is no compelling evidence that placement rather than type and intensity of instruction, combined with careful, frequent monitoring of student progress, has a significant effect on a student's progress (Hocutt, 1996), but including children with special needs in regular classrooms will hopefully increase the public's awareness and acceptance of individuals with chronic conditions. Although this has been found to occur (York et al, 1992), discrimination continues (Turner-Henson et al, 1994). Children with mild to moderate disabilities have been found to gain more from integrated classes than children with severe disabilities (Cole et al, 1990; Hocutt, 1996; Jenkins, Odom, and Speltz, 1989). Each child must be carefully assessed during the IEP process, and the classroom assignment best suited for each should be identified and evaluated over time (Box 5-4).

Box 5-4

Questions to Ask when Performing a School Assessment

1. What does the child know about the condition? How much of the care is the child responsible for?
2. Is the child's general health stable, improving, or worsening? Is the child terminally ill?
3. Are any classes or school activities contraindicated by the child's condition?
4. Is preferential seating in the classroom recommended?
5. What modifications in diet exist? Will the child be bringing his or her own lunch or will he or she be participating in the school meals program?
6. What physical restrictions and exercise limitations exist? How are they best managed at home? Are assistive devices required?
7. What medications and/or treatments does the child receive during the school day? Can dosage times be modified around school hours?
8. Does the child require counseling, special therapies (e.g., occupational, physical, or speech), adaptive equipment, or protective devices?
9. Does the child need assistance with any activities of daily living?
10. What precautions and first aid interventions should school personnel be familiar with? Does the child wear a medic-alert bracelet?

The Role of Health Professionals in Determining Special Education Services

Individualized Education Programs (IEP)

The IEP is the cornerstone of IDEA. The legislation requires that each child referred for special education follow a predetermined process to ensure compliance with the law in a timely manner (Figure 5-2). Each child must be evaluated by a

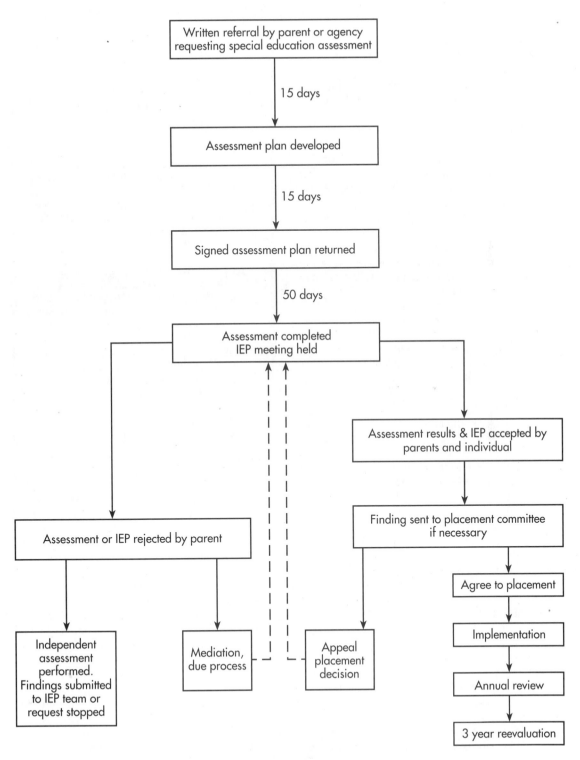

Figure 5-2 Identification procedure for Individualized Educational Program (IEP).

multidisciplinary team comprising appropriately chosen professionals (Box 5-5). This team is responsible for writing the IEP that contains specific educational goals and therapeutic strategies. Therefore the team must include the professionals needed to determine the best possible plan for the child. This team proposes the teaching environment for the child under the principle of "the least restrictive environment" with the knowledge of programs available in the school system. Their plan will also identify the related services (i.e., including the technological assistive devices) required to support the child's educational goals. Specific measurable goals and a timeline for attaining those goals are built into the plan. An IEP is reviewed annually, and a reevaluation must occur every 3 years. A review or reevaluation may occur sooner if requested by the parents, child, or teaching staff (Lipton, 1997). The IEP is a contract for services that must be provided and paid for by the school system (Reschly, 1996) (Box 5-6).

The primary care provider's role starts with early identification and assessment of children with disabilities, as well as "children at risk" for disabilities as part of the mandated "child find" regulations of IDEA. If the primary care provider identifies a child at risk, the family should be referred to the school district's special education office to determine the appropriate public agency to evaluate the child. Children in the birth to 2-year age range may be evaluated through a variety of agencies depending on the state's implementation strategy for Part C of the newly amended IDEA (Lipton, 1997).

In order to initiate the IEP process, the parents or caretakers must request a special education assessment in writing. A written letter by the primary care provider is critical because it provides medical documentation to evaluate and support that request. The IEP assessment plan is determined by this initial request, so it is important to identify all areas of delay or potential risk.

The primary care provider is part of the comprehensive multidisciplinary assessment process by providing health records and physical findings with parental consent to the IEP team. The primary care provider may participate in additional assessments or referrals to other specialists. Although the IEP team is responsible for explaining the assessment findings to the parents and child, the primary

---

Box 5-5

IEP Team as Required Under the Individual With Disabilities Education Act Amendments of 1997

1. The parents of the child
2. At least one regular teacher of the child
3. At least one special education teacher or provider of the child
4. A representative of the school district who is:
   a) qualified to provide or supervise the provision of special education
   b) knowledgeable about the general curriculum
   c) knowledgeable about the availability of the district's resources
5. An individual who can interpret the instructional implications of the evaluation results
6. At the discretion of the parent or the school district, others who have knowledge or special expertise regarding the child, such as a health care provider
7. When appropriate, the child or youth with the disability

Adapted from Lipton DJ, Individuals With Disabilities Education Act Amendments of 1997, Disability Rights Education and Defense Fund, Inc., 1997

---

care provider may be able to offer additional insight or interpretation. In many districts the school nurse is a member of the IEP team, especially for children who require an IHP as part of the IEP. School nurses, working with primary care providers, should oversee the development and management of the IHP.

The school district has 50 days to complete the assessment process and establish the educational plan. The primary care provider can be very helpful in reviewing the plan with the family to determine its appropriateness for the child. If the provider and family think that the plan is not sufficient to meet the child's developmental and cognitive needs, then it can be rejected and additional recommendations made to the IEP team. Recommendations supported by assessment findings or relevant literature are more likely to be accepted and incorporated

Components of an IEP

IEP forms vary from school district to school district but should all include the following information:

1. *Present Level of Performance*
☐ Describes student in positive way?
☐ Reflects parent concerns?
☐ *Include strengths and needs,
☐ State results of most recent evaluations, and
☐ Describe how disability affects involvement in general education program?

2. *Transition*
☐ *Before age 14, what needs to happen to prepare for future?
☐ *At age 14, a statement of classes needed to prepare for future?
☐ *By age 16, specific transition services, related services needs, and other agencies to be included?
☐ *Before age 18, what rights will transfer to the student?

3. *Annual Goals and Objectives/Benchmarks*
☐ Are they meaningful and attainable within 1 school year?
☐ *Do they allow student to be involved in and progress in the general class program?
☐ Are they clear on *what* student will do and *how, where,* and *when* he or she will do it?
☐ *Do they include positive behavioral supports, if needed?
☐ *Is it clear how progress will be measured?
☐ *Is it clear how parent will be informed of progress?

4. *Related Services, Supplementary Aids, and Supports Necessary*
☐ To help the child reach annual goals?
☐ *To progress in the general education program?
☐ *To participate with other students—disabled and nondisabled?

☐ *Specifics listed: start/finish dates? frequency? location, length of time for services?
☐ *Modifications for participation in standardized tests *or*
☐ *A statement of why a particular test is not appropriate and what will be used instead?

5. *Placement*
☐ Is placement decided *after* goals, objectives, and supports are agreed upon?
☐ Is placement in the *least restrictive environment?*
☐ *If student is *not* participating in all general education activities, is there an explanation why not?
☐ *Is IEP coordinated with general classroom schedules, activities, and programs?

6. *Instruction and Adaptations*
☐ Who does what?
    Special education teacher?
    General education teacher?
    Parents?
    Student?
    Specialists?
    Aides or others?
☐ When, where, and how often will IEP be carried out?
    Seating preferences?
    Individual or small group instruction as needed?
    Extra time to complete assignments?
    Assistive technology needs?
☐ When and how will progress be reviewed?
☐ How will necessary changes to the IEP be made?

*Changes in IEP regulations due to Public Law 105-17, 1997, Individuals With Disabilities Education Act Amendments of 1997.

Adapted from IEP Checklist Parents Educational Advocacy Training Center 20(2):16-17, 1998.

into the plan. The primary care provider should act as an advocate for the parents and child when there is evidence of inappropriate or incomplete planning by the IEP team (Committee on Children with Disabilities, 1992).

504 Accommodation Plans

Students whose disabilities are not severe enough to qualify for an IEP can still be eligible for services under Section 504 of the Rehabilitation Act. Under this section an individualized approach to meet the child's needs must be implemented. Strategies for classroom adaptation are written into an accommodation plan designed to meet the child's unique needs (Snyder, 1997).

Facilitating the School Experience

Many chronic conditions affect children's development—either directly or indirectly (i.e., by diminishing the child's opportunity to participate in developmentally appropriate activities) (see Chapter 2). An important developmental task of children at least 5 years old is to move beyond the family sphere into the school community, where academic achievement, social competence, and regular attendance are major goals.

Primary care providers can facilitate a child's adjustment to school. Although the school district is the lead agency for services provided in the school setting, school personnel often welcome the child's primary care provider to coordinate medical services. If the school district has a nurse assigned to oversee the health care services for children with chronic conditions, the primary care provider should establish a link with that individual so that changes in the child's condition or medical management can be easily communicated. The clinician can serve as a resource to the school by offering in-service education sessions on the child's health care needs, teaching specific therapy techniques, or demonstrating the appropriate use of assisted technology.

To best assist children, it is important to obtain a detailed history regarding their capabilities in performing daily living skills and assessing their stamina. This information is invaluable in helping children cope with limitations that may be encountered in school while helping them maintain independence.

Before initiating discussion with the school, it is important for primary care providers to seek the permission of the child and the family before releasing medical information to the school district or carrying on any dialog with school personnel. Although this will not be a problem for most families, establishing open communication with the school district may need to be explored. If a condition is mild and not visible, families may not want information about the condition conveyed to school personnel to prevent their child being labeled as "different." In other cases, families genuinely fear ostracism or reprisal from the school community. The family's wishes should be respected if at all possible; however, when withholding information about a child places that child at risk, the family must be counseled about the risks and benefits of disclosure, and appropriate legal action must be taken. For example, withholding information about an adolescent with uncontrolled epilepsy who is enrolling in driver's education is both dangerous and illegal.

Promoting the Child's Self-Concept

Developing a healthy self-concept is paramount if children with chronic conditions are to succeed in school and later activities. Many normative school activities (e.g., instruction in nutrition or sexuality) teach children health-promoting behaviors that can help build healthy self-concepts. Helping these children develop wholesome relationships and share their talents with other children is also beneficial; children who excel in a specific academic area or participate in sports and other extracurricular activities are more likely to be successful. Participating in these activities not only helps build self-esteem but also enhances other spheres of development (Walsh and Ryan-Wenger, 1992).

Unfortunately, developing the self-esteem of children with chronic conditions in the school setting is not without difficulty. These children are likely to be teased; many may experience bullying or even ostracism (Berstein and Watson, 1997). Children with chronic conditions will benefit from interventions to strengthen the coping abilities that help them deal constructively with the peer rejection, loneliness, or isolation resulting from such discriminatory practices (Turner-Henson et al, 1994). Incorporating social skills training into the child's educational plan is one way to help the child and family become more confident in their interactions with others and their use of appropriate behaviors when dealing with discrimination. School personnel can assist by dealing with inappropriate behavior of other students and developing an awareness of what it is like to have a chronic condition.

Parents, teachers, and school professionals need to acknowledge that children with chronic conditions experience the same developmental stressors as their peers and therefore need to be treated similarly and taught the same coping skills. Using a variety of techniques to help these children normalize their school experience will be beneficial to developing their self-concept (Walsh and Ryan-Wenger, 1992).

Administering Medications and Treatments

If medications are required during the school day, the general guidelines and criteria of each state and school district must be followed: (1) a legal prescriber must authorize the medication, (2) parents must give written permission for medication to be given, (3) the medication should be properly labeled, (4) the medication must be stored in a locked area, and (5) the school must document that the medication was administered. If it is likely that a child will need to take medications ordered on an as-needed basis, clearly defined protocols should be made for their administration.

Whenever possible, clinicians should alter treatment protocols to occur around school schedules for several pragmatic reasons. The child with a chronic condition wants to be considered normal. Requiring the child to go to the nurse for medications may be met with resistance, particularly in this era of "Safe and Drug-free Schools." Moreover, even in the best of circumstances, there may not be adequate time or qualified personnel within the school to administer medications or oversee treatments. As children enter adolescence, it is often appropriate to explore ways to help them develop self-care behaviors (e.g., self-medication, intermittent clean catheterizations, or testing blood glucose levels). Such activities will help children become more autonomous, which is an important developmental goal.

Promoting Mobility

Limited mobility is an issue for many students with chronic conditions. Mobility is affected by physical impairments, diminished strength, and fatigue. Regardless of the cause, limited mobility can affect students' ability to achieve and compete. Physical changes can limit some children from participating fully in gym, recess, sports, and afternoon activities (Ahmann and Rollins, 1995). In the worst case scenario, limited mobility will hinder children from participating in critical learning activities.

If mobility is a problem, it must be discussed and appropriate adaptations planned for and addressed in the child's educational planning meetings. Two major approaches are used to facilitate a child's mobility: structuring the environment and improving mobility. When choosing a school is an option, its physical layout (e.g., one floor, width of hallways, presence of elevators, location of bathrooms) needs to be considered. Providing the child with two sets of books, one for the classroom and one for home, eliminates the problem of transporting them. Scheduling classes close to one another and a study hall or lunch after physical education class gives the student more time to change and to avoid tardiness for the next class.

The student's mobility will be improved and normalization promoted if appropriate assistive devices are used. For example, an adolescent in a large high school may prefer to use a wheelchair when traveling long distances between classes rather than limiting the class schedule to classes that are near each other. Adaptive aids can help children write, reach books on library shelves, or respond to questions in the classroom. Schools have eliminated many physical obstacles while they conform with the Americans with Disabilities Act.

Managing Fatigue

It is important to set reasonable expectations for children. Fatigue is an integral part of many chronic conditions that is sometimes a symptom of the disease (e.g., in heart disease) and other times associated with time-consuming therapies (e.g., with cystic fibrosis) or a side effect of medications (e.g., those given for epilepsy). Fatigue may also occur as a result of induced physiologic changes, such as in children undergoing chemotherapy.

There are several strategies for reducing fatigue, most of which focus on structuring a child's educational experience in a way that is not physically taxing. For example, the child could be encouraged to use a tape recorder for note taking, serve as scorekeeper rather than participating in vigorous activity during physical education, or be assigned easy classroom chores such as sharpening pencils with an electric sharpener. Classes that are located close together require less travel and reduce fatigue, which is particularly important in large schools or those with several buildings.

Scheduling a study hall period immediately after lunch gives the child an opportunity to nap (ideally in a different setting) without missing class time. Another strategy is arranging the student's schedule so that the most important classes are either in the morning or in the afternoon; that way if only half-day sessions are possible, the child can still learn the important content. The homework demands of various courses should also be taken into account when planning a child's schedule. It is better to defer one class than to have children take on a rigorous schedule that sets them up for failure. Selected courses may be taken during summer school to lighten a child's academic load, which is ideally included in a child's academic plan because many schools have limited summer offerings.

Ensuring Safety

There are many safety issues to consider. Environmental safety is paramount. Ramps need to be installed where necessary, and electric adaptive equipment must be periodically inspected. A reserve generator must be available for children on life-sustaining equipment such as ventilators. Provisions for transporting a student with a physical disability during emergencies such as fires and earthquakes need to be determined and disseminated to all school personnel. School buses may need to be retrofitted with appropriate safety devices (e.g., seat belts or wheelchair locks) (Committee on Injury and Poison Prevention, 1993).

Many chronic conditions place children at greater risk for infection and illness. The school's policy on notifying parents of possible exposure to communicable diseases must be clarified. Depending on the child's chronic condition, specific areas of concern may include strep throat, measles, mumps, meningitis, hepatitis A and B, salmonella, or shigella infections (McMillan, 1995). Other chronic conditions such as asthma can be aggravated by chemicals used in chemistry class, cleaning fluids, chalk dust, animal fur, and other substances found in schools (Swanson and Thompson, 1994).

Disability may hinder participation in sports and place a child at higher risk for injury (Ahmann and Rollins, 1995). Appropriate safety equipment must be used, and there must be supervision. Strengthening exercises also help prevent injury.

School Absenteeism and Reentry

Parents must clearly communicate their expectations about school to their children and whenever possible facilitate their attendance. The more school absences a child experiences, the greater the risk of poor academic achievement (Walker and Jacobs, 1984); and studies indicate that school absences are significantly higher among children with chronic conditions (Newacheck and Halfon, 1998). Although all absences place a child at risk, frequent short-term interruptions are more disruptive than a single, longer absence (Perrin, 1992). Exacerbations in the child's condition, side effects from various interventions, fatigue, and health care appointments are the primary reasons for absenteeism (Passarelli, 1992). If psychosocial problems (e.g., behavior or family difficulties) coexist, however, a child is at greater risk for high absenteeism (Collins and LeClere, 1996). For example, parental guilt and anxiety can foster school phobia and subsequent absenteeism. Repeated absenteeism not only affects academic performance but also may create a downward spiral in a child's self-concept, peer relations, and subsequent family functioning.

Illness alone is rarely a suitable excuse for school failure. Families and professionals need to work together to reduce absenteeism. Whenever possible, health care visits should be scheduled around school hours. If this is impossible, several appointments should be scheduled on one day so that the child does not have to miss several half days of class.

If a prolonged absence is anticipated, parents must arrange for home instruction. School policies vary, and delays as a result of child ineligibility, poor coordination of services, or unavailable teachers may be encountered before homebound education is initiated. If schools are not approached before the requisite length of absenteeism (i.e., usually 2 to 4 weeks) is met, additional delays are likely to be encountered before services are arranged. Many schools, however, are willing to work with families in maintaining their child's education by providing homework assignments, communicating with hospital-based teachers, helping parents become informal tutors, and arranging for tutorial services to begin as soon as the child is eligible. If hospitalizations are frequent or prolonged absences are anticipated, a specific objective should be included in the child's educational plan to plan for uninterrupted schooling.

The decision to repeat a grade must be made with great care. This setback can cause feelings of shame, inadequacy, and inferiority; but the decision to remain in the same grade may also enhance feelings of success because the work requirements may be easier. New classmates provide a second chance to form friendships (Whaley and Wong, 1979).

Children who have had prolonged absences or disfigurement must successfully reenter school so that their development is not impeded. A positive experience of reentry can provide children with a sense of accomplishment and social acceptance, strengthen faltering self-esteem, and lessen maladaptive emotional responses to their condition (Chekryn, Deegan, and Reid, 1986). Primary care providers can help promote a smooth transition for such children by working with school nurses and helping the family proactively determine strategies to facilitate school reentry (Rabin, 1994). The two primary goals are to help the child and family anticipate situations they may encounter and to prepare teachers and classmates for the child's return.

One helpful approach to preparing the child for reentry is role playing, wherein primary care providers play the role of a classmate and children play themselves (Rabin, 1994). The purpose is to act out a variety of scenarios that may occur during the first day back at school so that the child can develop answers to potentially embarrassing questions or situations that may arise. Another useful strategy is to ask close friends to accompany the child and serve as a buffer upon the return to school. Parents may also bring the child for several "drop-in visits" or sponsor a "welcome back" class party designed to promote peer acceptance.

A variety of approaches can be used to help teachers and classmates adjust. A child may be encouraged to write a letter or record a videotape for classmates about the experience of being in the hospital or undergoing treatment, which is then shared with teachers or classmates several days before the child's return. Providing visual images of a child—either on videotape or in a snapshot—allows time for "sanctioned staring" or for classmates to ask questions or express their concerns without fear of recrimination. This is particularly important if the child has undergone major physical changes (e.g., alopecia secondary to chemotherapy or scarring from burns). Role-playing is another helpful strategy. Two classmates can act out the scenario, with the teacher or the primary care provider guiding the experience. Science projects, literature assignments, and video presentations can be used by teachers to promote understanding and acceptance within the child's peer group. Careful advance planning will improve the likelihood of a successful return to school for the child.

Educating the Terminally Ill Student

School is an appropriate activity for many children who are terminally ill because it provides opportunities for socialization and personal achievement (Davis, 1989). Depriving a child of such opportunities may cause increased stress. For children to have a successful school experience, several issues must be considered. First, the developmental level of the child and peer group must be considered in deciding on how the "who, what, where, and how" information about the child's condition is shared with the child, peers, school personnel, and other parents. Second, flexibility in planning the child's educational program is necessary if the condition deteriorates. Third, efforts to help the child maintain a positive self-concept and body image are important but may be difficult when a child begins to lose weight, cough productively, or have skin changes. Fourth, academic programming needs to be tailored for the child. For example, an adolescent enrolled in a college preparatory curriculum needs to be helped to develop achievable objectives rather than giving up all hope for the future (Davis, 1989). Finally, children who are dying often need to exhibit more control over their lives and environments. Whenever possible, efforts must be made to help children reach the goals that they have set for themselves.

It is not enough to focus attention only on the dying child and the family because many children have not had to confront death and dying and do not know how to act or the appropriate thing to say. Many of the strategies suggested in the section of this chapter on school reentry are equally appropriate for helping students deal with the death of a peer.

The effect that a dying child has on school personnel must be considered. The attitudes of school personnel toward illness and death, as well as their ability to individualize instruction, their concern or need to protect the dying child, and their fear of an emergency arising in the classroom, can influence their effectiveness (Davis, 1989). Flexibility and realistic expectations are needed if the school experience is to be successful for a child who is terminally ill.

Do Not Resuscitate Orders

Comprehensive planning for end-of-life care for a child with a terminal condition may include promulgating the family's wishes that the child not be resuscitated if a cardiac arrest occurs. A comprehensive approach to responding to do not resuscitate (DNR) orders in the school requires school personnel to develop a protocol to follow when a child with a DNR order attends school.

The National Education Association (NEA) (1994) developed guidelines for DNR orders in school (i.e., if a school district honors a DNR), emphasizing that a policy was *not* established. The NEA has suggested the following minimum conditions if a school board is to honor DNR: the request should be submitted in writing and be accompanied by a written order signed by the student's physician; the school should establish a team to consider the request and all available alternatives, and if no other alternative exists, to develop a medical emergency plan; staff should receive training; and staff and students should receive counseling. In its statement, the NEA delineated the following elements of the medical emergency plan: (1) the student's teacher specifies his or her actions if the student suffers a cardiac arrest or other life-threatening emergency; (2) other school employees who supervise the student receive briefing sessions; (3) the student wears an identification bracelet indicating the DNR order; (4) the parents execute a contract with the local emergency medical service and send a copy to the superintendent; and (5) the team reviews the plan annually.

In addition, individual states have DNR policies and laws and that govern the actions of emergency medical personnel actions when treating students (Miller-Thiel, 1998). These regulations are quite varied, but a summary is presented in Table 5-3. Schools should develop protocol for responding to DNR orders in accordance with NEA guidelines; state regulations; and in a spirit of collaboration, respect, and sensitivity. Parents, educators, support personnel, and members of the health care team must be committed to a process that is flexible and responsive to the changing needs of the child. Essential to this process are ongoing forums where parents and educators can discuss their concerns,

Table 5-3
State-by-State DNR Policy/Law Status for Emergency Medical Services

State	DNR School	School DNR Minors	Pending Law
Alabama	N	N	N
Alaska	Y	Y	IN
Arkansas	Y	Y	N
Arizona	N	N	N
California	Y	Y	N
Colorado	IN	IN	IN
Connecticut	Y	Y	N
Delaware	N	N	Y-school
District of Columbia	N	N	Y
Florida	Y	Y	IN
Georgia	N	N	N
Hawaii	Y	N	N
Idaho	Y	Y	N
Illinois	Y	Y	Y
Indiana	N	N	Lost '98
Iowa	N	N	N
Kansas	N	N	N
Kentucky	Y	N	N
Louisiana	N	N	N
Maine	Y	Y	Update
Maryland	Y	Y	IN
Massachusetts	Y	Y	4/1/98
Michigan	Y-Hospice	Y-Hospice	Y
Minnesota	N	N	Maybe
Mississippi	N	N	N

*Adapted from Miller-Thiel J: Do not resuscitate (DNR): state policies for at-home and in-school, Pediatr Nurs 24(6):599-601, 1998.
Y = *law or policy available*
N = *no law or policy or substantial stipulations are placed*
IN = *insufficient information*

share their values and preferences about how certain situations should be handled, and define or revise plans. Within these discussions, it is crucial to define the range of possible scenarios that are likely to occur for the child and to build contingency plans for how they should be handled (Rushton, Will, and Murray, 1995).

Summary

Primary care providers must not lose sight of the fact that schools provide opportunities for social, emotional, and cognitive development (Rabin, 1994). Primary care providers may assume the role of coordinator by bringing together the child, parents, peers, and school personnel and fostering open communication; but a team approach is the only way to guarantee that educational and health care needs are met (Davis, 1989). Innovative school health programs based on delivering primary care in the school and linking it to the school program should be encouraged.

References

Ahmann E and Rollins J: Family-centered care of the child with special needs. In Wong D, editor: Nursing care of infants and children, ed 5, St Louis, 1995, Mosby.

Ballard J: Public law 94-142 and section 504: understanding what they are and are not, Reston, Va., 1977, Governmental Relations Unit, The Council for Exceptional Children.

Berstein JY and Watson MW: Children who are targets for bullying, J Interpersonal Violence 12(4):483-498, 1997.

Brown v Board of Education, US Supreme Court 347 US 483, 1954.

Burns M and Thornan CB: Broadening the scope of nursing practice: federal programs for children, Pediatr Nurs 19(6):546-552, 1993.

Chekryn J, Deegan M, and Reid J: Normalizing the return to school of the child with cancer, Ped Oncol Nurses 3:20-24, 34, 1986.

Cole KN et al: Effects of preschool integration for children with disabilities, Exceptional Child 58:36-45, 1990.

Collins JG and LeClere FB: Health and selected socioeconomic characteristics of the family, Vital Health Stat 10 195(i-vi):1-85, 1996.

Committee on Children with Disabilities: Pediatrician's role in the development and implementation of an individual evaluation plan (IEP) and/or individual family service plan (IFSP), Pediatrics 89:340-342, 1992.

Committee on Children with Disabilities: Provision of related services for children with chronic disabilities, Pediatrics 92(6):879-881, 1993.

Committee on Injury and Poison Prevention: School bus transportation of children with special needs, AAP News 9(11), 1993.

Davis K: Educational needs of the terminally ill student, Issues Compr Pediatr Nurs 12:235-245, 1989.

Fox HB and McManus MA: Improving state Medicaid contracts and plan practices for children with special needs, Future Child 8(2):105-118, 1998.

Harrison BS, Faircloth JW, and Yaryan L: The impact of legislation and litigation on the role of the school nurse, Nurs Outlook 43:57-61, 1995.

Hocutt AM: Effectiveness of special education: is placement the critical factor? Future Child 6(1), 1996.

Igoe J: Personal communication, 1999.

Jenkins JR, Odom SL, and Speltz ML: Effects of social integration on preschool children with handicaps, Exceptional Child 55:311-320, 1989.

Krier JJ: Involvement of educational staff in the healthcare of medically fragile children, Pediatr Nurs 19(3):251-254, 1993.

Lipton DJ: Individuals with disabilities education act amendments of 1997, Berkeley, Calif, 1997 Disability Rights Education and Defense Fund, Inc.

Martin EW, Martin R, and Terman JD: The legislative and litigation history of special education, Future Child 6(1), 25-39, 1996.

McCarthy AM, Williams JK, and Eidahl L: Children with chronic conditions: educators' views, J Pediatr Health Care 10:272-279, 1996.

McMillan JA: Control of infections in schools, Pediatr in Rev 16:283-88, 1995.

Mills v Board of Education of the District of Columbia, US Court of Appeals 348F, Supp. 866, 1972.

Miller-Thiel J: Do not resuscitate (DNR): state policies for at home and in school, Pediatr Nurs 24:599-601, 1998.

National Education Association Executive Committee: Policy on do not resuscitate orders, June 1994, Washington, D.C., The Association.

Newacheck PW and Halfon N: Prevalence and impact of disabling chronic conditions in childhood, Am J Public Health, 88:610-617, 1998.

Palfrey JS et al: Providing therapeutic services to children in special educational placements: an analysis of the related services provisions of Public Law 94-142 in five urban school districts, Pediatrics 85(4):518-525, 1990.

Parette HP and Parette PC: Young children with disabilities and assistive technology: the nurse's role on multidisciplinary technology teams, J Pediatr Nurs 7:237-245, 1992.

Parrish TB and Chambers JG: Financing special education, Future Child 6:121-138, 1996.

Passarelli C: Case management of chronic health conditions of school-age youth. In Wallace HM et al, editors: Principles and practices of student health: school health, vol 2, Oakland, Calif, 1992, Third Party Publishing Co.

Passarelli C: School nursing trends for the future, J Sch Health 64(4):141-148, 1994.

Pennsylvania Association for Retarded Citizens v Pennsylvania, US Court of Appeals 343 F, 1972.

Perrin J: Developmental-behavioral pediatrics, ed 2, Philadelphia, 1992, W.B. Saunders.

Public Law 93-112: The Vocational Rehabilitation Act, Section 504, 29 USC, 45CFR, Washington, DC, 1973, US Government Printing Office.

Public Law 94-142: The Education for All Handicapped Children Act 20 USC Sec 11 404 [18], Washington, DC, 1975a, US Government Printing Office.

Public Law 94-142: The Education of the Handicapped Act 20 USC Sec 121a, 13[4], Washington, DC, 1975b, US Government Printing Office.

Public Law 94-142: The Education of the Handicapped Act 20 USC Sec 121a, 13[4], Washington, DC, 1975c, US Government Printing Office.

Public Law 94-142: The Education of the Handicapped Children Act 20 USC Sec 121a, 13[10], Washington, DC, 1975d, US Government Printing Office.

Public Law 99-457: The Education of the Handicapped Act Children Amendments of 1986, Washington, DC, 1986, US Government Printing Office.

Public Law 100-407: Technology-Related Assistance for Individuals with Disabilities Act of 1988, Washington, DC, 1988, US Government Printing Office.

Public Law 101-336: Americans with Disabilities Act of 1990, 42 USC 12101 et seq. Washington, DC, 1990, US Government Printing Office.

Public Law 101-476: The Individuals with Disabilities Education Act of 1990, Washington, DC, 1990, US Government Printing Office.

Public Law 102-119: The Individuals with Disabilities Education Act Revisions of 1991, Washington, DC, 1991 US Government Printing Office.

Public Law 105-17: Individuals with Disabilities Education Act Amendments of 1997, Codified at 20 USC 1401 et seq. Washington, DC, 1997 US Government Printing Office.

Rabin N: School reentry and the child with a chronic illness: the role of the pediatric nurse practitioner, J Pediatr Health Care 8:227-232, 1994.

Reschly DJ: Identification and assessment of students with disabilities, Future Child 6(1):40-53, 1996.

Rushton CH, Will J, and Murray M: To honor and obey: DNR orders in the schools, Pediatr Nurs 20(6):581-585, 1995.

Shalit R: Defining disability down, The New Republic, 16-22, August 25,1997.

Snyder M: Case management of the child with a learning disorder or ADHD. In Vessey JA, editor: The child with a learning disorder or ADHD: a manual for school nurses, Scarborough, Me, 1997, National Association of School Nurses.

Swanson MN and Thompson PE: Managing asthma triggers in school, Pediatr Nurs 20(2):181-184, 1994.

Terman DL et al: Special education for students with disabilities: analysis and recommendations, Future Child 6(1):4-24, 1996.

Turner-Henson A et al: The experiences of discrimination: challenges for chronically ill children, Pediatr Nurs 20(6):571-577, 1994.

Wagner MM and Blackorby J: Transition from high school to work or college: how special education students fare, Future Child 6(1):103-120, 1996.

Walker D and Jacobs F: Chronically ill children in school, Peabody J Educ 61:28-74, 1984.

Walsh M and Ryan-Wenger N: Sources of stress in children with asthma, J School Health 62(10):459-463, 1992.

Whaley LF and Wong DL, editors: Nursing care of infants and children, St Louis, 1979, Mosby.

York J et al: Feedback about integrating middle-school students with severe disabilities in general education classes, Exceptional Child 58:244-258, 1992.

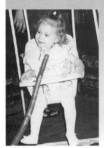

CHAPTER 6

Ethics and the Child with a Chronic Condition

Cindy Hylton Rushton and Teresa A. Savage

Decision Making along the Course of Chronic Conditions

The course of a chronic condition is likely to include diagnosis and treatment; periods of recovery, exacerbations, stability, or instability; and in some cases, deterioration and death. These phases are often punctuated by recurring ethical questions, including the following: (1) defining what constitutes a life worth living, (2) recognizing the threshold for certainty in diagnosis and treatment, (3) choosing a decision maker to decide about treatment or nontreatment, (4) determining the role of minors in making treatment decisions, (5) deciding whether to pursue experimental or innovative therapies, and (6) knowing how to resolve conflicts. The range of chronic conditions in childhood and adolescence is paralleled by the range of values held by people with chronic conditions or care givers of those with chronic conditions. Competing ethical obligations can create a set of problematic situations for children, families, and health care providers.

The Ethical Domain

Ethics is concerned with "what ought to be" and how individuals think about and discuss "what ought to be." Ethics is concerned with the behavior, choices, and character of individuals and groups. Ethical questions arise alongside—but differ from—fundamental social, legal, political, professional, and scientific questions. For example, public policies and laws (e.g., the death penalty) set boundaries for human behavior but do not necessarily correspond to an individual's sense of "what ought to be." It is within this context that ethical discourse occurs.

There are many ways of discerning the ethical dimensions of an issue or quandary. The process of discernment is complex and influenced by emotions, scientific facts, values, interpersonal relationships, culture, religion, the essence of who we are, and myriad situational factors—all of which converge to shape the way ethical questions are framed. Ethical questions arise because an individual is unsure of the right thing to do or the proper outcome to pursue. For example, primary care providers may be concerned about whether to offer an experimental treatment protocol to a family when the likelihood of altering the natural course of the child's condition is remote and pursuing such treatment will require the family to pay out-of-pocket. Ethical questions may also arise because there are genuine value conflicts about the right thing to do or the proper outcomes to pursue. For example, primary care providers and families may disagree about whether it is justified to continue aggressive treatment for a child with end-stage cystic fibrosis. The providers may reason that continued treatment is burdensome and will prolong death; in contrast, the parents may believe that extending life is the appropriate goal to be pursued—despite the burden endured by the child. In both instances, careful consideration of the judgments and the justifications that are used to defend one's position and behavior is warranted.

Ethical deliberation involves the process of discerning, analyzing, and articulating ethically defensible positions and then acting upon them. Ethical thinking provides a reasoned account of an ethical position and helps one move beyond intuition or emotions. The goal of ethical deliberation is not to achieve absolute certainty about what is right but to achieve *reliability* and *coherence* in behavior, choices, character, process, and outcomes.

Ethical theories and principles provide a foundation for ethical analysis and deliberation (Box 6-1), as well as a guide for organizing and understanding ethically relevant information in a dilemma or conflict situation. These theories and principles also suggest directions and avenues for resolving competing claims and supply reasons that justify moral action. Ethical principles are universal in nature but are *not* absolute. Each case involves particular principles and values integral to the decision-making process. One must balance the claims generated from competing principles relevant to a particular case. Moreover, factors such as family dynamics, the nature of relationships, contextual features, integrity, and faithfulness to commitments are also morally relevant to the decision-making process. Even when one chooses a morally justifiable course of action, there are always unmet obligations when resolving ethical dilemmas (i.e., a "moral remainder").

Ethical theories and principles must be applied systematically within the decision-making process. Ethical analysis is enhanced when a framework that provides a systematic process of decision making is used and mistakes by using only logic and reason are avoided (Box 6-2). In addition, because some decisions (e.g., those to withhold or withdraw certain therapies) help to determine the timing and consequences of death, other important social, ethical, and religious values come into play.

A Moral Framework for Decision Making

A specific framework provides a mechanism for individuals, families, and providers dealing with the ethical dimensions of difficult situations. For adults, a morally defensible framework for decision making is relatively straightforward and widely accepted (President's Commission for the Study of

---

Box 6-1

Normative Ethical Theories and Principles

Ethical Theories

Teleological theories—Determine an action to be right or wrong based on the consequences the action produces. For example, in utilitarianism the principle of utility (i.e., maximizing the good or minimizing harm) is the central criterion for action.

Deontological theories—Focus on doing one's duty. The intrinsic quality of the act itself or its conformity to a rule—not its consequences—determines whether an act is right or wrong.

Selected Ethical Principles

Beneficence—The duty to do good; to promote the welfare of the individual.

Nonmaleficence—The duty not to harm or burden.

Respect for Persons—Recognizing another person as sharing a common human destiny.

Derivative Principles

Autonomy—Self-determination.

Veracity—The duty to tell the truth

Fidelity—The duty to keep one's promise or word

Justice—Fairness. *Distributive justice* refers to the equitable distribution of benefits and burdens under conditions of scarcity and competition.

Adapted from Beauchamp TL and Childress JF: Principles of biomedical ethics, ed 4, New York, 1994, Oxford University Press.

Ethical Problems in Medicine and Biomedical and Behavioral Research, 1983) (Box 6-3). Consistent with the western view of autonomy, treatment options should promote the well-being of the individual according to that individual's understanding of well-being. When individuals lack the capacity to make choices for themselves, someone else must represent their particular values and preferences. Ethical decision making is a process with multiple contributors; it is a combination of the health

---

Box 6-2

Framework for Examining Ethical Conflicts

Questions to Consider:

1. What are the significant medical factors in the case?
2. What are the significant human factors in the case? (This may include relationships, contextual features, culture, religion, etc.)
3. What values/duties/rights are at stake for the individual? Are these values/duties/rights in conflict with others?
4. What is the ethical problem in this case? Which moral principles are in conflict?
5. What are the possible courses of action that could be pursued in this case? What are the potential consequences of each?
6. How do you weigh conflicts among the stakeholders' values, duties, rights, principles? Is it more important to preserve or protect some values, duties, rights, or principles than others? Justify your position.
7. Considering all of the above, what ought to be done in this case?
8. Prioritize the various courses of action.
9. What competing values might affect your willingness to take moral action?
10. What kinds of objections might be raised about your decision? How can you explain your decision in a way that addresses those objections?
11. Identify possible strategies for resolving the issue.

Adapted from Duckett et al, 1986.

Box 6-3

A Moral Framework for Decision Making

Beneficence
Balancing benefit and burden.

Respect for Persons
Informed consent.

Justice
Macro- and microallocation of resources. Individual vs society needs.

An ethic of care

---

provider's expertise on the available choices and the individual or surrogate's expertise on which choices best promote that individual's life goals and values. This decision-making process is also influenced by the family system, culture, religious and spiritual affiliations, and personal values and preferences (Grodin and Burton, 1988).

For children, ethical decision making is more complex because most lack the capacity to make informed, independent decisions. Children have not formulated the life goals and values upon which to base such decisions. Although the capac-

ity to be involved in decision making varies according to a child's level of maturity, it is generally assumed that children need surrogate decision makers (Committee on Bioethics, 1994). Decisions made on behalf of children lack a key feature of the moral framework for adults: an individual's unique assessment of his or her own well-being. Despite this, minors can be involved in meaningful ways in decisions about their own health care (see the section later in this chapter on respect for persons). The moral principles involved in adult decision making do, however, provide a valuable framework for making decisions on behalf of children (Committee on Bioethics, 1994).

Beneficence

The primary principles involved in decision making are beneficence (i.e., doing good) and its corollary nonmaleficence (i.e., avoiding or minimizing harm). Treatment options should include those that benefit the infant or child and clearly outweigh the associated burdens and harms. This "best-interest" standard is often used as a hallmark when making decisions for children; it establishes a presumption in favor of life because existence is usually required for other interests to be advanced. Generally, life should be saved when possible. When life cannot be saved or the chance of survival is minimal, however, burdensome treatment should not be provided (Levetown et al, 1994). Burdens for children with chronic conditions include repeated pain and suffering associated with invasive procedures, symptoms, or disability, as well as emotional distress caused by fear, immobilization, prolonged hospitalization, or isolation from family and friends. Decisions about a child whose chances of dying are great might reasonably focus on the comfort associated with dying instead of on therapies to prolong life.

An additional standard, the "relational potential" standard, has also been suggested as an adjunct to the "best interest" standard when balancing the benefits and burdens of various courses of action (McCormick, 1974). This standard focuses on the child's cognitive and intellectual capacities, the degree of neurologic impairment, the prognosis of reversing the neurologic condition, and whether the outcome of the condition can be altered through treatment or therapy. For example, infants or children who are permanently unconscious have no capacity to feel either pleasure or pain, so their "interests" are limited to prolonging biologic life. Because such children cannot be burdened in the usual sense and most of the reasons for treatment (e.g., better function, fewer symptoms, the opportunity for human relationships or greater opportunity to achieve life's goals) are gone, many would argue that treatment is not obligatory (Nelson et al, 1995). The Baby Doe regulations (PL 98-457, 1984), for example, regard permanent unconsciousness as a condition that does not require life-sustaining treatment; yet there are a wide range of views on the degree of neurologic impairment that justifies limiting or foregoing treatment.

The challenge for children, parents, and health care providers is to understand the unique meaning of the concepts of health, sickness, disability, suffering, care, and death for a child in a particular situation. The meaning that these concepts give to an individual's life is influenced by that individual's values, interests, aims, rights, and duties. A holistic understanding of a child's life, a recognition of important values that give direction to treatment decisions, and the tenor of the professional-client relationship evolve and change over time; therefore discovering the threshold for balancing benefits and burdens in a certain case may change as the child's condition changes. For example, the initial goals for a newborn with multiple congenital anomalies resulting in neurologic impairment and severe physical disability may be to understand the extent of the child's condition and to preserve life. In this instance, parents and professionals may agree to tolerate a high degree of burden to the child in order to diminish the uncertainty surrounding diagnosis and prognosis. However, 2 years later after the diagnosis and prognosis have been clarified, parents and professionals may have a different view of how much burden the child must tolerate to sustain life, especially when continued treatment will not alter the prognosis and may impose significant burdens.

Beneficence is promoted by helping the child and family construct a meaningful life by balancing the burdens of the condition with the positive dimensions of living. Beneficence is expressed by identifying individualized care outcomes that enhance the child's well-being (e.g., adequately managing symptoms, accommodating to limitations imposed by the chronic condition, and maximizing functional capacities). Therefore treatment interventions must be designed to contribute to the individualized goals that enhance quality of life and promote the child's sense of integrity despite the limitations related to the condition.

Parents and professionals must openly discuss the uncertainty in diagnosis and prognosis and explore the extent of certainty necessary for both parental and professional decision making. At times, the need for greater certainty of either parents or professionals may result in burdensome diagnostic evaluations that do not contribute to the child's well-being or outcome. Alternatively, parents may accept uncertainty when professionals are compelled to seek further evidence to support their recommendations. The dynamic nature of the condition's course may create special challenges for caregivers and parents. Ideally, a shared vision and a common understanding of the balance of benefit and burden that is acceptable for a certain child are created.

The introduction of experimental or innovative therapies for children with chronic conditions often raises ethical concerns. Primary care providers, children, and families must consider the balance of benefit and burden of experimental therapies. To address these challenging situations, parents and caregivers should engage in ongoing, open discussions about poorly tested therapies or experimental treatments. For example, when an innovative surgical procedure is considered for a young child with an orthopedic deformity, the health care provider must disclose the uncertainty surrounding its effectiveness.

Respect for Persons

A second principle involved in decision making is respect for persons. Respect for persons means respecting another person as sharing a common human destiny (Curtin, 1986). Adult decisions focus on the unique life goals and values of the individual out of respect for that individual and the integrity of each life. The uniquely human freedom of each person to create a meaningful life is highly valued. Even though children are neither autonomous nor self-determining, respect is still required because their lives also have unique meaning. To treat individuals with respect is to acknowledge and value who they are outside of a medical context, rather than to only treat them in accordance with how professional goals and values are advanced. Most children live in families that provide nurturance and care. The relationships that arise within families are inherently valuable to the well-being of children. To respect a child is to acknowledge the importance of the child's world and the relationships that are central to it. Unilateral decision making by health care professionals based solely on "medical indications" denies a child fullness of life and relationships that are also benefiting and sustaining.

A central problem associated with parental or other surrogate decisions is the inherent difficulty of judging the quality of a child's life and the benefits and burdens that are experienced. The child, family members, and health care providers may attach different meanings to the child's life. Although life is regarded as valuable, professionals and surrogate decision makers cannot consider the prolongation of life exclusively. Decisions need to benefit and respect the child as an individual but recognize that the child relies on the family for nurturance and physical care. The values that parents place on their parenting roles may make it difficult for them to separate the benefits and burdens of parenting a child with special needs from the benefits and burdens that the child experiences. These

decisions are even more complex for primary care providers as they attempt to discern what is best for the child in the context of the family. The choice of interventions can positively or negatively affect the comfort or ease with which a child lives.

Respect for others is enhanced and evidenced by nonjudgmental attitudes and behaviors. It is important to stress that being nonjudgmental does not mean relinquishing values or being blind or indifferent to personal principles. Instead, the goal is openness to different ways of viewing and acting upon personal commitments and life circumstances. An essential dimension of nonjudgmental behavior is not imposing personal judgments on others.

The standard of informed consent is derived from the principle of respect for persons. Autonomy (i.e., self-determination) is the central moral value expressed through the process of informed consent. Legally, informed consent requires disclosure, comprehension, and voluntary agreement or consent by the competent individual or surrogate. To every possible extent, relevant information about diagnosis and treatment—including a description of the nature and purpose of the treatment or procedure, the benefits and risks, the problems related to recovery, the likelihood of success, and alternative treatments—must be discussed with the surrogate and the child (Grodin and Glantz, 1994). The person giving consent (i.e., usually a parent) must be able to understand relevant information, to reason and deliberate according to his or her values and preferences and the perceived values and preferences of the child, as well as to communicate the choices to others. Finally, consent must be given voluntarily without coercion. The informed consent process must be evaluated as the child matures and altered as necessary to include the child's expressed decisions or concerns.

Justice

Justice pertains to fair and equal treatment of others. Therefore justice also refers to an individual's access to an adequate level of health care and the distribution of available health care resources. Caregivers promote the principle of justice by being fair in providing care and attending to children and their families. For example, the Code for

Nurses focus on delivery of care with respect for human dignity, which is not to be defined in terms of personal attributes, socioeconomic status, or the nature of an illness (American Nurses Association, 1985). This provision requires that a criterion (e.g., age, gender, wealth, religious beliefs, or social unacceptability) should not be a factor in deciding between individuals competing for the same treatment. This provision strives for genuine impartiality, equal respect for all persons, and refusal to create a hierarchy of individual worth. Prejudicial treatment on the basis of personal or other attributes is a violation of a moral norm and ideal precious to the nursing profession for generations.

Consistent with the ethical obligations of justice, children with chronic conditions are legally protected from discriminatory treatment by state and federal laws. Section 504 of the Rehabilitation Act of 1973 (PL 93-112) grants protection from discrimination based on disability, whereas the Individuals with Disabilities Education Act (IDEA) (PL 101-476) and its amendments (PL 105-17) guarantee access for children with disabilities to education by establishing a federal grant program to help states provide a free and appropriate public education to all children in need of special education (see Chapter 5). The Americans with Disabilities Act (ADA) (1990) gives civil rights protection to individuals with disabilities by guaranteeing equal opportunity to public accommodations, employment, transportation, state and local government services, and telecommunications. Such laws create important obligations for both parents and health care providers and must be considered within the ethical analysis of troubling cases.

Health policies for children with chronic conditions address some of the concerns encompassed in the principle of justice. These policies include strategies to avoid discrimination, stigmatization, and the exploitation of dependence. Strategies to support health insurance reform, delivery of family-centered service, access to employment and educational opportunities, as well as the community's role in supporting children and their families are consistent with a justice perspective.

Issues involving the just distribution of health care resources arise at two levels. The *macroallocation level* refers to the share of societal resources allocated to specific societal goods, such as health

care. Resources allocated to support the health, development, and education of children with chronic conditions are a reflection of society's values and willingness to recognize and address the unique circumstances and needs of these children. For example, proposed national health care reform legislation rarely includes habilitation-rehabilitation services for children. Furthermore, access to long-term care and other services (e.g., home nursing, some durable and nondurable equipment, and/or services for children without clear diagnoses) is usually limited. Eligibility is often restricted and based on income or physical, mental, or emotional disabilities. Additionally, by not establishing uniform eligibility requirements for Medicaid or the State Childrens Health Insurance programs (SCHIP) from state to state, children who depend on either of these insurance plans for support services and care in one state may not be able to obtain the same services if they move to another state. These issues reflect some of the challenges of devising a national health policy that supports the interests of children with chronic conditions.

Within health care, *macroallocation* refers to division of a resource (e.g., money) among various services (e.g., transplantation programs, critical care, or outpatient services) (Beauchamp and Childress, 1994). This issue is particularly relevant at the institutional level, where costs and priorities for allocating scarce resources are determined. In an era of cost containment and downsizing, institutions and programs providing specialized services to children with chronic conditions are particularly vulnerable. For example, providers may reason that the expenditures for specialized services for children with organ transplants consume a disproportionate share of the overall budget for pediatric care. They may conclude that more children can be helped if money is spent on preventive services. Such reasoning focuses on the consequences of actions by evaluating their utility based on how they can maximize the benefits and outcomes for the greatest number of children. Focusing on a single criterion such as utility may not account for other important moral values (e.g., protection of vulnerable populations or existing obligations toward those in the greatest need of services).

The term *microallocation* is applied at the individual level; these decisions involve determining the distribution of a specific resource. In general, the professional's main concern is for the individual, but the needs of others may impinge on an individual's care—especially during periods of shortages of human and material resources. Health care providers participate in microallocative decisions when determining which child needs the greatest amount of care, thereby limiting care to others perceived as less needy. Microallocation issues arise when resources are limited and there is not enough of a resource to provide for all who need it.

The ethical principles of beneficence and justice are central to issues of resource allocation and rationing. The principle of beneficence requires health care providers to help others and promote good. This principle is evident on two levels: the individual level and the societal level (Beauchamp and Childress, 1994). Each level includes different considerations about allocating limited resources. On the individual level, health care providers fulfill the duty of beneficence by allocating resources based on individual needs. Scarce resources are distributed to those with immediate needs without regard for the needs of other potential clients or the community at large. For example, when an infant is born with spina bifida, a cadre of medical, developmental, educational, and social resources are mobilized—regardless of socioeconomic status, cultural or religious heritage, or ability to pay. This initial commitment to provide equitable and fair services for all families may not be sustained. Cost constraints, lack of available resources, and accessibility of resources may limit services for some children as they mature.

Realizing beneficence at the societal level involves allocating resources based on the needs of society and considering the greatest good for the entire community—a utilitarian perspective. The focus shifts from crisis care and doing good for the individual to preventive care and actions that benefit society. This shift is particularly important for children with chronic conditions because greater emphasis on prevention may diminish the specialized services designed to meet their needs. As resources become scarce, difficult decisions must be made to balance the needs of individuals—especially those with chronic conditions—with the needs of society.

An Ethic of Care

Traditional ethical reasoning requires providers to ascertain the rights of the individual and weigh the ethical principles in order to resolve conflicting obligations. Applying ethical principles alone cannot resolve the clinical quandaries that arise during the care of a child with a chronic condition. The language and method used to analyze a particular case can either clarify or confound the situation. When the rights of children are held in opposition to the rights of their parents, for example, an adversarial tension can be established that may polarize discussion. In contrast, if it is recognized that most parents are motivated to promote their child's interests, such polarity may be avoided. Considering other aspects of the moral life (e.g., virtue and individual experience) may reduce adversarial tensions between the rights of children and their parents and allow for a more comprehensive appreciation of the attitudes, values, and moral commitments of decision makers within the context of family relationships. This perspective is often referred to as an ethic of care.

From the care perspective, the resolution of ethical quandaries is focused on the child's needs in the context of the family and the provider's corresponding responsibilities in the context of the provider-client relationship. Primary care providers can focus on the special circumstances and context of the specific situation in which moral action occurs instead of merely considering the individual's interests and preferences in isolation. That is, the uniqueness of individuals and the particular dynamics of their relationships are endorsed as essential components of moral decision making (Carse, 1991). Such a model supports efforts to help children and their families find unique meaning or purpose in living or dying and realize goals that promote a meaningful life or death.

From this vantage point, the values and expectations involved in certain roles and relationships are primary. Therefore being an advocate for a child with a chronic condition involves appreciating the relationships significant to the child and understanding how those relationships affect care. Children with chronic conditions develop an intricate web of relationships that support and sustain them throughout their lives. In keeping with a family-centered philosophy of care, families are viewed as essential partners in the treatment and care of a child. Professionals must recognize and respect these interconnections as central to the well-being of a child. A care perspective also emphasizes the interrelationships of the members of the health care team. Therefore it recognizes that nurses, physicians, and other care givers work collaboratively to advance the interests and goals of children with chronic conditions.

Ethical principles (e.g., beneficence, nonmaleficence, respect for persons, and justice) and an ethic of care provide a framework for approaching ethical questions that occur in clinical practice. It must also be acknowledged that although these are the most common, they may not be the only principles that are relevant to a particular case. The challenge for primary care providers is to discern how these and other principles can help illuminate the ethical issues and guide the resolution of competing obligations.

The Process of Decision Making

Shared Decision Making

Traditionally, a model of shared decision making is based on the assumption that decisions are shared between children (i.e., if capable), parents, and professionals. Treatment decisions must represent a combination of the individuals' expertise in order to select choices that best promote the life goals and values of the child. Parents do not have the expertise to act as surrogate health care professionals, and health care professionals cannot replace the expertise of parents. Shared decision making means that parents and professionals should agree about general treatment goals, but professionals should make decisions about which treatment modalities are necessary to advance the agreed-upon goals.

Endorsement of a model of shared decision making ideally means that parents and—if capable—children engage fully in the process by understanding the range of treatment possibilities and the consequences of each and sharing their goals, values, and aspirations in a meaningful way. Such a model goes beyond the legal requirements for disclosure, comprehension, and voluntary con-

sent (Gale and Franck, 1998). Although professionals theoretically embrace the ideal of shared decision making as the desired model of parent-professional decision making, it is rarely accomplished in reality (Gale and Franck, 1998).

The Role of Parents in Treatment Decision Making

Based on the moral framework of shared decision making described here, someone must represent the interests of the child. There is a strong presumption that parents should make judgments about the best interest of the child (Gale and Franck, 1998). Parents are appropriate surrogates because their strong bonds of affection and commitment are likely to yield the greatest concern for the well-being of their children. Parents are obligated to protect their children from harm and to do as much good for them as possible (Fletcher, 1983).

There is a direct connection between the well-being of parents and children; the identities of each are inextricably linked. For example, a woman who defines herself as a mother regards her own welfare partly in terms of the welfare of her child. Harm to the child constitutes personal harm to the mother. Such relationships are valuable to both parents and children, and society needs to limit its interference in this private realm (Caplan and Cohen, 1987). Furthermore, parents are identified as primary decision makers because of the importance of the family institution. Families play an essential role in maintaining the integrity of society. Children learn values of cooperation and commitment within the family context that can then be generalized to other members of society.

Parents must be involved in treatment decisions for their infants and children because there are lifelong consequences of these decisions. Parents will be responsible for the ongoing physical, emotional, medical, and financial care of the infant or child who survives with serious disabilities (Rushton and Glover, 1990; Savage, 1998) and will also live with the consequences of those decisions. Long after health care professionals have forgotten a case, the family will remember and have incorporated such momentous decisions into the fabric of their lives.

Limits of Parental Authority

Children are not only members of their immediate families but of the broader community, as well. A moral community shares an interest in the life and well-being of each member. There are certain community standards of best interest (e.g., preservation of life) that may override a family's interpretation of a child's best interest. Although there are compelling reasons to support the decision-making authority of parents, such authority is not absolute. The interests of the parents and the family must take a high priority but should not override the fundamental respect for the best interest of the infant or child (Doyal, Wilsher, 1994; Hastings Center Research Project on the Care of Imperiled Newborns, 1987).

Even when parents and professionals presume shared responsibility to promote the well-being of a child, there are times when parents should be disqualified as primary decision makers. This disqualification may be the result of incapacity or choosing a course of action that is clearly against the child's best interest (President's Commission, 1983). If a parent has a known psychiatric condition and is behaving irrationally or has a documented history of child abuse or neglect, the primary care provider may question parental capacity to advocate on behalf of the child. If there is a dispute about parental intentions or capacity to function as decision makers, it is incumbent that those who substitute another decision maker provide convincing evidence why the parents should be disqualified. For example, even though respect for religious beliefs is an important community value, so is the value of life. Although adults who are Jehovah's Witnesses can choose to forgo a lifesaving blood transfusion for themselves, they are often not permitted to make a similar decision for their children. Moreover, children are entitled to grow up and make independent assessments of their own religious beliefs.

In such circumstances health care providers must advocate for children and uphold the community standard of best interest. There will always be cases in which such assumptions are challenged; but these are likely to be few. Those who challenge parental motives and commitments must prove that parents should be disqualified as decision makers instead of having parents prove that their motives and commitments are authentic. Safeguards to protect the interests of children, families, and professionals will continue to be necessary and prudent (Rushton, 1994). Assessing when community standards should outweigh a family determination is extremely difficult.

Whether the disqualification of parents always requires court intervention is the source of much debate (Hastings Center, 1987; Mahowald, 1993; President's Commission, 1983). When parents are disqualified, a surrogate decision maker should know all relevant facts and be able to perceive and represent the feelings and interests of those involved. Surrogate decision makers should also be free of serious conflicts of interest that may bias a decision. A court-appointed guardian *ad litem* often serves as a surrogate decision maker.

The Role of Minors in Treatment Decision Making

Professionals who care for children and adolescents with chronic conditions are increasingly concerned about the role minors play in making decisions about their health care. Many adolescents experience catastrophic physical and mental problems associated with severe disabilities, malignancies, or cardiac, pulmonary, and hepatic organ disease without having the legal right to decide about their treatments.

As client advocates, primary care providers must be concerned with how to promote the interests of adolescents in decisions regarding their health care. The concerns of adolescents escalate when parents and primary care providers seem to disregard the adolescent's previously expressed preferences or embark on a course of treatment that is inconsistent with the adolescent's life goals and values. Many health professionals are questioning the adequacy of current decision-making models and searching for creative solutions, perhaps through the advent of advance directives for minors.

From a moral viewpoint, minors with decision-making capacities have a legitimate claim to be involved in decisions about their health care. This claim is based on a respect for persons that recognizes that adolescents and young adults can be self-determining and therefore should have a voice in their care and the extent of medical interventions provided. Such respect for them as individuals and members of families and society compels primary care providers to take their preferences seriously when treatment decisions are made. Moreover, adolescents' interpretations of the benefits and burdens of treatment should be considered.

The standards for determining the decision-making capacity of minors are the same as those for adults: (1) the ability to comprehend essential information about their diagnosis and prognosis, (2) the ability to reason about their choices in accordance with their values and life goals, and (3) the ability to make a voluntary informed decision, which includes being able to recognize the consequences of various courses of action (Midwest Bioethics Center Task Force, 1995; President's Commission, 1983). Based on our knowledge of conceptual development, most children do not reach this level of maturity until they are 11 or 12 years of age (Grisso and Vierling, 1978; White, 1994), although there is wide variation. These standards are straightforward, but applying them in clinical practice requires clinicians to be more skilled in systematically assessing and documenting the decision-making capacity of minors.

Despite the importance of self-determination and well-being in justifying the participation of minors in treatment decisions, there is another competing value at stake: the interests of parents in making decisions for their minor children. It has traditionally been assumed that minors require surrogates to make decisions for them. Parents are generally identified as the appropriate surrogates for their children and have been afforded considerable discretion in making treatment decisions. Currently, treatment decisions for adolescents are made through a joint determination by the physician and/or health care team and the parent or guardian for the child. Joint decisions to withhold or withdraw therapeutic interventions are difficult for both parents and health care providers to formulate. Parents may seek any possible intervention to prolong their child's life—regardless of the burden to be endured. Alternatively, they may wish to relieve their child's suffering by forgoing certain life-sustaining treatments. The physician and/or health care team and the parent or guardian may have a different agenda for either continuing or initiating

certain therapeutic interventions, or instead forgoing certain interventions. Yet both groups may interpret their decisions as being in the best interest of the child. Despite their assessments, neither group may truly understand the adolescent's perspective. In many cases, the adolescent may already understand the pain and consequences of the treatment options, including the finality of death. Unfortunately, parents and health care providers may be hesitant to consider adolescents as legitimate decision makers about medical treatment.

As the model of decision making enlarges to include a definitive role for minors with decision-making capacity, health care providers must recognize that such a departure will also challenge the traditional process of decision making and may create conflicts between minors and their parents. The potential for such moral and legal conflicts will necessitate the determination of a mechanism for resolving disputes.

Legal Viewpoint on the Role of Minors in Decision Making

The legal system has determined that adolescents in certain circumstances have specific rights and responsibilities associated with their decision-making capabilities for health care (Oberman, 1996). Emancipated minors are children under 18 years of age who are financially self-supporting and have renounced their parents' rights and responsibilities for caretaking (Black's Law Dictionary, 1990). Most states have legislation recognizing the rights and responsibilities of emancipated minors. Emancipation is rarely determined by the courts and is generally implied through factors such as marital status, pregnancy or parenthood, and financial self-sufficiency. Emancipated minors do not need parental consent for medical treatment and have rights similar to adults in refusing medical treatment (Oberman, 1996).

The courts have also classified some adolescents as mature minors in relation to their decision-making capacity for seeking and accepting health care interventions. Mature minors are at least 15 years of age and thought to have the capacity to understand the nature and risk of medical interventions. Adolescents classified as mature minors may consent to treatment that benefits them and does not involve any substantial risk (Oberman, 1996).

State statutes generally support a minor's (i.e., 14- to 17-year-old's) rights to consent to ordinary medical care. For example, some state statutes support the right of minors to consent to specific medical treatment (e.g., contraceptive therapies) without parental notification and consent; the right to consent to abortion, however, is complex and varied. The Omnibus Reconciliation Act of 1990, which is also called the Patient Self-Determination Act (PSDA) of 1990, supports the right of adults (i.e., at least 18 years old) admitted to health care facilities to accept or refuse medical treatment. This age limit is based on the belief that only adults have the capacity and the right to determine what should be done to their bodies—even if executing this right means implementing their right to die. It is crucial, however, that health care providers do not ignore the plight of thousands of adolescents (i.e., 12- to 17-year-olds) who face similar catastrophic and terminal conditions but are not given this legal right.

Although the PSDA was created for adults, the spirit of the PSDA provides an opportunity to examine the potential role of minors in their treatment decisions and ultimately their right to determine the circumstances of their death. It is likely that many young children and adolescents have the capacity to help make their own treatment decisions and determine what is in their best interest. There has been minimal guidance from the courts or from legislation on a minor's right to refuse life-saving medical care. In the few decisions that have been rendered, the application of the mature minor status was used to support the minor's decision-making capacity to refuse treatment and understand the consequences of this decision. Unfortunately, because there are minimal and vague legal guidelines available to support a minor's rights to refuse treatment, health care providers are reluctant to intervene and support the minor's decision to withhold treatment—especially if this opposes the parents' wishes.

Involving minors in decision making about treatment requires families and professionals to create a system that supports the participation of minors. Such a system must include comprehensive guidelines for assessment, intervention, and ongoing revision (McCabe et al, 1996).

Making Shared Decisions a Reality

Regardless of the child's age, the family's composition, or professionals' involvement, resolution of ethical concerns is supported by an authentic model of shared decision making that accommodates the diverse ways children and families choose to participate. To resolve ethical concerns, it is necessary to move beyond a procedural model of informed consent to an authentic partnership where parents, the child, and professionals create an alliance that promotes the child's interests. The foundation for this alliance is a mutual understanding of each other's aspirations and goals, perspectives on what makes life meaningful for the child, and concepts of benefit and burden. In addition, parents need to share their goals, values, and definition of being good parents; and professionals must share their uncertainties and boundaries of their professional responsibility.

Shared decision making requires a vision that results from collaboration and open, effective communication using language without technical terminology and jargon. One reason success in achieving shared decision making fails is that professionals may focus primarily on the decision itself, instead of on the process. Parents also may have difficulty separating emotions from facts. A revised model of shared decision making would focus more on the context of the situation—especially the relational dimensions, the parents' unique concept of good parenting, and the factors that mediate decision making—rather than on the decision itself.

Professionals must begin to appreciate the parents' perspective in decision making and not try to force them into a traditional, rational, stepwise model that is incongruent with their perspective. Therefore the goals of the parent-professional relationship, the outcomes of the process, and the process itself must be closely scrutinized. For example, if the goal of the relationship with families is to get them to see the world in the same way as the professional, then dissenting views cannot be articulated or respected. Parents should be engaged early in a variety of choices about their child's care, so that their involvement is not reserved for required consents for treatment or decisions about life-sustaining treatment. Parents need and want professionals to be partners in the care of their child—

regardless of the outcome—and want professionals to help them be good parents in the process. Therefore sharing in decision making must begin early in the management of the condition.

Authentic shared decision making does not mean that differences will not exist or that everyone will come to the same conclusion about when and how to advance the child's interests. Nor does it mean that all participants will have the same skills, abilities, or preferences. Shared decision making is a process in which differences are discussed, differing opinions are valued, and the quality of care ultimately provided to the child and family is enhanced.

Transition to Adulthood

In most states, people 18 years of age and older are legally responsible for giving or refusing consent for medical treatment. People with chronic conditions often continue to be treated by pediatric subspecialists into their 20s and 30s because children with these disorders (e.g., spina bifida) in the past did not survive into adulthood. Unfortunately, pediatric health care providers operate under a child-focused model of decision making and do not transition to an adult model when young adults are legally able and willing to serve as primary decision makers.

Many older adolescents and young adults demonstrate a sophisticated level of understanding of their conditions and treatment. Members of the health care team can honor the autonomy of older adolescents and young adults by preparing them to participate in decisions and acting upon their choices after the informed consent process (Committee on Bioethics, 1995; Rushton and Lynch, 1992; Weir and Peters, 1997). There are other older adolescents or young adults who—because of cognitive comorbidity or immaturity—do not have the capacity to make decisions. Although they may be legally competent because they have not been declared incompetent by the courts, their ability to reason may be legitimately questioned. An assessment of their decision-making capacity, specific to the decision, should be undertaken and documented. Traditionally, parents or guardians have retained decision-making authority in such circumstances. Clinicians must work to foster decision making within the family context. To avoid confusion, parents should be counseled to seek legal guardianship for adult sons or daughters who lack decision-making capacity. Unfortunately, the cost of doing so is prohibitive for some families. Persons who lack the capacity to make decisions (e.g., those with severe mental retardation) should be respectfully allowed to participate in the decision-making process. As with young children, every child should be afforded the opportunity to be prepared for medical interventions, to receive developmentally appropriate explanations, and to express preferences. The more important the decision in the life of the person, the greater the care in assessing that person's decision-making capacity pertinent to the specific decision. Health care providers must be familiar with their institution's policies on surrogate decision making for adults who lack decisional capacity.

Strategies for Ethical Decision Making

Increase Knowledge of Ethics, Laws, and Policies

Professionals can enhance their effectiveness in resolving ethical conflicts by seeking opportunities to enhance their knowledge of and skills in ethical analysis, as well as by identifying resources to assist them in resolving dilemmas. Furthermore, knowledge of legal, public, and professional policies is advantageous. In particular, primary care providers who care for children with chronic conditions should be aware of pertinent state statutes and case laws that may affect their health care. Primary care providers must be particularly aware of institutional policies on discontinuing life-sustaining treatment, if such policies exist, and participate in developing them if they do not. Institutional policies that permit information to be withheld from parents or effectively deny parental access to divergent medical opinions should also be examined and challenged.

Proactive Dialogue, Assessment, and Planning

Children with chronic conditions and their families often have a high level of personal interaction with primary care providers. Because many chronic conditions persist over a lifetime, there are many natural opportunities to examine, revise, or abandon various goals or dimensions of the treatment plan. With proactive planning, it is also possible and desirable to anticipate the ethical conflicts that accompany the treatment plan. Wharton and colleagues (1994) have developed a Child Health Advisory Plan, which is a clinical tool to assist parents and providers in engaging in a process to generate and support decisions that are in the child's best interest. Ongoing dialogue about these issues is essential for optimal planning and must not be reserved for crisis situations associated with acute episodes or illness, deteriorating conditions, or death.

Many children with chronic conditions and their families and providers will confront difficult decisions about treatment that will create significant moral tension. Questions about whether to use psychoactive medications to treat children with attention deficit hyperactivity disorder or to try an experimental protocol for treating cancer may arise. Such morally difficult decisions are best made when there is adequate time for education, discussion, and reflection. Therefore ethical issues should be anticipated, and discussions begun early.

Genetic Testing: Privacy and Confidentiality

As the Human Genome Project nears completion in the next decade, the use of genetic testing and—hopefully—successful techniques for preventing or curing genetic disorders will occur. It is likely that each person's entire genetic code will eventually be encrypted on a computer card that can be carried in a purse or wallet. By that time, thorny ethical and legal questions about informed consent and the privacy and confidentiality of genetic test results must be resolved.

In the meantime, technology has advanced to be able to identify many genetic disorders. Parents may be offered the opportunity to have genetic testing for themselves and their child in an attempt to diagnose their child's condition. When signs and symptoms indicate that a child may have a genetic disorder, the family may benefit by knowing the diagnosis, planning for the child's future needs, and

learning the probability of future children being affected. While parents may have an intense desire to discover their child's diagnosis, they may fear that their child will be stigmatized and discriminated against by insurance, school, and eventually employment. With the ever-changing financing system of health care, such parental fears may not be unfounded.

Federal legislation to prevent exclusion from health care coverage and discrimination in employment has been proposed, but it is not known if the final laws will be sufficient (Beckwith and Alper, 1998; Rothstein, 1998). Although the technique of obtaining a blood test or a buccal smear or performing a skin biopsy in the office may seem rather benign, the ramifications of the findings can have profound consequences on the child's and family's future. Primary care providers can guard the privacy and confidentiality of a child's medical information by developing and implementing institutional policies on informed consent for genetic testing, special disposition of test results, and special procedures for releasing medical records containing test results (i.e., to school, [Task Force on Confidential Student Health Information, 1999], insurers, and others). Many institutions currently have special procedures for tests (e.g., HIV) that protect a client from unwarranted disclosure of information. Presymptomatic genetic testing for adult-onset conditions (e.g., Huntington's disease or breast cancer) is not recommended for children (American Society of Human Genetics and American College of Medical Genetics, 1995). Until the thorny ethical and legal issues are resolved, clinicians working with children with chronic conditions and their families should stay abreast of genetic advances and applicable laws. Programs such as the Ethical, Legal, and Social Implications (ELSI, 1996) branch of the National Human Genome Research Institute provide leadership in this area (Box 6-4). Professional organizations may also provide information and advocacy on advances in genetics. Scanlon and Fibison (1995) offer guidance for providers in managing genetic information.

Strategies for Dealing with Conflict

Even when communication among children, parents, and professionals is optimal, conflicts arise. In fact, good communication may illuminate points of

---

Box 6-4

Selected Web Sites for Information on Ethics and Genetics

Alliance of Genetic Support Groups, Inc.
www.medhelp.org/geneticalliance/

*American Nurses Association**
www.nursingworld.org

American Society for Bioethics and Humanities
www.asbh.org

Center for Bioethics, University of Pennsylvania Medical Center
www.med.upenn.edu/~bioethic

Center for Clinical Ethics and Humanities in Health Care, University of Buffalo
wings.buffalo.edu/faculty/research/bioethics

Eubios Ethics Institute
www.biol.tsukuba.ac.jp/~macer/index.html

International Society of Nurses in Genetics (ISONG)
www.nursing.creighton.edu/isong

Kennedy Institute of Genetics, Georgetown University
adminweb.georgetown.edu/kennedy/

MacLean Center for Clinical Ethics at University of Chicago
CCME—mac4.bsd.uchicago.edu/ccme.html

Bioethics Online Service, Medical College of Wisconsin
www.mcw.edu/bioethics

National Bioethics Advisory Commission
bioethics.gov/cgi-bin/bioeth_counter.pl

National Library of Medicine
www.nlm.nih.gov/

National Reference Center for Bioethicsline
guweb.georgetown.edu/nrcbl/

*State nurses' association sites can be accessed here as well through the SNA Gateway.

---

real ethical dispute. Participants often prioritize values differently and employ different processes to reach morally defensible conclusions. Therefore activities that promote multidisciplinary sharing, analysis, and decision making in an atmosphere of openness, objectivity, and diversity can lead to more tolerance of others' views.

When moral disagreements occur, strategies for resolution include the following: (1) obtaining the most current factual information on points of controversy; (2) reaching a consensus about the language used for concepts or definitions; (3) agreeing on a framework of moral principles to guide discussions; and (4) engaging in a balanced discussion of the positive and negative aspects of a viewpoint.

Institutions can review difficult or disputed cases through institutional ethics committees and other means of efficiently accessing legal, governmental, and consultative services. An internal review process can serve several purposes, including: (1) verifying the facts of the case, (2) confirming the propriety of decisions, (3) resolving

disputes, or (4) making referrals to public agencies when appropriate. Institutional ethics committees are often consultants to staff and families experiencing ethical conflict. Multidisciplinary membership (i.e., including a parent) provides a broad representation of different viewpoints. In general, these committees are primarily consultative without any binding authority. The opportunity for uninvolved parties to assist in reviewing difficult cases, however, can provide constructive recommendations for resolution.

Mechanisms to resolve conflicts between minors and their parents must be developed as the process of involving minors in treatment decisions unfolds. Based on a model of family-centered care, mechanisms supporting individual self-determination within the context of the family system are necessary. Strategies will also be needed to support families as they allow their minor children to be more involved in decision making. Mechanisms for examining the decision-making patterns of families and the roles of children and parents in other types of decisions within the family are also necessary. Finally, strategies to prepare minors to participate in decisions about health care through community and/or school educational programs and as part of routine health care encounters are important prerequisites (McCabe et al, 1996; Weir and Peters, 1997).

Summary

The resolution of ethical conflicts requires that health care professionals recognize there is a moral problem, use a systematic process of moral reasoning, and take action. As a prerequisite to such analysis, primary care providers who care for children with chronic conditions and their families must examine their own values about the content and structure of treatment decisions. Such clarification is necessary to ensure that the ideal of authentic shared decision making becomes a reality.

References

American Association of School Health Task Force: Guidelines for protecting confidential records, The Association (in press).

American Nurses Association: Code for nurses with interpretive statements, Kansas City, 1985, The Association.

American Society of Human Genetics and American College of Medicine Genetics: Point to consider: ethical, legal, and psychosocial implications of genetic testing in children and adolescents, Am J Hum Genet, 57:1233-1241, 1995.

Americans with Disabilities Act of 1990, 42 USC 12101 et seq, 1990.

Beauchamp TL and Childress JF: Principles of biomedical ethics, ed 4, New York, 1994, Oxford University Press.

Beckwith J and Alper JS: Reconsidering genetic antidiscrimination legislation, J Law Med Ethics 26:205-210, 1998.

Black's law dictionary, ed 6, St Paul, 1990, West Publishing Co.

Caplan A and Cohen C: Ethics and the care of imperiled newborns: a report by the Hastings Center's research project on ethics and the care of imperiled newborns, Briarcliff Manor, NY, 1987, The Hastings Center.

Carse A: The voice of care: implications for bioethical education, J Med Philos 16:5-28, 1991.

Committee on Bioethics: Guidelines for forgoing life-sustaining medical treatment, Pediatrics 93(3):532-536, 1994.

Committee on Bioethics: Informed consent, parental permission, and assent in pediatric practice, Pediatrics 95:314-317, 1995.

Curtin L: The nurse as advocate: a philosophical foundation for nursing. In Chinn PI, editor: Ethical issues in nursing, Rockville, Md., 1986, Aspen Systems.

Doyal L and Wilsher D: Towards guidelines for withholding and withdrawing of life prolonging treatment in neonatal medicine, Arch Dis Child Fetal Neonatal Ed 70(1):F66-70, 1994.

Duchett et al: Ethics education project, 1986, Minneapolis, Univ. of Minnesota School of Nursing.

Ethical, Legal, and Social Interactions branch of the National Human Genome Research Institute: A review of the ethical, legal, and social implications research program and related activities: 1990-1995, 1996, Bethesda, Md., The Institute.

Fletcher JC: Ethics and trends in applied human genetics, Birth Defects 19(5):143-158, 1983.

Gale G and Franck LS: Neonatology: toward a standard of care for parents of infants in the neonatal intensive care unit, Crit Care Nurs 18(5):66-74, 1998.

Grisso T and Vierling L: Minors' consent to treatment: a developmental perspective, Professional Psychology 9:412-427, 1978.

Grodin M and Burton LA: Context and process in medical ethics: the contribution of family-systems theory, Family Systems Medicine 6:435-445, 1988.

Grodin M and Glantz LH: Children as research subjects: science, ethics and law, New York, 1994, Oxford University Press.

Hastings Center Research Project on the Care of Imperiled Newborns: Imperiled newborns: a report, Hastings Cent Rep 17(6):5-32, 1987.

Levetown MJ et al: Limitations and withdrawals of medical interventions in pediatric critical care, *JAMA,* 272(16):1271-1275, 1994.

Mahowald MB: Women and children in health care: an unequal majority, New York, 1993, Oxford University Press.

McCabe MA et al: Implications of the patient self-determination act: guidelines for involving adolescents in medical decision-making, J Adolesc Health 19(5):319-324, 1996.

McCormick R: To save or let die: the dilemma of modern medicine, JAMA 229(2):172-176, 1974.

Midwest Bioethics Center Task Force on Health Care Rights for Minors: Health care treatment decision-making guidelines for minors, Bioethics Forum 11(4):A1-A16, 1995.

Nelson LJ et al: Forgoing medically provided nutrition and hydration in pediatric patients, J Law, Med Ethics 23(1):33-46, 1995.

NIH-DOE Committee to evaluate the ethical, legal, and social implications program of the human genome project: Report of the joint NIH/DOE committee to evaluate the ethical, legal, and social implications program of the human genome project: 12 December 1996.

Oberman M: Minor rights and wrongs, J Law, Med Ethics 24(2):127-138, 1996.

Omnibus Reconciliation Act (Patient Self-Determination Act [PSDA]), Title IV, Section 4206, h12456-h12457, Congressional Record, October 26, 1990.

President's Commission for the Study of Ethical Problems in Medicine and Biomedical and Behavioral Research: Deciding to forgo life-sustaining treatment, Washington, DC, 1983, US Government Printing Office.

Public Law 93-112, Section 504 of the Rehabilitation Act of 1973, Washington, DC, 1973, US Government Printing Office.

Public Law 98-457, The Child Abuse Amendments 42 US Code, 101, Interpretative guidelines (45 CFR Part 1 1340.15 et eq.), Washington, DC, 1984, US Government Printing Office.

Public Law 101-476, Individuals with Disabilities Education Act (IDEA), Washington, DC, 1990, US Government Printing Office.

Rothstein MA: Genetic privacy and confidentiality: why they are so hard to protect, J Law, Med Ethics, 26:198-204, 1998.

Rushton CH: Ethical decision making: the role of parents, Capsules and Comments in Pediatric Nursing 1(2):1-10, 1994.

Rushton CH and Glover J: Involving parents in decisions to forgo life-sustaining treatment for critically ill infants and children, AACN Clin Issues Crit Care Nurs 1(1):206-214, 1990.

Rushton CH and Lynch MA: Dealing with advance directives for critically ill adolescents, Crit Care Nurse 12(5):31-37, 1992.

Savage TA: Children with severe and profound disabilities and the issue of social justice, Adv Pract Nurs Quart 4(2):53-58, 1998.

Scanlon C and Fibison W: Managing genetic information: implications for nursing practice, Washington, DC: American Nurses Association, 1995.

Task Force on Confidential Student Health Information: Guidelines for protecting confidential student health information: navigating a course through conflicting obligations, Kent, Ohio, 1999, American School Health Association.

Weir RF and Peters C: Affirming the decisions adolescents make about life and death, Hastings Cent Rep 22(6):29-40, 1997.

Wharton RH et al: Parental wishes regarding participation in critical health care planning for children with disabilities, Pediatr Res 35:47A, 1994 (abstract).

White BC: Competence to consent, Washington DC, 1994, Georgetown University Press.

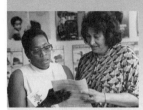

CHAPTER *7*

Financing Health Care for Children with Chronic Conditions

Judith A. Vessey

Sources of Funding

Today in the United States, care for children with chronic conditions is financed by complex methods that are generally categorized as follows: (1) private health insurance; (2) public programs (e.g., Medicaid, The State Children's Health Insurance Program [SCHIP], the Title V Program for Maternal and Child Health Services, and other federal and state categorical programs); (3) private, philanthropic sources; and (4) the family's own funds (Perrin, Shayne, and Bloom, 1993; Stein, 1997). A child's health care may be supported by one or a combination of these methods. The source of financial coverage depends on a number of factors, including the type of health condition, the family's socioeconomic status, the state and county of residence, the availability of a voluntary organization for the specific condition, and the availability of health care and legal personnel to advocate for the child's rights for specific sources of financial assistance.

Both private and public sources of funding for the general population have undergone and continue to undergo massive reforms to control costs of care while improving access to and quality of care. These reforms have had mixed results but are of particular interest to families and primary care providers of children with chronic conditions because they may be insensitive to the interests of children—especially those with chronic conditions (Garwick et al, 1998).

Major Financing Structures of Insurance

Fee-for-Service Plans

Historically, private and government insurance plans were *fee-for-service* (see Box 7-2 at the end of the chapter for definitions of italicized words) in design. Fee-for-service plans are insurance schemes that are separate from care-delivery systems and are determined by a variety of market forces, including custom, altruism, profit, and administrative costs. Three such examples are Blue Cross/Blue Shield, the major nonprofit associations; commercial health insurance offered by profit-making organizations; and traditional Medicaid. Benefits that are likely to be covered by fee-for-service plans are hospital room and board, miscellaneous hospital expenses, surgery, physicians' nonsurgical services rendered in a hospital, and outpatient diagnostic radiographic examination and laboratory expenses. Room and board in an extended care facility may be included when there is proof that continued medical—as opposed to custodial—care is required (Health Insurance Association of America [HIAA], 1994). Medicaid also covers a variety of ambulatory care and outpatient expenses, but such coverage is highly variable in private fee-for-service plans.

Managed Care Plans

Managed care is an integrated system of health insurance, financing, and service delivery functions that attempts to control and coordinate its enrolled members' use of health services in order to contain health expenditures, eliminate inappropriate care, and improve quality. In a managed care arrangement, the insured individual or family has access to selected providers who have agreed to furnish a defined set of health care services at a fee that is lower than usual. This is typically done through *prospective payment* and *capitation.* There are many types of managed care plans, including *health maintenance organizations (HMOs), preferred provider organizations (PPOs),* and *point-of-service (POS)* plans. There also are different models of HMOs such as: (1) the *staff model,* (2) the *group model,* (3) the *network model,* and (4) the *independent practice association (IPA).* Although services provided by managed care organizations (MCOs) are similar to those offered in fee-for-service plans, MCOs include preventive health services as a covered benefit because they have a strong financial incentive to keep their enrollees healthy.

In general, managed care plans operate by providing the insured with a list of providers enrolled with their plan. The insured chooses a primary care provider to go to for all routine care and encumbers little or no *out-of-pocket expenses.* To go outside the plan for care, the insured must pay a significantly higher share of the cost. The primary care provider may also suffer financially by referring the insured to more costly specialty services, especially those that are "out-of-plan." MCOs may restrict access to specialty health care in the interest of controlling overall health-plan costs. MCOs restrict access to pediatric specialty care by limiting referrals to selected specialty providers, requiring the family to bear a higher share of the total cost of out-of-plan services, and/or penalizing the primary care provider for referrals to specialists or subspecialists. In most capitation arrangements, the primary care provider is penalized by deducting the cost of specialty care from the overall profit of the plan or the fees paid to the provider, and either way of imposing restrictions may not be in the best interests of a child with a chronic condition. Because MCOs have limited lists of participating providers, the child's primary care provider or specialist may not be as knowledgeable about either the diagnosis or treatment of

rare conditions as a pediatrician or pediatric specialist. The child may be at further risk by not having easy access to approved ancillary health care services (e.g., physical therapy or in-home care) that may greatly enhance the quality of life for the child and family.

Managed care plans may use *service carve-outs* as a way of providing care to a historically difficult and expensive group of beneficiaries who are often referred to as *outliers.* Care for children with selected pediatric conditions, primarily those that are behavioral in nature, is handled under a separate managed health care contract that is often held by a different agency. Although carve-outs should theoretically provide higher levels of specialty care to populations formerly denied access to managed care (e.g., *population carve-outs*), they actually may further fragment care.

Parents of children with chronic conditions must carefully consider their health insurance options to choose the best coverage for their particular needs. Table 7-1 provides a guide for families to use in evaluating plans. Once the policy is obtained through employment or government agencies, attention must be given to filling out claims accurately and filing them promptly, working with a claims agent who understands the family's problems, and following up rejected claims with convincing evidence of the treatment or piece of equipment's importance to the child's well-being (Jones, 1985). The primary care provider can help the parents by supporting their legitimate insurance claims and completing the insurance forms accurately and on time.

Private Health Insurance

Private insurance remains the major method of financing health care in the United States, although small decreases in the percent of expenditures, as well as in the number of people covered, have been realized during the last decade. The role of private health insurance in paying the costs of care for children with chronic conditions is substantial but difficult to comprehend because of the variation in patterns of coverage and scope of benefits. Private health insurance is generally categorized by the method of reimbursement. Historically, most of

Table 7-1
Plan Features to Evaluate

Pediatric Services Covered	Extent of Coverage	In-Plan Cost Sharing	Out-of-Plan Cost Sharing
Pediatric Preventive Care Services			
Well child and adolescent visits, including developmental screening			
Immunizations			
Vision and hearing			
Dental care			
Health education			
Pediatric Primary and Other Services			
Physician services			
Hospital services			
Emergency services			
Surgical care			
Prescription medications			
Lab and radiographic services			
Pediatric Chronic Care Services			
Medical subspecialists and surgical specialty services			
Occupational, physical, speech, and respiratory therapy services			
Mental health and chemical dependency services			
Durable medical equipment, supplies and assistive technology devices			
Home health care			
Nutrition services and products			
Care coordination services			
Other			

Cost-Sharing Provisions and Catastrophic Protections	Amount
Annual premium	
Annual deductible	
Annual out-of-pocket cost limit	
Lifetime out-of-pocket cost limit	

Pediatric Provider Network Capacity	Yes	No
A. Are pediatricians included as primary care clinicians?		
B. Does the plan recruit physicians and other health professionals with expertise in the care of children with chronic conditions?		
C. Does the plan make exceptions to allow specialists to serve as primary care clinicians for certain children with complex conditions?		

From: Institute for Child Health Policy, Gainesville, Fla.; Website: http://www.ichp.edu/managed/materials/purchaser/pedserv.html.

Continued

Table 7-1
Plan Features to Evaluate—cont'd

Pediatric Services Covered	Extent of Coverage	In-Plan Cost Sharing	Out-of-Plan Cost Sharing

Pediatric Provider Network Capacity—cont'd

		Yes	No

D. Does the plan allow for shared management of children with chronic conditions between primary care physicians and subspecialists?

E. If the primary or specialty care provider of a child with a chronic condition is not in the plan's network, are exceptions made to reimburse the physician to ensure continuity of care?

F. Does the plan rely on pediatric—not adult—subspecialists to care for children with chronic conditions?

G. Does the plan have an up-to-date inventory that lists and describes pediatric professionals within the plan who are experts in the care of children with chronic conditions?

H. Does the plan include or contract with the following primary care pediatricians, pediatric medical subspecialists, and pediatric surgical specialists in the following areas? (If not, what alternative arrangements are used to ensure access to these pediatric subspecialists?)

    Adolescent medicine
    Allergy/immunology
    Anesthesiology
    Cardiology
    Child and adolescent psychiatry
    Critical care
    Dermatology
    Development/Behavioral medicine
    Emergency medicine
    Endocrinology
    Gastroenterology
    Genetics
    Hematology/Oncology
    Infectious disease
    Neonatology/Perinatology
    Nephrology
    Neurosurgery
    Ophthalmology
    Oral surgery
    Orthopedics
    Otolaryngology
    Pediatric surgery
    Plastic surgery

Table 7-1
Plan Features to Evaluate—cont'd

Pediatric Services Covered	Extent of Coverage	In-Plan Cost Sharing		Out-of-Plan Cost Sharing

Pediatric Provider Network Capacity—cont'd

		Yes	No	

Pulmonology
Radiology
Rheumatology
Urology
I. Does the plan include or contract with the following other pediatric specialty health professionals and facilities? (If not, what alternative arrangements are used to ensure access to these other pediatric specialty providers?)
    Nurses with pediatric expertise
    Child and adolescent psychologists
    Social workers with pediatric expertise
    Physical therapists with pediatric expertise
    Occupational therapists with pediatric expertise
    Speech therapists with pediatric expertise
    Respiratory therapists with pediatric expertise
    Home health providers with pediatric expertise
    Nutritionists with pediatric expertise
    Genetic screening and counseling services
    Care managers with pediatric expertise
    Dentists or orthodontists with pediatric expertise
    Hospitals and/or medical centers specializing in the care of children
J. Does the plan encourage coordination and integration of physical and mental health services for children with chronic conditions?
K. Does the plan include state-designated pediatric centers of care (e.g., perinatal, hemophilia, trauma, transplant care)?
L. Are multidisciplinary teams available for the care of children with chronic conditions through:
    Contracts with hospital outpatient departments that specialize in the care of children?
    Contracts with specialty pediatric clinics?
    Contracts with developmental centers?
    Other arrangements?
M. Do durable medical equipment vendors have the capacity to individualize and customize equipment for children?
N. Are the plan's utilization review and appeals processes performed by appropriate pediatric specialists and subspecialists?

these plans were fee-for-service, but over the last decade managed care has become the dominant organizational form (Ireys, Grason, and Guyer, 1996). A continuum of arrangements, varying by the onset of prepayment required and restriction to selected providers, are now available to consumers.

Fee-for-Service Plans

Despite the decreased availability of private fee-for-service arrangements, families of children with chronic conditions may prefer this type of coverage because there are few restrictions on choice of providers. In fee-for-service arrangements, the insured person usually pays a fee, or *deductible,* before insurance benefits are realized. The insured individual may also pay *coinsurance,* which is approximately 20% of physician, hospital, and other related fees. There is usually also a *stop-loss provision,* as well as a maximum lifetime benefit. Providers of care are reimbursed for services rendered based on schedules of usual and customary charges.

A study of private fee-for-service plans by Fox and Newacheck (1990) indicated that typical coverage included hospital care and physician services for diagnosis and treatment of illness or injury. Approximately 60% of plans covered some preventive services, and about 20% covered *case management.* Coverage was good for medical supplies and equipment, but other therapies (e.g., speech, occupational, or physical therapy) were less likely to be covered. Less than 10% of plans covered nutrition services. Long-term care was often covered with limitations placed on the number of in-home services or days of service. Home care was only approved if the care was tied to an immediately prior hospitalization. Of the plans surveyed, 69% had plans that included a comprehensive home-care benefit (i.e., including skilled nursing, home health aids, physical therapy, respiratory therapy, and medical social work). Mental health services also may be covered with limitations on the number of visits and the type of provider.

The problems faced by families who depend on fee-for-service private health insurance to finance care for a child with a chronic condition are evident by looking at the *exclusions* and limitations of the health care policies. The insurer usually does not pay for *preexisting conditions.* Thus if a family was not adequately covered before their child acquired the chronic condition, a fee-for-service plan will not often cover the medical expenses related to the chronic condition. Other common exclusions are payments for preventive health care, rehabilitation services and equipment, and expenses associated with the birth of an infant up to the first 30 days of life. Coverage for health needs defined as non-medical (e.g., special education, transportation to health care facilities, and home renovations needed to care for a child with a chronic condition) are rarely included in fee-for-service plans.

Separate from general health insurance policies are major medical expense policies that cover a broad range of catastrophic medical expenses. The cost of major medical insurance is controlled by sizable deductible fees and coinsurance fees for medical expenses that exceed the deductible. Maximum benefits are usually limited to $250,000 per person within a benefit period of 1 to 3 years, but there may be no limit to coverage within the benefit period (HIAA, 1994). Major medical plans are not necessarily advantageous for children with chronic conditions because their health care needs are likely to be long-term and repetitive and therefore do not fit into the designated structure (Jameson and Wehr, 1993).

Managed Care Plans

It is hard to evaluate the effectiveness of private managed care plans in providing care for children with chronic conditions because of their structural diversity and rapid evolution. The majority of MCOs, however, avoid *adverse selection* and do not actively enroll children with special needs or develop programs for them; service carve-outs are common (Ireys, Grason, and Guyer, 1996). Most plans do not actively restrict the enrollment of such children, but there is little incentive for them to do so.

Of the various types of private managed care plans, HMOs have the potential to provide more comprehensive services to children with chronic conditions because they may include: (1) comprehensive outpatient services including basic mental health care; (2) coverage for ancillary therapies; (3) home health services; (4) coverage for durable medical equipment, supplies, and prescription drugs; and (5) access to pediatricians and pediatric subspecialists, pediatric nurse practitioners, psychologists, nutritionists, and social service workers with expertise in various problems of living with a chronic condition (Fox, Wicks, and Newacheck, 1993). Other advantages are that preexisting conditions are generally not excluded, *co-payments* are small, and there may be no deductible or coinsurance provision.

Conversely, *gatekeeper* activities that restrict access to the best providers for a child's condition are a serious limitation of HMO plans. Moreover, a large number of services are excluded when a child goes out-of-plan, which may be very costly to the family. Out-of-pocket expenses can become a substantial burden, especially because many plans do not have a stop-loss provision (Fox, Wicks, and Newacheck, 1993). Although case management services are included, they are often ineffectual in providing higher quality care due to the other limitations.

Self-Insured Plans

Self-insured plans, whether they are fee-for-service or managed care, are not governed by the same laws as other private health insurance plans. They may offer even fewer benefits to children than other private insurance plans that are subject to the statutory and common law doctrines regulating insurance. Self-insured plans are governed by the Employee Retirement Income Security Act of 1974 *(ERISA),* which makes them exempt from state and federal insurance regulations and allows employers to establish, modify, and cancel employee medical benefits without state or federal interference (Jameson and Wehr, 1993). The children of employees on self-insured plans can be left without coverage for costly conditions, and their families have little legal recourse. ERISA protections are currently being challenged in a number of states.

Government Health Care Programs

There are public health care financing programs for individuals and families who do not have access to employer-based health insurance or cannot afford to purchase private insurance. These programs may be entirely supported by federal money or may be jointly administered and funded by the federal government and the states. States also may have revenue-sharing agreements with counties or other local health jurisdictions to provide financial coverage for health care through public revenue.

Those who do not have health insurance are not necessarily unemployed or living at or below the federal poverty level (FPL). In 1996, there were approximately 11 million uninsured children in the United States, although 90% of them lived in families with one working adult (Weigers, Weinick, and Cohen, 1998). Uninsured workers are usually employed in small businesses or are self-employed. Employed persons may lose health insurance if they or their family member acquires a chronic condition with high medical costs and the employer cancels the coverage. Employers also avoid the high cost of insuring their employees by relying on part-time workers or contracting work out to small firms, neither of which requires employers to offer insurance benefits. Undocumented residents are another group at risk for being uninsured. They may not wish to be identified as working in the United States and therefore may accept positions without health insurance coverage or other work-related benefits.

Medicaid

Medicaid (Title XIX of the Social Security Act) is a federal-state matching entitlement program that pays for medical assistance for selected needy populations. In 1996, Medicaid served approximately 18.7 million children, including 1.5 million with chronic conditions who comprise over 48% of the 36 million Medicaid recipients (US DHHS, HCFA, 1997a,b). Children's share of total Medicaid expenditures, however, is only $17.9 billion (i.e., approximately 15% of total expenditures). Medicaid is the largest public health care program in the United States and is administered by the Health Care Financing Administration (HCFA) within the US Department of Health and Human Services (US DHHS). It was established in 1965 and soon surpassed any other federally funded public health care program serving children. Medicaid guarantees eligible children a comprehensive package of health insurance benefits, which is generally more extensive than those of private insurance plans (Fox et al, 1997).

Medicaid programs vary among states. Within broad federal statutes and policies, each state: (1) establishes its own eligibility standards; (2) determines the scope of services; (3) sets payment rates; and (4) administers its own program. The complexity of Medicaid regulations accompanied by the state's latitude in designing programs has resulted in disparity among state plans. Eligibility for federal funds, however, requires states to provide Medicaid coverage for the following "categorically needy" groups: (1) children under 6 years of age and pregnant women whose family income is at or below 133% of the FPL; (2) children born before September 30, 1983 but under the age of 19 and with families with incomes at or below the FPL; (3) recipients of adoption assistance and foster care under Title IV-E of the Social Security Act; (4) Supplemental Security Income recipients (in most states); (5) pregnant women whose family income is below 133% of the FPL; and (6) special protected groups (i.e., typically individuals who lose their cash assistance due to increased work earnings or increased Social Security) for a limited period of time (US DHHS, HCFA, 1998a).

Prior to 1996, another group automatically eligible for Medicaid were those who met their state's requirements for Aid for Families with Dependent Children (AFDC), but the Temporary Assistance for Needy Families (TANF) program has replaced AFDC in all states. Although most persons covered by TANF will receive Medicaid, it is not required by federal law (US DHHS, HCFA, 1996a).

States have the option of providing Medicaid coverage to "categorically related" groups including but not limited to: (1) infants up to age 1 and pregnant women whose family income is no more than 185% of the FPL; (2) children under the age of 21 who meet their state's 1996 AFDC eligibility criteria; (3) children who are receiving care under home-and community-based waivers; (4) targeted low-income children covered under SCHIP (see section on SCHIP later in this chapter); and (5) medically needy persons (US DHHS, HCFA, 1998a). The medically needy program gives states the option to extend Medicaid eligibility to persons who would be eligible for Medicaid under other

criteria except that their income and/or resources are too high. Individuals may qualify immediately or may "spend-down" by incurring medical expenses that reduce their income to state-designated levels. If states choose to have a medically needy program, they must include services for medically needy children under age 19 and pregnant women. Legal resident aliens who entered the United States after August 22, 1996, are barred from receiving Medicaid for 5 years; the eligibility of other groups of legal resident aliens is an option left up to individual states (US DHHS, HCFA, 1998a).

It is very important that families of children with chronic conditions and their primary care providers are informed of the Medicaid service rights and entitlement programs of the state where the child resides. All states that receive funds from the Developmentally Disabled Assistance and Bill of Rights Act of 1978, the Protection and Advocacy for Mentally Ill Individuals Act of 1986, the Protection and Advocacy of Individual Rights Act of 1992, and the Technology-Related Assistance for Individuals with Disabilities Act of 1988 are required to have a protection and advocacy organization to inform persons with disabilities of their rights to payment for health care through Medicaid. Contact may be made through information from the local Medicaid office.

A full range of preventive-related and illness-related services are covered by Medicaid, including inpatient, outpatient, rural health clinic, and federally qualified health-center services; prenatal care; vaccines for children; physician, nurse practitioner, and midwife services; family planning services and supplies; laboratory and radiographic services; and skilled nursing services or home health care for those eligible. States also may choose to cover any of 34 other approved services, some of the more common of which are as follows: diagnostic services; rehabilitation and physical therapy services; optometrist services and eye glasses; prescribed medications and prosthetic devises; transportation; and facility services for the mentally retarded (US DHHS, HCFA, 1998a).

One program of particular importance to children is the Early Periodic Screening Diagnosis and Treatment Program (EPSDT), which is a preventive health program that was added to Medicaid in 1972 and amended in the 1989 Omnibus Budget

Reconciliation Act, PL 101-329 (1989). Although EPSDT enables children who are eligible for Medicaid to receive health screening, the 1989 revisions require states to establish standards for medical, vision, hearing, and dental screenings and further require services to be furnished at other than the medically necessary scheduled intervals to treat a suspected illness or condition. In addition, states must offer the necessary health services to correct or ameliorate a condition found in the EPSDT screen, whether or not such services are covered by the state plan.

Federal law (PL 101-329, 1989) further stipulates that children enrolled in Medicaid are entitled to case management, rehabilitative services, psychologic counseling, and recuperative and long-term residential care as deemed necessary by a primary care provider. States must now include in their Medicaid benefit package all ambulatory health care services offered to Medicaid beneficiaries receiving care in community and migrant health centers that are funded by the federal Public Health Services Act. The law also encourages the use of pediatric and family nurse practitioner services in rural health clinics by mandating states to cover their services as long as they are practicing within the scope of state law—regardless of whether they are supervised by or associated with a physician. Other provisions of Public Law 101-329 (1989) encourage the referral of mothers eligible for Medicaid and infants at nutritional risk to the Special Supplemental Food Program for Women, Infants, and Children (WIC), which is funded by the Department of Agriculture (US DHHS, HCFA, 1997a, b; 1998a).

In most states, eligibility for Medicaid for individuals and families is determined by the Department of Social Services in each county. Social workers in hospitals, public health, child welfare, and other human services agencies can help families with children with chronic conditions to determine if they are eligible for Medicaid coverage. Social workers can also help primary care providers to remain informed of health services that are covered by Medicaid. Receiving Medicaid coverage for health care does not preclude receiving assistance from other federal programs for services and equipment not covered by Medicaid.

Providers who are familiar with Medicaid law can advocate for families who may be denied services to which they are entitled. The provider should also know the local protection and advocacy staff and parent advocacy groups who stay abreast of issues regarding the various laws affecting both private and public health insurance plans and are able to protect the civil, legal, and service rights of children with chronic conditions.

Traditional Medicaid

Medicaid was originally fashioned along the same lines as private fee-for-service insurance and designed as a program of inclusion. That is, eligible families were able to seek care from any provider, and then Medicaid reimbursed willing providers at set rates for services rendered (Gurny, Baugh, and Reilly, 1992). There are nominal participation requirements, and each state oversees the statutes and regulations of provider participation (Stein, 1997).

During its first 25 years, Medicaid liberalized its criteria several times. The total number of children served increased as did the percent of medically needy children (i.e., from 6% to 11%) (Cartland, McManus, and Flint, 1993). For example, in order to meet the needs of children who are dependent on ventilators, parenteral nutrition, or other technologies that could not be discharged from the hospital without skilled nursing and other health services, the Medicaid Model Home and Community-Based Waiver was created. These services were initially authorized in 1981 in the Omnibus Budget Reconciliation Act, Section 2176 (PL 97-35). The purposes of the program are to reduce the cost of care to Medicaid that results from lengthy hospitalizations, as well as to avoid the unnecessary institutionalization of children by providing case management, homemaker services, home modifications, and other therapies.

Qualification for coverage and services for home care varies among states. States may remove parental income and assets as an eligibility consideration or may raise the Medicaid income standard. The eligible conditions may differ, and some states require that the child be discharged from an institution immediately before applying for the waiver (Leonard, Brust, and Choi, 1989). Primary care providers who wish to determine if this program is appropriate for a Medicaid-eligible or medically needy client and available in their state should request information from the state agency responsible for implementing the Medicaid program. The local protection and advocacy office (Protection and Advocacy, Inc., 1995) will also explain a family's rights to have a child cared for under home care Medicaid waiver programs and will help the family plead their case when a waiver is denied by the local Medicaid agency.

A major problem faced by traditional Medicaid programs is that provider reimbursement rates are often significantly lower than the prevailing rates in the community. In order to compensate for this, states may choose to reimburse obstetricians and pediatricians at rates that are higher than prevailing Medicaid rates. Such reimbursement would ideally enlist enough providers to serve eligible families and encourage them to accept these families into their practices and reduce visits to hospital emergency and/or outpatient departments for needed health care services (Cartland, McManus, and Flint, 1993). This provision met with limited success, however; states using a fee-for-service Medicaid structure also needed to address spiraling costs. In order to improve access and outcomes while reducing expenditures, states have begun adopting a managed care structure for administering Medicaid programs.

Medicaid Managed Care

As the costs of Medicaid rise, the majority of states are adopting certain strategies to conserve funds (US DHHS, HCFA, 1993). States are operating a variety of Medicaid demonstration programs under section 1115 waivers. This waiver program was designed by HCFA to allow states to develop innovative solutions to health and welfare problems and expand coverage to additional populations provided that they do not increase the proportion of federal spending (Holahan et al, 1995). States are using 1115 waivers to implement a variety of managed care plans for maternal-child health programs. To date, over 80% of states have 1115 waivers (US DHHS, HCFA, 1997 a,b).

These managed care plans are similar to the plans described earlier for private insurance. State Medicaid agencies sign service agreements with MCOs to provide Medicaid services. MCOs must operate against the backdrop of Medicaid and other relevant state and federal laws. The individual or family receiving Medicaid has access to selected MCOs and providers who have agreed to furnish a defined set of health care services using prospective capitated payment, which is paid by the state Medicaid agency. Unlike traditional Medicaid, recipients are generally separated from privately insured clients.

HCFA has provided guidelines for states to follow in designing and implementing managed care programs for persons with special needs (US DHHS, HCFA, 1998c). These nonmandatory guide lines request that states consider the following: (1) building understanding and support for the program from the grassroots level for value-based approaches to providing services; (2) adopting value-based purchasing strategies when buying specialized health services; (3) ensuring that enrollees with special needs can access provider networks offering quality services and expertise in a timely manner; (4) developing a systematic and objective evaluation scheme to measure the accountability of participating MCOs; (5) guaranteeing that the system of care can respond to the routine and unique medical and social needs of enrollees with special needs; and (6) selecting reimbursement strategies that adequately cover the costs of caring for these populations (US DHHS, HCFA, 1998c). Because Medicaid managed care is still relatively new, it is unclear if states will be able to successfully meet these objectives.

If the state plan is well-constructed, joining a managed care plan could benefit children with chronic conditions because a more comprehensive range of preventive health services and other therapies may be available and better coordinated than under the traditional Medicaid fee-for-service plan (Fox et al, 1997). There is evidence that some Medicaid managed care products restrict access to necessary specialty providers and services (Stein, 1997). The capitation rate may be too low to refer a child to pediatric specialty providers outside of the plan, and pediatric specialty providers and services may not be available within the plan. Benefit packages offered by HMOs contracted with Medicaid are generally less comprehensive than those under Medicaid fee-for-service plans because many optional services are eliminated (Fox et al, 1997; Fox, Wicks, and Newacheck, 1993). Prior authorization arrangements of these MCOs may be designed to restrict referrals to pediatric subspecialists and ancillary services, as well as to obtain durable medical equipment (Fox et al, 1997). As with private insurance MCOs, Medicaid-contracted MCOs have little incentive to establish link with community agencies (Lipson, 1997). Another problematic area is the relationship between Medicaid-contracted MCOs and the responsibility for and payment of health services provided to children with special needs by school districts under PL 101-476: IDEA (see Chapter 5). These MCOs also have little experience providing selected Medicaid-required services (e.g., transportation).

The Medicaid managed care programs of many states are in the earliest phases of implementation, so their ability to provide quality care for children with chronic conditions must be monitored in terms of quality, eligibility, cost efficacy, access to care, provider qualifications, and reimbursement levels (American Academy of Pediatrics, 1995; Newacheck et al, 1994; Perrin et al, 1994).

State Children's Health Insurance Programs (SCHIP or CHIP)

SCHIP (PL 105-100: Title XXI of the Social Security Act) enables states to expand insurance coverage to uninsured, low-income children through a program of matching funds. This program was included in the Balanced Budget Act of 1997 in response to the growing percentage of children without health insurance (US DHHS, 1997c). The increased number of uninsured children is due in part to legislative reform of AFDC, Medicaid, and SSI (Perrin, 1997). The goal of SCHIP is for states to provide health care coverage for all uninsured children in families with incomes below 200% of the FPL or 50% above their Medicaid eligibility level—whichever is higher.

SCHIP programs vary widely in structure and coverage because the federal government has given states considerable latitude to design their programs in accordance with their political and fiscal climates. All programs, however, provide assistance through the following broad mechanisms: (1) establishing or expanding a separate child health insurance program, (2) expanding the state's

Medicaid program, or (3) a combination of the two (PL 105-100, 1997). Medicaid expansion programs meet federal Medicaid program guidelines and benefits packages (see discussion earlier in this chapter). The federal government has established benchmarks for non-Medicaid–based programs that mirror those of health plans offered to state and/or federal employees (US DHHS, PL 105-100, 1997; HCFA, 1997c).

It is estimated that 16.9% of eligible children have a special health care need, so Title XXI legislation has wide-ranging implications for children with chronic conditions (Newacheck et al, 1998). The Maternal Child Health Policy Research Center has analyzed both the legislation and the state plans to assess how SCHIP will service children with special needs in terms of eligibility, benefits, plan design, and cost-sharing (Fox et al, 1998). They have found that the majority of states have retained the same eligibility thresholds for special needs children as for other eligible children, although states may adopt more liberal eligibility requirements for special needs children than for other enrollees (e.g., states may use the Social Security Administration's definition of "special needs" or choose a more inclusive definition). States then may choose to provide additional benefits to this population by selectively expanding the FPL (i.e., up to the designated maximum), using more liberal methodologies in determining the family's income, and/or shortening the designated period of uninsurance (Fox, Graham, and McManus, 1998).

Benefits offered by SCHIP plans may be inadequate for children with special needs. The benchmarks of the benefits set by federal legislation provide limited coverage for the many specialized services required by children with chronic conditions, which is reflected in the majority of non-Medicaid SCHIP programs. Limits are often imposed on services such as ancillary therapies, durable medical equipment, disposable supplies, home health care, and case management; although most programs provide coverage for basic primary care (Fox, Graham, and McManus, 1998). Mental health coverage is also highly variable, being expanded by some states and completely excluded by others. Despite these limitations, several states have adopted innovative approaches to augment available benefits for children with special needs under non-Medicaid plans. For example, some states are offering more comprehensive benefits packages or establishing linkages with other benefit packages, such as coordination with Title V services or other state and/or federal programs (Committee on Child Health Financing, 1998a; Fox, Graham, and McManus, 1998).

Plan arrangements for providing services vary widely. Medicaid-expansion plans mirror the fee-for-service or managed care arrangements of their state's Medicaid program. States with non-Medicaid plans have broad discretion in structuring the insurance plan using fee-for-service or capitation arrangements—with or without carve-outs for selected services. Establishing comprehensive health plans that specifically address these children's needs is another avenue that has been adopted. States may also establish separate requirements in the plan's structure to better address the needs of children with chronic conditions. For example, states enrolling children into MCOs may require participating MCOs to provide mechanisms to ensure that these children receive the necessary care required (e.g., providing access to pediatric specialty providers, allowing a specialist to be designated as the primary care provider, or guaranteeing out-of-plan access to specialty care). Despite these options, some state plans are silent on the issue of medical necessity. Measures of quality also vary dramatically among plans (Fox, Graham, and McManus, 1998).

State plans include a wide variety of cost-sharing requirements such as premiums, deductibles, co-payments, and/or coinsurance, although the level of cost-sharing is restricted in accordance with the family's income level. Because of the child's increased care needs, however, the level of cost-sharing required by families of children with chronic conditions is likely to be higher than the cost-sharing required by other families. In order to better meet the needs of children with chronic conditions, some states have made adjustments for this in their cost-sharing requirements for populations with special needs. Tracking SCHIP's 5% out-of-pocket limit may also be problematic for families because they are generally required to keep track of these expenditures and seek reimbursement. Despite these limitations, most states have designed plans with modest cost-sharing requirements for

children with special needs (Committee on Child Health Financing, 1998a; Fox, Graham, and McManus, 1998). Although most states have not structured their SCHIPs with special attention to the needs of children with chronic conditions, some have pursued innovative strategies in this area (Fox, Graham, and McManus, 1998). SCHIP is new, however, and changes in the enrollment eligibility, benefits, and structure of plans are likely. Because SCHIP is still evolving and each state's program is unique, practitioners are advised of the need to consult specific sources for their state.

Supplemental Security Income

The SSI program, which is Title XVI of the Social Security Act, was established by Congress in 1972 for aged, blind, and disabled adults and in 1976 for children under 16 years of age with disabilities. This program is based on the assumption that those with substantial disabilities and little income have increased costs of health care and daily living. Income support is provided to help recipients become as self-sufficient as possible within the limits of their disability. SSI does not pay directly for the health care costs of a child with a chronic condition, but its recipients are generally eligible to receive health care services through Medicaid (i.e., regardless of other state Medicaid eligibility requirements) and food stamps. It can be of great financial help to families to have their children with chronic conditions become eligible for SSI and thus receive Medicaid coverage for costly health care.

Eligible children are those who are U.S. citizens or nationals, have significant disabilities, and live in low-income households. Until 1990, children with disabilities were less likely than adults with disabilities to be eligible for SSI because children's impairments had to meet or equal those on a specified list of conditions designed for adults. This definition of disability for children seeking SSI was contested in the courts. On February 20, 1990, the Supreme Court upheld a lower court ruling that the policy for determining SSI eligibility for children was unfair and inconsistent with the statutory standards of comparable severity, and the regulations were changed. The definition of disability for children was again revisited in the 1996 Personal Responsibility and Work Opportunity Reconciliation Act (PL 104-193). The current definition is as follows: (1) a child must have a physical or mental condition that can be medically proven and results in marked and severe functional limitations; (2) the medically proven physical or mental condition(s) must last or be expected to last at least 12 months or expected to result in death; and (3) a child may not be considered disabled if he or she is working at a job that is considered substantial work (Social Security Administration [SSA] 1997). The law also changes the way certain pediatric developmental and behavioral problems are assessed. Today, the program limits its support to those children with severe developmental and behavioral problems (Doolittle, 1998; Perrin, 1997).

The child and adolescent SSI program continues to expand dramatically—from 297,00 enrollees in 1989 to 1,000,000 enrollees in 1996 (Kuhlthau et al, 1998; Perrin, et al, 1998). Despite the expansion of the program, selected children have lost their eligibility because of the new definition of disability adopted in 1996. They may, however, still be eligible for Medicaid. The eligibility requirements for SSI continue to be debated (Perrin, 1999).

The financial requirements for SSI eligibility are complex (SSA, 1999). The first requirement is that the applicant must be beneath the maximum income level. The amount of SSI paid to an individual and the administration of the program varies by state because states have the option of supplementing the payments. SSI rules allow families up to 200% of the FPL to enroll (Perrin et al, 1998). Twenty-eight states administer their own supplementary payments, and the recipients receive this payment separately from that of the federal program. Fifteen states elect to have the federal SSA issue the federal payment and the state supplement in one check; seven states offer no supplementation. Applications for SSI payments are made at district offices of the SSA, where supporting documentation on age, income, and assets is examined (SSA, 1999).

The second step in determining financial eligibility is to know the cash value of the applicant's resources, which for children involves determining the portions of the parents' income that are available to the child. The regulations must be carefully studied to understand how the amount of available income is calculated. In 1997, the maximum monthly federal SSI payment made to an individual in his or her own household with no other countable income was $484 (Perrin et al, 1998). Countable income, which is the amount of parental income determined to be available to the child or any income earned by the child, reduces this amount, and state supplements increase it.

Medicare's End-Stage Renal Disease Program

Medicare is authorized under Title XVIII of the Social Security Act. Children are generally not entitled to any health care benefits under Medicare because it provides health insurance protection for persons over 65 years of age and persons under age 65 who are collecting Social Security or Railroad Retirement Benefits. Children with end-stage renal disease, however, may be eligible to receive health care benefits to cover the costs of peritoneal dialysis or hemodialysis and related services in the hospital or home. This program is subject to change as Medicare moves towards adopting a managed care structure.

TRICARE: The Department of Defense Insurance Program

Traditionally, the Department of Defense provided health insurance to active duty personnel and their dependents, retirees, and other eligible individuals through the Civilian Health and Medical Program of the Uniformed Services (CHAMPUS). Military health care, however, has undergone significant reforms as the federal government responds to rising health care costs and the closing of military bases and hospitals. TRICARE is the new insurance plan offered by the Department of Defense. It provides coverage for essentially the same population as CHAMPUS, but is called TRICARE because it offers three managed care plans (US Department of Defense Military Health System, 1998).

The first option is TRICARE Prime, which is similar to an HMO. The majority of care comes from a military treatment facility and is augmented by the TRICARE contractor's preferred provider network. Provider choice is limited. Although there is no enrollment fee for active duty personnel and their families, others pay an annual fee. A primary care manager supervises and coordinates care, and appointments are guaranteed. There also is a point-of-service option. A small fee per visit to civilian providers will be assessed if the claimant is not from an active duty family (US Department of Defense Military Health System, 1998).

The second option is TRICARE Extra. In this preferred provider arrangement, participating individuals do not enroll but choose an authorized civilian network provider who agrees to accept a fee set by CHAMPUS. This option covers a discounted share of costs over TRICARE Standard (see next paragraph) if the client uses services within the network. This plan does not provide a primary care manager; provider choice is limited; and cost-sharing through deductibles and co-payment is required. To date, it is not universally available (US Department of Defense Military Health System, 1998).

The third option is TRICARE Standard, which is a fee-for-service option that is the same as the old CHAMPUS plan. This plan is widely available and allows an unrestricted choice of providers. There is no enrollment fee or primary care manager. Significant cost-sharing through deductibles and co-payments and balances for non-participating provider charges that exceed the insurance cap are imposed. The scope and structure of these three options vary as widely as their costs. Moreover, eligible individuals may seek additional coverage through TRICARE/CHAMPUS supplemental insurance policies (US Department of Defense Military Health System, 1998).

The effect of these plans on access to care for military dependents with chronic conditions is not yet known. Military organizations provide families of children with chronic conditions with information, financial assistance, and health care within the military community or through local community, state, and federal agencies. Health benefits advisors located on military bases facilitate access to both military and public programs in coordination with the multidisciplinary medical and social service support from the Army's Ex-

ceptional Family Member Program, the Air Force's Children Have Potential Program, and the Navy's Family Support Program. Eligible families with children with chronic conditions must choose the plan that best fits their needs after considering the issues of access to care, quality of care, overall out-of-pocket costs, other non-military insurance coverage, and the need for other services such as home care, durable medical equipment, drugs and supplies, or physical, occupational, or speech therapy.

Indian Health Service

The Indian Health Service (IHS) is an organization within the Public Health Service of the US Department of Health and Human Services. Its purpose is to ensure that a comprehensive health care delivery system is available to American Indians and natives of Alaska. Services include primary and tertiary care, rehabilitation services, health education, school-based services, mental health services, and other community and environmental health programs (US DHHS, INS, 1999). The IHS integrates health services delivered directly through IHS facilities with purchased Contract Health Services (CHS) from the private sector. CHS help pay for care when other sources (e.g., private insurance or SCHIP) are not available. Referrals for CHS funds are based on medical priorities and are not available in all instances.

The extent to which children with chronic conditions are well-served in this system depends on the staff at the local IHS unit's skill in determining the family's eligibility for third-party payment for health services, making appropriate referrals, and providing culturally sensitive counseling and education. The IHS interacts with other federal and state agencies and public and private institutions to develop ways to deliver health services, stimulate consumer participation, and apply resources. These resources include tribal-operated hospitals and health centers and rural and urban health programs that receive both state and federal funding and are subject to regulations of Medicaid, SCHIP, and private health care insurance (US DHHS, IHS, 1996a and b). Information on eligibility and the location and health care programs of the local IHS unit may be obtained from the IHS Headquarters in

Washington, DC, the Headquarters West in Albuquerque, or through one of 11 area service offices.

The Maternal and Child Health Block Grant: Title V

This federal-state program was established under Title V of the Social Security Act of 1935. The purpose of this block grant is to improve the health of mothers and children. It is administered by the Maternal Child Health Bureau (MCHB), which is a division of the Health Resources Service Administration (HRSA) of the US Department of Health and Human Services. The Maternal Child Health (MCH) Services Block Grant program has three categories: (1) formula block grants to all states and territories, (2) Special Projects of Regional and National Significance (SPRANS) Grants, and (3) Community Integrated Services (CIS) Grants. In order to meet its diverse mandate, it is organized into four divisions, two of which are of particular interest to primary care providers for children with special needs: the Division of Child, Adolescent, and Family Health, and the Division of Services for Children with Special Needs.

Title V legislation grew out of increased recognition at the turn of the century that the federal government should bear some responsibility for the well-being of mothers and children, and that federal assistance to state health departments would enable the states to provide needed services on the local level. MCHB's predecessor, the Children's Bureau, was established in 1912; and the Maternal and Infancy (The Sheppard-Towner) Act of 1920-1929 then set the precedents for federal assistance to states for services for pregnant women and for infants and children with disabilities or conditions that might lead to a disability. Although the Sheppard-Towner Act only survived briefly, states had the opportunity to establish a public health unit for mothers and children, improve birth registration, and increase public health nursing services. These positive experiences with federal support of state public health programs helped to lessen resistance to federal intervention in health care on the part of private practitioners of medicine and enabled passage of Title V (Lesser, 1985). Over time, expan-

sion in the number and variety of categorical services was realized (Stein, 1997).

In 1981, with passage of the Omnibus Reconciliation Act (PL 97-35), specific Title V programs were consolidated and continued as the MCH Services Block Grant. Control was returned to the states, and the federal government's role in organizing health services for mothers and children was diminished (Stein, 1997). The MCH Block Grant, as amended in 1989 (PL 101-329), continues the original purpose of the 1981 Act, but efforts of consolidation and state control eroded as congress began mandating categorical services as a requirement of funding. Provisions to strengthen connections between health services for mothers and children on Medicaid and its EPSDT program were included in these mandates. The 1989 MCH Block Grant legislation also specified connections between the infants' and children's immunization programs of the US Public Health Service, Centers for Disease Control (CDC); and the supplemental feeding program for low-income women, infants, and children (WIC) in the Department of Agriculture (US Code, 1989).

Today, the goals of the program are as follows:

1. Significantly reduce infant mortality;
2. Provide and ensure access to comprehensive perinatal care for women;
3. Provide and ensure access to preventive and primary child care services for children with and without special health care needs;
4. Increase the number of children appropriately immunized against disease;
5. Reduce adolescent pregnancy rates;
6. Prevent injury and violence; and
7. Meet nutritional and developmental needs of mothers, children, and families (US DHHS, HRSA, 1999).

Each state's share of the total allocation is based in part on the number of births and the percentage of the nation's low-income children residing in each state. A rural birth counts for twice as much as an urban birth, which is a concept that goes back to 1935 when children born in rural areas were more likely to be isolated from health services. Other determinants of a state's allocation are the amounts spent on Title V and other maternal and child health programs before 1981. The states are required to match each $4 of federal funds with $3 in cash or kind.

The MCH Block Grant also includes a program of discretionary grants that are financed by 15% of block grant funds for SPRANS. These discretionary programs are as follows:

- Maternal and Child Health (MCH) research.
- Training of health professionals for public health practice in MCH.
- Genetic disease testing, counseling, and information dissemination.
- Hemophilia diagnostic and treatment centers.
- Maternal and child health improvement projects.

States have some authority to prioritize how they will meet the goals of the program but are required to allocate 30% of Title V funds for children with special health care needs. No more than 10% of the state allocation may be spent on administrative costs.

MCH Block Grant Programs for Children with Special Health Care Needs

The program for children with special health care needs mandated by the Omnibus Reconciliation Act Title V legislation requires that federal funds and state matching funds be used to provide services for locating such children and providing medical, surgical, corrective, and other services, as well as establishing facilities for diagnosis and treatment for chronic conditions or conditions that may become chronic. States have different service delivery systems that are funded by this program. The delivery systems may provide services directly through program-funded clinics that are staffed by program providers, or they may be a source of reimbursement for services rendered in the private sector by medical specialists selected by the state program as qualified to offer services on a fee-for-service basis. Many states have elements of both systems (Ireys and Eichler, 1989).

In general, children likely to be eligible for care under this program have chronic conditions that are correctable (e.g., a range of orthopedic conditions, conditions requiring plastic or orthodontic reconstruction, eye and ear conditions that if untreated would lead to loss of vision or deafness, and other congenital anomalies that can be corrected or ameliorated with medical and surgical intervention). In addition to the eligible condition, most states require that the family income not exceed a specified amount. This amount varies according to family size and tends to be set at 100% to 200% of poverty. Another criterion for eligibility is often that the child's parents are legal residents of the county or state in which they apply for assistance. This makes some children of undocumented persons ineligible.

The covered benefits are as follows: (1) diagnostic services; (2) comprehensive treatment by the appropriate pediatric medical and surgical specialties, including nursing, social work, physical and other therapies; and (3) case management to enable the child and family to benefit from the multidisciplinary services. Case management includes the services of a professional who can evaluate the psychosocial needs of the family and approve authorized services and interpret them for the family. As states have received less money for this program, some case management has been taken over by persons trained on the job and supervised by the program administrator, nurse, or social work consultant. These persons are paid less than the health professionals but are able to approve authorized services and give advice on the location of such services. They generally do not provide other counseling.

Children with mental retardation, mental illness, and illnesses for which there is little curative or corrective intervention available are generally not eligible for this program. With the development of new therapies in recent years, however, some state programs have broadened the definition of a child with a chronic condition to include children with neoplasms, conditions of the nervous system, and endocrine and metabolic disorders. Primary care providers must continually update themselves on the conditions covered by the states in which they practice by consulting with the state office responsible for Title V programs. In most states, this office is located in the state health department but may be found in a university medical center, the state welfare department, or the state education department.

Genetic Services Program

Education, counseling, and medical referral for all genetic disorders mandated by Public Law 95-626,

Title XI of the Public Health Services Act 1978, are included in this program. The goal of this program is to establish genetic services as an integral component of comprehensive MCH services, particularly for underserved families. Emphasis is on helping states build an infrastructure for genetic services and integrate genetic services into managed care arenas, particularly for children with special needs (US DHHS, HRSA, 1998a). The program also supports the following: (1) the National Clearinghouse for Human Genetic Diseases for the collection and dissemination of informational materials; (2) a laboratory support program in hematology, cytogenetics, and biochemistry to develop laboratory standards, provide training, and conduct proficiency testing; and (3) a system to collect and analyze epidemiologic data on genetic disease.

There are no direct payments to families for genetic counseling, fetal diagnosis, and other services under this program. Clinics serving pregnant women and families of children with genetic diseases must seek third-party payment for their clients to be financially self-supporting. Screening programs for newborns exist in all states, but states differ in disorders screened. All states screen for phenylketonuria and hypothyroidism, but many states also screen for galactosemia and hemoglobinopathies. Other screening tests that may be offered are for maple syrup urine disease, homocystinuria, and biotinidase (Council of Regional Networks for Genetic Services [CORN], 1994).

Hemophilia Treatment Centers

The purposes of this program are to establish comprehensive hemophilia diagnostic and treatment centers for providing clinical services; training professional and paraprofessional personnel in research, diagnosis, social, and vocational counseling; and establishing comprehensive individual care plans for those affected with hemophilia. Once the center is established, third-party payment for services to individuals must be sought to enable the center to be financially solvent. Persons with hemophilia are represented by the National Hemophilia Foundation, which is a nationally coordinated health agency with local chapters to promote education and change the restrictive policies of third-party payment programs to better cover treatment (Hilgartner, Aledort, and Giardina, 1985).

Federal Programs for Individuals with Mental Retardation and Developmental Disabilities

Mental retardation is defined as significantly subaverage intellectual functioning with an IQ of 70 or below that exists concurrently with deficits in at least two areas of adaptive behavior and is manifested during the developmental period from birth to 18 years of age (Luckasson, 1992). The term *developmental disabilities* was introduced in the 1970s to enable children with cerebral palsy, epilepsy, autism, and learning disabilities to benefit from federal programs directed at children with mental retardation and other functional problems that inhibited their schooling, employment, and mobility in the community. By the 1980s the definition of developmental disabilities changed from the previous categories to a functional description. The new definition required a limitation in at least three of seven areas of major life activities: self-care, receptive and expressive language, learning, mobility, self-direction, capacity for independent living, and economic self-sufficiency (Braddock, 1987).

Third-party payment for preventive and illness care of children with mental retardation and developmental disabilities does not differ from that for other children with chronic conditions. Eligibility for private health insurance depends on parents' access to comprehensive health insurance through employment. Medicaid eligibility is determined on a state-by-state basis by household income in relation to the federal poverty guidelines and the Medicaid regulations. Eligibility for financial support of medical and surgical treatment through the MCH Block Grant, Title V, and Program for Children with Special Health Care Needs depends on family income, the state definition of an eligible condition, and access to other third-party payments of medical expenses.

The history of federal programs for individuals with mental retardation and developmental disabilities is reviewed by Braddock (1987) (Box 7-1). Care of children with such diagnoses was traditionally the responsibility of states and counties and voluntary associations. The programs for mothers and infants in Title V of the Social Security Act of 1935 were intended to prevent mental retardation, but the care and rehabilitation of these children were considered to be beyond the scope of Title V. Unless they have an eligible condition in addition to mental retardation, children with mental retardation have been excluded from these state programs

Funds for researching mental retardation, demonstrating services, and training personnel were provided by several congressional bills in the 1950s. In the early 1960s, President John F. Kennedy's panel on mental retardation contributed to the passage of Public Law 88-164, the Mental Retardation Facilities and Community Mental Health Centers Construction Act of 1963, thus beginning the modern era of the federal government's mental retardation and financial assistance programs. This law established research centers, a mental retardation branch at the National Institute of Child Health and Human Development, and 18 university-affiliated facilities for the provision of clinical services and training of personnel in the care of children with mental retardation.

Public Law 91-517, the Developmental Disabilities Services and Facilities Construction Act of 1970, extended services to individuals with cerebral palsy and epilepsy, as well as to those with mental retardation. To receive federal funds under this Act, states were required to establish developmental disabilities councils to promote coordinated planning and service delivery. Other significant legislation during this decade included the follow-

ing: (1) Public Law 92-603, the Social Security Amendments of 1972, which added Title XVI, Supplemental Security Income; (2) Public Law 92-223, the Social Security Amendments of 1971, which permitted the reimbursement for active treatment of those with developmental disabilities in intermediate care facilities (ICFs); (3) Section 504 of the Rehabilitation Act of 1973, which prohibited discrimination against individuals with developmental disabilities in any activity or place of employment receiving federal assistance; (4) Public Law 93-647, the Social Security Amendments of 1974, which consolidated social services grants to states under a new Title XX of the Social Security Act to provide them with funds to develop alternatives to institutional care; and (5) Public Laws 94-142, 99-457, and 101-476, Education for All Handicapped Children Act and its amendments, which ensure that children with developmental disabilities or any chronic illness would have access to public education in the least restrictive environment.

By the 1980s the definition of developmental disabilities required a limitation in at least three of seven areas, as previously described. The Omnibus Reconciliation Act of 1981 reduced federal funding of all social programs, and for several years there was no growth in developmental disabilities services. The Medicaid waiver program for home-based and community-based care, however, was included in the Omnibus Reconciliation Act to discourage the use of the more expensive intermediate care facilities.

In the area of civil rights legislation for all persons with disabilities—including those with mental retardation, the Americans with Disabilities Act, which was passed in 1990, extended federal protection in the private and public sectors in employment, transportation, public accommodations, and communication. This law required changes in physical plants to accommodate employees with disabilities; that buses, trains, subway cars, hotels, retail stores, and restaurants are accessible; and that ordinary telephones are equipped with telecommunications devices to enable hearing-impaired and voice-impaired persons to place and receive calls.

Given the complexity of both federal and state laws that govern the availability and accessibility of services for individuals with developmental disabilities, it is often difficult for families to know their rights in regard to treatment, education, and employment of a child with a developmental disability. Protection and Advocacy, Inc. provides advocacy and education for parents and primary providers who are determining the legal entitlements and service benefits for children with developmental and mental disabilities. *Rights Under the Lanterman Act* (Protection and Advocacy, 1994b) is an example of a manual written for parents that simply and concisely explains the service rights and entitlement programs for children and adults with developmental and mental disabilities in California. Other sources of information include social workers in agencies serving those with developmental disabilities, public health nurses in programs for children with special health care needs, teachers in special education programs in public schools, voluntary organizations for individuals with mental retardation and other diagnoses leading to developmental disabilities, and members of local developmental disabilities councils.

HIV/AIDS Bureau

This bureau, which is administered by HRSA, was formed in 1997 by consolidating Title IV programs for HIV Coordinated Services and Access to Research for Women, Infants, and Children with the Ryan White CARE Act, and AIDS Drug Assistance Program (ADAP) Titles I, II, III, and IV. Title IV programs focus on the development and operations of community-based primary health care and social service systems for children and women with HIV/AIDS. Funds are provided to communities for providing information and training, organizing and improve access to care, and linking clients to federally funded research. A new Adolescent Service Initiative seeks to identify and enroll teens into care (US DHHS, HRSA, 1998b).

Individuals with Disabilities Education Act

The Education for All Handicapped Children Act (PL 94-142, 1975) resulted from legal decisions establishing that children with disabilities had a constitutional right to a publicly funded education

in the least restrictive environment. This law and its amendments covered children aged 3 to 21 years. The Education for the Handicapped Amendments of 1986, Public Law 99-457, Part H, extended the benefits of Public Law 94-142 to handicapped children from birth to 2 years of age. This act designated funds for the development of a statewide comprehensive, coordinated, multidisciplinary interagency system to provide early intervention services. The Individuals with Disabilities Education Act (IDEA: PL 101-476) was passed in 1990.

IDEA defines disabled children as those who require special education and related services because they have a learning disability, mental retardation, emotional disturbance, or specified physical handicaps. Other services that must be provided if deemed necessary to the educational program are transportation, developmental, corrective, or other support services required for the child to benefit from education. These services may include speech and hearing therapy, psychologic services, physical and occupational therapy, recreation, counseling, social work, and nursing and medical services. Parents have the right to participate in planning their child's educational program and to appeal a school system's decision about their child's education. State education agencies are responsible for implementing the law. Programs supported by these laws are fully described in Chapter 5.

Future Trends in Financing Health Care for Children with Chronic Conditions

Families have four basic recommendations for improving services for their children with chronic conditions, as follows: (1) improving the quality of services; (2) decreasing barriers to services and programs; (3) improving the training that health care professionals, families, and members of the community receive about chronic conditions and their management; and (4) bettering the quality and availability of community-based services (Garwick et al, 1998). All of these recommendations are predicated on two factors: adequate financing and universality of care.

Unfortunately, accessing and financing children's health care—including care of children with chronic conditions—continues to become more fragmented. Less than two thirds of all children are covered by private health insurance, and this number continues to decline (Havens and Hannan, 1997). The presence or absence of health insurance is a powerful indicator of children's degree of access to care. Analyses suggest that the disparity in access between uninsured and insured children has worsened over the last decade (Newacheck et al, 1998), despite reform efforts of the way health care is organized, administered, financed, and delivered. The problems of accessing quality care are amplified in the pediatric special needs population.

All health insurance programs—public and private—are becoming increasingly complex as efforts are made to balance the quality and cost of care with access to services. New variations (e.g., capitating specialists, expanding carve-outs, and designating specialists as primary care providers) are being tested. Quality, comprehensive coverage by private health insurance companies has been a long-standing problem. The dilemma faced by health care providers and children's advocates is how to support the highest quality of pediatric care in a managed care environment.

In order to accomplish this objective, emphasis is placed on the development of *integrated service networks*. These organizations offer tremendous potential for meeting the special health care needs of children. Employers, insurance companies, and the government need to work toward more universal standards of eligibility and access, enhanced program consolidation and coordination, and improved continuity of care (Perrin, 1999).

Summary

Private and public programs and agencies for financing care for children with chronic conditions are examining ways to provide adequate health care while reducing the costs of care. The immediate future of health care for children with chronic conditions is marked by limitations in the choices of specialty providers and services. Primary care providers (i.e., both physicians and nurse practi-

tioners) will find that they are increasingly limited in their abilities to advocate for quality care for children in their case loads who have chronic conditions. Families will advocate for their children by joining together, becoming informed of their rights under the law, and using the legal system for access to care. Adding to the complexity of seeking health care for children with chronic conditions are the inequalities in implementing private and public health care programs among counties both within a state and among states. Access to private insurance is favorable for those who are steadily employed in large businesses or members of strong labor unions that can negotiate comprehensive benefit packages.

Primary care providers must be informed about how families of children with chronic conditions in their case loads are paying for care and about access to specialty services under the various payment plans so that families realize the benefits for which they are eligible. Referral for help in purchasing appropriate insurance or accessing a federal-state public benefit requires dedication and persistence on the part of the family and primary care provider and is crucial to implementing the care plan.

Useful References on Financial Coverage for Children with Chronic Conditions

Department of Health and Human Services Websites: www.mchb.hrsa.gov; www.hcfa.gov.medicaid; ww.hcfa.gov.init; www.ihs.gov

Griffiths B and Peterson RA: Families forward: health care resource guide for children with special health care needs, Madison, Wis., 1993, Center for Public Representation. For reprint permissions or ordering contact Publications Department, Center for Public Representation, 121 Pinckney St., Madison, Wis. 53703, or call 1-800-369-0388.

Kongstvedt PR: The managed health care handbook, ed 2, Gaithersburg, Md., 1993, Aspen Publishers, Inc.

Stein, REK: Health care for children. What's right, what's wrong, what's next, New York, 1997, United Hospital Fund of New York. For information write, Publications Program, United Hospital Fund, Empire State Building, 350 Fifth Avenue, 23rd Floor, New York, NY 10118-2399.

Box 7-2

Glossary of Italicized Words

Adverse selection: When a larger proportion of individuals with poorer health status enroll in specific plans or select specific options. Plans with a subpopulation of higher-than-average costs are adversely selected.

Capitation: A method of payment wherein a fixed amount per enrollee per month is paid to the provider to cover a specified set of services regardless of the actual services rendered.

Case management: A system of improving the quality of care while managing costs by monitoring and coordinating the delivery of health services to individuals with complex health problems.

Co-insurance: A method of cost-sharing in which the insurer and insured party share payment for an approved charge of covered services according to a predetermined specified ratio after payment of the deductible.

Co-payment: A method of cost-sharing in which the insured party pays part of the amount due on receiving services and the insurer pays the remaining portion.

Deductible: A method of cost sharing in which the insured party pays a predetermined amount with the insurance covering the balance.

ERISA: The Employee Retirement Income Security Act, which exempts self-insured health plans from state laws governing health insurance.

Exclusions: Populations or services that are not covered by an insurance plan.

Fee-for-Service: Plans in which the payer (i.e., either patients or insurers) agrees to pay the fee set by the provider after the service is provided.

Gatekeeper: An MCO employee who authorizes patient referrals for specialty care.

HEDIS: A standardized set of measures used in evaluating health plan performance.

Health Maintenance Organization (HMO): A managed care plan that integrates financing and delivery of a comprehensive set of health services to an enrolled population.

Group-Model HMO: An HMO that pays a medical group a negotiated, per capita rate that the group distributes among its providers, often as salary.

Independent Practice Association (IPA): An HMO that contracts with individual providers to provide services to enrollees as a negotiated per capita or fee-for-service rate. Providers may see other patients besides those enrolled in the HMO plan.

Network Model HMO: An HMO that contracts with several medical groups, often at a capitated rate.

Staff Model HMO: An HMO where providers practice solely as employees and provide services exclusively to HMO plan enrollees.

Integrated Service Networks (ISNs): Organizations that are accountable for the costs and outcomes associated with delivering a full continuum of health care services to a defined population. All necessary health services are provided for a fixed payment.

Out-of-Pocket Expense: Payments made by an individual for medical services, which may include direct payments to providers, deductibles, co-insurance, and for services not covered by the plan and/or charges in excess of the plan's limits.

Outliers: Cases with extremely long lengths of stay or extraordinarily high costs.

Point-of-Service Plan: A managed care plan that combines features of both prepaid and fee-for-service insurance. Enrollees decide whether to use network or non-network providers, generally with sizable co-payments for selecting the latter.

Population Carve-outs: A population carve-out provides health care to a designated population that is targeted or defined by a specific health condition.

Preexisting Condition Exclusion: A practice of some health insurers to deny coverage to individuals for a certain period for health conditions that already exist when coverage is initiated.

Preferred Provider Organizations (PPO): A health plan with a network of providers whose services are available to enrollees at lower cost than services of non-network providers.

Prospective Payment: A method of paying health care providers in which rates are established in advance. Providers are paid these rates regardless of the costs they actually incur.

Service Carve-outs: A set of specific services provided outside a mainstream plan.

Stop-Loss Provision: The amount that the enrollee must pay out-of-pocket in a calendar year before the plan pays 100% of further covered charge.

References

American Academy of Pediatrics: Medicaid managed care: can it work for children? Pediatrics 95(4):591-594, 1995.

Braddock D: Federal policy toward mental retardation and developmental disabilities, Baltimore, 1987, Paul H. Brookes.

Cartland JDC, McManus MA, Flint SS: A decade of Medicaid in perspective: what have been the effects on children, Pediatrics 91(2):287-295, 1993.

Committee on Child Health Financing: Implementation principles and strategies for title XXI (State Children's Health Insurance Program), Pediatrics 101(5):944-948, 1998a.

Committee on Child Health Financing: Principles of child health financing, Pediatrics 102:994-995, 1998b.

Council of Regional Networks for Genetic Services (CORN): National newborn screening report—1991, New York, July 1994, The Council of Regional Networks for Genetic Services.

Doolittle DK: Welfare reform: loss of supplemental security income (SSI) for children with disabilities, JSPN 3(1):33-44, 1998.

Fox HB and Newacheck PW: Private health insurance of chronically ill children, Pediatrics 85:50-57, 1990.

Fox HB, Wicks LB, and Newacheck PW: Health maintenance organizations and children with special health needs: a suitable match?, Am J Dis Child 147:546-552, 1993.

Fox HB et al: Medicaid managed care policies affecting children with disabilities: 1995 and 1996, Health Care Financing Review 18(4):23-36, 1997.

Fox HB, Graham RR, and McManus M: States' SCHIP policies and children with special health care needs, The Child Health Insurance Project. Maternal and Child Health Policy Research Center, 1998. Website: http://www.mchpolicy.org/issue4.html.

Garwick AW et al: Families' recommendations for improving services for children with chronic conditions, Arch Pediatr Adolesc Med 152:440-448, 1998.

Gurny P, Baugh DK, and Reilly TW: Payment, administration, and financing of the Medicaid program, Health Care Financing Review Suppl:285-301, 1992.

Havens DH and Hannan C: Children first: Expanding health insurance coverage for children, J Pediatr Health Care 11:85-88, 1997.

Health Insurance Association of America: Source book of health insurance data, ed 33, Washington, DC, 1994, Health Insurance Association of America.

Hilgartner MW, Aledort L, and Giardina PJV: Thalassemia and hemophilia. In Hobbs and Perrin, editors: Issues in the care of children with chronic illness, San Francisco, 1985, Jossey-Bass.

Holahan J et al: Insuring the poor through section 1115 Medicaid waivers, Health Aff 199-216, 1995.

Ireys HT, Grason HA, and Guyer B: Assuring quality of care for children with special needs in managed care organizations: roles for pediatricians, Pediatrics 98(2):178-185, 1996.

Ireys HT and Eichler RJ: Program priorities of crippled children's agencies: a survey, Public Health Rep 103:77-83, 1989.

Jameson E and Wehr E: Drafting national health care reform legislation to protect the health interests of children, Stanford Law and Policy Review 5(1):152-176, 1993.

Jones ML: Home care of the chronically ill or disabled child, New York, 1985, Harper & Row.

Kuhlthau K et al: High-expenditure children with supplemental security income, Pediatrics 102(3):610-615, 1998.

Leonard BJ, Brust JD, and Choi T: Providing access to home care for disabled children: Minnesota Medicaid Model Waiver Program, Public Health Rep 104:465-472, 1989.

Lesser AJ: The origin and development of maternal and child health programs in the United States, Am J Public Health 75:590-598, 1985.

Lipson DJ: Medicaid managed care and community providers: new partnerships, Health Aff 16(4):91-107, 1997.

Luckasson R, editor: Mental retardation: definition, classification and systems of support, ed 9, Washington, DC, 1992, American Association on Mental Retardation.

Newacheck PW et al: New estimates of children with special health care needs and implications for the State Children's Health Insurance Program, Washington, DC, 1998, Maternal and Child Health Policy Research Center.

Newacheck PW: Health insurance and access to primary care for children, New Engl J Med 338(8):513-519, 1998.

Newacheck PW et al: Children with chronic illness and Medicaid managed care, Pediatrics 93(3):497-500, 1994.

Perrin JM: Universality, inclusion, and continuity: implications for pediatrics, Pediatrics 103(4):859-863, 1999.

Perrin JM et al: State variations in supplemental security income enrollment for children and adolescents, Am J Public Health 88(6):928-931, 1998.

Perrin JM: The implications of welfare reform for developmental and behavioral pediatrics, J Dev Behav Pediatr 18(4):264-266, 1997.

Perrin JM et al: Health care reform and the special needs of children, Pediatrics 93(3):504-506, 1994.

Perrin JM, Shayne MW, and Bloom SR: Home and community care for chronically ill children, New York, 1993, Oxford University Press.

Protection and Advocacy, Inc: Rights under the Lanterman Act: service rights and entitlement programs affecting Californians with disabilities, revised ed, Sacramento, 1994, Protection and Advocacy, Inc.

Protection and Advocacy, Inc: Medi-Cal: service rights and entitlement programs affecting Californians with disabilities, Sacramento, 1995, Protection and Advocacy, Inc.

Public Law 88-164: The Mental Health Centers Construction Act of 1963.

Public Law 91-517: Developmental Disabilities Services and Facilities Construction Act of 1970.

Public Law 92-223: The Social Security Amendments of 1971.

Public Law 92-603: The Social Security Amendments of 1972.

Public Law 93-647: The Social Security Amendments of 1974.

Public Law 94-142: Education for all Handicapped Children Act, 1975.

Public Law 95-626: Title XI of the Public Health Services Act of 1978.

Public Law 97-35: Omnibus Budget Reconciliation Act of 1981, Section 2176.

Public Law 99-457: Education of the Handicapped Children Act, 1986.

Public Law 101-329: Omnibus Budget Reconciliation Act of 1989, Section 6403.

Public Law 101-476: Individuals with Disabilities Education Act, 1990.

Public Law 105-100: State Children's Health Insurance Program, Section 4901, 1997, HCFA.

Section 504 of the Rehabilitation Act of 1973.

Social Security Administration: A desktop guide to SSI eligibility requirements, Pub No 05-11001, 1999; Website: http://www.socialsecurity.gov/pubs/11001.html.

Social Security Administration: The definition of disability for children, Pub No 05-11053, 1997; Website: http://www.socialsecurity.gov/pubs/11053.html.

Social Security Administration: Annual statistical supplement to the social security bulletin, Washington, DC, 1994, US Government Printing Office.

Stein REK: Health care for children: what's right, what's wrong, what's next, New York, 1997, United Hospital Fund.

US Code: Congressional and administrative news, 1st Session, Public Laws, St. Paul, Minn., 1989, West Publishing.

US Department of Defense Military Health System: The history of champus and its evolving role in tricare, 1998; Website: http://www.tricare.osd.mil/factsheets/historyoftricare.htm.

US Department of Health and Human Services, Health Care Finance Administration: Fact sheet #1: link between Medicaid and temporary assistance for needy families, 1996a, Website: http://www.hcfa.gov.medicaid/wrfs1.htm.

US Department of Health and Human Services, Health Care Finance Administration: Fact sheet #2: link between Medicaid and SSI coverage of children under welfare reform, 1996b; Website: http://www.hcfa.gov.medicaid/wrfs2.htm.

US Department of Health and Human Services, Health Care Finance Administration: HCFA statistics: Populations, 1997a; Website: http://www.hcfa.gov.stats/hstats96/blustats.htm.

US Department of Health and Human Services, Health Care Finance Administration: National summary of Medicaid managed care programs and enrollment, 1997b; Website: http://www.hcfa.gov.medicaid/trends97.htm.

US Department of Health and Human Services, Health Care Finance Administration: State Children's Health Insurance Program, 1997c; Website: http://www.hcfa.gov/init/cht21new.htm.

US Department of Health and Human Services, Health Care Finance Administration: Brief summaries of Medicare and Medicaid, 1998a; Website: http://www.hcfa.gov/medicare/ormedmed.htm.

US Department of Health and Human Services, Health Care Finance Administration: Chapter 1—managed care, 1998b; Website: http://www.hcfa.gov/regs/subt_h.htm.

US Department of Health and Human Services, Health Care Finance Administration: Key approaches to the use of managed care systems for persons with special health care need, 1998c; Website: http://www.hcfa.gov/medicaid/smd%2Dsnpf.htm.

US Department of Health and Human Services, Health Resources and Services Administration: Genetic services program, 1998b; Website: http://www.mchb.hrsa.gov/genetics.htm.

US Department of Health and Human Services, Health Resources and Services Administration: Fact sheets: HIV/AIDS bureau, 1998c; Website: http://www.hrsa.gov/hab/OC/factsheet/hab.htm.

US Department of Health and Human Services, Health Resources and Services Administration: Maternal and child health bureau—overview, 1999; Website: http://www.mchb.hrsa.gov/overview.htm.

US Department of Health and Human Services, Indian Health Services: Regional differences in Indian health, Washington, DC, 1993, US Government Printing Office.

US Department of Health and Human Services, Indian Health Service: Comprehensive health care program for American Indians and Alaska Natives, 1999; Website: http://www.ihs.gov.

US Department of Health and Human Services, Health Care Financing Administration: National summary of state medicaid managed care programs, Baltimore, 1993, Medicaid Bureau, US DHHS.

Weigers ME, Weinick RM, and Cohen JW: Millions of American children still lack health insurance and face barriers to care, AHCPR 214:11-12, 1998.

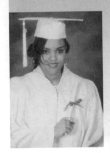

CHAPTER 8

Transitions to Adulthood

Kathleen J. Sawin, Ann W. Cox, and Stephanie G. Metzger

Transition planning for adolescents with chronic conditions is a much more prevalent issue for primary care providers than it has been in the past (Johnson, 1996). The life expectancy for youth with chronic conditions has dramatically increased in the last 20 years. Today more than 2 million young people between the ages of 10 and 18 years (i.e., 3.8% of our population) have some functional limitation due to chronic and disabling conditions, which is a 100% increase since 1960 (Blum and Garber, 1992; Newacheck and Halfon, 1998). Therefore more than a million young Americans with chronic conditions or disabilities will have transitioned to young adulthood by the year 2000.

An expanded Civil Rights Movement has demanded equal life options for individuals with disabilities and chronic conditions (Table 8-1). The most influential event in this movement has been the adoption of the Americans with Disabilities Act (ADA) of 1990. This act was designed to ensure that persons with disabilities have the same rights as those without disabilities: specifically, the right to a free public education and access to public transportation, clinics, restaurants, stores, and recreational facilities. The right to live in the community and hold a job are hallmarks of the ADA. The thrust of the legislation was to "normalize" life for persons with a disability. Discrimination against those with disabilities or chronic conditions in school, health care, or community living is prohibited. These changes make the concept of purposeful planned transition a priority for primary care providers (Johnson, 1996).

Outcome data suggest that youth with disabilities are not making the transition to a full adult life in the areas of education, employment, development of meaningful relationships, and independent community living. In a comprehensive longitudinal study of students with and without chronic conditions, school dropout rates for students with chronic conditions in ninth grade were greater than for their unaffected peers—a rate almost doubled in tenth grade and continued at an alarming rate even in twelfth grade (Pledgie, Tao, and Freed, 1998). Twenty percent of people with disabilities do not graduate from high school compared with only 9% of those without disabilities (NOD, 1998). Of those with disabilites who finished high school, the college graduation rates are less than half (Betz, 1998a). Unemployment rates of youth and adults with chronic conditions are reported to be from 50% to 71%, and the general population rates are currently 3% to 5%. Native American youth with chronic conditions have an even more difficult time with less than 30% employed or living independently (Schafer and Rangasamy, 1995). Of those unemployed with chronic conditions, 72% indicate that they would prefer to work. In addition, 34% of adults with disabilities have household incomes of $15,000 or less compared with only 12% of those without disabilities (1998, NOD), and many young adults with disabilities do not live independently after high school (Pledie, Tao, and Freed, 1998; USGAO, 1996).

Youth with disabilities are also at greater risk for acquiring other compromising behavioral morbidities. For instance, there is a higher than average prevalence of depression and attempted suicide with this population, reflecting the social isolation experienced by many youth with disabilities (Sawin et al, 1999). Substance abuse rates among persons with disabilities may be twice as high as those for the general population (Edelman, 1995) again with a disproportionate rate in minority communities (Schafer and Rangasamy, 1995). These co-morbidity outcomes make it more difficult to obtain an independent and fulfilling adult life.

Unsuccessful transition to adult life has become a concern to health professionals, educators,

Table 8-1
Recent Legislation Affecting the Transition to Adulthood for Youths with Chronic Conditions

American with Disabilities Act of 1990	Prohibits discrimination against persons with disability in employment, public accommodations, and public services.
Rehabilitation Act—1992 and 1998 Amendments of the 1973 Act	Strengthens the focus on employment for youths with disabilities, expanded eligibility criteria, and expanded customer choice.
Section 504 of Rehabilitation Act	Prohibits discrimination for those with disabilities by any program or agency receiving federal funds. Mandates equal opportunity to participate in or receive services from programs or activities and requires accommodations necessary to participate.
Individuals with Disabilities Education Act Amendments (IDEA) of 1997 (PL 105-17)	Modified earlier transition planning requirements by lowering the age that schools must initiate transition planning and services to 14 years
Carl D. Perkins Vocational and Applied Technology Education Act Amendments of 1997 (PL 104-134)	Helps provide vocational and/or technical education programs and services to youths and adults. Funds go to local education agencies and postsecondary institutions to provide educational opportunities for students with disabilities.
School to Work Opportunities Act of 1994 with 1998 amendments (PL 103-239)	Support to build high school learning systems to prepare students for further education and careers.
Title XIX of the Social Security Act Medicaid Amendments Home and Community-based Services Waiver (PL 97-35), 1990	Provides funds to support community services that enhance community living options.
Community Supported Living Arrangements (CSLA) (PL 101-508), 1990	Promotes development of statewide systems of individual supported living.
Supplemental Security Income (SSI) and Social Security Disability Insurance (SSDI)	Provides income benefits for youths (over 18 years of age) with substantial disabilities and low income. Parental income is not considered. Usually provides Medicaid benefits.

and community activists, and barriers to optimal transition have been identified. The ultimate goal of transition planning is to provide comprehensive health, education, and vocational services that are seamless, coordinated, developmentally appropriate, and psychosocially sound (Blum, 1995). The educational community and health care providers, directed by the 1997 revision to the Individuals with Disabilities Education Act (IDEA), have begun to initiate transitional planning for youth with chronic conditions during middle school. All of the assessment and counseling interactions—both formal and informal—need to focus on developing skills in adolescents that enhance competency, autonomy, and responsibility, which are all necessary to make transition successful (Blum, 1995). Attainment of competency requires time for maturation and training and therefore must begin early and build over time. The primary care provider has a

significant role to play in the purposeful endeavor of transition.

Adolescence: A Universal Time of Change

The central developmental task during adolescence is achieving a sense of personal identity based on adaptation to a new physical, cognitive, and social self (Orr, 1998). Youth with chronic conditions and disabilities confront obstacles similar to those experienced by all adolescents living and growing up in our complex and pluralistic society, but they encounter additional challenges associated with the demands and restrictions of their conditions. Primary health care providers must be aware of both the typical and condition-based challenges encountered by youth with a chronic illness or disability in order to effectively support their need for autonomy as they transition into adulthood.

Adolescence is one of the most fascinating and complex periods of transitions in an individual's life. It is a time of accelerated growth and change second only to infancy, as well as expanding horizons, self discovery, and emerging independence. This metamorphosis from childhood to adulthood can extend a full decade and in many ways encompasses a series of multiple transitions from early to late adolescence.

All adolescents, including youth with chronic conditions or disability, must meet the same fundamental requirements if they are to grow up to be healthy, constructive adults. The Carnegie Council on Adolescent Development (1995, pp. 10-11) summarizes these competencies as follows:

- Finding a valued place in a constructive group;
- Learning how to form close, durable human relationships;
- Feeling a sense of worth as a person;
- Achieving a reliable basis for making informed choices;
- Knowing how to use the available support systems;
- Expressing constructive curiosity and exploratory behavior;
- Finding ways of being useful to others; and
- Believing in a promising future with real opportunities.

While striving toward these outcomes, youth experience an array of interconnected challenges that are related to the following: (1) the biological changes of puberty that result in reproductive capacity and new social roles, (2) the movement toward psychologic and physical independence from parents, and (3) the search for friendship and belonging among peers.

Today's youth are growing up in a climate marked by dramatic changes in American families; less time spent with adults; changing work expectations; earlier reproductive capacity but later marriage and financial independence; dominance of electronic media; and a more diverse, pluralistic society (Carnegie Council on Adolescent Develop-

ment, 1995). The result is that a series of new morbidities plague adolescents: higher rates of suicide, depression, reported abuse (Schoen et al, 1997), earlier experimentation with drugs (Lynch and Bonnie, 1994), earlier sexual activity (Alan Guttmacher Institute, 1994), inadequate learning (National Center for Education Statistics, 1994), and more health-damaging behavior (Johnson, O'Malley, and Bachman, 1995). Today, younger adolescents exhibit many of the risky behaviors that were once associated with middle and late adolescence.

Youth with chronic conditions or disability find that the integration of their chronic condition or disability with their self-identify only reinforces a sense of being "different" at a time when "sameness" is desired. Further, the physiologic changes of maturation may influence the actual management of a chronic condition (e.g., in diabetes or asthma), and social role expectations may be inconsistent with cognitive ability (e.g., with mental retardation). The challenges of puberty, autonomy, personal identity, sexuality, education, and vocational choices may all be influenced by physical or mental abilities, pain, medical setbacks, forced dependence, and perceived prognosis (Blum et al, 1993). Key developmental parameters of early and mid-to-late adolescence are provided in Table 8-2, along with the associated implications of chronic conditions or disability. These implications are generic in nature because specificities of conditions are addressed in subsequent chapters. The heterogeneity of youth with chronic conditions or disabilities implies that primary providers must take the time to know the individual's and family's uniqueness.

Understanding Transition

Clinicians and researchers studying transition (Bridges, 1994; Cowan and Hetherington, 1991; Schumacher and Meleis, 1994; Selder, 1989) propose that transition is a process—not an event. Bridges (1994, p. 5) defines it as "the psychological process people go through to come to terms with the new situation. Change is external, transition is internal." For life changes to be described as transitional, they must involve both a qualitative internal shift (i.e., how people understand and feel about themselves and the world) and an exter-

Table 8-2

Key Developmental Parameters and Associated Implications of Chronic Conditions

Adolescent Developmental Stage	Typical Developmental Parameters	Chronic Illness/Disability Implications
Early Adolescence (generally 11 to 14 years of age)	***Rapid physical growth***—particularly sensitive to their changing bodies. ***Sexual maturation***—initiation of the biologic changes of puberty; new social roles reinforced. ***Relationships***—shift from family to peer groups as source of security and status; intense need to belong to a group, usually of the same sex. ***Cognitive***—generally remain in concrete operational thought. ***Self-concept/esteem***—described in terms of physical features and likes; less tolerant of deviations from the "norm." ***Health issues***—nutrition, acne, smoking, alcohol consumption; homicide from firearms has more than doubled in this age group; increase in reported victims of child abuse and neglect. ***Career awareness***—typically begin thinking about the future.	Certain developmental and disease conditions can alter rate of physical growth. Primary providers need to address these with youth and their families. In some conditions sexual maturation is early and menstruation is accelerated by several years. Anticipate interaction of sex hormones with other medication and counsel accordingly. Education regarding emerging sexuality and consequences of resultant choices is essential. Social isolation is a critical issue. Encourage group peer activities at and away from home. Teens are eager for information about their development and need accurate information about chronic conditions or disabilities—especially implications for sexuality and fertility. Respectfully deal with their many questions and concerns. At risk for some health consequences. Reported to have higher risk for victimization due to desire to "fit in." Career awareness activities are often overlooked by youths with disabilities. Have high and realistic expectations and communicate these.
Middle-Late Adolescence (generally 15-21 years of age)	***Physical growth***—continued physical growth but at a slower rate; strength and endurance increase. ***Sexuality***—sexual maturation and/or experimentation heightened; sexual development typically completed by 16 years of age; intimate sexual relationships develop. ***Relationships***—achieving psychologic independence from parents becomes particularly important; peer relationships become central. Although family relationships are changing, they remain important. ***Cognitive skills***—rapid growth and increasingly comprehend abstractions; movement into formal operational and abstract thinking.	Physical activity may be limited by certain conditions or disabilities; alternate means of physical activity must be provided. Information on risks associated with sexual activity is needed. Contraception explored, and implications of interactions with other medications are provided. If sexual maturation is delayed, this must be addressed with adolescent. In many settings, because of age and/or physical development, appropriate social skills are expected. Even individuals who are developmentally and/or cognitively disabled must be taught appropriate public behavior.

Continued

Table 8-2
Key Developmental Parameters and Associated Implications of Chronic Conditions—cont'd

Adolescent Developmental Stage	Typical Developmental Parameters	Chronic Illness/Disability Implications
Middle-Late Adolescence (generally 15-21 years of age)—cont'd	*Self-concept/esteem*—increasing individuation with some diminishing of peer influence; self is defined by including interpersonal traits and abstract categories. *Health issues*—experimentation with alcohol, cigarettes, and illicit drugs increases. Unintentional injury, homicide, and suicide are leading causes of morbidity and mortality. Exposure and/or participation in violence may arise. Females report higher incidence of depression than males. *Career*—planning emphasizes examination of own interests, aptitude abilities, and occupational aptitudes.	Youth vary in their ability to assume independence activities due to skills, cognition, or the complexity of the condition, but every effort should be made to foster choice in decisions related to health condition. Address strengths and encourage positive self-concept. There are some particularly dangerous interactions between prescribed medications and other drugs and substances. Additional nutritional education is particularly relevant because youth with limited mobility can be overweight and experience resultant complications. Abuse and victimization is higher in youth with disabilities than nondisabled peers. Emphasis should be on developing self-sufficiency skills, vocational and career decisions, and future planning. Active transition planning in health care, employment, and independent living must begin.

nal visibility of this change reflected in a reorganization of personal competence and roles and/or relationships with significant others (Cowan and Hetherington, 1991). Bridges (1994) describes stages of transition, proposing that the starting point for a transition is the ending one must make to leave the old situation behind and indicates that even good transitions begin with "having to let go of something." After "letting go," individuals enter into a "neutral zone" where the work of transition, creativity, renewal, and development occurs. This neutral zone between the old sense of identity and the new sense of self, however, is a place of some anxiety, uncertainty and confusion. As individuals successfully transition, new beginnings are created.

A review of the transition literature from 1986 to 1992 identified the following four categories of transitions: (1) developmental, (2) situational,

(3) health and/or illness, and (4) organizational (Schumacher and Meleis, 1994). In addition, this review delineated the process and outcome of transition as a powerful determinant of an enhanced sense of subjective well-being, role mastery, and the well-being of relationships, which enables the individual to function with increased confidence and skill in future challenges (Schumacher and Meleis, 1994; Younger, 1991).

Adolescents with chronic conditions enter into developmental, health and/or illness, and potentially situational transitions. Primary care providers are in an excellent position to assess the factors associated with the quality of the transition experience and intervene with adolescents and families to optimize outcomes. To do this effectively, primary care providers need to understand the family and individual factors that can moderate the transitional process.

Family Factors that Moderate Transition

The family is a constant factor in all transition endeavors working to prepare youth to consider options, set goals, develop the skills to work with service agencies and bureaucracies, find and use community support services and solve problems to shape their lives and environments (Hallum, 1995). Primary care providers have an opportunity to facilitate parent practices to reduce stress in the family and facilitate independence in youth.

The adolescent transitional years are stressful for all parents—but especially for those whose dependents have severe disabilities. According to Hallum (1995), families whose adolescents do not become as independent as expected report high levels of stress. The transition to independent living may be delayed by several years for youth with severe disabilities. In such situations, families must advocate for their adolescents to achieve supported living arrangements. Families with youth who have severe physical or cognitive limitations and who plan to remain in the family home face increasing responsibility as school eligibility terminates and family members' daily care responsibilities increase. Often resources to employ other caregivers are limited in the community (Hallum, 1995). These families need support and resource information to connect them with independent living centers and other community programs that offer alternative options and respite care. Families of youth who need continual supervision also must consider developing plans for custody and financial arrangements to ensure ongoing supervision when parents die or are unable to provide care. Medicaid-financed homes and daycare programs for adults with disabilities are scarce, so many parents must continue to care for their adult children at home. Advocates for people with mental retardation have recently filed class action suits to require states to provide housing and daycare services to these people or risk losing state Medicare funding (Associated Press, 1999).

In a qualitative study, young adults with disabilities reported several family themes associated with effective transitions (Powers, Singer, and Todis 1996). These successful young adults indicated that their families did the following: (1) treated them as typical children and adolescents, (2) expected them to participate fully in family responsibilities, (3) gave them nonpreferential treatment, (4) facilitated their participation in leisure activities, (5) focused on their strengths, (6) discussed their disability with them, and (7) assisted them in accommodating challenges. These young adults valued family experiences and discussions that allowed them to develop skills, participate in risk taking, and cope with social rejection. These youth perceived that their family was a safe and nurturing environment where competence was developed.

Providers need to assess family knowledge and family behaviors that facilitate the development of competence. Primary care providers working with families of youth with chronic conditions should begin to talk to parents about strategies that foster effective transition into adulthood when the affected child is still young. Many parents of children with chronic or disabling conditions have difficulty "letting go" and encouraging independence and may see their children as vulnerable. Early discussions on the importance of fostering autonomous decision-making skills and independence in the activities of daily living may help parents realize the importance of assisting their child to build the necessary skills for a successful transition into adulthood.

Factors Moderating Individual Transition

Cognitive ability, personal philosophy of self-competence, ability to solve problems, degree of autonomy, and peer relationships are all factors that influence an adolescent's ease and success in the transition to adulthood.

Cognitive Ability

Cognition plays a major role in transition planning. Self-sufficiency assumes the cognitive abilities necessary to carry out the education, employment, and management of health care and community living (Sawin et al, 1999). An adolescent's developmental abilities and age need to be considered in individual planning. If cognition is moderately or significantly impaired, families or advocates must increase their participation in the planning and implementation of the transition plan (Sawin et al, 1999). Many people with significant cognitive disabilities, however, can be competent, self-determined individuals (Wehmeyer, 1996). Achieving this goal may require individual skill building, alteration of the environment and interaction patterns, and use of available supports. Youth with cognitive disabilities must be afforded the basic rights that accompany the belief that all people are worthy of respect and dignity (Wehmeyer, 1996).

At the age of 18 all youth obtain the legal right to make decisions about life activities. When cognition is impaired, legal guardianship of a young adult should be considered and pursued by family members. Once the age of majority is reached, medical, school, and financial information, as well as consent to treatment, is not accessible to others without the youth's or guardian's permission. It is important to be clear about access to information and consent of the individual, family, school, primary care provider, and other agencies involved. Youth can determine access to information unless a court finds otherwise. Issues of information sharing should be openly discussed with youth and their families; a plan should be created as youth near the age of 18 years (Sawin et al, 1999).

Self-Competence

All transition programs are built on the assumption that youth are being educated to develop self-competence. Self-competence is thought to be a function of two domains: skills or efficacy and a sense of well being (Powers, Singer, and Sowers, 1996), and comprises self-determination, self-advocacy, assertiveness, coping, and self-esteem. Activities, experiences, and programs should be designed to develop self-competence and each of its components.

Problem Solving and Autonomy

Studies of youth with chronic conditions have identified that problem solving and autonomy skills are related to positive health outcomes (Blum et al, 1991; Johnson, 1996; Sawin and Marshall 1992). Interestingly, many youth with disabilities have limited experience making basic life decisions, much less decisions about health care (Hallum, 1995; Johnson 1996; Sawin, Metzger, and Pellock, 1996). Knowledge about health care, the specific chronic condition, and experience in making decisions are prerequisites for making decisions about health. By practicing decision-making in other ar-

eas (e.g., what clothes to purchase, how to wear your hair, what to do with friends, or how to budget money), youth will gain confidence through experience (Hallum, 1995). Without these basic decision making skills, choices related to health care are not possible. Because all problem solving is context based, experience is essential to solving potential health care dilemmas. Simple choices (e.g., whether to take medication with applesauce or jello) should be given as early as developmentally possible so that gradual movement to making all choices about health care management is made (Sawin et al, 1999).

Specific interventions to enhance autonomy through skill development have been described by practitioners at the University of Virginia, who developed an autonomy project based around an "interpretive interview" and "teaching physical" that focused on teaching youth about the effects of their condition (Hostler et al, 1989). Evaluations indicated that significant gains in knowledge and autonomy were achieved with this interactive approach. A second approach was developed by the Spina Bifida Association of Kentucky. The Transition to Independence Project developed a series of workbooks for youth and their parents that focused on youth making more decisions and taking charge. The program curriculum is well-developed and could be useful for the development of school-based systematic transition programs (Denniston and Enlow, 1995; Hardin, 1995a and 1995b). HealthPACT, which was developed at the University of Colorado Office of School Health, is a prototypic consumer-oriented, health-education program that prepares youth to communicate with health professionals and actively participate in their care (Igoe, 1994). This program also prepares providers for shared decision making. A fourth program, TAKE CHARGE, is designed to systematically promote self-determination and functional competence by reducing learned helplessness and promoting motivation and self-efficacy expectations. This comprehensive program has components of skill development, the role of mentors, and peer and parental support. Recent qualitative and quantitative evaluations support the effectiveness of this program to promote self-determination (Powers et al, 1996).

Few research projects have examined the effect of interventions targeting enhanced autonomy of youth with chronic conditions in health or adaptation outcomes, but two are notable: one in the school setting and one in the health care setting. Magyary and Brandt (1996) developed and evaluated a school-based self-management program for youth with chronic health conditions. The intervention involved peer groups, cognitive and/or behavioral intervention, and parental support groups. The evaluation showed that youth in the intervention group had improved self-responsibility with higher therapeutic adherence. Although the youth-reported intervention effects began to fade after several months, parental reports indicated that important effects remained.

Pless and associates (1994) evaluated the effect of nursing support on youth with a wide variety of chronic conditions and their families by using a clinical trial with random assignment. The intervention consisted of at least 12 contacts by a nurse over a 1-year period with focus on fostering family coping and independence. The nurses covered the effect of the condition on the youth and families, behavioral issues, and issues related to school performance, parenting, and family relationships. These nurses helped families see their situations differently by increasing their knowledge, facilitating family problem solving, and identifying and obtaining resources and services that met family needs. When compared with the control group using several standardized measures, the intervention group had improved adjustment and was less dependent, anxious, and depressed. This effect was the most positive for the 8- to 16-year-old age group.

Peer Relationships

Establishing meaningful friendships with others is the hallmark of successful social interaction. Friendships are the basis for the social, emotional, and practical support needed to become truly integrated into society and are one measure of success in community integration (Traustadottir, 1993). The social skills necessary for successful peer relationships are the ability to read both verbal and nonverbal cues from others, make judgments about those cues, and respond in a socially appropriate manner. These social skills can be hard for many

individuals with learning disabilities or neurodevelopmental deficits to learn. Social expectation for displays of affection, caring, anger, and frustration must be learned in adolescence if not acquired during childhood. Social immaturity, restricted social lives, and lack of social skills may all be present in youth with chronic conditions (Blum et al, 1991). Transition plans must aggressively identify mechanisms for integrating youth with chronic conditions with their peers in educational, recreational, sports, and social activities. Adults who have made successful transitions report that peer and inclusion activities are fundamental to achieving independence (Powers, Singer, and Todis, 1996).

Sexuality

Sexuality is a basic component of a full, adult life. Developing an identity as a sexual being is a universal developmental task of adolescents and young adults and should not be confused with sexual activity. Youth with chronic conditions are sexual beings with desires and interests similar to those of their unaffected peers, yet society often views and treats them as asexual. This can have disastrous consequences for youth (i.e., from being uneducated about sex and vulnerable to exploitation to feeling they have to prove their sexuality through risky behaviors) (Cox and Sawin, 1999). A survey of parents of youth with chronic conditions identified that 24% to 34% of women with sensory conditions (vision and hearing) dropped out of school on account of pregnancy or childbearing issues. Thus issues of sexuality can pose major threats to the transition plan if overlooked (Blum, 1997; Sawin, 1998; Spencer, Fife, and Rabinovich, 1995; Suris et al, 1996; USDHSS, 1992).

For a successful transition, sex education should start with a focus on the physical changes of puberty integrated with alterations caused by the youth's condition (Blum, 1994). Discussions over time should include abuse and pregnancy prevention, access to reproductive health care, and responsible sexual decision making. Youth, particularly females in this population, are at high risk for sexual and substance abuse (American Academy of Pediatrics, 1996b; Lollar, 1994; Nosek, 1995; Sobsey, 1994). Early sex education is important for youth with chronic conditions because of their high risk for sexual abuse and pregnancy (Spencer, Fife, and Robinovich, 1995). Unfortunately, issues of sexuality for children and youth with chronic conditions are not routinely addressed by health care providers or other transition team members (Blum, 1991; Blum, 1997; Nosek et al; 1994; Sawin, 1998).

Condition-specific information is critical. For example, it is important for youth with spina bifida, who have a very high incidence of latex allergy, to avoid latex condoms. Likewise, women with spinal cord injuries may not be good candidates for oral contraceptives due to their high risk for deep vein thrombosis (Sawin, 1998). Young women with epilepsy treated with anticonvulsants have an increased risk of fetal anomalies if the type and dose of the medications are not altered before conception. It is also important to realize that seizure medication can interact with some oral contraceptives, decreasing their effectiveness (Santillli, 1996). All young women of childbearing age should be taking a multivitamin with .4 mg of folic acid. Because women with spina bifida, epilepsy, and diabetes have an increased risk of bearing an infant with neural tube deficits, it is especially important for these women to take a multivitamin and have preconception counseling (Cox and Sawin, 1999). Neurological deficits (e.g., those due to spinal cord injury, spina bifida, or muscular dystrophy and musculoskeletal limitations, such as those associated with severe juvenile rheumatoid arthritis or individuals with a high degree of spasticity) may limit some sexual positions or practices (Metzger, 1999; Sawin, 1998). Alternative strategies for sexual gratification must be openly discussed.

Transition Planning for Health Care

The majority of adolescents with chronic conditions receive their health care in the pediatric primary care setting. It is the responsibility of the pediatric primary care provider to facilitate the transition from child-centered to adult-centered health care. This responsibility is identified and supported by both by the American Academy of Pediatrics (1996a) and the Society of Adolescent Medicine (Blum et al, 1993). The primary care

provider often initiates and facilitates the transition for youth with chronic conditions by helping the adolescent and family to develop competency in condition self-management (i.e., including knowledge and self-care skills, health care maintenance, and prevention of secondary or associated conditions).

Condition Self-Management

In order to begin the transition to adult health care, adolescents must have a basic understanding and awareness of their condition or disability. Each contact with the adolescent is an opportunity to assess self-care knowledge and to provide further education. The need for knowledge was underscored in a Hostler and associates' study (1989) of 44 adolescents between the ages of 11 and 14 with physical disabilities. The study found that 57% were unable to discuss or explain their disability, 90% were unable to describe therapy goals and medication usage, and 50% were unable to name the medications they were taking or the reason for taking them.

Primary care providers need to have a wide range of educational materials in multiple formats and be open to exploring new ways for youth to acquire the knowledge necessary to build self-management skills. The Internet is a powerful source of information that can be used to encourage knowledge acquisition. Adolescent chat lines for specific conditions are increasing and may be accessible sources of support and information for many teens. Web TV is relatively inexpensive and is being used to provide health-related information on a variety of subjects. Adolescents and their parents must be cautioned about the accuracy of information from the Internet and encouraged to discuss what they learn with health care providers. In addition, Internet safety (e.g., privacy) needs to be addressed. Agencies or organizations with a broad focus (e.g., the March of Dimes) can often be a source of program support for other educational materials. Additional avenues for education include conferences sponsored by disability agencies, health camp experiences, and mentoring by an adult with a similar condition or disability.

The primary care provider must assist adolescents in developing age-appropriate self-care skills for health promotion and condition management (i.e., knowing their condition and its management in detail and knowing how to use the health care system to address their needs).

Developing self-care skills to manage chronic health conditions must begin as early as developmentally feasible and be emphasized as the child approaches adolescence. Self-care skills include all activities of daily living (e.g., dressing, toileting, feeding), use of medical prosthesis or equipment, administration of medication, health promotion activities, prevention of secondary conditions, and how to access health care services. Table 8-3 provides a developmental checklist for acquisition of needed self-care skills. Cappelli, McDonald, and McGrath (1989) found that a skills questionnaire was a better predictor of successful transition than age and that questions such as, "Do you take your medicines without someone having to remind you?" and "When you are not feeling well, who usually phones the clinic or doctor?" were especially helpful in predicting transition outcome. Primary care providers may find the in-depth "Transition Health Care Assessment Guide" developed by The California Healthy and Ready to Work Project (www.cahrtw.org) useful (Betz, 1998b).

Close evaluation of the development of self-care skills is critical. Familiarity with language and procedures may make young and middle adolescents with chronic conditions seem more knowledgeable or sophisticated than they really are. The gradual transfer of responsibility for complex self-care is optimal but can be overwhelming for young adolescents striving to assume total responsibility for managing their condition (Vessey and Miola, 1997). Moreover, it can lead to poor condition outcomes (Giordano et al, 1992). The "drivers license" model is a useful analogy for establishing self-care responsibility. That is, youth drive under supervision for a prolonged period. Even after new drivers get a license, many parents often restrict them to familiar routes and provide them with a way of obtaining help in unexpected or complex situations. If youth are driving long distances or to unfamiliar territory, parents intervene by providing discussions on how to manage unforeseen occurrences. Parents often reassess the skill of the driver and, if major deficits occur, arrange additional training or supervision. Even when an adolescent with a chronic condition masters a skill, occasional help

or a holiday from selected responsibilities helps maintain the commitment necessary for care of a chronic condition (Sawin et al, 1999).

Adolescents unable to care for themselves need to develop the ability to supervise others caring for them. There is little in the literature, however, on how to teach adolescents or families to recruit, train, evaluate and hold attendants or personal care providers accountable—critical skills for youth in transition who need assistance in activities of daily life. In addition, service animals may be a reasonable resource for youth who are not functionally independent. Such resources and an array of technological resources must be explored when considering transition planning for adolescents who are not independent in activities of daily living (Sawin et al, 1999).

Health Care Maintenance

The development of a condition-specific health care maintenance plan for adults is an important part of transition planning. Key issues include nutrition, exercise, dental care, safety, injury prevention, substance abuse, and mental health. Although these goals are the same for all adolescents making the transition into adulthood, adaptations and accommodations must be made for individuals with cognitive impairments, impaired mobility, and altered physiologic states. For example, planning for the transition to an adult dental care provider needs to include issues of spasticity, latex allergy, and decreased cognition or behavioral difficulties if any exist.

Youth with chronic conditions are generally at greater risk for substance abuse and mental health issues, and focused attention is appropriate. Multiple reviews of the literature have concluded that having a chronic condition is not a cause of psychiatric illness in either individuals or families. Youth and their families, however, do have more psychosocial and adaptive issues that can be severe (Faux, 1998). A person with a disability has a higher risk of abusing alcohol and other drugs than a person without a disability. Rates of abuse in persons with disabilities range from 15% to 30%, which is well above the national average (SARDI, 1995). Most youth with chronic conditions are on two or more prescription medications. The dangers

Table 8-3
Developmentally Based Skills Checklist

Stage of Adolescence	Health Promotion and Condition Management	Medications, Supplies, and Other Equipment	Health Care System
Early, 11 to 14 years	• Knows simple anatomy, physiology, and pathology. • Able to tell health care provider what's wrong. • Discusses diagnosis and management plans with parents and providers. • Knows name(s), dates, and significance of any chronic illness and significant injuries. • Can perform appropriate first aid. • Knows CPR. • Knows any allergies and can outline avoidance and emergency treatment actions. • Takes responsibility to monitor chronic condition and quickly notify parents of any new developments. • Manages aspects of chronic condition in predictable or common situations, accessing consultation for family or other resource people in unfamiliar situations. • If assistance with ADLs needed, can identify needs and preferences and knows the tasks to be carried out by others. • Has opportunity to develop decision making and has responsibilities at home. • Knows about basic money management (e.g., function of checking and saving account) and manages small personal resources.	• Knows names of medication taken, dose, reason, expected response. • Is aware of amount of regularly taken medication remaining in container and alerts parents or caregiver when low. • Understands the difference between illicit drugs and medications. • Takes medications for chronic condition correctly. • Knows use and care of equipment and/or supplies and can notify parents when problems occur.	• Knows the difference in kinds of health care providers (e.g., obstetrician vs. optometrist). • Knows date and reason of next health appointment. • Knows where primary care providers and specialists are located and how to contact them.
Middle, 15 to 17 years	• Knows date of last menstrual period (girls) and keeps record on personal or family calendar (i.e., may be early task for females with early onset menses).	• Calls pharmacy to reorder own meds or calls own provider about need for refill.	• Makes own health care appointments.

Reprinted with permission from Sawin KJ et al: Transition planning for youth with chronic conditions: an interdisciplinary process, *N Acad Pract For 1*(3): 183-196, 1999. Adapted from: Vessey J and Miola ES: Teaching adolescents self-advocacy skills, *Pediatr Nurs 23*(1); 53-56, 1998. With information from Hallum A: Disability and the transition to adulthood: issues for the disabled child, the family, and the pediatrician, *Curr Prob Pediatr 25*(1): 12-50, 1995; and Sawin K: Health care concerns for women with physical disability and chronic illness. In Youngkin E and Davis M, editors: *Women's health: a primary care clinical guide*, ed 2, Stamford, Conn., 1998, Appleton & Lange.

Table 8-3
Developmentally Based Skills Checklist—cont'd

Stage of Adolescence	Health Promotion and Condition Management	Medications, Supplies, and Other Equipment	Health Care System
Middle, 15 to 17 years —cont'd	• Knows the basics of own health history, including family history. • Knows year of last tetanus shot. • Knows about TSE and BSE; performs regularly. • Manages chronic conditions in less predictable situations. Seeks consultation when needed. Requires minimal day-to-day supervision. • Can plan ahead to anticipate problem areas and generate options. • If assistance with ADL is needed, knows care well enough to direct others in what he or she is unable to do. • Has increasing responsibility in family. • Has a savings or checking account and manages it with supervision from parents if needed.	• Knows the difference between generic and proprietary medications • Selects own medications for minor illnesses (e.g., URI, headaches). • Orders new supplies or equipment with supervision. Can reorder these materials independently. • Arranges for transportation to get medication and/or supplies or for appointments.	• Knows basic facts of own health insurance. Knows limitations and issues for insurance in ordering supplies and/or medications and other equipment.
Late, 18 to 21 years	• Manages stable chronic condition independently. Uses parents and/or professionals to get advice regarding complex situations but makes management decisions. • Participates in discussions regarding adult health care options. • Understands the connection between mind, body, and spirit in health and illness. • Engages in healthy lifestyle activities; chooses healthful foods, exercises regularly, avoids caffeine, tobacco, illicit substances, gets adequate amount of sleep. • If assistance for ADL is needed, participates in the hiring, supervision, and termination of attendant caregiver.	• Independently manages medication, assessment and repair of any equipment, and pays for or arranges payment for medication and/or supplies.	• Understands the complexities of own health insurance plan. • Understands effect of change in employment and/or school status on insurance options. • Keeps updated file of own health records. • Takes responsibility to initiate contact with providers when transition to new living or educational environment occurs.

of prescription drug abuse and mixing prescriptions with alcohol or other street drugs are often overlooked by the adolescent, parents, professionals, and friends (Hallum, 1995; Sawin, 1998). Even when adolescents ask about the possible interaction of their prescribed medication with recreational drugs, the answers are often not readily available. Just having access to a "no-nonsense" discussion of the potential interactions of street and prescription drugs, as well as the legal consequences of illicit drug use is often useful to adolescents (Kaufman, 1995). When referral is necessary, it must be made to a professional with training and compassion for the struggles and transition needs of youth with chronic or disabling conditions. The "dual diagnosis" must be addressed in any counseling program.

Prevention of Secondary Disabilities

The prevention of secondary disabilities must be a major theme of each health care transition plan. This prevention is accomplished by the following: (1) aggressively addressing health maintenance and condition-specific primary prevention issues, (2) aggressively addressing condition-specific management issues, (3) facilitating the development of a philosophy of self-competence in the adolescent, and (4) identifying condition-specific, high-risk issues and developing a plan for early recognition of the need for treatment and specific management plans (Farley et al, 1994).

The coordinated effort to address secondary conditions in cerebral palsy and spina bifida is an example of such an integrated approach. In 1994, a "state of the science" conference was initiated by the US Department of Health and Social Services, the Centers for Disease Control and Prevention (CDC), and two voluntary organizations: the United Cerebral Palsy Association and the Spina Bifida Association of America. This cooperative effort addressed the wide range of physical, psychosocial, and social "secondary problems" of youth with disabilities when appropriate prevention efforts are not factored into care. Most important was the transition to independent living as a young adult (Sawin et al, 1999). A model for accentuating preventive strategies in high-

risk populations was developed, and strategies to prevent secondary conditions (i.e., ranging from impaired mobility, pain, and spasticity to reproductive issues and adjustment concerns) were shared. The conference proceedings delineate a proactive approach toward developing a state of well-being for young adults (Lollar, 1994).

Access to Health Care as an Adult

Health care providers need to initiate and coordinate referral to an adult-focused health care system. The American Academy of Pediatrics (1996a) recommends that in "some cases" pediatricians with skills in the health care needed by certain youth may provide care into adulthood. One of the barriers to an effective transition to adult care is the perception among many pediatric primary care providers that there is a lack of knowledgeable, sensitive providers in the adult health care system to care for adult survivors of congenitally acquired conditions. The focus must be on consulting with adult specialists to enable them to address the needs of young adults with chronic conditions—not on keeping them in the pediatric health care system.

Health Insurance Issues

The quality and amount of health care available to transitioning adolescents may be adversely affected by insurance limitations and a lack of coordinated case management. Insurance coverage becomes an issue as youth transition into adulthood and are no longer covered by their parents' insurance or federal and state programs established for care of children. One study reported that 25% of young adults and adolescents with disabilities were without insurance (McManus, Newacheck and Greaney, 1990). If an individual has a high health care risk, lack of insurance may be a major barrier to fully independent living (Johnson, 1996). Once a young adult leaves school, parental insurance is usually terminated. The cut-off age for students still in school varies by policy, but almost no coverage exceeds age 25 years. Youth in college can access the student health center for primary care but may need to have another source of inpatient coverage. Most medical plans for college students, however, have a preexisting condition clause that eliminates eligibility for many.

Youth can opt to continue parental insurance through the COBRA insurance program. This program allows youth to retain parental insurance with the same coverage for 18 months, but the cost is high. Youth in some states can join a "high-risk" insurance plan supplemented by the state, but this option is also costly and usually has no sliding scale for income. Options for individuals to "buy into" either a high risk insurance or Medicaid plan on a sliding-fee scale are being proposed by some legislators on both the national and state levels (Johnson, 1996). Families and health care providers must advocate for innovative insurance options that would support optimal transition outcomes and ensure continued health care.

Further complicating the loss of personal insurance is the termination at a specific age of supplemental benefits available in most states through block grant programs (e.g., Title V programs) for children with special health care needs. Federal block grants give states financial resources to provide specialty clinical services and supplemental fiscal support for families with children with special health care needs. These programs were created as a "health care safety net" for at risk children and families and cease at age 21 years. Eligible youth may apply for Supplemental Security Income (SSI) or Social Security Disability Insurance (SSDI), which usually come with automatic Medicaid benefits. Employment, however, may result in loss of eligibility and termination of financial and medical benefits (see Chapter 7). Thus youth in transition may lose the medical support available from the state and not be able to access any other type of insurance. Even if insurance is available to youth in transition, the benefits may be severely restricted—especially for therapies important to youth with mobility, communicative, or psychologic challenges. If services are provided, they are often limited in amount and duration (American Academy of Pediatrics, 1996a), which is a problem that may be accentuated if an individual uses a managed care organization with limited resources and restricted referral options.

Transition Planning in The School System

Although the focus of transition planning in the health care system is accessing adult health care services, the focus in the school system is preparing individuals for life in the community and meaningful employment. The Individuals with Disabilities Education Act (IDEA) is the only federal legislation that requires a planning process to enable students with disabilities to achieve a smooth, gradual, and planned transition to community life. The legislation defines transition services as follows:

> . . . a coordinated set of activities for a student, designed with an outcome oriented process that promotes movement from school to post-school activities including secondary education, vocational training, integrated employment (including supported employment) continuing and adult education, adult services, independent living and community participation. A coordinated set of activities shall be based upon the individual student's needs, taking into account the student's experiences, level of employment, post-school adult living objectives and when appropriate, acquisition of daily living skills and a functional vocational evaluation (National Information Center for Children and Youth with Disabilities, 1997).

The transition provisions were set forth in the 1990 reauthorization of IDEA that required schools to develop individualized transition plans (ITPs) for students 16 years of age with a chronic condition or disability. IDEA 1997 (PL105-17) modifies transition planning by requiring that each student's IEP contains a statement of transition service needs beginning at age 14 years. Students with chronic or disabling conditions who are not eligible for special education and therefore do not have an IEP can and should receive transition services under Section 504 of the Rehabilitation Act. Students with chronic health conditions (e.g., diabetes or asthma) often have transition services addressed in their Individual Health Service Programs (IHPs). These 504 plans and IHPs should address transition service needs starting at 14 years of age. Neither 504 plans nor IHPs have legal mandates for transition planning, even though it is a recommended practice. Primary care providers may need to advocate for appropriate school-based services for youth who do not have a legal mandate for transition planning in the school. Working in conjunction with the school nurse in advocating and planning services is most effective. Educational transition teams often overlook the health care issues that must be addressed for successful planning. If health care issues are not adequately addressed, a successful transition into postsecondary education or full-time employment, community living, and self-sufficiency will be jeopardized.

Postsecondary Education

The statistical profile of college students with disabilities reveals that in the 1992-1993 school year, 9.2% of all freshmen reported having some type of disability compared with 2.6% in 1978. The percentage of freshmen with disabilities who reported a learning disability more than doubled from 1988, increasing from 15.3% to 32.2% (Henderson, 1995). More than half of all freshmen with disabilities are students with hidden disabilities (i.e., learning, health, etc.) and freshmen who reported having disabilities were more likely than their nondisabled peers to be older men, from lower income families, and significantly concerned about financing their college education. Many received financial aid from Vocational Rehabilitation funds and were more interested in education and technical fields than in business. Many used special support programs offered at colleges and reported having been influenced by a role model and /or mentor to go to college.

Plans for a transition from high school to college should be reflected in an IEP, IHP, or 504 accommodation plan. There are schools around the country that are especially noted as having strong support programs for those with chronic conditions (Back to School, 1996). Youth—especially those with severe physical disabilities—may find the extensive educational, health, recreational, and social support services of these universities helpful. Almost all colleges and universities have an Office of Disabled Student Services. Contacting this office before applying to determine available services is

often useful. Some students are unwilling to identify themselves as having a chronic condition or disability because of the stigma associated with differences in our society. Students should be encouraged to use all services available to them to enhance their potential for success.

As with other college students, financial considerations are important. Early consultation in high school with the Division of Rehabilitation Services can determine if a student is eligible for any educational or support services. Services vary across states, and early consultation is important because staff in all agencies have a heavy caseload. Youth and their parents must be clear about what services are available and then vigorously pursue them.

A major source of information about postsecondary education is The HEATH Resource Center of the American Council on Education, which is the national clearinghouse on postsecondary education for individuals with disabilities. Support from the US Department of Education enables the Center to serve as a resource for exchange of information about educational support services, policies, procedures, adaptations, and opportunities at American campuses, vocational-technical schools, and other postsecondary training entities. In operation since 1984, HEATH offers a multitude of resource papers, monographs, guides, and directories focusing on a broad range of disability-related topics such as accessibility, career development, classroom and laboratory adaptations, financial aid, independent living, transition resources, training and postsecondary education, vocational education, and rehabilitation. Providers should encourage youth and their families to access this information via the public library or Internet early in the planning process. At a minimum, youth and families need to ask basic questions about a school. Useful questions proposed by HEATH are outlined in Box 8-1.

Some universities have preenrollment programs for students with severe disabilities—especially those who will need attendant care (Sawin, 1983). The focus of the health providers in these situations is evaluation of the attendant care needs of the student, as well as—and more importantly—the student's independent ability to teach others to provide the necessary care. Each student must determine if health care should be transferred from

---

Box 8-1

Useful Questions in Assessing a Postsecondary Education Environment

What are the medical and health needs of this young adult?

Will a plan for health care transition need to be developed?

What factors would be included in the health component of the transition plan?

When should the health transition process be initiated?

How will the chronic illness affect this individual?

How does the chronic illness affect this youth's educational process?

How does the chronic illness affect this individual's living environment?

How does the chronic illness affect activities of daily living?

Disclosure

Should the individual disclose the chronic illness when applying to colleges or other postsecondary training institutions? To whom? When?

What laws are in place to protect the rights of people with disabilities? How do they relate to young adults with chronic illness?

Accommodations

What educational or environmental accommodations or modifications will need to be in place to increase independence?

What accommodations are postsecondary educational institutions required by law to provide?

If this individual needs additional accommodations or modifications, who will pay for them?

How can this individual assess the ability of the postsecondary institution and the surrounding community in meeting his or her needs?

Locating Resources

When should financial, medical, and support service resources begin?

Who can assist at the postsecondary site?

Whose responsibility is it?

Adapted from Edelman A: Maximizing success: transition planning for education after high school for young adults with chronic illness, Information from HEATH 15(1): 3.

---

their home community to either the college health care center or a local speciality provider or if the community provider should be maintained. Access to emergency health care must always be evaluated, and youth should have a copy of all critical health care records with them if they are far from their usual sources of health care.

Vocational Training and The Transition to Work

The 1992 Amendments to the Rehabilitation Act of 1973 (PL 102-569) strengthened the role of vocational rehabilitation to work collaboratively with special education in preparing youth for transition into adult life while they are in school. Having already initiated the independent living movement with the 1986 amendments, the Rehabilitation Act of 1992 addressed the needs of youth and young adults for personal assistant services, supported employment opportunities, and a broad range of assistive technology (Johnson, 1996; Wehman, 1992). The 1998 amendments reinforce that employment is the intended outcome of vocational rehabilitation services. Most high school students identified as having a disability intend to enter the workforce upon leaving school but face many employment barriers. Wagner and Blackorby (1996) studied data from the National Longitudinal Transition Study of Special Education Students and identified factors that contributed to the outcomes for youth who were in special education. They found that students from low-income households experienced the worst post-school outcomes; students with sensory or motor disabilities benefited the most from special education; and concentrated vocational education (i.e., several courses focusing on a specific area)—as opposed to one course from a variety of concentrations—yielded higher employment and income rates. Even with vocational courses, however, outcomes for employment were still low when compared with those of youth not in special education.

The major resource for youth making the transition to work is the Vocational Rehabilitation Service in their state. The changes in the Rehabilitation Act in 1993 and 1998 strengthened the focus on employment and changed the criteria for service. The only criterion is that the adolescent would benefit from employment, and the definition of employment has been broadened to include supported employment (Johnson, 1996). The act also provides technological resources and personal assistance services if necessary to provide assistance in activities of daily living on or off the job. Even with these resources, however, the transition to work is often problematic. Early referral to vocational support services and conveying the expectation that work, in some form, is an expected outcome must be the focuses of the home, school, and health care communities.

Transitioning from Home to Community Living

The transition to independent living is difficult for many youth and young adults with cognitive, physical, and emotional disabilities to achieve because necessary support systems are not readily available. Youth with chronic unstable health conditions find this transition particularly difficult if they have not developed the skills necessary to manage their conditions and solve problems associated with their condition and limited functional capacity.

Several recent legislative initiatives have given communities the impetus to develop supports for young adults who want to study, work, and live as independently as possible in the community. These initiatives include the Americans with Disabilities Act (ADA) of 1990 (PL 101-336), the 1992 Amendments to the Rehabilitation Act of 1973 (PL 102-569), the Home and Community Based Services (HCBS) waiver, and the Community Supported Living Arrangement (CSLA) of 1990 (PL 101-508) amendments to Medicaid. These programs are often underfunded, however, and there

are often insufficient resources available in the community to meet the needs of youth and adults with disabilities who seek independence.

The ADA is considered civil rights legislation for individuals with disabilities. School, health care, and community segregation are now considered discriminatory, and institutionalization is discouraged (Johnson, 1996). This law has encouraged funding to shift toward more integrative approaches to community living. In order to fulfill its promise of equal rights to accessing public transportation, public and private services, recreational activities, independent living and competitive employment, the focus must be in the community. The 1992 amendments to the Rehabilitation Act of 1973 (PL 102-569) earmarked funds for support services to strengthen options for independent or supported living. These options include personal assistant services and a broad range of assistive technology (Johnson, 1996; Wehman, 1992).

Finally, two amendments to the Medicaid program have systematically provided funding mechanisms to support community living for young adults with chronic conditions or disabilities. The first, the Home and Community Based Services (HCBS) Waiver, which was first enacted in 1982, has gained momentum and is rapidly replacing Title XX as the major source of federal funding for community services (Braddock et al, 1995). Although originally intended to support the movement of individuals from institutional care to residential care, this program now finances case management, homemakers, home health aides, personal care, residential habilitation, day habilitation, respite care, transportation, supported employment, adapted equipment, and home modification. The second ammendment, which is a relatively new program, the Community Supported Living Arrangements (CSLA), promotes the development of statewide systems of individualized supported living (Braddock et al, 1995). The support services available through these two programs are critical for many youth and young adults with disabling conditions making a transition to the community.

If young adults with chronic conditions or disabilities are to be successful living independently, they must have the social skills—including the skills necessary to make appropriate decisions about their health and activities of daily living, as well as the technical skills or assistance to actually meet their daily needs for physical care, communication, and transportation. Most youth with chronic conditions and those with mild degrees of disability negotiate the road to community living much like youth without disabilities. Youth with moderate to severe degrees of functional disability will have more difficulty.

Learning to be as independent as possible with activities of daily living does not mean doing things without help or modification. On the contrary, distinguishing between when and how much assistance is needed is indicative of mature decision-making for many young persons with chronic conditions or disabilities. Ideally, the development of self-help skills that began at home and continued throughout school was geared toward the ultimate goal of independent living. These skills include personal hygiene; domestic skills; transportation; safety; financial management including banking, purchasing, spending; and seeking and developing meaningful leisure activities (Axelson and Jackson, 1997; Hallum, 1995; Klein, 1992; Wehman, 1992).

Coordination of Transition Planning

Families report not only frustration with obtaining a coordinated transition plan but also confusion about where to get assistance (Johnson, 1996; Stevenson, Pharoah, and Stevenson, 1997). Care coordination across systems (i.e., family, school, employment, community and health care) and communication among providers, transition team members, and the family are essential to providing a smooth transition to adulthood. Families usually try to coordinate the transition process, but the primary care provider may facilitate the process and communication across systems. When an individual's health problems are significant, the primary care proivder may need to assume a leadership role in the transition process. In order to facilitate the plan, the primary care provider must know the needs of the adolescent and family; the agencies and team members involved; and the family, school, community, and health care resources available.

When the family is articulate and knowledgeable and can access resources, the primary care provider may only need to coordinate health information and referrals to community health agencies. Primary care providers may provide health information on a regular basis for school transition team conferences and be available as needed for consultation. If there is a significant health component to the transition plan, the primary care provider may actually be the case manager or can be the team leader while a specialty provider is the case manager. All transition team members—including the adolescent and family—must work toward similar goals to achieve a smooth transition to the adult health care system.

As adulthood approaches, primary care providers must encourage youth and their families to address future planning for education, health care, employment, and community living options with referrals to appropriate resources. In preparation for adulthood, the primary health care provider has an obligation to do the following: (1) educate and inform adolescents of their conditions, including future expectations and preventive health care; (2) encourage parents to adopt parenting styles that support the transition to independent adulthood; (3) recognize and plan for opportunities to support young adults' autonomous decision-making regarding health care, building on the strengths of the individual; (4) convey a positive attitude about the potential of young adults and provide information to agencies or people who can help them reach their full potential; (5) be knowledgeable about the evolving community system of supports and legal mandates for services; (6) help individuals access appropriate health care services and function as a consultant to adult providers when necessary; (7) advocate at the legislative level for insurance coverage and community services to enable individuals to live as full and healthy adult lives as possible; and (8) advocate for appropriate and comprehensive transition services that integrate systems of care and educational, health, community, and family resources.

Resources for Youth and Their Families

Denniston S and Enlow C: Making choices: a journal workbook for teens and young adults with spina bifida that provides opportunities for making choices about their lives, Louisville, Ky., 1995, Spina Bifida Association of Kentucky's Transition to Independence Project.

Farwisk AW and Millar HE: Promoting resilience in youth with chronic conditions and their families, Vienna, Va., 1996, Maternal and Child Health Bureau, Health Resources and Services Administration, US Public Health Service. Available from the National Maternal and Child Health Clearinghouse, 2070 Chain Bridge Road, Suite 450, Vienna, Va. 22182-2536.

Hardin P: Building skills: a guide for parents and professionals working with young people who have spina bifida, Louisville, Ky., 1995a, Spina Bifida Association of Kentucky's Transition to Independence Project.

Hardin P: Becoming the me I want to be: a guide for youth with spina bifida and their parents, Louisville, Ky., 1995b, Spina Bifida Association of Kentucky's Transition to Independence Project.

HEATH: Resources paper for readers with chronic illness, their parents and counselors; (202) 884-3203.

Information for Parents of High School Students with Disabilities in Transition to Adult Life, Minneapolis, 1993, Parent Advocacy Collaboration for Education Resources (PACER) Center. This is a practical workbook to prepare youth to participate as productive members of their own IEP meeting. Many other transition materials are also available. The center has an extensive catalogue that may be helpful to families; 1-800-848-4912.

Kaufman M: Easy for you to say: questions and answers for teens living with chronic illness or disability, Toronto, 1995, Key Porter Books.

Kriegsman KH, Zaslow EL, and D'Zmura-Rechsteiner MA: Taking charges: teenagers talk about life and physical disability, Bethesda, Md., 1992, Woodbine House. Available from the American Spina Bifida Association; a much acclaimed primer for older school-age and teenage patients.

SARDI: Substance abuse and students with disabilities: little known facts, Dayton, Ohio, 1995, Wright State University. Available from Wright State University, School of Medicine, SARDI, PO Box 927, Dayton, Oh 45401; (513) 259-1384.

Shapiro JP: No pity: people with disabilities forging a new civil rights movement, New York, 1993, Random House.

Organizations and Agencies

National Council on Disability (NCD): An independent federal agency that makes recommendations to the President and Congress on issues affecting 54 million Americans with disabilities. The NCD is composed of 15 members appointed by the President and confirmed by the Senate. Its overall purpose is to promote policies, programs, practices, and procedures that guarantee equal opportunity for all individuals with disabilities—regardless of the nature or severity of the disability—and to empower individuals with disabilities to achieve economic self-sufficiency, independent living, and inclusion and integration into all aspects of society. http://www.ncd.gov/

National Transition Alliance: Mission is to ensure that youth with disabilities—including those with severe disabilities—acquire skills and knowledge, gain experience, and receive the services and supports necessary to achieve successful results post-school. www.dssc.org/nta

National Organization on DisABILITY: Promotes full and equal participation for the 54 million U.S. men, women, and children with disabilities in all aspects of life. www.nod.org

Parent Training and Information Centers (PTI), Technical Assistance to Parents Program (TAPP): National network of parent-run projects that address information, advocacy, and consultation to education and health care providers. Of the 71 projects, one such program, the Parenting Educational Advocacy Training Center in Fairfax, Va. provides links to almost every disability organization. www.peatc.org

HEATH Resource Center: National Clearinghouse on Postsecondary Education for Individuals with Disabilities. Located at One Dupont Circle, Suite 800, Washington, DC 20036-1193. It is a clearinghouse that collects and disseminates information on postsecondary education and offers support services, position papers, resources, and training.

National Information Center for Children and Youth with Disabilities (NICHCY): Provides information and referral on all disability issues (also available in Spanish). www.nichcy.org

Several national demonstration projects are currently funded by the Maternal Child Health Bureau (MCHB). These programs will test new health care transition models that can be replicated throughout the nation. Many have produced or are developing useful materials for primary care providers. Providers can contact the MCHB (http://www/mchb.hrsa.gov/chcnmc.html) for information on these programs or contact the programs directly:

California—UCLA-affiliated program at the Southern California Transition Center: "Healthy and Ready to Work." http://www.cahrtw.org

Iowa—Consortium of Iowa Child Health Specialty Clinics, Iowa UAP, Iowa Creative Employment Options, Adolescent Transition: "Healthy and Ready to Work." http://www.iowaceo.com

Kentucky—Collaborative public-private effort between States Children's Special Health Care Needs (CSHCN), Title V, Early Intervention, Vocational Rehabilitation, and Shriners Hospitals. CHOICES (Childrens' Health Care Options Improved through Collaborative Efforts and Services) Transition Project; choices001@aol.com

Louisiana—The Human Development Center (HDC), Louisiana State University: "Healthy and Ready to Work."

Maine—Department of Human Services, Bureau of Health, Division of Community and Main Adolescent Transition Partnership.

Massachusetts—Division for Children with Special Health Care Needs (DCSHCN) Initiative for Youth with Disabilities (MIYD).

Minnesota—PACER Center, a parent training and information center, www.pacer.org

Ohio—Lighthouse Youth Services, Inc. with Work and Rehabilitation Center of Greater Cincinnati, Inc. Hamilton County Adolescent Transition Project, lighthou@ix.netcom.com

References

Alan Guttmacher Institute: Sex and America's teenagers, New York, 1994, The Institute.

American Academy of Pediatrics, Committee on Children with Disabilities and Committee on Adolescence: Transition of care provided for adolescents with special health care needs, Pediatrics, 98(6):1203-1206, 1996a.

American Academy of Pediatrics: Sexuality education of children and adolescents with developmental disabilities, Pediatrics 97(2):275-278, 1996b.

Associated Press: Parents with retarded children file lawsuit over long wait for care, San Francisco Chronicle, March 20, 1999.

Axelson P and Jackson P: Transition for adolescence to adulthood. In Vessey J, editor: The child with a learning disorder or ADHD: a manual for school nurses, Scarborough, Me., 1997, National Association of School Nurses.

Back to school, Sports 'n Spokes 11-17, May/June 1996.

Betz CL: Adolescent transitions: a nursing concern, Pediatr Nurs 24(1)23-29, 1998a.

Betz CL: Facilitating the transition of adolescents with chronic conditions from pediatric to adult health care and community settings, Issue Comp Pediatr Nurs 21:97-115, 1998b.

Blum RW: Overview of transition issues for youth with disabilities, Pediatrician 18:101-104, 1991.

Blum RW: Adolescents with chronic conditions and their families: the transition to adult services. In Hostler SL, editor: Family-centered care: an approach to implementation, Charlottesville, Va., 1994, The University of Virginia.

Blum RW: Transition to adult health care: setting the stage, J Adolesc Health 17:3-5, 1995.

Blum RW: Sexual health contraceptive needs of adolescents with chronic conditions, Arch Pediatr Adolesc Med 151(3):290-297, 1997.

Blum RW et al: Transitions from child-centered to adult-care systems for adolescents with chronic conditions: a position paper of the Society of Adolescent Medicine, J Adolesc Health 14(7):570-576, 1993.

Blum RW and Garber J: Chronically ill youth. In McAnarney ER et al, editors: Textbook of adolescent medicine, Philadelphia, 1992, W.B. Saunders.

Blum RW et al: Family and peer issues among adolescents with spine bifida and cerebral palsy, Pediatrics, 88:280-285, 1991.

Braddock D et al: The state of the states in developmental disabilities, Washington, DC, 1995, American Association on Mental Retardation.

Bridges W: Transitions—making sense of life's changes, Reading, Mass., 1994, Addison-Wesley.

Cappelli M, MacDonald NE, and McGrath PL: Assessment of readiness to transfer to adult care for adolescents with cystic fibrosis, Children's Health Care, 18:218-221, 1989.

Carnegie Council on Adolescent Development: Great transitions: preparing adolescents for a new century, New York, 1995, The Council.

Cowan PA and Hetherington M, editors: Family transitions, Hillsdale, NJ, 1991, Lawrence Erlbaum Associates.

Cox A and Sawin KJ: The school nurse. In DeFur S and Patton J, editors: The relationship of school-based services to the transition process, Austin, Tx, 1999, Pro-Ed.

Denniston S and Enlow C: Making choices: a journal workbook for teens and young adults with spina bifida that provides opportunities for making choices about their lives, Louisville, Ky., 1995, Spina Bifida Association of Kentucky's Transition to Independence Project.

Edelman A: Maximizing success: transition planning for education after high school for young adults with chronic illness, Washington, DC, 1995, HEATH Resource Center.

Farley T et al: Secondary disabilities in Arkansans with spina bifida, European Journal of Surgery 40:39-40, 1994.

Faux SA:.Historical overview of responses of children and their families to chronic illness. In Broome ME et al, editors: Children and families in health and illness, Thousand Oaks, Calif., 1998, Sage Publications.

Giordano BP et al: The challenge of transferring responsibility for diabetes management from parent to child, J Pediatr Health Care 6(5 pt 1):235-239, 1992.

Hallum A: Disability and the transition to adulthood: issues for the disabled child, the family, and the pediatrician, Current Problems in Pediatrics 25(1):12-50, 1995.

Hardin P: Building skills: a guide for parents and professionals working with young people who have spina bifida, Louisville, Ky., 1995a, Spina Bifida Association of Kentucky's Transition to Independence Project.

Hardin P: Becoming the me I want to be: a guide for youth with spina bifida and their parents, Louisville, Ky., 1995b, Spina Bifida Association of Kentucky's Transition to Independence Project.

Henderson C: College freshmen with disabilities: a statistical profile, Washington, DC, 1995, HEATH Resource Center.

Hostler SL et al: Adolescent autonomy project: transition skills for adolescents with physical disabilities, CAC 18:12-18, 1989.

Igoe JB: School nursing, Nurs Clin North Am 29(3):443-458, 1994.

Johnson CP: Transition in adolescents with disabilities. In Capute A and Accardo P, editors: Developmental disabilities in infancy and childhood, ed 2, Baltimore, Md., 1996, Paul H. Brookes Publishing Company.

Johnson LD, O'Malley PM, and Bachman JG: National survey results on drug use from the Monitoring the Future study, 1975-1994, Rockville, Md., 1995, National Institute on Drug Abuse.

Kaufman M: Easy for you to say: questions and answers for teens living with chronic illness or disability, Toronto, 1995, Key Porter Books, Ltd.

Kelly A: The primary care provider's role in caring for young people with chronic illness, J Adolesc Health 17:32-36, 1995.

Klein J: Supporting people with disabilities to live in their own homes. In Nisbet J, editor: Natural supports in school, at work, and in the community for people with severe disabilities, Baltimore, Md., 1992, Paul H. Brookes.

Lollar DJ, editor: Preventing secondary conditions associated with spina bifida or cerebral palsy, Washington, DC, 1994, Spina Bifida Association of America.

Lynch BS and Bonnie RJ: Growing up tobacco free: Preventing nicotine addiction in children and youth. Washington, DC, 1994, National Academy Press.

Magyary D and Brandt P: A school-based self-management program for youth with chronic health conditions and their parents, Canadian Journal of Nursing Research 28(4):55-77, 1996.

McManus MA, Newacheck PW, and Greaney AM: Young adults with special health care needs: prevalence, severity, and access to health services, Pediatrics 86:674-682, 1990.

Metzger SG: Individual with disabilities. In Youngkin et al, editors: Pharmacotherapeutics: a primary care clinical guide, Stamford, Conn., 1999, Appleton & Lange.

National Center for Education Statistics: The condition of education, 1994, Washington, DC, 1994, US Government Printing Office.

National Information Center for Children and Youth with Disabilities: The IDEA amendments of 1997, News Digest 26, Washington, DC, 1997, The Center.

Newacheck PW and Halfon N: Prevalence and impact of disabling chronic conditions in childhood, Am J Public Health 88(4):610-617, 1998.

National Organization on Disability (NOD): National Organization on Disability/Harris Survey of Americans with disabilities, website: www.NOD.org.

Nosek MA et al: Wellness models and sexuality among women with physical disabilities, Journal of Applied Rehabilitation Counseling, 25 (1):50-58. 1994.

Nosek MA: Sexual abuse of women with physical disabilities, Physical Medicine and Rehabilitation: State of the Art Reviews, 9(2):487-501, 1995.

Orr DP:. Helping adolescents toward adulthood, Contemp Pediatrics 15(5):55-76, 1998.

PEATC: IDEA 97: a checklist for effective IEPs, The PEATC Press 2(2)16-17, 1998.

Pledgie TK, Tao Q, and Freed C: Documenting the need for transition services at an earlier age, Work, a Journal of Prevention, Assessment and Rehabilitation 10(1):15-19, 1998.

Pless ID et al: A randomized trial of a nursing intervention to promote the adjustment of children with chronic physical disorders, Pediatrics 94:70-75, 1994.

Powers LE, Singer GH, and Sowers JA:. Self-competence and disability. In Powers L, Singe G, and Sowers JA, editors: On the road to autonomy, promoting self-competence in children and youth with disabilities, Baltimore, Md., 1996, Paul H. Brookes.

Powers LE, Singer GH, and Todis B: Reflections on competence, perspectives on successful adults. In Powers L, Singer G, and Sowers JA, editors: On the road to autonomy, promoting self-competence in children and youth with disabilities, Baltimore, Md., 1996, Paul H. Brookes.

Powers LE et al: TAKE CHARGE: a model for promoting self-determination among adolescents with challenges. In Powers L, Singer G, and Sowers JA, editors: On the road to autonomy, promoting self-competence in children and youth with disabilities, Baltimore, Md., 1996, Paul H. Brookes.

Santilli N, editor: Managing seizures disorders, Landrover, Md., 1996, Lippincott-Ravin.

SARDI: Substance abuse and students with a disability, Information from HEATH, October/November 1995, 5-6.

Sawin KJ: Assisting the adolescent with disabilities through a college health program, Nurs Clin North Am 18(2):257-274, 1983.

Sawin KJ: Health care concerns for women with physical disability and chronic illness. In Youngkin E and Davis M, editors: Women's health: a primary care clinical guide, ed 2, Stamford, Ct., 1998, Appleton and Lange.

Sawin KJ et al: Transition planning for youth with chronic conditions: an interdisciplinary process, National Academies of Practice Forum 1(3):183-186, 1999.

Sawin KJ and Marshall J: Developmental competence in adolescents with an acquired disability, Rehabilitation Nursing Research Journal 1:41-50, 1992.

Sawin KJ, Metzger S, and Pellock J: The experience of living with epilepsy from an adolescent and parent's perspective, Epelilepsia 37(suppl 5):86, 1996.

Schoen C et al: The health of adolescent boys: Commonwealth Fund survey findings, New York, 1998, Louis Harris and Associates, Inc.

Schoen C et al: The Commonwealth Fund survey of the health of adolescent girls, New York, 1997, Louis Harris and Associates, Inc.

Schafer MS and Rangasamy R: Transition and Native American youth: a follow up study school leavers on the Fort Apache Indian Reservation, Journal of Rehabilitation 61(1):60-65, 1995.

Schumacher KL and Meleis AI: Transitions: a central concept in nursing, IMAGE: Journal of Nursing Scholarship 26(2)119-127, 1994.

Selder F: Life transition theory: the resolution of uncertainty, Nursing and Health Care 10:437-451, 1989.

Sobsey D: Violence and abuse, Baltimore, Md., 1994, Paul H. Brookes.

Spencer A, Fife R, and Rabinovich C: The school experience of children with arthritis: coping in the 1990s and transition into adulthood, Pediatr Clin North Am 42(5):1285-1298, 1995.

Stevenson CJ, Pharoah PO, and Stevenson R: Cerebral palsy-the transition from youth to adulthood, Developmental Medicine and Child Neurology 39:336-342, 1997.

Suris JC et al: Sexual behavior of adolescents with chronic disease and disability, J Adolesc Health 19(2):124-131, 1996.

Traustadottir R: The gendered context of friendships. In Amado A, editor: Friendships and community connections between people with and without developmental disabilities, Baltimore, Md., 1993, Paul H. Brookes.

US Department of Health and Human Services, Maternal and Child Health Bureau: Moving on: transition from child-centered to adult health care for youth with disabilities, Washington, DC, 1992, The Bureau.

United States General Accounting Office (USGAO): Report to the chairman, subcommittee on employer-employee relations, Committee on Economic and Educational Opportunities, House of Representatives. People with disabilities: federal programs could work together more efficiently to promote employment (publication no. GAO/HEHS 96-126), Washington, DC, 1996, US Government Printing Office.

Vessey J and Miola ES: Teaching adolescents self-advocacy skills, Pediatr Nurs 23(1):53-56, 1997.

Wagner MM and Blackorby J: Transition from high school to work or college: how special education students fare, Special Education for Students with Disabilities 6(1):103-119, 1996.

Wehman P: Life beyond the classroom: transition strategies for young people with disabilities, Baltimore, Md., 1992, Paul H. Brookes.

Wehmeyer J: Self-determination for youth with significant cognitive disabilities, from theory to practice. In Powers L, Singer G, and Sowers J, editors: On the road to autonomy, promoting self-competence in children and youth with disabilities, Baltimore, Md., 1996, Paul H. Brookes.

Younger JB: A theory of mastery, Adv Nurs Science 14(1):76-89, 1991.

part 2 two

CHRONIC CONDITIONS

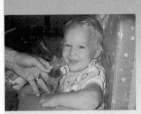

CHAPTER 9

Asthma

Gail Kieckhefer and Marijo Ratcliffe

Etiology

The exact etiology of asthma remains equivocal. Although a familial tendency has long been recognized, environmental factors are also thought to contribute to the presence of clinically recognized asthma. Asthma has been characterized as obstructive airway disease caused primarily by bronchoconstriction (i.e., smooth muscle contraction), but over the last decade the roles and mechanisms of inflammation and mucous secretion have become increasingly recognized (Colton and Krause, 1997).

The current definition of asthma includes the following three components:

1. Airway inflammation,
2. Airway obstruction that can be partially or completely reversed, and
3. Increased (hyperreactivity) airway responsiveness to stimuli (Colton and Krause, 1997).

Asthma episodes have at least two types of offending triggers: (1) inflammatory triggers (e.g., allergens, chemical sensitizers, viral infections); and (2) noninflammatory triggers (e.g., dust, cold air, and other irritants). Inflammatory triggers are considered asthmogenic insofar as they cause asthma by increasing the frequency and severity of airway smooth muscle contraction and enhance airway responsiveness through inflammatory mechanisms. Noninflammatory triggers cause a bronchospastic response that may become more severe depending upon the existing level of responsiveness in the airway.

Within the first 10 to 20 minutes of the initial response phase when a trigger is encountered, an acute reaction will occur when an antigen binds to the specific immunoglobulin-E surface on the mast cell and a cell mediator (e.g., histamine) is released. Intercellular chemical mediators such as leukotrienes are also released (Frost and Spahn, 1998). This early response causes bronchospasm even though inflammatory mediators are involved and can spontaneously remit within 60 to 90 minutes. When treatment is required, however, a bronchodilator (e.g., a b_2-adrenergic agonist) is effective as a result of the underlying pathophysiology of bronchospasm.

During the late-phase response, which may occur a few hours later, the initial bronchospastic reaction has moderated and the cellular phase of inflammation will peak up to 12 to 24 hours later. This response is most likely due to the early phase stimulation of chemotactic factors that recruit inflammatory cells (e.g., activated lymphocytes, eosinophils and neutrophils) to the submucosa of the large and small airways. Histamine and other mediator levels then increase again, adding to the bronchospastic component in addition to the inflammatory reaction. This response can cause a continuing cycle with both inflammatory and bronchospastic components requiring treatment with antiinflammatory and b_2-adrenergic medications.

Airway hyperreactivity to stimuli is noted in all children with asthma but is particularly correlated with individuals experiencing a late-phase response. "The degree of hyperresponsiveness also correlates with the severity of asthma, as measured by reduced airway caliber and the amount of medication required to control symptoms" (Cockroft, 1990). Therefore a child with asthma may have heightened sensitivity to nonallergic stimuli, which will more readily exacerbate the airway obstruction. This airway responsiveness may persist for weeks to months. The nature of the child's response—early, late, or dual (i.e., early and late)—and the severity of the long-term hyper-responsive phase will direct therapeutic modalities. The chronic inflammation may in turn lead to progressive airway remodeling, which will affect both airway smooth muscle and connective tissue (Chernik and Boat, 1998).

Incidence

Respiratory disease remains the major cause of hospitalization in young children. Cumulative prevalence rates of wheezing in young children range from 30% to 60%, with two recent U.S. reports of 4.5% of children under 17 years having diagnosed asthma (Halfon and Newacheck, 1993; Silver et al, 1998). When recurrent wheezing is considered in addition to formal diagnosis, prevalence increases to over 8% (Silver, Crain and Weiss, 1998). With even more liberal criteria, others quote 15% or higher prevalence rates in school-age children (Cypcar, Stark, and Lemanske, 1992; Redding et al, 1995).

Reports on the incidence of asthma indicate an increase in the diagnosis over the past decade, with an even greater increase in reported morbidity and mortality (Rachelefsky, 1995). Whether the increase in asthma is the result of a rise in the disease or in improved diagnostic screening is unknown, however many children with typical asthmalike symptoms of cough, shortness of breath, and wheezing are underdiagnosed (Redding et al, 1996). Asthma is more common in boys than girls, with a ratio of 2:1.5 until puberty. It has been postulated that infant males may have smaller airways than females; younger children also have smaller caliber airways and chest walls. These and other factors may contribute to early wheezing in young children (Stein and Martinez, 1999).

A longitudinal prospective study of 1246 newborns in Tucson, Arizona revealed that 60% of children with wheezing illnesses in the first 3 years of life stop wheezing by 6 years of age. It has been suggested that these children have transient conditions that do not lead to lifelong problems with asthma and allergies. Persistent wheezing after 6 years of age, however, was associated with maternal history of asthma, atopy, and maternal smoking. The latter was a risk factor for all children who wheezed—whether only in the first 3 years or after 6 years of age. Continuing future assessments through this prospective study may enable a better understanding of the development of asthma and allergies (Martinez et al, 1995).

Clinical Manifestations at Time of Diagnosis

Many children with asthma initially present with wheezing associated with or following an upper respiratory infection (URI). Other conditions that may lead to the diagnosis of asthma include recurrent pneumonia, sinusitis, chronic cough in the absence of wheezing, and persistent nocturnal cough or wheeze. In children and teenagers, decreased ability to exercise with complaint of shortness of breath, chest pain or pressure, and a history of cough or wheeze after exercise are indicative of exercise-induced bronchospasm (EIB) (Box 9-1).

Because children have a variety of symptoms with asthma, other diseases must be ruled out. Children who have recurrent pneumonia or sinusitis—even with no evidence of malabsorption—should have a quantitative pilocarpine ionophoresis (i.e., sweat chloride test) for cystic fibrosis (see Chapter 18). In young children, monophonic expiratory wheezing or expiratory stridor—which are sometimes difficult to distinguish from one another—may indicate foreign body aspiration, tracheal

---

Box 9-1

Clinical Manifestations

I. Symptoms
  - Cough
  - Wheezing
  - Nocturnal cough and wheeze
  - Recurrent pneumonia and/or sinusitis
  - Shortness of breath on exercise (EIB)
II. Family history
III. Pattern recognition
  - Follows URI or exercise
  - Seasonal presentation
IV. Response to therapy

compression, stenosis, tracheomalacia, or bronchomalacia. Referral to a pulmonologist or otolaryngologist for bronchoscopy may be necessary for diagnosis.

Usually the diagnosis of asthma is made when a child has been seen repeatedly for wheezing or coughing episodes, especially when there is a positive family history of asthma or the episodes are responsive to bronchodilator therapy. Many children seen during acute exacerbations of asthma have a history of upper respiratory infection (URI). Symptoms typically include a 2- to 3-day history of rhinitis and slight fever. As these common URI symptoms persist, a cough or wheeze or both begin. Some children respond more quickly to asthma triggers, so exacerbations occur within a short period after exposure. These children may have tachypnea, increased use of accessory muscles (e.g., nasal flaring, retractions), and a prolonged expiratory phase or wheeze or both. Children with sternocleidomastoid retraction and supraclavicular indrawing most often have severe airway obstruction and need rapid assessment of their cardiorespiratory status—including pulse oximetry if available in the office setting—and interventions immediately initiated. Observations regarding degree of dyspnea, retractions, body position, use of abdominal muscles to expel air, and mental status should also be noted. Auscultation for adventitious sounds will elicit the following and represent increasing airway obstruction: prolongation of the expiratory phase, expiratory wheeze, inspiratory and expiratory wheeze, and absence or distancing of breath sounds, which is an ominous sign indicative of little air exchange and possible impending respiratory arrest (Provisional Committee on Quality Improvement, 1994).

Treatment

The current approach to asthma treatment reflects the understanding that airway inflammation seems to be evident in most phases of the illness. Although therapy must be individualized to the particular child, it is now recognized that prevention of symptoms due to underlying inflammation must be treated in addition to treatment of the acute symptoms due to bronchoconstriction (Box 9-2).

Prevention of airway remodeling through appropriate and timely antiinflammatory treatment may help to preserve the child's pulmonary function and activity tolerance as an adult.

In the treatment of the child with asthma, the primary goal is to allow the child to live as normal a life as possible. The child should be able to participate in normal childhood activities, experience exercise tolerance similar to peers, and attend school to grow intellectually and develop socially. Treatments to obtain these goals should be blended into family schedules, and if possible, side effects should minimally interfere with achievement of goals. The 1997 NIH Expert Panel Report II (EPR-II) articulates current best practices on the diagnosis and comprehensive management of asthma (NHLBI, 1997) and should guide decision making. Because knowledge is rapidly expanding in this area, primary care providers must regularly review updated online reports on management strategies.

Shared Management

Educating the family and maturing child to become effective partners with the primary care provider in the day-to-day management of asthma is a primary treatment goal (NHLBI, 1997; Rachelefsky, 1995). Instruction in shared management is a necessary

Box 9-2

Treatment

Shared Management Programs
 I. NHLBI Asthma Education Program
 II. Educational components (see Box 9-3)
 III. Lifelong learning
 IV. Treatment plans
   A. Recognition of early warning signs
     Treatment appropriate to level of severity
       Mild intermittent
       Mild persistent
       Moderate persistent
       Severe persistent
   B. Management of chronic condition
 V. Medications
   A. Long-term controllers
   B. Quick relievers (i.e., rescue medications)

cornerstone in regular health care and requires age-appropriate sharing of responsibilities among family members and the primary care provider. The purposes of shared management education are to help prevent episodes of asthma exacerbation, minimize the severity of episodes that cannot be prevented, enhance the family's ability to understand and implement treatment strategies, and provide healthy responses to life changes that may be necessitated by asthma.

Family education in shared management should promote a sense of teamwork. The foundations should be laid early at diagnosis, with primary care providers drawing families into treatment decisions as their basic knowledge and skills increase.

Individual providers or community organizations recruiting families from a variety of providers have offered formal education programs and developed and extensively tested curricular guides for several programs, which are useful, relatively inexpensive, and easy to implement (Howell, Flaim, and Lung, 1992). Other approaches have successfully used games and camp experiences, most commonly coupled with a formal education program. But consistent with the EPR-II, the primary care provider should play a central role with the family in ensuring a comprehensive mix of ongoing educational experiences for the family and child.

Most asthma education programs contain information on the basic pathophysiology of asthma exacerbation and information on controlling triggers, knowing early warning signs that signal the onset of a problem, managing an exacerbation (i.e., including when to contact the primary care provider), knowing strategies for relaxation and controlled breathing, altering medications according to set guidelines, and solving problems. Programs have shown effectiveness in reducing child and family anxiety, increasing asthma management behavior, improving school attendance, and reducing costly emergency room and hospital use. Before a program is implemented or a child is referred to a program, the primary care provider must review the program to ensure it is consistent with the provider's treatment philosophy; know whether it is an individualized or group approach; and identify the age, child, and type of family for whom the program has previously worked best. When the provider is knowledgeable about the shared man-

agement program and can reinforce learning during routine health care visits with the family, a true child-parent-provider partnership is enhanced to ultimately improve the child's overall health status.

Education must be viewed in the context of lifelong learning. Changes in the child's and family's capabilities and in treatment modalities necessitate ongoing evaluation and provision of further education. This ongoing education helps ensure that as the family gains experience in managing the child's asthma, the depth of their knowledge and skills is enhanced and keeps pace with treatment guidelines.

When the diagnosis of asthma is made during an acute exacerbation, the family first needs education on immediate care, signs of improvement or deterioration that require immediate contact with the provider, immediate environmental changes that could be implemented, and action and side effects of medications being taken. Once the crisis has passed, the provider will want to plan with the family for ongoing, comprehensive asthma education. Families have noted that it takes them up to a year to gain any sense of ease with the full perspective of asthma management. The components of an asthma education program suggested by the EPR-II are listed in Box 9-3.

Specific treatment modalities will depend on the age of the child, severity of disease, medication tolerance, and the ability of the child or family to implement the treatment regimen. A detailed history is necessary when various medications and schedules are considered. The frequency and severity of the episodes will direct intermittent vs. con-

---

Box 9-3

NHLBI Asthma Education Program

Educational Components
- Basic facts about asthma
- Roles of medications
- Skills: inhaler/spacer/holding chamber use
- Self-monitoring
- Environmental control measures
- When and how to take rescue actions

tinuous treatment. Children who quickly develop severe airway obstruction when exposed to a trigger must immediately initiate an action plan of treatment. Identification of triggers helps in developing a plan for avoidance, pretreatment with medications before exposure (e.g., exercise-induced asthma), or initiating treatment with early symptomatology (e.g., begin rescue medication such as bronchodilators, an anti-inflammatory agent, or oral prednisone with signs of respiratory tract infection). Clearly documenting presenting or persistent symptoms over time helps to identify specific components and grading of severity of asthma. Children living in households where individuals smoke may need more intense treatment (Abulhosn et al, 1997).

Treatment of a Child with Asthma

Because asthma is a chronic disease with episodic symptoms, asthma management entails treatment based on the needs or severity of the child's underlying airway pathology. The following four categorizations of asthma severity are currently used: mild intermittent, mild persistent, moderate persistent, and severe persistent (Tables 9-1 and 9-2) These categories are adapted from the EPR-II for severity categorization, description, and treatment. The section detailing therapeutic considerations provides guidance to "step up treatment" if asthma remains uncontrolled or "step down" treatment after control has been achieved (NHLBI, 1997).

Timely treatment of an asthma exacerbation requires recognition of early warning signs of an acute exacerbation in a child and treatment appropriate to the level of severity. These early warning signs may be unique to a particular child (e.g., tickle in the throat, frequent yawning or sighing) or may be fairly common symptoms (e.g., a cough especially at night, tightness in the throat with URI symptoms of a runny nose and congestion, and a decreased peak expiratory flow rate [PEFR] if the child can perform this maneuver). Later symptoms usually include wheezing, shortness of breath, and chest pain or tightness.

Children with mild intermittent asthma need a written action plan to implement in times of exacerbation. Children with persistent asthma need a written daily management plan, as well as a writ-

ten action plan to begin during acute exacerbations. After reviewing the child's usual early warning signs with the primary care provider, parents can be instructed to evaluate their child's respiratory rate, breathlessness, use of accessory muscles, alertness and color and have a mutually agreed upon individualized plan of action to initiate treatment of the exacerbation (NHLBI, 1997). For example, an exacerbation treatment plan might be as follows: (1) begin or increase albuterol medication up to every 4 hours at home, (2) start oral steroid "burst" at prescribed dose if symptoms are not improved after first step of action plan, and (3) notify primary care provider of progress. This type of action plan is meant to reduce the severity and the length of the exacerbation, so that emergent medical care is not needed (Stemple and Redding, 1992).

If the symptoms do not respond to home management, the child will need further evaluation and treatment in a primary care provider's office—if appropriate monitoring and treatment equipment are available—or in an emergency room or hospital setting. These settings offer the added ability to monitor the child's air movement, oxygenation and/or blood gases, administer oxygen as needed, perform spirometry, monitor cardiac and respiratory status continually, and give medications frequently in a controlled environment. Delineated treatment modalities for management of all four severity categorizations of asthma are available to facilitate decision making in any setting (Kemper, 1997; NHLBI, 1997; Rachelefsky, 1995).

Medications

Asthma therapy has changed to reflect the need to focus on reducing the inflammatory processes and combining bronchodilatory medications with anti-inflammatory medications during acute exacerbations. Several types of medications are currently used (Box 9-4). For quick relief, "rescue" medications of short-acting, inhaled b_2-agonists, anticholinergics, and/or systemic corticosteroids are used. A wider array of long-term controller medications includes inhaled or systemic corticosteroids, cromolyn sodium and nedocromil, long-acting b_2-agonists, methylxanthines, and leukotriene modifiers (NHLBI, 1997).

Table 9-1
Asthma Severity Categorization: Infants and Children <5 Years—Therapeutic Considerations

Severity	Long-Term Control	Quick Relief
STEP 1 Mild Intermittent	No daily medicine needed.	• Bronchodilator as needed for symptoms <2 times a week. Intensity of treatment will depend upon severity of exacerbation. Use either: —inhaled short-acting b_2-agonist by nebulizer or face mask and spacer/holding chamber. or: —Oral b_2-agonist for symptoms. • With viral respiratory infection: —bronchodilator q 4 to 6 hours up to 24 hours (longer with physician consult) but, in general, report no more than once every 6 weeks. —consider systemic corticosteroid if current exacerbation is severe OR if patient has history of previous severe exacerbations.
STEP 2 Mild Persistent	Daily antiinflammatory medication. One of the following: • Cromolyn (nebulizer) is preferred; or MDI or nedocromil (MDI only) tid-qid. • Infants and young children usually begin with a trial of cromolyn or nedocromil. or • Low-dose inhaled corticosteroid with spacer/holding chamber and face mask.	• Bronchodilator as needed for symptoms (see STEP 1).
STEP 3 Moderate Persistent	Daily antiinflammatory medication. One of the following: • Medium-dose inhaled corticosteroid with spacer/holding chamber and face mask. Once control is established, • medium-dose inhaled corticosteroid and nedocromil. or: • Medium-dose inhaled corticosteroid and long-acting bronchodilator (theophylline).	• Bronchodilator as needed for symptoms (see STEP 1) up to 3 times a day.
STEP 4 Severe Persistent	Daily antiinflammatory medicine • High-dose inhaled corticosteroid with spacer/holding chamber and face mask. • If needed, add systemic corticosteroids 2 mg/kg/day and reduce to lowest daily or alternate-day dose that stabilizes symptoms.	• Bronchodilator as needed for symptoms (see STEP 1) up to 3 times a day.

Notes:
Gain control as quickly as possible, then decrease treatment to the least medication necessary to maintain control. Gaining control may be accomplished by either starting treatment at the step most appropriate to the initial severity of the condition or by starting at a higher level of therapy (e.g., a course of systemic corticosteroids or higher dose of inhaled corticosteroids).
A rescue course of systemic corticosteroid (prednisolone) may be needed at any time and step.
• In general, use of short-acting b_2-agonist >3 or 4 times in 1 day or regular use on a daily basis indicates the need for additional therapy.
• It is important to remember that there are very few studies on asthma therapy for infants.
The stepwise approach presents guidelines to assist clinical decision making. Asthma is highly variable, so clinicians should tailor specific medication plans to the needs and circumstances of individual patients.
• Consultation with an asthma specialist is recommended for patients in this age group requiring STEP 3 or STEP 4 care. Consider consultation for patients in this are group requiring STEP 2 care.
↓ Step down: Review treatment every 1 to 6 months. If control is sustained for at least 3 months, a gradual stepwise reduction in treatment may be possible.
↑ Step up: If control is not achieved, consider step up. But first: review patient medication technique, adherence, and environmental control (i.e., avoidance of allergens or other precipitant factors).

Table 9-2
Asthma Severity Categorization: Children >5 years*

Severity	Description	Therapeutic Considerations for the Treatment of Asthma: Adults and Children >5 Years
STEP 1† Mild Intermittent	Symptoms ≤2/weeks; asymptomatic; brief exacerbations. Nighttime symptoms ≤2/month. FEV_1 or PEF >80% predicted; PEF variability <20%.	• No daily medication needed. • Use inhaled short-acting b_2-agonist as needed for symptoms. If short-acting b_2-agonist is needed more than twice a week, the child should be moved to the next step of care.
STEP 2† Mild Persistent	Symptoms >2/week but <1/day. Exacerbations may affect activity. Nighttime symptoms >2/month. FEV_1 or PEF ≥80% predicted, PEF variability 20 to 30%.	• Add inhaled corticosteroid (low doses), cromolyn, or nedocromil. (Children usually begin with cromolyn or nedocromil.) • Sustained-release theophylline is a nonpreferred alternative. Leukotriene modifiers may also be considered for children ≥12 years of age. Use a spacer/holding chamber and rinse mouth after inhalation to limit local and systemic toxicity from inhaled corticosteroids.
STEP 3† Moderate Persistent	Daily symptoms; daily use of inhaled short-acting beta$_2$-agonists. Exacerbations affect activity. Exacerbations ≥2/week. Nighttime symptoms >1/week. FEV_1 or PEF >60% to <80% predicted, PEF variability >30%.	• Use either an inhaled corticosteroid (medium dose) OR an inhaled corticosteroid (low-medium dose) AND a long-acting bronchodilator (inhaled preferred)‡ or, if needed. • Inhaled corticosteroids (medium-high dose) AND long-acting bronchodilator (inhaled preferred)‡ • Salmeterol (Serevent), a long-acting inhaled b_2-agonist, is a maintenance medication not to be used to reverse acute symptoms or exacerbations. Use a short-acting b_2-agonist for these events. Salmeterol may be beneficial especially for nighttime symptom control. Prevention of inhaled corticosteroid dose escalation has been demonstrated. Patients should be instructed not to stop antiinflammatory therapy even though their symptoms may improve with salmeterol. Salmeterol should not be used more than twice a day.
STEP 4† Severe Persistent	Continual symptoms; limited physical activity; frequent exacerbations; frequent nighttime symptoms. FEV_1 or PEF ≤60% predicted, PEF variability >30%.	• Use inhaled corticosteroid (high-dose) AND a long-acting bronchodilator (inhaled preferred)‡ AND oral corticosteroid tablets or syrup long-term. • Short course of systemic steroids may be used to establish control. For long-term, use the lowest effective dose of systemic steroid possible and consider alternate-day dosing to minimize toxicity.

*Adapted from the National Heart, Lung, and Blood Institute: Expert panel report II: guidelines for the diagnosis and management of asthma, National Institutes of Health publication 97-4051:45-48, 1997.
†Use short-acting inhaled b_2-agonist as needed for symptoms.
‡Long-acting bronchodilator; long-acting inhaled b_2-agonist, long-acting b_2-agonist tablets or sustained-release theophylline.

For most children the first medication chosen for symptomatic treatment of an acute exacerbation is a quick-acting b_2-adrenergic agent such as albuterol, which inhibits the early phase bronchospastic response. All b_2-adrenergics can cause increased heart rate and may cause tremor of the fingers or hands. Hyperactivity, irritability, and sleeplessness are also noted by some parents of young children. Using an air compressor with an updraft nebulizer to deliver a b_2-adrenergic med-

> ## Box 9-4
> # Medications
>
> ### Long-Term Control Medications
> *Corticosteroids*
> Most potent and effective antiinflammatory medication currently available. Inhaled form is used in the long-term control of asthma. Systemic corticosteroids are often used to gain prompt control of the disease when initiating long-term therapy.
>
> - **Cromolyn sodium and nedocromil:** Mild-to-moderate antiinflammatory medications. May be used as initial choice for long-term control therapy for children. Can also be used as preventive treatment prior to exercise or unavoidable exposure to known allergens.
> - **Long-acting beta₂-agonists:** Long-acting bronchodilator used concomitantly with antiinflammatory medications for long-term control of symptoms, especially nocturnal symptoms. Also prevents exercise-induced bronchospasm (EIB).
> - **Methylxanthines:** Sustained-release theophylline is a mild-to-moderate bronchodilator used principally as adjuvant to inhaled corticosteroids for prevention of nocturnal asthma symptoms. May have a mild antiinflammatory effect.
> - **Leukotriene modifiers:** Zafirlukast, a leukotriene receptor antagonist, or zileuton, a 5-lipoxygenase inhibitor, may be considered an alternative therapy to low doses of inhaled corticosteroids or cromolyn or nedocromil for
>
> children at least 12 years of age with mild persistent asthma, although further clinical experience and study are needed to establish their roles in asthma therapy.
> - **Montelukast:** Available as a QD 5 to 10 mg chewable tablet for children at least 6 years of age. It has been shown to be clinically effective in mild-moderate persistent asthma as a steroid sparing adjunct and for exercise-induced symptoms (Stohlmeyer, 1998).
>
> ### Quick-Relief Medications
> *Short-acting beta₂-agonists*
> Therapy of choice for relief of acute symptoms and prevention of EIB.
>
> - **Anticholinergics:** Ipratropium bromide may provide some additive benefit to inhaled beta₂-agonists in severe exacerbations. May be an alternative bronchodilator for children who do not tolerate inhaled beta₂-agonists.
> - **Systemic corticosteroids:** Used for moderate-to-severe exacerbations to speed recovery and prevent recurrence of exacerbations.
>
> Asthma Severity Categorization: Children >5 years (see Table 9-1)
>
> Asthma Severity Categorization: Infants and Children <5 years (Table 9-2)

ication is common; but children as young as 4 years of age may be able to use a metered dose inhaler (MDI, or puffer) if a spacer is used with it. A spacer is a chamber that attaches to the MDI, allowing the medicine to be puffed into the chamber. The child can then inhale from the spacer to receive the medication, which avoids having to coordinate compressing the MDI while slowly inhaling. Dry powder inhalers (DPIs), which involve inhaling a powdered form of the medication but do not require a coordinated effort like an MDI, are now being used to deliver a variety of medications. Delivery devices are also now being altered to reduce environmental chlorofluorocarbons (CFCs). Because of the wide variety of delivery devices

available—each with unique steps to activate, providers should diligently review the directions for proper use.

Nebulized treatments offer several advantages, including the following: (1) direct deposition of aerosolized medication in the respiratory tract, (2) decreased side effects, (3) better delivery than an MDI when the tidal volume is reduced during an acute episode, and (4) the ability to mix b_2-adrenergic medications with other medications (e.g., cromolyn sodium or atropine). Oral syrups containing b_2-adrenergic agents are also available but cause hyperactivity in many children. For convenience, some older children prefer to take a pill rather than use an MDI, and therapeutic adherence may be improved if adolescents are given this choice.

When a child experiences EIB, either a b_2-agonist or an antiinflammatory agent (e.g., cromolyn) can be used to block the symptoms that inhibit the child's continued exercise. These agents should be taken approximately 15 minutes before participation in scheduled exercise. Serevent (Salmeterol xinafoate), a long acting b_2-agonist, is administered via an MDI or DPI twice daily (i.e., approximately 12 hours apart) for individuals experiencing daily asthma symptoms—especially nocturnal symptoms—and those who need long-lasting protection against exercise-induced symptoms. Severent, however, is only for routine use and not for treatment of exacerbations. The addition of short-acting b_2 medications such as albuterol is still required for intervening symptoms (Mirgalia de Guidudici et al, 1995).

Leukotriene modifiers are a relatively new class of medications that attempt to intervene earlier in the inflammatory cascade. Montelukast, a leukotriene inhibitor, is approved for children 6 years of age as opposed to zafirlukast and zileuton, which are approved for ages 12 and older (Frost and Spahn, 1998). Montelukast decreases arachidonic acid metabolites, leading to inflammatory mediator release of leukotrienes, which activate neutrophils and eosinophils, produce mucus, and constrict airways. Further investigation regarding the use of montelukast as a steroid sparing medication for use with atopic children and children with EIB is under way (Stohlmeyer, 1998).

Antiinflammatory agents are used as the first-choice preventive medication for asthma because they inhibit both the early and the late phase response. These agents are best known as mast cell stabilizers but may have other inhibitory effects on inflammatory cells. Cromolyn delivered by nebulizer or MDI is given two to four times daily. One treatment per day is not sufficient for maintenance therapy. Cromolyn is compatible for delivery by a hand-held nebulizer when mixed with b_2-adrenergics or anticholinergics. Nedocromil is another nonsteroidal, antiinflammatory medication that is unique in chemical structure and appears to have a synergistic effect with inhaled steroids (Mosby, 1998). Nedocromil inhibits the release of inflammatory chemotactic and smooth muscle-contracting mediators from eosinophils, neutro-

phils, and mast cells. It has been more effective than cromolyn with regard to antigen and exercise-induced symptoms in some individuals and should be considered as part of a preventive therapeutic plan. Although usually well-tolerated, the most significant disadvantage to nedocromil has been its undesirable taste, so it is best administered with a spacer to minimize this effect. Recommended dosage is two puffs qid or tid initially, which, based on the response, may then be reduced to bid (Mosby, 1998).

Corticosteroids inhibit the late phase asthmatic response and are used to treat inflammation and edema associated with asthma. Children who do not responding adequately to b_2-adrenergics and cromolyn will require long-term inhaled corticosteroid therapy. Triamcinolone acetate and beclomethasone have long been used as inhaled corticosteroids. Budesonide and fluticasone are two other inhaled corticosteroids that appear to reduce airway obstruction, as well as reduce the number of inflammatory cells in the airways and the number of asthma exacerbations (Mosby, 1998). Both are highly potent corticosteroids that have lower systemic bioavailability as measured by plasma cortisol levels compared with the currently prescribed inhaled medications (Fabbri et al, 1993). One advantage of budesonide is that it can be nebulized for children under 4 or 5 years of age who are unable to reliably use an MDI with a spacer and must take oral steroids for antiinflammatory effects. Nebulized budesonide, however, is awaiting FDA approval in the United States. Fluticasone is available in three different concentrations and in both MDI and DPI devices.

Children on long-term asthma therapy may require systemic corticosteroid treatment when severe asthma exacerbations occur. Children who need corticosteroid therapy more than once every 6 weeks to manage symptoms may require a daily or every other day treatment program with systemic corticosteroids (NHLBI, 1997) and require evaluation of the need for long-term controller therapy. Reevaluation is needed every 3 to 4 months. By 4 to 6 years of age, children may be able to use inhaled corticosteroids via MDI with a spacer or other device and reduce their need for systemic treatment. Spacers with masks are also an option for children under 4 years of age who need inhaled steroids. Children using a spacer with inhaled steroids should always rinse their mouth and spit and wipe the facial area that was covered by the mask after use to prevent development of thrush.

When a child is receiving continuous systemic corticosteroid therapy, complications may occur. Such complications include development of a cushingoid appearance, growth suppression, eye abnormalities (e.g., glaucoma or cataracts), osteoporosis with development of pathologic vertebral fractures, hypertension, glycosuria, menstrual disturbances, and peptic ulceration. At each visit a thorough interval history is necessary to determine any adverse effects from corticosteroid therapy. In addition, growth and blood pressure should be monitored at each well-child visit. Other tests (e.g., urinalysis or ophthalmic examination) are indicated when a child is on long-term, high-dose corticosteroid therapy. Referral to the pulmonary-allergy specialist is warranted when adverse side effects of corticosteroid therapy are detected.

In order to prevent problems with growth suppression, impaired bone mineralization, or an effect on the hypothalamus-pituitary-adrenal (HPA) axis, whenever possible, the dose of both oral, inhaled and topical corticosteroids should be adjusted to the lowest level necessary to maintain asthma symptom control. An awareness of cumulative corticosteroid effects must be maintained even with children on medium- to high-dose inhaled corticosteroids (Heuck et al, 1998).

Anticholinergic agents (e.g., ipratropium bromide) block cholinergic reflex bronchoconstriction and may be most useful in children with bronchitic symptoms of increased mucous secretion when used with b_2-agonists and or anti-inflammatory agents. These agents, however, are not particularly helpful against allergic challenges and neither block late-phase response nor inhibit mediators from mast cells. Ipratropium bromide is the only anticholinergic drug currently approved for treatment of airway disease. Delivery of ipratropium is by MDI or nebulizer and can be mixed with albuterol and cromolyn sodium for the convenience of providing three medications with one aerosol treatment. Side effects include dry mucous membranes, cutaneous flush, and fever. Behavioral and neurologic symptoms can occur with central nervous system toxicity (Zorc, Ogborn, and Pusic, 1998).

Some children may benefit from the addition of theophylline if asthma is not controlled by anti-inflammatory and b_2-adrenergic agents. Methylxanthines in combination with b_2-adrenergics work synergistically to produce bronchodilation and may improve control of nocturnal asthma symptoms in particular. A high level of provider and family monitoring is necessary, however. Metabolism of theophylline varies among individuals and age groups, as does serious toxicity with possible permanent CNS side effects; therefore the dose must be individually adjusted by monitoring theophylline levels in the blood. For children in the ambulatory setting, a level of 15 µg/ml should be the upper limit because theophylline metabolism is affected by many factors, and this level provides a safe buffer if the theophylline level rises. Some children have a therapeutic response with as low of a level as 5 µg/ml and will not need an increase in their maintenance dose (Chernik and Boat, 1998).

Theophylline levels should be initially obtained after 2 to 4 days because a steady state is reached in an average of 40 hours in adults (Mosby, 1998). Levels also must be rechecked at least every 6 to 12 months. The theophylline dose may need to be significantly adjusted and levels rechecked when there are signs of toxicity or when the child experiences persistent or recurring asthma episodes on maintenance medications or is acutely ill. Side effects of theophylline include nausea, hyperactivity, and restlessness. Signs of toxicity that indicate an immediate need to determine the theophylline level include severe headaches, abdominal pain, vomiting, or any combination of these. Seizures are also a sign of severe toxicity and require immediate intervention and hospital admission.

Recent and Anticipated Advances in Diagnosis and Management

There is increasing thought that delayed diagnosis and undertreatment of childhood asthma may contribute to increased pulmonary dysfunction in adults (Warner, Naspitz, and Cropp, 1998). Thus health service researchers are testing new models of care that not only aggressively treat asthma in children but also actively seek to identify undiagnosed children. In addition to free running methods, self-report on standardized questions linked to video scenario displays are useful in identifying school-age and adolescent populations experiencing the burdens of asthma symptoms but not yet diagnosed or under treatment (Redding et al, 1998). With more research the EPR-II (NHLBI, 1997, p. 3b-3) approaches of either starting with high-dose therapy and stepping down or gradually stepping up therapy may be further explicated.

New medications and delivery devices continue to be developed and tested. Single-isomer b_2-agonists (e.g., levalbuterol) may be added to formularies. All CFC-based MDIs should soon be replaced. Devices such as the portable Smartmist Respiratory Management System (ARADIGM), which coordinates delivery with inhalation and provides visual feedback on a child's accurate performance, may become common. Computerized monitoring devices, such as the Air Watch Asthma Monitor or LifeChart (ENACT Health Management Systems, Inc.), which can store and transmit PEF and FEV_1 cumulative results and provide a 30-day summary, will soon be readily available. Then they must be investigated for their effect on client outcomes.

Families increasingly acknowledge their concurrent use of alternative therapies (Andrews et al, 1998; Malthouse, 1997). More research examining the short- and long-term outcomes of alternative therapies and their joint use with mainstream protocols is necessary.

Associated Problems (Box 9-5)

Allergies

All children who have allergies do not have asthma, but the majority of children with asthma have allergies. These allergies can be in the form of atopic dermatitis or allergic rhinitis. Allergic triggers may include foods such as peanuts or, less frequently, cow's milk, soy, egg, wheat, fish, and powder used with latex products (Kelso, 1998; Mahan and Arlin, 1992). Animal dander, pollens from trees, grasses, weeds, or a variety of other substances (e.g., feathers, lamb's wool, and house dust mites) are also common allergens. If there is a strong history of allergic reactions associated with respiratory symptoms, testing to determine specific problematic allergens may be beneficial. Avoid-

---

Box 9-5
Associated Problems

Additional allergies
Aspirin sensitivity
Gastrointestinal reflux

---

ance techniques and allergy immunotherapy may then be helpful. Antihistamines for treatment of allergic rhinitis may also help relieve the postnasal drip that can accompany sinusitis symptoms, which can trigger an asthma episode (Zacharisen and Kelly, 1998).

Medications

Aspirin and nonsteroidal antiinflammatory agents may precipitate an asthma episode in adults and possibly in children. Although aspirin is rarely indicated in children, these substances should be avoided and parents taught about reading over-the-counter drug labels because aspirin can be combined with other substances in certain drugs—especially cold remedies. Leukotriene modifiers may be useful in preventing aspirin idiosyncratic reactions (Frost and Spahn, 1998).

Gastroesophageal Reflux

Gastroesophageal reflux (GER) is found in many children with chronic lung disease. Reflux of gastric secretions into the esophagus can initiate a vagal response with an increased production of airway secretions. Theophylline is known to increase gastric secretion and decrease esophageal pressure and thus may aggravate GER in some children. Management of GER includes upright positioning following thickened feedings for infants and use of medications that reduce acidity or increase gastric motility.

Prognosis

The mild to moderate asthma of many children can be controlled with effort from the child, family, and health provider. Some children will have refractory asthma, which may be caused by poor implementation of the treatment plan, severe labile asthma, or corticosteroid resistance. Psychosocial difficulties in families also can complicate asthma and its management. Chronic uncontrolled asthma may lead to persistent airway inflammation and airway remodeling. Although some children seemingly outgrow their asthma, some who experience a disappearance of symptoms during the teen years or early adulthood will have symptoms return and/or increase in severity with age (Weiss, 1995).

Mortality from asthma is increasing again after a slight fall from 1989 to 1990. Death rates have increased in all age groups with the highest mortality occurring in African-Americans and the greatest proportional increase in the 10- to 14-year-old age group (Sly, 1994). Many factors may contribute to the increased rate of reported mortality, including increased severity of the disease, undertreatment or misuse of pharmacologic treatment, failure to recognize severity of asthma symptoms, delay in initiating treatment, and psychosocial factors.

PRIMARY CARE MANAGEMENT

Health Care Maintenance

Growth and Development

There is evidence that asthma is not outgrown; persistent changes remain in the pulmonary tract of adults with asthma who have been free of symptoms for many years. Therefore asthma must be considered a chronic condition that may affect growth and development throughout life. As always, it is essential that the practitioner consistently measure height and weight and record these measurements on the child's growth grid. Any major deviation from the population norms (i.e., less than the 10th or above the 90th percentile) or departure (i.e., two or more zones) from the child's individualized curve should be noted and assessed in further detail. Smaller alterations may need to be monitored. During a series of acute exacerbations of asthma, the primary care provider may note a plateau or small drop in weight; but with improvement in health status, catch-up growth should oc-

cur. If it does not occur, the cause of the weight loss should be further explored. Genetic, social, and nutritional factors that are potentially unassociated with asthma must be considered.

Investigators continue to explore whether asthma has a direct influence on growth. It has been associated with delay in the onset of puberty (Reid, 1992), but controversy remains on the extent to which medications used to treat asthma may also diminish growth velocity (Crowley et al, 1995). Of asthma medications, corticosteroids are most frequently associated with delayed growth. Controversies remain about the possible effect on growth of the dose and frequency of administration of even inhaled corticosteroids (Brook, 1998; Heuck et al, 1998). Primary care providers should be concerned if a prepubescent or pubescent child uses inhaled steroids more than 12 puffs per day or a medium- to high-dose of inhaled corticosteroids. Concern might necessitate reevaluation of the comprehensive management regimen (NHLBI, 1997). Although the adolescent growth spurt may be slightly delayed, with optimal management of the disease, maximal height attainment is thought to be possible in children with asthma. The better the daily management and control of acute exacerbations, the more likely full height will be obtained at the age-appropriate time.

Standard infant, child, and adolescent assessment tools are appropriate for use in assessing development (see Chapter 2). Research has documented both normal and delayed development in children with asthma, with delayed development not necessarily related to the physiologic severity of the asthma but to the imposed limitations placed on a child's experiences (Taylor and Newacheck, 1992). Limitations typically involve reductions in physical activity and social experiences, including day care and school attendance. Therefore practitioners should encourage normalization of experiences whenever possible to reduce the unnecessary negative effect on development.

If there are instances when normal experiences must be discouraged to avoid specific asthma triggers, primary care providers should assist parents and children to identify alternative experiences that could provide developmental stimulation. For example, if the child cannot play competitive soccer because of grass allergy, the child and family should be helped to identify an alternate sport, such as basketball or swimming allow the child to exercise and participate in a competitive team sport and provide the opportunity to engage in an age-appropriate social and skill-building activity. Without normalized experiences a child's self-image, self-esteem, perception of bodily control, and overall level of health are likely to be reduced and anxiety, fear, and dependent behavior increased (Creer et al, 1992). If these feelings and/or behaviors develop, consultation with or referral to a mental health practitioner should be considered.

Parents and children may limit strenuous activity because of repeated exacerbations or fear of exacerbations. If such limitations are often placed, the primary care provider should assist family members in building an exercise habit into their daily routine and devising a treatment plan that supports such activity, which will help avoid a sedentary life pattern that may lower the child's sense of physical accomplishment and result in unwanted weight gain.

Unnecessary limitation of a child's activity may be particularly harmful because children connect activity with health and may limit activity even further, possibly producing a downward spiral of self-perception. Integration of children into sports programs has been associated with positive clinical outcomes. Helping a child find an enjoyable sport should be a significant goal for primary care providers.

There are reports of impaired cognitive development in children with repeated brief school absences. Similar impairment has been linked to some medications used to manage asthma, but the demonstrated negative effect of medications on cognitive capabilities is not universal and still being investigated. Prevention and swift, adequate management of exacerbations will reduce the number and length of school absences, thus limiting what is thought to contribute most to the impairment of cognitive development.

Diet

Today's children and families eat many meals away from home, so dietary restrictions could effect family habits. Sulfites, which were previously used to enhance the appearance of many fresh foods, have been implicated in severe asthma exacerbations in some children. Although sulfite levels and uses have decreased, the FDA has ruled that foods containing sulfites must be clearly labeled. Sulfites can still be found in processed potatoes, shrimp, dried fruits, molasses, nonfrozen lemon and lime juices, and labeled bulk preparations of fruits and vegetables (Rachelefsky, 1995). There are no other special dietary requirements for children with asthma unless a child has concurrent food allergies. When food allergies are present, primary care providers must be familiar with alternative sources of the nutrients in the eliminated foods. If local grocery stores do not carry the alternative food sources, health food stores, dairy councils, or American Lung Association affiliates may be of assistance in locating the necessary items. Alternatively, primary health care providers may refer families to a local dietitian for consultation. When a child has multiple food allergies, such referral is critical.

Safety

All age-appropriate family safety precautions must also be considered for the child with asthma. Primary care providers should furnish anticipatory guidance in this area and be familiar with age-typical risks. Equipment and medications used to prevent or treat asthma exacerbations in the home may present additional concerns for safety.

Electrical burns are possible when equipment (e.g., nebulizers) is run in the child's presence. Infants and young children should never be left alone where they can reach the equipment, cord, or open socket. School-age children and adolescents should be properly instructed in the safe use of electrical equipment and should demonstrate their use to parents or the primary care provider before being encouraged to use the equipment independently.

Medications kept in the home must be safely stored in their original containers in a locked location that is inaccessible to infants and young children. Because children will ultimately need to develop age-appropriate responsibility for medication administration, families will need help to evaluate how to do this safely.

Practitioners can help parents identify their child's developmental capabilities and limits for safely assisting in the medication regimen by providing age-normative suggestions. For example, when a child is an infant or toddler, the parents must speak about the medications as such—not as candy. With maturation, toddlers can be taught how to help take medicine from a spoon or hold the nebulizer mask to assist in therapy. Preschool-age children typically have the manual dexterity to take part in the medicinal therapy by helping parents pour the medication or, in the parent's presence, take the capsule from the container. Young, school-age children may be asked to get the medication and take it in the presence of a parent. When older school-age children can tell time, they can assume greater responsibility to prompt the parent when the medication is needed, get the medication, take the medication in the parent's presence, and return it to its proper storage place. School-age children should also become increasingly responsible for taking needed medication while at school. Parents can monitor and encourage safe and knowledgeable use by discussing or having a child count and record on a calendar the number of times medication was taken as required. As a child grows to adolescence, more autonomy should be given for independently purchasing, taking, and replenishing both routine and prn medication. Parents need to be reminded, however, that one consistent finding in successful adolescent adherence to prescribed regimens is the continued support and age-appropriate assistance of their parents. This support is not shown by "doing for" or "nagging" adolescents but by demonstrating faith in their capabilities and offering assistance with any problems that arise. Thus parents can maintain an interested, interdependent attitude to best assist an adolescent in growing in the shared management of asthma (Vessey and Miola, 1997).

There has been concern about the safe use of inhaled medications by persons of all ages. This concern is greatest for children too young to fully appreciate temporal relationships. Although inhaled medications are considered safe and uniquely effective in directly delivering a therapeutic dose of medication to the target organ, their use by children must be monitored by the family and the primary care provider. The child's skill in using the inhaler should be observed at each visit with the practitioner. Even many adults have difficulty in this maneuver. Up to 50% of children who do not receive such monitoring and corrective prompting for proper technique do not use the inhaler effectively. Use of spacers with MDIs for all age groups lessens these problems and enhances proper medication deposition. New, breath-activated devices may also help.

With age and increasing time spent away from parents, children must independently recognize when their treatment is not as effective as expected and seek the assistance of their parent or another adult. An episode that does not respond to treatment in the manner expected may herald a particularly severe exacerbation requiring medical assistance. Simple mnemonic devices are helpful in this regard. A rhyme of "twice is nice but three needs more than me" could be a mnemonic device used to teach children their individual asthma plan (i.e., they can try their quick-relief inhaler twice, but if symptoms persist and they feel the need to use it a third time, they should discuss it with a parent or health care provider). In addition to mnemonics, however, is the need for a written action plan for daily long-term control, as well as a plan to be implemented if an acute exacerbation begins.

Immunizations

The most recent recommendations of the Committee on Infectious Diseases (1997) should guide immunization decisions. Although it has been suggested by some that vaccination with live virus vaccines may lead to airway inflammation and therefore increased hyperresponsivity in children with asthma, the standard schedule of immunizations is recommended. Accordingly, guidelines for live-virus vaccination of children receiving corticosteroids are as follows:

- Topical therapy: Administration of topical corticosteroids, either on the skin or in the respiratory system (i.e., by aerosol of corticosteroids), usually does not result in immunosuppression that would contraindicate administration of live-virus vaccines. If clinical or laboratory evidence of systemic immunosuppression results from their prolonged application, however, live-virus vaccines should not be given until corticosteroid therapy as been discontinued for at least 1 month.

- Low or moderate doses of systemic corticosteroids given daily or on alternate days: Children receiving less than 2 mg/kg per day of prednisone or its equivalent or less than 20 mg or more daily if they weigh more than 10 kg can receive live-virus vaccines while on treatment.
- High doses of systemic corticosteroids given daily or on alternative days for less than 14 days: Children receiving 2 mg/kg per day or more of prednisone or its equivalent or 20 mg or more daily if they weigh more than 10 kg, can receive live-virus vaccines immediately after discontinuation of treatment. Some experts, however, would delay immunization until 2 weeks after corticosteroid therapy has been discontinued if possible (i.e., if the child's condition allows temporary cessation).
- High doses of systemic corticosteroids given daily or on alternate days for 14 days or more: Children receiving 2 mg/kg per day or more of prednisone or its equivalent or 20 mg or more daily if they weigh more than 10 kg should not receive live-virus vaccines until steroid therapy has been discontinued for at least 1 month (Committee on Infectious Diseases, 1997, p. 52).

If a child has egg sensitivity, treatment equipment for anaphylactic reactions should be readily available in the office and the child should be observed for up to 90 minutes after immunization.

Although infants and children with asthma may have signs of respiratory infection more often, these signs alone—in the absence of specific contraindication—should not be the basis for deferring immunizations (Committee on Infectious Diseases, 1997). Inadequate immunization with subsequent risk of infection is of great concern. Individualized assessment of the child with respiratory symptoms, including progressive signs of pulmonary dysfunction, should guide decisions about immunization. Delayed immunizations should be rescheduled as soon as possible. Special brief appointments (e.g., when the child is afebrile) may be needed to ensure adequate immunization during early childhood.

Children with asthma may experience complications with influenza (e.g., increased wheezing, fluctuating theophylline levels, bronchitis, pneumonia, increased school absences, and increased medical care visits). Therefore, despite recent or current prednisone bursts, children with asthma should annually receive an influenza vaccine after the age of 6 months (Committee on Infectious Diseases, 1997; Fairchok et al, 1998). The subviron (split) vaccine is given to children under 13 years of age in the fall before influenza season. Children without prior vaccination may require two doses to develop a satisfactory antibody response. If a child has had a related strain vaccine previously, one dose is thought to be adequate to confer protection. Children with severe, anaphylactic reactions to chicken or eggs generally should not receive the immunization given the risk, the need for yearly vaccination, and the availability of chemoprophylaxis (Committee on Infectious Diseases, 1997). Before 6 months of age and in the presence of contraindications to influenza vaccination, alternative treatment methods should be considered. These methods include immunization of contacts or treatment of influenza with amantadine or rimantadine if the child is over 1 year of age (Committee on Infectious Diseases, 1997). The influenza vaccine may be given at the same time as measles-mumps-rubella (MMR), DTP or DTaP, Varivax Hepatitis A and B, and oral polio vaccines. Pneumococcal immunization is not recommended.

Screening (Box 9-6)

Vision: Routine screening is recommended unless the child is taking daily high-dose corticosteroids because these drugs are known to cause inflammatory changes, cataracts, and glaucoma. If abnormal findings are identified during an eye examination the child should be referred to an ophthalmologist.

Hearing: Routine screening is recommended.

Dental: Routine screening is recommended.

Blood pressure: Blood pressure should be evaluated at each visit if the child is on b_2-adrenergic agents and/or corticosteroids are used regularly.

Box 9-6

Screening

Routine childhood screening
Vision—see text
Hearing—routine
Dental—routine
Blood pressure—see text
Urinalysis—see text
Tuberculosis—routine

Condition-specific screening
Lung function
Spirometry
Peak expiratory flow rate
Theophylline levels
Allergic triggers

Hematocrit: Routine screening is recommended.

Urinalysis: Routine screening is recommended unless the child is taking high-dose corticosteroids daily, which may cause glycosuria. If glycosuria is present the child should be referred to a pulmonary allergy specialist for evaluation.

Tuberculosis: Routine screening is recommended.

Condition-Specific Screening

Lung Function   Monitoring lung function is essential to assess immediate function, as well as to identify long-term trends. Pulmonary function testing should be done to establish lung function baseline levels when a child is well. Referral to a specialist for spirometry in children with moderate or severe disease may be warranted to monitor lung function and thus direct appropriate treatment. Spirometry, recording the forced expiratory flow in 25 to 75 seconds (FEF 25-75) and the forced expiratory flow in 1 second (FEV), assesses severity of airway obstruction. Table 9-3 lists pulmonary function norms.

Spirometry tests are recommended at initial assessment, with treatment changes and stabilization and minimally every 1 to 2 years after that. Peak flow meters are more commonly used in the primary care office to measure the greatest rate of air flow during a forced exhalation. This measurement is labeled the peak expiratory flow rate (PEFR). PEFR, however, is effort-dependent and only reflects large airway function. Thus if a child is obviously in respiratory distress or unwilling to cooperate, a PEFR may not be obtainable. Measurements of PEFR over time will establish an individual's baseline personal best effort for continuous assessment and may or may not reflect average expected PEFR values listed in Table 9-3. PEFR should not be expected to replace spirometry measurements.

Children who cannot or will not recognize airway obstruction or those with very labile asthma can use a home peak flow meter to monitor their asthma. Indeed, most primary care providers advocate the systematic use of peak flow meters for all children with moderate to severe asthma (NHLBI, 1997). These meters are inexpensive, fairly easy to use, and provide a detailed record of airway reactivity in the morning and evening. These objective data are used to individualize the child's treatment plan—often in the form of a three-zone action plan (Table 9-4). These meters can help the child, family, and provider decide when to initiate early treatment and to evaluate the response to treatment.

Theophylline Levels   Because theophylline preparations come in quick-release (i.e., every 6 to 8 hours), sustained-release (i.e., every 8 to 12 hours), or ultra–sustained-release (i.e., every 24 hours) forms, monitoring theophylline levels is determined by the preparation or reason for the level. In general, it is best to follow the manufacturer's guidelines for measuring theophylline levels. The level should be drawn at the same time (e.g., always 4 hours after the dose of a sustained-release preparation) to ensure consistency in level monitoring. In the case of suspected theophylline toxicity, levels should be ordered immediately (Table 9-5).

Allergic History   A biannual review of possible environmental allergens and irritants is helpful. In addition to identification of asthma triggers, this review provides a time to discuss other health issues (e.g., parent or adolescent smoking, avoidance of triggers, dust control, or desirability of allergy skin testing). Asthma shared-management education can

Table 9-3
Pulmonary Function Norms

Height		FVC (L)				
cm	in	Boys	Girls	FEV$_1$ (L)	PEFR (L/min)	FEF 25-75 (L/sec)
100	39.4	1.00	1.00	0.70	100	0.90
102	40.2	1.03	1.00	0.75	110	0.99
104	40.9	1.08	1.07	0.82	120	1.08
106	41.7	1.14	1.10	0.89	130	1.16
108	42.5	1.19	1.19	0.97	140	1.25
110	43.3	1.27	1.24	1.01	150	1.34
112	44.1	1.32	1.30	1.10	160	1.43
114	44.9	1.40	1.36	1.17	174	1.51
116	45.7	1.47	1.41	1.23	185	1.60
118	46.5	1.52	1.49	1.30	195	1.69
120	47.2	1.60	1.55	1.39	204	1.78
122	48.0	1.69	1.62	1.45	215	1.86
124	48.8	1.75	1.70	1.53	226	1.95
126	49.6	1.82	1.77	1.59	236	2.04
128	50.4	1.90	1.84	1.67	247	2.12
130	51.2	1.99	1.90	1.72	256	2.21
132	52.0	2.07	2.00	1.80	267	2.30
134	52.8	2.15	2.06	1.89	278	2.39
136	53.5	2.24	2.15	1.98	289	2.47
138	54.3	2.35	2.24	2.06	299	2.56
140	55.1	2.40	2.32	2.11	310	2.65
142	55.9	2.50	2.40	2.20	320	2.74
144	56.7	2.60	2.50	2.30	330	2.82
146	57.5	2.70	2.59	2.39	340	2.91
148	58.3	2.79	2.68	2.48	351	3.00
150	59.1	2.88	2.78	2.57	362	3.09
152	59.8	2.97	2.88	2.66	373	3.17
154	60.6	3.09	2.98	2.75	384	3.26
156	61.4	3.20	3.09	2.88	394	3.35
158	62.2	3.30	3.18	2.98	404	3.44
160	63.0	3.40	3.27	3.06	415	3.52
162	63.8	3.52	3.40	3.18	425	3.61
164	64.6	3.64	3.50	3.29	436	3.70
166	65.4	3.78	3.60	3.40	446	3.78
168	66.1	3.90	3.72	3.50	457	3.87
170	66.9	4.00	3.83	3.65	467	3.96
172	67.7	4.20	3.83	3.80	477	4.05
174	68.5	4.20	3.83	3.80	488	4.13
176	69.3	4.20	3.83	3.80	498	4.22

Adapted from Polgar G and Promadhar V: Pulmonary function testing in children: techniques and standards, Philadelphia, 1971, W.B. Saunders.

Table 9-4
Zone Action Plan

Zone	PEFR (Best or predicted for age)	Action
Green	80% to 100%	All clear, continue regular management plan
Yellow	50% to 80%	Caution, implement action plan predetermined with primary care provider
Red	50% or less	Medical alert, implement action plan predetermined with primary care provider; if PEFR does not return to yellow or green zone, call provider

Table 9-5
Factors Affecting Serum of Theophylline Levels

	Factors increasing serum levels due to decreased clearance	Factors decreasing serum levels due to increased clearance
Age	Infants	12 months to 12 years
Medications	Erythromycin—alone or in combination	Phenobarbital
	Azithromycin (Zithromax)	Phenytoin (Dilantin)
	Clarithromycin (Biaxin)	Rifampin (Rifadin)
	Cimetidine (Tagamet)	
	Oral contraceptives	
	Propanolol (Inderal)	
	Carbamazepine (Tegretol)	
	Zileuton (Zyflo)	
Illnesses	Liver or heart dysfunction	
	Acute viral illnesses	
Other	Obesity	Cigarette or marijuana smoking
	Fever for over 24 hours	

be updated at this time to ensure an increasingly mature understanding of the condition and its management.

Common Illness Management
(Box 9-7)

Differential Diagnosis

Wheezing

It is well known that all wheezing is not asthma, so when a child presents with recurrent or persistent cough or wheeze, other diagnoses should be considered. Such diagnoses include foreign body aspi-

ration (particularly in the infant or toddler); vocal cord dysfunction; infections (e.g., bronchitis, bronchiolitis, or pneumonia); other underlying airway diseases (e.g., cystic fibrosis or bronchiectasis); structural abnormalities (e.g., a vascular ring); or aspiration as a result of a primary swallowing disorder, GER, or secondary to underlying neuromuscular disease.

Respiratory Infections

Viral respiratory infections are the most common cause of exacerbations of asthma in children. Treatment is usually supportive and parents need to know to give antipyretics for fever if indicated and provide extra fluids, as well as that a change in asthma therapy medications may be necessary. For

---

Box 9-7

Differential Diagnosis

Wheezing—may not be asthma only

Respiratory infections—trigger asthma exacerbation

Vomiting and diarrhea—may indicate theophylline toxicity

Headache—may indicate sinusitis or theophylline toxicity

Fever—not associated with asthma unless underlying infection present

---

example, the child who only receives cromolyn sodium via nebulizer for long-term asthma control may need to temporarily add albuterol to the nebulized treatments for quick relief of cough or wheeze during an exacerbation.

Vomiting and Diarrhea

Children with asthma who present with vomiting should be evaluated for theophylline toxicity if they are on theophylline preparations, especially if the vomiting is associated with headache or stomachache. When gastroenteritis occurs in a child with asthma, the usual supportive care is required. The child should remain on the usual asthma therapy but may have difficulty with oral medications because of vomiting and may be at increased risk for mucus plugging if dehydration occurs. Controlling the respiratory symptoms with nebulized medications and providing extra fluids should be considered. Hospitalization may be necessary if the child's asthma worsens, medications cannot be tolerated orally or by nebulizer, or fluid intake is extremely reduced.

Headache

Sinusitis can present as a headache, especially if associated with complaints of purulent nasal drainage, foul breath odor, or nighttime cough. Because sinusitis can trigger an asthma episode, there may also be increased wheezing. When diagnosed, sinusitis must be treated aggressively and early to minimize the occurrence of asthma exacerbations. The common cold and symptoms of allergic rhinitis do not, however, require antibiotic treatment.

If a child with asthma (on a theophylline preparation) presents with complaint of headache, theophylline toxicity should be ruled out especially if gastrointestinal upset, stomachache, and vomiting are also occurring.

Fever

Asthma exacerbations are not associated with fever unless there is an underlying infection (e.g., sinusitis, pneumonia, or otitis media). The cause of the fever must be evaluated by the usual methods. Increased fluids should be given to keep the child hydrated and to avoid mucus plugging, which can occur with asthma. In a child taking a theophylline preparation, a febrile viral illness may alter metabolism necessitating a theophylline level.

Drug Interactions

Several factors cause theophylline levels to rise or fall and should be considered when a child's overall health care plan is assessed (see Table 9-5). Medications that affect theophylline clearance should be avoided, or the theophylline dose should be appropriately adjusted and levels monitored. Zafirlukast inhibits the cytochrome P-450 isoenzyme system, which interacts with other drugs metabolized by this system. Warfarin, phenytoin, carbamazepine, and erythromycin interactions are known, but those of cisipride, cyclosporin, calcium channel blockers, and astemizole are yet unknown, though monitoring is advised (Frost and Spahn, 1998). Because zileuton is metabolized by the cytochrome P-450 isoenzyme system, similar monitoring is advised. It is known that zileuton coadministration with theophylline approximately doubles the serum theophylline levels, necessitating a reduction in the dose (Frost and Spahn, 1998).

Cough suppressants should generally be avoided because they may mask asthma signs or symptoms and delay diagnosis and appropriate treatment. Cough suppressants are occasionally helpful to control nighttime or continuous postviral cough in which coughing itself is a trigger for increased cough because of irritation of the trachea and bronchi. In these cases, over-the-counter cough medicines are probably inadequate for cough control.

Antihistamines are now available without medical prescription and may be helpful in relieving allergic rhinitis. Antihistamines are thought not to contribute to drying or inspissation of secretions in well-hydrated children. A history of a child's use is important in planning a treatment regimen. More recently developed second generation antihistamines have the advantage of little or no sedation.

Children with asthma are often atopic and receive topical steroids in addition to inhaled steroids. Therefore the provider must be aware of the potential cumulative effects.

Developmental Issues

Sleep Patterns

The sleep of young children is often disrupted during asthma exacerbations. Even when an exacerbation is not evident, a child may routinely awaken and cough during the night or early morning hours. This tendency for early morning problems probably represents the normal circadian rhythm in airway caliber and steroid production (Meijer, 1998). Because the symptom pattern represents an exaggeration of existing bronchial hyperresponsivity, optimizing daytime control and reducing environmental irritants in the sleeping room minimizes the symptoms. Persistent difficulty may necessitate an evening dosage of a short-acting theophylline preparation (DuBuske, 1994), long-acting time-release theophylline preparation, long acting b_2 medications, or leukotriene modifiers in school-age children or adolescents.

Parents have reported that some medications disrupt their children's sleep, but systematic documentation is scarce. Most providers attempt an alternative medication regimen if the sleep disturbance does not resolve within 1 or 2 weeks of beginning a medication. Young children find a nighttime ritual soothing. Primary care providers should help parents establish a bedtime ritual that is relaxing and can be easily implemented by the family. A consistent bedtime is also helpful because frequent deviation of more than 30 minutes may cause difficulty in both settling a child and sleep onset.

Toileting

Toileting needs are typically not altered by a child's asthma. Bowel and bladder training is achieved at the expected ages. Clinicians have noted that a small proportion of children experience problems with enuresis when taking theophylline preparations, possibly because of its diuretic action. The exact incidence, however, is undocumented. If standard behavioral interventions are not effective in eliminating enuresis, most primary care providers seek an alternative medication regimen to manage the asthma. Constipation could occur if the child becomes dehydrated during exacerbations.

Discipline

Parents may report that it is difficult to deal with discipline for fear of upsetting the child and initiating an asthma exacerbation. Because children with asthma may experience some degree of bronchospasm with intense crying, parental concern is understandable. Crying cannot be entirely avoided, but parents should be reassured that most discipline can be implemented by rewarding desirable behaviors, if this is done routinely and begun early in a child's life. Inconsistent limit setting for undesirable behavior only confuses children and makes it more difficult for them to learn and internalize the limits chosen by the parents.

Another parental concern is that the child's irritability, refusals, or acting-out behavior is caused by illness or medications. Medications and illness may influence the child's behavior, but consistency of expectations is of greater importance. Blaming the illness or medication does not remove the necessity to help a child develop behaviors desired by the family and social networks. A child will ultimately need to develop a strong sense of internal control to effectively participate in self-management. Early consistent positive expectations set by the parents will form the foundation for a child's later self-discipline and sense of mastery and control. Avoiding discipline early in a child's life will not make the ensuing years more pleasant for parents or help the child in learning socially expected behaviors. Thus primary care providers should initiate discussion about positive discipline early during an infant's first year of life, assuring parents that with time this issue should become less burdensome as the child is able to verbally express emotion without excessive crying leading to bronchospasm.

Child Care

Most families find it necessary to use child care services on a regular or sporadic basis. Having a child with asthma should not prohibit the use of child care. Because URIs trigger exacerbations of asthma in many children under 5 years of age, a smaller day care with less chance of exposure to these infections may reduce the number of illnesses. Parents should evaluate the child care environment for any known triggers. Licensed daycare centers should prohibit exposure to second-hand smoke and are evaluated for cleanliness, molds or mildew, and animals. If unlicensed, private or in-home daycare arrangements do not need to meet state requirements, so parents must evaluate for known or common triggers. With proper communication and explanation, child care can be safely accomplished with a responsible, interested caretaker. Whether child care is at a center or is home based, provided by a relative, neighbor, or professional, information must be shared by parents to ensure success.

Parents must be responsible for providing all relevant information to the caretaker; that is, what triggers the child's asthma, early warning signs of an impending asthma episode, what the caretaker should do first, and what should be done next if the last action is not effective, how the parent and other responsible parties (i.e., including health care provider) can be reached, and what information must be passed on to emergency personnel if they are called. The best way to provide this information is in a written format. A laminated card with detailed instructions on one side and the primary care provider's name and telephone number on the reverse side has proved helpful for many families.

If the child care provider is to give any treatments, the parent must demonstrate the procedures and observe the provider's repeat performance. In addition, center-based programs may require written prescriptions from the primary health care provider and written permission of the parent for the child care provider to perform the treatment. Parents must maintain close contact with the child

care provider to learn about changing triggers, medications, or early warning signs. Anyone in repeated contact with the child who observes responses to treatments should also relay that information to the parent. This information can then be integrated into the overall routine reevaluation of the treatment plan. Any treatment changes should be immediately related to the child care provider so that a consistent approach is provided to the child regardless of setting. Frequent and open communication is the key to successful child care arrangements.

Schooling

Surveys of children with asthma report an average of 18 days lost from a typical 180-day school year (Redding et al, 1995). These days are often scattered throughout the year. This pattern of frequent, brief absences has been thought to be more harmful to academic progress than infrequent long absences, and efforts should be made to avoid this tendency.

Parents report that communicating with school personnel is essential but often difficult. Many fears and misconceptions about children with asthma still exist in the general public. Many teachers do not recognize a cough as a symptom of asthma. They may believe the child has an infectious disease that restricts school attendance. Teachers and administrators may attempt to limit the child more than the parents or primary care provider believes necessary—especially in regard to sports participation. With proper therapy and education, only those children with severe asthma should consider limitations (American Academy of Pediatrics Committee on Sports Medicine and Fitness, 1994). With appropriate warm-up, pacing, hydration, and preventive pharmacologic therapy, almost all children with asthma will be able to participate in sports activities.

Scheduling an annual parent-teacher conference to discuss the child's current treatment regimen is essential. Teachers and sports coaches should have the same written information suggested for child care providers. In addition, the teacher should be informed the child's skills for shared management. The school nurse may provide support to the parent during annual conferences and should have a copy of the child's written routine and emergency plan. Provider-prescribed emergency medications that may be needed should be given to the nurse or designate. If school personnel hesitate to assume this responsibility, the parents or primary care provider should discuss with them their legal responsibility to allow all children access to medications they need to enable school attendance. Mutual problem solving is essential to finding a workable solution.

Fitting in with school peers and maintaining positive peer relationships are essential to the child's full development. Parents can actively arrange peer gatherings, encourage the child to join clubs or organizations, and allow the child age-appropriate independence in visiting friends to ensure social experiences. Friends may question why the child is taking medications or has special equipment in the home. Simple explanations about the child's asthma should be given with the assurance that asthma is not contagious. This might also be done in school as a class presentation with the teacher's assistance. Parents are encouraged to discuss their child's asthma with parents of their child's peers so that all may have an honest understanding of the child's condition and abilities, as well as of any temporary limitations or needs for treatment. The American Lung Association's program, "Open Airways," for school age children is available from local chapters.

Sexuality

As noted earlier, sexual development may be delayed if the asthma has not been adequately controlled to allow regular growth. Systemic corticosteroids historically have been associated with delay in sexual development because of their effect on the adrenal glands and corticosteroid production. Current treatment regimens that rely on either inhaled corticosteroids or an oral corticosteroid every other day with morning dosage schedules appear to have reduced the adverse effect on general and sexual growth patterns.

If an adolescent becomes sexually active and wishes to use contraceptives, drug interactions must be considered. It is known that oral contraceptives may interfere with the breakdown of theophylline, thus increasing the likelihood of toxicity.

As new asthma management drugs are developed, their effect on the efficacy of any pharmacologic means of birth control must be explored.

Transition into Adulthood

As youths with asthma enter adulthood, it is important that they continue to increase and periodically update their understanding of asthma and its management with the goal of achieving complete control. Reviewing and updating the education might take place before a move to college or a switch in primary care providers. If persons with a history of moderate to severe asthma are currently without symptoms, they should be reminded to inform their new provider of this history because symptoms may return later in life. Maintaining a smoke-free work environment is essential. Some vocations that involve inhaled irritants or allergens and overexposure to known triggers (e.g., work with laboratory animals, cleaning fluids, bakery or painting products) may be best avoided.

Special Family Concerns and Resources

Because of the familial nature of asthma, some family members express guilt during the child's exacerbations. Parents should be reminded that there is nothing they could have done to prevent asthma and that in regard to acute exacerbations, hindsight is always better than foresight. Eliminating all exacerbations may be an ideal but impossible goal to achieve. A more realistic goal is to limit the number and extent of problems and to learn something about prevention or management from each episode.

If many family members have a history of asthma, the family may retain outdated beliefs and habits regarding the treatment of asthma. The primary care provider must respect the family history but also stress new knowledge and discuss the development of new therapies to encourage the family to take advantage of current information.

Given the familial nature of asthma, cultural and ethnic considerations are important. In the United States, minority ethnicity and poverty continue to be linked to increased prevalence, reduced access to care, lower quality of care, and reduced implementation of recommended care with subsequent higher risks of morbidity and mortality. Primary care providers need to consider their role in changing this reality. Providers must be child advocates to reduce environmental exposures of children to causes of asthma and its exacerbation (e.g., smoke, preterm birth, housing with poor ventilation, mold and mildew, early URI). Providers can continue to support policies and legislation that ensure universal access to health care. Exploring values, beliefs, and health practices of the families should enable the creative primary care provider to individualize critical elements of practice guidelines with the individual family. This individualization may help to ensure the greatest acceptance and implementation of the recommended care by tailoring the management program to the cultural realities of the child and family. It is within the ongoing trusting relationship of the family and caregiver that further information regarding cultural beliefs and practices can be discussed.

Most parents express ambivalence about long-term medication regimens. Although most parents acknowledge the effectiveness of these regimens, most also hold the belief that long-term medication—especially steroids—can be harmful to their child. Helpful approaches for supporting parents include acknowledging and discussing these common feelings while presenting the fact that the most detrimental effects of asthma seem to come from poor management. It is also useful to reinforce that the program will continue to be tailored to their child while trying to decrease medication to the minimum amount needed for control.

Asthma disrupts the life of the child's primary caretaker, who is most often the mother. This disruption is marked when the child is young but can be minimized by actively involving the other parent or another family member in concrete, daily management tasks.

Smoking by a family member continues to be associated with increased asthma flare-ups (Abulhosn, 1997), but changing the smoking habits of family members is difficult. When advising families to eliminate smoke from their child's environ-

ment, the practitioner should convey resources for smoking cessation. In severe cases, in-home smoking can be viewed as child endangerment. Parents must be reminded to only smoke outside (i.e., not in another room, near an open window, or in car) and wear a "smoking jacket" (i.e., an outer layer to prevent smoke retention on clothes).

Resources

Primary care providers should become familiar with the local offices of national organizations (see the list that follows) to identify community-based services in local areas that can complement their health care services. Many of these community-based services have programs that are useful to children and parents in managing day-to-day effects of asthma. These programs typically offer education about asthma and training in shared management skills for the child and parents.

If the primary care provider's practice is large enough, educational programs for similar-aged children with asthma have been effectively implemented in private practices. A well-stocked lending library of reading materials on asthma helps parents and children learn how to manage asthma. Practitioners must provide families with information on how to obtain these materials for their own use. Many Internet resources of high quality, up-to-date information are now easily accessed from public libraries or home computers.

Selected Information Materials

Self-management curricular guides:
From Asthma and Allergy Foundation of America: Asthma Care Training for Kids (ACT).

From the American Lung Association: Super Stuff: Open Airways for Schools.

Media:
From American Lung Association: A is for Asthma (VHS), 1998. Also available in Spanish.

From KidSafety America: Asthma, Asthma: You Can't Stop Me and At Ease with Asthma VHS (1998). KidSafety America, 4750 Chino Ave., Suite D, Chino, Calif.; (909) 902-1340.

Organizations:
Allergy and Asthma Network/Mothers of Asthmatics, Inc.; (800) 878-4403; http://www.podi.com/health/aanma.

Summary of Primary Care Needs for the Child with Asthma

HEALTH CARE MAINTENANCE
Growth and development
Prolonged or systemic use of steroids may affect growth; must be monitored carefully.

Delayed adolescent growth is associated with poor control with exacerbations or chronic oral corticosteroids.

Delayed development is only noted when unnecessary limitations are imposed on the child.

Impaired cognitive development is most clearly linked to repeated school absences.

Diet: Children may have allergies to sulfites or foods.

Safety: Electrical burns are possible from nebulizers or steamers.

Medication safety varies with developmental age.

Caution is needed on repeated use of quick-relief medications if improvement not achieved.

Adherence is an issue with adolescents.

Immunizations: Routine immunizations are recommended.

Caution is necessary with use of live virus vaccines in children on systemic or long-term steroids.

If a child has documented egg sensitivity, vaccines using other media must be considered.

Influenza vaccine is recommended for children over 6 months of age. Pneumococcal immunization is not currently recommended.

Screening
Vision: Routine screening is recommended unless daily high-dose corticosteroids are taken, which may result in cataracts or glaucoma, then referral to ophthalmologist is required for complete eye examination.

Hearing: Routine screening is recommended.

Dental: Routine screening is recommended.

Blood pressure: Should be evaluated at each visit due to possible sympathetic stimulation from medications or corticosteroids.

Hematocrit: Routine screening is recommended.

Urinalysis: Routine screening is recommended unless daily doses of corticosteroids are taken, which may result in glycosuria. If glycosuria is present, refer to physician for reevaluation of asthma management.

Tuberculosis: Routine screening is recommended.

Condition-specific screening
Corticosteroid therapy: Additional assessments are necessary to monitor glycosuria, osteoporosis, blood pressure, cataracts, glaucoma, and growth delay.

Lung function tests: Testing of PEFR should be done at each primary care office visit and on a routine schedule in the home based on individualized management plan. Spirometry should be done every 1 to 2 years.

Theophylline levels: Should be monitored with change in therapy, growth, and illness.

Allergy testing: Skin testing may be indicated depending on history and therapy response.

COMMON ILLNESS MANAGEMENT
Differential diagnosis
Recurrent or persistent cough or wheeze: Rule out infection, aspiration, structural anomalies, and cystic fibrosis.

Viral respiratory infections: URI may require change in asthma therapy to prevent or modify exacerbation of asthma.

Gastrointestinal symptoms: Rule out theophylline toxicity and GER.

Headache: Rule out theophylline toxicity and sinusitis.

Fever: Not associated with asthma alone. When fever is present, prevention of dehydration is important to prevent mucus plugs.

Continued

Summary of Primary Care Needs for the Child with Asthma—cont'd

Drug interactions

Antihistamines are not contraindicated.

Leukotriene modifiers of some types affect or are affected by the cytochrome P-450 isoenzyme system, thus several drug interactions documented and others suspected.

Medications such as erythromycin, cimetidine, zileuton or oral contraceptives will raise theophylline levels.

Phenobarbital will decrease theophylline levels.

Cough suppressants may mask symptoms of asthma.

Developmental Issues

Sleep patterns: Exacerbation may interfere with sleep.

It is important to reduce environmental allergens in sleep area.

If medications disturb sleep, an alternative regimen should be tried.

Toileting: Toileting is routine.

Few children experience enuresis while on theophylline.

Discipline: Concern over discipline initiating asthma attack.

Rewarding desirable behavior should be encouraged.

The influence of medication and illness on behavior is often a concern of parents and needs discussion.

Consistency of expectation is important.

Child care: Evaluate child care environment for known or common triggers.

Child care workers must be provided with information on asthma triggers, early warning signs of asthma, a written action plan for treatment, emergency contacts, and medications used in day care.

Schooling: Repeated school absences may interfere with academic performance.

School personnel must be educated to evaluate child's symptoms and use of medications.

School personnel need a written copy of the asthma action plan.

Encourage participation in asthma education programs if available.

Enhancing the child's strengths in all areas will support peer acceptance.

Sports participation should be maintained.

Sexuality: Sexual development may be delayed in severe cases or with prolonged corticosteroid use.

Oral contraceptives may interfere with breakdown of theophylline.

Transition to adulthood

Assume complete responsibility for asthma management.

Update knowledge and mature shared management roles.

Inform new primary care provider.

Discuss vocational issues.

Special family concerns

Familial nature of asthma may contribute to outdated beliefs of treatment.

Parents may be ambivalent regarding long-term medication regimens.

Smoking in home is detrimental to children with asthma. Parents who smoke need support and assistance in quitting.

Ethnic minority and poverty have been linked with increased prevalence, morbidity, and mortality.

System changes to improve access to care are necessary.

American Academy of Allergy, Asthma, and Immunology; (800) 822-ASTHMA; http://www.aaaai.org.

American Association for Respiratory Care; (972) 243-2272; http://www.aarc.org.

American College of Allergy, Asthma, and Immunology; (800) 842-777; http://allergy.mcg.edu.

American Lung Association; (800) LUNG-USA; http://www.lungusa.org.

American Pharmaceutical Association; (202) 628-4410; http://www.aphanet.org.

American Thoracic Society; (212) 315-8700; http://thoracic.org.

Asthma and Allergy Foundation of America; (800) 7-ASTHMA; http://www.aafa.org.

National Asthma Education and Prevention Program; (301) 251-1222; http://www.nhlbi.nih.gov/nhlbi/lung/lung.htm.

US Environmental Protection Agency; (800) 296-1996; http://www.epa.gov/ozone.

Internet:

NHLBI, Expert Panel Report II: Guidelines for the Diagnosis and Management of Asthma; http://www.nhlbi.nih.gov/nhlbi/lung/asthma/prof/asthgdln.htp

References

Abulhosn RS et al: Passive smoke exposure impairs recovery after hospitalization for acute asthma, Arch Pediatr Adolesc Med 151:135-139, 1997.

American Academy of Pediatrics Committee on Sports Medicine and Fitness: Medical conditions affecting sports participation, Pediatrics 94(5):757-760, 1994.

Andrews L et al: The use of alternative therapies by children with asthma: a brief report, J Paediatr Child Health 34:131-134, 1998.

Brook CDG: Short stature never killed anybody, J Pediatr 133(5):591-592, 1998.

Chernik V and Boat TF: Kenaig's disorders of the respiratory tract in children, ed 6, Philadelphia, 1998, W.B. Saunders.

Cockroft DW: Airway hyperresponsiveness in asthma, Hosp Pract 1:111-129, 1990.

Colten HR, Krause JE: Clinical implications of basic research: Pulmonary inflammation—a balancing act, NEJM 336(15):1094-1096, 1997.

Committee on Infectious Diseases: Report of the committee on infectious diseases, ed 23, Elk Grove Village, Ill., 1997, American Academy of Pediatrics.

Committee on Sports Medicine and Fitness: Medical conditions affecting sports participation, Pediatrics 94(5):757-760, 1994.

Creer TL et al: Behavioral consequences of illness: childhood asthma as a model, Pediatrics 90(suppl 5):808-815, 1992.

Crowley S et al: Growth and the growth hormone axis in children in prepuberty with asthma, J Pediatr 126(2):297-303, 1995.

Cypcar N, Stark J, and Lemanske R: The impact of respiratory infections on asthma, Pediatr Clin North Am 31(6):1259-1276, 1992.

DuBuske LM: Asthma: diagnosis and management of nocturnal symptoms, Compr Ther 20(11):628-639, 1994.

Fabbri L et al: Comparison of fluticasone propionate with beclomethasone dipropionate in moderate to severe asthma treated for 1 year, international study group, Thorax 48(8):817-823, 1993. Comment in Thorax 49(4):385, 1994.

Fairchok MP et al: Effect of prednisone on response to influenza virus vaccine in asthmatic children, Arch Pediatr Adolesc Med 152:1191, 1998.

Frost DA and Spahn JD: The leukotriene modifiers: a new class of asthma medication, Contemp Pediatr 15(12):95-107, 1998.

Halfon N and Newacheck PW: Childhood asthma and poverty: differential impacts and utilization of health services, Pediatrics 91(1):56-61, 1993.

Heuck C et al: Adverse effects of inhaled budesonide (800 mg) on growth and collagen turnover in children with asthma: a double-blind comparison of once-daily versus twice-daily administration, J Pediatr 133(5):608-612, 1998.

Howell H, Flaim T, and Lung C: Patient education, Pediatr Clin North Am 39(6):1333-1361, 1997.

Kelso JM: Latex allergy, Pediatr Ann 27(11):736-739, 1998.

Kemper KJ: A practical approach to chronic asthma management, Contemp Pediatr 14(8):86-106, 1997.

Mahan KL and Arlin M: Food, nutrition and diet therapy, ed 8, Philadelphia, 1992, W.B. Saunders.

Malthouse S: Homeopathic remedies for asthma, Canadian Family Physician 43:1917, 1997.

Martinez FO et al: Asthma and wheezing in the first 6 years of life, New Engl J Med 3:133-138, 1995.

Meijor GG: The pathogenesis of nocturnal asthma in childhood, Clin Exp Allergy 28(8):921-926, 1998.

Mirgalia de Giududici M et al: Salmeterol vs. theophylline in asthmatic children, Respir Crit Care Med 151(4):A270, 1995.

Mosby: Mosby's GenRx—the complete reference for generic and brand drugs, ed 8, St Louis, 1998, Mosby.

National Heart, Lung and Blood Institute: National Asthma Education and Prevention Program Expert Panel Report II Guidelines for the Diagnosis and Management of Asthma, National asthma education program expert panel report II, US Department of Health and Human Services, Publication No 97-4051A, 1997, US Government Printing Office.

Provisional Committee on Quality Improvement: Practice parameter: the office management of acute exacerbations of asthma in children, Pediatrics 93:119-126, 1994.

Rachelefsky GS: Asthma update: new approaches and partnerships, J Pediatr Health Care 9(1):12-21, 1995.

Redding GJ et al: Prevalence and impact of diagnosed asthma among primary school children, Am J Resp Crit Care Med 4:A540, 1995a.

Redding GJ et al: Prevalence and impact of diagnosed asthma among primary school children, Am J Resp Crit Care Med 151(94):A363, 1995b.

Redding GJ et al: Functional impact and health care utilization of middle school students with diagnosed and undiagnosed asthma, Amer J Resp Crit Care Med 4:A540, 1996.

Redding GJ et al: Prevalence of asthma among Native American children, Pediatr Research 48(4 Pt 2): 335A, 1998.

Reid M: Complicating features of asthma, Pediatr Clin North Am 39(6):1327-1341, 1992.

Silver et al: Burden of wheezing illness among U.S. children reported by parents not to have asthma, J Asthma 35(5):437-443, 1998.

Sly RM: Changing asthma mortality, Ann Allergy 73(3):259-268, 1994.

Stein R and Martinez F: Mechanisms of disease in childhood asthma. In Taussig L and Landau L, editors: Pediatric respiratory medicine, St Louis, 1999, Mosby.

Stempel DA and Redding GJ: Management of acute asthma, Pediatr Clin North Am 39:1311-1325, 1992.

Stohlmeyer L: Montelukast: a new medication for pediatric asthma management, Pediatr Pharmacol 6:324-328, 1998.

Taylor WR and Newacheck PW: Impact of childhood asthma on health, Pediatrics 90(5):657-662, 1992.

Vessey JA and Miola B: Teaching self-advocacy skills to adolescents, Pediatric Nursing 23:53-56, 1997.

Warner J, Naspitz C, and Cropp G, editors: Third international pediatric consensus statement on the management of childhood asthma, Pediatr Pumlonol 25:1-17, 1998.

Weiss S: Early childhood asthma: what are the questions: long-term outcome, Am J Respir Crit Care Med 151 (suppl 6):S1-S42, 1995.

Zacharisen MC and Kelly KJ: Allergic and infectious pediatric sinusitis, Pediatr Ann 27(11):759-766, 1998.

Zorc JJ et al: Ipratropium bromide: what role does it have in asthma therapy?, Contemp Pediatr 15(4):81-94, 1998.

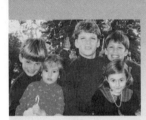

CHAPTER 10

Autism

Maureen Sheehan

Etiology

Autism was initially described by Leo Kanner in 1943, who thought that children with autism were of normal intelligence and the product of cold and distant parenting. His description of the 11 children he studied focused on their social impairment and, to a lesser extent, their insistence on "sameness" (Kanner, 1943). Autism is currently recognized as a triad of impairments in the areas of communication, social interactions, and imagination, as represented by restricted interests, activities, and stereotyped behaviors (Wing, 1997).

Results of family and twin studies suggest genetic involvement in the etiology of autism (Smalley and Collins, 1996). Compared with an incidence rate of 1 to 2 in 1,000 children, siblings of children with autism have autism at a rate of 3% to 5% (Smalley and Collins, 1996), which may be an artificially low rate of recurrence of familial autism because many parents with one child with autism decide not to have more children (Folstein and Piven, 1991). By only considering the rate of recurrence of autism in siblings born after the child with autism, the risk of autism in subsequent children increases to 8.6% (Ritvo et al, 1989), which represents a 50- to 100-fold increase in the expected prevalence of autism in siblings (Folstein and Piven, 1991). Three twin studies report a concordance rate of 36% to 91% among monozygotic twins and a 0% concordance rate among dizygotic twins (Harris JC, 1995). Because the concordance rate among identical twins was less than 100% and identical twins with autism were not always affected to the same degree, there may be some environmental and/or genetic interaction (Rapin and Katzman, 1998). Studies of family members found that family members and twins without autism were more likely to have cognitive difficulties,

social deficits, language abnormalities, and affective and anxiety disorders (Folstein and Piven, 1991). These problems were mild but bear some resemblance to the core deficits of autism.

Evidence to date suggests genetic heterogeneity with variable expression and interaction with nongenetic factors as an etiological basis for autism (Bailey, Phillips, and Rutter, 1996; Harris, 1995; Rapin, 1997; Rapin and Katzman, 1998). The mode of inheritance is unknown. Because of the profound deficits of autism, vertical transmission is unlikely, which makes dominant inheritance patterns difficult to assess (Rapin and Katzman, 1998). It is possible that genetic anticipation with expansion of trinucleotide repeats may be involved (Harris, 1995; Rapin and Katzman, 1998).

Numerous studies have identified pre-, peri-, and neonatal factors that have occurred in children with autism. The problems observed (e.g., vaginal bleeding, hypertension, use of prescription medication, nonvertex presentation, and hyperbilirubinemia) have not been consistently seen, are not specific to autism, and cannot be used to either predict or prevent autism (Nelson, 1991). Piven and colleagues (1993) found no association between these factors after accounting for maternal parity. Other studies provide evidence that the minor obstetrical complications observed were more likely to be the result of preexisting fetal developmental anomalies than the cause of them (Bailey et al, 1996; Harris JC, 1995).

Neuropathologic studies have been done on the brains of 35 people who had autism. These studies have found abnormalities in the hippocampus, amygdala, septum, mammillary bodies, and the cerebellum—areas important to processing social and environmental information that appear to be abnormal in persons with autism (Bauman, 1996; Bristol et al, 1996). The differences found in these areas of the brain indicate a developmental disorder before 30 weeks gestation that is expressed when the limbic circuits fail to grow and develop normally (Bristol et al, 1996). This pathologic process is thought to continue into adulthood, as evidenced by the larger than expected brains of children with autism and the atrophy found in the brains of adults with autism (Kemper and Bauman, 1998; Rapin and Katzman, 1998). The significance of these findings is not clear because there is no evidence that these findings are specific to, or occur universally in, autism (Bristol et al, 1996).

Neuroimaging results have been contradictory (Bailey et al, 1996). Magnetic resonance imaging (MRI), positron emission tomography (PET), and single-photon emission computed tomography (SPECT) studies have all found abnormalities in children with autism but the studies have been done with very few subjects and often without controls. As yet, there is no clinical significance to their findings. Electroencephalographic (EEG) studies in a number of individuals with autism provide further evidence of abnormal brain development (Bailey et al, 1996), but there is no singular EEG pattern exclusive and universal to autism.

The most consistent neurochemical finding in autism is hyperserotoninemia (Rapin and Katzman, 1998). Because of the frequency of sleep disorders in children with autism, melatonin abnormalities have been hypothesized (Rapin and Katzman, 1998). Levels of dopamine, norepinephrine, endogenous opioids, and cortisol may play roles in the behavioral symptoms of autism (Harris JC, 1995; Rapin and Katzman, 1998). To date, all biochemical research is speculative.

Incidence

Autism was considered to be a rare condition, affecting as few as two to five in 10,000 children (Gillberg, 1998). Recent estimates, however, suggest that autism is much more common. Current prevalence estimates range from one to two in 1,000 children (Rapin and Katzman, 1998). This rate puts autism on a par with Down syndrome as one of the most common developmental disabilities. The Autism Society of America estimates there are over 1.5 million people in the United States with some form of autism, and as many as 115,000 of them may be children (Rapin, 1997).

The reasons for the apparent increase in the incidence of autism are not clear. Although it is possible that there has been an actual increase in the prevalence of autism, the reported increase is more likely a reflection of increased identification. As specific behavioral criteria for a diagnosis of autism have been delineated by the American Psychiatric Association (DSM-IV) (1994) and the World Health Organization (ICD-10) (1994), a wider spectrum of children and adults with autism has been identified.

Autism is found in all ethnic and socioeconomic groups. It is more common in boys than in girls (e.g., in an approximate 3:1 ratio) and in children who have relatively mild autism (Bryson, 1996). In children with more severe disabilities, the ratio of boys to girls is much closer to 1:1 (Bauer, 1995a).

Clinical Manifestations at the Time of Diagnosis

The fourth edition of the *Diagnostic and Statistical Manual of Mental Disorders* has established a set of diagnostic criteria with which to make the diagnosis of autism (APA, 1994). (Box 10-1). The principal symptoms of autism fall into three categories: delayed communication skills (both verbal and nonverbal); impaired social interactions; and restricted play, activities, and interests (Rapin, 1997). The majority of children with autism have cognitive deficits and other symptoms, such as stereotypical motor behaviors, self-injurious behaviors, and paradoxic reactions to sensory stimuli (Rapin, 1997). Although autism may present in infancy as a lack of attention, interest in objects instead of faces, and social inhibition, most children with autism are diagnosed as toddlers (i.e., between their first and third birthdays).

Delayed Communication

Expressive language delay in a child is generally the primary concern that parents bring to the attention of pediatric primary care providers (Lainhart

Box 10-1

Clinical Manifestations

Delayed or absent communication
Expressive language delay
Receptive language delay

Impairment of social interaction
Avoidance of eye contact
Fascination with objects rather than people
Interactions revolve around obtaining desired
    objects rather than emotional responses

*Restrictive and repetitive behavior, interests,
and activities*
Organizes toys, rather than manipulates them
Throws tantrums when repetitive behaviors are
    interrupted
Hand-flapping, twirling, toe-walking,

Resistance to changes in schedule or environment
Narrow Food Preferences
Auditory Hypersensitivity

and Piven, 1995; Siegel, 1996). As children near their second birthday, parents express concern that they are not yet talking because many children with autism do not speak their first words until after their second birthday (Bauer, 1995a). Hearing impairment must be ruled out through audiologic evaluation. Brainstem auditory evoked response testing may be necessary if the audiologic evaluation is inconclusive or cannot be performed due to behavioral factors; 20% of children with autism may also have some degree of hearing impairment (Minshew, 1991).

Young children with autism also will have impaired receptive language (Harris JC, 1995). Such children may be unable to recognize their own name, follow simple commands, and may seem oblivious to the speech of others. Some children with autism have verbal auditory agnosia (i.e., word deafness) and cannot decode speech (Rapin, 1997). Children who cannot understand speech are generally unable to acquire functional spoken language.

About half of all children with autism develop language, although it is often remarkable for a number of unusual features. Spoken words may be unintelligible. When words are intelligible, they may be strung together in nonsensical phrases or jargon (Harris JC, 1995). The speech of children with autism may consist largely of echolalia; preoccupation with certain topics; and perseverative repetition of phrases, questions, rhymes, and/or content obtained from the television, radio, or movies (Bauer, 1995a; Harris JC, 1995; Rapin, 1997). Echolalia is present in about 80% of people with autism who develop speech (Sigman and Capps, 1997). Pronoun reversal (e.g., a child uses "you" when the correct pronoun is "I") also occurs (Harris JC, 1995). In addition, children with autism often speak in high-pitched voices with markedly impaired intonation and prosody (i.e., appropriate stress in their patterns of speech) (Rapin, 1997; Sigman and Capps, 1997). These children are often unable to use intonation and prosody to either convey meaning in their speech or derive meaning from the speech of others (Sigman and Capps, 1997).

Nonverbal communication is limited. Children with autism may not point to engage the attention of their caretakers but may take the hand of their caretaker and move it to the desired object (Sigman and Capps, 1997). This hand-leading behavior is almost never seen in normal children. Normal babies point before they can walk and talk (Siegel, 1996). Hand-leading develops after walking at a time when many children with autism are still unable to point but most normal children can use pointing and vocalizations to obtain what they want (Siegel, 1996). Children with autism may have difficulty shaking their head "no" and using hand and facial gestures to add meaning to their utterances (Bauer, 1995a). These deficits in nonverbal expression are mirrored in the difficulties people with autism have in attending to and interpreting the nonverbal communications of those around them.

Impairment in Social Interaction

The deficits in social interaction set autism apart from other developmental and language disorders. These deficits are difficult for parents to quantify and describe (Siegel, 1996). Children with autism may demonstrate an aversion to being cuddled (Harris JC, 1995). They may avoid prolonged direct eye contact and ignore others in their environment, leading them to be described as "withdrawn" and "in their own world" (Harris JC, 1995; Siegel, 1996). When a child with autism chooses to interact with someone else, it is often to obtain some object rather than to receive an emotional response (Siegel, 1996). Siegel refers to this as "instrumental" relating. This fascination with objects rather than people can be tenacious and difficult to interrupt—both at home and in the provider's office and can also lead parents to view their child as serious, goal-directed, focused, and intelligent rather than socially deficient (Siegel, 1996).

Restrictive and Repetitive Behavior, Interests, and Activities

Children with autism frequently demonstrate odd, perseverative, stereotypic behaviors, such as hand flapping, twirling objects, rocking, head banging, and toe-walking (Bauer, 1995a). They may repeatedly flick light switches on and off, show a fascination with running water or flushing toilets, or collect unusual objects such as bits of string or paper (Tonge, Dissanayake, and Brereton, 1994). These children will often ignore new toys (Siegel, 1996). If they do play with a toy, they tend to focus on just one aspect of the toy and often on a feature that is not germane to the toy's intended use. Given a group of toys, a child with autism will organize them in some fashion but not manipulate them imaginatively. For example, given a collection of little toy cars, a child with autism will line them up but not pretend to drive them. A child with autism may play with a spinning top seemingly endlessly. Parents may initially be pleased with their child's ability to engage in a single activity for many minutes or even hours and view this as a sign of maturity and above-average intellect. When attempts to interrupt the child's play are met with a tantrum, parents may begin to recognize the child's play as aberrant.

Most children with autism are very resistant to changes in their schedule and environment (Siegel, 1996). Rearranging furniture, accidentally break-

ing a household object, or interrupting regularly scheduled television programming may all cause extreme distress in a child with autism. Children with autism also often demonstrate very narrow food preferences (Lord, Rutter, and Le Couteur, 1994). These children may be hypersensitive to certain sounds such as sirens or vacuum cleaners (Bauer, 1995a; Lord et al, 1994). Self-injurious behaviors (e.g., hand-biting and severe head-banging) and unusual fears of seemingly benign objects may also be seen (Bauer, 1995a; Lord et al 1994)

Treatment

Just as there is no cure for autism, there is no one treatment that works for every child (Box 10-2). As the genetic and/or neurobiologic basis for the deficits of autism has become more apparent, approaches to treatment have focused on the specific symptoms of autism. A comprehensive treatment plan for a child with autism must include both education and behavior management and, often times, pharmacological treatment (Bauer, 1995b). This comprehensive treatment must be planned, coordinated, and delivered by a multidisciplinary team that includes the child's parents; primary care provider; school personnel; psychiatrist; and behavioral, speech, and occupational therapists as needed.

Box 10-2

Treatment

Developed by multidisciplinary team specializing in autism
One-to-one discrete trial learning
Behavior management
Early intervention programs
Speech and language therapy
Special education support focused on specific symptoms
Pharmacologic intervention as adjunctive therapy
Alternative therapies

Early Intervention

Early intervention (i.e., between the ages of 2 and 4 years) has been shown to improve children's level of functioning and decrease the frequency of aberrant behaviors (Howlin, 1998). Therapeutic education during the preschool years takes advantage of the child's most rapid period of development and greatest degree of brain plasticity. This type of early treatment can result in some children with autism, who are cognitively intact and no longer meet the criteria for autism by the school-age years (Rapin and Katzman, 1998). What form this intervention should take is a matter of some debate. Many clinicians in the field of autism recommend that preschoolers with autism receive 40 hours a week of one-to-one discrete trial learning based on the methods used by Lovaas in the Early Intervention Project (Siegel, 1996). Parents are now implementing early intervention programs with their child at home under the direction of a behavior therapist (Sheinkopf and Siegel, 1998), which is expensive and very time- and energy-consuming. Parents are increasingly turning to their school districts for help with one-to-one early intervention and often meeting with resistance, resulting in litigation (Gresham and MacMillan, 1998).

Other early educational approaches include therapeutic preschools with a developmental approach, behavioral one-on-one interventions in an academic setting rather than at home, and preschools that use the Treatment and Education of Autistic and Related Communication-Handicapped Children (TEACCH) approach, (Cohen, 1998). This approach relies primarily on group instruction and extensive teaching through visual means to compensate for the verbal deficits of children with autism (Cohen, 1998).

Behavioral Management

Behavioral management is an essential part of the treatment plan for a child with autism and should begin as soon after diagnosis as possible, before problematic behaviors are deeply entrenched. Parents may be reluctant to set the firm limits that even a very young child with autism requires to prevent the establishment of inappropriate behaviors. As Howlin (1998) describes, parents can be reminded that removing a screaming 3-year-old from a store

is embarrassing, but removing a screaming 13-year-old may be impossible.

Pharmacological Intervention

Medication is not a substitute for appropriate education and behavioral management but may be a useful adjunct and enable a child to make full use of other therapies. Medications are generally used to treat targeted, specific symptoms of autism. Medication is most often used to reduce self-injurious and aggressive behaviors, attention deficits, hyperactivity, compulsive behavior, psychotic symptoms, and affective lability (Harris JC, 1995). The primary care provider may want to consult a child psychiatrist, pediatric neurologist, and/or personnel from developmental disorders clinics for their expertise about new antiepileptic and psychoactive medications that may be useful in treating specific behaviors. No medication has ever been shown to be efficacious with all children with autism, but many can make some symptoms better or have a paradoxical effect (Bauer, 1995b) (Table 10-1).

Methylphenidate (Ritalin) and dextroamphetamine (Dexedrine) are stimulants that may decrease hyperactivity and increase attention. In children with autism, however, these drugs may increase attention to the one thing to which the child is already overattending (Siegel, 1996). Ritalin frequently increases hyperactivity in children with autism or has a "rebound" effect that causes children to be more active when the dose has worn off (Siegel, 1996).

Fluoxetine (Prozac) has been shown to improve behavior, cognition, language, affect, and social skills in some children with autism (DeLong, Teague, and Kamran, 1998; Fatemi et al, 1998). Not all children treated responded, however, and some had increases in hyperactivity. DeLong and colleagues (1998) reported that a response to fluoxetine in their subjects correlated with a family history of a major affective disorder (i.e., bipolar disorder or major depression).

Carbamezapine (Tegretol or Carbatrol) and valproate (Depakene or Depakote) are two antiepileptic drugs that also have mood stabilization effects. Parents must be cautioned to report any symptoms of liver toxicity or thrombocytopenia that their

Table 10-1
Medications used for Autism*

Stimulants

Medication	Dose	Indications	Side Effects
Methylphenidate (Ritalin)	2.5 mg bid, increase by 5 mg/wk; MDD = 60 mg	ADHD Low impulse control	Precipitation of tics Overattention Hyperactivity Anorexia
Dextroamphetamine (Dexedrine)	2.5 mg qd, increase by 2.5 mg/wk; MDD = 40 mg	ADHD Low impulse control	Precipitation of tics Overattention Hyperactivity Anorexia

Antidepressants

Buspirone (Buspar)	7.5 mg bid, increase by 15 mg/wk; MDD = 60 mg	Anxiety Aggression	Rare

Neuroleptics

Haloperidol (Haldol)	0.05 to 0.5 total mg/day bid or tid, increase by 0.25 mg/wk; MDD = 6 mg/day	Agitation Aggression Severe behavior problems Preoccupations	Extrapyramidal symptoms Sedation Tardive dyskinesia Neuroleptic malignant syndrome
Risperidone (Risperdal)	0.25 mg qd, increase by 0.25 mg/wk; MDD = 2 mg/day, divided bid	Agitation Aggression Stereotypical behaviors Preoccupations	Sedation Weight gain Few to no extrapyramidal symptoms Neuroleptic malignant syndrome
Olanzapine (Zyprexa)	Consult with child psychiatrist	Agitation Aggression Preoccupations	Few to no extrapyramidal symptoms

Mood Stabilizers

Carbamezpine* (Tegretol or Carbatrol) and Valproate (Depakote)	See Chapter 21	Labile moods	Hepatotoxicity Thrombocytopenia Rash Appetite changes

Sedative Agents

Diphenhydramine (Benadryl)	12.5 to 50 mg	Sedation	Paradoxical agitation
Chloral hydrate	25 mg/kg, may repeat once	Sedation	Paradoxical agitation
Amitriptyline (Elavil)	0.1 mg/kg	Sedation	Tachycardia Arrhythmia EKG before giving

*For antiepileptic drugs, see Chapter 21.
bid, twice a day; MDD, mean daily dose; qd, every day; qod, every other day; tid, three times a day.

child exhibits. A complete blood count (CBC), aspartate aminotransferase (AST), and alanine aminotransferase (ALT) must be obtained before initiating therapy, after reaching the maintenance dose, and then semiannually.

Haloperidol (Haldol) and thioridazine (Mellaril) were traditionally the neuroleptics used to treat aggressive and self-injurious behavior in children with autism, but both can cause dyskinesias and extrapyramidal symptoms. The new generation of neuroleptics, which includes risperidone (Risperdal), are now being tested and used in children with autism. As with all other medications, the response is variable, but some children achieve a marked reduction in the targeted symptoms of aggressive behavior and extreme behavior management problems (Findling, Maxwell, and Wiznitzer, 1997; Nicolson, Awad, and Sloman, 1998; Schreier, 1998).

Children with autism often require sedation for medical and dental procedures. Many medications used for sedation, however, produce paradoxic effects in children with autism (Sigman and Capps, 1997). Primary care providers may want to work with parents to give test doses of agents such as chloral hydrate and diphenhydramine (Benadryl) at home before attempting to use them for sedation for a medical or dental procedure. Haloperidol (Haldol) has also been used but presents the risk of neuroleptics. Children taking haloperidol must be monitored for the development of extrapyramidal symptoms and neuroleptic malignant syndrome. Administering a dose of diphenhydramine simultaneously with haloperidol can prevent extrapyramidal symptoms. Amitriptyline (Elavil) is the most sedative antidepressant used in children with autism (Shlafer, 1993). Amitriptyline is contraindicated in children with preexisting cardiac disease. Because tricyclic antidepressants (e.g., amitriptyline) can potentially cause hypotension, tachycardia, and arrhythmias, children should have a normal EKG before receiving this drug.

Other medications that have been used with children with autism are buspirone (Buspar) and propranolol (Inderal) for anxiety and aggression, clomipramine (Anafranil) for ritualistic behavior, lithium for severe mood lability, clonidine (Catapres) for compulsive behavior, and naltrexone (Trexan) for self-injurious behavior and hyperac-

tivity (Harris, 1995; Howlin, 1998; Siegel, 1996). All of these medications, however, lack research using double-blind, controlled trials to truly determine their efficacy in autism.

Alternative Therapies

A number of alternative treatments for autism are available. Megadose vitamin B_6 and magnesium are used to improve speech and behavior (Rimland and Baker, 1996) but can cause diarrhea and peripheral neuropathy so their use should be monitored by a care provider. Dietary treatments include gluten-free and/or dairy-free diets (Rimland and Baker, 1996). Intravenous immunoglobulin administration to 10 children with autism only led to significant improvement in one child, who reverted to his previous autistic behavior when treatment was stopped (Plioplys, 1998). The wearing of ambient transitional lenses has been reported to decrease behavior problems (Kaplan, Edelson, and Seip, 1998). In 1998 the Committee on Children with Disabilities of the American Academy of Pediatrics published a statement on the use of auditory integration training and facilitated communication for autism that concluded that these treatments are only warranted as part of research protocols. The Committee, however, did encourage primary care providers to obtain and review information about alternative treatments to help families evaluate their efficacy and safety.

Recent and Anticipated Advances in Diagnosis and Management

There are numerous questions about autism that are in need of investigation. The precise etiology of autism remains unclear, but many different possibilities are being explored. This exploration may reflect the lack of a sound theoretic foundation for the central deficits of autism on which researchers can base their hypotheses.

In an attempt to find the biologic basis of autism, researchers are examining genetic, neuropathologic, and neurochemical mechanisms. The anticipated completion of the Human Genome Project early in the twenty-first century may yield insights into the suspected genetic heterogeneity of autism.

Many people with autism have normal MRI scans. It is possible that MRI technology is not yet sensitive enough to discover the subtle abnormalities that may be present in autism (Courchesne, 1991). PET imaging has begun to identify abnormalities of brain metabolism in individuals with autism. As the use of PET is expanded to people with autism, understanding of the connection between the brain and behavior should be enhanced (Happé and Frith, 1996), which, in turn, should lead to insights into the cognitive and behavioral disturbances of autism.

The fields of biostatistics and epidemiology are pioneering new methodologies that obviate the need for costly and difficult-to-complete prospective, longitudinal studies. With these methodologies, it may be possible to accurately determine whether subtypes of autism with different etiologies, courses, and/or responses to treatment exist (Bristol et al, 1996).

Psychopharmacology may be the answer to some of the most troubling manifestations of autism. The new generation of antipsychotic medications, primarily risperidone and olanzapine, has been especially effective in reducing the negative symptoms associated with schizophrenia (e.g., social withdrawal, apathy, lack of motivation, and anhedonia) (Hostetler, 1998; Pickar, 1996). Perhaps these medications will also reduce these symptoms in people with autism. Some child psychiatrists have had some success with olanzapine in reducing behavioral outbursts and aggressive behavior in children with autism (Lotspeich and Shaw, 1998). Future research in psychopharmacology using systematic, double-blind, placebo-controlled studies of medications that will benefit individuals with autism is needed (Hellings et al, 1996).

Associated Problems (Box 10-3)

Mental Retardation

Children with autism may have intelligence quotients (IQs) ranging from profound retardation to superior intelligence. Approximately 75% of people with autism are mentally retarded, and 20% to 25% have IQs in the normal to near normal range

---

Box 10-3
Associated Problems

Mental retardation
Epilepsy
Tuberous sclerosis
Fragile X syndrome
Psychiatric disorders

(Bryson, 1996; Harris JC, 1995). Children with autism usually have higher non-verbal than verbal IQ scores, and testing must be done by an experienced psychologist who can work with the child's potential negativity, distractibility, and comprehension difficulties (Harris JC, 1995). Because a child's cognitive ability can help predict the child's future course and outcome, accurate assessment of a child's IQ provides the child's family with important information for treatment planning (Bailey et al, 1996).

Epilepsy

Of people with autism, 20% to 25% have been reported to develop epilepsy, with the peak onset of seizures during adolescence (Bailey et al, 1996; Harris JC, 1995). The risk of developing epilepsy is slightly higher in individuals with autism who are also profoundly retarded, which is consistent with the incidence of epilepsy in people who are profoundly retarded (Bailey et al, 1996). Because of the high incidence of epilepsy in children with autism, primary care providers should not hesitate to obtain an electroencephalogram (EEG) if parents report any behavior that could be seizures. Primary generalized, complex partial, atypical absence, and other types of seizures—alone or in combination—have all been reported (Rapin, 1997) (see Chapter 21).

Tuberous Sclerosis

Tuberous sclerosis, a neurocutaneous syndrome, is found in 3% to 9% of individuals with autism (Bailey et al, 1996), which is the most significant association of a known, genetically determined medical condition (Lainhart and Piven, 1995). The primary care provider should thoroughly examine the skin of any child with autistic symptoms to look for the hypopigmented macules (i.e., ash-leaf spots) characteristic of tuberous sclerosis (Coleman and Gillberg, 1985).

Fragile X Syndrome

Over the past decade, the estimated rate of autism associated with fragile X syndrome has dropped from 16% to 2.5% (Bailey et al, 1996) (see Chapter 22). Although many individuals with fragile X syndrome may exhibit some autistic traits (e.g., poor eye contact and vocal perseveration), relatively few meet the DSM-IV criteria for a diagnosis of autism (Harris JC, 1995; Lainhart and Piven, 1995).

Psychiatric Disorders

A number of psychiatric conditions, including attention deficit hyperactivity disorder (see Chapter 28), obsessive-compulsive disorder, and affective disorders (e.g., depression) may exist with autism (Tonge et al, 1994). Adolescents and adults with autism have a slightly higher risk of developing symptoms of psychosis, such as hallucinations or paranoia (Mauk, 1993).

Other Conditions

There have been reports of other conditions associated with autism. Phenylketonuria; intrauterine rubella and cytomegalovirus infection; lactic acidosis; purine disorders; autosomal and sex chromosome anomalies; and Williams, Möbius, Sotos and other syndromes have all been found with autism (Bauer, 1995a; Gillberg and Coleman, 1996; Harris, 1995; Lainhart and Piven, 1995). These associations, however, are all statistically weak and hampered by the very small number of cases involved (Lainhart and Piven, 1995).

In a review of the literature on autism and medical disorders, Gillberg and Coleman (1996) concluded that the rate of associated medical conditions was between 11% and 37%. This rate includes both the relatively common conditions of tuberous sclerosis and fragile X syndrome, as well as the very rare conditions listed in the previous paragraph. The more comprehensive the medical and neuropsychiatric examinations, the more likely an associated problem will be discovered. Primary care providers must be alert to signs and symptoms of these disorders in children diagnosed with autism and obtain electroencephalography, neuroimaging, and metabolic and chromosome testing as needed. When possible, treatment of the comorbid condition often results in an improvement in the child's autistic symptoms. In addition, information about associated problems—even when a problem cannot be treated—can be important for genetic counseling and educating the family about their child's diagnosis and prognosis (Gillberg and Coleman, 1996).

Prognosis

The outcome for children with autism, similar to the expression of the syndrome itself, varies. At one end of the spectrum are individuals with average or high cognitive abilities who have attended college, have careers, and can live independently. The majority of children with autism, however, have an IQ in the moderately retarded range (Harris JC, 1995).

The development of useful language by the age of 5 years is an important prognostic factor (Harris JC, 1995). Approximately one half of children with autism will not develop usable language (Mauk, 1993). Young children who demonstrate joint attention behaviors (i.e., communication signals such as pointing to direct someone's attention to an experience they want to share) are more likely to have better language skills. Children without language—either verbal or sign—by the age of 5 years are likely to not attain socially usable language skills. They function poorly socially and remain dependent as adults. A nonverbal IQ less than 50 in combination with the absence of meaningful speech by 5 years old is currently predictive of serious deficits that will be lifelong (Bauer, 1995b).

The natural course of autism often varies over time. It is unclear if children with autism present with symptoms during the first year of life. Most parents first report differences in a child's communication, social, and play skills during the second year of life. Children with milder autism, however, may not be diagnosed until school age. Many parents report that the behavior of children with autism is particularly problematic during the preschool years (Tonge, Dissanayake, and Brereton, 1994). With intensive interventions, these children may experience an improvement in their symptoms as they enter the school-age years. With the onset of puberty, many of a child's disturbed behaviors may reappear and then fade somewhat in adulthood (Wing, 1997).

Increases in behavioral disturbances (e.g., self-injurious, aggressive, obsessive, and anxious behaviors) have been reported in adolescence (Bryson, 1996). This decline in functioning may be due to hormonal influences, the onset of other coexisting conditions, a response to increased demands, or their own increased awareness of their limitations (Tonge, Dissanayake, and Brereton, 1994).

Approximately two thirds of young adults with autism will be unable to work or live on their own (Bauer, 1995b). Even adults with average intelligence and academic achievement may have such serious social and judgment deficits that living completely independently is impossible (Rapin and Katzman, 1998). The one caveat to this rather grim picture is that these results are from adults not generally exposed to early, intensive, and continual therapeutic education and treatment. As research on autism continues and findings are put into clinical practice, more children may be able to function independently when they reach adulthood.

PRIMARY CARE MANAGEMENT

Health Care Maintenance

Growth and Development

Perhaps the most challenging aspect of monitoring the growth and development of a child with autism is enlisting the child's cooperation. Before a child's visit to the provider, consultation with the parents regarding the child's behavioral symptoms, fears, and likes can give the provider information to make the child's visit a success (Seid, Sherman, and Seid, 1997). With the parents' permission, the provider may also find it useful to talk with the child's teacher and/or behavioral therapist about the best ways to approach the child (Seid et al, 1997). Together, the provider and the parents can devise a plan for the examination that will help the provider and child begin to form a working relationship and

lead the provider from the child's most to least favorite parts of the exam. A flexible unhurried approach is best. A reward at the completion of the exam can be planned, available, and referred to during the examination as necessary. Because many children with autism are highly distractible, time spent in the waiting room with other children and parents can leave them overstimulated and unable to fully cooperate. Therefore many providers find it best to schedule a child with autism as the first morning or afternoon appointment.

Children with autism may have their growth affected by disease symptomatology and/or pharmacologic therapies. Weight gain and height increases may falter as the result of decreased caloric intake secondary to restricted food preferences. The use of stimulant medication can decrease a child's appetite. Conversely, valproic acid can result in unwanted weight gain because of its appetite-stimulating effect. Parents should be educated about the possible affects on the child's growth and encouraged to monitor the child's growth and consult with a provider if there are concerns. Children with risk factors for altered growth should be measured every 6 months.

As many as 25% of people with autism have head circumferences above the 97th percentile (Bailey et al, 1996; Happé and Frith, 1996). Head circumferences should be measured until the age of 5 years and annually if a child also has tuberous sclerosis. It is not clear if this phenomenon is a result of some underlying neuropathology in autism, a marker of the stage of gestation at which autism might originate, or—less likely—a contributing factor to autism (Happé and Frith, 1996).

Children with autism generally develop normally or with differences too subtle to detect until 12 to 18 months of age (Mauk, 1993). Between 18 and 30 months of age, the child's parents and primary care provider notice a language delay (Rapin, 1997). As soon as the diagnosis of autism is considered, the child should be referred for a multidisciplinary developmental evaluation that includes thorough neuropsychologic, speech, and language testing (Harris JC, 1995; Siegel, 1996). Primary care providers should not delay this referral in the hope that the child will "outgrow" a language delay.

The success of a child's treatment for autism is measured empirically. Therefore the child will need to be annually reevaluated by the multidisciplinary team during the first few years of treatment and then every few years after. These evaluations will serve as the basis for treatment planning. Many health insurance plans—both publicly and privately funded—are reluctant to pay for neuropsychologic testing. Primary care providers must advocate for a child and family in pursuing appropriate referrals and payment for them.

Diet

Throughout the lifetime of a child with autism, parents, teachers, therapists, and providers are faced with decisions about when and when not to accommodate the child's insistence on sameness (Cohen, 1998). There is no one right answer for every child and family. Each family, with the help of their child's provider, should assess their own values, needs, and level of tolerance and make decisions accordingly.

Many children with autism have feeding and eating difficulties (Mauk, 1993). Adequacy of dietary intake should be evaluated at each well child visit. An excessive adherence to routine and an abhorrence of changes in the environment may lead children with autism to reject their parents' efforts to provide them with a balanced diet. These children may have periods when they eat only one or a few foods (Wing, 1997). It seems that the hypersensitivity of some children with autism to smell, taste, and touch results in the rejection of certain foods and food textures (Rapin, 1997; Sigman and Capps, 1997). Some of these difficulties may be ameliorated through the interventions of the child's behavioral therapist. If the child insists upon using certain dishes and cups for eating, the provider may advise the parents to have multiple sets of the preferred items. A daily multivitamin supplement is recommended to ensure adequate vitamin and mineral intake. Parents of children taking valproic acid should be encouraged to provide them with plenty of low-calorie, low-fat snacks and water—instead of juice or soda.

Safety

The parents of children with autism are faced with a number of safety issues that arise from the cognitive and behavioral deficits of autism. Because of their poor judgment and lack of impulse control,

children with autism must be supervised at all times. Children with autism often do not generalize information from one experience to another. Therefore it may take years for a child with autism to learn to avoid dangerous situations; and many will never learn. Their ability to recognize a potentially dangerous activity (e.g., tree climbing) is usually far behind their chronologic age and gross motor capabilities (Sigman and Capps, 1997). Children with autism have been known to swallow an entire bottle of medication in the time it takes a parent to turn away and answer the telephone. In a study of the long-term outcomes of 163 adolescents and young adults with autism, Ballaban-Gil, Rapin, and associates (1996) found that three of their subjects had died—including one from drowning. In the publication of the results of this study, Rapin also reports personal knowledge of two other young children with autism who had drowned (Ballaban-Gil et al, 1996). Morbidity and mortality can be the result of momentary lapses in supervision.

Child-proofing the home of a child with autism is essential. Medications must be out of reach and securely locked. Other dangerous objects (e.g., knives and matches) must be kept out of reach. Hot stoves and liquids present a constant danger to children with autism.

Children with autism may develop self-injurious behaviors such as head-banging, hand-biting, and scratching or picking at their skin (Siegel, 1996). Some of these behaviors may be gentle and are probably self-stimulatory (Siegel, 1996). Other self-injurious behavior, however, can cause significant bodily harm, and parents must stop this behavior even if the child becomes aggressive. Parents of children with self-injurious behavior must work with the child's primary care provider and autism treatment team to devise a plan for responding to this behavior. This plan may include pharmacotherapy. Self-injurious behaviors are extremely upsetting to parents, so they will need a great deal of support and assistance as they attempt to manage and prevent these behaviors.

The presence of self-injurious behaviors is complicated by an apparent decreased sensitivity to pain in many children with autism (Rapin, 1997). That is, they may fail to respond with tears or a painful outcry to painful stimuli (e.g., a hot stove or laceration). They often fail to approach their parents for comfort when they have been injured. Because of their lack of communication and social skills, the only sign that a child with autism is in pain may be an exacerbation of their autistic symptomatology. The provider must pay attention to parental reports that their child's behavior is different for no apparent reason because this may be the only clue that the child has suffered an injury.

The parents of children with autism and epilepsy should follow the safety measures prescribed for children with epilepsy. Most importantly, a child with epilepsy should never be allowed to take a bath or be around bodies of water without supervision because a seizure while bathing or playing in water while unsupervised can be fatal

Immunizations

Children with autism should be vaccinated following the schedule recommended by the American Academy of Pediatrics. Because of their insensitivity to pain and inability to report discomfort, they may be given acetaminophen prophylactically 1 hour before and periodically for 24 hours following the administration of vaccinations.

Children with autism who also have epilepsy should be vaccinated following the guidelines of the American Academy of Pediatrics for children with neurologic disorders (see Chapter 21).

Screening

Vision: A child with autism needs a thorough ophthalmologic examination at the time of diagnosis to look for the ocular signs of tuberous sclerosis, hypopigmented spots in the iris, and choroid hamartomas. Following this initial screening, routine screening is recommended.

Hearing: Following an initial evaluation by an audiologist to rule out hearing loss as a cause of communication delay, routine screening is recommended.

Dental care: Routine screening is recommended. Children with autism who are also taking phenytoin (Dilantin) for epilepsy are prone to development of gum hyperplasia and need to have their gums checked at least semiannually. Referral to a dentist familiar with treating children with developmental disabilities is essential. Some children with autism will not be able to tolerate routine dental screening and dental work without sedation.

Blood pressure: Routine screening is recommended. Children with autism may take clonidine (Catapres) to either treat a concomitant tic disorder or decrease hyperactivity and improve attention. Clonidine can cause both hypo- and hypertension. Blood pressure should be monitored before initiation of therapy. Lowering the dose of clonidine or stopping it completely must be done very slowly with blood pressure monitoring after each dose change. A rapid decrease in the clonidine dose can precipitate potentially dangerous rebound hypertension (Shlafer, 1993).

Hematocrit: Routine screening is recommended. Children with autism who are taking carbamezapine (Tegretol or Carbatrol) or valproic acid (Depakene or Depakote) should have complete blood counts (CBCs) with platelets and AST and ALT done before initiation of therapy and after establishment of the maintenance dose. These tests should be repeated annually and should also be done if the child develops symptoms of thrombocytopenia or liver dysfunction (e.g., unusual bruising or petechiae, unusual bleeding, jaundice, or hepatomegaly).

Urinalysis: Routine screening is recommended.

Tuberculosis: Routine screening is recommended.

Common Illness Management

Differential Diagnosis (Box 10-4)

Because of their social, communication, and cognitive deficits, most children with autism cannot accurately report symptoms of illness to their parents or providers. Parents or caretakers of children with autism are the experts on their child's baseline behavior and level of functioning (Seid et al, 1997). Regression in a child's skills or a negative change in behavior is often the first indication that a child with autism is ill (Tonge et al, 1994). Therefore it is important for primary care providers to listen carefully to parental reports of children who are not behaving in their customary ways. Head-banging or other self-injurious or aggressive behaviors may suddenly begin as a response to a painful illness such as otitis media (Cohen, 1998).

Injury

Children with autism are at high risk for injury. The frequency of accidental injury may obscure the occurrence of nonaccidental injury that can result from caretaker fatigue and the extremely trying and sometimes dangerous behavior of a child with autism. Self-injurious behaviors (e.g., hand-biting and head-banging) can also cause injuries that may require both treatment of the injury and behavioral and pharmacologic intervention to prevent further injury.

Seizures

Children with autism may have any one of the various types of seizures: simple or complex partial seizures, absence, or generalized tonic and/or clonic seizures. Children who manifest signs of seizure activity (e.g., rhythmic jerking, stiffening, staring with unresponsiveness to physical stimulation, and eye fluttering or deviation) should have an EEG at a diagnostic laboratory experienced in obtaining EEGs in children. An abnormal EEG indicates the need for referral to a pediatric neurologist (see Chapter 21).

Medication Side Effects

Although there are no routinely prescribed medications for children with autism, many affected children take medications for controlling seizures and/or behavioral disturbances. Primary care providers should know what medications a child is taking and the common and adverse side effects and signs of toxicity of each. Although these medications will have been prescribed by the child's neurologist or psychiatrist, parents will call the primary care provider first if the child develops nausea and vomiting, ataxia, lethargy, tremor, or other potential symptoms of toxic drug levels. It is up to primary care providers to be aware of what medications, if any, a child is taking and the possible ramifications of their use.

Drug Interactions

The use of erythromycin in children taking carbamazepine (Tegretol or Carbatrol) should be avoided. Erythromycin increases carbamazepine blood levels, which can result in toxicity (see Chapter 21 for other antiepileptic drug interactions). Priapism is a potential adverse side effect of trazodone (Desyrel), so it should be used cautiously in postpubertal males (Shlafer, 1993).

Developmental Issues

Sleep Patterns

From infancy on, many children with autism will have difficulty falling and staying asleep (Coleman and Gillberg, 1985; Harris JC, 1995; Rapin, 1997; Wolff, 1991). Many children with autism seem to need less sleep than other children their age and refuse naps, fall asleep late, and awaken during the night and stay awake for long periods (Siegel, 1996). As they get older, children with autism may repeatedly attempt to leave their room at night, causing parents to take them into their bed (Siegel, 1996). This disturbing sleep pattern may be related to altered amounts of neurotransmitters, particularly serotonin (Coleman and Gillberg, 1985).

Sleep disturbances may respond to behavioral intervention. Children with autism need highly structured bedtime rituals (Siegel, 1996) and may need a parent at their bedside until they fall asleep. Because they may awaken and get out of bed during the night, their rooms must be safe and free of objects with which the children could harm themselves. Some children with autism learn to play alone in their room, even in the dark (Siegel, 1996).

The door of the room must be secured, however, so that a child cannot wander about the house and engage in potentially dangerous behavior. A Dutch door is a useful alternative for some families. Parents will need reassurance that this aberrant sleep pattern is not unusual for their child and that it is fine for the child to be awake and playing at night.

Sleep disturbances are not particularly amenable to medication (Harris JC, 1995). Many of the typical sedatives used with children (e.g., chloral hydrate and diphenhydramine [Benadryl]) can have paradoxic effects in children with autism. When given as part of the bedtime ritual, trazodone (Desyrel) may help the child both fall asleep and stay asleep (Siegel, 1996). A child receiving a neuroleptic or tricyclic antidepressant for behavioral symptoms may derive some sedative effect from it if given in the evening. Trazodone is a better alternative than neuroleptics or tricyclic antidepressants only used to promote sleep because of it has fewer side effects. Trazodone should be taken with food to promote absorption. Research has begun on the use of melatonin to improve the quantity and quality of sleep. There is no evidence, however, that it helps without highly structured and consistent bedtime routines used simultaneously (Lord, 1998).

Toileting

Children with autism are often very difficult to toilet train (Wolff, 1991). Children with performance IQs below the equivalent of 30 months of age are generally not ready for toilet training, and parents should be advised not to initiate toilet training until this performance level is obtained (Siegel, 1996). Children with autism do not respond to many of the standard toilet training strategies parents use (e.g., being encouraged to imitate the parent or wear "big kid underwear") but can often be toilet trained by using a behavioral approach with food as a reward (Siegel, 1996).

Toilet training should be initiated by taking the child to the bathroom at set times when the child is mostly like to urinate. These times include soon after getting up in the morning, after meals and snacks, before and after going to school, and before going to bed. It is helpful if all the child's caretakers work on toilet training together, using a very structured and consistent approach and including the same language and rewards. Parents should be advised that toilet training can take months or even longer if a child has both autism and mental retardation.

Discipline

Discipline is an all-day, every day affair with children with autism. As questions arise about appropriate discipline, providers will want to consult with the child's treatment team. A highly structured and consistent environment is necessary for a child to learn socially appropriate behavior and refrain from dangerous behavior. The use of positive reinforcers (e.g., play with favorite objects and food) is essential. Time-out for negative behaviors can also be employed if positive reinforcement is not totally successful (Harris, 1995). Negative reinforcement, such as a firm "No" and restraint or removal from the situation, may be necessary for potentially dangerous or self-injurious behaviors, but parents should be warned that children with autism do not readily generalize from one situation to another and often only attend to one very specific component of a situation (Cohen, 1998). In certain situations, parents may feel the need to discipline their child with autism even when they are not sure that the child will understand the discipline. For example, Harris (1994) relates the story of a mother who sent her daughter with autism for a time-out after she broke her brother's favorite toy. Although she knew her daughter might not learn from the time out, she thought it was important for her son to see his sister receive appropriate consequences for her actions.

Child Care

There are two types of child care that may be essential for children with autism: traditional child care during the hours the child's parents are working and respite care (i.e., care provided so that the child's parents may have time away from the constant responsibility of caring for their child with autism).

Children with autism are often easily overstimulated and can respond by withdrawing into self-stimulatory behaviors. They generally cannot interact with peers without teaching and supervision from adults. For these reasons, large-group child care is inadvisable unless a child has an accompanying aide to ensure that the child is appropriately occupied. Small, family daycare arrangements can work well (Siegel, 1996). The daycare provider must be educated about the special behavior training and safety needs of the child with autism and willing to take on the challenge of integrating the child into activities with other children.

Therapeutic after-school programs are increasingly becoming available for school-age children with autism and may be covered under the related services clause of IDEA (see Chapter 5). These programs feature a low staff-to-child ratio and activities designed to teach social skills and appropriate public behavior. Although some children with autism can be fully included in regular after-school programs, many find these programs too unstructured and unpredictable.

Respite care is sometimes provided in the home by a trained respite care worker. Out-of-home respite care is provided by a licensed worker in the worker's home or in a group home designed to provide short-term respite care (Harris, 1994). The primary care provider can be instrumental in referring the family to local respite services. Parents may be reluctant to use these services because they are fearful that their child will not be adequately cared for and that their need for respite services is a reflection on their parenting. The provider can reassure the parents that by taking care of themselves and the other children in the family, they will have more energy with which to meet the needs of their child with autism. Respite care is also excellent practice for the transition to living away from home that many children with autism make in young adulthood.

Schooling

The most significant treatment for autism is early and intense education to improve the child's communication, self-care, social skills, and behavior (Mauk, 1993; Rapin, 1997). All children with autism fall under the province of federal legislation for children with disabilities (see Chapter 5). School services that are available to children with autism vary widely (Sigman and Capps, 1997). Infants and toddlers are eligible for early intervention programs provided by state services for children with developmental disabilities. Preschool and school-age children with autism may be offered educational programs ranging from full inclusion in a standard classroom with an aide to time divided between a regular classroom and special resources (e.g., speech therapy) to placement in a special day class solely for children who qualify for special education.

Throughout a child's school years, parents need to participate in Individualized Family Service (IFSP) or Individualized Education Plan (IEP) meeting. During these meetings the child's school placement is determined. Parents must carefully evaluate all alternatives for their child, choose the one that they and the treatment team feel is most appropriate, and be prepared to present the reasons for their choice at the planning meeting because federal law neither guarantees the best education for the child nor adequately funds programs to provide the highest standard of care (Siegel, 1996). Parents will want to consider adding augmentative communication methods (e.g., pictures, sign language, or computers) to their child's program if the child has not developed language by the age of 5 or 6 years (Howlin, 1998).

The recent movement to full inclusion of all children in standard public schools may have an effect on educational services for children with autism (Bristol et al, 1996). Although some parents would like their children to be fully included, others argue that the resources available to a child with autism in a standard classroom can be very limited (Bauer, 1995b). Some children with autism will find the stimulation of a public school class of 20 to 30 or more students overwhelming. Parents often seek the advice of their child's primary care provider while they evaluate various school options.

One of the key roles for the primary care provider of a child with autism is making the clinical, educational, and management needs of the child clear to the school district and other agencies involved in therapeutic interventions with the child (Bauer, 1995b). In particular, providers may need to advocate for early intervention for preschoolers with autism (Bauer, 1995b). Parents, with support from health professionals, must advocate for the services necessary to maximize the child's potential.

Sexuality

Children with autism must be taught appropriate behaviors regarding their sexuality that are tailored to their developmental level and told about the particularly inappropriate behaviors they may exhibit. Because of their cognitive, communication, and social deficits, children with autism will not necessarily independently learn behaviors such as refraining from masturbating or undressing in public and shutting the door when using the bathroom. Ruble and Dalrymple (1993) found that 90% of individuals over the age of 9 years with autism had been taught specific rules about private behavior. Methods used included repetition, redirection, positive reinforcement, and modeling. The parents of the individuals in this study reported that almost two thirds of their children had touched their private parts in public and approximately one quarter had removed clothing in public and/or masturbated in public. There was no significant difference in the frequency of these behaviors between individuals with autism who were verbal and high-functioning and those without language who were low-functioning. Primary care providers can work with parents to identify problematic sexual behaviors and solicit help from the child's treatment team in developing a plan to ameliorate them. No research indicates that teaching children with autism about their sexuality encourages the development of aberrant behaviors, although many parents fear this (Konstanareas and Lunsky, 1997). The provider can reassure parents that many children with autism display inappropriate sexual behaviors but that these behaviors can be dealt with using the behavior management techniques for nonsexual behaviors. To prevent the development of inappropriate behaviors, parents should be guided to teach their children very specific and concrete rules about acceptable and unacceptable sexual behavior.

Transition into Adulthood

Children with autism grow up to be adults with autism. The majority of those who have cognitive deficits in addition to autism will require lifelong care, support, and supervision (Lainhart and Piven, 1995; Wing, 1997). These services may in-

clude residential placement, sheltered workshop employment, continued education, and behavioral management (Ballaban-Gil et al, 1996; Wing, 1997). In their follow-up study of 102 children with autism, Ballaban-Gil and associates found that 69% continued to experience behavior problems in adolescence and adulthood. Over 90% of these individuals with autism still had social deficits. Despite one third of the children having near-normal to normal intelligence, only 11% of the adults had jobs—and all were menial. Previous follow-up studies done in the United States and Europe found even smaller proportions of the adults employed. As treatment of autism improves, so should these statistics. The persistent social deficits of autism (e.g., poor judgment in social situations, limited conversation skills, and impaired problem-solving) preclude most adults with autism from independent employment and marriage. Work that involves little social interaction and concrete and repetitive tasks may be the most suitable (Harris JC, 1995).

The parents of children with autism must be encouraged and counseled by their child's primary care provider to plan for the child's future. Education is mandated for children with significant disabilities until they are 22 years of age. At that time, the parents and treatment team will need to help the adult with autism in make the transition from school to sheltered or supervised work through a public or private community agency. Those few individuals able to attend college will still need a great deal of support and assistance with organization and planning. The end of mandated education may also be an appropriate time for a young adult to enter residential placement. Planning for this and locating a suitable home with an opening can take years. In early adolescence, the child's primary care provider should guide parents to begin exploring their options.

Finally, the pediatric primary care provider must help the parents find adult primary care for their child. As increasing numbers of children with developmental disabilities grow to adulthood and live and work in the community, family and adult providers will need to learn how to care for individuals who are often nonverbal and have continuing behavioral disturbances.

Special Family Concerns and Resources

Receiving a diagnosis of autism is intensely painful for most families. It often is months or even years from the time a toddler's delayed speech development is first recognized until the final diagnosis of autism is made. During this time, parents may have heard from several different providers in various specialties, including the child's primary care provider, that something is wrong with their child and it might be autism. The wait for the final diagnosis can be agonizing and delays implementation of appropriate interventions. Because there is no biologic marker for autism, the diagnosis is made based on neuropsychologic testing, careful history-taking, and observation of the child's behavior. This relatively subjective way of diagnosing such a serious and lifelong condition is often difficult for parents to understand. Primary care providers can play a crucial role in educating parents about the diagnosis, how it is determined, and the treatments that are available.

As families raise their child with autism, they will often meet professionals and lay people who view autism as a psychiatric disorder engendered by deficient mothering. Families will hear unkind remarks about their child's behavior and poor social skills and be given conflicting advice about how their child should be parented, treated, and educated. They will often have to struggle with school systems and after-school programs that are not designed to meet the special needs of a child with autism. Parents will need to educate all those who interact with their child about autism, their child's individual case, and the latest advances in the field of autism. In addition to educating parents, primary care providers will need to be open to receiving information from the parents about their child and the subject of autism in general.

Parenting a child with autism can be a tremendous physical, emotional, and financial challenge. A great deal of time and energy may be directed toward the child with autism and away from other relationships and family members—especially siblings (Harris, 1994; Tonge et al, 1994). Siblings may be embarrassed or afraid of the behavior of their sibling with autism and thus reluctant to bring friends home (Harris, 1994). Primary care providers can direct families to support groups, social services, and organizations that can address these issues.

Organizations

Autism Society of America
  7910 Woodmont Avenue, Suite 650
  Bethesda, Md. 20814-3015
  (800) 3-AUTISM
  http://www.autism-society.org
CAN (Cure Autism Now)
  5225 Wilshire Blvd., Suite 503
  Los Angeles, Calif. 90036
  (213) 549-0500
  http://www.canfoundation.org
NAAR (National Alliance for Autism Research)
  414 Wall St., Research Park
  Princeton, N.J. 08540
  (609) 430-9160 or (888) 777-NAAR
  http://www.naar.org

Information

Clinic for the Behavioral Treatment of Children
  (O. Ivar Lovaas, Director)
  Department of Psychology
  128A Franz Hall, PO Box 951563
  University of California
  Los Angeles, Calif. 90095-1563
  (310) 815-2319
Division TEACCH
  The Division for Treatment and Education of Autistic and Related Communication Handicapped Children
  University of North Carolina, Chapel Hill
  School of Medicine
  310 Medical School, Wing E, CB 7180
  Chapel Hill, N.C. 27599-7180
  (919) 966-2174
  http://www.unc.edu/depts/teacch/teacch.htm
The Family Connection
  Beach Center on Families and Disability
  31111 Haworth Hall
  University of Kansas
  Lawrence, Kan. 66045
  (800) 854-4938
  http://www.lsi.ukans.edu/beach/beachp.htm

Summary of Primary Care Needs for the Child with Autism

HEALTH CARE MAINTENANCE
Growth and development

Height and weight are usually within normal range but may be altered by medication side effects or restricted food preferences.

Measure head circumference annually until age 5 years. If child also has tuberous sclerosis, annual measurement of head circumference should continue after age 5 years.

Delayed language development usually noticed between 18 and 30 months of age.

Do not delay referral for diagnostic evaluation.

Diet

Child's insistence on sameness may affect food intake.

Well-balanced diet encouraged.

Multiple vitamin supplements may be indicated.

Valproic acid may cause increased hunger and excessive weight gain.

Safety

Risk of injury increased due to lack of impulse control, inability to generalize safety rules from one situation to another, and motor abilities more advanced than judgment.

Self-injurious behavior can result in injury due to increased pain tolerance and inability to communicate injury.

Diagnosis of acute and chronic medical conditions can be delayed by child's inability to report symptoms.

Children with autism and epilepsy must follow safety guidelines for children with epilepsy, including no unsupervised baths or swimming.

Immunization

Routine schedule is recommended.

Children with autism and epilepsy should follow the guidelines for children with epilepsy.

Screening

Vision: Routine screening after initial ophthalmological examination to look for signs of tuberous sclerosis.

Hearing: Routine screening after initial audiology evaluation which may include brainstem auditory evoked response testing.

Dental: Routine dental care is recommended. Children on phenytoin therapy require more frequent dental care for gum hyperplasia.

Sedation for dental care of the child with autism may be necessary.

Blood pressure: Routine screening is recommended.

Children on clonidine therapy require blood pressure monitoring before initiation of therapy and with all dosage changes.

Hematocrit: Routine screening is recommended.

Children on carbamezapine or valproate therapy should have CBC with platelets done before initiation of therapy, after establishment of maintenance dose, and annually thereafter.

Urinalysis: Routine screening is recommended.

Tuberculosis: Routine screening is recommended.

COMMON ILLNESS MANAGEMENT
Differential diagnosis

Communication and cognitive deficits make assessment difficult.

Change in behavior can indicate injury or illness.

continued

Summary of Primary Care Needs for the Child with Autism—cont'd

COMMON ILLNESS MANAGEMENT—cont'd
Differential diagnosis—cont'd

Injury: Cause of injury, accidental injury, self-injury, and nonaccidental injury must be determined and appropriate intervention identified.

Seizures: Seizure activity must be differentiated from repetitive or stereotypical behaviors.

Medication side effects.

Drug interactions

Erythromycin can increase plasma levels of carbamazepine.

Developmental issues

Sleep Patterns: Difficulty falling asleep and staying asleep is common.

Highly structured, consistent bedtime rituals are a necessity.

Sleep disturbances are not often amenable to standard mild sedatives.

Bedroom must be thoroughly child-proofed and secured so children cannot wander out alone or harm themselves at night.

Toileting: Training is often delayed.

Child must have performance IQ of 30 before training should be attempted.

Structured, behavioral approach with reward system is usually needed.

Mimicking parental behavior usually not effective.

Discipline: Highly structured and consistent approach is necessary.

Continuous discipline is necessary because children with autism do not readily generalize from one situation to another.

Concrete positive reinforcement (e.g., food) is essential.

Negative reinforcement may be needed for dangerous behavior.

Child Care: Family daycare or therapeutic child care setting is recommended.

After-school care may be covered under the related services clause of IDEA.

Respite care can be important for primary caretaker and other family members.

Schooling: Early, intense intervention, which may include 1:1 teaching, is often needed and most effective.

Families will need support during the IEP process to advocate for their child.

Parents must choose from range of options from full inclusion to self-contained schools for children with autism.

Sexuality: Appropriate sexual behavior must be taught.

Specific and concrete rules about sexuality are necessary.

Transition to adulthood

Most adults with autism require life-long care, support, and supervision.

Work that involves concrete and repetitive tasks and little social interaction may be most suitable.

Parents need to plan for child's future, including finding appropriate adult primary care.

Special family concerns

Diagnosis is made relatively subjectively, so it can be hard to comprehend.

Lack of understanding of autism in the community contributes to lack of supportive services.

Siblings and others may be afraid of and/or embarrassed by behavior of child with autism.

References

Committee on Children With Disabilities: Auditory integration training and facilitated communication for autism, Pediatrics 102(2 Pt 1):431-433, 1998.

American Psychiatric Association: Diagnostic and statistical manual of mental disorders, ed 4, Washington, DC, 1994, The Association.

Bailey A et al: Autism: towards an integration of clinical, genetic, neuropsychological, and neurobiological perspectives, J Child Psychol Psychiat 37(1):89-126, 1996.

Ballaban-Gil K et al: Longitudinal examination of the behavioral, language, and social changes in a population of adolescents and young adults with autistic disorder, Pediatr Neurol 15(3):217-223, 1996.

Bauer S: Autism and the pervasive developmental disorders, part 1, Pediatr Rev 16(4):130-136, 1995a.

Bauer S: Autism and the pervasive developmental disorders, part 2, Pediatr Rev 16(5):168-176, 1995b.

Bauman ML: Brief report: neuroanatomic observations of the brain in pervasive developmental disorders, J Autism Dev Disord 26(2):199-203, 1996.

Bristol MM et al: State of the sciences in autism: report to the national Institutes of Health, J Autism Dev Disord 26(2):121-154, 1996.

Bryson SE: Brief report: epidemiology of autism, J Autism Dev Disord 26(2):165-167, 1996.

Cohen S: Targeting autism, Berkeley, Calif., 1998, University of California Press.

Coleman M and Gillberg C: The biology of the autistic syndromes, New York, 1985, Praeger Publishers.

Courchesne E: Neuroanatomic imaging in autism, Pediatrics 87(5 pt 2):781-790, 1991.

DeLong GR, Teague LA, and Kamran MM: Effects of fluoxetine treatment in young children with idiopathic autism, Dev Medicine and Child Neurology 40:551-562, 1998.

Fatemi SH et al: Fluoxetine in treatment of adolescent patients with autism: a longitudinal open trial, J Autism Dev Disorders 28(4):303-307, 1998.

Findling RL, Maxwell K, and Wiznitzer M: An open clinical trial of risperidone monotherapy in young children with autistic disorder, Psychopharmacol Bull 33(1):155-159, 1997.

Folstein SE and Piven J: Etiology of autism: genetic influences, Pediatrics 87(5 pt 2):767-773, 1991.

Gillberg C and Coleman M: Autism and medical disorders: a review of the literature, Dev Med Child Neurol 38:191-202, 1996.

Gillberg C: Neuropsychiatric disorders, Curr Op Neurol 11:109-114, 1998.

Gresham FM and MacMillan DL: Early intervention project: can its claims be substantiated and its effects replicated?, J Autism Dev Disord 28(1):5-13, 1998.

Happé F and Frith U: The neuropsychology of autism, Brain 119:1377-1400, 1996.

Harris JC: Developmental neuropsychiatry: assessment, diagnosis, and treatment of developmental disorders, vol II, Oxford, 1995, Oxford University Press.

Harris SL: Siblings of children with autism, Bethesda Md., 1994, Woodbine House.

Hellings JA et al: Sertaline response in adults with mental retardation and autistic disorder, J Clin Psychiatry 57(8):333-336, 1996.

Hostetler C: Comparison of the atypical antipsychotics, lecture given at Purdue University, 1998, Website: www.iupui.edu/~bcarlste/atypsych.html.

Howlin P: Practitioner review: psychological and educational treatments for autism, J Child Psychol Psychiatry 39(3):307-322, 1998.

Kanner L: Autistic disturbances of affective contact, The Nervous Child 2:217-250, 1943.

Kaplan M, Edelson SM, and Seip JL: Behavioral changes in autistic individuals as a result of wearing ambient transitional prism lenses, Child Psychiatry Hum Dev 29(1):65-76, 1998.

Kemper TL and Bauman M: Neuropathology of infantile autism, J Neuropathol Exp Neurol 57(7):645-652, 1998.

Konstantareas MM and Lunsky YJ: Sociosexual knowledge, experience, attitudes, and interests of individuals with autistic disorder and developmental delay, J Autism Dev Disord 27(4):397-413, 1997.

Lainhart JE and Piven J: Diagnosis, treatment, and neurobiology of autism in children, Curr Opinion Pediatr 7:392-400, 1995.

Lord C: What is melatonin? Is it a useful treatment for sleep problems in autism? J Autism Dev Disord 28(4):345-346, 1998.

Lord C, Rutter M, and Couteur AL: Autism diagnostic interview-revised: a revised version of a diagnostic interview for caregivers of individuals with possible pervasive developmental disorders, J Autism Dev Disord 24(5):659-685, 1994.

Lotspeich L and Shaw R, personal communication, 1998.

Mauk JE: Autism and pervasive developmental disorders, Child Dev Disabil 40(3):567-587, 1993.

Minshew N: Indices of neural function in autism: clinical and biologic implications, Pediatrics 87(5 pt 2): 774-780, 1991.

Nelson KB: Prenatal and perinatal factors in the etiology of autism, Pediatrics 87(5 pt 2):761-766, 1991.

Nicolson R, Awad G, and Sloman L: An open trial of risperidone in young autistic children, J Am Acad Child Adolesc Psychiatry 37(4):372-376, 1998.

Pickar D: Facts about Risperdal, Helpline fact sheet of the National Alliance for the Mentally Ill, 1996, Website: www.nami.org/helpline/riperidone.htm

Piven J et al: The etiology of autism: pre-, peri- and neonatal factors, J Am Acad Child Adolesc Psychiatry 32(6):1256-1263, 1993.

Plioplys AV: Intravenous immunoglobulin treatment of children with autism, J Child Neurol 13:79-82, 1998.

Rapin I and Katzman R: Neurobiology of autism, Ann Neurol 43:7-14, 1998.

Rapin I: Autism, New Engl J Med 337(2):97-104, 1997.

Rimland B and Baker SM: Brief report: alternative approaches to the development of effective treatments for autism, J Autism Dev Disord 26(2):237-241, 1996.

Ritvo E et al: The UCLA-University of Utah epidemiologic survey of autism: prevalence, Am J Psychiatry 146:194-199, 1989.

Ruble LA and Dalrymple NJ: Social/sexual awareness of persons with autism: a parental perspective, Arch Sex Behav 22(3):229-240, 1993.

Schreier HA: Risperidone for young children with mood disorders and aggressive behavior, J Child Adolesc Psychopharmacol 8(1):49-59, 1998.

Seid M, Sherman M, and Seid AB: Perioperative psychosocial interventions for autistic children undergoing ENT surgery, Int J Pediatr Otorhinolaryngology 40:107-113, 1997.

Sheinkopf SJ and Siegel B: Home-based behavioral treatment of young children with autism, J Autism Develop Disord 28(1):15-23, 1998.

Shlafer M: The nurse, pharmacology, and drug therapy: a prototype approach, ed 2, Redwood City, Calif., 1993, Addison-Wesley.

Siegel B: The world of the autistic child, Oxford, 1996, Oxford University Press.

Sigman M and Capps L: Children with autism, Cambridge, Mass., 1997, Harvard University Press.

Smalley SL and Collins F: Brief report: genetic, prenatal, and immunologic factors, J Autism Dev Disord 26(2):195-198, 1996.

Tonge BJ, Dissanayake C, and Brereton AV: Autism: fifty years on from Kanner, J Paediatr Child Health 30:102-107, 1994.

Wing L: The autistic spectrum, Lancet 350:1761-1766, 1997.

Wolff S: Childhood autism: its diagnosis, nature, and treatment, Arch Dis Child 66(6):737-741, 1991.

World Health Organization: International classification of diseases, 10th rev, Geneva, 1994, The Organization.

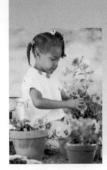

CHAPTER 11

Bleeding Disorders

Susan Karp

Etiology

Hemophilia and von Willebrand's disease are the most common inherited bleeding disorders resulting from deficiencies or abnormalities of specific coagulation proteins. The von Willebrand protein is activated when the endothelium is damaged. This protein promotes formation of an initial platelet plug by enabling platelet adhesion. Multiple coagulation proteins, including those that are deficient in hemophilia, are critical components of the secondary or intrinsic hemostatic mechanism that is activated when collagen fibers are exposed in a damaged blood vessel. These proteins are required for the formation of the final fibrin clot (Hoyer, 1994; Roberts et al, 1998).

Hemophilia

Hemophilia involves a defect in the intrinsic hemostatic mechanism (Figure 11-1). Factor VIII deficiency (e.g., classic hemophilia, hemophilia A) accounts for approximately 75% to 80% of hemophilia cases, whereas factor IX deficiency (e.g., Christmas disease, hemophilia B) accounts for 20% to 25% of such cases (Crudder, 1998; Soucie, Evatt, and Jackson, 1998). Less common factor deficiencies exist but are not specifically discussed in this chapter. Severity of hemophilia is defined by the percentage of activity of the deficient coagulation protein (Table 11-1).

Hemophilia is inherited in an X-linked pattern. Most frequently, female carriers pass the disorder to their sons. The severity of hemophilia remains constant within families, although clinical symptoms may vary based on lifestyle and treatment regimens. Approximately 30% of all hemophilia cases are sporadic (e.g., negative prior family history) (Hoffman and Roberts, 1995). A woman is considered to be an obligate carrier if hemophilia has been diagnosed in either her father, two of her sons, or one son and one other relative. Carriers of hemophilia A or B are expected to have, on average, factor VIII or IX levels that are approximately 50% of normal. Because of lyonization, however, some carriers have very low factor levels with resultant symptoms of excessive or unusual bleeding—particularly menorrhagia (Kadir et al, 1998; Kadir et al, 1999), which validates the need for determination of factor VIII/IX coagulant levels—even in obligate carriers.

von Willebrand's Disease

Generally a mild bleeding disorder, von Willebrand's disease is closely related to hemophilia. The von Willebrand protein's primary action is to facilitate platelet adhesion (see Figure 11-1). This protein also helps to stabilize factor VIII; and when von Willebrand's protein is deficient, the amount of circulating active factor VIII may also be reduced (Ewenstein, 1997; Nichols and Ginsburg, 1997).

Three main variants of the disorder exist (Ewenstein, 1997; Federici, 1998; Nichols and Ginsburg, 1997). In the most common variant, type I, the total amount of the protein is decreased and both large and small forms (i.e., multimers) of the von Willebrand protein are present. Inheritance of type I is autosomal dominant. In type II the large and intermediate multimers are absent in the plasma and platelets. The potential for thrombocytopenia with use of desmopressin in type IIB, in which the large multimers are absent in the plasma, should be noted (Mannucci, 1997). Type III is a severe autosomal recessive form of the disorder marked by the absence of detectable von Willebrand protein.

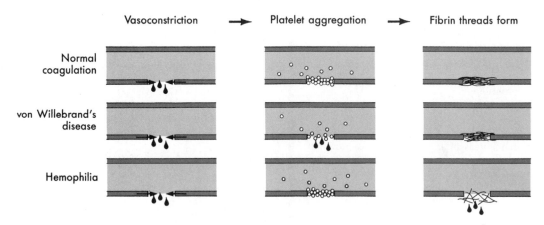

Figure 11-1   Comparison of the defect in hemophilia and von Willebrand's disease with normal coagulation after a break in a vessel wall. Defect in von Willebrand's disease is in platelet aggregation. Defect in hemophilia is in fibrin thread formation.

Table 11-1
Severity of Hemophilia

Severity	Factor VIII and IX Coagulant Activity (%)	Frequency and Type of Bleeding
Severe	<1	By school age, several bleeding episodes that require treatment often occur each month. Bleeding may be spontaneous or the result of injury.
Moderate	1 to 5	Frequency of bleeding is variable. Spontaneous bleeding is less common.
Mild	>5	Bleeding is generally only a result of trauma or surgery.

Note that normal factor VIII and IX coagulant levels are generally 50% to 150% (.50 to 1.5 U/dl) but vary slightly between laboratories.

Incidence

Hemophilia occurs in all ethnic groups, with an incidence of 1 in 5,000 live male births. (Soucie, Evatt, and Jackson, 1998). Although the true incidence of von Willebrand's disease is not known, it is thought to be the most common inherited bleeding disorder. Many scientists estimate that von Willebrand's disease is present in more than 1% of the general population (Ewenstein, 1997; Nichols and Ginsburg, 1997). Many cases are not diagnosed because of the mild nature of many of the symptoms.

Clinical Manifestations at Time of Diagnosis

When a newborn has a family history of hemophilia, circumcision, heel sticks, and intramuscular immunizations and injections should ideally be delayed until a definitive diagnosis is made. Vitamin K may be given subcutaneously instead of intramuscularly to reduce the risk of hematoma development. Diagnosis is performed prenatally or by using cord or peripheral blood to test factor levels.

By 12 to 18 months of age, most children with severe hemophilia are diagnosed because of posi-

Clinical Manifestations at the Time of Diagnosis

Hemophilia
- Bleeding following circumcision and/or heel stick
- Excessive bruising
- Hematomas after venipuncture or minimal injury
- Bleeding from the umbilical cord stump
- Intracranial bleeding
- Cephalohematoma
- Prolonged oral bleeding (i.e., after frenulum tear, dental extraction, tooth loss)
- Hemarthrosis (i.e., generally not the first symptom)

von Willebrand's Disease
- Prolonged or repeated epistaxis
- Prolonged or excessive menstrual bleeding
- Gastrointestinal bleeding

tive family history or unusual bleeding (Box 11-1) (Onwuzurike, Warrier, and Lusher, 1996). Before diagnosis, parents may be questioned about child abuse because of excessive bruising. Diagnosis in infancy most commonly occurs because of a positive family history, which is confirmed by cord blood coagulation assays, intracranial hemorrhage, excessive bruising with hematomas, cephalohematoma, or bleeding following circumcision and venipuncture (Conway and Hilgartner, 1994). Bleeding from the umbilical cord stump may be indicative of factor XIII deficiency (Hoffman and Roberts, 1995).

Intracranial hemorrhage may be life-threatening and occurs in 1% to 5% of newborns with moderate to severe hemophilia; one half of these newborns develop neurologic deficits (Michaud et al, 1991). Michaud and colleagues (1991) recommend that male newborns of known carriers not diagnosed prenatally be tested for hemophilia by cord or peripheral blood sampling. If a child has a positive prenatal diagnosis of hemophilia by cord blood analysis, they also recommend follow-up with computerized tomography (CT) or ultrasonography in the first 24 hours of life, even after cesarean section. Cesarean section is not routinely recommended in nontraumatic deliveries (Medical and Scientific Advisory Council [MASAC], 1998). Although factor VIII levels generally rise above 50% during pregnancy, carriers whose baseline levels are below 50% may be at particular risk for postpartum hemorrhage. Factor IX levels do not rise significantly in pregnancy, and carriers with low levels of factor IX are more likely to need hematologic support with delivery (Giangrande, 1998). The inheritance pattern for hemophilia is shown in Figure 11-2.

Children who first show signs of bleeding later in childhood or in adolescence more often have mild to moderate hemophilia. A frequent misconception is that all children with hemophilia can bleed to death from a typical childhood cut or scratch. They may, however, demonstrate joint bleeding (i.e., hemarthrosis); muscle hematomas; excessive postoperative bleeding; or excessive or prolonged oral bleeding following frenulum tears, lost deciduous teeth, tooth eruption, and dental extractions (DiMichele, 1998; Hoyer, 1994; Venkateswaran et al, 1998).

von Willebrand's disease is commonly manifested by bleeding from the mucous membranes. Although epistaxis is most frequently noted, excessive oral, gastrointestinal (GI), and menstrual bleeding also occur (Ewenstein, 1997). Diagnostic testing is often requested when there is a positive family history of the disorder or when an increased partial thromboplastin time is obtained during routine preoperative screening. Because the levels of the von Willebrand protein and factor VIII vary over time, coagulation testing may need to be repeated to establish a diagnosis (von Willebrand Working Party, 1997). Despite the relatively high incidence of this disorder, it is not often diagnosed because the common symptoms of epistaxis and heavy menstrual bleeding are often not brought to medical attention.

Hemophilia Carrier Testing

A single performance of carrier testing for hemophilia using a factor VIII coagulant-to-antigen ratio has an accuracy rate of 80% to 90% (Jandl, 1996).

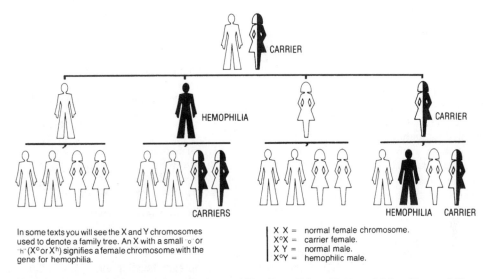

In some texts you will see the X and Y chromosomes used to denote a family tree. An X with a small "o" or "h" (X° or X^h) signifies a female chromosome with the gene for hemophilia.

X X = normal female chromosome.
X°X = carrier female.
X Y = normal male.
X°Y = hemophilic male.

Figure 11-2 Inheritance pattern for hemophilia. (From Eckert EF: Your child and hemophilia, New York, 1990, The National Hemophilia Foundation.)

The use of DNA testing to detect carriers has an estimated accuracy of 95% to 99%, depending on the number of probes used; it is expensive and requires blood samples from multiple family members, including an affected male (Dardik et al, 1996; Gupta and Bianchi, 1996). A factor VIII inversion is a genetic defect found in approximately 50% of people with severe hemophilia A and occurs when the distal end of the X chromosome containing part of the factor VIII gene flips over so that the factor VIII message is interrupted by irrelevant genetic material. If an affected male has this inversion, all female relatives who are carriers will also have it. This inversion test has 100% accuracy (Naylor et al, 1996; Vnencak-Jones et al, 1996). Carrier testing for factor IX hemophilia using DNA probes is also available (Young et al, 1996).

Prenatal diagnosis may be performed by amniocentesis as early as 13 to 16 weeks' gestation, by chorionic villus sampling at 8 to 12 weeks' gestation, or by fetal blood sampling (i.e., using percutaneous umbilical blood sampling) at 18 to 20 weeks' gestation. Male fetuses can be diagnosed as having hemophilia in utero by the use of DNA probes or the inversion test. If a percutaneous umbilical blood sampling is performed, the hemophilia diagnosis is made by means of a specialized test called factor VIII or factor IX clotting antigen (Dardik et al, 1996; Aledort et al, 1998).

Treatment

Comprehensive Care

The standard of care in hemophilia is a collaborative interdisciplinary approach facilitated by local hemophilia treatment centers (HTCs). These centers, which are funded in part by the federal government, provide comprehensive management of inherited coagulation disorders. The core team consists of a pediatric hematologist, nurse coordinator, and social worker. A genetic counselor and physical therapist are other integral team members. A pediatric dentist and orthopedic surgeon provide consultative services. With the advent of human immunodeficiency virus (HIV), HTCs have also been mandated by the government to either provide or procure comprehensive management for clients exposed to HIV. Individuals exposed to hepatitis C are often seen by a liver specialist. Services of the HTC include interdisciplinary comprehensive evaluations, counseling and support services, carrier detection, access to new technology treatment products through clinical trials, and instruction on home infusion (Cahill, 1996; Jandl, 1996).

All children and adolescents with hemophilia and von Willebrand's disease should receive regular comprehensive evaluations at the nearest HTC. The frequency of these evaluations should be every 6 months to 1 year, depending on the severity of the child's bleeding disorder, use of prophylaxis, and immune status. At these visits, children and their families are routinely seen by the members of the interdisciplinary team. The family and primary care provider receive updated information on the status of a child's health and development, treatment options, and readiness for home therapy. HTCs work closely with primary care practioners to provide comprehensive, coordinated, and accessible care for day-to-day management of pediatric health care.

General Guidelines of Treatment

The goals of treatment are to rapidly initiate clotting when bleeding occurs, prevent bleeding during high-risk procedures, and in many persons with moderate or severe hemophilia, to prevent joint bleeding through prophylactic infusions of factor concentrate (Box 11-2).

The treatment product of choice should be decided by consulting with the child's hematologist (Table 11-2). This information should be updated at least yearly to incorporate changes in available technology. It has been shown that CD4 counts may be more stable in persons with HIV who use affinity purified factor concentrates than in those who use intermediate purity concentrates (Hoots and Canty, 1998). This information should be considered when recommending factor concentrates for a child's use (MASAC, 1998).

Some families who are not on home therapy keep a supply of the preferred concentrate in their home refrigerators to expedite treatment of their child in local emergency rooms. Factor concentrate does not need to be kept at school unless infusions are performed there.

Box 11-2

Treatment

- Comprehensive treatment programs at HTCs
- Factor replacement products (see Table 11-2)
- Desmopressin acetate (vWd and mild hemophilia)
- Prophylactic factor treatment (hemophilia)
- Estrogen therapy (vWd) for women
- Oral antifibrinolytic agents
- Topical hemostatic agents
- Physical therapy
- Surgery (e.g., synovectomy, joint replacement)

Significant head trauma or bleeding into the iliopsoas muscle (retroperitoneal), hip, GI tract, neck, or posterior pharynx are bleeding episodes that frequently require hospital admission and hematologic consultation. Such consultation is also recommended for bleeding that requires more than two treatments (i.e., concern that an inhibitor may be developing) and when there is any doubt about the need to treat an injury or bleeding episode. When there is doubt, however, it is safest to provide treatment if a bleeding episode is suspected (Furie, Limentani, and Rosenfield, 1994; Hoffman and Roberts, 1995; Hoyer, 1994).

School personnel and families often ask providers to recommend first-aid measures to be instituted while a child is waiting for evaluation and possible infusion. For soft tissue, joint, and muscle bleeding, elevating the affected area and applying an elastic bandage and ice may help to reduce swelling. The child should be allowed to fully rest the affected joint (Duthie et al, 1994). Firm pressure applied over a clean dressing is often sufficient to stop bleeding from surface lacerations in children with both hemophilia and von Willebrand's disease. Firm pressure applied to the nares is recommended for nose bleeding. Universal precautions must be used whenever blood or body secretions are encountered. Although ice may help to reduce the superficial swelling from a head hematoma, it should never replace a medical evaluation because intracranial bleeding is unaffected by its application.

Text continued on p. 223

Table 11-2
Factor VIII Products Licensed in the United States

Ultrapure Recombinant Factor VIII Products

Product Name	Manufacturer	Method of Viral Depletion or Inactivation	Specific Activity† (IU/mg protein), Final Product	Specific Activity† (IU/mg protein), Discounting Albumin	Hepatitis Safety Studies in Humans with this Product
Recombinate	Baxter	Immunoaffinity chromatography	16-19	>3000	Yes
Kogenate	Bayer	Immunoaffinity chromatography	8-30	>3000*	Yes
Broctate	Baxter (distributed by Centeon)	Immunoaffinity chromatography	16-19	>3000	Yes
Helixate	Bayer (distributed by Centeon)	Immunoaffinity chromatography	8-30	>3000*	Yes

Immunoaffinity Purified (Very High Purity) Factor VIII Products Derived from Human Plasma

Product Name	Manufacturer	Method of Viral Inactivation	Specific Activity† (IU/mg protein), Final Product	Specific Activity† (IU/mg protein), Discounting Albumin	Hepatitis Safety Studies in Humans with this Product	Hepatitis Safety Studies in Humans with Another Product, but Similar Viral Inactivation Method
Monoclare P	Centeon	1. Immunoaffinity chromatography 2. Pasteurization (60° C, 10h)	approx. 5-10	>3000	Yes	Yes

*Representative sample from in-process materials prior to addition of albumin.
†Note: The degree of product purity is reflected by the specific activity of factor VIII (units/mg protein). Because most factor VIII concentrates, including recombinant factor VIII, have human serum albumin added as a stabilizer, most persons look at the specific activity discounting albumin. Recombinant clotting factor preparations are referred to as "ultrapure."
‡Does not contain albumin.

Continued

Table 11-2—cont'd
Factor VIII Products Licensed in the United States

Immunoaffinity Purified (Very High Purity) Factor VIII Products Derived from Human Plasma—cont'd

Product Name	Manufacturer	Method of Viral Inactivation	Specific Activity† (IU/mg protein), Final Product	Specific Activity† (IU/mg protein), Discounting Albumin	Hepatitis Safety Studies in Humans with this Product	Hepatitis Safety Studies in Humans with Another Product, but Similar Viral Inactivation Method
Hemofil M	Baxter	1. Immunoaffinity chromatography 2. Solvent detergent (TNBP/Triton X-100) 3. Heat (25° C ≥10h)	approx. 2-11	>3000	Yes	No
Monam M	Manufactured by Baxter for American Red Cross (ARC) from ARC-collected plasma	1. Immunoaffinity chromatography 2. Solvent detergent (TNBP/Triton X-100) 3. Heat (25° C ≥10h)	approx. 2-11	>3000	No	Yes

Intermediate Purity and High Purity Factor VIII Products Derived from Human Plasma (Containing von Willebrand Factor)

Product Name	Manufacturer	Method of Viral Inactivation	Specific Activity† (IU Factor VIII/mg protein), Final Product	Specific Activity† (IU Factor VIII/mg protein), Discounting Albumin	Efficacy Studies in Humans for von Willebrand Disease	Hepatitis Safety Studies in Humans with this Product	Hepatitis Safety Studies in Humans with Another Product, but Similar Viral Inactivation Method
Alphanate	Alpha	1. Affinity chromatography 2. Solvent detergent butyl phosphate (TNBP and polysorbate 80) 3. Heat (80° C 72h)	approx. 8-30	corrected specific activity of 77	Yes	No	Yes

Product Name	Manufacturer	Method of Viral Inactivation	Specific Activity† (IU Factor VIII/mg protein), Final Product	Specific Activity† (IU Factor VIII/mg protein), Discounting Albumin	Hepatitis Safety Studies in Humans with this Product	Hepatitis Safety Studies in Humans with Another Product, but Similar Method	Efficacy Studies in Humans for von Willebrand Disease
Koate-HP	Bayer	Solvent detergent (TNBP and polysorbate 80)	approx. 9-22	50	No	Yes	No
Humate P	Centeon Pharma (Marberg, Germany)	Pasteurization (60° C, 10h)	approx. 1-2	—	Yes	No	Yes

Porcine Factor VIII

Product Name	Manufacturer	Method of Viral Inactivation	Specific Activity (IU/mg protein), Final Product	Hepatitis Safety Studies in Humans with this Product	Hepatitis Safety Studies in Humans with Another Product, but Similar Method
Hyate C	Speywood	None	>50	No (but no report of transmission of human viruses)	No

Continued

Table 11-2—cont'd
Factor VIII Products Licensed in the United States

Recombinant Factor IX Products

Product Name	Manufacturer	Method of Viral Depletion or Inactivation	Specific Activity† (IU/mg Protein), Final Product‡	Hepatitis Safety Studies in Humans with this Product	Hepatitis Safety Studies in Humans with Another Product, but Similar Viral Inactivation Method
BeneFix	Genetics Institute	1. Affinity chromatography 2. Ultrafiltration	>200	Yes	No

Coagulation Factor IX Products Derived from Human Plasma

Product Name	Manufacturer	Method of Viral Depletion or Inactivation	Specific Activity (IU/mg Protein), Final Product	Hepatitis Safety Studies in Humans with this Product	Hepatitis Safety Studies in Humans with Another Product, but Similar Viral Inactivation Method
AlphaNine SD	Alpha	1. Dual affinity chromatography 2. Solvent detergent (TNBP and Polysorbate 80) 3. Nanofiltration	approx. 229 ± 23	Yes	Yes
Mononine	Centeon	1. Immunoaffinity chromatography 2. Sodium thiocyanate 3. Ultrafiltration	>160	Yes	No

Factor IX Complex Concentrates Derived from Human Plasma

Product Name	Manufacturer	Method of Viral Inactivation	Specific Activity (IU/mg Protein), Final Product	Hepatitis Safety Studies in Humans with this Product	Hepatitis Safety Studies in Humans with Another Product, but Similar Viral Inactivation Method
Konyne 80	Bayer	Dry heat (80° C, 72h)	approx. 1.25	No	Yes
Proplex T	Baxter	Dry heat (68° C, 144h)	approx. 3.9	No	No
Profilnine SD	Alpha	1. Solvent detergent (TNBP and polysorbate 80)	approx. 4.5	No	Yes
Bebulin VH	Immuno (distributed by Baxter)	Vapor heat (10h, 60° C, 1190 mbar pressure plus 1 h, 80° C, 1375 mbar)	approx. 2	Yes	No

Activated Factor IX Complex Concentrates Derived from Human Plasma

Product Name	Manufacturer	Method of Viral Depletion or Inactivation	Specific Activity (IU/mg Protein), Final Product	Hepatitis Safety Studies in Humans with this Product	Hepatitis Safety Studies in Humans with Another Product, but Similar Viral Inactivation Method
Autoplex T	Baxter (distributed by Nabi)	Dry heat 68° C, 144h)	approx. 5	No	No
FEIBA VH	Immuno (distributed by Baxter)	Vapor heat (10h, 60° C, 1190 mbar plus 1h, 80° C, 1375 mbar)	approx. 0.8	No	Yes

Continued

Table 11-2—cont'd
Factor VIII Products Licensed in the United States

Desmopressin Formulations Useful in Disorders of Hemostasis

Product Name	Manufacturer	Distributed in United States By	Formulation	Recommended Dosage and Administration
DDAVP (injection)	Ferring AB (Malmo, Sweden)	Rhone-Poulene-Rohrer	For parenteral (IV) or SQ use, 4 µg/ml in a 10-ml vial or 15 µg/ml in a 1-ml or 2-ml vial	1. 0.3 µg/kg mixed in 30 ml normal saline solution infused slowly over 30 minutes IV 2. 0.4 µg/kg subcutaneously May repeat after 24 hours
Stimate (Nasal spray)	Ferring AB	Centeon	Nasal spray, 1.5 mg/ml. The metered dose pump delivers 0.1 ml (150 µg) per acutation. The bottle contains 2.5 ml with spray pump capable of delivering 25 150-µg doses or 12 300-µg doses	In patients weighing <50 kg, one spray in one nostril delivers 150 µg. For those weighing >50 kg, give one spray in each nostril (total dose 300 µg). May repeat after 24 hours.

Hemophilia Treatment

Compared with fresh frozen plasma and cryoprecipitate, clotting factor concentrates revolutionized the treatment of hemophilia in the early 1970s because of their ease of administration, fewer allergic side effects, and the ease of home storage. Each vial of these factor concentrates contains the plasma of thousands of donors. Prior to 1986, production methods did not inactivate HIV. There have been neither seroconversions in viral safety studies of the concentrates that are currently available nor seroconversions to HIV, hepatitis B, or hepatitis C using products that are currently available (Mannucci, 1995; MASAC, 1998; Teitel, 1998).

Large amounts of extraneous proteins in earlier products led to the development of higher purity products using affinity purification techniques. The newest technologic advance in factor replacement is the use of recombinant DNA to manufacture recombinant factor VIII concentrates. These factor VIII products are not entirely plasma-free because they are stabilized using albumin (Teitel, 1998; UK Haemophilia Centre Directors Organization Executive Committee, 1997).

Advanced technologic products for factor IX were generally available a few years after similar factor VIII concentrates were introduced (see Table 11-2). The newest factor IX product is a recombinant product produced from genetically engineered cells. No plasma products are used in the manufacturing process (Adamson et al, 1998; White, Beebe, and Nielsen, 1997).

In addition, there are two types of plasma-derived factor IX products available for use: prothrombin-complex concentrates, which are also known as factor IX-complex concentrates, and coagulation factor IX products. The prothrombin-complex concentrates contain clotting factors II, VII, IX, and X and are thrombogenic when given often and in large doses. The coagulation factor IX products contain only factor IX and do not induce thrombosis. Therefore children who are having surgery, have experienced trauma, or are having a severe bleeding episode and require factor IX therapy more than once a day for several days in a row, should be treated with one of the coagulation factor IX products or recombinant factor IX. There have been no reported cases of thrombosis with these products (Jandl, 1996; MASAC, 1998; UK Hae-

mophilia Centre Directors Organization Executive Committee, 1997).

Unfortunately, a number of children were reported to have developed severe allergic reactions in association with the development of a factor IX inhibitor after a median number of 11 exposure days to factor IX. The median age of these children was 16 months (Warrier et al, 1997). These reactions did not occur with any specific brand of factor IX, but all of the children had either a complete deletion or major derangements of the factor IX gene. The study investigators suggest that the first 10 to 20 infusions of factor IX be given in a medical setting where the child can be monitored.

Desmopressin acetate (DDAVP) is also effective in raising the levels of factor VIII in many children with a mild factor VIII deficiency (Mannucci, 1997; MASAC, 1998). The benefits of DDAVP include relatively few major side effects and the lack of viral contaminants because it is not derived from human blood. DDAVP is discussed in greater detail in reference to von Willebrand treatment options.

A number of studies have documented that prophylactic factor treatment can reduce the incidence of chronic hemophilic synovitis and joint damage when begun as early as 1 to 2 years of age; when begun at a later age, such treatment may prevent further deterioration even when arthropathy is present (Aledort et al, 1994). Some dosing schedules are 20 to 40 units/kg/dose administered 3 times each week for children with hemophilia A and 25 to 40 units/kg/dose administered 2 to 3 times each week for children with hemophilia B (Ljung, 1998; Lusher, 1997; Rodriquez-Merchan, 1997).

The use of implanted venous access devices (IVAD) has been helpful when prophylactic or frequent treatment is needed in children with poor venous access. IVADs have been used successfully in many children with hemophilia, but the incidence of line sepsis and clotting has reportedly been relatively high in children with hemophilia (Geraghty and Kleinert, 1998; Perkins et al, 1997).

Studies have shown that as many as 20% to 30% of persons with factor VIII deficiency will develop an inhibitor (i.e., antibody) to infused factor VIII (Ehrlich et al, 1998). The level of inhibitor severity is measured in Bethesda units. Most persons who will develop an inhibitor do so at an early age, after an average of 9 treatment days. A much smaller percentage (i.e., less than 5%) of persons with factor IX deficiency will develop an inhibitor (Brettler, 1995). Many inhibitors are transient, or levels may be so low as to be clinically insignificant, but half of persons with inhibitors develop significant inhibitors and cannot be treated with conventional factor VIII or IX therapy. Treatment options include immune tolerance regimens, high doses of certain factor concentrates that can bypass part of the standard clotting cascade, porcine factor VIII, and recombinant factor VIIa (Brettler, 1995; DiMichele, 1998; Hay, 1995; Sallah, 1997; White and Roberts, 1996). The use of immune tolerance regimens is becoming a more commonly accepted and desirable option. These treatment regimens call for large doses of factor VIII or IX to be given daily in an effort to suppress or eradicate the inhibitor. When laboratory measurements indicate that suppression has been achieved, the frequency of administration and dose of factor concentrate can be tapered. Success rates have been reported at 60% to 90% (Brackmann, Oldenburg, and Schwaab, 1996; DiMichele, 1998; White and Roberts, 1996). Immune tolerance therapy is extremely costly, often requires use of an implanted venous access device, and necessitates a great deal of compliance from the family.

The unit of measurement for products that replace the deficient factor protein is calculated in international units of factor VIII or IX activity. Choice of a particular dose is based on the type of hemophilia, the child's weight, the severity of the bleeding episode, the halflife of the chosen product, and occurrence or bleeding in a chronically affected joint (Table 11-3). Repeat doses may be given if significant improvement has not occurred (DiMichele, 1998; Rickard, 1995).

Treatment is initiated as soon as a bleeding episode is identified. For bleeding in a joint, treatment may begin when a child notices tingling in the joint. Many children have come to know this as the first indicator of oozing blood in that area. For some children, mild swelling, mild pain, or loss of range of motion of a joint may be the first recognizable indicators. In other children with high pain tolerances or little self-awareness of bodily changes, the bleeding episode may not be recognized until there is severe swelling, major limitation of joint motion, and severe pain. Joint and bone radio-graphic examinations are generally not needed unless the child has a history of trauma and a broken bone is suspected. Treatment is usually given on demand as soon as bleeding is identified but may be given prophylactically to facilitate healing when bleeding is recurrent or severe or before high-risk procedures (e.g., surgery, dental extractions, and physical therapy of a chronically affected joint).

Vials of factor concentrate come in various sizes with varying numbers of factor units per vial. When a child is prescribed a specific dose of factor (i.e., expressed in factor VIII or IX units), this is considered a minimum dose and the child should be given the number of whole vials at minimum that provide the desired dose without discarding any of the factor. This minimum dosing is due to the high cost of the medication and the lack of adverse sequelae from a dose slightly higher than that originally prescribed. Most concentrates may be given by slow intravenous (IV) push over 5 to 10 minutes. Because most of these concentrates are blood products, those who reconstitute the lyophilized factor should always wear gloves and dispose of supplies that contact the factor in approved infectious waste containers.

High-purity products, such as the recombinant and affinity purified factor VIII and IX concentrates, may cost two times as much as the intermediate-purity products. A school-aged child with severe hemophilia who is on prophylactic therapy may use close to 150,000 units of factor VIII or IX per year (Szucs et al, 1998); a 1-year supply of recombinant costs more than $150,000 (Cardinale, 1998).

von Willebrand's Disease Treatment

The standard treatment for this disorder encompasses both synthetic and plasma-derived products. Primary care providers are urged to consult with the child's hematologist and the National Hemophilia Foundation for the most current recommendations (MASAC, 1998).

Desmopressin acetate (see Table 11-2), which is a synthetic analog of vasopressin, is the treatment of choice for persons with von Willebrand's disease—excluding those with subtypes IIB and III (Ewenstein, 1997). Although the mechanism of action is not completely understood, it is thought that desmopressin releases stores of factor VIII and the

Table 11-3
Assessment and Treatment of Common Bleeding Episodes*

Site of Bleeding	Signs and Symptoms	Treatment
Subcutaneous and/or soft tissue	Mild: not interfering with ROM, not enlarging	Ice, Ace wrap
	Moderate: occurring in wrist, volar surface of forearm, plantar surface of foot; interferes with ROM or is enlarging	Ice, splint/Ace wrap FVIII 20-30 U/kg or desmopressin† FIX 30-50 U/kg
	Severe: pharyngeal; areas listed in "moderate" category accompanied by change in neurologic signs	Admit to hospital FVIII 50 U/kg and follow-up doses FIX 80-100 U/kg and follow-up doses
Joint	Earlier: moderate swelling, mild to moderate pain, warmth, stiffness, limited motion	Rest, splint/crutches FVIII 20-25 U/kg or desmopressin† FIX 30-50 U/kg
	Later: tense swelling, moderate to severe pain, marked decrease in ROM; hip bleeding; limited abduction or adduction	Rest, splint/crutches PT plan May need repeat doses FVIII 30-40 U/kg FIX 40-50 U/kg Ultrasound follow-up for hip bleed
Muscle	Mild: swelling does not greatly affect ROM, mild discomfort	Rest, crutches, PT plan Ice, splint/Ace wrap FVIII 20-30 U/kg or desmopressin† FIX 30-40 U/kg
	Severe: swelling with neurologic changes, decreased ROM	Rest, splint/Ace wrap PT plan FVIII 50 U/kg and follow-up doses FIX 80-100 U/kg and follow-up doses
	Iliopsoas: abdominal, inguinal, or hip area pain, limited hip extension, numbness from nerve compression	Strict bed rest/hospitalization Will need repeat doses FVIII 50 U/kg FIX 80-100 U/kg
Nose	Mild: 10 min	Pressure to nares
	Severe: prolonged or recurrent	Collagen hemostat fibers and nasal pack vWd: desmopressin, EACA FVIII 20 U/kg or desmopressin† FIX 40 U/kg
Oral areas	Dental extractions; frenulum, tongue, or lip bleeding	Topical hemostatic agent EACA (caution with PCCs) May need follow-up doses May need hospitalization if hard to control or severe anemia vWd: desmopressin FVIII 30-40 U/kg or desmopressin FIX 50-100 U/kg

Modified from: Rickard, 1995; DiMichele, 1998; Furie, 1994; Jandl, 1996.
Note: Specific dosages may vary for individual patients; consult with the child's hematologist.
*ROM, range of motion; FVIII, factor VIII hemophilia; FIX, factor IX hemophilia; U/kg, units of factor VIII or IX per kilogram (factor concentrate vial contain a given number of FVIII or FIX activity units); PT, physical therapy; vWd, von Willebrand's disease; EACA, antifibrinolytic: e-aminocaproic acid; cryo, cryoprecipitate.
†Desmopressin may be used if, after a test dose, the child with mild hemophilia has achieved a factor VIII coagulant level equal to the level that would be achieved after the recommended dose of factor VIII concentrate. Example: For a moderate soft tissue bleed in the calf, a dose of 20-30 U/kg should raise a child's factor VIII level to 40% to 60%. If after desmopressin the child reached a peak of only 25%, it is likely desmopressin would not be beneficial.

Continued

Table 11-3
Assessment and Treatment of Common Bleeding Episodes*—cont'd

Site of Bleeding	Signs and Symptoms	Treatment
Gastrointestinal system	Abdominal pain, hypotension, blood in emesis, tarry or bloody stools, weakness	Hospitalization likely VWd: desmopression/FVIII product with high level vWd FVIII 50 U/kg and follow-up doses FIX 100 U/kg and follow-up doses
Central nervous system	Head, neck, or spinal injury; presence of blurred vision, headaches, vomiting, unequal pupils, change in speech or behavior, drowsiness; if no symptoms yet significant injury, treat and observe	Hospitalization and immediate consult with hematologist depending on injury CT scan vWd: desmopressin/FVIII product with high level vWd factor FVIII 50 U/kg for at least 1 wk FIX 80-100 U/kg for at least 1 wk May require f/u prophylaxis if positive MRI or CT
Urinary tract	Gross hematuria (bright red to brown); if clots present, more likely to infuse with factor concentrate	Push oral fluids, rest Prednisone (2 mg/kg/day, maximum 60 mg/day) for 5 days Factor concentrate/DDAVP EACA contraindicated

Follow-up: By daily telephone contact or office visits through resolution of bleeding episode. If family is on home therapy, they should have telephone or office consultation if head, neck, or throat injury occurs; if more than 2 treatments are needed; or if bleeding occurs in hip, iliopsoas muscle, or urinary tract.

von Willebrand protein from the endothelial lining of the blood vessels. Stores may be depleted, however (see Table 11-2), if treatment is repeated more often than every 24 hours (Jandl, 1996; Mannucci, 1997). The intravenous dosage is 0.3 mcg/kg diluted in 30 to 50 ml of normal saline infused over 30 minutes.

Use of this medication for various bleeding episodes depends on the rise in coagulation protein activity after a test dose. Peak response is generally obtained 30 minutes after IV infusion is complete. Individuals should have a test dose of this product to determine response before using it therapeutically. The response varies among individuals, and if an individual is a candidate for this therapy should be determined before it is used for a bleeding episode. Individuals tend to show consistency in the degree of response over time. Desmopressin has also been given subcutaneously at a slightly higher dose with good results in some children (Ewenstein, 1997; Mannucci, 1997; Von Willebrand Working Party, 1997).

A concentrated intranasal form of desmopressin is now available as Stimate Nasal Spray (Ferring AB) (1.5 mg/ml). The peak effect of this form is obtained 1 hour after administration. Studies have shown significant clinical response with the use of this intranasal form in children with mild hemophilia A and von Willebrand's disease who responded well to the intravenous form. If a child has had prior desmopressin testing with the intravenous form, repeat laboratory testing with the intranasal form is still indicated before clinical use (Ewenstein, 1997; Mannucci, 1997). It should be noted that the less-concentrated DDAVP Nasal Spray (Ferring AB) (0.1 mg/ml) is ineffective in treating these bleeding disorders.

Desmopressin has an antidiuretic effect, so children and parents must be cautioned to limit fluid intake for the remainder of the day that the drug is administered (Jandl, 1996).

If a blood product is needed to control bleeding in children with von Willebrand's disease, virally inactivated intermediate-purity factor VIII concentrates containing von Willebrand factor are preferable to cryoprecipitate, which cannot be virally inactivated (Mannucci, 1997; MASAC, 1998; Menache and Aronson, 1997).

Estrogens may be useful in the management of excessive menstrual and other types of bleeding in women because they can increase levels of factor VIII and the von Willebrand protein (Aledort, 1998; Jandl, 1996).

Oral Antifibrinolytic Agents

Children with hemophilia and von Willebrand's disease often have oral bleeding that requires additional medication to keep the clot stable once it has formed. Because of the presence of digestive enzymes in the saliva that lyse fibrin clots, an antifibrinolytic agent should be given orally for 7 to 10 days or until the site of oral bleeding has completely healed (Hilgartner and Corrigan, 1995; Hoffman and Roberts, 1995; Radivoyevitch, 1996). The only such agent currently available is epsilon aminocaproic acid (Amicar) (see Table 11-2).

Topical Hemostatic Agents

Collagen hemostat (Avitene) fibers can be applied to nasal packing or salt pork pledgets to control epistaxis or at the site of frenulum tears or tooth extraction. When nasal packing is used, it is generally left in place for 24 to 36 hours to promote stable clot formation. Nosebleeds can often be diminished by using petroleum jelly or antibiotic ointment in the nares or humidification of room air. Less conventional topical agents have been used successfully in the treatment of oral bleeding. Moistened tea bags containing tannic acid may provide local hemostasis. Fibrin glue has been used to promote local hemostasis in some circumcisions (Jackson et al, 1996); cryoprecipitate is the source of fibrinogen in this treatment.

Pain Management

Uncontrolled bleeding into a joint or muscle can produce significant pain. Prompt replacement of the deficient coagulation protein is the most effective way to prevent significant pain and relieve current pain. Mild pain may be treated with acetaminophen (not aspirin), ice, and elevation of the affected extremity. If pain is moderate or severe, acetaminophen with codeine every 4 to 6 hours is recommended. Pain medication is generally not necessary after the first day of factor replacement. Continued pain may suggest ineffective control of bleeding because of inadequate dosing of the factor concentrate, development of an inhibitor, or synovitis. Pain caused by irritation of the synovial lining may be more effectively treated with a nonsteroidal antiinflammatory agent. These agents should be used with caution, however, because they can cause GI bleeding secondary to interference with platelet aggregation (DiMichele, 1998).

Physical Therapy

Splinting and immobilization for 1 to 2 days after acute bleeding often aid resolution of the episode. A resting splint that places the extremity in a comfortable position is recommended for night use for up to several days following a significant hemarthrosis to prevent further bleeding during sleep. Following severe bleeding or prolonged immobilization, a physical therapy program should be prescribed to enable children to achieve their baseline range of motion and regain muscle mass. Factor replacement is often needed with vigorous physical therapy (Buzzard, 1997; Duthie et al, 1994; Gilbert and Radomisli, 1997).

Surgical Intervention

Destruction of a joint secondary to repeated bleeding episodes can result in significant pain, decreased strength and range of motion, and an impaired ability to use the affected extremity. Several orthopedic procedures have been successful in individuals with hemophilia and can provide them with significantly reduced joint pain and greater range of motion and endurance. Open synovectomy is successful in reducing pain and bleeding episodes, but mobility is often lost and progression of the arthropathy continues. Arthroscopic synovectomy reduces the pain and frequency of bleeding episodes without loss of mobility (Duthie et al, 1994; Gilbert and Radomisli, 1997). Injection of a radioactive isotope into the affected joint to eradicate abnormal synovium, which is a less-invasive procedure, has been successful in improving range of motion and decreasing bleeding episodes in individuals who are not surgical candidates (Fernandez-Palazzi, 1998; Siegel et al, 1994). Once a child is fully grown and the epiphyseal plates are closed, total joint replacements—particularly of the knee—have been quite successful in individuals with hemophilia, as measured by increased function and decreased pain and frequency of bleeding episodes (Heeg et al, 1998).

Anticipated Advances in Diagnosis and Management

Attainment of a cure for hemophilia has been explored through liver transplantation and gene-insertion therapy. Liver transplantation has been found to cure both hemophilia A and B because both factors VIII and IX are synthesized in the liver. Liver transplantation, however, is both an extremely costly and high-risk procedure and requires immunosuppressive therapy for life. In the future, successful gene insertion therapy may provide a cure for hemophilia or at least convert persons with severe hemophilia to a milder form of the disorder. Research is underway to find the best vector for gene expression and define the best animal model for research (Connelly and Kaleko, 1998).

Associated Problems (Box 11-3)

Anemia

Anemia can occur as a result of slow, persistent oozing from the mouth or nose or bleeding or pooling of blood in muscle hemorrhages. In persons with von Willebrand's disease, excessive or prolonged menstrual bleeding or persistent or recurrent epistaxis can result in anemia.

Neurologic Problems

Intracranial hemorrhage is the most frequent cause of death in children with hemophilia (Dietrich et

---

Box 11-3
Associated Problems

- Anemia
- Neurologic deficits from intracranial hemorrhage, bleeding around spinal column, compartment syndrome compression of nerves
- Airway obstruction as a result of bleeding
- Hepatitis
- Gastrointestinal bleeding
- HIV
- Arthropathy and/or arthritis
- Genitourinary bleeding

---

al, 1994; Jandl, 1996). Intracranial hemorrhage also can result in spastic quadriplegia and developmental delay. In some cases of intracranial bleeding, no known prior injury is identified. Therefore any injury or neurologically related symptom should be treated aggressively. There may be significant intracranial bleeding without the presence of a "goose egg" because the most significant bleeding occurs from internal shearing of the brain and cranium. The presence of a hematoma, however, indicates that the cranium may have met with significant force. Because of the high risk of rebleeding after intracranial bleeding, prophylactic factor treatment is continued for an extended period of time. Those with von Willebrand's disease also are at increased risk for this type of bleeding. Bleeding within or around the spinal column can also produce enough pressure to cause neurologic damage. Compartment syndrome resulting from nerve compression may occur after untreated bleeding into the forearm or calf (DiMichele, 1998; Jandl, 1996).

Respiratory Problems

Posterior pharyngeal bleeding, which increases the potential for asphyxia, can result from a traumatic throat culture, bronchoscopy, or dental extractions or deep injection of anesthetic without pretreatment with factor concentrates or desmopressin. Intubation should only be attempted after pretreatment with factor concentrate.

Hepatitis/Gastrointestinal Problems

In the past, exposure to blood products resulted in a high incidence of infection with hepatitis B and C in the population with hemophilia. Approximately 75% of those with hemophilia have been exposed to hepatitis B; the majority have developed immunity, but approximately 8% are chronic carriers. Of the individuals with hemophilia, 80% to 90% have been exposed to hepatitis C (Blanchette et al, 1994; Kasper, 1996; Rockstroh et al, 1996). With the use of the hepatitis B vaccine series, the incidence of hepatitis B has been greatly reduced. In addition, the factor products currently on the market are considered to have a negligible risk of hepatitis transmission as a result of current screening and processing methods (MASAC, 1998).

A new combination therapy that uses subcutaneous alfa-interferon 2b in combination with oral ribavirin has been successful having an undetectable serum HCV RNA level after completion of treatment, improving liver histology as detected by liver biopsy, and/or decreasing sodium aminotransferase in as many as 61% of individuals treated for as long as 48 weeks. Unfortunately, the side effects of this therapy often include severe anemia, flulike symptoms, and severe psychiatric symptoms, so some individuals need to discontinue treatment before completing the full course (McHutchison et al, 1998; Davis et al, 1998). It has been found that HIV-induced immune dysfunction may increase hepatitis C replication and promote an increased incidence of liver disease and liver failure in individuals coinfected with HIV and hepatitis C (Rockstroh et al, 1996).

Bleeding into the GI tract may occur in children with von Willebrand's disease and in those with hemophilia. The fragile mucous membrane-lined digestive system is prone to bleeding that can result from ulcers, gastritis, hemorrhoids, rectal fissures, and endoscopic procedures. This type of bleeding should be considered when there is an unexplained drop in hemoglobin levels or abdominal pain.

Immunologic Problems

Approximately 50% of those exposed to untreated factor concentrates between 1978 and 1985 (i.e., approximately 9,200 persons) have developed HIV infection. Approximately 2,500 of those individu-

als were still alive in 1998 (Crudder, 1998; Rosenberg and Goedert, 1998). The incidence of HIV infection in persons with von Willebrand's disease who were exposed to cryoprecipitate is much lower, however, because of the decreased risk with exposure to single-donor units.

Musculoskeletal Problems

The normally smooth synovial lining of a joint produces synovial fluid that with the cartilage serves as a shock absorber for the joint (Figure 11-3). The synovium is also supplied with many blood vessels. When bleeding into a joint ceases with the administration of the deficient coagulation protein, enzymes clear away the blood from the synovial fluid. These enzymes, however, do not seem to focus their destruction solely on the unwanted blood cells; they begin to eat away at the smooth synovial lining, producing breaks in the surface that can make it easier for bleeding to recur in that joint. Eventually they may destroy the cartilaginous surface of the bones. The nonintact synovial lining can cause the synovium to produce abnormal amounts of fluid in an inflammatory response known as synovitis. Even when actual bleeding into the joint does not occur, the joint may become swollen and stiff. Synovitis is differentiated from a hemarthrosis by its gradual onset, mild or absent pain, and fuller range of motion. The more blood that accumulates in the joint capsule, the more enzymes that are released. This destructive process can ultimately lead to severe osteoarthritic-like conditions and joint contractures. A single hip hemarthrosis can produce aseptic necrosis of the femoral head if bleeding is not fully resolved. When bleeding recurs in a specific joint, it may be referred to as a "target joint" (Duthie et al, 1994). Thus a strong case is made for early detection and treatment of bleeding episodes and ultimately for the use of prophylactic treatment for children with severe hemophilia (Aledort et al, 1994; Rodriquez-Merchan, 1997).

Genitourinary Problems

If a boy has bleeding into the testicle that is not treated promptly, future fertility and maintenance of a patent urinary tract may be compromised. This type of bleeding can result from performing bi-

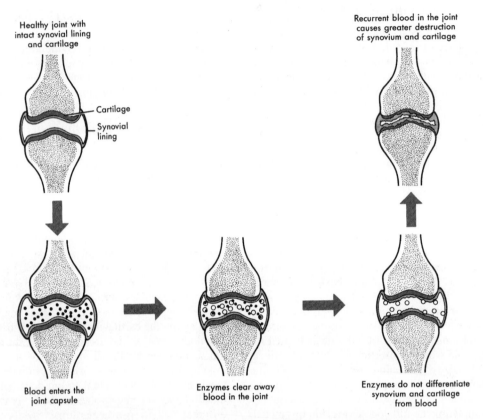

Healthy joint with
intact synovial lining
and cartilage

Cartilage

Synovial
lining

Blood enters the
joint capsule

Enzymes clear away
blood in the joint

Enzymes do not differentiate
synovium and cartilage
from blood

Recurrent blood in the joint
causes greater destruction
of synovium and cartilage

Figure 11-3   Progression of joint destruction in hemophilia.

cycle stunts or taking part in vigorous play on a rocking horse or playground toy.

Hematuria occurs most commonly in adolescents with hemophilia, is usually of short duration and not a result of trauma, and often stops spontaneously. Clots can sometimes cause renal or ureteral obstruction with temporary renal colic and, at times, hydronephrosis. Treatment with epsilon aminocaproic acid (Amicar) should be avoided during periods of hematuria because of the risk of developing clots in the genitourinary system (Hoffman and Roberts, 1995).

Prognosis

The major factors contributing to morbidity in hemophilia are neurologic sequelae of intracranial bleeding, disability from chronic joint disease (arthropathy), liver disease secondary to hepatitis, and HIV infection. Intracranial bleeding that occurs at or soon after birth may result in spastic quadriplegia and brain damage, whereas bleeding that occurs later in life may affect the achievement of developmental milestones. Because of the availability of clotting factor concentrates, disabling arthropathy in childhood is now much less common. Those who are affected by it, however, often have visible deformities, increased school absenteeism, and difficulty finding suitable employment. Before the use of heat-treated concentrates, approximately 75% to 90% of those treated were exposed to hepatitis B, with 5% to 10% becoming chronic carriers It is also believed that 90% of those who received untreated products have been exposed to hepatitis C. The incidence of hepatitis should decrease with the use of more highly purified products and the hepatitis B vaccine. The rate of HIV infection among adolescents with hemophilia in the United States in 1997 was 3% (Crudder, 1998). The lower incidence reflects that fact that there have been very few HIV seroconversions since 1986, so many individuals have now reached adulthood. In addition, many individuals with hemophilia and HIV have died.

By the early 1980s, the life expectancy of individuals with hemophilia approached that of the general population (Walker et al, 1998). HIV-related disease is the leading cause of death in persons with hemophilia, accounting for 51% of deaths in 1997 (Crudder, 1998). In those not affected with HIV, however, the leading cause of death is bleeding, especially from intracranial hemorrhage (Jandl, 1996).

Data regarding morbidity and mortality of persons with von Willebrand's disease are not readily available, but because of the generally mild nature of the disorder, life expectancy is thought to be normal. The relatively small number of individuals infected with HIV or hepatitis through infusions of cryoprecipitate have a decreased life expectancy.

PRIMARY CARE MANAGEMENT

Health Care Maintenance

Growth and Development

Monitoring a child's weight is especially important because obesity places added stress on joints and muscles. Limb length may be increased by bony overgrowth of the epiphysis from chronic arthropathy. Gait disturbances caused by scoliosis may predispose individuals with hemophilia to joint or muscle bleeding.

A thorough baseline and ongoing assessment of developmental parameters and neurologic status is useful in follow-up for head trauma and screening of potentially undiagnosed or unreported intracranial bleeding. Normal development is anticipated unless there is a history of intracranial bleeding.

Diet

It is especially important for children with bleeding disorders to meet the recommended requirements for protein and calcium intake because of their role in bone and muscle formation. A nonconstipating diet may prevent the rectal bleeding that can occur when hard stools are passed. When a child has mouth bleeding, a soft diet and avoidance of foods that are hot or have sharp edges (e.g., chips) and straws (i.e., because the sucking action can disturb the clot) are recommended.

Safety

Protection against head injury is of primary importance. A protective helmet for children with hemophilia who are learning to walk may reduce the risk of head injury. Knee pads may be used for toddlers prone to knee hematomas. From the time they start to walk, children at risk for hemarthroses should wear high-top leather sneakers and shoes. Walkers are never recommended for young children but may be particularly hazardous for children with bleeding disorders. Care must also be taken that the child is safely strapped in when using portable swings.

Contact sports (e.g., football, soccer, hockey, wrestling, boxing, and competitive basketball) are strongly discouraged because of the increased chance of head trauma. Appropriate physical activity is encouraged, however, to maintain strong muscles that promote joint stability and normal social adjustment. Swimming is an ideal aerobic activity. Although recommended for all children, helmets are particularly important for those with bleeding disorders when riding bikes or scooters or using roller skates and/or blades. Knee and elbow pads are also recommended for roller skating and/or blading and skateboarding.

Use of a medical identification emblem that includes diagnosis, treatment product, and blood type is required for safety. Infants can have the emblem pinned to their car seats or jackets when traveling. Older children who grow up wearing an emblem become accustomed to it. A wallet identification card may be used if a child or adolescent refuses to wear the emblem. Medical information should be checked yearly and updated as necessary.

Families participating in a home infusion program should follow accepted guidelines for infection control, including the use of gloves to mix and administer factor concentrates and the disposal of infectious wastes in approved containers that are disposed of appropriately.

Immunizations

Routine injectable vaccines should be given subcutaneously when possible because intramuscular injections may cause muscle bleeding. When any injectable vaccine is given, the following interventions can help to prevent hematoma development: applying firm pressure to the site for 5 minutes after injection, using a 25-gauge needle, and using a factor concentrate before intramuscular injection.

The hepatitis B vaccine series is recommended for all children likely to be exposed to blood products. If an at-risk child did not receive the vaccine as an infant, the vaccine should be administered immediately and again at 1 month and 6 months after the first dose (Lemon and Thomas, 1997; National Digestive Diseases Information Clearinghouse, 1997).

Hepatitis A vaccine has been recommended for use in individuals with bleeding disorders who are at least 2 years of age and seronegative for the hepatitis A virus. The recommendations are currently a two-dose series for adults (i.e., the vaccine is again administered 6 to 12 months later) and a two- or three-dose series for children at least 2 years of age (i.e., again administered 1 and 6 months later [for the three-dose series]). The number of dosages for children depends on the vaccine brand and dose per vial (Centers for Disease Control and Prevention, 1996; National Digestive Diseases Information Clearinghouse, 1997; Shouval, 1998).

Screening

Vision: Following an eye injury, referral to an ophthalmologist is recommended, with follow-ups until resolution is obtained. Otherwise, routine office screening and attention to the fundal examination are sufficient. Individuals with HIV should have yearly eye exams to screen for CMV.

Hearing: Routine screening is recommended.

Dental: Invasive dental procedures can often be prevented through careful oral hygiene (i.e., including flossing under parental supervision), fluo-ride treatments, and regular dental evaluations. An initial dental evaluation is recommended at 2 to 3 years of age, in part to help the child establish a positive relationship with the dentist, as well as to impress upon parents the importance of preventive care. Pediatric dentists with expertise in the management of persons with bleeding disorders are often associated with the local hemophilia treatment center. If necessary, local dentists can manage most procedures with consultation from the hemophilia treatment center. The hemophilia treatment center should be consulted about whether prophylactic treatment with factor concentrate or desmopressin is necessary for routine dental cleaning or anesthetic infiltrates close to the gumline for a particular child. For dental extractions, desmopressin or factor concentrate plus an antifibrinolytic is recommended (Boyd et al, 1994; Jandl, 1996). If a child has an implantable port, external venous catheter, or joint replacement, some treatment centers advocate the use of subacute bacterial endocarditis (SBE) antibiotic prophylaxis (see Chapter 17).

Blood pressure: Routine screening is recommended.

Hematocrit: Annual screening for anemia is recommended. Nosebleeds that are short in duration but occur frequently may not be regularly reported by families and may lead to significant anemia. If venipuncture is required, a 23-gauge butterfly needle should be used and firm pressure applied to the site for at least 5 minutes to prevent hematoma formation. Trauma may be reduced if a skilled pediatric phlebotomist performs venipuncture.

Urinalysis: An annual urinalysis is recommended to screen for microscopic hematuria.

Tuberculosis: Routine screening is recommended. No factor pretreatment is needed for tine or purified protein derivative (PPD) skin testing.

Condition-specific screening: Children who have received any blood products in the past year should have liver function studies performed. A factor VIII or IX inhibitor screen should also be performed for those with hemophilia and is usually performed during comprehensive evaluations at the hemophilia treatment center. HIV antibody testing with pre- and posttest counseling is recommended for adolescents exposed to blood products before

1986 who have not previously been tested. Arterial blood samples should only be drawn after pretreatment with factor concentrate.

Common Illness Management

Differential Diagnosis

Headaches and Head Injury

Intracranial bleeding must be ruled out whenever there is a history of injury within the past several days, focal headaches, or vomiting without GI distress. A computed tomographic (CT) scan is often helpful in ruling out intracranial bleeding. If either significant history or physical symptoms are present, however, providers in consultation with the hemophilia team often treat a child with factor concentrate or desmopressin prophylactically to achieve a 100% factor VIII or IX level. This conservative approach is often adopted because of the serious implications of a delay in diagnosis. Therapy may cease after the resolution of symptoms if scans remain normal. If bleeding is documented, the child would need hospitalization and factor replacement regularly for several weeks or longer.

Visual Disturbance

In the presence of acute changes in visual acuity, it is necessary to rule out intraocular bleeding by performing a thorough funduscopic examination. Documented bleeding, ocular injury, or persistent visual changes, however, warrant referral to an ophthalmologist.

Fever

When children with IVADs develop a fever, blood cultures should be drawn and intravenous antibiotics started until the cultures are shown to be negative. These indwelling devices present a significant risk for infection even in children whose immune systems are not suppressed.

If pretreated with factor concentrates or desmopressin, children with hemophilia may have lumbar punctures—if required for a sepsis work-up—performed safely (Jandl, 1996).

Sore Throat

If a throat culture is indicated, extreme caution must be exercised because of the potential for posterior pharyngeal bleeding. A throat culture should not be attempted in an uncooperative child. If streptococcal pharyngitis is suspected, a course of penicillin should be initiated based on history and physical findings.

Mouth Bleeding

Although oral bleeding may not appear profuse in children with hemophilia, persistent slow oozing can cause a significant drop in hemoglobin levels. Topical measures and antifibrinolytics alone are often not sufficient to control bleeding well. In most cases, factor replacement or the use of desmopressin is also required. Rebleeding can be prevented with a soft diet and avoidance of placing straws, hot foods, chips, and toys in the mouth.

Abdominal Pain

Primary care practitioners should have a high suspicion of GI bleeding with acute abdominal pain or a significant drop in hemoglobin levels in the absence of other bleeding in children with hemophilia or von Willebrand's disease. Testing stool or emesis for blood can easily be done in the office as a screening tool. In hemophilia, iliopsoas bleeding (i.e., a combination of the iliacus muscle [origin, iliac fossa; insertion, greater trochanter] and psoas muscle [origin, thoracic and lumbar vertebrae; insertion, lesser trochanter]) can cause pain in the abdomen or in the inguinal area. Psoas bleeding can result in a large amount of blood loss and nerve damage that necessitates hip joint replacement in some men in later life. Hospital admission and aggressive treatment with factor is often required for iliopsoas and GI bleeding.

Gait Disturbance

Gait disturbance may be the result of bleeding in or around the ankle, knee, hip, or iliopsoas muscle. Inability to fully extend the hip and, later, leg paresthesias are characteristics of iliopsoas bleeding. Ultrasonography is useful for confirmation. Bleeding into the hip socket, which is rare in children, is characterized by limitation of hip abduction and adduction. Hospital admission is often required for severe hip or iliopsoas bleeding.

Dysuria and Hematuria

Pressure within the urinary tract can cause dysuria. Testicular bleeding, however, must be ruled out. Bleeding into the testicular area is often quite pronounced with obvious bruising and swelling. Hospitalization may be required for aggressive therapy and bed rest. Hematuria may be spontaneous and directly related to the bleeding disorder. Whenever bleeding occurs, however, its origin within the urinary tract and any potential infection should be considered. Increased fluid intake, bed rest, and avoidance of antifibrinolytic agents, which may cause obstructive clots, are routinely recommended as part of a treatment plan. The benefits of treatment with factor concentrate or corticosteroids, however, are debated among clinicians.

Heavy Menstrual Bleeding

Women who are carriers of hemophilia or have von Willebrand's disease may have heavy menstrual flow, resulting in anemia. Once other causes have been ruled out, these women may benefit from treatment with estrogen therapy in the form of oral contraceptives or intranasal DDAVP.

Numbness, Tingling, and Pain

Compression of nerves caused by deep or superficial hematomas should be suspected in individuals with changes in sensation or focal pain. Bleeding in or near the calf, spine, buttock, iliopsoas muscle, and volar surface of the forearm can lead to neurologic changes.

Drug Interactions

All products that contain aspirin are contraindicated. Caution should also be exercised with prolonged use of other medications that can affect platelet aggregation (e.g., nonsteroidal antiinflammatory agents). Because of the proliferation of over-the-counter medications, a list of those that can affect bleeding may soon be obsolete. It is more helpful to educate parents on how to read medication labels (e.g., choosing those with aceta-

minophen over those with acetylsalicylic acid) and enlist the help of the pharmacist when they are in doubt about the use of a particular product.

Developmental Issues

Sleep Patterns

Standard developmental counseling is advised. Parents are often advised to pad their child's crib rails to prevent bruising. Crib side rails should be lowered and pillows placed on the floor below as soon as the child begins to crawl out of his or her crib.

Toileting

Standard developmental counseling is advised.

Discipline

Some families tend to overprotect children with a bleeding disorder and may be more strict with unaffected siblings. Positive disciplinary techniques that are age- and developmentally appropriate and do not include physical punishment should be recommended for all children. Pulling a child with a bleeding disorder by the arm is a specific action that may result in serious shoulder bleeding and radial head subluxation. Primary care providers should evaluate the disciplinary style of the parents and offer counseling on alternative discipline measures if potentially injurious methods are used. Families should be counseled about the use of non-contact limit-setting measures (e.g., time-outs, distraction, and activity limitations).

Child Care

Contact with the proposed source of child care can help allay fears and clarify the caretaker's responsibilities with regard to the prevention and management of bleeding episodes. Hemophilia treatment center personnel or the primary care provider may provide this service. It is helpful to emphasize that early recognition of bleeding (e.g., mild swelling or slight change in range of motion) and rapid access to medical evaluation and treatment are of primary importance for children with hemophilia. Spontaneous bleeding may occur, however, despite diligent safety efforts. Child care providers should be discouraged from trying to make treatment decisions without the input of the parents, which is especially important when seemingly mild head "bumps" occur. To find the safest environment possible, parents may be encouraged to seek out sources of child care that have smaller numbers of children per provider, protective ground cover under outside activity spaces, and a staff willing to learn about the special needs and activity requirements of a child with a bleeding disorder. Some facilities may be fearful of admitting children with bleeding disorders because of their fear of liability. Health care providers can provide education and help allay concern.

Schooling

Teachers, school nurses, and athletic coaches should be informed of a child's bleeding disorder. Families and children may be reticent to disclose the diagnosis to others for fear of discrimination because of the connection between hemophilia and HIV. School personnel are more often concerned with prevention of bleeding (which may not be possible), emergency management, and HIV infection. Many HTCs offer school visits by the program's nurse coordinator and social worker. These educational visits are most helpful upon entrance to a new school and should be done with the permission and—ideally—participation of the child and parents. It is not uncommon for children and adolescents with hemophilia to encounter peer disbelief that the disability and the need for crutches or a sling created by an acute bleeding episode can resolve in 1 to 2 days.

Alterations in body image and self-esteem may be precipitated by chronic joint arthropathy or limitations on physical activity caused by the bleeding disorder. From the time of diagnosis, parents may be assisted in guiding their child toward skills, careers, and sports that place less stress on joints and are not associated with high rates of injury. It is critical that children have activities and skills at which they can excel. The advent of prophylaxis has enabled more "normal" active play without the fear of increased injury and bleeding.

Children with learning problems resulting from intracranial bleeding must be fully evaluated and provided with appropriate support.

Sexuality

Safe-sex counseling (i.e., including decision-making skills; values clarification; and instruction in the use of condoms to prevent transmission of HIV, hepatitis B and C, and other sexually transmitted diseases) should be offered to all adolescents. Some adolescents who test HIV-antibody positive may avoid sexual relationships because of fear of rejection once their status is known to a potential partner.

The genetic counselor at the HTC first interacts with children with basic education on the inheritance of the bleeding disorder and eventually includes a discussion of reproductive options.

Transition into Adulthood

The transition from adolescence to adulthood can be particularly stressful for some individuals with bleeding disorders. When they approach adulthood, such individuals have their comprehensive HTC medical care transferred from the pediatric hematology service to the adult hematology service. Some young men experience feelings of anger and rejection because of the need to develop relationships with new providers and sever nurturing relationships they have had with the pediatric team since infancy. This is usually the time when the responsibility for medical care is transferred from the parents to the young adult. Choice of college may also be influenced by the availability of specialized medical care in the area, and choice of career may be influenced by physical limitations.

As adolescents make the transition to adulthood, they may no longer be eligible for medical coverage under their parent's policy and may have difficulty finding coverage that will accommodate their disorder. In many states, there are special programs that cover individuals with hemophilia, or individuals may be eligible for a federal government program (e.g., Medicare, Medicaid, or Supplemental Security Income [SSI]) as a result of disability.

Special Family Concerns and Resources

If a child with a bleeding disorder has excessive bruising before and after diagnosis, parents often encounter questions about suspected child abuse from health care providers or stares from friends, relatives, teachers, and strangers. Compounding the parents' distress may be guilt regarding the inheritance of the bleeding disorder.

It is difficult for parents to cope with their inability to prevent bleeding episodes despite diligent efforts to prevent injury. Fear of injury to the infant may even interfere with parent-infant bonding. When a child requires an infusion of blood products to stop bleeding, parents often continue to question the viral safety of the product despite current data on product safety (Saviolo-Negrin et al, 1999).

Reimbursement for high-priced factor replacement has become an area of real concern as adults and, in some cases, children reach the maximum lifetime amount of insurance reimbursement.

Different racial and ethnic groups may have varying feelings about and experiences of disability and chronic illness. As a result, individuals with hemophilia may receive little understanding from their own ethnic community and may even encounter racial bias in the delayed diagnosis of a hemarthrosis (e.g., an African-American man presenting with a swollen joint may be assumed to be having a sickle cell episode instead of being treated with a prompt infusion of factor concentrate). In many Asian cultures, it is a sign of weakness to tell others about an illness or disease. Many Latinos are hesitant to join organized support networks for their disorder because they fear stigmatization. Women are another minority group in whom the effect of bleeding disorders or carrier status has been overlooked.

Organizations

The National Hemophilia Foundation (116 West 32nd Street, 11th floor, New York, NY, 10001 [212] 328-3700 and [800] 424-2634) and its local chapters disseminate information on recent advances in therapy not only for hemophilia and von Willebrand's disease but also for HIV infection. Active members of the foundation include consumers, families, and health care providers at HTCs. The local chapters provide educational programs and support services to meet the members' needs.

HTCs also provide educational programs and support groups for individuals with bleeding disorders and their families. A list of HTCs is available from the National Hemophilia Foundation in New York or from local National Hemophilia Foundation chapters.

Summary of Primary Care Needs for the Child with Bleeding Disorders: Hemophilia and von Willebrand's Disease

If a child or adolescent with a bleeding disorder also has an HIV infection, please see additional guidelines given in Chapter 24.

HEALTH CARE MAINTENANCE
Growth and development

Developmental screening should be done as a follow-up for head trauma or screening for undiagnosed or unreported intracranial bleeding.

Diet

Adequate protein and calcium intake is of particular importance because of the role of both in bone and muscle formation.

Obesity should be avoided because it places extra stress on joints.

Safety

A protective helmet may be recommended for children who are learning to walk to reduce the risk of head injury. Use of a helmet is controversial because it restricts peripheral vision.

Knee pads in the pants of toddlers may decrease knee hematomas.

High-top sneakers and shoes (i.e., not canvas type of shoes) are recommended for children at risk for hemarthroses from the time they start to walk.

Summary of Primary Care Needs for the Child with Bleeding Disorders: Hemophilia and von Willebrand's Disease—cont'd

Participation in noncontact sports should be encouraged.

The child should wear a medical identification emblem that includes information regarding diagnosis, treatment product, and blood type. The information should be updated annually.

Activities that increase the chance of testicular bleeding—particularly in boys with moderate or severe hemophilia—should be discouraged.

Families participating in a home infusion program should follow accepted guidelines for universal precautions and disposal of infectious wastes.

Immunizations

Some sources recommend that the hepatitis A and B, DPT, and HIB vaccines be given intramuscularly, despite risk of bleeding, whereas other sources recommend giving all immunizations subcutaneously.

Hepatitis A vaccine is recommended for persons at least 2 years of age.

Some children may require factor replacements before immunization injections if given intramuscularly.

Injectable vaccines should be given with a 25-gauge needle.

Firm pressure should be applied over the immunization site for 5 minutes. Ice may be applied after pressure.

Because of potential contact with family members who may have hemophilia and HIV infection, an inactivated polio vaccine may be needed. Inactivated vaccine is also indicated when the child is untested for HIV but has been exposed during risk years.

Screening

Vision: Examination for eye injury should be done by an ophthalmologist. Routine office screening with attention to funduscopic examination is recommended.

Hearing: Routine screening is recommended.

Do not curette wax aggressively.

Dental: Teeth should initially be evaluated at 2 to 3 years of age, followed by regular routine examinations. Hygiene should include flossing under supervision. Factor replacement or desmopressin is recommended for regional blocks; an antifibrinolytic should be added for dental extractions.

Blood pressure: Annual screening is recommended.

Hematocrit: Annual screening is recommended.

Use a 23-gauge butterfly needle for venipuncture in persons of any age.

Urinalysis: Annual screening for microscopic hematuria is recommended.

Tuberculosis: Routine screening is recommended.

Condition-specific screening: If blood product has been received in the past year, a factor VIII or IX inhibitor screen (i.e., specifically for persons with hemophilia) and liver function studies are indicated. HIV antibody testing with pre- and postcounseling is recommended for those exposed to blood products before 1986 if not previously performed.

COMMON ILLNESS MANAGEMENT
Differential diagnosis

Headaches and head injury: Rule out intracranial bleeding, especially with concurrent vomiting and absence of GI symptoms.

Visual disturbance: Rule out intraocular bleeding.

Fever: If indwelling venous access device is present, blood cultures must be drawn and intravenous antibiotics started.

Sore throat: Throat cultures present a risk for posterior pharyngeal bleeding. Cultures should not be taken from an uncooperative child.

continued

Summary of Primary Care Needs for the Child with Bleeding Disorders: Hemophilia and von Willebrand's Disease—cont'd

Mouth bleeding: Mouth bleeding often requires factor replacement in addition to topical measures and antifibrinolytic agents.

Abdominal pain: Rule out GI bleeding. Rule out iliopsoas muscle bleeding with groin pain and decreased hip extension.

Gait disturbance: Rule out bleeding in and around the ankle, knee, hip, and iliopsoas muscle. Rule out scoliosis.

Dysuria and hematuria: Rule out testicular bleeding, renal or ureteral bleeding, and infection.

Heavy menstrual bleeding: May occur in hemophilia carriers or women with von Willebrand's disease. DDAVP or estrogen therapy may be helpful.

Numbness, tingling, and pain: Rule out nerve compression caused by bleeding.

Drug interactions: Products that contain aspirin are contraindicated.

Prolonged use of other substances that can affect platelet aggregation (e.g., nonsteroidal anti-inflammatory agents) should be avoided.

DEVELOPMENTAL ISSUES

Sleep patterns

Standard developmental counseling is advised. Safety of sleeping environment must be assessed.

Toileting

Standard developmental counseling is advised.

Discipline

Recognize the potential for overprotection of the affected child and the use of deferential disciplinary methods when compared with unaffected siblings.

Pulling a child by the arm may result in shoulder joint bleeding.

Physical punishment may result in internal bleeding.

Parents should be counseled about use of time-outs and other nonphysical methods of limit setting.

Child care

Contact with the proposed source of care by the primary health care provider or hemophilia treatment center staff is often useful to allay fears and clarify responsibilities with regard to prevention and management of bleeding episodes and trauma. The importance of early recognition and treatment of bleeding should be stressed.

Recognize that the child care provider may have fears regarding potential HIV infection.

Schooling

School visits are most helpful on enrollment in a new school and ideally include the child and parent or parents.

Because of the difficulty in understanding acute onset and resolution of bleeding episodes, peer acceptance may initially be poor.

Acknowledge potential fear of HIV infection among school personnel, and educate regarding transmission.

Recognize potential alterations in body image and self-esteem because of chronic joint arthropathy or limitations on physical activity.

Intracranial bleeding may result in learning problems.

Sexuality

Delay circumcision until the child with a positive family history is screened for a bleeding disorder.

Safe-sex counseling is recommended to prevent sexually transmitted diseases.

Summary of Primary Care Needs for the Child with Bleeding Disorders: Hemophilia and von Willebrand's Disease—cont'd

Transition into adulthood

The transfer of medical care from a pediatric center to an adult hemophilia center may be difficult.

Educational and career opportunities may be restricted because of physical limitations and the need to be near a treatment center.

Obtaining health care coverage for a bleeding disorder may be difficult and may limit employment opportunities. Individuals may be eligible for SSI if disabilities are significant.

SPECIAL FAMILY CONCERNS

Child abuse may be suspected.

Parents may experience guilt regarding hereditary nature of a bleeding disorder.

The fear of injury to an infant may decrease parent-infant bonding.

Parents may fear the inability to prevent bleeding episodes despite attempts to prevent injury.

The potential for undiscovered HIV and hepatitis C infection may be a concern.

The family may experience uncertainty regarding the viral safety of blood products.

Insurance problems may occur as children and adults reach lifetime maximum amounts of reimbursement.

References

Adamson S et al: Viral safety of recombinant factor IX, Sem Hematol 35(suppl 2):22-27, 1998.

Aledort L et al: A meeting held in London, 12-13 January, 1998, to discuss bleeding disorders in women, Haemophilia 4:145-154, 1998.

Aledort L et al: A longitudinal study of orthopaedic outcomes for severe factor-VIII-deficient haemophiliacs, J Intern Med 236:391-399, 1994.

Blanchette V et al: Hepatitis C infection in patients with hemophilia: results of a national survey, Transfus Med Rev 8:210217, 1994.

Boyd D et al: Recent advances in the management of patients with haemophilia and other bleeding disorders, Dent Update 6:254-257, 1994.

Brackmann H, Oldenburg J, and Schwaab R: Immune tolerance for the treatment of factor VIII inhibitors—twenty years' "Bonn Protocol," Vox Sanguinis 70(suppl 1):30, 1996.

Brettler D: Inhibitors of factor VIII and IX, Haemophilia 1(suppl 1):35-39, 1995.

Buzzard B: Physiotherapy for prevention and treatment of chronic hemophilia synovitis, Clin Orthop 343:42-46, 1997.

Cahill M: Hematologic problems in pediatric patients, Semin Oncol Nurs 12:38-50, 1996.

Cardinale V, editor: 1998 Drug topics red book, Montvale, NJ, 1998, Medical Economics Co.

Centers for Disease Control and Prevention: Prevention of hepatitis A through active or passive immunization: recommendations of the Advisory Committee on Immunization Practices, MMWR 45:12-14, 1996.

Connelly S and Kaleko M: Hemophilia A gene therapy, Haemophilia 4:380-388, 1998.

Conway J and Hilgartner M: Initial presentations of pediatric hemophiliacs, Arch Pediatr Adolesc Med 148:589-594, 1994.

Crudder S: 1997 National summary of hemophilia patients, Centers for Disease Control and Prevention, private communication, 1998.

Dardik R et al: Current strategy for genetic analysis of haemophilia A families, Haemophilia 2:11-17, 1996.

Davis G et al: Interferon alfa-2b alone or in combination with ribavirin for the treatment of relapse of chronic hepatitis C, N Engl J Med 339:1493-1499, 1998.

Dietrich A et al: Head trauma in children with congenital coagulation disorders, J Pediatr Surg 29:28-32, 1994.

DiMichele D: Immune tolerance: a synopsis of the international experience, Haemophilia 4:568-573, 1998.

DiMichele D and Neufeld E: Hemophilia: a new approach to an old disease, Hematol Oncol Clin No Amer 12:1315-1344, 1998.

Duthie R et al: The management of musculoskeletal problems in the haemophilias, ed 2, New York, 1994, Oxford University Press.

Ehrlich H et al: Comparison of high responder inhibitor frequency in recent studies of previously untreated patients with hemophilia A, Thromb Hemostat 97:242-243, 1998.

Eickhoff H et al: Control of the synovium in haemophilia, Haemophilia 4:511-513, 1998.

Ewenstein B: von Willebrand's disease, Ann Rev Med 48:525-542, 1997.

Federici A: Diagnosis of von Willebrand's disease, Haemophilia 4:654-660, 1998.

Fernandez-Palazzi F: Treatment of acute and chronic synovitis by non-surgical means, Haemophilia 4:518-523, 1998.

Furie B, Limentani S, and Rosenfield C: A practical guide to the evaluation and treatment of hemophilia, Blood 84:3-9, 1994.

Giangrande P: Management of pregnancy in carriers of hemophilia, Haemophilia 4:779-784, 1998.

Geraghty S and Kleinert D: Use and morbidity of venous access devices in patients with hemophilia, J Intrav Nurs 21:70-75, 1998.

Gilbert M and Radomisli T: Therapeutic options in the management of hemophilic synovitis, Clin Orthop 343:88-92, 1997.

Gupta G and Bianchi D: DNA diagnosis for the practicing obstetrician, Obstet Gynecol Clin N Am 52:243-247, 1996.

Hay C: Factor VIII inhibitors, Haemophilia 1(suppl 2):16-17, 1995.

Heeg M et al: Total knee and hip arthroplasty in hemophilic patients, Haemophilia 4:747-751, 1998.

Hilgartner M and Corrigan J: Coagulation disorders. In Miller D and Baehner R, editors: Blood diseases of infancy and childhood, St Louis, 1995, Mosby.

Hoffman M and Roberts H: Hemophilia and related conditions—inherited deficiencies of prothrombin (factor II), factor V, and factors VII-XII. In Beutler E et al, editors: Williams hematology, ed 5, New York, 1995, McGraw-Hill.

Hoots K and Canty D: Clotting factor concentrates and immune function in haemophilia patients, Haemophilia 4:704-713, 1998.

Hoyer L: Hemophilia A, N Engl J Med 330: 38-47, 1994.

Jackson M et al: Fibrin sealant: current and potential clinical applications, Blood Coagul Fibrinolysis 7: 737-746, 1996.

Jandl J: Disorders of Coagulation. In: Blood: textbook of hematology, ed 2, New York, 1996, Little Brown and Co.

Kadir R et al: Assessment of menstrual blood loss and gynaecological problems in patients with inherited bleeding disorders, Haemophilia 5:40-48, 1999.

Kadir R et al: Quality of life during menstruation in patients with inherited bleeding disorders, Haemophilia 4:836-841, 1998.

Kasper C: Hereditary plasma clotting factor disorders and their management, Los Angeles, 1996, Los Angeles Orthopaedic Hospital.

Lemon S and Thomas D: Vaccines to prevent viral hepatitis, N Engl J Med 163:196-204, 1997.

Ljung R: Prophylactic treatment in Sweden—overtreatment or optimal model, Haemophilia 4:409-412, 1998.

Lusher J: Prophylaxis in children with hemophilia, is it the optimal treatment? Thromb Hemostat 78:726-729, 1997.

Mannucci P: Desmopressin (DDAVP) in the treatment of bleeding disorders: the first 20 years, Blood 90:2515-2521, 1997.

Mannucci P: Viral safety of plasma derived and recombinant products used in the management of hemophilia A and B, Haemophilia 1(suppl 1):14-20, 1995.

McHutchison J et al: Interferon alfa-2b, alone or in combination with ribavirin as initial treatment for chronic hepatitis C, N Engl J Med 339:1485-1492, 1998.

Medical and Scientific Advisory Council of the National Hemophilia Foundation (MASAC): Recommendations concerning neonatal intracranial hemorrhage and post partum hemorrhage (Medical Advisory #311), New York, 1998, National Hemophilia Foundation.

Medical and Scientific Advisory Council of the National Hemophilia Foundation (MASAC): Recommendations concerning the treatment of hemophilia and related bleeding disorders (Medical Advisory #312), New York, 1998, National Hemophilia Foundation.

Medical and Scientific Advisory Council of the National Hemophilia Foundation (MASAC): Recommendations concerning the treatment of von Willebrand disease (Medical Advisory #314), New York, 1998, National Hemophilia Foundation.

Menache D and Aronson D: New treatments of vwd: plasma derived vwd factor concentrates, Thromb Hemostat, 78:566-570, 1997.

Michaud J et al: Intracranial hemorrhage in a newborn with hemophilia following elective cesarean section, Am J Pediatr Hematol Oncol 13:473-475, 1991.

National Digestive Diseases Information Clearinghouse: Vaccination for hepatitis A and B, NIH Publication No. 97-4245, 1997.

Naylor J et al: A novel DNA inversion causing severe hemophilia A, Blood 87:3255-3261, 1996.

Nichols W and Ginsburg D: Von Willebrand's disease, Rev Mol Med 76:1-10, 1997.

Onwuzurike N, Warrier I, and Lusher J: Types of bleeding seen during the first 30 months of life in children with severe hemophilia A and B, Haemophilia 2:137-140, 1996.

Perkins J et al: Use of implantable venous access devices (IVADs) in children with hemophilia, J Pediatr Hematol Oncol, 19:339-344, 1997.

Radivoyevitch M: Hemophilia and EACA, Oral Surg Oral Med Oral Pathol Oral Radiol Endod 82:118, 1996.

Rickard K: Guidelines for therapy and optimal dosages of coagulation factor for treatment of bleeding and surgery in haemophilia, Haemophilia 1(suppl 1):8-13, 1995.

Roberts H et al: Newer concepts of blood coagulation, Haemophilia 4:331-334, 1998.

Rockstroh J et al: Immunosuppression may lead to progression of hepatitis C virus-associated liver disease in hemophiliacs coinfected with HIV, Am J Gastroenterol 91:2563-2568, 1996.

Rodriquez-Merchan E: Pathogenesis, early diagnosis, and prophylaxis for chronic hemophilic synovitis, Clin Orthop 343:6-11, 1997.

Rosenberg P and Goedert J: Estimating the cumulative incidence of HIV infection among persons with haemophilia in the United States of America, Stat Med 17:155-168, 1998.

Sallah S: Inhibitors to clotting factor, Ann Hematol 75:1-7, 1997.

Saviolo-Negrin N et al: Psychological aspects and coping of parents with a hemophilic child: a quantitative approach, Haemophilia 5:63-68, 1999.

Shouval D: Vaccines for prevention of viral hepatitis, Haemophilia 4:587-594, 1998.

Siegel J et al: Hemarthrosis and synovitis associated with hemophilia: clinical use of P-32 chromic phosphate synoviorthesis for treatment, Radiology 190:257-261, 1994.

Soucie J, Evatt B, and Jackson D: Occurance of hemophilia in the United States, Am J Hematol 59:288-294, 1998.

Szucs T et al: Resource utilization in haemophiliacs treated in Europe: results from the European study on socioeconomic aspects of haemophilia care, Haemophilia 4:498-501, 1998.

Teitel J: Safety of coagulation factor concentrates, Haemophilia 4:393-401, 1998.

United Kingdom Haemophilia Centre Directors Organization Executive Committee: Guidelines on therapeutic products to treat hemophilia and other hereditary coagulation disorders, Haemophilia 3:63-77, 1997.

Venkateswaran L et al: Mild hemophilia in children: prevalence, complications and treatment, J Pediatr Hematol Oncol 20:32-35, 1998.

Vnencak-Jones C et al: Analysis of factor VIII gene inversion mutations in 166 unrelated hemophilia A families: frequency and utility in genetic counseling, Haemophilia 2:18-23, 1996.

Von Willebrand Working Party of the United Kingdom Haemophilia Centre Directors' Organization: Guidelines for the diagnosis and management of von Willebrand's disease, Haemophilia 3(suppl 2):1-8, 1997.

Walker I et al: Causes of death in Canadians with hemophilia 1980-1995, Haemophilia 4:714-720, 1998.

Warrier I et al: Factor IX Inhibitors and anaphylaxis in hemophilia B, J Pediatr Hematol Oncol 19:23-27, 1997.

White G, Beebe A, and Nielsen B: Recombinant factor IX, Thromb Hemost 78:261-265, 1997.

White G and Roberts H: Treatment of factor VIII inhibitors—a general overview, Vox Sang 70(suppl 1):21-22, 1996.

Young J et al: Prenatal and molecular diagnosis of hemophilia B, Am J Hematol 52:243-247, 1996.

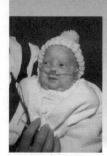

CHAPTER 12

Bronchopulmonary Dysplasia

Kayla Harvey

Etiology

Bronchopulmonary dysplasia (BPD) was first described by Northway, Rosan, and Porter (1967) in a review of chest radiographs of premature infants who were treated with positive pressure ventilation and oxygen for respiratory distress syndrome (RDS). When the disease was first described, a four-stage radiographic classification was used.

Philip (1975) broadened the definition to include nonradiographic findings and management, including the following: (1) institution of positive pressure ventilation within the first week of life for a minimum of 3 days; (2) clinical findings of tachypnea, rales, and retractions persisting beyond 28 days of life; (3) an oxygen requirement to maintain arterial oxygen pressure (PaO_2) above 55 mm Hg for more than 28 days; and (4) chest radiographs showing persistent strands of densities with normal and hyperlucent areas in bilateral lung fields.

As advances in the study, diagnosis, and treatment of BPD progress, these early classification systems are used less often. Today, BPD might be described as "classic" or "late" BPD. BPD is often used interchangeably with the term *chronic lung disease* (CLD) and is usually classified as mild, moderate, or severe.

Respiratory failure at birth is critical to the etiology of classic or severe BPD because it requires treatment with supplemental oxygen and mechanical ventilation (Hazinski, 1998). Respiratory failure may be a result of several causes but is most often due to RDS (Hazinski, 1998). Other contributing conditions to the development of BPD include hyaline membrane disease, meconium aspiration, congenital heart disease, patent ductus arteriosus, fluid overload, pulmonary air leak, and edema in newborns (Bancalari and Sosenko, 1990).

Rozycki and Kirkpatrick (1993) describe BPD pathogenesis in the following sequence: (1) exposure to damaging stimuli (e.g., barotrauma and oxygen); (2) local cellular damage and death from oxygen radicals and lung stretch; (3) mediators initiate the inflammatory process; (4) persistent alveolitis; (5) proliferation of fibroblasts with subsequent fibrosis; and (6) epithelial metaplasia and inflammation followed by smooth-muscle hypertrophy. Figure 12-1 outlines the pathogenesis of BPD.

Risk factors that are key indicators of infants prone to develop BPD include lung immaturity, oxygen toxicity, positive pressure ventilation with lung stretch, inflammation, infection, and family history of asthma (Ghezzi et al, 1998; Hazinski, 1998).

Current perspectives on CLD suggest that it is a complex disorder resulting from more than lung injury associated with oxygen toxicity and barotrauma. Studies on premature infants indicate that inflammation plays a key role in the development of CLD (Groneck et al, 1994). Specific microbes (e.g., ureaplasma urealyticum and chlamydia trachomatis) have been implicated along with high levels of inflammatory mediators (e.g., interleukin-8) in the bronchial secretions of premature infants (Groneck et al, 1994). Moreover, the presence of patent ductus arteriosus (PDA) further contributes to the development of significant CLD. Left-to-right shunting of blood flow through a PDA increases pulmonary blood flow and lung fluid. This process interferes with normal lung mechanics and gas exchange. The combination of neonatal infection and a PDA appears to be a significant risk factor for the development of CLD (Gonzalez et al, 1996). CLD represents a wide spectrum of clinical entities that are not completely understood and results from a variety of insults and predisposing factors.

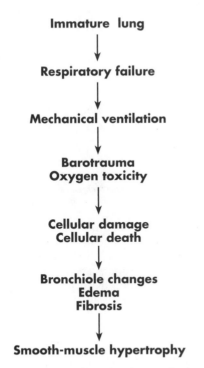

Immature lung

↓

Respiratory failure

↓

Mechanical ventilation

↓

Barotrauma
Oxygen toxicity

↓

Cellular damage
Cellular death

↓

Bronchiole changes
Edema
Fibrosis

↓

Smooth-muscle hypertrophy

Figure 12-1   Outline of pathogenesis of BPD.

Incidence

BPD may be associated with chronic pulmonary dysfunction, recurrent hospitalization, increased incidence of developmental disabilities, growth delay, and even death (Barrington and Finer, 1998; Fillmore and Cartlidge, 1998). An estimated 7000 to 10,000 new cases of BPD are diagnosed each year (Hoekstra et al, 1991). BPD is the leading cause of CLD in infants in the United States (Rojas et al, 1995). Parker, Lindstrom, and Cotton (1992) reported a 22% rise in the incidence of BPD in the past decade, but the reported incidence of BPD varies because there is not a consistent definition of the disease. As medical technology progresses, the increase in BPD may be a result of an increase in the survival of premature and very low birth weight (e.g., less than 1500 gm) newborns (Parker, Lindstrom, and Cotton, 1992). It is estimated that 75% of infants with BPD are very low birth weight (Hazinski, 1998).

The classic form of BPD or severe CLD is less common with the use of surfactant and prenatal steroids. As a result, a milder form of CLD has emerged as a major entity in the population of high-risk premature infants (Rojas et al, 1995). These infants usually present with a need for ventilatory support initially for poor respiratory effort but are often quickly weaned from the ventilator after a few hours to days of support at low pressures and low oxygen concentration. Therefore these infants can avoid the initial lung insults of barotrauma and oxygen toxicity. Some of these infants have progressive deterioration, however, despite their early success. Complications such as patent ductus arteriosus (PDA) and/or infection appear to trigger lung function deterioration in the group of infants with mild CLD (Gonzalez, et al, 1996; Pierce and Bancalari, 1995).

Clinical Manifestations at Time of Diagnosis

Clinical manifestations of BPD vary depending on the age of the child at onset and the severity of the disease. The severity can range from a child having some pulmonary symptoms that require bronchodilator treatment and diuretics to a child requiring a tracheostomy and mechanical ventilatory support for prolonged periods of time in the hospital and at home (Box 12-1).

An infant with BPD displays significant alteration in lung mechanics. Compliance is diminished by a combination of the following: (1) fibrosis secondary to alveolar injury; (2) increased lung fluid as a result of damage at the alveolar-capillary membrane; and (3) overdistention because of injury to alveolar-supporting structures, which causes airway collapse and subsequent air-trapping (Ackerman, 1994). An increase in airway resistance is found secondary to fibrosis, airway edema, and bronchoconstriction (Ackerman, 1994). The combination of decreased lung compliance and increased airway resistance produces clinical findings such as tachypnea, wheezing, and increased work of breathing. Fluid leak from cellular damage is manifested as inspiratory and expiratory rales.

┌─────────────────────────────────┐
│ **Box 12-1** │
│ **Clinical Manifestations** │
│ │
│ Tachypnea │
│ Retractions │
│ Rales │
│ Wheezing │
│ Cyanotic episodes │
│ Activity/handling intolerance │
│ Abnormal chest radiograph │
│ Poor growth │
└─────────────────────────────────┘

┌─────────────────────────────────┐
│ **Box 12-2** │
│ **Treatment** │
│ │
│ Synthetic surfactant │
│ Systemic steroids │
│ Supplemental oxygen │
│ Diuretics │
│ Bronchodilators │
│ Antiinflammatories │
│ "Tincture of time" │
└─────────────────────────────────┘

Chest radiographs of infants with BPD reveal increased interstitial markings, including cystic changes or fine, lacy densities with or without hyperinflation (Alpert, Allen, and Schidlow, 1993). The degree of abnormality in radiographs of children at 1 month of age can provide some insight for prognosis (Greenough, 1990). Scoring systems for chest radiographs have been developed to correlate films with respiratory support and create a standardization for comparison of severity among infants with BPD (Weinstein, 1994).

An abnormal respiratory examination is the key finding in the diagnosis of BPD (Figure 12-2). On visual examination, the respiratory rate may be elevated by as much as 20 to 30 breaths/minute above the baseline for a child's age. With respiratory distress, the primary care provider will observe a prolonged exhalation with increased use of abdominal and accessory muscles. Umbilical or inguinal hernias may occur as a result of increased abdominal pressure from high airway resistance and use of accessory muscles (Hazinski, 1998).

Other clinical manifestations of the preterm infant with BPD include poor gas exchange, bronchospasm, mucus plugging, and poor physical growth. Cyanosis and activity intolerance with feeding and handling are common findings (Hazinski, 1998). Ultimately the task of breathing robs these infants of precious calories needed for physical growth and development.

Treatment

The BPD process is initiated through cellular injury to the immature lung (Box 12-2). Infants born before 28 to 32 weeks' gestation have an insufficient amount of pulmonary surfactant. Surfactant is a lipoprotein that lowers the surface tension of the air-alveolar surface and allows lung expansion, thus maintaining the patency of the alveoli and preventing atelectasis. Synthetic surfactant given in the first 24 hours of life has been shown to decrease neonatal mortality but not significantly reduce the incidence of BPD (McColley, 1998). Some studies have analyzed the outcome of surfactant use in the first 12 hours as prophylaxis in high-risk infants and as treatment for infants with known RDS. Outcomes indicate surfactant use as treatment can reduce medical costs for large infants by decreasing complications and the length of time they need ventilatory support (Jobe, 1993). The early use of surfactant in very small premature infants significantly reduces mortality (Jobe, 1993).

Additionally, use of systemic steroids in the first 12 days of life has had a positive effect on accelerating the lung maturation of high-risk premature infants. Infants ranging from 700 to 1500 gm with severe RDS who were given both surfactant and dexamethasone in the first 12 hours required less mechanical ventilation and supplemental oxygen (Rastogi et al, 1996).

Treatment also focuses on enhancing the infant's natural healing process, thereby avoiding further complications often associated with BPD. A "tincture of time" is the primary force that leads to stabilization of BPD. In the interim, support is employed until physiologic maturation of lung tissue can support oxygen needs. Such treatment modalities include oxygen therapy, diuretics, bronchodilators, and corticosteroids.

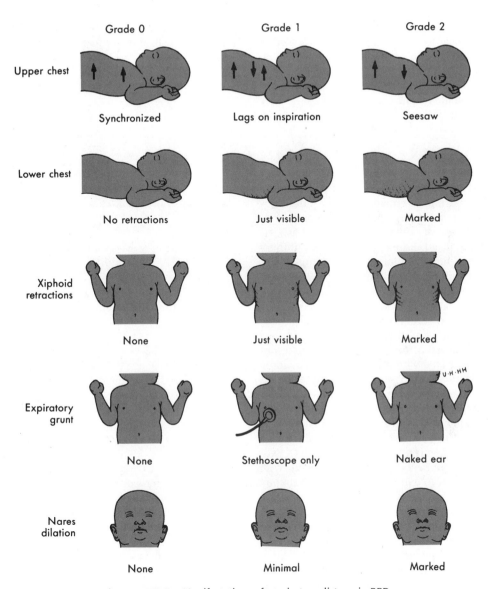

	Grade 0	Grade 1	Grade 2
Upper chest	Synchronized	Lags on inspiration	Seesaw
Lower chest	No retractions	Just visible	Marked
Xiphoid retractions	None	Just visible	Marked
Expiratory grunt	None	Stethoscope only	Naked ear
Nares dilation	None	Minimal	Marked

Figure 12-2 Manifestations of respiratory distress in BPD.

Oxygen

The need for supplemental oxygen varies with the severity of lung dysfunction. Infants who require oxygen after hospital discharge rarely require more than 1 to 2 L/min via nasal cannula. Children on oxygen must be followed at frequent intervals to assess for hypoxia by physical examination and oxygen and carbon dioxide readings. These read-ings can ideally be obtained via pulse oximeter or transcutaneous oxygen monitoring instead of via arterial blood samples. Oxygen and carbon dioxide measurements must be done during periods of rest and activity to accurately determine a child's con-tinuing supplemental oxygen needs (Hazinski, 1998). When the child appears clinically stable, is gaining weight, and is not anemic, gradual weaning from oxygen is initiated by the neonatal pulmonary team. A typical weaning schedule is presented in Table 12-1. To avoid significant oxygen desaturation during sleep, a child with BPD should continue nighttime supplemental oxygen until daytime oxygen saturation equals or exceeds 92% in room air (Hazinski, 1998).

Diuretics

Diuretics are often used in the care of infants with BPD. These medications correct fluid retention, prevent fluid overload, decrease pulmonary resistance, and increase pulmonary compliance (Box 12-3) (Brem, 1992). Furosemide (Lasix) is a commonly used diuretic effective in eliminating excess fluid in the lungs that accumulates as a result of a disruption in lymph drainage and increased capillary permeability (Kugelman et al, 1997). In moderate to severe BPD, potassium sparing spironolactone (Aldactone) and chlorothiazide (Diuril) are often needed for additional diuresis. Because of the potential electrolyte imbalance associated with diuretic therapy, children with BPD must have serum electrolyte values monitored and are often given potassium chloride supplements. Serum electrolytes should be monitored monthly with supplements adjusted to maintain chloride above 92 mEq/L and potassium above 3.5 mEq/L (Ackerman, 1994). Nutritional requirements must be balanced with fluid restriction to avoid overloading the already stressed cardiopulmonary system.

Inhaled furosemide has been evaluated on a sample of neonates with severe BPD (Kugelman et al, 1997). Researchers hoped to improve gas exchange and pulmonary mechanics while sparing neonates the electrolyte imbalance that is often caused by systemic furosemide. The therapy was proven safe, but its efficacy was no different than the placebo (Kugelman et al, 1997). It has been suggested, however, that the study dose of 1 mg/kg may be too low to cause an effect via inhalation.

Bronchodilators

Infants with BPD may be predisposed to bronchial hyperreactivity and bronchospasm from neonatal lung injury and hyperplasia of smooth muscle

Table 12-1
Weaning a Patient from Supplemental Oxygen: Sample Schedule

Time	Amount of Oxygen (per min)
At hospital discharge	0.5 L at all times
1 month after discharge*	0.5 L during feedings and sleep; 0.25 L when awake
2 months*	0.25 L at all times
3 months*	0.25 L during feedings and sleep; room air when awake

From Hazinski TA: Bronchopulmonary dysplasia. In Kendig EL: Kendig's disorders of the respiratory tract in children, Philadelphia, 1998, W.B. Saunders.
*Assumes clinical stability, adequate weight gain, and proof of adequate oxygen saturation (intervals may vary).

(Hazinski, 1998; Rush and Hazinski, 1992). Bronchodilator therapy is used to reduce the effects of bronchoconstriction by relaxing smooth muscle in the airways. The outcome of this therapy is improved gas exchange through a decrease in airflow resistance and gas trapping (Fok et al, 1998). A positive response from this therapy is clinically shown by a decrease in wheezing, coughing, or supplemental oxygen requirements.

Machines used to administer aerosolized medications can be cumbersome and inconvenient. Spacer devices have become a portable alternative for older children and adults with airway obstruction. Studies on infants indicate that a spacer with a mask is an effective means of administering aerosolized bronchodilators (Fok et al, 1998).

Three categories of bronchodilators are beta-adrenergic agonists (albuterol), anticholinergics (ipratropium [Atrovent]), and methylxanthines (theophylline). Albuterol is commonly used via inhalation at a dose of 0.02 to 0.1 ml/kg/dose (maximum 0.5 ml) every 4 to 6 hours depending on response and disease severity (Ackerman, 1994). Use of nebulized ipratropium bromide (Atrovent) in combination with albuterol can enhance pulmonary function in infants with BPD. Ipratropium bromide antagonizes muscarinic receptors in the airways, resulting in bronchodilation (Benitz and Tatro, 1996). Theophylline is an oral bronchodilator that also stimulates respiratory drive; however, it has

---

Box 12-3

Diuretics Used to Treat BPD

Furosemide (Lasix)
1 to 4 mg/kg/dy in 1 to 2 divided doses.

Chlorothiazide (Diuril)
30 to 40 mg/kg/dy in 2 divided doses.

Spironolactone (Aldactone)
2 to 4 mg/kg/dy in 1 to 2 divided doses.

Data from The Harriet Lane handbook, ed 14, St Louis, 1996, Mosby. The Pediatrics Drug Handbook, 1996. Benitz WE and Tatro D: The pediatric drug handbook, ed 3, St Louis, 1996, Mosby.

---

many side effects, including feeding intolerance, tachycardia, irritability, diarrhea, increased gastroesophageal reflux (GER), and lowered seizure threshold (The Harriet Lane Handbook, 1996; Benitz and Tatro, 1996). As a result, the role of theophylline in bronchodilator therapy is diminished, but it may be indicated in infants with BPD with apnea of prematurity.

Antiinflammatories

Systemic corticosteroids have been used in the acute and chronic phases of BPD disease. Steroid treatment with dexamethasone has been effective in weaning infants with BPD from mechanical ventilation during hospitalization (Rastogi, 1996). Corticosteroids can reduce pulmonary edema and inflammation in the small airways, as well as potentiate the effects of bronchodilators (Benitz and Tatro, 1996). Prednisone (i.e., 1 to 2 mg/kg) given for 3 to 5 days can be effective for acute exacerbations. Watterberg and Scott (1995) speculate that infants with BPD have a decreased ability to secrete cortisol in response to stress, which leaves them more vulnerable to inflammatory lung injury. Infants with severe BPD may require a prolonged course of corticosteroids with a slow tapering of the drug treatment over weeks. A common weaning schedule is a gradual decrease in dosage every 3 to 7 days followed by a change in frequency to every other day at twice the daily dose (Truog, 1993;

Kountz, 1989). Infants using this type of therapy are at risk for adrenal suppression and should receive an increase in their usual steroid dose during significant biophysical stressors (e.g., moderate-severe infection or surgical procedures) (The Harriet Lane Handbook, 1996).

The use of inhaled corticosteroids (ICS) for infants with BPD has increased. Studies evaluating the efficacy and safety of nebulized steroids in infants and children with BPD revealed that those treated were hospitalized for fewer days and had an ability to decrease oral corticosteroid therapy (Cloutier, 1993; Konig et al, 1992).

Bronchopulmonary disease is often associated with asthma. Research on children with asthma using ICS (via MDI with spacer) has revealed consistent efficacy in the reduction of airway inflammation. Concern about long-term effects on growth, however, has prompted further evaluation of the use of ICS in prepubertal children. A review of 30 studies revealed that children using relatively high doses of ICS for 7 to 12 months had documented growth suppression of 1.0 to 1.4 cm/year (Welch, 1998). It is unclear how to apply this information to infants using ICS and whether the growth suppression will be permanent or temporary. It is clear, however, that ICS have systemic bioavailability and should be used cautiously.

Cromolyn sodium (Intal) is an inhaled, nonsteroidal antiinflammatory that can be beneficial to infants and children with BPD (Ackerman, 1994; Truog, 1993). Cromolyn sodium reduces airway hyperreactivity by preventing the release of inflammatory mediators into the airways. Cromolyn sodium (20 mg) given via inhalation 2 to 4 times a day may be indicated for an empirical trial in infants with a significant reactive airway disease (Rush and Hazinski, 1992).

Recent and Anticipated Advances in Diagnosis and Management

In an effort to decrease the incidence of BPD, giving antenatal steroids to pregnant women at high risk for preterm delivery has become more common. There seems to be a correlation between intrauterine inflammation and subsequent development of BPD in the fetus (Ghezzi et al, 1998). Specifically, high levels of interleukin-8 may be a risk factor of an infant developing BPD (Ghezzi et al, 1998). Controlled trials indicate that treatment with antenatal steroids is successful in reducing the incidence of death and RDS in preterm infants by about 50% (Battin et al 1998; Crowley et al, 1993).

Respiratory syncytial virus (RSV) infection causes significant mortality and morbidity in infants with BPD. Researchers have found that administering immunoglobulins specific to RSV decreases the incidence and severity of RSV infection in children with BPD (Groothuis et al, 1993). Subsequently, intravenous respiratory syncytial virus immune globulin (RSV-IGIV; RespiGam) was made available to infants with BPD in the winter of 1996-1997 (PREVENT study group, 1997). Monthly infusions of RespiGam, however, proved cumbersome. A synthetic formulation of the monoclonal antibody for RSV called palivizumab (Synagis) was developed and approved for intramuscular injection for at-risk infants in the winter of 1998-1999 (The Impact Study Group, 1998).

Continuous negative extrathoracic pressure (CNEP) has been studied as an alternative to traditional invasive positive pressure ventilation for neonatal respiratory failure (Samuels et al, 1996). Researchers hoped to achieve a decrease in lung trauma with the use of noninvasive ventilation, but the incidence of pneumothorax, effects on cerebral blood flow, and skin maceration in the infants receiving CNEP indicates that this mode of ventilation requires further study (Samuels et al, 1996).

Some clinicians speculate that supplementing deficient nutrients in premature neonates can prevent BPD. Vitamin E (for reduction of oxygen-free radicals) and vitamin A (to promote healing) have been given to infants considered to be at high-risk for BPD without uniform success (Rozycki and Kirkpatrick, 1993). Further research is needed to investigate treatment modalities that will reduce the severity of BPD.

Medical and technologic advances in neonatology have resulted in an increase in the survival rates of very low birth weight infants (i.e., less than 750 g), thus contributing to the increased incidence of BPD (Jacob et al, 1998). Prevention of premature births through improved prenatal care is the key to decreasing the incidence of BPD. Several

***

Box 12-4

Treatment that May Decrease the Incidence of CLD in High-Risk Infants

Prenatal steroids (maternal)
Early surfactant
Postnatal steroids
Less aggressive ventilator management
Early PDA closure
Conservative fluid management

From Bancalari E: Bronchopulmonary dysplasia: then and now. Presented at the American Thoracic Society Conference, Chicago, May 1998.

***

changes in the early treatment of high-risk premature infants and their mothers have resulted in a shift in CLD severity. Therefore the practice of antenatal steroids, early use of surfactant, systemic steroids, PDA closure, less aggressive ventilator management, and conservative fluid management may have contributed to the decreased incidence of severe BPD (Box 12-4).

Associated Problems (Box 12-5)

Airway Complications

Structural damage to an infant's premature respiratory tree often occurs as a result of endotracheal intubation and positive pressure ventilation (Alpert, Allen, and Schidlow, 1993). Upper airway anomalies (i.e., including subglottic stenosis, granuloma, tracheal scarring, and polyp formation) can occur immediately after extubation or as a late presentation (Hazinski, 1998). Infants presenting with homophonous wheezing, hypoxia, and bradycardia (i.e., cyanotic "BPD spells") should be evaluated for lower airway anomalies such as tracheomalacia and bronchomalacia (Alpert, Allen, and Schidlow, 1993, Hazinski, 1998).

Infants who require prolonged ventilatory support and infants who develop respiratory failure from an upper airway obstruction need a tracheostomy. Children with a tracheostomy are now

> ## Box 12-5
> ### Associated Problems
>
> Airway complications
> Infection
> Poor growth and nutrition
> Gastroesophageal reflux
> Cardiac conditions
> Neurodevelopmental complications
> Seizures
> Ophthalmologic sequelae
> Renal conditions
> Rickets
> Stoma care
> Otitis media/sinusitis

often cared for at home. The most frequent complications are infection of the tracheostomy, obstruction by secretions, or accidental decannulation. Parents and primary care providers must be competent in tracheostomy care. This includes the knowledge and skills necessary for maintaining tracheostomy patency, caring for the stoma, and changing tracheostomy tubes.

Airways of infants with BPD exhibit significant loss of cilia and denudation of their lining, resulting in the absence of the normal cleansing abilities of the lung (Hazinski, 1998). Daily chest physiotherapy (CPT) and postural drainage help mobilize secretions so they can be removed from the airway by coughing or suctioning if an artificial airway is present. During a viral or bacterial illness, secretion production increases and more frequent CPT and drainage may be necessary.

Infection

Infants with BPD are at increased risk of lower respiratory tract infections in the first year of life (Furman et al, 1996). Infection is the major cause of rehospitalization, late morbidity, and mortality in children with BPD (Groothuis, 1993). Therefore early evaluation and close follow-up are recommended for children with BPD with any upper respiratory illness or cold. Community-acquired viruses can exacerbate BPD by making hypoxia, edema, bronchoconstriction, and secondary bacter-

ial infection worse (Hazinski, 1998). Treatment to stabilize such episodes includes an increase in supplemental oxygen, extra doses of diuretics, and administration of aerosolized bronchodilators (Hazinski, 1998). Broad-spectrum antibiotic treatment and a septic work-up may be indicated for a febrile infant with BPD. Nasopharyngeal aspirate for immunofluorescence may be helpful in identifying particularly harmful viruses such as RSV, adenovirus, and influenza.

Poor Growth and Nutrition

Growth patterns in children with BPD depend on the nutritional status and the severity of the lung disease. Growth retardation in infants with BPD most commonly occurs as a result of an inability to match caloric intake with energy expenditure (Rozycki and Kirkpatrick, 1993). The combination of fluid restrictions, frequent respiratory infections, and an elevated metabolic rate often results in poor weight gain (Hazinski, 1998). Feeding disorders (e.g., oral aversion) can occur in infants with BPD as a result of exposure to negative oral stimuli (e.g., endotracheal tubes and suctioning) and deprivation of positive oral feeding and/or sucking experiences (Alpert, Allen, and Schidlow, 1993). Furthermore, infants with BPD who have labored breathing while at rest often have difficulty coordinating their rapid respirations, sucks, and swallows (Truog, 1993). Other potential causes of growth failure in infants with BPD include hypoxemia, heart failure, gastroesophageal reflux, and rickets of prematurity (Alpert, Allen, and Schidlow, 1993).

Early in treatment, total parenteral nutrition is often necessary, followed by supplementation of breast or bottle feedings with gavage feedings. In infants with severe BPD and feeding problems, a gastrostomy tube may be necessary. Caloric requirements are high (i.e., up to 150 to 200 kcal/kg per day). Most infants require formula with a caloric concentration of at least 24 to 30 kcal/30 ml (1 oz) to achieve optimal catch-up growth (Ackerman, 1994; Hazinski, 1998). Formula may be fortified with vegetable oil, triglycerides, or glucose polymers to increase the calories per ounce (Hazinski, 1998). In addition, formulas with higher protein, calcium, phosphorus, and zinc may contribute to more linear growth, lean body mass, and bone mass (Mueller, 1998).

As a result of a high risk for growth delay, some infants with BPD benefit from a comprehensive evaluation by a nutritional specialist. In one study, risk factors associated with growth failure included low socioeconomic status, postdischarge days of illness, and "suspect" development (Johnson et al, 1998). Management strategies should be implemented to ensure adequate energy intake, parental support and/or education, and feeding therapy needs.

Gastroesophageal Reflux

Gastroesophageal reflux (GER) is a common gastrointestinal dysfunction seen in children with BPD that is caused by an incompetent lower esophageal sphincter that allows acidic gastric contents to pass back into the esophagus. Symptoms of GER include emesis, apnea, bradycardia, recurrent pneumonia, delayed growth, and esophagitis (Armentrout, 1995). Abnormal lung mechanics leading to abnormal pressure gradients between the chest and abdomen may contribute to the occurrence of GER in infants with BPD (Hazinski, 1998). Esophageal pH probe monitoring over 18 to 24 hours is used to confirm the diagnosis of GER (Alpert, Allen, and Schidlow, 1993; Armentrout, 1995). Theophylline decreases the tone of the lower esophageal sphincter and should therefore be avoided in infants with both BPD and GER. Ranitidine (Zantac) and cimetidine (Tagamet) help to buffer the acidity of the stomach after meals and decrease episodes of bronchospasm caused by gastric content irritation. If these medications are not effective in controlling symptoms, metoclopramide (Reglan) and cisapride (Propulsid) should be considered to promote gastric emptying and prevent residual reflux (see the section on drug interactions later in this chapter). Thickening food with rice cereal and using reflux precautions (e.g., keeping head of bed elevated 30 degrees with infant in prone position) may help (Armentrout, 1995), although the efficacy of such precautions is now being questioned. If symptoms and the clinical picture do not demonstrate any improvement, Nissan fundoplication surgery is the last option (Armentrout, 1995).

Cardiac Conditions

Chronic cardiac changes persist in children with BPD who have suffered numerous hypoxic insults or have been maintained at a low PaO_2. Pulmonary vasoconstriction occurs in response to alveolar hypoxia, which results in pulmonary hypertension (Hazinski, 1998). The main treatment of pulmonary hypertension is supplemental oxygen (Ackerman, 1994). Maximum pulmonary vasodilation occurs when oxygen saturation is maintained at between 92% and 95%. Progression of pulmonary hypertension can lead to right ventricular hypertrophy, cor pulmonale, and congestive heart failure (Alpert, Allen, and Schidlow, 1993). Congestive heart failure can present as unexplained weight gain and significant liver enlargement (i.e., a .7-cm span) (Alpert, Allen, and Schidlow, 1993). Refractory hypoxemia or sudden fluctuations in PaO_2 may indicate a cardiac defect (Alpert, Allen, and Schidlow, 1993). PDA, incompetent foramen ovale, or septal defects can cause congestive heart failure or pulmonary hypertension (Alpert, Allen, and Schidlow, 1993; Hazinski, 1998). Diagnostic tests (i.e., including echocardiogram and cardiac catheterization) are used to confirm cardiac complications.

Neurodevelopmental Complications

Children with BPD are at high risk for developmental delays. All aspects of development can be affected: physical, cognitive, language, and sensorimotor skills. Mild gross motor sequelae (i.e., including hypotonia, hypertonia, and delayed motor development) are often seen in the first year of life (Piecuch, Leonard, and Cooper et al, 1997). Intraventricular hemorrhage, periventricular leukomalacia, or echodensity in the newborn period is predictive of a poor developmental outcome (Ackerman, 1994; Wilson-Costello, 1998). Regular assessment with early intervention involving a physical and/or occupational therapist and a developmental specialist or neurologist is necessary for optimal development (Ackerman, 1994). Regular screening exams for vision and hearing are important in a population prone to retinopathy of prematurity (ROP) and recurrent ear infections. A history of CLD seems to add significant risk for poor school performance that is often associated with very low birth weight infants (Farel et al, 1998).

Seizures

Hypoxic insults and intraventricular hemorrhages occurring in the newborn period predispose an infant to seizures. Even with anticonvulsant therapy the onset of new seizures can be triggered at any time by an infection with a high fever or a hypoxic insult. Children with BPD who have not had a seizure for at least 1 year with electroencephalograms (EEGs) free of epileptiform activity can be considered for weaning of anticonvulsants (see Chapter 21).

Ophthalmologic Sequelae

The incidence of ROP has decreased as the toxic effects of oxygen have become known. Prematurity, however, remains one of the strongest risk factors for ROP (Holmstrom et al, 1998). Central blindness can occur with repeated incidence of severe hypoxia and severe intraventricular hemorrhage. All infants weighing less than 1500 g or under 28 weeks gestational age should be screened for ROP (Oh and Merenstein, 1997). Infants with BPD who are diagnosed with ROP should be followed closely by an ophthalmologist because of their risk for strabismus and amblyopia (Oh and Merenstein, 1997).

Renal Conditions

One half of infants with BPD who receive chronic furosemide (Lasix) therapy will develop renal calcification (Hazinski, 1998). Infants on IV furosemide for over 2 weeks should have a renal ultrasound (Greenough, 1990). Thiazides (Diuril) decrease calcium excretion and may help prevent nephrocalcinosis (Alpert, Allen, and Schidlow, 1993). If renal stones are identified, furosemide should be discontinued as soon as possible to allow the calcium to reabsorb.

Rickets

Infants with BPD often develop rickets secondary to prolonged parenteral nutrition and difficulty absorbing calcium and phosphorus. The population most at risk for rickets are infants with a birth weight less than 1000 g. Long-term furosemide administration can also contribute to a negative calcium balance, thus inhibiting normal bone formation. This condition is reversible with dietary management and use of alternate diuretics (e.g., spironolactone and hydrochlorothiazide) (Alpert, Allen, and Schidlow, 1993).

Stoma Problems

Children with tracheostomy tubes are at risk for irritation around the tracheostomy stoma. Secretions that ooze from tracheostomy stomas may irritate the skin. Meticulous regular care to the tracheostomy stoma generally maintains skin integrity. Fastening tracheostomy ties too tightly can cause skin lacerations on the neck. A small, premeasured protective patch of skin barrier may be placed over the laceration to allow it to heal without continued direct contact with the tracheostomy ties or the flange of the tracheostomy tube.

Some children may develop areas of granulation tissue on and around the tracheostomy stoma. If left unattended, the tissue will continue to grow and can impede or block insertion of the tracheostomy tube into the stoma. The tissue occasionally forms a tight band around the tracheostomy stoma. Applying silver nitrate to the site will promote shrinkage and eliminate tissue. In extreme cases a child must be referred to an otorhinolaryngologist for possible surgical excision under anesthesia. Similar difficulties with granulation tissue occur with gastrostomy stomas, and the same treatment applies. Leakage of feeding around the gastrostomy tube irritates the skin on the abdomen. The cause of such leakage is usually mechanical. Some families are instructed to change gastrostomy tubes on a regular basis because over time the stomach acid alters the integrity of the tube within the stomach.

The primary care provider should examine the tube to determine its type and how it is inserted. Foley catheters, Malecot tubes, and gastrostomy button devices may be used as gastrostomy tubes. Some tubes may be placed securely with a fluid-inflated balloon. The amount of fluid in the balloon should be documented in the discharge plan. If the amount in the balloon is less than the prescribed amount, it can contribute to leakage. It is important to ensure that the internal balloon is pulled up close to the internal abdominal wall to prevent leakage. When leakage is persistent, some practitioners insert a larger tube into the stoma. This technique is controversial because over time the stoma expands and the problem will recur. The less the tube is manipulated, the longer the stoma will remain intact. Secure fastening procedures can minimize movement of the gastrostomy tube.

Otitis Media/Sinusitis

The same bacteria that colonize the lower airways often colonize the upper airways and precipitate upper respiratory infections. Recurrent otitis media is often seen in this population and results in the need for antibiotic prophylaxis or placement of bilateral myringotomy tubes or both. Hearing loss can occur as a result of chronic infection and chronic intravenous use of furosemide and aminoglycosides.

The risk of sinusitis is greater in children with CLD and those who have required or continue to require nasogastric tube feedings because the tube is a place for bacteria to seed and interferes with normal defenses in the lining of the epithelium. With sinusitis, there is a persistent unilateral or bilateral off-colored drainage from the nares. Postnasal drainage results in coughing and throat clearing, especially after a child awakes. Severe sinusitis causes coughing throughout the day and is unrelieved by bronchodilator therapy or frequent suctioning of an artificial airway. Radiographs of the sinuses confirm the presence of infection and degree of involvement. Oral antibiotics taken for at least 3 weeks clear most infections, but prolonged therapy may be needed to treat severe cases.

Prognosis

Survival rates and outcomes are steadily improving for infants with BPD. Expert medical care is now available for these infants through easier access to tertiary care personnel. Improvements in prenatal care and technologic advances in diagnostic and treatment techniques have improved the outcome

for infants with BPD. Improved survival rates are seen in infants at 26 to 28 weeks gestational age with the use of antenatal steroids, surfactant, and dexamethasone (Battin et al, 1998).

Even with these new advances, mortality is approximately 25% for infants with BPD (Ackerman, 1994). Ventilator parameters (e.g., peak inspiratory pressure and ventilator rate) on day 28 of life may be predictive of survival outcomes in infants with severe BPD (Gray et al, 1993). Higher peak inspiratory pressure (e.g., >20) and ventilator rate (e.g., >40) were associated with the death of infants requiring prolonged ventilation (Gray et al, 1993). Duration of oxygen requirement also may be a predictor of outcomes. Infants who required oxygen beyond 36 weeks gestational age had more days of readmission for respiratory problems and a lower mean developmental quotient at 18 months of age (Gregoire et al, 1998). In addition, toddlers with a history of BPD were twice as likely to require hospitalization in the first 2 years of life than were toddlers without BPD (Gross et al, 1998).

For infants with BPD who survive, growth and developmental delay improve over time. When compared with their peers as young children, adolescents, and young adults, however, the effects of BPD appear to linger. Infants and children with BPD have a lower mean weight and less subcutaneous tissue than their peers (Robertson et al, 1992). Reduced height and weight (i.e., 25% to 35% of these children are below the 10th percentile) can persist into middle childhood and adolescence (Robertson et al, 1992; Vrlenich et al, 1995). Catch-up growth of a child's head circumference in the first year of life may predict neurodevelopmental outcome. Hack and colleagues (1991) found that infants with subnormal head growth at 8 months of age had poor academic performance, lower IQs, and fewer speech-language skills at 8 to 9 years of age. For children without perinatal CNS insult, however, the neurodevelopmental outcome was good. By age 10 to 12 years, more than 60% of children with BPD were developmentally normal. Other outcome studies of infants with BPD show that they have poorer motor outcome at age 3 years than unaffected infants.

Overall, school age children with a history of BPD demonstrated academic delays when compared with their peers (Robertson et al, 1992).

Assessments often reveal attention deficit disorders, perceptual-motor integration problems, and language delays (Leonard and Piecuch, 1997). Longitudinal studies of extremely low birth weight infants reveal that despite increased nursery survival over the past 15 years, there has not been an increase in neurodevelopmental morbidity (Pine et al, 1995).

Although the effects of BPD on the respiratory system diminish in time, 70% of adolescents with BPD demonstrate continued airway obstruction and 52% have persistent airway hyperreactivity (Ackerman, 1994). One study evaluated 7-year-olds with a history of BPD and found that they had more airway obstruction evidenced by reduction of forced vital capacity, forced expiratory flow, and midflows (Gross et al, 1998). Infants who required supplemental oxygen for at least 1 month after term had a significant degree of gas trapping at 1 year of age (Jacob et al, 1998). There may be a difference, however, in long-term pulmonary function in infants with milder CLD. There is limited follow-up data of pulmonary function in this group, but it appears that the abnormalities are less pronounced and tend to improve during the first 3 years of life (Bancalari, 1998).

PRIMARY CARE MANAGEMENT

Health Care Maintenance

Growth and Development

Length and/or height, weight, and head circumference measurement (i.e., corrected for gestational age) should be obtained and plotted monthly while a child is hospitalized and with each subsequent ambulatory care visit (Trachtnenbarg and Golemon, 1998). Growth measurements taken before a child is discharged from the hospital help establish growth trends in the newly discharged infant. Even minor illness in children with BPD may result in weight loss because of their high caloric needs.

The head shape of a premature infant often appears boxy, and the head circumference must be measured and recorded carefully on standardized growth curves for premature infants or corrected for gestational age and plotted on National Center

for Health Statistics graphs. The corrected age should be used for 2 years or until the sutures are normally fused. If the head circumference percentile is significantly higher than the weight or height percentile, the possibility of intraventricular hemorrhage or poor nutritional status with head sparing is suggested (Gardner and Hagedorn, 1992). Careful physical examination and documentation of caloric intake should indicate if a cranial ultrasound is needed.

Developmental screening by the primary care provider can be accomplished using the child's corrected age and standard screening tools. Even with correction for prematurity, these infants often exhibit a developmental lag during the first year of life. Most infants with transient developmental delays test normal after they are 1 year of age. If developmental delays are significant or persist after the first year of life, the child should be referred for further assessment and therapeutic intervention. Early intervention for children who are high-risk and control of secondary pulmonary problems offer the best prospect for optimal long-term prognosis.

Diet

The high caloric requirements caused by prematurity and the increased work of breathing with BPD require creative ways of providing adequate nutrition in an appealing, tasteful manner that does not require a high expenditure of energy for consumption or create fluid overload in a compromised infant. It is important for the primary care provider to regularly assess weight gain and evaluate nutritional needs. It is beneficial to maintain contact with the nutritionist from the discharging hospital and ask for assistance in maintaining adequate caloric intake. As previously mentioned, children with severe BPD or feeding problems may require supplemental feedings via gavage or gastrostomy tube.

The introduction of solid foods is generally initiated between 4 and 6 months of corrected age or when an infant weighs 6 to 7 kg. Oral-tactile hypersensitivity as a result of oral trauma from the passage of nasogastric or orogastric tubes, endotracheal tubes, or repeated suctioning may make it difficult for a child to adequately feed. Early recognition of the problem and intervention by trained health care providers (i.e., nurses, a speech pathologist, or occupational therapist) can facilitate feeding and decrease parental frustration and feelings of failure (see Chapter 2).

Safety

Children with BPD who are tethered by oxygen or ventilator tubing require close supervision. Respiratory equipment should have alarm systems because freespirited toddlers will wander beyond the length of the tubing. Restricted and supervised areas of play must be set up to create a safe environment for recreation. Children should be supervised at all times to prevent them from manipulating dials on their support equipment. Some devices have safety covers of control dials.

Children with tracheostomy tubes need virtually continuous observation. If they are not directly attended by caregivers, a noninvasive monitoring system with an oxygen saturation or apnea monitor should be in place. An accidental decannulation can cause death or serious physical and developmental sequelae. Security of the tracheostomy tube ties should be assessed every 4 to 8 hours and readjusted if more than one finger can be inserted between the tracheostomy ties and the child's neck. Family members should be taught CPR before the child is discharged from the hospital.

Families with toddlers must be warned against the insertion of small toys into ventilator tubing and artificial airways. When insufficiently supervised or educated, playful siblings can contribute to accidental airway decannulations and equipment disconnections. Older school-aged and adolescent children can be instructed to observe and intervene with specified responsibilities in emergency or routine situations.

Oxygen is a highly flammable gas and must be used with caution in the home. Parents and caretakers must be taught necessary safety precautions. The implementation of these safety measures should be evaluated whenever a home visit is made (Table 12-2).

Table 12-2
Safe Use of Oxygen at Home

Safety Guidelines	Rationale
Secure oxygen tank in upright position. Keep oxygen tanks at least 5 ft from heat source and electrical devices (e.g., space heaters, heating vents, fireplaces, radios, vaporizers, and humidifiers).	Oxygen tanks are highly explosive; if a horizontally positioned tank explodes, the rapid release of oxygen can catapult it through animate (e.g., human bodies) and inanimate (e.g., walls) objects.
Ensure that no one smokes in the room or in the area of the oxygen tank.	Smoking increases the risk of fire, which could cause the tank to explode; escaped oxygen would feed the fire.
Use lemon-glycerin swabs to relieve dryness around the child's mouth; avoid oil or alcohol-based substances (e.g., petroleum jelly, vitamin A and D ointment, baby oil).	Both alcohol and oil are flammable and increase the risk of fire.
Have the child wear cotton garments.	Silk, wool, and synthetics can generate static electricity and cause fire.
Keep a fire extinguisher readily available.	It is necessary to put out fire immediately.
Turn off both volume regulator and flow regulator whenever oxygen is not in use.	If the volume regulator is on when oxygen is turned on, the child might receive a rapid, forceful flow of oxygen in the face that could be frightening and uncomfortable.
	Oxygen leakage, which might not be detected because oxygen is odorless, can cause fire.

From Hagedorn MI and Gardner SL: Physiologic sequelae of prematurity: the nurse practitioner's role, part 1: respiratory issues, J Pediatr Health Care 3:288-297, 1989.

The primary care provider should review the use of aerosol cans and open flames in the home with the family. Fumes and smoke cause increased irritation to already sensitive airways and present a fire hazard if oxygen is in use. Caregivers and visitors should be warned against smoking in the home and around the child.

Consideration for safety with the use of electrical equipment should be part of the preparation for discharge from the hospital. Safety concerns should also be reinforced by the primary care provider. All medical equipment should be electrically grounded. Extension cords should not be used unless approved by the home care equipment vendor.

Before a child is discharged, contact with emergency services should be established. Contacts include fire, ambulance, police, electric, and telephone services. The contacts should be reviewed with families to reinforce required actions. The inadvertent omission of an essential contact may be identified, thus avoiding needless anxiety or lack of attention in a true emergency.

Immunizations

Infants with BPD should receive all standard immunizations at the appropriate chronologic age (Committee on Infectious Disease, 1997). Hepatitis B immunization is usually given to preterm infants at discharge if they weigh 2 kg or more or at 2 months of chronologic age (Committee on Infectious Disease, 1997). Because of prolonged hospitalizations and recurrent illnesses, however, the immunization schedules of infants with BPD are often delayed. Before immunizations are initiated in the primary care office, hospital records should be reviewed to determine if any immunizations were administered during hospitalization. If an infant has a history of uncontrolled seizures, pertussis may be withheld until the seizures are controlled, or diphtheria and tetanus vaccines may be given without pertussis (see Chapter 21). Infants and children with chronic BPD are at highest risk for serious morbidity with pertussis infection, so pertussis vaccination should not be withheld without cause.

The subviron influenza vaccine should be administered to children over 6 months of age with BPD and their caretakers during the fall or early winter months (Committee on Infectious Disease, 1997). The pneumococcal vaccine is recommended at 24 months of age (Committee on Infectious Disease, 1997).

Synagis (palivizumab) should be given as an IM injection once a month through the RSV season (usually Oct/Nov to April/May). This injection is indicated for infants 2 years of age or younger with a diagnosis of BPD who require some form of respiratory therapy in the 6 months prior to RSV season (Impact, 1998). Synagis does not interfere with MMR or the varicella vaccine as previously seen with respiratory syncytial virus immune globulin (RSV-IVIG [RespiGam]) (Committee on Infectious Disease, 1998).

Screening

Vision: Evaluations for ROP should be done by a pediatric ophthalmologist every 2 or 3 months during the child's first year of life. If there is a question of blindness, a visual evoked-response test can be requested. Routine eye examinations with Hirschberg, cover test, tracking, and fundoscopic examinations should be done at each primary care visit to follow the common problems of myopia and strabismus. Surgical correction for strabismus is often required.

Hearing: Infants with BPD are at risk for hearing loss as a result of prematurity and the IV administration of furosemide, corticosteroids, and aminoglycosides. A basal auditory evoked-response (BAER) test should be completed before discharge from the hospital, and routine screening for hearing should be conducted with each primary care visit. If recurrent otitis media is a problem, regular audiometric examinations should be conducted to identify hearing impairment and speech delays. Speech delays can be anticipated in children with long-term tracheostomies.

Dental: Routine dental care is recommended. Orally ingested ferrous sulfate may stain teeth, but this can be remedied with good dental hygiene. Daily tooth brushing may be a challenge for parents because of a child's oral defensiveness. Primary care providers can recommend using toothettes or foam-tipped brushes, which are softer, and baking soda instead of toothpaste because of its milder taste.

Blood pressure: Blood pressure should be measured with every visit and routinely followed to detect early signs of progressive cardiac disease, pulmonary hypertension, or renal dysfunction.

Hematocrit: Premature infants are more susceptible to iron deficiency anemia than full-term infants and must be followed closely during their first year of life. Hematocrit values should be checked monthly for the first 6 months of life and bimonthly for the following 6 months. Anemia of prematurity may be further aggravated by erosive gastroesophageal reflux and frequent blood tests. Children with chronic hypoxia may have elevated hemoglobin and hematocrit values.

Urinalysis: Routine screening is recommended.

Tuberculosis: Routine screening is recommended.

Condition-Specific Screening

Chest radiographic films: Chest radiographic studies should be ordered upon discharge from the hospital to establish lung disease severity and then annually for evaluation and with acute illness as clinically indicated.

Pulmonary function tests: Infant pulmonary function tests should be done upon discharge from the hospital to establish lung disease severity and then annually for evaluation and with acute illness as clinically indicated.

Common Illness Management

Differential Diagnosis (Box 12-6)

Respiratory distress: Respiratory distress is a common cause of urgent visits to the primary care practitioner. A child should be assessed for an elevated respiratory rate, increased work of breathing with substernal and intercostal retractions, nasal flaring, and a change in baseline breath sounds. Oxygenation can be quickly and accurately assessed via pulse oximetry if available in the office. Activity level and appetite may decrease. The child

---

Box 12-6
Differential Diagnosis

Respiratory Distress
Pneumonia (viral-bacterial)
Pulmonary edema
Congestive heart failure
Cardiac defect
Bronchospasm

Cough
Sinusitis
Gastroesophageal reflux (GER)
Reactive airways
Pulmonary edema
Pertussis
Respiratory syncytial virus (RSV)

Gastrointestinal Disturbances (e.g., emesis, feeding intolerance, diarrhea)
Antibiotic therapy
Theophylline toxicity
Gastroesophageal reflux (GER)
Formula density intolerance
Gastroenteritis

Fever
Otitis media
Sinusitis
Respiratory tract infection
Urinary tract infection
Septicemia

Skin-Mucosa Changes
Candida dermatitis
Oral thrush

BPD Unresponsive to Therapy
Wilson-Mikity syndrome
Pulmonary interstitial emphysema
Congenital heart disease
Pulmonary hemorrhage
Viral pneumonia
Cystic fibrosis
Pulmonary lymphangiectasia

should also be assessed for sources of infection (e.g., a viral illness). Children dependent on respiratory support (e.g., oxygen, aerosolized bronchodilators, or mechanical ventilation) may require an increased level of support to reverse hypoxia and hypercarbia during this period of respiratory workload.

A chest radiograph will determine if a child has atelectasis, aspiration pneumonia, an infectious pulmonary process (e.g., viral-bacterial pneumonia), or increased pulmonary fluid. Respiratory distress with wheezing or prolonged expiratory phase that resolves after bronchodilator treatment indicates bronchospasm.

Significant respiratory distress in the infant with severe BPD may be cardiac in origin. Pallor, diaphoresis, and tachypnea may indicate congestive heart failure. Evaluation with an ECG will reveal right and left ventricular hypertrophy. A heart murmur in an infant with severe BPD necessitates an immediate cardiologic consultation to rule out patent ductus, foramen ovale, or septal defects.

An infant with diagnosed BPD will occasionally not respond to treatment as expected. If unresponsiveness occurs, other respiratory disorders related to the neonatal period should be considered. Several conditions that may mimic BPD in infants, including the following: (1) Wilson-Mikity syndrome, which presents as increasing respiratory distress in the premature infant at 2 to 6 weeks of life, although cystic changes make it pathologically different from BPD; (2) pulmonary interstitial emphysema, which appears similar to stage III BPD on radiographs; (3) congenital heart disease with left-to-right shunting, which can result in respiratory failure secondary to pulmonary edema; (4) pulmonary hemorrhage that causes complete opacification on chest radiographs, mimicking stage II BPD; (5) viral pneumonia; (6) cystic fibrosis, which may present with respiratory distress and abnormal radiographs similar to BPD; and (7) congenital pulmonary lymphangiectasia, which is an overgrowth of the lung lymphatic vessels that shows mottling and hyperinflation on chest radiographs at birth.

Cough: Cough in an infant with BPD can indicate several possible processes. A productive, persistent, or moist cough without changes in lung sounds or chest radiographs may indicate sinusitis. Intermittent dry cough that is more pronounced af-

ter feedings and when the infant is supine may result from undiagnosed or poorly controlled reflux. Cough associated with increased activity may indicate undertreated reactive airway disease. A new cough in combination with tachypnea and crackles without evidence of infection often indicates pulmonary edema. Sudden onset of a staccato cough—with or without apnea—that interferes with feedings may indicate pertussis. If this cough is accompanied by copious, clear rhinorrhea, RSV should be considered.

Fever: If an infant's body temperature persists above 101° F for more than 24 hours despite antipyretic administration, the primary care provider should consider further work-up with a complete blood cell count, secretion culture, and possible chest radiograph. The outcome of the culture and sensitivity test will determine the antibiotic of choice and the route of administration (i.e., either enteral or intravenous). An infant with BPD who exhibits a toxic or septic appearance should also have a blood culture drawn to rule out septicemia. Otitis media and sinusitis often cause fever in infants with BPD, and their upper respiratory tract processes can lead to lower respiratory tract infection.

Gastrointestinal disturbances: Disturbances such as diarrhea, nausea, emesis, and feeding intolerances are common in infants with BPD. Gastrointestinal disturbances may be associated with a respiratory infection, antibiotic therapy, theophylline toxicity, feeding intolerance to formulas, or a change in osmotic load as a result of changes in caloric density of the formula. If these reasons have been reviewed and diarrhea persists, a stool specimen should be obtained to rule out bacterial or viral etiology. Frequent emesis may indicate gastroesophageal reflux. Hydration status must be monitored to avoid dehydration. The child may need to be hospitalized for fluid management.

Skin-mucosa changes: Candida infections are often contracted after a course of antibiotic treatment or prolonged systemic steroid treatment. The warm, moist surfaces of the body, including diaper areas, oral mucosa, tracheostomy and gastrostomy stomas, are most sensitive. Practicing good skin hygiene and keeping the skin dry prevent the spread of the rash. Topical treatment with antifungal creams such as Nystatin is also indicated.

Nystatin suspension also is the treatment for oral thrush.

Drug Interactions

Cough suppressants are not recommended for children with BPD; the cause of the cough should be evaluated and treated. Likewise, antihistamines are not recommended for children with artificial airways. The drying effect can thicken airway secretions, presenting the potential for plugging of the smaller peripheral airways and the tracheostomy tube.

Theophylline is a commonly used bronchodilator. If doses are missed, the blood level and resulting effectiveness of the medication may be significantly altered. Theophylline may cause a number of adverse GI side effects, including gastric irritability, nausea, and vomiting, but these can be prevented by administering certain preparations with food. If a child is already difficult to feed, this adds an additional challenge. Theophylline levels are altered by some commonly used medications, and serum levels must be checked often when these medications are prescribed. (See Chapter 9 for additional asthma drug interactions.)

Cisapride (Propulsid) is often prescribed for GER for its promotility effects on the GI tract. The manufacturer, however, sent out mailings to clinicians with a few reports of adverse events manifesting as cardiac arrhythmia in infants taking Propulsid. Providers should confirm that an EKG has been completed and is stable on infants taking Propulsid. There are also several medications that are contraindicated when taking Propulsid including theophylline and macrolides (Benitz and Tatro, 1996; The Harriet Lane Handbook, 1996).

Developmental Issues

Sleep Patterns

Most hospitals preparing to discharge a child with BPD attempt to arrange the child's care to provide for several hours of undisturbed sleep at night. The primary care provider should determine if there has been any change in the child's status as a result of the schedule adjustment. For example, bronchodilator treatments and CPT may be extended from 6 to 8 hours to promote the child's and parents' sleep. If schedules for home life have not been restructured, this is an appropriate time to discuss the schedule with the family and gradually implement changes.

The infant's and parents' sleep patterns may be altered because of the monitors placed in the home for children who require mechanical ventilation, receive oxygen therapy, or have a history of apnea. The primary care provider should inquire about the frequency of alarms and determine what type of alarm is appropriate for the child's condition. Readjustment of alarm limits may be warranted if false alarms are frequent; the limits are set within the physiologic range of the child's heart and respiratory rate. With increasing frequency, the pulse oximeter is the preferred monitor because of its simplicity of use and accuracy of measurement.

It is important to determine how audible the monitor alarm is to the family. If the alarm is so loud that it is very disturbing, the monitor can be placed on a cloth to absorb sound. If the sound is not sufficiently audible, the primary care provider can recommend a commercially available intercom system.

Toileting

Delayed bowel and bladder training may be a result of prolonged hospitalization, prematurity, or neurodevelopmental delay. The use of diuretics or theophylline may make bladder training more difficult because of increased frequency of urination. Parents must be helped to identify cues that indicate a child's developmental readiness for toilet training.

Discipline

Children with technologic support learn quickly that the sounding of alarms and monitors immediately summons a caregiver. Purposeful disconnections can easily become an attention maneuver. The child and family should be educated with regard to potential risks.

Parents need support and guidance from the primary care provider to recognize that their children need reasonable, consistent discipline. Primary care providers can help families develop consistent responses and discipline approaches that can be used by numerous caregivers (i.e., including parents, siblings, therapists, and nurses). Approaches should be based on the child's cognitive and developmental—not chronologic—age.

Child Care

Children requiring mechanical ventilation often have the support of nursing care during the night that is reimbursed by third-party payers. Children who have an artificial airway may or may not have this coverage, depending on third-party payer guidelines.

Children who do not require technologic support may not qualify for supportive care through insurance. This can present a problem for families who have limited budgets and cannot afford private, in-home baby-sitters. Regular daycare services are not recommended because of the increased exposure to infections (Takala et al, 1995).

Traditional well-child daycare centers are not equipped or trained to care for a child who is medically fragile (Fewell, 1993). There have been a few medical daycare centers created by individuals or agencies that employ skilled nurses to provide high-quality child care. Primary care providers can help families explore child care options. Hospital discharge programs often incorporate additional family members or neighbors into the teaching plans if requested.

The primary care provider should review the family support systems to determine if the systems are satisfactory to the well-being of the child and family. Nursing care should be used to provide support for families during activity-intensive periods of the day. Time without nursing support can be scheduled to incorporate activities and responsibilities within the context of the family structure and routine.

There is increasingly an awareness of the need for medical daycare facilities that provide services for children requiring supportive treatments. Funding may be supported by insurance. The number of operating facilities is small, but the availability should increase as the need intensifies.

Schooling

All children with BPD should have a thorough developmental evaluation. Plans should be established for outpatient follow-up either at a community-based education center or within the home (i.e., in accordance with Public Laws 99-457 and 101-476). Parents will need ongoing support as the child grows and develops.

On entering the school system, a child may notice differences in physical build and exercise endurance. Body image and peer acceptance may become an issue. Children with attention deficit hyperactivity disorder or those who are put in special classes for learning disabilities may have difficulty developing social skills (see Chapter 28). Increased absences during the winter season because of respiratory tract infections may further disrupt the school routine. Parents may develop separation anxiety from concern for their loss of control of their "fragile" child.

Primary care providers can assist in the transition from home to school by providing school personnel with specific instructions about the child's medical conditions and medications. Each school has a policy regarding medication administration during school hours. The ultimate goal is to encourage children with special needs to take responsibility for self-care.

Sexuality

There are no specific sexuality problems related to BPD. Children with physical and developmental delays and handicaps will need referrals and follow-up appropriate to their needs. The earliest survivors of BPD are now approximately 30 years of age, and to date no difficulties in the area of sexuality have been documented.

Children with BPD generally become adults with asthma. For women with a history of BPD, pregnancy brings a certain degree of stress on the respiratory system. Airway inflammation and bronchoconstriction should be controlled so both mother and baby receive an adequate oxygen supply

(National Institute of Health [NIH] Executive Summary, 1997). Inhaled bronchodilators and anti-inflammatories are considered safe for pregnant women (NIH, 1997).

Transition to Adulthood

Pulmonary dysfunction is common in adolescents and adults with a history of BPD. Airway obstruction, airway hyperreactivity, and hyperinflation persist in a significant percentage of persons with BPD (Ackerman, 1994). Anticipatory guidance that includes environmental control and possible future needs for asthma therapy is suggested. Vocational counseling on environmental irritants in the workplace (i.e., secondhand cigarette smoke, construction dust or particles, pollens, and factory smoke) and their relationship to asthma should be provided. A yearly influenza vaccine is recommended for individuals with BPD. An educational review of the pathophysiology of airway disease, medication action and indication, use of a peak flow meter and an MDI or aerochamber, and signs and symptoms of distress that warrant immediate medical attention is essential during adolescence and young adulthood for older individuals to assume self-care.

Special Family Concerns

Education and Discharge Planning

Discharge planning ideally starts several weeks before the anticipated discharge date. Family members who will be caregivers must attend teaching sessions and hands-on practice sessions with the hospital nurses and therapists in order to safely care for the infant when at home.

Basic respiratory assessment skills, which include counting a breathing rate during sleep and recognizing fluid overload (puffiness), retractions, flaring, and color changes, are essential for families to monitor their infants at home. Family members should have a basic understanding of the pathophysiology of BPD, its chronic nature, and the need for close follow-up. Caregivers at home should understand the infant's high nutritional needs and appreciate the infant's low respiratory reserve. CPR

instruction must be provided before a child is discharged from the hospital. The family must be able to demonstrate use of any medical equipment that will be in the home (i.e., oxygen, apnea monitor, and nebulizer and/or compressor).

Family members and friends should practice good hand washing and when ill avoid contact with the infant. Environmental control of airway irritants can be maximized in the home. A smoke-free, pet-free home without mold or mildew and with minimal dust is ideal.

Financial Responsibilities

Most third-party payers—including Medicaid—fund the cost of equipment and rehabilitative and nursing needs. Significant variations exist, however, among plans. The financial strain created by numerous visits from medical and rehabilitative care practitioners (McAleese, Knapp, and Rhodes, 1993; Miller et al, 1998) can stress family budgets. Equipment such as mechanical ventilators, compressors, and monitors increase the use of electricity. Calls to physicians, therapists, vendors, and nursing services increase telephone bills. Some utility companies have programs for families with special needs. Other hidden costs (e.g., medications, special formulas, corrective glasses, rehabilitative equipment, and higher electricity and heat bills) can create further financial burden (Miller et al, 1998). Loss of parental wages because of a leave of absence from work in order to care for a fragile infant cause families additional financial burden.

Privacy

The increased amount of people in the home environment (i.e., including nurses, vendors, respiratory therapists, and rehabilitative therapists) can seriously limit family privacy. When the family appears capable of assuming care safely and voices concerns about the lack of privacy and the needs of the child are stabilized, the primary care provider, in conjunction with the pediatric respiratory team, can suggest decreasing some of this support.

Once a child has been discharged from the hospital, the reality of the developmental delay may become apparent. Families will need ongoing emotional support to face and adjust to this problem.

Summary of Primary Care Needs for the Child with Bronchopulmonary Dysplasia

HEALTH CARE MAINTENANCE

Growth and development

Height and weight are below average in the majority of children—even at 2 years of age.

Plot head circumference, height, and length corrected for gestational age with each visit. Review caloric intake for adequacy.

Developmental delay is often seen during the first year of life. Continued delays may be seen in children of very low birth weight or with a history of severe BPD. Learning disabilities are often evident during school years.

Diet: Adequate caloric intake is important for optimal lung repair and growth and development.

Difficulties may arise with oral motor function. Oral feedings may need to be supplemented with enteral feedings.

Early referral to a pediatric nutritionist can prevent long-term problems.

Safety: Beware of accidental decannulations and disconnections from respiratory support.

Oxygen should be used with caution in the home.

Electrical safety requires grounded equipment.

Establish emergency service contact before a child is discharged from the hospital.

Immunization

Many children are delayed in receiving immunizations because of prolonged hospitalization.

Children should be immunized according to a routine schedule based on chronologic—not gestational—age.

Hospital records must be reviewed.

Pertussis vaccine should only be withheld with just cause because of the high risk of significant morbidity with active disease in children with BPD. Use acellular pertussis if appropriate.

Inactivated polio vaccine may be administered in the hospital before discharge.

Influenza vaccine is recommended yearly for children with CLD.

Pneumococcal vaccines are recommended.

Screening

Vision: Children should be evaluated by a pediatric ophthalmologist every 2 to 3 months during the first year of life to rule out ROP. Cover test should be done and tracking ability screened at each visit.

Myopia and strabismus are common and must be followed in the primary care office and by a pediatric ophthalmologist.

Hearing: A BAER test should be done before discharge from the hospital.

There is a risk of hearing loss because of prematurity and medications.

Age-appropriate screening should be done at each office visit.

Audiometry screening should be done with recurrent, serous otitis media.

Speech delays are anticipated in children with tracheostomies.

Dental: Routine screening is recommended.

Hypoplastic and discolored teeth are common.

Oral defensiveness may make dental hygiene difficult.

Blood pressure: Blood pressure should be taken at each visit. Children with abnormal blood pressure findings should be referred to a pulmonologist.

Hematocrit: Because of prematurity, iron deficiency anemia is common.

Hematocrit screening must be done frequently during the first year of life.

Chronic hypoxia may cause elevated hemoglobin levels.

Urinalysis: Routine screening is recommended.

Tuberculosis: Routine screening is recommended.

Continued

Summary of Primary Care Needs for the Child with Bronchopulmonary Dysplasia—cont'd

Condition-specific screening

Chest radiograph: Radiographic examinations of the lung should be done at discharge and then annually and as needed per clinical indication.

Pulmonary function tests: Pulmonary function tests should be done at discharge, annually and as necessary per clinical indication.

COMMON ILLNESS MANAGEMENT

Differential diagnosis

Respiratory distress: Rule out bacterial or viral infection, atelectasis, pneumonia, bronchospasm, pulmonary edema, heart failure, and sinusitis. Consider RSV infections from November to March.

Cough: Rule out sinusitis, GER, reactive airway disease, pulmonary edema, pertussis and RSV.

Fever: Rule out otitis media, sinusitis, upper or lower respiratory tract infection, urinary tract infection, and septicemia.

Rule out respiratory tract infection, otitis media, and viral infection.

Gastrointestinal disturbances: Consider feeding intolerances, bacterial and viral infections, GER, or theophylline toxicity.

Skin: For skin problems around tracheostomy and gastrostomy stomas and diaper areas, consider candida infection and cellulitis.

Drug interactions

Theophylline interacts with other medications (see Chapter 9).

Cough suppressants may mask an underlying condition and are not recommended.

Do not use antihistamines with children with tracheostomy tubes because of the thickening of airway secretions.

Developmental issues

Sleep patterns: Attempt to evaluate the child's schedule of care to decrease disturbances and provide for the whole family.

Evaluate functioning of monitors.

Toileting: Delayed bowel and bladder training may occur as a result of prolonged hospitalization and the use of diuretics and theophylline.

Discipline: Children should receive discipline appropriate to their developmental level of understanding.

A consistent plan should be followed.

Child care: Recommend that children not supported by oxygen and mechanical ventilation attend home or small daycare centers to reduce exposure to infection.

Children with mechanical support may be eligible for nursing support from third-party payers.

Schooling: Help family with developmental evaluations and planning early intervention programs.

Assist families with adjustment to developmental delays.

Sexuality: Care is routine unless associated problems warrant additional care.

Transition to adulthood: Abnormal pulmonary function frequently persists into adulthood. Counsel regarding possible environmental irritants in workplace or school. Review and educate concerning disease process and management.

Special family concerns

Financial responsibilities are great even with insurance coverage.

There may be a lack of privacy in the home because of the need for medical caregivers.

Developmental outcome is uncertain. The potential for developmental delay and persistent medical problems result in great emotional strain on parents.

The primary care provider can assist with investigation of appropriate educational and rehabilitative programs.

Resources

Exceptional Parent Magazine
PO Box 3000
Denville, N.J. 07834
1-800-562-1973
www.eparent.com

Parents of Prematures
PO Box 3046
Kirland, WA 98083-3046
Publishes monthly newsletter.

Parents of Preemies, support group:
http://abilene.com/armc/wwwboard/messages/39.html

Mary Searcy's Resources for Parents of Preemies
Exhaustive list of resources for parents of preemies:
http://Members.aol.com/MarAim/preemie.htm

American Association for Premature Infants (AAPI)
National advocacy organization:
http://www.aapi.online.org

American Lung Association
1-800-586-4872
www.LungUSA.org

Special needs organizations (i.e., SSI, Medically Fragile Programs)
mailing list by state for parents of children with special needs:
http://www.comeunity.com.special_needs/speclists.html

Message board for CLDs
http://www.cheshire-med.com/programs/pulmrehab/forum/cldforum.html

References

Ackerman VL: Bronchopulmonary dysplasia. In Loughlin GM and Eigen H, editors: Respiratory disease in children: diagnosis and management, Baltimore, Md., 1994, Williams & Wilkins.

Alpert BE, Allen JL, and Schidlow DV: Bronchopulmonary dysplasia. In Hilman B, editor: Pediatric respiratory disease: diagnosis and treatment, Philadelphia, 1993, W.B. Saunders.

Armentrout D: Gastroesophageal reflux in infants, Nurs Pract 20:54-63, 1995.

Bancalari E and Sosenko I: Pathogenesis and prevention of neonatal CLD: recent developments, Pediatr Pulmonol 8:109-116, 1990.

Bancalari E: Bronchopulmonary dysplasia: then and now. Presented at the American Thoracic Society conference, Chicago, May 1998.

Barrington KJ and Finer NM: Treatment of bronchopulmonary dysplasia, a review, Clin Perinatol 25(1):177-202, 1998.

Battin M et al: Has the outcome for extremely low gestational age (ELGA) infants improved following recent advances in neonatal intensive care? Am J Perinatol 15(8): 469-477, 1998.

Benitz WE and Tatro D: The pediatric drug handbook, ed 3, St Louis, 1996, Mosby.

Brem AS: Electrolyte disorders associated with respiratory distress syndrome and bronchopulmonary dysplasia, Clin Perinatol 19:223-232, 1992.

Cloutier MM: Nebulized steroid therapy in bronchopulmonary dysplasia, Pediatr Pulmonol 15:111-116, 1993.

Committee on Infectious Disease: Report of the committee on infectious disease, ed 24, Elk Grove Village, Ill., 1997, American Academy of Pediatrics.

Committee on Infectious Diseases and Committee of Fetus and Newborn: Prevention of respiratory syncytial virus infections: indications for the use of palivizumab and update on the use of RSV-IVIG, Pediatrics 102(5):1211-1216, 1998.

Crowley P et al: The effects of corticosteroid administration before preterm delivery: an overview of the evidence from controlled trials, Br J Obstet Gynaecol 50:515-525. 1993.

Farel AM et al: Very-low-birthweight infants at seven years: an assessment of the health and neurodevelopmental risk conveyed by CLD, J Learn Disabil 31(2):118-126, 1998.

Fewell RR: Child care for children with special needs, Pediatrics 91:193-198, 1993.

Fillmore EJ and Cartlidge PH: Late death of very low birthweight infants, Acta Paediatr 87(7):809-810, 1998.

Fok TF et al: Randomized crossover trial of salbutamol aerosol delivered by metered dose inhaler, jet nebuliser, and ultrasonic nebuliser in CLD, Arch Dis Child Fetal Neonatal Ed 79(2):100-104, 1998.

Furman L et al: Hospitalization as a measure of morbidity among very low birth weight infants with CLD, J Pedatr 128:447, 1996.

Gardner SL and Hagedorn MI: Physiologic sequelae of prematurity: the nurse practitioner's role, J Pediatr Health Care 6:263-270, 1992.

Ghezzi F et al: Elevated interleukin-8 concentrations in amniotic fluid of mothers whose neonates subsequently develop bronchopulmonary dysplasia, Eur J Obstet Gynecol Reprod Biol 78(1):5-10, 1998.

Gonzalez A et al: Influence of infection on patent ductus arteriosus and CLD in premature infants #1000 gms, J Pediatr 128:470-478, 1996.

Gray PH et al: Prediction of outcome of preterm infants with severe bronchopulmonary dysplasia, J Paediatr Child Health 29:107-112, 1993.

Greenough A: Bronchopulmonary dysplasia: early diagnosis, prophylaxis, and treatment, Arch Dis Child 65:1082-1088, 1990.

Gregoire MC et al: Health and developmental outcomes at 18 months in very preterm infants with bronchopulmonary dysplasia, Pediatrics 101(5):856-860, 1998.

Groneck P et al: Association of pulmonary inflammation and increased microvascular permeability during the development of bronchopulmonary dysplasia: a sequential analysis of inflammatory mediators in respiratory fluids of high-risk preterm neonates, Pediatrics 93(5):712-718, 1994.

Groothuis JR et al: Prophylactic administration of respiratory syncytial virus immune globulin to high-risk infants and young children, N Engl J Med 329:1524-1530, 1993.

Gross SJ et al: Effect of preterm birth on pulmonary function at school age: a prospective controlled study, J Pediatr 133(2):171-172, 1998.

Hack M et al: Effect of very low birth weight and subnormal head size on cognitive abilities at school age, N Engl J Med 325:231-237, 1991.

The Harriet Lane handbook, ed 14, St Louis, 1996, Mosby.

Hazinski TA: Bronchopulmonary dysplasia. In Kendig: Kendig's disorders of the respiratory tract in children, Philadelphia, 1998, W.B. Saunders.

Hoekstra RE et al: Improved neonatal survival following multiple doses of bovine surfactant in very premature neonates at risk for respiratory distress syndrome, Pediatrics 88:10-18, 1991.

Holmstrom G et al: Neonatal risk factors for retinopathy of prematurity—a population-based study, Acta Ophthalmology Scand, 76(2):204-207, 1998.

Impact-RSV Study Group: Palivizumab, a humanized respiratory syncytial virus monoclonal antibody, reduces hospitalization from respiratory syncytial virus infection in high-risk infants, Pediatrics 102(3):531-537, 1998.

Jacob SV et al: Long-term pulmonary sequelae of severe bronchopulmonary dysplasia, J Pediatr 133(2):193-200, 1998.

Jobe AH: Drug therapy: pulmonary surfactant therapy, N Engl J Med 328(12):861-868, 1993.

Johnson DB, Cheney C, and Monsen ER: Nutrition and feeding in infants with bronchopulmonary dysplasia after initial discharge: risk factors for growth failure, J Am Diet Assoc 98(6):649-656, 1998.

Konig PK et al: Clinical observations of nebulized flunisolide in infants and young children with asthma and bronchopulmonary dysplasia, Pediatr Pulmonol 13:209-214, 1992.

Kountz DS: An algorithm for corticosteroid withdrawal, Clin Pharmacol 39:250-254, 1989.

Kugelman A et al: Pulmonary effect of inhaled furosemide in ventilated infants with severe bronchopulmonary dysplasia, Pediatrics 99(1):71-75, 1997.

Leonard CH and Piecuch RE: School age outcomes of low birth weight preterm infants, Sem Perinatol 21:240-253, 1997.

McAleese KA, Knapp MA, and Rhodes TT: Financial and emotional cost of bronchopulmonary dysplasia, Clin Pediatr 393-400, 1993.

McColley SA: Bronchopulmonary dysplasia: impact of surfactant replacement therapy, Pediatr Clin North Am 45(3):573-586, 1998.

Miller VL et al: A analysis of program and family costs of case managed care for technology-dependent infants with bronchopulmonary dysplasia, J Pediatr Nurs 13(4):244-251, 1998.

Mueller DH: Timeliness of codifying nutrition ABCDE's for BPD, J Pediatr 133(3):315-316, 1998.

National Institutes of Health Executive Summary: Management of asthma during pregnancy, National Asthma Education Program, National Heart, Lung and Blood Institute, National Institutes of Health, Washington DC, 1997, US Government Printing Office.

Northway WH, Rosen RC, and Porter DV: Pulmonary disease following respiratory therapy of hyaline membrane disease, N Eng J Med 267:357-368, 1967.

Oh W and Merenstein G: Fourth edition of the guidelines for perinatal care: summary of changes, Pediatrics 100(6):1021-1022, 1997.

Parker RA, Lindstrom DP, and Cotton RB: Improved survival accounts for most, but not all, of the increase in bronchopulmonary dysplasia, Pediatrics 90:663-668, 1992.

Philip AG: Oxygen plus pressure plus time: the etiology of bronchopulmonary dysplasia, Pediatrics 55:44-50, 1975.

Piecuch RE et al: Outcomes of infants born at 24-26 weeks gestation (part 2), Obst Gynecol 90:809-814, 1997.

Pierce MR and Bancalari E: The role of inflammation in the pathogenesis of bronchopulmonary dysplasia, Pediatr Pulmonol 19:371-378, 1995.

PREVENT Study Group: Reduction of respiratory syncytial virus hospitalization among premature infants and infants with bronchopulmonary dysplasia using respiratory syncytial virus immune globulin prophylaxis, Pediatrics 99:93-99, 1997.

Rastogi A et al: A controlled trial of dexamethasone to prevent bronchopulmonary dysplasia in surfactant-treated infants, Pediatrics 98(2):204-210, 1996.

Robertson CMT et al: 8-year school performance, neurodevelopmental and growth outcome of neonates with bronchopulmonary dysplasia: a comparative study, Pediatrics 89:365-372, 1992.

Rojas MA et al.: Changing trends in the epidemiology and pathogenesis of neonatal CLD, J Pediatr 126:605-610, 1995.

Rozycki HJ and Kirkpatrick BV: New developments in bronchopulmonary dysplasia, Pediatr Ann 22:532-538, 1993.

Rush MG and Hazinski TA: Current therapy of bronchopulmonary dysplasia, Clin Perinatol 19:563-590, 1992.

Samuels MP et al: Pediatrics 98(6):1154-1160, 1996.

Takala AK et al: Risk factors for primary invasive pneumococcal disease among children in Finland, JAMA 273:859-864, 1995.

Trachtenbarg DE and Golemon TB: Office care of the premature infant: part II: common medical and surgical problems, Am Fam Physician 57(10):2383-2390, 1998.

Truog WE: Bronchopulmonary dysplasia: issues in long-term management, J Resp Diseases 14:130-145, 1993.

Vrlenich LA et al: The effect of bronchopulmonary dysplasia on growth at school age, Pediatrics 95:855-859, 1995.

Watterberg KL and Scott SM: Evidence of early adrenal insufficiency in babies who develop bronchopulmonary dysplasia, Pediatrics 95:120-125, 1995.

Welch MJ: Inhaled corticosteroids and growth in children, Pediatr Ann 27(11):752-758, 1998.

Weinstein MR: A new radiographic scoring system for bronchopulmonary dysplasia, Newborn Lung Project, Pediatr Pulmonol 18(5):284-289, 1994.

Wilson-Costello D et al: Perinatal correlates of CP and other neurologic impairments among LBW children, Pediatrics 102:315-322, 1998.

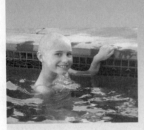

CHAPTER 13

Cancer

Mary Alice Dragone

Etiology

An estimated 8700 children are diagnosed with cancer annually in the United States (American Cancer Society, 1998). Cancer results when the body fails to regulate cell production. A proliferation and spread of abnormal cells then occurs, which—if left unchecked—may lead to death of the host. Common sites of malignancy in children include the blood and bone marrow, bone, lymph nodes, brain and central nervous system (CNS), kidneys, and soft tissues (Table 13-1).

The specific causes of childhood cancers are poorly identified. It is hypothesized, however, that genetic and environmental influences play a role in the expression of malignancies (Ross and Davies, 1998; Sandler and Ross, 1997).

Incidence

The overall incidence of malignancy in children under 15 years of age is approximately 13.6:100,000 per year (Ries et al, 1998). Leukemia and CNS tumors account for the majority of pediatric malignancies. A comparison of the incidence of the various childhood malignancies in the United States (see Table 13-1) illustrates a wide variation depending on site.

Clinical Manifestations at Time of Diagnosis

The signs and symptoms of a malignant disease depend on the interval between time of origin and diagnosis, as well as the type and location of the tumor. In general, cancer may manifest in one of the following three ways: (1) as a mass lesion, (2) with symptoms directly related to the tumor, or (3) with nonspecific symptoms. The presence of a mass lesion should alert the primary care provider to the possibility of a malignancy after benign conditions (e.g., constipation and a distended bladder) have been ruled out (Kucera et al, 1997). A biopsy of other lesions should be taken in a timely manner to rule out malignancy. Symptoms related directly to the tumor may include bone pain, limping, unexplained bleeding, bruising or petechiae, morning headache and vomiting, hematuria, pallor, swelling of the face or neck, white spot in pupil (leukocoria), airway or urinary tract obstruction, or endocrinologic symptoms from hormone production by the tumor. Nonspecific symptoms include weight loss, diarrhea, low-grade fevers, malaise, or failure to thrive (Box 13-1).

Prompt referral to a pediatric cancer treatment center ensures that specimens for staging are properly obtained and the child is enrolled in multiinstitutional treatment studies. The initial work-up is crucial to the accurate and timely establishment of a diagnosis. One large study of the "lag times" to diagnosis of pediatric solid tumors found that older children and those with Ewing's sarcoma and osteosarcoma had much longer "lag times" than young children and those with other tumors (Pollock, Krischner, and Vietti, 1991). Children with neuroblastoma had the shortest "lag time". After a thorough history and physical examination and laboratory tests, the work-up may include nuclear-radiological examinations, ultrasound, bone marrow aspirate-biopsy or lumbar puncture, depending on the type of tumor suspected and the most frequent sites for metastases.

Whenever a biopsy is being considered, the primary care provider should consult an oncology treatment center before proceeding. Accurate staging is increasingly dependent on molecular genetics and the immunocytochemistry of initial diagnostic materials processed in specialty laboratories (American Academy of Pediatrics Section on

Text continued on p. 272

Table 13-1
Common Pediatric Cancers

Type	Site	Incidence (ages 0-14)	Etiology	Signs/Symptoms	Treatment
Leukemia	Bone marrow	3.8 per 100,000 children per year	*For ALL and AML:* Genetic factors Chromosomal abnormalities (trisomy 21, Bloom's syndrome, Fanconi's anemia, AT*) Familial predisposition (ALL-infant identical twins) Environmental factors Ionizing radiation Chronic chemical exposure Use of alkylating agents for treatment of malignant disease (AML) Possible viral infection	*For ALL and AML:* Pallor Fatigue, headache Fever, infection Purpura, bruising Organomegaly Bone pain	Combination chemotherapy CNS prophylaxis Radiation therapy (for high risk cases) Intrathecal chemotherapy
Acute lymphoblastic leukemia (ALL)					
Acute myelogenous leukemia (AML)					Combination chemotherapy CNS prophylaxis Single-agent intrathecal chemotherapy Bone marrow transplant in first remission
Central Nervous System		3.2 per 100,000 children per year	*For all CNS cancers:* Genetic factors Heritable disease (NF*, VHL*, LFS*) Familial		
Infratentorial Medulloblastoma	Cerebellum/brainstem Midline cerebellar			Early Decreased academic performance Fatigue	Anticonvulsants, if symptoms present Treatment of hydrocephalus

Incidence data modified from Gurney JG et al: Incidence of cancer in children in the United States, sex, race, and 1-year age-specific rates by histologic type, Cancer 75:2186, 1995.
Ries LA et al, editors: SEER cancer statistics review, 1973-1995, Bethesda Md, 1998, National Cancer Institute, Table XXVII-I.
*GI, gastrointestinal; NF, neurofibromatosis; AT, ataxiatelangiectasia; VHL, von Hippel-Lindau; LFS, Li-Fraumeni syndrome (a germ line mutation of the p53 tumor suppressor gene).
Additional sources: Brodeur GM et al: Biology and genetics of human neuroblastoma, J Pediatr Hematol Oncol 19:93-101, 1997.
Clericuzio CL and Johnson C: Screening for Wilms tumor in high-risk individuals, Hematol Oncol Clin North Am 9:1253-1265, 1995.
Haller J: Aids-related malignancies in pediatrics, Radiol Clin North Am 35:1517-1538, 1997.
Horowitz ME et al: Ewings sarcoma family of tumors. In Pizzo P and Poplack D, editors: Principles and practice of pediatric oncology, Philadelphia, 1997, Lippincott-Raven, pp 831-864.
Link MP and Eilber F: Osteosarcoma. In Pizzo [as above] pp 889-920.
Wexler LH and Helman LJ: Rhabdomyosarcoma and undifferentiated sarcoma. In Pizzo [as above]. pp 799-830.

Continued

Table 13-1
Common Pediatric Cancers—cont'd

Type	Site	Incidence (ages 0-14)	Etiology	Signs/Symptoms	Treatment
Central Nervous System—cont'd					
Infratentorial —cont'd					
Ependymoma	Ependymal lining of ventricular system or central canal of spinal cord		Environmental factors Chronic chemical exposure	Personality changes Intermittent headache	Corticosteroids Shunting Surgical resection (if operable)
Brainstem glioma	Brainstem		Ionizing radiation Other primary malignancies Exogenous immunosuppression	Late Morning headache Vomiting Diplopia/visual changes Brainstem/cerebellar Deficits of balance/ positioning	Radiation therapy Chemotherapy for some tumors Bone marrow transplant in rare cases
Supratentorial Astrocytomas	Ventricles, midline diencephalous, cerebrum			Supratentorial Nonspecific headache Seizures Hemiparesis	
Craniopharyngioma Gliomas Pineoblastoma or germ cell tumors	Sella turcica Visual pathway Pineal region				
Non-Hodgkin's Lymphoma		1.0 per 100,000 children per year			
Lymphoblastic lymphoma	Usually generalized Anterior mediastinum Lymph nodes Bone marrow		*For all Non-Hodgkin's lymphomas:* Immunodeficiency (HIV) Exogenous immunosuppression Viral-associated with Epstein-Barr virus	Generally rapid progression Lymphoblastic lymphoma Dysphagia, dyspnea Swelling of neck, face, upper extremities Supradiaphragmatic lymphadenopathy	Treatment of emergent symptoms Multiagent chemotherapy CNS prophylaxis

Type	Incidence	Location	Etiology	Clinical Manifestations	Treatment
Small noncleaved lymphoma Burkitt's lymphoma Non-Burkitt's lymphoma		Abdomen Bone marrow Lymph nodes		Respiratory distress Small noncleaved lymphoma Abdominal pain or swelling Change in bowel habits Nausea/vomiting GI* bleeding Intestinal perforation (rarely) Inguinal/iliac adenopathy Intussusception	Treatment of emergent symptoms and tumor lysis syndrome Multiagent chemotherapy CNS prophylaxis
Large cell lymphoma		Lymph nodes Cutaneous lesions Mediastinum Abdomen Head, neck		Large cell lymphoma As cited earlier, depending on site	Multiagent chemotherapy
Hodgkin's Lymphoma	0.4 per 100,000 children per year	Single lymph node or lymphatic chains Mediastinal mass Spleen	Genetic factors Familial predisposition Environmental influence Iatrogenic or acquired immunodeficiency (HIV, AT*) Infectious etiology (Epstein-Barr virus)	Lymphadenopathy Organomegaly Fatigue Anorexia/weight loss/fever	Splenectomy, if surgical staging Multiagent chemotherapy Radiation therapy
Neuroblastoma	1.1 per 100,000 children per year	Anywhere along the sympathetic nervous system chain Most commonly Abdomen Adrenal gland Paraspinal ganglion Thorax Neck	Genetic factors Autosomal dominant inherited predisposition in some children Familial predisposition Associated with fetal alcohol syndrome and fetal hydantoin syndrome	Dependent on primary site, site of metastases Metastases present in 70% of cases at diagnosis (especially in bone marrow) Presence of a mass (abdomen, thoracic, cervical, pelvic, liver)	Treatment of emergent symptoms Surgery (staging excision of tumor, evaluation of treatment) Radiation therapy Combination chemotherapy Bone marrow transplant, in some cases

Continued

Table 13-1
Common Pediatric Cancers—cont'd

Type	Site	Incidence (ages 0-14)	Etiology	Signs/Symptoms	Treatment
Neuroblastoma—cont'd				Symptoms from compression of mass (Horner's syndrome, edema of upper and lower extremities secondary to vascular compression, hypertension caused by compression of renal vasculature, cord compression symptoms [paresis, paralysis, bowel/bladder dysfunction]) Diarrhea from vasoactive intestinal peptides produced by tumor cells Skin or subcutaneous nodules (infants only) Nonspecific symptoms (fever, weight loss, failure to thrive, generalized pain) Rarely syndrome of opsoclonus-myoclonus	
Soft Tissue Sarcomas Rhabdomyosarcoma Undifferentiated sarcoma	Head and neck (most common) Abdomen Anywhere in body	0.9 per 100,000 children per year	*For both sarcomas:* Genetic factors Associated with NF*, LFS*, and Beckwith-Wiedeman Environmental factors Parental use of recreational drugs Possible viral etiology	*For both sarcomas:* Dependent on location and size of tumor	*For both sarcomas:* Surgical removal (if feasible) Radiation therapy for residual tumor Multiagent systemic chemotherapy

	Location	Incidence	Etiology	Clinical Manifestations	Treatment
Kidney					
Wilms' tumor (nephroblastoma, renal embryoma)	Unilateral, bilateral	0.8 per 100,000 children per year	Genetic factors Associated with aniridia, NF*, Beckwith-Wiedemann, hemihypertrophy, Denys-Drash syndrome Familial predisposition Environmental factors Chronic chemical exposure (hydrocarbons/lead)	Asymptomatic mass Malaise, pain Microscopic or gross hematuria Hypertension	Complete surgical excision (if bilateral, nephrectomy of more involved site, excisional biopsy/partial nephrectomy of smaller lesion in remaining kidney) Multiagent chemotherapy Radiation therapy
Bone Tumors					
Osteosarcoma	Long bones of extremities	0.8 per 100,000 children per year	Genetic factors Familial predisposition (hereditary retinoblastoma) Environmental factors Ionizing radiation Use of alkylating agents	Pain over involved area with or without swelling (often 3-6 mo. or longer)	Multiagent chemotherapy Surgical excision of tumor with limb salvage or amputation if extent of disease or location does not allow complete excision
Ewing's sarcoma	Bones of the extremities and central axis		Possible genetic factors No strong or consistent association with constitution of chromosomal abnormalities or congenital diseases	In presence of metastatic disease nonspecific symptoms (fatigue, anorexia, weight loss, intermittent fever, malaise)	Localized radiation therapy (Ewing's sarcoma)
Retinoblastoma	Eye	0.5 per 100,000 children per year	Genetic factors Gene mutation (nonhereditary) Autosomal dominant (all bilateral retinoblastoma and 15% of unilateral)	Leukocoria (cat's eye reflex) Squint Strabismus Orbital inflammation	Surgery (resection, enucleation with extensive disease; salvage of one eye attempted in bilateral disease) Radiation therapy Chemotherapy (usually palliative)

Box 13-1

Clinical Manifestation at Time of Diagnosis

- Mass lesion, particularly in abdomen
- Lymph node enlargement that is unresponsive to antibiotic therapy or accompanied by nonspecific symptoms
- Unexplained bruising, bleeding, or petechiae
- Pallor and fatigue
- Unexplained or persistent fevers
- Recurrent infection
- Bone pain or limping
- Morning headache with vomiting
- Swelling in the face or neck
- White spot in pupil (leukocoria)
- Hematuria
- Airway or urinary tract obstruction
- Nonspecific symptoms: weight loss, diarrhea, failure to thrive, malaise, low-grade fevers

---

Box 13-2

Treatment

- Surgery
  Biopsy
  Resection
  Palliation
- Chemotherapy
- Radiation
- Bone marrow or blood stem cell transplantation
- Immunotherapy

Hematology/Oncology, 1997). Prompt referral to a pediatric cancer treatment center will allow a child to be enrolled in multiinstitutional treatment studies.

Treatment

Cancer treatment involves the concurrent or sequential use of surgery, chemotherapy, radiation therapy, bone marrow or blood stem cell transplantation, and immunotherapy (Box 13-2).

State-of-the-art treatment is provided by multiinstitutional cooperative study groups and some specialty cancer treatment centers. These centers generally employ a multidisciplinary approach combining the expertise of physicians, advanced practice nurses, social workers, art and child life therapists, and other specialists. The National Cancer Institute sponsors two groups that register over 94% of children under 15 years of age with cancer in the United States for treatment: the Children's Cancer Group (CCG) and the Pediatric Oncology Group (POG) (Ross et al, 1996). These two groups will merge in the year 2000, becoming the Children's Oncology Group. Children under 15 years of age are equally represented in these groups regard-

less of race (Bleyer et al, 1997). Only 25% of adolescents ages 15 to 19, however, are represented in any pediatric or adult cooperative group sponsored by the National Cancer Institute (Bleyer et al, 1997). Adolescents' lack of equal access to national clinical trials requires further analysis of the effect on survival and quality of life.

A child's treatment protocol, determined by the type of cancer and the extent of disease, consists of a schedule and combination of therapies shown to be effective in treating the condition. A particular disease protocol may have several treatment regimens ("arms"), which are based on an accepted standard treatment with slight variations. Because no protocol regimen is known to be more effective than another, ongoing research investigates various therapies that maximize treatment efficacy while minimizing toxicity. Before a child is assigned to a particular protocol, informed consent is obtained from the parents and, if appropriate, the child. If a child is treated on a research protocol, the family may elect to withdraw the child from the study at any time and have the child treated according to standard therapy.

Surgical intervention is used to: (1) obtain a biopsy specimen, (2) determine the extent of disease, (3) remove primary or metastatic lesions, (4) evaluate previously unresectable tumors, (5) provide a "second look" to evaluate the effects of chemotherapy and radiation on partially or nonresected tumors, and (6) relieve symptoms. Surgical procedures are also used to place indwelling venous access devices and to displace organs outside of the radiation field (e.g., ovaries during pelvic irradiation).

The goal of chemotherapy is to interrupt the cell cycle of proliferating malignant cells while minimizing the damage to normal cells. In combination chemotherapy, different drugs are used to disrupt the cell cycle at different phases, which increases the exposure of the malignant cells to cytotoxic agents. The route of chemotherapy administration includes oral, intramuscular, intravenous, intrathecal, and intraventricular routes. Although most intravenous infusions have traditionally been administered in the hospital setting, certain agents lend themselves to safe administration in the home (Close et al, 1995). Eligibility for home infusion often depends on stable utilities in the home, parental reliability, and few side effects during an in-hospital trial of the agent.

Chemotherapeutic agents may be either cycle phase specific or nonspecific. Cell-cycle specific drugs kill cells only in a certain stage of the cell's development and are most effective on rapidly growing cells. Along with malignant cells, the cells of the bone marrow, hair follicles, and intestinal epithelium are susceptible to damage from these drugs. Cell-cycle nonspecific drugs kill cells regardless of their stage of development. They act on dormant as well as dividing cells. Chemotherapeutic agents are further classified by their mechanism of action. The major classifications include alkylating agents, antimetabolites, vinca alkaloids, antibiotics, and corticosteroids. Side effects and toxicities vary depending on the specific agent (Table 13-2).

Radiation therapy is often used in conjunction with surgery and chemotherapy. Radiation causes breakage of DNA strands, thus inhibiting cell division. The goal of radiation therapy is to destroy the cancer cells while minimizing complications and long-term sequelae. The role of radiation therapy may be definitive, adjunctive, or palliative. Definitive treatment is given with curative intent to a tumor on which a biopsy has been performed or that has been partially resected. In adjunctive radiotherapy, a primary tumor—although totally resected—is at risk for a local recurrence. This area is then treated with a lower dose of radiation than what would be given to control the tumor without surgery. Palliative radiotherapy is used to relieve symptoms of incurable disease after more conservative methods have proved ineffective.

Some children with CNS tumors benefit from hyperfractionated radiation delivery. This method uses smaller individual doses of radiation two or more times daily instead of the usual daily dose to affect more of the rapidly dividing tumor cells. Overall, the total dosage of radiation used is higher. Early studies of its use in individuals with brain tumors have not shown greater toxicity (Heideman et al, 1997); but long-term studies are needed to detect late effects.

The tumor's response to radiation depends on the type of tumor, the type and dose of radiation delivered, and the size of the area irradiated. These factors also influence the type and severity of side effects and long-term sequelae. Many side effects are similar to those of chemotherapy but, rather than a systemic response, the side effects are generally related to the irradiated area. They include nausea and vomiting, diarrhea, mucositis, cataracts, skin changes, neurocognitive deficits, and growth and endocrine abnormalities (Kalapurakal and Thomas, 1997).

The use of immunotherapy in the treatment of cancer is one of the newest available treatment modalities. Donors of bone marrow or blood stem cells come from three sources: the affected person (autologous), an identical twin (syngeneric), or another histocompatible or incompatible donor (allogeneic). It encompasses both cytokines (interleukins, interferons, tumor necrosis factor) and monoclonal antibodies. This therapy stimulates the body's natural immune system and has the potential to selectively target and destroy malignant cells. Immunotherapy has been more completely studied in adults and is currently being applied to children with cancer (Baquiran, Dantis, and McKerrow, 1996; Farrell, 1996; Karius and Marriott, 1997; Cheung, 1997).

Bone marrow or blood stem cell transplantation is used in treating some cases of relapsed ALL, AML, neuroblastoma, and lymphoma and is being investigated for use in recurrent Ewing's sarcoma and brain tumors. Hematopoietic stem cells for transplantation come from either bone marrow, peripheral blood, or umbilical cord blood (Appelbaum, 1997; Ravindranath et al, 1996; Secola, 1997). In some institutions, transplantation is the initial therapy of choice for children with high-risk (having clinical and laboratory features at diagnosis that are known to have a poor prognosis) ALL and AML. This procedure allows for potentially lethal doses of chemotherapy and radiation to be given to rid the body of all malignant cells. The

Text continued on p. 280

Table 13-2
Summary of Chemotherapeutic Agents Used in the Treatment of Childhood Cancers*

Agent/Administration	Side Effects and Toxicity	Comments and Specific Nursing Considerations
Alkylating Agents	All alkylating agents: Azospermia, ovarian failure Secondary malignancy (AML)	Sperm banking, egg donation, if feasible
Mechlorethamine (nitrogen mustard, Mustargen) IV	N/V§ (0-2 hrs later) (severe) BMD‖ (2-3 wks later) Alopecia Local phlebitis Mucositis Anaphylaxis (rare)	Vesicant†
Cyclophosphamide (Cytoxan, CTX) PO, IV	N/V (4-12 hrs later) (severe at high doses) BMD (7-10 days later) Alopecia Hemorrhagic cystitis Severe immunosuppression Stomatitis (rare) Hyperpigmentation Transverse ridging of nails Cardiac toxicity (high dose) Pulmonary fibrosis (high dose) Syndrome of inappropriate secretion of antidiuretic hormone (SIADH)	BMD has platelet-sparing effect Give dose early in day to allow adequate fluids afterward Force fluids before administering drug and for 2 days after to prevent chemical cystitis; encourage frequent voiding even during night Warn parents to report signs of burning on urination or hematuria Mesna given with high doses to protect bladder Mesna causes false ketonuria
Ifosfamide (IFEX) IV	N/V (moderate) BMD (7-10 days later) Alopecia Renal tubular damage (Fanconi-like syndrome) Hemorrhagic cystitis Peripheral neuropathy Encephalopathy	See cyclophosphamide above Mesna is given with all doses to protect the bladder
Busulfan (Myleran) PO	N/V (mild) BMD (11-30 days later) Excessive dryness of skin and mucous membranes Gynecomastia (rare) Pulmonary fibrosis (long-term therapy)	Pulmonary function tests
Melphalan (Alkeran, L-PAM) PO, IV	Severe BMD (14-21 days later, lasting 5-6 weeks) N/V Mucositis Diarrhea Alopecia Hypersensitivity reaction	Take PO on empty stomach Hydrate well for 24 hrs after close

Sources: Renick-Ettinger A: Chemotherapy. In Foley G, Fochtman D, and Mooney K, editors: Nursing care of the child with cancer, Philadelphia, 1993, WB Saunders, pp 81-116.
Balis F, Holcenberg J, and Poplack D: General principles of chemotherapy. In Pizzo P and Poplack D, editors: Principles and practice of pediatric oncology, Philadelphia, 1997, Lippincott-Raven, pp 215-272.
*Table includes principal drugs used in the treatment of childhood cancers. Other chemotherapeutic agents may be employed in treatment regimens.
†Vesicants (sclerosing agents) can cause severe cellular damage if even minute amounts of the drug infiltrate surrounding tissue. These drugs must be given through a free-flowing intravenous line. The infusion is stopped *immediately* if any sign of infiltration (pain, stinging, swelling, or redness at needle site) occurs. Additional interventions for extravasation vary.
‡IV, intravenous; IT, intrathecal; PO, by mouth; IM, intramuscular; SC, subcutaneous.
§N/V, nausea and vomiting. Mild = <20% incidence; moderate = 20% to 70% incidence; severe = >75% incidence.
‖BMD, bone marrow depression.
¶Abbreviations stand for chemical compound.
**Emergency drugs include oxygen and parenteral preparations of epinephrine 1:1000, diphenhydramine or similar antihistamine, aminophylline, corticosteroids, and vasopressors.

Table 13-2

Summary of Chemotherapeutic Agents Used in the Treatment of Childhood Cancers*—cont'd

Agent/Administration	Side Effects and Toxicity	Comments and Specific Nursing Considerations
Alkylating Agents—cont'd		
Procarbazine (Matulan) PO	N/V (moderate) BMD (3-4 weeks later) Lethargy Dermatitis Myalgia Arthralgia Diplopia Stomatitis Neuropathy Alopecia Diarrhea Amenorrhea	CNS depressants (phenothiazines, barbiturates) enhance central nervous system symptoms Monoamine oxidase (MAO) inhibition sometimes occurs; therefore all other drugs are avoided unless medically approved; red wine, fava beans, broad bean pods, tea, coffee, cola, cheese, banana are to be avoided Give medication in evening to reduce nausea
Dacarbazine (DTIC) IV	N/V (especially after first dose) (severe) BMD (3 weeks later) Alopecia Flulike syndrome Burning sensation in vein during infusion (not extravasation)	Vesicant (less sclerosive) Must be given cautiously in individuals with renal dysfunction Decrease IV rate or use cold pack on IV site to decrease burning
Carmustine (BCNU) IV	N/V (2-6 hours later) (severe)	Prevent extravasation; contact with skin causes brown spots
Lomustine (CCNU) PO	BMD (3-4 weeks later) Burning pain along IV infusion (usually due to alcohol diluent) BCNU—flushing and facial burning on infusion —pulmonary infiltrates and/or fibrosis	Oral form—give on empty stomach Reduce IV burning by diluting drug and infusing slowly via IV drip Crosses blood-brain barrier Check pulmonary function tests
Antimetabolites		
Cytarabine (Ara-C, Cytosar, Cytosine arabinoside) IV, IM, SC,‡ IT	N/V (within 2 hours of IT dose) (mild-severe dose dependent) BMD (7-14 days later) Mucosal ulceration Hepatitis (usually subclinical) Conjunctivitis (high dose) ARA-C syndrome: fever, myalgia, malaise, rash 6-12 hr after administration Neurotoxicity with high doses	Crosses blood-brain barrier Use with caution in individuals with hepatic dysfunction Corticosteroid ophthalmic drops to prevent conjunctivitis
Mercaptopurine (6-MP, Purinethol) PO, IV	N/V (mild) Stomatitis BMD Dermatitis Elevated liver enzymes	6-MP is an analog of xanthine; therefore allopurinol (Zyloprim) delays its metabolism and increases its potency, necessitating a lower dose (⅓ to ¼) of 6-MP

Continued

Table 13-2
Summary of Chemotherapeutic Agents Used in the Treatment of Childhood Cancers*—cont'd

Agent/Administration	Side Effects and Toxicity	Comments and Specific Nursing Considerations
Antimetabolites—cont'd		

Methotrexate (MTX, Amethopterin) PO, IV, IM, SQ, IT. May be given in conventional doses (mg/m^2) or high doses (g/m^2)	N/V (moderate-severe at high doses)
	Diarrhea
	Mucosal ulceration (2-5 days later)
	BMD (10 days later)
	Dermatitis
	Photosensitivity
	Alopecia
	Hepatitis (fibrosis)
	Elevated liver enzymes
	Nephropathy
	Pneumonitis (fibrosis)
	Neurologic toxicity with high doses and IT use—arachnoiditis, leuko-encephalopathy, seizures
		Side effects and toxicity are dose-related
		Potency and toxicity increased by reduced renal function, salicylates, sulfonamides, and aminobenzoic acid; avoid use of aspirin and ibuprofen
		High dose therapy:
		  Citrovorum factor (folinic acid or leuco-vorin) decreases cytotoxic action of MTX; used as an antidote for overdose and to enhance normal cell recovery following high-dose therapy; avoid use of vitamins containing folic acid during MTX therapy unless prescribed by physician
		IT therapy:
		  Drug *must* be mixed with preservative free diluent
		  Report signs of neurotoxicity immediately

6-Thioguanine (6-TG) PO	N/V (mild) BMD (7-14 days later) Stomatitis Dermatitis Liver dysfunction	Side effects are unusual
5-Fluorouracil (5-FU, Fluorouracil) IV	N/V (moderate) BMD (9-14 days later) Dermatitis Stomatitis Alopecia Hyperpigmentation of nail beds	Take at least 2 hours before or after food
Plant Alkaloids		
Vincristine (Oncovin, VCR) IV	Neurotoxicity—paresthesia (numb-ness), ataxia, weakness, foot drop, hyporeflexia, constipation (ady-namic ileus), hoarseness (vocal cord paralysis); abdominal, chest, and jaw pain Fever N/V (mild) BMD (minimal; 7-14 days later) Alopecia SIADH	Vesicant Report signs of neurotoxicity because this may necessitate cessation of drug Individuals with underlying neurologic problems may be more prone to neuro-toxicity Monitor stool patterns closely; administer stool softener Excreted primarily by liver into biliary sys-tem; check bilirubin before administra-tion

Table 13-2
Summary of Chemotherapeutic Agents Used in the Treatment of Childhood Cancers*—cont'd

Agent/Administration	Side Effects and Toxicity	Comments and Specific Nursing Considerations
Plant Alkaloids—cont'd		
Vinblastine (Velban) IV	Neurotoxicity (same as for vincristine but less severe) N/V (mild 4-12 hours later) BMD (especially neutropenia; 7-14 days later) Alopecia	Same as for vincristine
Etoposide, (VP-16 Ve-Pesid) PO, IV	N/V (mild) BMD (7-14 days later) Alopecia Hypotension with rapid infusion Diarrhea May reactivate erythema of irradiated skin (rare) Allergic reaction with anaphylaxis possible Secondary malignancy (AML)	Give slowly via IV drip over at least 1 hr with child recumbent Have emergency drugs available at bedside** Vital signs with blood pressure every 15 minutes during infusion
Teniposide (VM-26) IV	BMD (3-14 days later) Alopecia N/V Hypotension with rapid infusion Mild neurotoxicity Hypersensitivity reaction with anaphylaxis possible	Irritant Have emergency drugs available at bedside
Paclitaxel (Taxol) IV	BMD (10 days later) N/V during infusion "Stocking-glove" peripheral neuropathy Mucositis Bradycardia Alopecia	Monitor frequently Premedicate with corticosteroids and antihistamines Avoid PVC bags and tubing
Antibiotics		
Dactinomycin (Antinomycin D, Cosmegen, ACT-D) IV	N/V (0-6 hours later) (moderate-severe) BMD (especially platelets; 2-3 weeks later) Mucosal ulceration Abdominal cramps Diarrhea Anorexia (may last few weeks) Alopecia Acne Erythema or hyperpigmentation of previously irradiated skin Fever Malaise	Vesicant Enhances cytotoxic effects of radiation therapy but increases toxic effects May cause serious desquamation of irradiated tissue

Continued

Table 13-2
Summary of Chemotherapeutic Agents Used in the Treatment of Childhood Cancers*—cont'd

Agent/Administration	Side Effects and Toxicity	Comments and Specific Nursing Considerations
Antibiotics—cont'd		

Doxorubicin (Adriamycin, ADR) IV	N/V (moderate)
	Stomatitis
	BMD (7-14 days later)
	Local phlebitis
	Alopecia
	Cumulative-dose toxicity includes
	    Cardiac abnormalities
	    ECG changes
	    Heart failure
	Hyperpigmentation of nailbeds
	Secondary malignancy (AML) when used in high doses with cyclophosphamide
		Vesicant (extravasation may *not* cause pain)
		Use only sterile distilled water as a diluent
		Observe for any changes in heart rate or rhythm and signs of failure; follow echocardiogram or MUGA (multiple gated uptake) scan
		Cumulative lifetime dose must not exceed 450 mg/m^2
		Warn parents that drug causes urine to turn red (for up to 12 days after administration); this is normal, not hematuria

Daunomycin (Cerubidine, Daunorubicin) IV	Similar to doxorubicin	Similar to doxorubicin

Bleomycin (Blenoxane) IV, IM, SC	Allergic reaction—fever, chills, hypotension, anaphylaxis
	Fever (nonallergic)
	N/V (mild)
	Stomatitis
	Cumulative dose effects include
	    Skin—rash, hyperpigmentation, thickening, ulceration, peeling, nail changes, alopecia
	    Lungs—pneumonitis with infiltrate that can progress to fatal fibrosis
	Raynaud's syndrome
		Should give test dose (IM) before therapeutic dose administered
		Have emergency drugs at bedside
		Hypersensitivity occurs with first one to two doses
		May give acetaminophen before drug to reduce likelihood of fever
		Concentration of drug in skin and lungs accounts for toxic effects
		Cumulative lifetime dose no >400 units
		Pulmonary function test as baseline and in follow-up

Idarubicin (Ida) IV	(Similar to Doxorubicin)	(Similar to Doxorubicin)
Hormones		
Corticosteroids (prednisone, prednisolone, dexamethasone) Prednisone—PO; Prednisolone—PO, IV; Dexamethasone—PO, IV, IM	Moon face, mood changes, increased appetite, insomnia Immunosuppression Aseptic necrosis Pancreatitis Psychiatric disorders Amenorrhea Trunk obesity Muscle wasting and weakness Osteoporosis Poor wound healing Gastric bleeding Hypertension Diabetes mellitus Growth failure Acne	Explain expected effects, especially in terms of body image, increased appetite, and personality changes Monitor weight gain Recommend moderate salt restriction May need to disguise bitter taste (crush tablet and mix with syrup, jam, ice cream or other high-flavored substance; use ice to numb tongue before administration; place tablet in gelatin capsule if child can swallow it) Observe for potential infection sites; usual inflammatory response and fever are absent Test stools for occult blood Monitor blood pressure Test blood for sugar and urine for acetone Observe for signs of abrupt steroid withdrawal; flulike symptoms, hypotension, hypoglycemia, shock

Table 13-2
Summary of Chemotherapeutic Agents Used in the Treatment of Childhood Cancers*—cont'd

Agent/Administration	Side Effects and Toxicity	Comments and Specific Nursing Considerations
Enzymes		
Asparaginase (L-ASP, Elspar) IM, IV	Allergic reactions (including anaphylactic shock) Fever N/V (mild) Anorexia Weight loss Fibrinogenemia Liver dysfunction Hyperglycemia (transient) Renal failure Pancreatitis Somnolence, lethargy	Have emergency drugs at bedside Record signs of allergic reaction (urticaria, facial edema, hypotension, or abdominal cramps) Normally, BUN and ammonia levels rise as a result of drug—not evidence of liver damage Check urine for sugar and ketones; treat with insulin as needed Check PT, PTT, fibrinogen—may need fresh frozen plasma Check amylase levels
PEG-Asparaginase (Oncaspar) IM	See Asparaginase	See Asparaginase Lower incidence of hypersensitivity reaction than use of native asparaginase
Other Agents		
Cisplatin (Platinol) IV	Renal toxicity (severe) N/V (1-6 hours later) (severe) BMD (2-3 weeks later) Ototoxicity Neurotoxicity (similar to that for vincristine) Nephrotoxicity-induced electrolyte disturbances, especially hypomagnesemia, hypocalcemia, hypo kalemia, and hypophosphatemia Anaphylactic reactions may occur	Renal function (creatinine clearance) must be assessed before giving drug Must maintain hydration before and during therapy (specific gravity of urine is used to assess hydration) Mannitol may be given IV to promote osmotic diuresis and drug clearance Monitor intake and output Monitor for signs of ototoxicity (e.g., ringing in ears) and neurotoxicity; report signs immediately; ensure that routine audiogram is done before treatment for baseline and routinely during treatment Do not use aluminum needle; reaction with aluminum decreases potency of drug Monitor for signs of electrolyte loss (i.e. hypomagnesemia—tremors, spasm, muscle weakness, lower extremity cramps, irregular heartbeat, convulsions, delirium) Have emergency drugs at bedside
Carboplatin (Paraplatin) IV	N/V BMD Ototoxicity (rare) Neurotoxicity Electrolyte disturbance: decreased sodium, potassium, calcium, magnesium Renal toxicity Anaphylaxis	As for Cisplatin

donor's marrow or blood stem cells replace the child's destroyed marrow and after engraftment should produce the donor's nonmalignant functioning cells.

An autologus transplantation may be used when there is no available histocompatible donor, the tumor is not in the marrow, or the marrow can be purged of all tumor cells. In allogeneic transplantation, the donor is preferably a tissue identical relative of the child, most often a sibling.

Bone marrow and blood stem cell transplantation is a promising treatment modality for certain malignancies in children. It must be realistically viewed, however, in terms of the potentially fatal toxicities, developmental sequelae, and psychosocial and financial effects on the child and family.

Recent and Anticipated Advances in Diagnosis and Management

Increasingly, cytogenetic studies have linked specific chromosomal changes with specific tumors or identified inherited genetic abnormalities that place persons at risk for developing cancer. One example is the identified loss of the p53 or tumor suppressor gene (i.e., through a germ-line mutation) that places an individual at risk for the development of specific types of cancer. Additionally, more biologic tumor markers (i.e., substances on the surfaces of tumor cells that identify them as malignant) have been identified to assist in the diagnosis and staging of tumors, as well as in determining a response to therapy. Polymerized chain reaction (PCR) is increasingly used to detect minimal residual cancer cells with greater sensitivity (Sievers and Loken, 1995). Advances in molecular genetics will help to refine prognostic groupings by identifying specific cell types in tumors that are associated with higher or lower rates of cure.

Treatment with chemotherapy is continuously being refined through the efforts of multiinstitutional and cooperative studies. Choice of agents, dosage, timing, and route of administration are more selective to increase effectiveness and decrease late effects of therapy. Future advances in chemotherapy will address the potential reversal of multidrug resistance in tumor cells (Balis, Holcenberg, and Poplack, 1997).

Advances in radiation therapy include hyperfractionated radiation dosing (discussed earlier) and stereotactic irradiation or radiosurgery. The latter uses CAT scans to focus radiation in a three-dimensional space to more specifically target the tumor. This highly focused radiation is typically delivered by photo-beams from cobalt 60 sources (Gamma Konfer, Elekta Corp., Atlanta, GA) or linear accelerators (Corn et al, 1997; Heideman et al, 1997; Kun, 1997). Although these delivery systems show promise, they are currently known to be beneficial for a relatively small number of children with brain tumors.

Bone marrow and blood stem cell transplant is being applied to more types of tumors and is being used as "rescue" therapy when very high doses of chemotherapy are needed to treat recurrent tumors. The source of hematopoietic stem cells has broadened to include peripheral stem cells and umbilical cord blood in addition to bone marrow. Autologous stem cell transplantation is now being considered more frequently—even in children at risk for the presence of residual malignant cells in the stem cells to be transplanted (Sanders, 1997; Secola, 1997).

As previously mentioned, immunotherapy is an exciting new addition to the multimodal treatment approach to curing childhood cancer and modifying treatment toxicities.

The ability of interferon to prolong the cell cycle would allow other agents to destroy a greater number of cells. It is hoped that the use of interleukins will modulate the body's natural immune system response (Wheeler, 1996). Interleukin-2 shows the potential for destroying tumor cells while leaving nonmalignant cells intact. Tumor necrosis factor (TNF) disrupts the vascular supply to tumor cells resulting in hemorrhagic necrosis. Monoclonal antibodies bind to specific antigens located on tumors and inform immune cells to destroy the tumor cells. The side effect common to most of the therapies described above is a flulike syndrome consisting of fever, chills, headache, fatigue, and muscle aches.

Colony stimulating factors (CSFs) are cytokines that stimulate the body's production of different types of hematopoietic cells. For example, G-CSF stimulates the production of granulocytes (G); GM-CSF stimulates the production of both granulocytes (G) and macrophages (M); and erythropoietin stimulates the production of red blood cells. These substances have helped to reduce the bone marrow suppressive toxicities of chemotherapy.

The newest area of exploration in cancer treatment is gene therapy. It is hoped that the transfer of genes may repair one or more genetic defects in a tumor cell, act as a drug delivery system, spare normal tissue from the cytotoxic effects of chemotherapy, and may label normal cells or tumor cells to assist monitoring the effectiveness of current therapy. Most clinical trials in gene therapy are currently limited to children with advanced malignancies (Adams and Emerson, 1998; Alavi and Eck, 1998; Brenner, 1997; Lea, 1997).

Associated Problems (Box 13-3)

Vascular Access

Children receiving prolonged, intensive treatment are required to endure frequent venipunctures for laboratory tests, chemotherapy, administration of blood products, antibiotic therapy, and nutritional support. These children are often aided by the placement of a long-term indwelling central venous access device (VAD), which helps minimize the trauma of frequent needle sticks and vein irritation from the chemotherapy. Access devices include tunnelled catheters and subcutaneous (SC) implanted ports.

Tunnelled catheters are single, double, or triple lumen silicone catheters with a Dacron (DuPont) felt cuff that anchors the catheter under the skin and provides a barrier to infection. Tunnelled catheters have an internal and external portion, whereas SC ports are totally implanted below the skin with the catheter tip at the junction of the superior vena cava and the right atrium. Venous access is achieved by puncturing the skin above the reservoir and passing a specially designed needle through the silicone membrane into the port receptacle (Hadaway, 1995; Winslow, Trammell and Camp-Sorrell, 1995). Topical anesthetics may be applied to port sites before accessing to reduce discomfort and fear.

The patency of all long-term VADs is maintained through periodic flushing with heparinized saline. Care of these lines is taught to the child (when appropriate) and parents. Complications of indwelling VADs include infection, occlusion of

---

Box 13-3

Associated Problems

- **Vascular access:** most children require the use of indwelling central VADs
  All lumens must be cultured if any fever
  SBE prophylaxis for dental procedures
- **Nausea and vomiting:** use antiemetics before and after chemotherapeutic administration, NOT on an "as needed" (i.e., prn) basis
- **Anorexia and weight loss:** monitor weight regularly, early intervention
- **Bone marrow suppression:**
  Hemoglobin < 7 to 8 g/dl, consider transfusion
  Platelets < 10,000 to 20,000, consider transfusion
  ANC < 500, high risk for infection
  Possible use of erythropoietins for treatment of anemia and GCSF or GMCSF neutropenia
- **Infection:** blood cultures for all fevers IV antibiotics for fever and neutropenia or for any child with an implanted central venous access device
- **Alopecia**
- **Late effects:** See Table 13-3

---

the catheter due to thrombus and fibrin formation, damage to the external portion of the catheter, and rarely, cardiac tamponade (Korones et al, 1996; Rumsey and Richardson, 1995).

Because a child with cancer is at risk for profound neutropenia as a result of therapy, prompt and aggressive treatment of infection at the catheter site is necessary. Most exit site infections can be cleared with oral and topical antibiotics; but tunnel infections and septicemia require IV antibiotics and possible catheter removal (Dillon and Wiener, 1997).

Therapy-Related Complications

Nausea and Vomiting

Nausea and vomiting are common side effects of chemotherapy and radiation. Nausea and vomiting can have profound physiologic and psychologic effects on the child receiving therapy (Hockenberry-Eaton and Kline, 1997). Problems including dehydration, chemical and electrolyte imbalances, and decreased nutritional intake can lead to decreased compliance or termination of treatment.

The mechanisms involved in nausea and vomiting are complex, and no single drug will consistently control these side effects. The situation is further complicated by the wide variation in response of the individual child to both the chemotherapeutic agent and the antiemetic. The antiemetic should be given before nausea and vomiting occur and should be continued until the symptoms have resolved. Nausea and vomiting related to the chemotherapy generally will not last longer than 48 hours after chemotherapy administration.

Serotonin antagonists have a significant role in the management of nausea and vomiting in children. Ondansetron (Zofran) and Granisetron (Kytril) inhibit the binding of serotonin to receptors in both the central nervous system and the gastrointestinal system. These medications do not cause drowsiness and rarely cause extrapyramidal side effects (Betcher et al, 1997). Adjunctive methods such as progressive relaxation and guided imagery have had some positive effects when combined with antiemetic medications (Fessele, 1996).

Anorexia and Weight Loss

During therapy, anorexia and weight loss are common and can be attributed to both the disease and its treatment. The psychologic impact of cancer and the tumor's metabolic influence can contribute to weight loss. Treatment-induced nausea and vomiting, as well as changes in taste acuity may lead to food aversion. Therefore the child's weight must be closely monitored throughout treatment. Oral supplements and, in some cases, nasogastric or gastrostomy feedings (Mathew et al, 1996) or hyperalimentation may be necessary.

Bone Marrow Suppression

Bone marrow suppression is another side effect of chemotherapy and radiation. Leukopenia, thrombocytopenia, and anemia usually begin within 7 to 10 days after drug administration, with the nadir (i.e., the point at which the blood cell counts are the lowest) occurring at approximately 14 days. The marrow then recovers by 21 to 28 days. The exact time of the nadir varies depending on the specific chemotherapeutic agent. Close monitoring is necessary to determine the extent of marrow suppression.

Leukopenia refers to the presence of a low number of all white blood cells (WBCs), whereas neutropenia refers specifically to a low neutrophil cell count. Neutrophils are the body's main defense against bacterial infection. It is necessary to determine the absolute neutrophil count (ANC) (Box 13-4) because the incidence and severity of infection are inversely related to an ANC < 500. Infections are a major life-threatening complication of cancer and its treatment (Chanock and Pizzo, 1997).

There are several precautions that can be taken to reduce the risk of infection. Good handwashing techniques by the child, the parents, and the caregivers are paramount to reducing the spread of pathogens. Good personal hygiene by the child, which includes thorough dental care, is also important. A child with neutropenia should avoid individuals who are ill, crowded situations, and anyone with a communicable disease, especially chickenpox. Rectal temperatures and suppositories should also be avoided because abrading the rectal mucosa increases the risk of introducing bacteria into the bloodstream.

Guidelines for transfusion are based on laboratory parameters and clinical symptoms. The child

---

Box 13-4

Calculation of Absolute Neutrophil Count (ANC)

White blood count (WBC) = 7400 (also expressed as 7.4 k/UL; $7.4 \times 10^3/mm^3$)
Neutrophils (poly. segs) = 40%
Nonsegmented neutrophils (bands) = 12%

Step 1: Determine total percent neutrophils (poly. segs + bands)
40% + 12% = 52% (0.52)
Step 2: Multiply WBC by % neutrophils
ANC = 7400 × 0.52
ANC = 3848 (normal)

WBC = 900 (0.9 k/UL; $0.9 \times 10^3/mm^3$)
Neutrophils (poly. segs) = 7%
Nonsegmented neutrophils (bands) = 7%
Step 1: 7% + 7% = 14% (0.14)
Step 2: ANC = 900 × 0.14
ANC = 126 (severely neutropenic)

who is thrombocytopenic may require transfusions of platelets because of the risk of serious hemorrhage. Transfusion is recommended if the platelet count is less than 10,000 to 20,000 and/or in the presence of bleeding. In a child whose hemoglobin level is less than 7 to 8 g and/or who is symptomatic (i.e., shortness of breath, headache, or dizziness), a transfusion is usually indicated (Webb and Anderson, 1997).

To reduce the risk of transfusion-acquired infections and graft vs. host reactions, blood products should be CMV-seronegative, irradiated, and leukocyte depleted for CMV-negative patients. If the child is a potential candidate for allogeneic bone marrow transplant, discourage directed donations of platelets and red cells from first degree relatives to reduce the risk of sensitizing the child to a potential bone marrow donor (Barnard, Feusner, and Wolff, 1997). Granulocyte and granulocyte-macrophage colony-stimulating factors (GCSF/GM-CSF) may be used in high risk children to reduce the severity and duration of neutropenia (American Society of Clinical Oncology, 1996; Vase and Armitage, 1995).

Hair Loss

A distinguishing therapy-related complication is alopecia. A generally temporary condition, it results from damage to the hair follicles by chemotherapy and radiation. Although the hair usually regrows after therapy, the texture and color may be slightly different. Cutting the child's hair into a shorter style may help to reduce some distress when the hair begins to fall out. Younger children and some adolescents prefer to cover their heads with colorful hats, baseball caps, and scarves. Adolescent girls are more likely to consider the use of wigs.

Late Effects

As the survival rates continually improve, the long-term effects of therapy are becoming evident. The goal of therapy is not merely improving survival but also reducing physiologic and developmental morbidity. A growing body of knowledge indicates that both chemotherapy and radiation have adverse effects on normal tissues that may not be manifested for months or years after therapy. The development of second malignancies, impaired growth, diminished cognitive functioning, and organ damage are the areas of greatest concern. Factors that appear to influence the development of late effects include the child's age and stage of development at the time of diagnosis, the primary tumor and extent of involvement, and the therapy used.

Secondary malignant neoplasms (SMN) are found with greater frequency in children with a genetic predisposition based on the primary tumor or as a result of chemotherapy and radiation therapy. The highest rate of SMN occurs in children with hereditary retinoblastoma. There may also be an increased risk of SMN in persons with the genetic forms of Wilm's tumor (bilateral), neuroblastoma, and other embryonal tumors. In children with Hodgkin's disease treated with radiation and chemotherapy, there is an increased incidence of SMN—especially AML and solid tumors including breast cancer (Bhatia et al, 1996). Treatment with alkylating agents and etoposide increases the risk of AML. Concurrent use of dose intensive anthracyclines with cyclophosphamide has been associated with an increased risk of SMN (Blatt, Copeland, and Bleyer, 1997).

Children receiving treatment directly to the CNS are at risk for negative neurologic and intellectual sequelae. Neurotoxicity is related to the number and sequence of treatment modalities used. The impact of late effects on the various organ systems is described in Table 13-3.

Relapse

Despite the advances in treatment of childhood cancer, some children will experience a relapse of their disease. Relapse, like diagnosis, is a crisis period for the family. It poses a challenge for the oncology team because the best methods of treatment were used at diagnosis. Relapse often requires more experimental modes of treatment. The primary care provider in cooperation with the oncology team can support the family—and especially the child—through this difficult time.

Death

There may come a time when all possible viable treatment options have been exhausted. The care of the child moves from focusing on a cure to providing comfort and as much quality time as possible. The collaboration between the primary care provider and the oncology team can be invaluable

Text continued on p. 290

Table 13-3
Adverse Effects of Antineoplastic Therapy Upon Body Systems

Body System	Adverse Effects	Causative Agent	Time Interval	Signs and Symptoms	Predisposing Factors	Preventive/ Diagnostic Measures
Cardiovascular system	Cardiomyopathy	Anthracycline chemotherapy Cyclophosphamide (high dose) Irradiation of mediastinum	Weeks to months	Abrupt onset of congestive heart failure; tachycardia; tachypnea; edema; hepatomegaly; cardiomegaly; gallop rhythms; pleural effusions; dyspnea	Increased risk with age <15 years and females Anthracycline therapy; especially lifetime cumulative dose of ≥550 mg/m^2	Careful monitoring with chest radiograph film ECG, Echocardiogram, MUGA scan Observation for shortness of breath, weight gain, edema Partial shielding of mediastinum Treatment with antiinflammatory agents Pericardial stripping
	Chronic constrictive pericarditis	Irradiation of mediastinum	Few months to years	Chest pain; dyspnea; fever; paradoxic pulse; venous distention; friction rub; Kussmaul's sign	Mediastinal radiation Most common with doses of 4000-6000 cGy	
Pulmonary system	Pneumonitis followed by pulmonary fibrosis	Pulmonary irradiation Bleomycin, BCUU, high-dose cytoxan	2-12 months following radiation	Increased dyspnea; decreased exercise tolerance; pulmonary insufficiency	Increased risk with Large lung volume in radiation field Therapy during period of pulmonary infection Concomitant mediastinal irradiation Chemotherapeutic agents that act as radiation sensitizers Doses > 4000 cGy	Careful monitoring of status with physical examination, chest radiograph, and pulmonary function tests High-dose corticosteroids for severe cases Yearly influenza vaccine Pneumovax Avoid smoking Encourage frequent rest periods
Hematopoietic system	Long-term suppression of bone marrow function	Extensive irradiation of marrow-containing bones Chemotherapy	Months to years following therapy	Fall in WBC and platelet counts; hypoplastic/aplastic bone marrow aspirates; diminished uptake of radioisotopes;	Radiation doses: 3000-5000 cGy in older individuals Concomitant use of chemotherapy	Limitation of areas of marrow irradiated Monitoring of child's status with periodic bone marrow aspirates and peripheral blood cell counts

System / Late effect	Causative treatment	Time of occurrence	Signs and symptoms	Predisposing factors	Management
Alterations in immune system	Bone marrow transplant Splenectomy		predisposition to infection		Pneumococcal vaccine and penicillin if splenectomized. Monitoring of child's status with periodic blood counts and tests of immune response
Gastrointestinal system Hepatic fibrosis-cirrhosis	Chemotherapy	Months to years following therapy	Persistent elevation of liver function tests after cessation of therapy; hepatomegaly; cirrhosis; jaundice; spider nevi	Daily low doses of methotrexate by mouth for long periods. Long-term use of 6-mercaptopurine	Monitor child's status with liver function tests. Perform liver biopsy if liver function test results remain persistently abnormal. Avoid concomitant use of radiation sensitizers
Chronic enteritis	Radiation therapy	Months to years following therapy	Pain, recurrent vomiting; diarrhea; malabsorption syndrome; weight loss	Radiation doses >5000 cGy. Children with previous abdominal surgery. Chemotherapy with radiation sensitizers (actinomycin and adriamycin)	Careful monitoring of height and weight. Supportive therapy when symptoms develop, including low residue, low-fat, gluten and milk-free diet
Kidney and urinary tract Nephritis Acute and chronic	Radiation to renal structures CCNV, BCUU, chemotherapy	Acute: 6-12 months following therapy Chronic: months to years following therapy	May appear as benign or malignant hypertension. Acute: rapid decrease in renal function with BUN, proteinuria, anemia, hypertension, signs of congestive heart failure	Renal radiation of 2000-3000 cGy. Combined use of radiation and chemotherapy	Periodically monitor renal status during and after therapy, with blood pressure readings, urinalysis, and CBC, BUN, and creatinine. Radiation-induced hypertension spontaneously resolves when damage is unilateral

Continued

Sources: Bhatia S et al: Breast cancer and other second neoplasms after childhood Hodgkin's disease, N Engl J Med 334:745-751, 1996.
Blatt J, Copeland D, and Bleyer A: Late effects of childhood cancer and its treatment. In Pizzo P and Poplack D, editors: Principles and practice of pediatric oncology, Philadelphia, 1997, JB Lippincott, pp 1303-1329;
Hobbie W et al: Late effects in long term survivors. In Foley G, Fochtman D, and Mooney K, editors: Nursing care of the child with cancer, Philadelphia, 1993, WB Saunders, pp 466-496.
Krischer J et al: Clinical cardiotoxicity following anthracycline treatment for childhood cancer: The Pediatric Oncology Group experience, J Clin Oncol 15:1544-1552, 1997.
Oberfield S et al: Endocrine late effects of childhood cancers, J Pediatr 131:537-541, 1997.
Román J et al: Growth and growth hormone secretion in children with cancer treated with chemotherapy, J Pediatr 131:105-112, 1997.
Schwartz C et al: Survivors of childhood cancer: assessment and management, St Louis, 1994, Mosby.

Table 13-3
Adverse Effects of Antineoplastic Therapy Upon Body Systems—cont'd

Body System	Adverse Effects	Causative Agent	Time Interval	Signs and Symptoms	Predisposing Factors	Preventive/ Diagnostic Measures
Kidney and urinary tract—cont'd				Chronic: persistence of above or insidious development of anemia, azotemia, proteinuria, hypertension; may lead to chronic renal failure or cardiovascular damage		Once progressive renal failure develops, treatment is supportive
	Chronic hemorrhagic cystitis	Chemotherapy: Cytoxan and Ifosfamide	Months to years	Sterile, painful hematuria; urinary frequency	Pelvic irradiation >4000 cGy Inadequate hydration of chemotherapy patients	Techniques to reduce bladder exposure during radiation therapy Frequent emptying of bladder during and 24 hrs after therapy Adequate hydration before, during, and after chemotherapy Concomitant use of MESNA with chemotherapy Treatment of bladder hemorrhage with formalin instillation and/or fulguration of bleeding sites
	Tubular dysfunction	Cytoxan and Ifosfamide		Low magnesium; Low phosphorus; glycosuria	None	Magnesium and phosphorus supplements
Musculoskeletal system	Impaired skeletal growth	Irradiation of skeletal structures and abdomen	Months to years following treatment	Growth retardation; reduction in sitting height; scoliosis; altered growth of facial skeleton	Effect of spinal irradiation to vertebral bodies in doses 1000-2000 cGy dependent on age of child; known damage > 2000 cGy	Careful monitoring of child's status with growth charts, radiographic studies, sitting and standing height Dose radiation reduction during periods of rapid growth

	Cause	Onset	Signs	Details	Management
Delayed or arrested tooth development	Irradiation of maxilla or mandible; Chemotherapy	Months to years	Teeth are small with pale enamel; malocclusion	Unilateral radiation results in asymmetric deformities; Symmetric growth delay during periods of chemotherapy; Radiation during period of dental growth and development	Dental examinations every 6 months; Good oral hygiene including flossing; Fluoride prophylaxis
Endocrine system					
Thyroid gland dysfunction	Irradiation of thyroid gland, brain, and total body irradiation	Months to years	Hypothyroidism; may be asymptomatic and have abnormal thyroid function; nodular abnormalities	Reported with varying radiation doses: 2500-7000 cGy	Monitor thyroid function with T3, Free T4, and TSH; Hormonal replacement therapy for all patients with abnormal thyroid tests
Injuries to gonads	Irradiation of gonads; Chemotherapy (alkylating agents)	Months to years	Infertility; sterility; hormonal dysfunction, azoospermia, teratogenic during first trimester of pregnancy	Testicular radiation; ovarian radiation; Chemotherapy damage dependent on drug used, dose, duration of therapy, child's sex, and age	Tanner staging yearly; Protection of testes/ovaries from radiation field; Gonadal dysfunction from chemotherapy may be reversible; Males (14 y.o.) check LH, FSH, testosterone levels; Females (12 y.o.) check LH, FSH, estradiol levels
Decreased growth rate	Irradiation of cranium and/or spine; Total body irradiation; Chemotherapy	Months to years	Reduction in height percentile or growth rate	Radiation therapy at younger age and dose of ≥3000 cGy to Brain; Spinal irradiation at >3500 cGy; Total body irradiation at >1000 cGy	After completion of therapy, check standing and sitting heights 1-2 times each year; Thyroid function tests, bone age, and growth hormone testing to be considered if growth rate declines

Continued

Body System	Adverse Effects	Causative Agent	Time Interval	Signs and Symptoms	Predisposing Factors	Preventive/ Diagnostic Measures
Nervous system	Peripheral sensory or motor neuropathies	Irradiation of peripheral nerves; chemotherapy (Vincristine, VP-16, cisplatin)	Months to years	Deficit in function Pain Decreased tendon reflexes	Radiation doses: 5500-12,000 cGy Chemotherapy with vinca-alkaloids	Careful monitoring of patient status during and after therapy Vinca-alkaloid damage may be diminished or reversed by reducing or withholding therapy
	Central neuroendocrine dysfunction of hypothalamic pituitary axis	Cranial irradiation; chemotherapy	Months to years	Growth hormone deficiency Panhypopituitarism with short stature; hypothyroidism; Addison's disease	Dependent on dose of radiation, age of child, and concomitant use of chemotherapy Younger children who receive >2400 cGy at greatest risk	Careful monitoring of patient status with growth charts, Tanner staging, Bone age at 9 yr then yearly to puberty Thyroid, hormone, insulin, and cortisol measurement may be necessary Treatment with replacement of deficient hormones
	Encephalopathy	Cranial irradiation; chemotherapy	Months to years	May be asymptomatic but demonstrate abnormalities on head CAT* scans May have overt symptoms ranging from lethargy, somnolence, dementia, seizures, paralysis, and coma	Cranial radiation alone or with concomitant chemotherapy Frequency increased with chemotherapy Less damage with cranial radiation <1800 cGy Younger children more vulnerable	Monitor patient status with careful physical examination, head MRI/ CAT* scans, psychometric testing Reduce chemotherapy dose when preclinical radiographic findings appear
	Intelligence deficits and/or neuropsychologic dysfunctions	Radiation therapy, chemotherapy	Months to years	Abnormal psychologic tests with deficits in perceptual behavior, language development, and learning abilities Personality changes	More common in younger children, those who received cranial irradiation > 1800 cGy and concomitant chemotherapy	Careful monitoring with periodic neurocognitive/psychologic evaluations Early intervention with multidisciplinary approach and specialized education programs

Secondary malignancy (multiple systems)					
Leukemia, especially AML	Alkylating agents Adriamycin Etoposide Irradiation of mediastinum	Years	Leukopenia Anemia Thrombocytopenia Fever Bone pain	Damage may occur in all individuals who receive CNS prophylactic or therapeutic cranial radiation and/or chemotherapy Hodgkin's lymphoma as primary malignancy	Monitor CBC
Thyroid cancer	Irradiation of mediastinum spine, head, or neck		Palpable mass/nodule Anterior cervical adenopathy	Younger age at time of radiation therapy	If thyroid nodule present obtain thyroid scintiscan, tests of thyroid function. Biopsy or bone needle aspiration of nodule or node
Breast cancer	Irradiation of mediastinum, spine, or chest wall		Palpable mass	More common with >2000 cGy to mantle area Genetic form of Wilms' tumor or Hodgkin's disease as primary malignancy	Teach adolescents to do breast self-examination Consider baseline mammogram in early 20s May consider chemoprevention for Hodgkin's survivors in the future
Bone and soft tissue tumors	Irradiation of bone or soft tissue		Mass Pain	Retinoblastoma as primary malignancy especially if treated with radiation or bilateral	

*CAT, Computerized Axial Tomography; MRI, Magnetic Resonance Imaging during this time. Families often seek guidance and support in making decisions that they can live with long after the child's death. Knowledge of the community- and hospital-based hospice programs in their area can be beneficial in meeting many of the home care and support needs of families. All families need reassurance that they will not be abandoned at this time and that multidisciplinary resources will be made available to them as required.

Prognosis

The prognosis of a malignancy is dependent on the age of the child, primary site, extent of the disease, and cell type. Over the past 20 years dramatic advances have been made in the treatment and potential cure of children with cancer (Table 13-4). The current figures estimate an overall 5-year disease-free survival of 72% for pediatric cancers in general (American Cancer Society, 1998).

PRIMARY CARE MANAGEMENT

Health Care Maintenance

Growth and Development

Although growth retardation secondary to chemotherapy often resolves when therapy is complete, it may persist for some children (Román et al, 1997). The effect of radiation, however, can be permanent. Radiation affects growth by damaging the epiphyseal plates of the long bones and the glands that are responsible for growth-related hormone production. A child's growth should be followed on a standardized growth curve, with growth patterns examined over time rather than as isolated measurements. Preferably both sitting and standing heights should be obtained. Growth rates should be followed every 1 to 3 months during therapy and for the first year after therapy; then measurements should be taken every 6 months until linear growth is completed. Because of the risk of significant

Table 13-4
Trends in Survival of Children with Malignant Disease

	Relative 5-Yr Survival Rates (%)						
			Yr of Diagnosis				
Site	1960-1963*	1970-1973*	1974-1976†	1977-1979†	1980-1982†	1983-1985	1986-1993†
All sites	28	45	55.1	61	65	68	72‡
Acute lympho-cytic leukemia	4	34	53.4	67	70	69	80‡
Acute myeloid leukemia	3	5	16.1	26§	21§	32§	37‡
Wilms' tumor	33§	70§	74.1	77	86	86	92‡
Brain and nervous system	35	45	54.5	57	55	62	61‡
Neuroblastoma	25	40	48.6	53	53	54	65‡
Bone	20§	30§	51.9§	52§	54§	59§	64‡
Hodgkin's disease	52§	90	80.4	83	91	90	94‡
Non-Hodgkin's lymphomas	18	26	42.3	51	62	70	73‡
Soft tissue	38§	60§	60	69	65	76	73‡

From Landis SH et al: Cancer statistics. CA, 48:6-30, 1998.
*Rates are based on End Results Group data from a series of hospital registries and one population-based registry.
†Rates are from the SEER program based on data from population-based registries in Connecticut, New Mexico, Utah, Iowa, Hawaii, Atlanta, Detroit, Seattle, Puget Sound, and San Francisco-Oakland. Rates are based on follow-up of patients through 1993.
‡The difference in rates between 1974-1976 and 1986-1993 is statistically significant ($p < 0.05$).
§The standard error of the survival rate is between 5 and 10 percentage points.

weight loss, weight should also be monitored at each visit.

Primary care providers can play an invaluable role in providing anticipatory guidance for parents about the developmental changes children with cancer will experience. Children with cancer are often limited in their opportunities to develop independence and autonomy. The limitations come from restrictions placed by treatment regimens, therapy-related complications, and protective parents.

Ongoing developmental assessment should be performed during and after therapy. Early identification and intervention are important in assisting the child in maintaining age-appropriate development. Neuropsychologic testing is recommended within the first 2 years after completion of therapy for children receiving cranial radiation. Age-standardized tests should be used to measure intellectual ability, visual perception, visual-motor and motor skills, language, memory and learning, academic achievement, and behavior and social functioning (see Chapter 2). Neuropsychologic testing may need to be repeated to diagnose long-term effects.

Diet

Maintaining adequate nutrition while a child is receiving treatment is challenging because of the child's anorexia. Well-balanced, nutritious meals should be offered. Small, frequent meals may often be more appealing than the standard three meals each day. High-calorie, high-protein snacks may also be helpful.

Children receiving corticosteroids often experience an increased appetite and weight gain, but because corticosteroids usually are administered for limited amounts of time, such symptoms generally are of short duration. Nutritious foods low in sodium should be encouraged.

Constipation and diarrhea are frequent side effects of chemotherapy. Constipation may be relieved by increasing the child's fluid intake and encouraging high-fiber foods and fruits. A stool softener or laxative may be necessary, especially with vincristine therapy. Enemas and suppositories should be avoided, especially if the child is neutropenic. Diarrhea should be monitored closely and the child evaluated for signs and symptoms of dehydration.

Parents will often inquire about the use of herbs, special diets, or other dietary interventions to speed the recovery of the blood cell counts or combat the tumor. Any supplement or major dietary change should be viewed in terms of its potential to interact with chemotherapeutic agents. The primary care provider can acknowledge and support the parents' desire to help their child while providing access to information that puts the cost and potential benefits of such treatments in perspective.

Safety

Safety issues for a child with a malignant disease involve balancing normal participation in daily activities with taking appropriate precautions imposed by the treatment of a malignant disease. For the safety of all children, chemotherapeutic agents must be stored securely out of reach. Thorough handwashing should follow the handling of any chemotherapeutic agent. Pregnant women should avoid contact with the chemotherapeutic agents and the urine of children on chemotherapy. If circumstances make this impossible, gloves should be worn to avoid direct contact with the medication. Unused portions of chemotherapeutic drugs should be returned to the dispensing pharmacy for disposal with other potent chemicals.

External tunnelled VADs must have a clean dressing applied to the exit site and the line secured to the chest to minimize any excessive tension of the catheter. Needles, syringes, and other supplies used to maintain the line should be stored properly out of reach of children. Needles should be disposed of carefully, without recapping, in an approved container.

Children with external tunnelled VADs should avoid lake or ocean swimming and hot tubs to reduce the risk of infection. They should also have an extra padded clamp available in case of damage to the catheter lumen.

If the child should have a significant fall or head injury, blood cell counts should be checked to determine the platelet count and the possible need for transfusion. Contact sports may be discouraged if the platelet count is less than 100,000.

Many of the chemotherapeutic agents will alter the skin's tolerance for sun exposure. It is important that children on chemotherapy take extra caution in using a *p*-aminobenzoic acid (PABA)-free sunblock whenever prolonged sun exposure is anticipated. It is best to avoid sun exposure during midday. If the child has alopecia, a hat and sunblock should be worn to protect the scalp.

The primary care provider can play a key role in helping the child and family set realistic expectations and limitations on activities. Limitations are influenced by immunosuppression, hematologic compromise, or extremity dysfunction because of peripheral neuropathy induced by chemotherapy or as a result of amputation or limb salvage procedures.

Immunizations

Because of the immunosuppressive nature of treatment, the child's immune system may not be able to mount a response to vaccinations. Normal immunologic response usually returns between 3 months and 1 year after discontinuing immunosuppressive therapy (Committee on Infectious Diseases, 1997). Because there is some variation in immunization recommendations among cancer treatment centers, it is best to consult with the child's oncology team for specific guidance. The child recovering from a bone marrow transplant presents a special situation. Immunizations should be given according to the schedules and protocols established by the transplant center (Somani and Larson, 1995).

Diphtheria, Tetanus, and Acellular Pertussis (DTaP)

The DTaP vaccine may safely be given at standardly scheduled times although immunogenicity may be reduced. The vaccine may be delayed if treatment will end shortly after the vaccine is due. Because titers to diphtheria, tetanus, and pertussis may fall as a result of therapy, booster doses are recommended 6 to 12 months after therapy is complete (Hastings, Goes, and Wolff, 1997; Hovi et al, 1995).

Poliovirus

Children should not receive the Sabin (live) oral polio vaccine once therapy has been initiated and also for the first year off therapy. Siblings of the child should receive the Salk (inactivated) polio vaccine until the child has been off therapy for 1 year because the polioviruses are transmissible to the child who is immunocompromised (Committee on Infectious Diseases, 1997; Hastings, Goes, and Wolff, 1997).

Measles, Mumps, and Rubella (MMR)

The MMR vaccine is contraindicated in children receiving chemotherapy and for the first year off therapy. Many children lose protective titers after administration of chemotherapy. Hastings, Goes, and Wolff (1997) recommend that children be immunized 1 year after therapy is complete and every 10 years thereafter. If the child is directly exposed to someone with a documented case of measles and the child is seronegative for the rubeola antibody, the child should receive prophylactic γ-globulin at a dose of 0.5 ml/kg, with a maximum dosage of 15 ml (Committee on Infectious Diseases, 1997). Siblings may receive the MMR vaccine without any special precautions.

Haemophilus Influenzae Type B

The *Haemophilus influenzae* type B vaccine may be given according to the standard schedule for children with ALL or solid tumors who are in maintenance therapy. If the vaccine is received during therapy, a booster dose is recommended 1 year after therapy is complete (Hastings, Goes, and Wolff, 1997). Children diagnosed with Hodgkin's disease should be immunized at least 7 to 10 days before starting chemotherapy or undergoing a splenectomy. A booster dose is recommended 3 to 5 years after completing therapy.

Hepatitis B

The vaccine for hepatitis B is recommended for children who are unimmunized according to the standard schedule. Titers should be checked to document an adequate antibody response (Hastings, Goes, and Wolff, 1997). It has been suggested that children receive twice the usual recommended dose as a three-shot series in order to establish an adequate antibody response (Hovi et al, 1995).

Varicella Exposure Prophylaxis and Vaccination

If a child who is seronegative for antibody to the varicella virus or who has not been vaccinated has a direct exposure to a person with active chickenpox or to a person who develops lesions within 48 hours of the contact, the child must receive varicella-zoster immune globulin (VZIG). This vaccine is available with a physician's order through the regional distribution centers of the American Red Cross Blood Services and should be administered within 48 to 96 hours of exposure. The dose of VZIG is 125 units/10 kg, with a maximum dosage of 625 units. Once a child is exposed to chickenpox, the child must be isolated from other children who are immunocompromised from day 10 to day 28 following the exposure.

According to the Committee on Infectious Diseases (1997), children with malignancies should not routinely receive the live attenuated varicella vaccine. Use of the vaccine may be considered, however, for children with ALL who have been in remission for at least 1 year and who have an absolute lymphocyte count over 700. If the child develops a rash within 4 to 5 weeks of vaccine administration, vaccine associated varicella should be ruled out. Hastings, Goes, and Wolff (1997) recommend a booster dose 3 months after the first with follow-up titers several months after the vaccine to document response. They also suggest yearly titers and a third dose if titers fall. In addition, the vaccine should not be administered within 5 months of the administration of blood products or any form of immune globulin. Vaccination of these children is being coordinated under research protocols, and specific recommendations may vary between treatment centers. Transmission of vaccine type of varicella from healthy children to their immune-compromised siblings has not been documented (Gershon, 1995).

Other Immunizations

Children with Hodgkin's disease should receive the pneumococcal and meningococcal vaccines before splenectomy or splenic irradiation. Booster doses of these polysaccharide vaccines should be given in 2 to 3 years and then every 5 to 6 years (Hastings, Goes, and Wolff, 1997). Additionally, these children should be maintained on twice daily penicillin, daily amoxicillin, or daily erythromycin to prevent bacterial infection. (Committee on Infectious Diseases, 1997).

Although there is limited research to validate the efficacy of giving routine influenza vaccines to either the child with a malignant disease or to their families, many centers do recommend vaccine use for children and their families during therapy and for up to 1 year off therapy. Persons at risk for pulmonary fibrosis may also benefit from using the vaccine throughout their lives.

Screening

Vision

Routine vision screening is advised. A recurring brain tumor may manifest as impaired visual acuity caused by ocular nerve compression or increased intracranial pressure or as blurred vision caused by papilledema. There may be ptosis, visual disturbances, and sixth cranial nerve dysfunction with recurrent orbital rhabdomyosarcoma. Two classic signs of recurrent retinoblastoma are the white eye reflex in place of the normal red reflex and strabismus. Cataracts are also a late effect of radiation therapy. In addition, vincristine and vinblastine may cause ptosis that can interfere with vision.

Hearing

Routine screenings of hearing is advised. Unilateral hearing loss may indicate the presence of a mass. Children receiving radiation or cisplatin or both are at increased risk for hearing loss (Landier, 1998); evaluation by an audiologist every 6 to 12 months is recommended.

Dental

Routine dental care is advised during treatment and after therapy. Both radiation therapy and chemotherapy place a child at risk for stomatitis, dental caries, and periodontal disease. Dental work requiring manipulation of the oral tissues should be avoided if the ANC is less than 1000 or the platelet count is less than 50,000. All children with central VADs having dental manipulation should receive antibiotic prophylaxis to prevent subacute bacterial endocarditis, as recommended by the American Heart Association (Altman and Wolff, 1997; Dajani et al, 1997) (see Chapter 17 for SBE guidelines). Daily brushing with a soft-bristled brush and flossing are recommended when the ANC is over 500, the platelet count is over 100,000, and stomatitis is not present. Daily fluoride rinses may be indicated in children with a high potential for caries. Good oral hygiene is important in preventing stomatitis and infection. In the presence of low blood cell counts or stomatitis, cleansing with a mild solution of sodium bicarbonate using a gauze pad or sponge is recommended. A 0.12% chlorhexidine gluconate mouthwash helps to prevent infection (Groncy, Udin, and Ablin, 1997; Hockenberry-Eaton and Kline, 1997).

Blood Pressure

Blood pressure should be measured at every visit because of possible hypertension from corticosteroids, potential renal toxicity of many chemotherapeutic agents, and cardiac toxicities from anthracyclines.

Hematocrit

Because of frequent hematologic analyses, routine hematocrit screening is not necessary while a child is on therapy. After therapy, routine screening is recommended.

Urinalysis

Routine urinalysis is advised because it may reveal RBCs in children with bladder or kidney tumors. Late effects of radiation therapy may include proteinuria. Children receiving cyclophosphamide (Cytoxan) may experience hemorrhagic cystitis, although symptoms may occur months to years after the drug has been discontinued. Particular care is required to screen for and treat urinary tract infections in children who have undergone a nephrectomy.

Tuberculosis

Routine screening for tuberculosis of children off therapy is advised. Children receiving therapy may be anergic to skin testing. The placement of controls (e.g., *Candida* and diphtheria-tetanus [dT]) will help assess the individual's responsiveness. A chest radiograph may be necessary if skin testing is unsuccessful.

Children receiving immunosuppressive therapy are at risk for tuberculosis. Children with a significant exposure to tuberculosis should receive 12 months of therapy with isoniazid (Hastings, Goes, and Wolff, 1997).

Condition-Specific Screening

The primary care provider must keep in mind the possibility of abnormalities because of disease recurrence or the long-term effects of treatment (see Table 13-3). Screening for these complications

should be done in consultation with either the pediatric oncology team or other subspecialty team.

Common Illness Management

Differential Diagnosis (Box 13-5)

Fever

The presence of fever (i.e., 38.3° C or 101° F) adds a critical dimension to diagnosis and treatment in the face of neutropenia. If adequate therapy is not initiated promptly, the result could be life-threatening. The first step in evaluating a fever is obtaining a complete blood cell count (CBC) with differential to determine if the child is neutropenic, blood cultures from all central VAD lumens, and cultures from other potential sites of infection as indicated by the history and physical exam. Obtaining a chest radiograph is not indicated in the absence of respiratory symptoms (Korones, Hussong, and

---

Box 13-5

Differential Diagnosis

Fever
- Bacterial, viral, fungal, or protozoal infection
- Site: blood, VAD, nasopharynx, skin, joints, perineal, perirectal areas

Gastrointestinal Symptoms
- Diarrhea: infectious causes or chemotherapy induced
- Constipation: vinca alkaloids (paralytic ileus)
- Vomiting: chemotherapy-induced, anticipatory

Headache
- Increased intracranial pressure due to a mass lesion or shunt malfunction
- CSF leak with recent history of lumbar puncture

Pain
- Tumor-related due to compression of nerves or invasion of bone
- Treatment-related: mucositis, dermatitis, neurotoxicity, phantom limb pain, infection
- Procedure-related: bone marrow, lumbar puncture, venipuncture

Gullace, 1997). The physical exam should focus on the skin, nose, sinuses, pharynx, catheter site, joints, perineal and perirectal areas (Wolff et al, 1997).

The febrile child with a central VAD should have aerobic and anaerobic blood cultures obtained peripherally and from each lumen of the catheter or port. Parenteral broad-spectrum antibiotics are initiated and later modified based on culture and sensitivity results. If after 48 to 72 hours, the ANC is over 500, the cultures are negative, and the child is afebrile, antibiotics may be stopped. If the cultures are positive, a full 10- to 14-day course of antibiotics should be administered (Wolff et al, 1997).

Admission to the hospital for treatment is generally required for the febrile neutropenic (i.e., ANC < 500) child. In selected cases of moderate neutropenia (i.e., ANC 200 to 500), however, the child may be treated as an outpatient with daily examination by the oncologist (Mustafa et al, 1996; Wolff et al, 1997). After cultures are obtained, parenteral broad-spectrum antibiotics should be started immediately. Antibiotic choice is based on suspected organism and institutional-regional patterns of antibiotic resistance.

Viral Infections

The human viruses most frequently affecting children with malignant diseases are herpes simplex virus (HSV), varicella-zoster virus (VZV), and cytomegalovirus (CMV). Treatment of HSV infections in children with cancer is dependent on the site and severity of the infection but is most often with Acyclovir (250 mg/m^2 every 8 hours).

In the event that the child contracts a primary (chickenpox) or secondary (shingles) VZV infection, Acyclovir (500 mg/m^2 every 8 hours) should be administered intravenously immediately and continued for at least 7 days or until all lesions have crusted. Vigorous hydration and monitoring of BUN and creatinine during Acyclovir treatment is needed to prevent renal toxicity of the drug.

An acute CMV infection may present with fever, hepatosplenomegaly, retinitis, pneumonia, colitis, CNS manifestations, and a rash. Antiviral therapy for CMV includes the use of gancyclovir and immune globulin intravenously.

Other Infections

Candidiasis and aspergillosis are the two most common fungal infections in children with malignant diseases. Candidiasis is more common and can involve the oral mucosa, GI tract, urinary tract, bone, lungs, and, less frequently, the blood. Meticulous oral care and prompt identification of lesions help to reduce morbidity from oral candidiasis. Prophylactic oral care regimens may include baking soda or normal saline mouth rinses, 0.12% chlorhexidine gluconate, or antifungal suspensions or troches. Once an oral infection is documented, systemic oral antifungal agents may be used. Aspergillosis is seen most frequently in the respiratory tract, GI tract, and brain. Amphotericin B is the most effective drug for systemic fungal infection; however, it has potent side effects.

The child who is immunocompromised and at risk for *Pneumocystis carinii* may take trimethoprim/sulfamethoxazole (Septra, Bactrim) prophylactically. The usual dose is 150 mg/m^2 divided and given twice daily for 3 days each week. The prophylaxis is continued for approximately 6 months after the completion of therapy. In children who cannot tolerate Septra or Bactrim, daily oral dapsone or monthly aerosolized or intravenous pentamidine may be used (Committee on Infectious Diseases, 1997). Pneumonitis is the most common clinical manifestation of *Pneumocystis carinii*. Symptoms include a dry cough, fever, tachypnea, cyanosis, and respiratory distress. Onset may be acute (few days) or insidious (months). All significant infections in children who are immunocompromised should be managed by the oncology specialist.

Gastrointestinal Symptoms

Nausea, vomiting, and diarrhea, which are common side effects of cancer treatment, may be difficult to distinguish from infections caused by bacteria, protozoa, viruses, or *Clostridium difficile* toxin. The primary care provider must establish the relationship of the symptoms to the administration of chemotherapy or radiation. During these periods, it is important to monitor fluid intake and avoid dehydration, especially in children who are currently receiving chemotherapy. In some cases IV fluid replacement and antiemetics may be necessary. Stool cultures will help to identify an infectious source of diarrhea. Blood chemistry values, especially BUN, creatinine, AST, and ALT, must be monitored closely to avoid damaging vital organs from concentrated levels of the chemotherapeutics and from delayed excretion as a result of dehydration. Many families are taught how to administer antiemetics and IV hydration at home.

Vinca alkaloids predispose children to the development of constipation. If dietary intervention is not successful, supplementation with a stool softener or laxative will be needed to prevent paralytic ileus. This is most often needed when frequent repeated doses of vincristine are used. Suppositories and enemas should not be used without consultation with the oncology team because of the potential risk of infection related to reduced WBC counts.

Headaches

Headache pain, which is usually benign late in childhood and adolescence, is indicative of serious underlying difficulties in young children. Morning headaches associated with vomiting and minimal nausea should always arouse suspicion of increased intracranial pressure caused by a mass lesion or shunt malfunction in a child with a brain tumor. Headaches following a lumbar puncture, which resolve with lying down, may be caused by a slow cerebrospinal fluid leak. This type of headache is best treated by bed rest and adequate hydration. While taking a thorough history, the primary care provider should note onset, any precipitating factors or symptoms, location, severity, and what, if any, medication gives relief. A thorough neurologic examination is imperative. Many headaches may be treated at home with acetaminophen and rest; but if the headache symptoms are unrelieved by medication or there is any change in vision or neurologic function, immediate evaluation is necessary.

Pain

Pain in children is often difficult to assess and requires understanding of normal child development and age-appropriate verbal and behavioral cues. Most importantly, keep in mind that children rarely fabricate the presence of pain. The child with cancer poses additional challenges because of the multiple etiologies of pain, which may result from the malignancy, treatments, or procedures (e.g., bone marrow and spinal tap).

Tumor-related pain occurs with direct tumor invasion of the bone, impingement of the tumor on nervous tissue, or metastatic lesions. Compression of the spinal cord by a tumor may result in back pain and is accentuated by maneuvers such as coughing, sneezing, and flexion of the spine (Alt-man, Schechter, and Weisman, 1997). Immediate evaluation is imperative because an untreated cord compression can rapidly progress to irreversible neurologic damage. Treatment-related pain can occur from mucositis, infection, radiation-induced dermatitis, neurotoxicity from chemotherapy (vincristine), abdominal pain, or phantom limb pain following the amputation of a limb (Collins and Berde, 1997). Management of disease-related pain relies on pharmacologic and behavioral approaches. Systematic assessment of the child's pain is needed to design an optimal plan.

Pain resulting from procedures is greatly reduced with the use of conscious sedation (e.g., using a combination of a sedative [midazolam, promethazine, chlorpromazine] and an opioid [fentanyl, morphine, meperidine]). Some children who experience great psychologic or physical pain during procedures may benefit from the use of short-acting general anesthetics.

Topical anesthetics are used in combination with sedation to reduce procedural pain. EMLA (Astra), a eutectic prilocaine-lidocaine cream, is applied at least 1 hour prior to the planned procedure (Gimenez et al, 1996). It is available as a cream or patch. Numby Stuff (Iomed), a relatively new product, delivers lidocaine into the skin using a low-level electric current from a battery-powered dose control unit. Topical anesthesia for procedures is achieved in 7 to 15 minutes.

Nonpharmacologic therapies to reduce pain and distress include distraction, guided imagery, and hypnosis. Art and play therapy can also assist children and adolescents in coping with the loss of control and pain associated with invasive procedures (Council, 1998).

Drug Interactions

Children receiving therapy need to avoid aspirin-containing products because they impair platelet function. Acetaminophen is generally recommended; however, its use during periods of neutropenia is discouraged because it may mask a fever. Multivitamins high in folic acid should be avoided because of the interference of folate with methotrexate. Vitamins low in folic acid are acceptable. Because of the number of drugs a child may be taking for therapy and the possibility of interaction, it is advisable that the primary care provider contact the pediatric oncology team before prescribing additional medications.

Developmental Issues

Sleep Patterns

Disturbances in sleep patterns are common. The extent to which the child is affected will depend on the age at diagnosis, medication schedules, the frequency of hospitalizations, and the general coping patterns of the child. Maintaining a consistent bedtime ritual whenever possible provides security during a time when many things are disrupted. Parents should also be encouraged to accept transitional objects (e.g., a teddy bear or favorite blanket) because these may help the child with sleep during periods of hospitalization.

Toileting

Diarrhea and constipation may occur with certain chemotherapy agents. Toilet training may be delayed or regression may occur if treatment occurs during the toddler or preschool period.

Discipline

Discipline for the child with cancer should be the same as for all children. A consistent approach in establishing expectations and setting limits is important to the child's sense of security. The parents should be supported in maintaining normal patterns of discipline, although they may initially be ambivalent about disciplining their child who is ill. Consistency in discipline among siblings is also important (Lauria et al, 1996).

Child Care

The intensity of certain phases of therapy may make regular day care both impractical and potentially harmful to the child with cancer because of the increased risk of acquiring some infectious diseases in these settings. When a child has begun less intensive therapy, a home or small group situation is recommended because it minimizes exposure to the various common pediatric illnesses. The caretaker must be educated about (1) the child's disease

and instructed to notify the family immediately of any fever, signs and symptoms of infection, or increased bruising or bleeding; (2) reporting any communicable illness—especially chickenpox—in the other children; and (3) any medication or oral chemotherapeutic agent that must be administered during child care hours. In addition, the importance of good handwashing should be emphasized, especially before and after toileting, food preparation, and meals.

Schooling

With advances in the treatment of children with cancer, more children are surviving into adulthood. The child who is too ill to participate in the regular classroom should be enrolled in a home study program. The role of health care providers, parents, and educators is to work as a team to assist the child in returning to school as soon after diagnosis as is medically possible. The return to school provides a sense of normalcy and contributes to the child's sense of hopefulness (see Chapter 5).

The child's school reentry must be carefully planned. To enhance the child's participation in school activities and prevent discrimination, anticipatory guidance should include attention to the balance between special precautions that need to be taken for the child's safety, learning needs, and avoidance of overprotectiveness (Hersh et al, 1997). This can be achieved by mutual respect between parents and school personnel, a willingness to provide needed resources such as homebound education, and advocacy on the part of parents and the oncology team to educate school personnel as to the special needs created by hospitalizations, chemotherapy-induced side effects, and long-term sequelae of surgery, radiation, and chemotherapy on learning abilities.

Establishing an individualized educational program (IEP) can help define and anticipate the special needs of the child. The teachers and the school staff must be informed of the child's illness and implications that will influence attendance, social interaction, educational capacity, and the restrictions or special needs dictated by medical care. Early recognition of learning disabilities will enhance prompt assessment and intervention.

It is recommended that, with the family's and child's permission, the child's classmates be taught about the child's illness at an appropriate developmental level. The child will also need to be prepared to answer classmates' questions. The primary care provider can provide the family with support and resources to help ease the transition into school. (See Chapter 5.)

Sexuality

The child with cancer often struggles with an alteration in body image because of hair loss, weight loss or gain, or disfiguring surgery. A major task of these children is learning to deal with this change, be it temporary or permanent. This is especially true in adolescents who, in addition to treatment, may or may not be experiencing the normal pubertal changes. Ongoing monitoring of the child's development through the use of Tanner staging is important. Failure to progress through the stages warrants referral to a pediatric endocrinologist.

A young woman on chemotherapy may experience delayed development of secondary sexual characteristics and amenorrhea. After the cessation of therapy, development often occurs and the menses will begin. Fertility status of children surviving childhood malignancies varies depending on the type and extent of treatment. Transposition of ovaries from the radiation field has been shown to help preserve ovarian function (Pieters, 1997). It appears that treatment with chemotherapy does not increase the risk of congenital anomalies in the offspring of childhood cancer survivors (Green et al, 1997). Ongoing long-term follow-up is required.

Sperm banking should be offered to pubescent males, if feasible, before therapy because sterility and mutagenicity can occur from cancer treatment. Ongoing assessment of appropriate sexual development and functioning (e.g., libido, impotence) is important. Hormone replacement may be necessary if there is a deficiency. Peer support groups are often helpful in helping adolescents to deal with issues of sexuality and body image.

Transition into Adulthood

Because most children diagnosed with cancer are surviving into adulthood, pediatric cancer centers are attempting to create follow-up or "late effects" clinics that meet the needs of young adults or are

referring them to adult oncologists who have remained current on issues specific to childhood cancer survivors. Follow-up including the same multidisciplinary approach used during treatment would benefit the young adult (MacLean et al, 1996).

The protections provided by Americans With Disabilities Act of 1990 apply to persons with cancer—whether it is cured, controlled, or in remission. The Department of Defense generally does not allow cancer survivors to enlist but has provided waivers on a case-by-case basis when the individual has been off therapy with no recurrence for 5 years. To avoid job discrimination, it is advisable for young adults to apply for jobs for which they are clearly qualified, be honest with employers' questions but not volunteer a prior cancer history, and supply a letter from their primary care provider about prognosis and life expectancy if a question arises (Monaco, Smith, and Fiduccia, 1997). Health insurance through large employers is much less likely to create a barrier to coverage than individual or small business policies.

Special Family Concerns and Resources

Advances in medicine that have led to improved survival rates of children with cancer have also brought problems of chronic uncertainty. The uncertainty faced by families centers around the basic issue of the child's survival. Family concerns often reflect the phase of treatment they are experiencing. In the beginning, uncertainty is focused on whether or not remission will be obtained. If remission is achieved, will it be long-term or will relapse occur? If relapse occurs, will the child enter remission again or die? At the end of treatment, families struggle with ambivalent feelings; they are grateful for the end of therapy yet fearful of the loss of their "safety net" of frequent contact with providers and the end of drugs that have maintained remission (Chanock et al, 1997).

The goal of members of the health care team must be to help families cope with uncertainty—not to focus on the unlikely goal of removing that uncertainty (Lauria et al, 1996). Learning to cope with uncertainty is important to the health and well-being of all family members. Support for the child and family must be ongoing, not only at diagnosis but also long after completion of therapy or death of the child.

At diagnosis, parents often feel incredible guilt for not having brought the child to medical care sooner or for not being a more vocal advocate if providers did not realize the significance of the symptoms. The pediatric oncology team tries to support families through this difficult time by allowing opportunities for individual and family counseling. Siblings of the child with cancer benefit from an understanding of what happens during clinic and hospital visits and from interventions directly addressing their need for communication and support (Zeltzer et al, 1996).

Compliance becomes an issue when the child or adolescent's chemotherapy consists primarily of oral medications taken at home. Several factors including confusion about parental vs. adolescent responsibilities, denial of the illness, and a loss of control may have an effect on adolescent noncompliance (Hersh et al, 1997). Compliance in younger children usually encompasses a parental inability to get them to take the medication because of its taste or form or because of the timing of doses (Lau et al, 1998). There are many innovative methods that can be shared with parents if they express their difficulties in administering the chemotherapy.

Cultural issues related to how individuals regard and prepare for death are of particular interest in the care of children with cancer. In Korea, for example, dying outside of the home is considered very undesirable, which has implications for the importance of home care for these children who are terminally ill. With regard to the caretaking of children who are ill, mothers most commonly take on this responsibility in Korea, Japan, and many Hispanic families, whereas in China, fathers often assume this role when the child is ill (Martinson et al, 1995). At an appropriate time, assessing such issues as the family's feelings about disclosure of information to the child, caretaking responsibilities, death rituals, and comfort with asking questions and voicing concerns and disagreement with health care providers is important.

The financial burden of a catastrophic illness is of monumental concern to the family. It not only affects the current financial status of the family but also has far-reaching implications for the child's future insurability. Insurance companies and health maintenance organizations (HMOs) vary in their reimbursement of medications and procedures they deem to be experimental. All of these factors place a tremendous amount of stress on an already taxed family unit.

Numerous local, regional, and national organizations provide information and educational resources about childhood malignant diseases. Local hospitals and cancer centers often provide support groups for family members. Informal parent-to-parent interactions based on the sense of having a common understanding of parenting a child with cancer can be a powerful source of support. Identifying local resources will provide a much-welcomed service to these families.

Organizations

American Cancer Society, 1599 Clifton Rd, NE, Atlanta, Ga. 30329. (800)ACS-2345 or (404)320-3333; www.cancer.org. This is a volunteer organization offering educational programs, family services, rehabilitation support, and referral to local and regional resources.

Cancer Information Service, National Cancer Institute, Blair Bldg, Rm 414, 9000 Rockville Pike, Bethesda, MD 20892. (800)4CANCER; www.cancernet.nci.nih.gov. This is a network of regional information centers that provides personalized answers to cancer-related questions from individuals, families, the general public, and health care professionals. This organization also provides referral to local and regional resources.

Candlelighters Childhood Cancer Foundation, Inc, 7910 Woodmont Ave, Suite 460, Bethesda, Md. 20814. (800)366-2223 or (301)657-8401; www.candlelighters.org. This is an international organization of parents whose children have had cancer. This organization provides guidance and emotional support through local chapters, information, and referral to local and regional resources.

Leukemia Society of America, 600 Third Ave, New York, NY 10017. (800)955-4572 or (212) 573-8484; www. leukemia.org. This is a volunteer organization offering educational programs, information, financial assistance, and referral to local and regional resources.

***Summary of* Primary Care Needs for the Child with Cancer**

HEALTH CARE MAINTENANCE

Growth and development

Slowing of growth because of chemotherapy and radiation.

Closely monitor weight; child is at risk for significant weight loss because of disease and treatment and is also at risk for weight gain due to steroids.

Periodic developmental screening to assess for age-appropriate behaviors.

Neuropsychologic testing for children who received cranial radiation.

Diet

Maintain an adequate diet. Offer small frequent meals if the child is experiencing anorexia. Low-sodium foods should be given to children on corticosteroid therapy. Increase fluid intake and high-fiber foods for constipation. Monitor diarrhea closely.

Safety

Ensure proper handling of chemotherapeutic agents at home and proper maintenance and protection of indwelling venous access devices.

Check platelet count after significant fall or head injury. May need platelet transfusion.

Minimize roughhousing and discourage contact sports if the platelet count is less than 100,000. Because of photosensitivity, protect the child from sun. Use PABA-free sunblock.

Immunizations

No live virus vaccines while on therapy or for the first year off therapy.

Some centers recommend administering killed vaccines if the child is scheduled to receive them by age; booster doses, however, may be needed after therapy is complete. Other centers do not give killed vaccines until child has been off treatment for 6 months.

Siblings and household contacts should not receive live polio vaccine because of transmissibility to child who is immunocompromised.

Siblings and household contacts may receive MMR vaccine.

The varicella vaccine, although not routinely recommended for children with malignancies, is available for use in some children with ALL who have been in remission for at least 1 year.

Children recovering from bone marrow transplantation require special consideration in determining immunization schedule and protocol.

Children with Hodgkin's disease should be vaccinated with the pneumococcal and *H. influenzae* type B conjugate vaccines before splenectomy or splenic irradiation.

Screening

Vision

Routine screening is recommended. Thorough assessment is warranted if visual abnormalities are detected.

Hearing

Routine screening is recommended. Children receiving ototoxic drugs should have regular evaluations by an audiologist.

Dental

Routine screening is recommended. A CBC count should be done before an appointment to verify adequate ANC, platelet count. Meticulous oral hygiene is necessary to prevent infections. Oral SBE prophylaxis is needed for children with central VADs.

Blood pressure

Blood pressures should be taken at each visit to evaluate for hypertension as a result of drug toxicity.

Hematocrit

Hematocrit testing is routine and is done off therapy. It is done as needed while the child is on therapy. Critical levels are ANC less than 500, platelets less than 20,000, and hemoglobin less than 7 to 8 g/dl.

Urinalysis

Urinalysis is routine. Protein may be observed after radiation therapy, or hematuria may be seen after cyclophosphamide/ifosfamide therapy. Special caution should be taken when only one kidney is present.

Summary of Primary Care Needs for the Child
with Cancer—cont'd

Tuberculosis

Tuberculosis screening is routine and is done off therapy. Possible anergic status requires use of a control if tested on therapy.

Condition-specific screening

Close assessment is required for signs and symptoms of late effects of therapy or recurrence of malignancy (see Table 13-3).

HEALTH CARE MAINTENANCE
COMMON ILLNESS MANAGEMENT
Differential diagnosis

Fever

Rule out neutropenia and infection. Do septic work-up as warranted. Prompt intervention is required with neutropenia or the presence of central VAD.

Viral and other infections

VZIG required within 96 hours of exposure if the child does not have antibodies to varicella or has not been immunized. Acyclovir is given intravenously for chickenpox in the immunosuppressed individual. Rule out dissemination of disease.

Give *Pneumocystis carinii* prophylaxis.

Gastrointestinal symptoms

For chemotherapy-induced constipation, ensure adequate hydration and begin stool softeners or laxatives as needed. Avoid suppositories and enemas.

For nausea and vomiting, determine the relationship to chemotherapy and radiation; rule out viral and bacterial infection. Give hydration fluid and antiemetics as needed.

Headaches

Perform a thorough neurologic examination. Consider possibility of a brain tumor, CNS involvement, sinusitis, and lumbar puncture cerebrospinal fluid leak.

Pain

Determine the source of pain; rule out cord compression.

Premedicate for procedures.

Drug interaction

No aspirin-containing products should be given. Acetaminophen is recommended except in times of neutropenia to avoid masking a fever.

Low folic acid multivitamins may be taken. Consult with the oncology team before prescribing additional medication because of the risk of drug interaction.

DEVELOPMENTAL ISSUES
Sleep patterns

Disturbances are common. Maintain consistent bedtime schedule and routine whenever possible. A transitional object may increase security during hospitalization.

Toileting

Standard developmental counseling is advised. Regression may occur.

Discipline

Use normal patterns of discipline; it is important to maintain consistency for all siblings.

Child care

Generally a small group setting is better than a large group to minimize exposure to infections. The caretaker should know the signs and symptoms that pose a concern.

Schooling

The child should return to school as soon as possible. Ongoing communication between primary care providers and teachers is necessary. Education of school staff and classmates is crucial. Assist the family in developing an IEP. Periodically assess for school problems and learning disabilities. If the child is unable to participate in a regular school program, arrange for home tutoring.

Sexuality

Give support for altered body image. Assess for appropriate Tanner staging. Sperm banking may

Continued

Summary of Primary Care Needs for the Child with Cancer—cont'd

be an option before an adolescent male begins chemotherapy or radiation.

Transition into adulthood

Need to transition care from pediatric oncology center to adult oncology center knowledgable on long-term survival of children with cancer.

Primary care providers may be of assistance in employment situations, if requested by client, by providing factual information concerning prognosis.

SPECIAL FAMILY CONCERNS

Dealing with chronic uncertainty.
Insurance and catastrophic financial effects.
Address needs of siblings.

References

Adams S and Emerson S: Gene therapy for leukemia and lymphoma, Hematol Oncol Clin North Am 12:631-648, 1998.

Alavi J and Eck S: Gene therapy for malignant glioma, Hematol Oncol Clin North Am 12:617-629, 1998.

Altman A, Schechter N, and Weisman S: The management of pain. In Ablin A, editor: Supportive care of children with cancer, Baltimore, 1997, Johns Hopkins University Press, pp 155-174.

Altman A and Wolff L: The prevention of infection. In Ablin A, editor: Supportive care of children with cancer, Baltimore, 1997, Johns Hopkins University Press, pp 1-12.

American Academy of Pediatrics Section on Hematology/-Oncology: Guidelines for the pediatric cancer center and role of such centers in diagnosis and treatment, Pediatrics 99:139-141, 1997.

American Cancer Society: Cancer facts and figures—1998, Atlanta, 1998, The American Cancer Society.

American Society of Clinical Oncology: Update of recommendations for the use of hematopoietic colony-stimulating factors: evidence-based clinical practice guidelines, J Clin Oncol 14:1957-1960, 1996.

Appelbaum F: Allogeneic hematopoietic stem cell transplantation for acute leukemia, Semin Oncol 24:114-123, 1997.

Balis F, Holcenberg J, and Poplack D: General principles of chemotherapy. In Pizzo P and Poplack D, editors: Principles and practice of pediatric oncology, Philadelphia, 1997, Lippincott-Raven, pp 215-272.

Baquiran D, Dantis L, and McKerrow J: Monoclonal antibodies: Innovations in diagnosis and therapy, Semin Oncol Nurs 12:130-141, 1996.

Barnard D, Feusner J, and Wolff L: Blood component therapy. In Ablin A, editor: Supportive care of children with cancer, Baltimore, 1997, Johns Hopkins University Press, pp 37-46.

Baysinger M et al: A trajectory approach for the child/adolescent with cancer, J Pediatr Oncol Nurs 10, 133-138, 1993.

Betcher D et al: Chemotherapy-induced nausea and vomiting. In Ablin A, editor: Supportive care of children with cancer, Baltimore, 1997, Johns Hopkins University Press, pp 144-154.

Bhatia S et al: Breast cancer and other second neoplasms after childhood Hodgkin's disease, N Engl J Med 334:745-751, 1996.

Blatt J, Copeland D, and Bleyer WA: Late effects of childhood cancer and its treatment. In Pizzo P and Poplack D, editors: Principles and practice of pediatric oncology, Philadelphia, 1997, Lippincott-Raven, pp 1303-1330.

Bleyer WA et al: National cancer clinical trials: children have equal access; adolescents do not, J Adol Health 21:366-373, 1997.

Bleyer WA: Equal participation of minority patients in U.S. national pediatric cancer clinical trials, J Pediatr Hematol Oncol 19:423-427, 1997.

Brenner M: The applications of gene transfer to pediatric malignant disease. In Pizzo P and Poplack D, editors: Principles and practice of pediatric oncology, Philadelphia, 1997, Lippincott-Raven, pp 375-384.

Brodeur G et al: Biology and genetics of human neuroblastoma, J Pediatr Hematol Oncol 19:93-101, 1997.

Chanock S and Pizzo P: Infectious complications of patients undergoing therapy for acute leukemia: current status and future prospects, Semin Oncol 24:132-140, 1997.

Chanock S et al: The other side of the bed: what caregivers can learn from listening. In Pizzo P and Poplack D, editors: Principles and practice of pediatric oncology, Philadelphia, 1997, Lippincott-Raven, pp 1267-1282.

Cheung N: Principles of immunotherapy. In Pizzo P and Poplack D, editors: Principles and practice of pediatric oncology, Philadelphia, 1997, Lippincott-Raven, pp 323-342.

Clericuzio C and Johnson C: Screening for Wilms tumor in high-risk individuals, Hematol Oncol Clin North Am 9:12533-1265, 1995.

Close P et al: A prospective, controlled evaluation of home chemotherapy for children with cancer, Pediatrics 95:896-900, 1995.

Collins J and Berde C: Management of cancer pain in children. In Pizzo P and Poplack D, editors: Principles and practice of pediatric oncology, Philadelphia, 1997, Lippincott-Raven, pp 1183-1199.

Committee on Infectious Diseases: Report of the committee on infectious diseases, ed 24, Elk Grove Village, Ill., 1997, American Academy of Pediatrics.

Corn B et al: Stereotactic radiosurgery and radiotherapy: new developments and new directions, Semin Oncol 24:707-714, 1997.

Council T: Art therapy with pediatric cancer patients. In Malchiodi C, editor: Medical art therapy with children, Philadelphia, 1998, Jessica Kingsley Publishers, pp 75-94.

Dajani A et al: Prevention of bacterial endocarditis: recommendations by the American Heart Association, Circulation 96:358-366, 1997.

Dillon P and Weiner E: Venous access devices in children. In Ablin A, editor: Supportive care of children with cancer, Baltimore, 1997, Johns Hopkins University Press, pp 217-227.

Farrell M: Biotherapy and the oncology nurse, Semin Oncol Nurs 12:82-88, 1996.

Fessele K: Managing the multiple causes of nausea and vomiting in the patient with cancer, Oncol Nurs Forum 23:1409-1415, 1996.

Gershon A: Varicella vaccine: its past, present and future, Pediatr Infect Dis J 14:742-744, 1995.

Gimenez J et al: Anesthetic efficacy of eutectic prilocaine-lidocaine cream in pediatric oncology patients undergoing lumbar puncture, Ann Pharmacother 30:1235-1237, 1996.

Green D et al: Birth defects and childhood cancer in offspring of survivors of childhood cancer, Arch Pediatr Adolesc Med 151:379-383, 1997.

Groncy P, Udin R, and Ablin A: Mouth care. In Ablin A, editor: Supportive care of children with cancer, Baltimore, 1997, Johns Hopkins University Press, pp 210-216.

Gurney JG et al: Incidence of cancer in children in the United States, Sex-, race- and 1-year age-specific rates by distologic type, Cancer 75:2186-2195, 1995.

Hadaway L: Comparison of vascular access devices, Semin Oncol Nurs 11:154-166, 1995.

Haller J: AIDS-related malignancies in pediatrics, Radiol Clin North Am 35:1517-1538, 1997.

Hastings C, Goes C, and Wolf L: Immunization of the child with cancer. In Ablin A, editor: Supportive care of children with cancer, Baltimore, 1997, Johns Hopkins University Press, pp 12-22.

Heideman R et al: Tumors of the central nervous system. In Pizzo P and Poplack D, editors: Principles and practice of pediatric oncology, Philadelphia, 1997, Lippincott-Raven, pp 633-698.

Hersh S et al: Psychiatric and psychosocial support for the child and family. In Pizzo P and Poplack D, editors: Principles and practice of pediatric oncology, Philadelphia, 1997, Lippincott-Raven, pp 1241-1266.

Hobbie W et al: Late effects in long-term survivors. In Foley G, Fochtman D, and Mooney K, editors: Nursing care of the child with cancer, Philadelphia, 1993, WB Saunders, pp 466-496.

Hockenberry-Eaton M and Kline N: Nursing support of the child with cancer. In Pizzo P and Poplack D, editors: Principles and practice of pediatric oncology, Philadelphia, 1997, Lippincott-Raven, pp 1209-1228.

Horowitz M et al: Ewing's sarcoma family of tumors. In Pizzo P and Poplack D, editors: Principles and practice of pediatric oncology, Philadelphia, 1997, Lippincott-Raven, pp 831-864.

Hovi L et al: Impaired response to hepatitis B vaccine in children receiving anticancer chemotherapy, Pediatr Infect Dis J 14:931-935, 1995.

Kalapurakal J and Thomas P: Pediatric radiotherapy, Radiol Clin North Am 35:1265-1280, 1997.

Karius D and Marriott M: Immunologic advances in monoclonal antibody therapy: Implications for oncology nursing, Oncol Nurs Forum 24:483-494, 1997.

Korones D et al: Right atrial thrombi in children with cancer and indwelling catheters, J Pediatr 128:841-846, 1996.

Korones D, Hussong M, and Gullace M: Routine chest radiography of children with cancer hospitalized for fever and neutropenia, Cancer 80:1160-1164, 1997.

Krischer J et al: Clinical cardiotoxicity following anthracycline treatment for childhood cancer: the Pediatric Oncology Group experience, J Clin Oncol 15:1544-1552, 1997.

Kucera E et al: Imaging modalities in pediatric oncology, Radiol Clin North Am 35:1281-1300, 1997.

Kun L: General principles of radiation therapy. In Pizzo P and Poplack D, editors: Principles and practice of pediatric oncology, Philadelphia, 1997, Lippincott-Raven, pp 289-322.

Landier W: Hearing loss related to ototoxicity in children with cancer, J Pediatr Oncol Nurs 15:195-206, 1998.

Landis SH et al: Cancer statistics, 1998, CA Cancer J Clin 48:6-29, 1998.

Lau R et al: Electronic measurement of compliance with mercaptopurine in pediatric patients with acute lymphoblastic leukemia, Med Pediatr Oncol 30:85-90, 1998.

Lauria M et al: Psychosocial protocol for childhood cancer, Cancer 78:1345-1356, 1996.

Lea D: Gene therapy: current and future implications for oncology nursing practice, Semin Oncol Nurs 13:115-122, 1997.

Link M and Eilber F: Osteosarcoma. In Pizzo P and Poplack D, editors: Principles and practice of pediatric oncology, Philadelphia, 1997, Lippincott-Raven, pp 889-920.

MacLean W et al: Transitions in the care of adolescent and young adult survivors of childhood cancer, Cancer 78:1341-1344, 1996.

Martinson I et al: Impact of childhood cancer on Korean families, J Pediatr Oncol Nurs 12:11-17, 1995.

Mathew P et al: Complications and effectiveness of gastrostomy feedings in pediatric cancer patients, J Pediatr Hematol Oncol 18:81-85, 1996.

Monaco GP, Smith G, and Fiduccia D: Pediatric cancer: Advocacy, legal, insurance, and employment issues. In Pizzo P and Poplack D, editors: Principles and practice of pediatric oncology, Philadelphia, 1997, Lippincott-Raven, pp 1367-1382.

Mustafa M et al: A pilot study of outpatient management of febrile neutropenic children with cancer at low risk of bacteremia, J Pediatr 128:847-849, 1996.

Oberfield SE et al: Endocrine late effects of childhood cancers, J Pediatr 131:S37-S41, 1997.

Pieters R: Side effects of radiation therapy in children and their prevention and management. In Ablin A, editor: Supportive care of children with cancer, Baltimore, 1997, Johns Hopkins University Press, pp 118-143.

Pollock B, Krischner J, and Vietti T: Interval between symptom onset and diagnosis of pediatric solid tumors, J Pediatr 119:725-732, 1991.

Ravindranath Y et al: Autologous bone marrow transplantation versus intensive consolidation chemotherapy for acute myeloid leukemia in childhood, N Engl J Med 334:1428-1434, 1996.

Renick-Ettinger A: Chemotherapy. In Foley G, Fochtman D, and Mooney K, editors: Nursing care of the child with cancer, Philadelphia, 1993, WB Saunders, pp 81-116.

Ries LA et al: SEER cancer statistics review, 1973-1995, Bethesda, Md, 1998, National Cancer Institute.

Román J et al: Growth and growth hormone secretion in children with cancer treated with chemotherapy, J Pediatr 131:105-112, 1997.

Ross J et al: Geographical analysis of cases from the pediatric cooperative clinical trials groups, Cancer 77:201-207, 1996.

Ross J and Davies S: Childhood cancer etiology: recent reports, Med Pediatr Oncol 30:143-146, 1998.

Rumsey K and Richardson D: Management of infection and occlusion associated with vascular access devices, Semin Oncol Nurs 11:174-183, 1995.

Sanders J: Bone marrow transplantation in pediatric oncology. In Pizzo P and Poplack D, editors: Principles and practice of pediatric oncology, Philadelphia, 1997, Lippincott-Raven, pp 357-374.

Sandler D and Ross J: Epidemiology of acute leukemia in children and adults, Semin Oncol Nurs 24:3-16, 1997.

Schwartz et al: Survivors of childhood cancer: Assessment and management, St Louis, 1994, Mosby.

Secola R: Pediatric blood cell transplantation, Semin Oncol Nurs 13:184-193, 1997.

Sievers E and Loken M: Detection of minimal residual disease in acute myelogenous leukemia, J Pediatr Hematol Oncol 17:123-133, 1995.

Somani J and Larson R: Reimmunization after allogeneic bone marrow transplantation, Am J Med 98:389-398, 1995.

Vase J and Armitage J: Clinical applications of hematopoietic growth factors, J Clin Oncol 13:1023-1035, 1995.

Webb I and Anderson K: Transfusion support in acute leukemias, Semin Oncol 24:141-146, 1997.

Wexler L and Helman L: Rhabdomyosarcoma and undifferentiated sarcomas. In Pizzo P and Poplack D, editors: Principles and practice of pediatric oncology, Philadelphia, 1997, Lippincott-Raven, pp 799-830.

Wheeler V: Interleukins: the search for an anticancer therapy, Semin Oncol Nurs 12:106-114, 1996.

Winslow M, Trammell L, and Camp-Sorrel D: Selection of vascular access devices and nursing care, Semin Oncol Nurs 11:167-173, 1995.

Wolff L et al: The management of fever: In Ablin A, editor: Supportive care of children with cancer, Baltimore, Md., 1997, Johns Hopkins University Press, pp 23-36.

Zeltzer L et al: Sibling adaptation to childhood cancer collaborative study: Health outcomes of siblings of children with cancer, Med Pediatr Oncol 27:98-107, 1996.

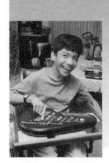

CHAPTER 14

Cerebral Palsy

Wendy M. Nehring

Etiology

Cerebral palsy, a condition first described by Dr. George Little in 1861, is an umbrella term used to define a group of nonprogressive disorders that cause aberrant movement and posture secondary to central nervous system (CNS) damage or insult in the early periods of brain development (Mutch et al, 1992). Cerebral palsy is described by both motor and anatomic groupings. Etiologically, it is a set of multifactorial disorders that are diverse in clinical presentation.

The classification system developed by Minear (1956) remains in use today. The four types of motor dysfunction seen in children with cerebral palsy are spastic, dyskinetic, ataxic, and mixed. Each of these types is then divided anatomically or by the number of extremities involved. Each category carries a different set of characteristics and prognoses (Box 14-1). Some health care professionals have started classifying cerebral palsy more succinctly according to the area of the brain affected (e.g., pyramidal [spastic] and extrapyramidal [primarily athetoid]) (Capute and Accardo, 1996) or more broadly according to muscle behavior or movement (Pellegrino and Dormans, 1998a). Young (1994) has stated that these terms may be presumptive or controversial, so the traditional classification model is used in this chapter.

Spastic

Spasticity describes the presence of increased muscle tone, which is noted through the passive range of motion of a joint. Characteristics of spastic or pyramidal cerebral palsy include persistent primitive reflexes, exaggerated stretch reflexes, positive Babinski reflex, ankle clonus, and later development of contractures. This form of cerebral palsy is most distinctly divided by the extremities involved and affects approximately 70% to 80% of people

with cerebral palsy. Damage occurs to the motor cortex and pyramidal tracts in the brain (Gersh, 1998a; Pellegrino and Dormans, 1998a).

Spastic diplegia affects all of the extremities, but the lower extremities are affected more than the upper (Pellegrino, 1997; Pellegrino and Dormans, 1998a). Spastic diplegia is often seen in premature and low birth weight infants and is related to cerebral asphyxia with or without the presence of an intraventricular hemorrhage and hydrocephalus. In mild cases, the condition may not be recognized until the child is school-aged. Spastic diplegia cerebral palsy occurs in 25% to 35% of the cases of cerebral palsy (Capute and Accardo, 1996; Pellegrino, 1997; Pellegrino and Dormans, 1998a).

Spastic quadriplegia is characterized by a dysfunction of the four extremities—sometimes the legs are more affected—and often of the musculature surrounding the trunk and the mouth, pharynx, and tongue. In a few rare cases, three limbs can be affected (i.e., triplegia). Spastic quadriplegia is the most common form associated with cerebral palsy, however, and is diagnosed in premature and low birth weight infants who have had severe asphyxial insults. Medical complications, seizures, mental retardation, and sensory impairments are often associated with quadriplegic cerebral palsy. Quadriplegia occurs in 40% to 45% of the cases of cerebral palsy (Capute and Accardo, 1996; Pellegrino, 1997; Pellegrino and Dormans, 1998a).

Spastic hemiplegia is characterized by a motor dysfunction on one side of the body with the upper extremity more affected than the lower extremity. This form of cerebral palsy is seen in low birth weight infants with a past episode of asphyxiation but can also result from a congenital vascular malformation or embolism causing postnatal brain damage. Periventricular leukomalacia is often found on an MRI. Medical complications, sensory impairments, and growth retardation are often present. Spastic hemiplegia occurs in approximately tone coordination by the CNS, which results from insult to the basal ganglia or extrapyramidal tracts. This category of cerebral palsy accounts for 10% to 15% of all cases of cerebral palsy. The two forms of dyskinetic cerebral palsy are athetoid and dystonic (Pellegrino and Dormans, 1998a).

Athetoid cerebral palsy has been associated with neonatal kernicterus and is the most common subtype of dyskinetic cerebral palsy (Palmer and Hoon, 1995). With prompt and aggressive management of hyperbilirubinemia in the first days of life, the incidence of cerebral palsy from this etiology has markedly decreased. Low birth weight and perinatal asphyxia are now more important risk factors (Capute and Accardo, 1996). Athetoid cerebral palsy is a result of damage to the basal ganglia and is characterized by chorea (i.e., jerky, rapid, and random movements) and athetosis (i.e., writhing and slow movements). Auditory impairment, dysarthria, and mental retardation are often associated with this type of cerebral palsy (Capute and Accardo, 1996).

Dystonic cerebral palsy is characterized by slow and twisting abnormal movements of the trunk or extremities that may involve abnormal posturing. In other words, with a voluntary change in position, the extremity moved shifts into an abnormal position and stays in that position (Pellegrino, 1997; Pellegrino and Dormans, 1998a).

30% to 40% of all cases of cerebral palsy (Capute and Accardo, 1996; Palmer and Hoon, 1995; Pellegrino and Dormans, 1998a).

Double hemiplegia occurs when both sides of the body are affected and is caused by damage or insults to both hemispheres of the brain. The difference between this diagnosis and spastic quadriplegia is that the upper extremities are more affected than the lower (Capute and Accardo, 1996).

Dyskinesic

Dyskinesia represents the second motor dysfunction group and is characterized by abnormal involuntary movements after the initiation of a voluntary movement and may show an inherited genetic pattern (Fletcher and Marsden, 1996). Children with this form of cerebral palsy often display rigid muscle tone when awake and normal or decreased muscle tone when asleep. This aberrant positioning is a result of the inadequate regulation of muscle

Ataxic

The third motor dysfunction group of cerebral palsy is ataxia. Neurologic damage is present in the cerebellum. Ataxia includes a range of conditions marked by the degree of muscle tone and coordination of movements and balance. These conditions can range from ataxic to hypotonic to atonic. Children with ataxia walk with an unstable, wide-based gait and have some difficulty trying to move a hand or arm voluntarily and/or timing such movement. Increased or decreased muscle tone may be present (Pellegrino, 1997; Pellegrino and Dormans, 1998a). The incidence of this type of cerebral palsy is approximately 5% to 10% (Palmer and Hoon, 1995; Pellegrino and Dormans, 1998a).

Mixed

The final motor dysfunction group of cerebral palsy is the mixed group, in which more than one type of motor pattern is found as a result of many defects to various areas of the brain. The term *mixed* is also used when no one motor pattern is dominant. Spasticity and dyskinesia can exist either alone or together (Pellegrino, 1997; Pellegrino and Dormans, 1998a).

The etiology of cerebral palsy may be due to a number of risk factors. Sometimes a cause for the diagnosis of cerebral palsy is never clearly identified. The possible causes are delineated by the period of time when the insult to the brain may have occurred in a child's life. In Table 14-1 the causes of cerebral palsy are listed according to the following time periods: prenatal, labor and delivery, perinatal, childhood (i.e., postnatal), and other. During the prenatal period, both maternal and gestational risk factors are included.

Parity alone is not a risk factor for cerebral palsy, but the incidence of cerebral palsy is increased with multiple births (Yokoyama, Shimizu and Hayakawa, 1995). Pharoah and Cooke (1997) discussed the vanishing-twin syndrome. This hypothesis concerns the increased risk for cerebral palsy in the surviving twin when the other twin dies late in gestation in monochorionic twin pregnancies. Further epidemiologic study is needed.

Incidence

The incidence of cerebral palsy is approximately 1.4 to 3 per 1000 live births (Dabney, Lipton, and Miller, 1997; Pellegrino, 1997). More specific findings from the 1988 National Health Interview Survey are found in Table 14-2. The 1992-1994 National Health Interview Survey does not specify specific conditions, such as cerebral palsy. Instead chronic conditions are grouped by diagnostic categories (Newacheck and Halfon, 1998; Newacheck and Taylor, 1992). The incidence of cerebral palsy in the United States has remained steady or has slightly increased since 1970 (see Table 14-2), mainly because of the decrease in incidences of kernicterus contrasted with the increase in very low birth weight and premature infants who survive (Lorenz et al, 1998). Lower rates of cerebral palsy have also been noted in mothers who received magnesium sulfate during pregnancy for tocolysis and preeclampsia. Further clinical study into the causes of cerebral palsy, however, is warranted (Hirtz and Nelson, 1998; Nelson, 1996; Schendel et al, 1996).

The specific prevalence of cerebral palsy is 2 per 1000 children at 3 years of age, with 10% of the cases being postnatal. Approximately 5000 infants born every year will be diagnosed with cerebral palsy. An additional 1,200 to 1,500 children are identified during the preschool years (Capute and Accardo, 1996; Pellegrino and Dormans, 1998a; United Cerebral Palsy Associations, 1996).

Clinical Manifestations at Time of Diagnosis

The three major elements leading to diagnosis of cerebral palsy are as follows: (1) a motor deficit with nonprogressive signs and symptoms; (2) failure of a child to reach normal motor milestones; and (3) CNS abnormality (Pellegrino and Dormans, 1998b). Diagnosis of cerebral palsy is based on an assessment of the child's developmental, functional, and physical abilities. If possible, medical history helps identify the cause of cerebral palsy. One or more forms of brain imagery are also done to aid in the diagnosis. When parents have related concerns, it is important for primary care providers to rule out other neurologic problems in conjunction with specialty consults. The diagnosis of cerebral palsy is not given until after the child is 2 years of age because early muscle and motor tone abnormalities may signify another neurodevelopmental problem. Moreover, some children who first present with risk factors of cerebral palsy no longer have them after 24 months of age. This change is especially true in cases of prematurity, although other communication and learning problems may persist (Pellegrino, 1997; Pellegrino and Dormans, 1998a).

Parents are often the first to discover a child's delayed or nonexistent attainment of motor milestones at the appropriate time and to bring this finding to the attention of their primary care provider. Specific signs noted by the practitioners include poor head control and clenched hands after 3 months of age, no side protective reflexes after 5 months of age, extended Moro and atonic neck reflexes past 6 months of age, no parachute reflex after 10 months of age, crossing of the midline to reach objects before 12 months of age, hand preference before 18 months of age—sometimes as early as 6 months, and/or leg scissoring in late infancy or

Table 14-1
Causes of Cerebral Palsy

Time Period	Causes
Prenatal (44%)	**Maternal:** Diabetes or hyperthyroidism Malnutrition Seizure disorder or mental retardation Infections Incompetent cervix Bleeding Polyhydramnios Previous child with developmental disabilities Previous premature birth Previous fetal loss Medication use (e.g. thyroid, estrogen, or progesterone) **Gestational:** Chromosomal abnormalities Genetic syndromes Teratogens Rh incompatibility Infections Congenital malformations Fetal development abnormalities Problems in placental functioning
Labor and Delivery (19%)	**Labor and delivery complications:** Premature delivery Prolonged rupture of membranes Fetal heart rate depression Abnormal presentations Long labor Preeclampsia Asphyxia
Perinatal (8%)	**Prematurity and associated problems:** Sepsis and/or CNS infection Seizures Interventricular hemorrhage (IVH) Periventricular encephalomalacia (PVL) Meconium aspiration Days on mechanical ventilation Persistent pulmonary hypertension in newborn Intrauterine growth retardation Low birth weight
Childhood/Postnatal (5%)	**Brain injury:** Meningitis/encephalitis Toxins Traumatic brain injury Infections
Unknown (24%)	

Adapted from Gersh E: What is cerebral palsy? In Geralis E, editor: Children with cerebral palsy: a parent's guide, ed 2, Bethesda, Md., 1998a, Woodbine House.

Hagberg B, Hagberg G, and Olow I: The changing panorama of cerebral palsy in Sweden, 1984-1970; II: analysis of the various syndromes, ACTA Paediatr Scand 64:193-202, 1975.

Murphy DJ, Hope PL, and Johnson A: Neonatal risk factors for cerebral palsy in very preterm babies: case-control study, Brit Med J 314:404-408, 1997.

O'Shea TM, Klinepeter KL, and Dillard RG: Prenatal events and the risk of cerebral palsy in very low birth weight infants, Am J Epidemiol 147:362-369, 1998.

Pellegrino L: Cerebral palsy. In Batshaw ML, editor: Children with disabilities, ed 4, Baltimore, Md., 1997, Paul H. Brookes.

Pellegrino L and Dormans JP: Definitions, etiology, and epidemiology of cerebral palsy. In Dormans JP and Pellegrino L, editors: Caring for children with cerebral palsy: a team approach, Baltimore, Md., 1998a, Paul H. Brookes.

Pinto-Martin JA et al: Cranial ultrasound prediction of disabling and nondisabling cerebral palsy at age 2 in a low birth weight population, Pediatrics 95:249-254, 1995.

Table 14-2
Prevalence Rates of Cerebral Palsy in Children under 18 Years of Age Based upon the 1988 National Health Interview Survey

National prevalence	1.8/1000
Prevalence in children under 10 years of age	2.2/1000
Prevalence in children 10 to 17 years of age*	1.2/1000
Prevalence in boys	2.0/1000
Prevalence in girls*	1.5/1000
Prevalence in Caucasians	1.9/1000

*Standard error exceeds 30% of the estimate value.
Adapted from Newacheck PW and Taylor WR: Childhood chronic illness: prevalence, severity, and impact, Am J Pub Health 82:364-371, 1992.

the early toddler period. These signs can appear in one or both sides (DeLuca, 1996; Pellegrino, 1997). An assessment of normal and abnormal muscle tone is outlined in Box 14-2.

Other behavioral manifestations during infancy that may be indicative of cerebral palsy include irritability, a weak cry, poor sucking ability with tongue thrust, excessive sleep patterns, and little interest in surroundings. Infants may also sleep in a rag doll or floppy position or in an arched and extended position (i.e., opisthotonos). Later signs include "bunny hopping" (i.e., when crawling, the legs are brought forward together after the hands and arms are advanced) and "W sitting" (Capute and Accardo, 1996; Pellegrino and Dormans, 1998a). Children may also show signs of toe walking, crouched gait, foot deformity, flat foot, unequal leg length, and/or walking on the outer aspects of the feet (DeLuca, 1996). A summary of the clinical manifestations of cerebral palsy is found in Box 14-3, and an example of scissoring is shown in Figure 14-1.

Treatment

The goals of treatment of children with cerebral palsy are designed to maintain mobility and maximize joint range of motion, as well as to optimize muscle control and balance and the ability to communicate and to perform activities of daily living. The orthopedic goals of treatment specific for nonambulatory children are to prevent hip dislocation, provide assistance with the activities of daily life,

---

Box 14-2

Assessment of Tone in Infants

Normal tone
Infant moves well against gravity and lacks high or low tone characteristics.

Low tone
Infant lacks tone to move against gravity and resistance to passive movement; has low tone postures (e.g., supine-lying with arm abducted and/or legs abducted in a frogged position) or decreased movement.

High tone
Infant becomes stiff when moving against gravity; the neck or extremities resist passive movement; infant has hypertonic head reactions (e.g., hyperextension of the neck when rolling over and/or head pushing when supine or when pulled to sitting position); infant has high tone posturing (e.g., increased extension of the head when supine-lying, retracted shoulder girdle, and lordosis of the back of extended lower extremities).

---

and help them develop good sitting posture (Dabney, Lipton and Miller, 1997). Treatment should always be individualized and developmentally appropriate to the type and severity of the cerebral palsy (Pellegrino, 1997). A summary of the forms of treatment used in cerebral palsy is in Box 14-4.

During infancy and toddlerhood, when most presumptive diagnoses take place, the first line of treatment involves physical and occupational therapy. The aim of these therapies is to enhance motor development and minimize the development of contractures (Pellegrino, 1997). For example, strength training has also been used with good results (Damiano and Abel, 1998).

More recently, physical therapists have used neuromuscular electrical stimulation in tandem with standard active and passive therapies to improve joint mobility, control muscle movement and strength, and reduce spasticity. Neuromuscular electrical stimulation has not been found useful for every muscle group but has been used successfully in muscle groups responsible for achieving task-

Box 14-3

Clinical Manifestations of Cerebral Palsy

Delayed or absent motor milestones
Poor head control
Clenched fists after 3 months
Prolonged primitive reflexes
Hand preference before 18 months
Irritability
Weak cry
Poor sucking ability with possible tongue thrust
Prolonged sleeping patterns
Hypo- or hypertonia
Lack of interest in the environment
Scissoring of the legs, clasped knife appearance
Asymmetries of movement
"Bunny hopping"
"W sitting"
Toe walking
Crouched gait
Foot deformity
Flat foot
Unequal limb length
Walking on outer aspects of feet

Adapted from Capute AJ and Accardo PJ: Cerebral palsy: the spectrum of motor dysfunction. In Capute AJ and Accardo PJ, editors: Developmental disabilities in infancy and childhood, vol. II: the spectrum of developmental disabilities, ed 2, Baltimore, Md, 1996, Paul H. Brookes.

DeLuca PA: The musculoskeletal management of children with cerebral palsy, PCNA 43:1135-1150, 1996.

Gersh E: What is cerebral palsy? In Geralis E, editor: Children with cerebral palsy: a parent's guide, ed 2, Bethesda, Md., 1998a, Woodbine House.

Pellegrino L: Cerebral palsy. In Batshaw ML, editor: Children with disabilities, ed 4, Baltimore, Md., 1997, Paul H. Brookes.

Pellegrino L and Dormans JP: Definitions, etiology, and epidemiology of cerebral palsy. In Dormans JP and Pellegrino L, editors: Caring for children with cerebral palsy: a team approach, Baltimore, Md., 1998a, Paul H. Brookes.

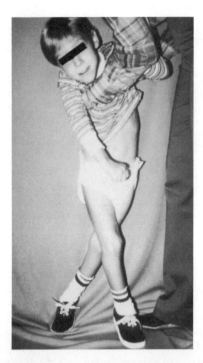

Figure 14-1   An example of scissoring in a young boy. (From Canale ST and Beaty JH: Operative pediatric orthopaedics, ed 2, St Louis, 1995, Mosby.)

oriented activities (Rose and McGill, 1998; Steinbok, Reiner and Kestle, 1997).

From the preschool years through adolescence, the aim of a treatment program is to help a child with cerebral palsy function optimally in the classroom. Gross motor skills, muscle control, balance, and coordination are needed for sitting and moving. Fine motor skills, muscle control, and coordination are needed for writing and holding materials. Motor, cognitive, and language skills also are needed for self-care activities. Independent ambulation may be decreased in adolescents using an orthotic device because of contractures, a lack of motivation, or weight gain (Pellegrino, 1997; Pellegrino and Dormans, 1998a).

Orthotic devices, which include braces and splints, usually accompany therapy when it alone no longer helps the child. Orthotic devices are used to provide stability to the joints, maintain the optimal range of motion of the joints, prevent the occurrence or progression of contractures, and control involuntary movements. The most common types of orthoses are the short leg brace, the hand brace, and the molded ankle-foot orthosis (MAFO), which is worn inside the shoe. Other types of adaptive equipment include boards for positioning a child (e.g., on his or her side or in the prone or supine posi-

Box 14-4

Treatments for Cerebral Palsy

Therapies
Physical
Method programs (e.g., Bobath)
Neuromuscular electrical stimulation
Occupational
Speech

Orthotic Devices
Braces
Splints
Casting

Adaptive Equipment
For functional use (e.g., eating utensils)
Switches
Computers
Boards
Scooters and tricycles
Wheelchairs

Surgery
Orthopedic-corrective (e.g., tendon transfers, muscle lengthening)
Neurologic (e.g., neurectomies)
Selective dorsal rhizotomy

Medications (for)
Spasticity
Pain
Constipation
Urinary tract infections
Upper respiratory infections
Decubitus
Other secondary complications and conditions

Special Education
Early intervention programs
Specialized learning programs and support services in school

tions), scooters, tricycles, and wheelchairs. In severe cases, wheelchairs and gait trainers are constructed and molded for an individual child (Figure 14-2) (Pellegrino, 1997). In each case, the orthosis is designed for a child and altered as the child grows or the condition changes.

Surgery for cerebral palsy is not an early choice of intervention. Both orthopedic and neurologic forms of surgery have been performed, but orthopedic surgery is not usually performed until after a child is 7 or 8 years old. A child attains independent ambulation by this age if independence is at all possible. Orthopedic surgery is performed to achieve greater leg movement and gait control, as well as to correct any extremity deformities. Orthopedic surgery is done to correct hip subluxation or dislocation and spinal deformities (e.g., scoliosis), to promote muscle balance and joint stabilization, and to reduce spasticity through muscle lengthening and tendon transfers (Pellegrino, 1997; Pellegrino and Dormans, 1998a).

Neurosurgery is done less frequently. The results of cerebellar and spinal cord stimulation for spasticity and stereotactic thalamic lesioning techniques to control abnormal movements have been mixed (Pellegrino, 1997).

Selective dorsal rhizotomy is still performed on a number of children with cerebral palsy. The best results have been obtained when prematurity is the cause of the cerebral palsy. Athetosis, extensive rigidity, and decreased strength and balance, however, are contraindications for this procedure (DeLuca, 1996). Increased studies have been done examining the effectiveness of selective dorsal rhizotomy, primarily in children with diplegic cerebral palsy (Buckon et al, 1995; Craft et al, 1995; Houle et al, 1998; McLaughlin et al, 1998; Thomas et al, 1997; Wright et al, 1998). The outcome of this surgical procedure is controversial; researchers have found both positive and negative results. Positive results included improvements in tasks requiring attention and cognition (Craft et al, 1995), gross motor function (Wright et al, 1998), and bladder function (Houle et al, 1998). Craft and colleagues (1995) cautioned that even with positive findings, a direct link to the procedure could not be proven. McLaughlin and associates (1998) found no differences between an intensive physical therapy program and the same program with selective dorsal rhizotomy. Thomas and colleagues (1997) also found no significant gait improvement 2 years after the procedure. Further study is needed to look at the long-term effects of selective dorsal rhizotomy on the symptomatology of cerebral palsy, including its effects on activities of daily life (Wright et al, 1998). In the meantime,

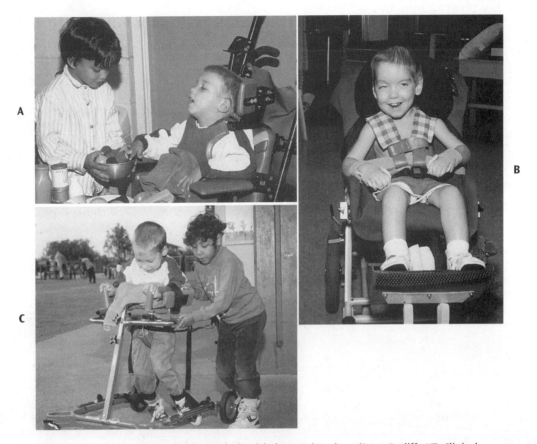

Figure 14-2   **A** and **B,** Individualized wheelchair. **C,** Gait trainer. (From Ratliffe KT: Clinical pediatric physical therapy, St Louis, 1998, Mosby.)

the primary care provider, surgeon, parents, and child should carefully discuss the risks and benefits.

Medications are usually unsuccessful in controlling symptoms, especially in children with ataxic and dyskinetic forms of cerebral palsy. Dantrolene sodium (Dantrium), baclofen (Lioresal Oral and Intrathecal [after 4 years of age]), diazepam (Valium), phenol and alcohol blocks, and botulinum toxin injections have been helpful in reducing spasticity (Im and McDonald, 1997). Ambulation may also improve with continuous intrathecal baclofen infusion. The effect of these drugs is individual, and at necessary doses their side effects have created further problems in many children (Albright et al, 1998; Bodensteiner, 1996; DeLuca, 1996; Gerszten, Albright, and Berry, 1997; Rawlins, 1998).

Along with an interdisciplinary health plan, which is mandatory for children with cerebral palsy, an accommodation plan or individualized educational program (IEP) is also necessary. Children must also have special support services throughout their developing years. (See Chapter 5 for more information on daycare and school issues and needs).

Recent and Anticipated Advanced in Diagnosis and Management

Cranial ultrasounds (Wilson-Costello et al, 1998), as well as MRIs to identify pathogenesis (Okumura et al, 1997), seem to facilitate early diagnosis of cerebral palsy in low birth weight and premature infants. Documentation of the effects of medications, specifically continuous intrathecal baclofen infusion on spasticity and ambulation, will further the continued efforts to improve the quality of life in children with cerebral palsy. Moreover, growth charts for children with cerebral palsy should be developed within the next decade (Stevenson, 1996). The use of magnesium sulfate during pregnancy to reduce the incidence of neurologic impairment, including cerebral palsy in premature infants, is perhaps of most interest today (Hirtz and Nelson, 1998; Nelson, 1996; Schendel et al, 1996). Randomized clinical studies are yet to be completed.

Associated Problems

Secondary conditions usually coexist and may include cognitive impairments (i.e., mental retardation or learning disabilities), seizures, sensory impairments (i.e., language and speech, vision, or hearing), motor problems, feeding issues, bowel and bladder problems, pulmonary infections, decubitus, dental problems, and behavioral and emotional problems (Box 14-5) (Capute and Accardo, 1996; Pellegrino and Dormans, 1998a). Plans for treatment, education, and habilitation must consider a child's individual presenting symptomatology and complaints. Secondary conditions may be acute, chronic, or transitory.

Cognitive Impairments

Learning disabilities or mental retardation frequently occurs in children with cerebral palsy. Mental retardation is usually most profound in children with spastic quadriplegia and least profound with hemiplegia, wherein over 60% of the children have a normal IQ. Of the children with spastic quadriplegia, diplegia, and extrapyramidal and mixed type of cerebral palsy, 50% to 60% also have mental retardation. Even if a child's IQ is normal, perceptual impairments and learning disabilities often exist; any associated speech articulation problems, however, should not be misconstrued as mental retardation (Capute and Accardo, 1996; Gersh, 1998a; Pellegrino, 1997; Pellegrino and Dormans, 1998a). For example, children with hemiplegia also have perceptual and attentional problems, with children with left hemiplegia ex-

periencing more perceptual problems and inattention than children with right hemiplegia (Katz, Cermak, and Shamir, 1998).

Seizures

Approximately 25% to 50% of children with cerebral palsy will also experience seizures. Seizures are most commonly seen in children with spastic quadriplegia and hemiplegia and are less common in children with dyskinesias and ataxia. Generalized tonic-clonic and minor motor types of seizures are the most common (Capute and Accardo, 1996; Palmer and Hoon, 1995; Pellegrino, 1997; Pellegrino and Dormans, 1998a). (See Chapter 21 for a further discussion of seizure disorders.)

Speech Impairments

The same muscle tone problems that make it difficult for children with cerebral palsy to move also create oral-motor problems. Limitations in trunk movements and positioning may limit lung capacity, which is needed for strength in speaking both clearly and loudly. Problems in articulation, dysarthrias, are caused by muscle tone deficiencies (Gersh, 1998a). In recent years, computers and adaptive equipment (e.g., switches) have allowed individuals with speech problems to dramatically improve their communication (Figure 14-3).

Sensory Deficits

Children with cerebral palsy may develop a number of visual problems, including refractive error, strabismus, amblyopia, cataracts, retinopathy of prematurity, and cortical blindness. The majority of all children with cerebral palsy develop strabismus (Gersh, 1998b); about 75% develop some form of refractive errors (i.e., most often farsightedness), and approximately 25% with hemiplegia develop homonymous hemianopsia (the inability to see toward the affected side) (Palmer and Hoon, 1995).

A small percentage of children with cerebral palsy have hearing impairments (5% to 15%). The hearing loss is either sensorineural (i.e., damage to the auditory nerve and/or the inner ear) or, more commonly, conductive (i.e., as a result of anatomic abnormalities and/or frequent otitis media). Hearing impairments further add to speech and commu-

---

Box 14-5

Problems Associated with Cerebral Palsy

Cognitive
Learning disabilities
Mental retardation

Seizure Disorders

Language and Speech Disorders
Articulation
Vocal strength and quality
Language processing

Vision
Refractive errors
Strabismus
Amblyopia
Cataracts
Retinopathy of prematurity
Cortical blindness
Homonymous hemianopsia (Hemiplegia)

Hearing
Conductive
Sensorineural

Other Sensory
Tactile hyper- or hyposensitivity
Dyspraxia
Balance and movement problems
Proprioception difficulties
Stereognosis

Motor
Prolonged primitive reflexes
Absence of protective reflexes
Delayed motor milestones
Hip subluxation and dislocation
Scoliosis
Contractures

Feeding and Eating Problems
Chewing, sucking, and swallowing deficits
Drooling

Hypoxemia
Fatigue
Under- and overweight
Gastroesophageal reflux
Aspiration

Bowel
Constipation
Encopresis

Urinary
Bladder control
Urinary retention
Urinary tract infections

Dental
Malocclusions
Enamel defects and caries
Gum hyperplasia (with phenytoin)

Pulmonary
Respiratory infections
Pneumonia

Skin
Decubitus
Latex allergy

Behavioral and Emotional
Behavioral disorders
Attention deficit disorder, with and without hyperactivity
Self-injurious behaviors
Depression
Autism
Growth failure
Other

nication delays (Gersh, 1998b; Palmer and Hoon, 1995).

As a result of damage to the parietal lobe of the brain, children with cerebral palsy have deficits in other sensory functions. These deficits may include tactile hypersensitivity or hyposensitivity, dyspraxia (i.e., difficulty in using one's senses to plan movements), balance difficulties, and problems with proprioception and movement (Gersh, 1998a).

Motor Impairments

Successful attainment of motor milestones is always delayed in children with cerebral palsy. Some

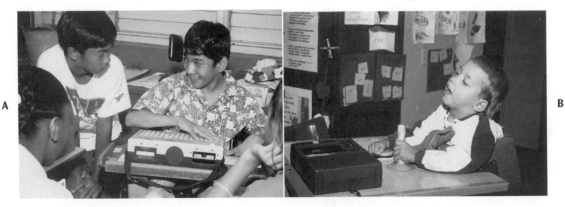

Figure 14-3   **A,** Child using an augmentative communication device. **B,** Child using a switch-activated tape player to sing along with music. (From Ratliffe KT: Clinical pediatric physical therapy, St Louis, 1998, Mosby.)

children's primitive reflexes persist and protective reflexes never develop, thus permanently blocking their ability to ambulate. Poor muscle tone and control often lead to secondary physical problems (e.g., hip dislocation, scoliosis, and contractures), which create further motor impairment and other medical problems related to basic physiologic functioning. In the worst-case scenario, these impairments are life-threatening.

Hip Dislocation, Scoliosis, and Contracture

Subluxation and dislocation of the hip are common in children with cerebral palsy (Figure 14-4). Subluxation occurs in approximately 25% of children with spastic cerebral palsy, and children bedridden with spastic quadriplegia are especially at risk. Complications can include further motor impairment, positioning difficulties, pain, chronic arthritis, scoliosis, and hygienic concerns (Gersh, 1998b).

Scoliosis can result from unequal muscle tension resulting from the cerebral palsy or from poor posture or positioning in seating and recumbent positions. The degree of scoliosis directly coincides with the amount of spasticity and neurologic damage present. The prevalence of scoliosis varies from 5% to 65% (Dabney, Lipton, and Miller, 1997; Gersh, 1998b).

Shortening and misalignment of the muscles can be created by a constant pull of tight muscles

or spasticity or by diminished muscle use, which may lead to contractures. Contractures in the lower extremities are most often seen in children with spastic quadriplegia and diplegia. Contractures in the upper extremities are most commonly found in children with spastic hemiplegia (Gersh, 1998b).

Feeding and Eating Problems

Feeding and eating difficulties are common in children with cerebral palsy primarily as a result of orofacial muscle impairments. Compromised cardiopulmonary functioning, as well as poor muscle tone (i.e., either hypertonic or hypotonic) in the neck, shoulders, and trunk, can impede the process of eating. Specifically, muscle tone and function deficits create problems with sucking, chewing, and swallowing. Increased drooling and gastroesophageal reflux may also occur. Feeding and eating disabilities are most often seen in children with athetoid type of cerebral palsy.

Bowel Problems

Constipation is a common and often chronic condition in children with cerebral palsy. Low muscle tone or spastic abdominal muscles can prevent contractility and pressure to adequately advance and empty the bowel contents. Further reasons for constipation include: lack of exercise; inability to sense the signals of a bowel movement; painful

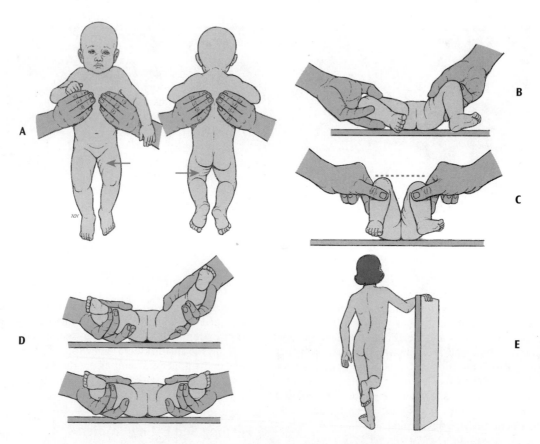

Figure 14-4   Signs of developmental dysplasia of the hip. **A,** Asymmetry of gluteal and thigh folds. **B,** Limited hip abduction, as seen in flexion. **C,** Apparent shortening of the femur, as indicated by the level of the knees in flexion. **D,** Ortolani click (if infant is under 4 weeks of age). **E,** Positive Trendelenburg sign or gait (if child is weight bearing). (From Wong DL et al: Whaley and Wong's nursing care of infants and children, ed 6, St Louis, 1999, Mosby.)

defecations; inadequate fluid intake; a diet lacking in fruits, vegetables, and fiber; medications; a fear of toileting; poor positioning on the toilet; and behavior problems (Gersh, 1998b). Bowel incontinence can also occur in cerebral palsy. Good dietary and bowel management is imperative.

Urinary Problems

Problems with bladder control and urinary retention that occur in cerebral palsy are often the result of neurologic insults (Mayo, 1992). Cognitive disabilities may reduce a child's ability to sense bladder fullness and signals to urinate. A combination of incomplete bladder emptying, infrequent void-

ing, severe fluid restriction, and urinary reflux increase the likelihood of frequent urinary tract infections (Dorval, 1994), as do chronic constipation, improper perineal hygiene, and motor impairments. Overall, children with cerebral palsy are three times as likely to have urinary tract infections than the general population (Gersh, 1998b). Prompt medical treatment of urinary tract infections is imperative.

Dental Problems

Malocclusions commonly occur in children with cerebral palsy as a result of orofacial muscle tone deficiencies. An over- or underbite can affect chewing and speech. Tooth enamel defects also occur frequently and if untreated may lead to dental caries. Children who have seizures and take phenytoin may experience hyperplasia (i.e., excessive growth of the gums). Problems with gum disease and oral hygiene can occur (Gersh, 1998b). Other medications taken for spasticity (e.g., sedatives or barbiturates) can reduce the amount of saliva, increasing the propensity for dental caries (Leibold, 1994).

Pulmonary Effects

Alterations in positioning caused by abnormal muscle tone and spasticity, immobility, scoliosis, and contractures can affect pulmonary function and place children with cerebral palsy at a higher risk for respiratory infections (e.g., pneumonia). When respiratory infections occur, they often linger beyond the usual period because many children have difficulty coughing and blowing their nose. Aspiration and gastroesophageal reflux can also cause pneumonia. Knowing the warning signs of respiratory infection and pneumonia is important for health professionals and families because pneumonia is the leading cause of death in children with cerebral palsy (Evans and Alberman, 1990; Gersh, 1998b). Children with severe dysphagia who show abnormal respiratory rates and fatigue during feeding are likely hypoxemic (Rogers et al, 1993).

Skin Problems

Skin breakdown leading to raw and excoriated skin and decubiti is a common problem in children affected by cerebral palsy—especially when mobility is compromised. Thorough skin assessment and protection of bony prominences while a child is seated or recumbent is necessary. Prompt and aggressive treatment of any evidence of skin breakdown is necessary.

Latex Allergy

An association between cerebral palsy and latex allergy has recently been reported. Primary care providers should be mindful of the risk for anaphylaxis if a child has had repeated surgeries and ventriculoperitoneal shunts (Delfico et al, 1996).

Behavioral and Emotional Problems

As a result of exaggerated and prolonged existence of primitive reflexes—especially the startle reflex, infants and children with cerebral palsy overreact to the mildest amounts of stimulation. As a result of the many problems associated with cerebral palsy, these children easily become tired, frustrated, and demanding and uncooperative (Urbano, 1992). Approximately 20% of children with cerebral palsy may also develop attention deficit hyperactivity disorder (Gersh, 1998a). Increased reports of depression in adolescents with cerebral palsy have also been reported.

Prognosis

Prognosis, similar to treatment, depends on the type and severity of the cerebral palsy. In general, the more extremities involved, the worse the prognosis (Pellegrino, 1997; Pellegrino and Dormans, 1998a). In the 1988 National Health Interview Survey, 89.2% of the respondents with cerebral palsy indicated that they were limited in their ability to conduct everyday activities as a result of cerebral palsy. Yet approximately 75% of the same respondents to this survey indicated that they never or rarely were bothered by their conditions, which suggests that these individuals adjusted well to their diagnosis (Newacheck and Taylor, 1992).

Prognosis is also specifically discussed in terms of independent ambulation. If primitive reflexes are generally still present at 12 months of age and the protective reflexes are not yet present or the child has not walked by 6 to 7 years of age, the child will not ambulate independently (Pellegrino and Dormans, 1998a). The locomotor prognoses based on attainment of selected motor milestones are located in Table 14-3 (dePaz, Burnett, and Braga, 1994).

Although most children with cerebral palsy live to be adults, their projected lifespan is less than that of the overall population with variable causes for this difference. Children with spastic quadriplegia who are bedridden with many associated conditions may not survive beyond age 30 years mainly because of complications of immobility (United Cerebral Palsy Research and Educational Foundation, 1995). Overall, reduced survival is associated with the presence of other significant diseases

Table 14-3
Prognosis for Independent Ambulation Based on Selected Motor Milestones

Prognosis and Developmental Milestone	Time in Months
Head Balance:	
Good	< 9 months
Guarded	9 to 20 months
Poor	> 20 months
Sitting:	
Good	< 24 months
Guarded	24 to 36 months
Poor	> 36 months
Crawling:	
Good	< 30 months
Guarded	30 to 61 months
Poor	> 61 months

Adapted from dePaz AC Jr, Burnett SM, and Braga LW: Walking prognosis in cerebral palsy: a 22-year retrospective, Dev Med Child Neurol 36:130-134, 1994.

(Plioplys et al, 1998) and significantly decreased self-care skills (Strauss and Shavelle, 1998).

PRIMARY CARE MANAGEMENT

Health Care Maintenance

Growth and Development

Growth retardation does not occur in all cases of cerebral palsy. Children who are nonambulatory or have spastic quadriplegia or seizures are shorter in height than peers of the same age (Stevenson et al, 1994). Growth hormone deficiency may be another factor in growth retardation, but more study is needed (Coniglio, Stevenson, and Rogol, 1996). Children with spastic quadriplegia and those who are nonambulatory are generally thinner than peers of the same age. A study of 171 infants and children from 10 months to 16 years of age found that all of the subjects' weights and heights were below the 5th percentile for their age and sex, and that 30% had triceps skinfold measurements below the 3rd percentile. When nutritional factors were con-trolled, growth retardation continued across time. It appears that the etiology of cerebral palsy, along with associated problems, contributes largely to growth retardation (Stevenson et al, 1994). Growth rates for children with cerebral palsy, however, are unknown (Stevenson, 1996). A goal of 10% weight for height is often reasonable (Palmer and Hoon, 1995).

Obtaining accurate measurements for height and weight can be challenging if a child experiences motor difficulty and has contractures. When height cannot be measured in either a standing or recumbent position, the upper arm length (UAL) and lower leg length (LLL) measurements are adequate. Figure 14-5 shows how to estimate height from segmental measures. Accurate measuring also monitors changes in spasticity, tone, contracture, and scoliosis (Morse, 1998). Tricep and subscapular skinfold thicknesses should also be obtained (Stevenson, 1998; Stallings et al, 1995). Growth charts for children with cerebral palsy are anticipated in the next decade. Weight may be recorded from a standing position on a standardized scale or while the child is sitting or supine on a chair or hammock scale (e.g., Hosey). Primary care providers may most easily obtain an accurate weight by having a parent hold the child and step on the scale and then subtracting the parent's weight (Stevenson, 1996).

An interdisciplinary team is needed to longitudinally follow the development of a child with cerebral palsy. Periodic assessments of the child's mental, motor, language, self-care, and emotional development is warranted. There are many general and specific screening instruments that can be used by primary care providers and should be an important part of a child's care (see Chapter 2) (Urbano, 1992). The most widely used general screening tool is the Denver Developmental Screening Test II (DDST II), which should only be used for screening and is not practical after the child has been diagnosed with cerebral palsy (Pellegrino, 1997).

Assessment of a child's cognitive status is important due to the presence of mental retardation in 25% to 60% of children with cerebral palsy (Gersh, 1998b), as well as physical limitations and speech and language problems that may make determining a child's true cognitive abilities difficult. Standardized intelligence tests for infants and children are appropriate, but someone experienced in examin-

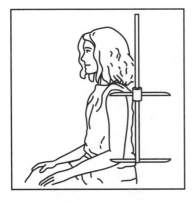
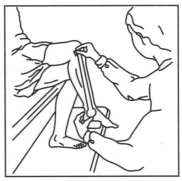
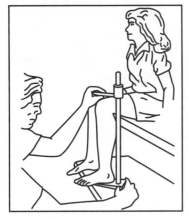

Estimation of Stature in Centimeters

Age 0 to 12
$(4.35 \times UAL) + 21.8$
$(3.26 \times TL) + 30.8$
$(2.68 \times KH) + 24.2$

Age 6 to 13
White male $(2.32 \times KH) + 48.51$
Black male $(2.18 \times KH) + 39.60$
White female $(2.15 \times KH) + 43.31$
Black female $(2.02 \times KH) + 46.59$

UAL = upper arm length
TL = tibia length
KH = knee height

Figure 14-5 Estimation of stature from segmental measures. (Redrawn from Stevenson RD: Measurement of growth in children with developmental disabilities, Dev Med Child Neuro 38:855-860, 1996.)

ing children with motor and language delays should be obtained for this assessment.

Motor assessment is most often completed by the physical or occupational therapist. Videotaping of a child's movements, in combination with computer analysis, has greatly enhanced the abilities of the physical therapist and physiatrist to plan and treat motor deficits and complications.

Speech and language problems can be screened by using, for example, the Preschool Language Scale or the Denver Articulation Screening Examination. There are also specific screening tools that assess a child's receptive and expressive language ability (see Chapter 2). Primary care providers must accurately assess parental reports of language skills, however, because parents often overestimate the number of spoken words by counting grunts and partial words. A speech therapist is the best person to assess language skills. Because of the many feeding and eating problems in infancy, a language assessment should be done in conjunction with a nutritional assessment when solid foods are introduced at about 6 months of age.

Self-care skills should be assessed throughout childhood and adolescence during the history-taking part of each primary health care visit. This assessment can be done through an interview, a questionnaire, or a standardized test (e.g., Functional Independence Measure for Children [WeeFIM] or the Pediatric Evaluation of Disability Inventory) (Campbell, 1996). How quickly children adjust to a new communication strategy or device may be indicative of their cognitive level (Willard-Holt, 1998).

Emotional development is another important area for periodic assessment. Although there are a number of available instruments that measure self-concept and self-esteem, a good discussion with a trusted health professional is usually adequate for obtaining an understanding of how a child is coping at home, school, and other environments.

Diet

Undernutrition is most often seen during infancy in children with cerebral palsy. After any medical reasons for such difficulty are determined, further problems must be assessed. Exercises to improve facial muscle tone can be initiated. If a child has trouble controlling the jaw or keeping the mouth closed, external assistance or supports can be applied. Children may also have oral tactile defensiveness and require a program of desensitization to different textures and a food plan developed around the foods that they will eat. Other children do not feel the food or drink in their mouths, so most of the food or liquid falls out of the mouth, creating skin problems. These children may also drool excessively.

Nutritional status often improves over time as a result of improved oromotor, gross and fine motor skills; general improvement in health status; and better nutritional intake. Decreased independent mobility in late childhood and adolescence can even lead to a child being overweight (Anderson, 1998; Gersh, 1998b).

As a result of hypersensitivity, infants may need to try different nipples until one is found that they prefer. The size of the nipple hole may also need to be increased if thickened formula is prescribed. Motor problems may inhibit a child from being an independent feeder. Adaptive equipment can be designed for a growing child at each developmental stage. Most importantly, bottle feeding or baby foods should not be forced upon an infant because there is a high risk for aspiration—a risk that is lifelong for children with severe cerebral palsy (Anderson, 1998; Leibold, 1994). A nutritionist and an occupational therapist can suggest ways to help a child with oromotor difficulties and supplement the diet to ensure a child receives adequate calories (Anderson, 1998).

Some children with severe cerebral palsy may eventually need a feeding tube surgically inserted in the stomach. A child's oral feeding ability, degree of malnutrition, and health complications (i.e., respiratory distress) during feeding must be carefully assessed, however, before a permanent tube is placed. A temporary nasogastric tube can be prescribed during an acute illness. In any event, careful lifelong monitoring of a child's feeding abilities and nutritional status is critically important in cerebral palsy.

Safety

Children with motor impairments and seizure disorders are at increased risk for injury. Special concern should be taken when physical activities, car seats, and environmental surroundings are chosen for children with cerebral palsy. Children with cerebral palsy may not be restricted in the type of physical activity (e.g., canoeing), but adult supervision is needed. Seizure precautions and helmets may be necessary for children with seizure disorders. Car seats should be appropriately padded and positioned to protect a child's head—especially if head control is an issue, extremities, and skin. These precautions apply to any seating arrangement. A child's environment should be free of sharp edges in case of unexpected falls and roomy enough for the child to maneuver. If the child is in a wheelchair, the home environment should be accessible. Some engineers are specially trained to suggest adaptations to homes, daycares, or schools to make them more wheelchair accessible. Home emergency plans should account for a child in a wheelchair, and local police and fire departments should be alerted.

Immunizations

Pertussis: Children with seizure disorders are at increased risk of seizure after receiving the pertussis vaccine. The risks and benefits of administering the pertussis vaccine when a child is at risk for seizures should be explained to the family, and the acellular form of the vaccine may be given in conjunction with tetanus and diphtheria (Committee on Infectious Diseases, 1997). Children with cerebral palsy who do not have seizures should maintain the regular schedule.

Measles: Children with a seizure disorder are also at risk for a seizure after receiving the measles vaccine in the form of the MMR. Because of the complications of measles, the high probability of contracting measles, and the unlikelihood of having a seizure after the immunization is administered, however, the standard schedule for measles vaccination should be followed (Committee on Infectious Diseases, 1997).

Chicken pox (varicella): Children with cerebral palsy should be immunized against varicella. For children with severe cerebral palsy in whom complications of the disease could be life-threatening, prophylactic treatment of varicella exposure with oral acyclovir could be recommended over the vaccine or varicella-zoster immunoglobulin to prevent the disease (Committee on Infectious Diseases, 1997; Huang, 1995).

Haemophilus influenzae **type B:** The standard schedule for the *Haemophilus influenzae* type B (Hib) vaccine should be followed for children with cerebral palsy. This schedule is especially pertinent for these children because of the increased risk for respiratory infections.

Influenza vaccine: Children with cerebral palsy are at risk for complications of influenza. Influenza vaccines and chemoprophylaxis should be given to children with cerebral palsy living in institutions during epidemics of influenza A (Committee on Infectious Diseases, 1997). Although the Committee on Infectious Diseases of the American Academy of Pediatrics does not recommend the influenza vaccine for all children with cerebral palsy, children who are severely affected and experience repeated respiratory infections would benefit from the yearly vaccine.

Other immunizations: Children with cerebral palsy should receive immunizations for mumps, rubella, hepatitis B, polio, and rotavirus as recommended (Committee on Infectious Diseases, 1997).

Screening

Vision: A pediatric ophthalmologist should periodically assess the eyes of children with cerebral palsy due to the many types of visual impairments that may occur. Vision can also be screened each time the child comes for a primary care visit. When performing a visual acuity test, children with motor problems may have difficulty showing which way an E points and those with speech problems may have difficulty naming the letters. Allen cards may be useful for screening.

Glasses often are prescribed for refractive errors. Contact lenses are contraindicated in children with cerebral palsy because their motor impairments inhibit placement and removal of the lenses. Glasses should be placed correctly on a child's face, and adaptive equipment (e.g., velcro straps) may be recommended for comfortable and correct placement. Patching and surgery may be recommended for other vision complications associated with cerebral palsy (e.g., strabismus and amblyopia) (Gersh, 1998b).

Hearing: A pediatric audiologist should regularly check the hearing of a child with cerebral palsy. For specific diagnostic information, an audiologist will use a tympanometer and evoked response audiometry. An otolaryngologist also may assess hearing loss along with the audiologist. Otitis media should be treated with antibiotics, and middle-ear fluid should be treated with decongestants; if both conditions become chronic, surgical placement of myringotomy tubes can be performed (Gersh, 1998b).

Children with sensorineural hearing loss may be fitted with a hearing aid. A speech therapist may join the assessment team when the hearing aid is placed to facilitate language development through words or signs (Gersh, 1998b). Proper maintenance and use of hearing aids by children and families will help a child to optimally interact with the environment.

Dental: Children with cerebral palsy need a dentist who has experience with children with movement and motor disorders. The environment of the dentist's office must be accessible, with a chair that allows for easy transfer from a wheelchair if the child uses one. The chair must also protect fragile skin and support spastic extremities (Leibold, 1994). Children with cerebral palsy should visit the dentist at least every 6 months, and more often if a child also has a seizure disorder and is taking phenytoin (Dilantin) for the prevention or early treatment of gum hyperplasia (Gersh, 1998b). Sedation may be necessary for children with severe spasticity.

Sealants are recommended for teeth with enamel defects. Malocclusions can be prevented through oromotor exercises to improve muscle tone around the oral cavity. An interdisciplinary team consisting of the nutritionist, occupational therapist, and speech-language pathologist can plan exercises to reduce the oral reflexes that can lead to development of over- or underbites. This team can also address drooling problems and help a child to swallow saliva and keep the tongue in the mouth. If drooling persists, surgery may be warranted (Gersh, 1998b). Adaptive equipment (e.g., an altered toothbrush or a washcloth for washing the teeth) may be appropriate (Gersh, 1998b).

Blood pressure: Routine screening is recommended.

Urinalysis: Routine screening is recommended. If a child has frequent urinary tract infections, a referral to a pediatric urologist may be necessary.

Hematocrit: Routine screening is recommended.

Tuberculosis: Routine screening is recommended.

Condition-Specific Screening

Motor and movement problems: A motor assessment should be done at each primary care visit. Body alignment and positioning; passive and active range-of-motion; and signs of hip dislocation, spinal deformities, contractures, and movement patterns (e.g., gait disturbances) should be assessed and measured when appropriate (Blackman, 1997). Goniometric measurements of the joint mobility and motion of the knee and ankle can assist in screening for abnormalities in tone (Pinto-Martin, Torre, and Zhao, 1997). Dormans (1993) provides an excellent format for orthopedic assessment in an article on the orthopedic management of children with cerebral palsy. Use of radiographs and MRIs may be needed for further diagnosis. Palisano and his associates (1997) have developed a five-level classification system for gross motor function in children with cerebral palsy that is included in the appendix of their article. Additional examination of the reliability and validity of the classification system for children under 2 years of age is needed. Correct management and follow-through by the child and family are necessary to prevent the development of further complications.

Common Illness Management

Differential Diagnosis

Fever: Children experience many febrile episodes in their lives as a result of the many viruses and bacteria that are present in their environment. Children with cerebral palsy are prone to respiratory and urinary tract infections and may also get gastrointestinal infections. In each of these infections, fever is usually an accompanying symptom. Children with cerebral palsy must be seen by a primary care provider if they are under 6 months of age, have had a fever over 38.6° C for 3 or more days without symptoms, appear acutely ill with undefined symptoms, or have had a seizure(s) with a fever. A physical assessment and laboratory work need to be done by the primary care provider at this time for an accurate diagnosis and treatment.

Children with severe cerebral palsy may have impaired immune function resulting from neurologic insult, and thus a minor illness may manifest into a more severe condition if treatment is not started promptly (Dorval, 1994). Regular follow-up by the primary care provider is essential.

Respiratory tract infections: Children with cerebral palsy are susceptible to upper and lower respiratory tract infections, namely otitis media, sore throats, rhinorrhea, sinusitis, and influenza. Asthma is more prevalent in premature infants with cerebral palsy. Routine management of these problems is warranted with careful monitoring of the resolution of the infection. Sometimes these infections are not resolved with one round of antibiotics and complications can occur (e.g., additional hearing loss from a case of otitis media). Referral to a specialist may be recommended.

Pain with an infection is difficult to assess in children with severe cerebral palsy. For example, the typical sign of pulling on the ear for an ear infection may not be present. Parents are often able to discern subtle signs in their child (e.g., increased irritability, decreased energy, less vocalizations, increased drooling) or to think that the child is just not acting like him or herself. Children can also be asked "yes" or "no" questions to identify the source of pain. If a child uses a communication system, signs or symbols can be used to describe pain. Children's pain scales (e.g., the Wong Faces Scale) can be used by primary care providers to further assess a child's pain.

It is important to stress the high probability of pneumonia occurring after an initial upper respiratory infection or bout of influenza in children with severe cerebral palsy. Pneumonia can also be caused by aspiration and gastroesophageal reflux. Careful monitoring must be done to prevent a life-threatening situation. Children with cerebral palsy are unable to expectorate well and handle increased secretions. Dehydration can easily occur after a few days of fever. Hospitalization may be suggested as a preventive measure to ensure close observation of any changes in a child's health status. If a child is being cared for at home, parents must understand the importance of the treatment plan and be instructed to contact their primary care provider if the condition worsens.

Urinary tract problems: Common problems are incontinence, urgency, frequency, and retention. Urinary tract infections also occur more frequently in children with cerebral palsy. The age of the child and any communication problems may impede the obtainment of detailed information on pain or other symptoms experienced by the child. A urinalysis and urine cultures must be ordered if there is any suspicion of a urinary tract infection or the cause of the fever or other symptoms cannot be identified. After one or two urinary tract infections have been diagnosed and treated in a child with cerebral palsy, the parents and primary care provider may be better able to identify the signs and symptoms associated with this condition in the child. This information is especially important in a child who is nonverbal and should be recorded in the child's chart for further reference.

Standard antibiotic therapy for urinary tract infections is recommended when a diagnosis is made. Additional comfort measures (e.g., increased fluid intake, perineal hygiene after voiding, increased rest, and taking acetaminophen based on body weight) can be ordered. Follow-up is imperative after a urinary tract infection and should include a urine culture 2 to 3 days after initiation of the antibiotic to assess its effect. Follow-up urine cultures after the course of antibiotics are also necessary. If recurrent urinary tract infections occur, referral to a pediatric urologist is recommended.

Gastrointestinal problems: Parents may note that a child has abdominal pain, straining with hard stools, rectal bleeding, soiled underwear, and a distended, hard abdomen when constipated. Documenting the signs and symptoms of this problem in infants or nonverbal children is especially important. Increased fluids, exercise, and a healthy diet with additional fiber is recommended. A bowel management program designed by an interdisciplinary team may be needed if constipation is a

chronic problem. A program of stool softeners, laxatives, suppositories, and enemas can be prescribed, as well as suggestions for proper positioning and seating on the toilet. The effectiveness of the program should be closely monitored and recorded. A pattern for bowel elimination should be initiated and maintained. Urinary tract infections and impactions are complications of chronic constipation. Constipation is a very difficult chronic problem to deal with when a child is immobile and has a poor appetite. Bowel management programs must be individualized and evaluated periodically.

Drug Interactions

Medications may be prescribed to reduce spasticity or other disease-associated conditions (e.g., infections, seizures, and constipation). Common medications used to reduce spasticity include diazepam (Valium), dantrolene sodium (Dantrium), and baclofen (Lioresal). Dantrolene sodium should be started at 1 mg/kg twice a day and gradually increased until positive results are seen without exceeding 100 mg four times per day. Also, baclofen should be started at 5 mg three times per day and increased until good results are found without exceeding 60 mg/day. Botulinum toxin, although used most often for focal dystonia, is being tested for use in treating spasticity (Albright, 1996; Dabney, Lipton, and Miller, 1997; Wollack and Nichter, 1996). Baclofen has recently been administered intrathecally in children with severe spasticity with good efficacy (Gersh, 1998a). Furthermore, nerve blocks have been used with alcohol, phenol, lidocaine, bupivacaine, or procaine with variable effects on decreasing spasticity (Pellegrino, 1997). No major side effects or drug interactions have been found with these medications. Anticonvulsants are used to treat seizures, antibiotics are given for infections, and laxatives are used for constipation. A discussion of the drug interactions for seizure medications is included in Chapter 21. The occurrence of constipation must be examined for its cause—whether because of diet or as a side effect of medications such as anticonvulsants or iron. Overall, drug interactions need to be assessed when a child with cerebral palsy is receiving multiple medications, but no specific drug interactions have been found with the medications used for spasticity.

Developmental Issues

Sleep Patterns

A clinical manifestation of cerebral palsy in infancy is prolonged sleeping patterns. A variety of other sleeping problems may also exist with cerebral palsy. Kotagal and associates (1994) found that obstructive and central sleep apnea can occur in children with severe cerebral palsy. Another problem may be severe hypoxemia during sleep, which may require a sleep apnea monitor. A neutral body position (i.e., with the neck and head slightly flexed) is encouraged during sleep. Bolsters or wedges can be used to facilitate appropriate positions. A side-lying position should be used for children who drool so that excessive fluid can drain out of the mouth instead of down the throat, which may cause choking.

Toileting

If children with cerebral palsy are able to be toilet trained, then—like any other children—they will give their parents clues of their physical and neurologic readiness. The potty chair or toilet must adequately support the child's body and minimize the risk of skin breakdown from extended sitting. The child's feet must be able to touch the floor to assist the abdominal muscles in pushing. Special potty chairs can be made, or current chairs can be adapted. A physical or occupational therapist can inform the parents if a chair with the adaptations is acceptable. Diapers are available for individuals of all ages and sizes (Anderson, 1998).

Discipline

Parents often discipline children who have special health and developmental needs differently than they do their siblings. As a result of their special needs and possible past health care emergencies, parents are often reluctant to discipline a child with cerebral palsy. Parents must be consistent in disciplining all of their children; both parents should agree with the type of discipline; and the discipline should be developmentally appropriate for a child's mental age.

Child Care

Many child care programs today include children both with and without chronic conditions. Parents of a child with cerebral palsy must be aware that the risk for infection is greater in settings where children are together (e.g., in daycare) (Committee on Infectious Diseases, 1997), and that issues of safety and accessibility are important to consider.

Schooling

Children with cerebral palsy may need to use different augmentative communication systems (e.g., communication boards, computers, and keyboard voice synthesizers). Adaptive equipment for communicating, seating, writing, and reading may be needed and should be obtained. Occupational, physical, and speech therapy, as well as adaptive physical education, are often needed and individually planned for either group or individual sessions. An aide may be required to help a child with cerebral palsy with personal needs. Of the children with hemiplegic cerebral palsy, 25% develop a condition called homonymous hemianopsia, in which the child can see straight ahead but not to the affected side. Diagnosis of this condition is important for classroom seating arrangements (Gersh, 1998a; Pellegrino and Dormans, 1998a). Transportation to and from school, transfer needs between classrooms, and emergency health and safety plans must also be arranged with school personnel.

Today most children with cerebral palsy participate in inclusive education. Special attention must be paid to a child's cognitive ability and social integration into the regular classroom by assisting the child with peer relationships and self-esteem. Primary care providers can assess the school situation and performance during well-child visits.

During the junior high and high school years, children with cerebral palsy can be enrolled in vocational or college preparation programs, depending on career interests and/or the presence and degree of mental retardation. Adolescents with cerebral palsy may also experience renewed social problems during these years as they cope with adolescent self-esteem and contemplate life after school. Work and social opportunities are not as prevalent in the adult years as they are during childhood for individuals with special health and developmental needs. Adolescents often experience depression when faced with the stigma of their condition and rejection in social situations. School performance also may decrease. Parents and professionals should look for signs that might alert them to these psychosocial issues during adolescence and offer support and professional counseling where needed.

Sexuality

Social isolation, chronic low self-esteem, and a poor body image can affect the development of intimate relationships. Sexuality education can be provided by a health care professional or an educator at school to help the adolescents develop a positive self-esteem and body image. Role modeling and exposure to social situations can be planned and executed (Carmody, Brown, and Roth, 1991; Wadsworth and Harper, 1993). During their adolescent years, children do not often discuss sexuality and their feelings with parents. Therefore peers, other adults, and support groups should be available to help adolescents with cerebral palsy with these issues. In some cases, referral to a sexuality counselor may be needed.

Female adolescents should begin to receive gynecologic care if they are sexually active. Because of spasticity, contractures, and/or poor muscle control, a woman's position for such an exam should be adapted, and she may require assistance in positioning menstrual pads or tampons. An annual pelvic ultrasound can be done by the physician for baseline data. Pregnancy is possible for women with cerebral palsy. Abnormal births can occur at an increased rate over the general population, but 90% of the births are normal (Winch et al, 1993).

Transition to Adulthood

The transition to adulthood in children with cerebral palsy must address medical care, equipment needs, communication, activities of daily life, mobility, nutrition, vocational decisions, transportation, housing, and social needs. Throughout life, optimal independence should be encouraged and learned helplessness avoided. Independence and self-advocacy should be stressed during the transitional period between adolescence and adulthood. Adolescents with cerebral palsy need to take an active role in choosing a primary care provider and health care interdisciplinary team. Their participation in decision making about dietary choices, medications, surgical interventions if needed, and adaptive equipment is important.

Vocational decisions should be discussed, and plans for successful employment should be determined. When deciding upon a site for college or work, the physical layout, wheelchair accessibility, availability of personal aides, housing, and repair shop for wheelchairs and any other adaptive equipment must be considered and resources identified. Independence in the use of public transportation should be planned. Individuals with mild cerebral palsy may be able to drive. Independent living or assisted living arrangements must be discussed; and individuals should be placed on waiting lists if living outside the home is desired. Social needs, including activities consistent with an individual's abilities, planned social programs, and opportunities to develop successful relationships, should be met. Most importantly, adolescents making the transition to adulthood must participate to the greatest possible extent in decisions about their lives.

Special Family Concerns and Resources

In incidences of mild cerebral palsy, the effects on the family may be minimal or nonexistent. Parents of children with severe cerebral palsy usually experience chronic sorrow when their child does not achieve the developmental milestones that other children without this condition achieve. Hirose and Ueda (1994) found that infancy was the most stressful time for mothers and that the period from toddlerhood to adolescence was most stressful for fathers. Respite care is highly recommended to give families time away from the constant responsibilities of caring for a child with cerebral palsy.

Siblings are also affected. In a study of sibling interactions with children with cerebral palsy, researchers found that the children with cerebral palsy were unassertive and passive in their play behaviors and unaffected siblings learned and exhibited more nurturing, directive, and extroverted behaviors (Dallas, Stevenson, and McGurk, 1993a and 1993b).

There are no specific cross-cultural or religious concerns for children with cerebral palsy, although a stigma based on the diagnosis is attached to all families. The visibility of this condition may create more of a stigma in some cultures than in others.

Resources

A variety of local, state, and regional services for children with cerebral palsy exist. Appropriate resources and organizations are usually listed in the local yellow pages of the telephone directory, under "Social Services and Organizations." Several books and organizations can also offer assistance to families and professionals:

Books:

Dormans JP and Pellegrino L: Caring for children with cerebral palsy, Baltimore, Md., 1998, Paul H. Brookes. Available from Paul H. Brookes Publishing Co., PO Box 10624, Baltimore, Md 21285-0624.

Finnie NR: Handling the young child with cerebral palsy at home, ed 3, Woburn, Mass., 1997, Butterworth-Heinemann. Available from Butterworth-Heinemann Publishing, 225 Wildwood Ave., Woburn, Mass. 01801.

Geralis E, editor: Children with cerebral palsy: a parent's guide, Bethesda, Md., 1998, Woodbine House. Available from Woodbine House, 6510 Bells Mill Rd., Bethesda, Md. 20817.

Miller F and Bachrach SJ: Cerebral palsy: a complete guide for caregiving, Baltimore, Md., 1998, Johns Hopkins University Press. Available from Johns Hopkins University Press, PO Box 19966, Baltimore, Md. 21211.

Campbell SK, Palisano RJ, and Vander Linden DW, editors: Physical therapy for children, Philadelphia, 1994, W.B. Saunders. Available from W.B. Saunders, The Curtis Center, Independence Square West, Philadelphia, Pa. 19106.

Organizations:

United Cerebral Palsy Associations, Inc.
1660 L Street NW, Suite 700
Washington, DC 20036
(800)776-0414 (national office), (202)842-1266 (voice/tt), (800)776-0414 (fax);
ucpnatl@http://www.ucpa.org

American Academy for Cerebral Palsy and Developmental Medicine
6300 North River Road, Suite 727
Rosemont, Ill. 60018-4226
(847) 698-1635, (847) 823-0536 (fax);
woppenhe@ucla.edu, http://accpdm.org

United States Cerebral Palsy Athletic Association (USCPAA)
200 Harrison Avenue
Newport, RI 02840
(401) 848-2460, (401) 848-5280 (fax);
uscpaa@mail.bbsnet.com, http://www.uscpaa. org

DisABILITY Information and Resources
Provides information on products, services, computer accessibility, home automation and environmental control, governmental and legislative disability information, legal advice and advocacy, sports, travel, recreation, and assistive technology.
http://www.eskimo.com/~jlubin/disabled/

Summary of Primary Care Needs for the Child with Cerebral Palsy

HEALTH CARE MAINTENANCE

Growth and development

Undernutrition in infancy often leads to growth retardation.

Different techniques should be used to get height, arm and leg lengths, and skinfold measurements.

Weights may be attained via standing or sitting scales or recumbent lifts.

Overweight conditions may occur in adolescence if mobility decreases.

Delayed development in motor and communication skills is common.

Developmental strengths and weaknesses must be assessed and recorded.

Mental retardation and seizure disorders inhibit intellectual development.

Diet

Infants can have difficulty with sucking, swallowing, and chewing; so assessment should be done early.

Drooling and aspiration can also be problems.

Nutritional concerns may be lifelong, and placement of a gastrostomy tube may be warranted in severe cases.

Referral to a nutritionist is needed.

Summary of Primary Care Needs for the Child with Cerebral Palsy—cont'd

Safety

Children are at risk for injury as a result of spasticity, muscle control problems, delayed protective reflexes, and potential seizures.

Positioning and adaptive equipment are often required.

Immunizations

If the etiology for seizure activity is unknown, the pertussis vaccine may be deferred or an acellular vaccine used when age appropriate.

The measles vaccine should be given as scheduled.

Haemophilus influenzae type B (Hib) vaccine and other immunizations should be given as scheduled.

Children with cerebral palsy are at risk for complications of influenza and varicella.

Fever management is necessary to decrease the possibility of febrile seizures.

Screening

Vision: A pediatric ophthalmologist should be seen during infancy because of the likelihood of vision problems.

Vision should be checked for acuity, refractive errors, strabismus, retinopathy of prematurity, and cataracts.

Hearing: Referral to a pediatric audiologist may be necessary during infancy to check for hearing problems and loss.

Both sensorineural and conductive hearing loss is possible.

Routine screening for conductive hearing problems and loss should be done.

Dental: Children should be evaluated by a dentist experienced with children with motor problems every 6 months.

Proper dental hygiene is needed.

Administration of phenytoin may cause hyperplasia of the gums; proper preventive care and early treatment of this condition is important.

Blood pressure: Routine screening is recommended.

Urinalysis: Routine screening is recommended.

A referral to a pediatric urologist may be needed if the child has chronic urinary tract infections.

Hematocrit: Routine screening is recommended.

Tuberculosis: Routine screening is recommended.

Condition-specific screening: A motor assessment, including assessment for scoliosis, hip dislocation, and contractures, should be done at every well-child visit.

COMMON ILLNESS MANAGEMENT

Differential diagnosis

Fever: Management of fever is routine.

Respiratory tract infections: Respiratory infections should be promptly treated. Pneumonia may be life threatening to children with severe cerebral palsy. Follow-up is important.

Urinary tract infections: Treatment for urinary tract infections should be prompt, and follow-up is essential. Urinary tract abnormalities may also be present.

Gastrointestinal problems: Constipation is a chronic problem for many children. A bowel management program may be needed.

Drug interactions: No medications are routinely prescribed, except if a seizure disorder is also present.

Developmental issues

Sleep patterns: Correct positioning is needed during sleep because sleep apnea can occur.

Toileting: Adaptive equipment is often needed for correct positioning on the toilet. Bladder and bowel training may be delayed.

Discipline: It is important that consistent and age-appropriate discipline measures be taken.

Child care: Careful planning must be undertaken in choosing the best child care arrangements, especially regarding issues of safety, accessibility, health care needs, and increased rates of infection.

Continued

***Summary of* Primary Care Needs for the Child
with Cerebral Palsy—cont'd**

Schooling: Use IEPs and inclusive class-rooms. Specialized services and therapies for each child must be procured. Adaptive equipment and computers enhance a child's ability to learn.

Behavioral and school problems can occur in adolescence as a result of poor esteem and body image.

Sexuality: Opportunities for social activities should be arranged. Transportation needs are important to consider.

Opportunities for same sex and opposite sex relationships are needed. Classes in social interaction and sexuality may be needed.

Gynecological exams should begin for women with adaptations to the normal positioning.

Reproductive issues should be discussed.

Transition to adulthood: A child's independence and self-advocacy should be promoted.

Future residential and vocational plans need to be addressed.

Special family concerns

Respite care meets a family's needs.

Effects on individual family members must be assessed and addressed. Special support groups are available for fathers and siblings.

Family stigmas may be perceived.

References

Albright AL: Baclofen in the treatment of cerebral palsy, J Child Neurol 11:77-83, 1996.

Albright AL et al: Infusion of intrathecal baclofen for generalized dystonia in cerebral palsy, J Neurosurg 88:73-76, 1998.

Anderson S: Daily care. In Geralis E, editor: Children with cerebral palsy: a parent's guide, ed 2, Bethesda, Md., 1998, Woodbine House.

Blackman JA: Medical aspects of developmental disabilities in children birth to three, ed 3, Gaithersburg, Md., 1997, Aspen Publishers.

Bodensteiner JB: The management of cerebral palsy: subjectivity and a conundrum, J Child Neurol 11:75-76, 1996.

Buckon CE et al: Assessment of upper-extremity function in children with spastic diplegia before and after selective dorsal rhizotomy, Dev Med Child Neurol 38:404-408, 1995.

Campbell SK: Quantifying the effects of interventions for movement disorders resulting from cerebral palsy, J Child Neurol 11(suppl 1):S61-S70, 1996.

Capute AJ and Accardo PJ: Cerebral palsy: the spectrum of motor dysfunction. In Capute AJ and Accardo PJ, editors: Developmental disabilities in infancy and childhood, vol. II: the spectrum of developmental disabilities, ed 2, Baltimore, Md, 1996, Paul H. Brookes.

Carmody MA, Brown M, and Roth SP: Perspectives: a case study, Information Plus 2:1-3, 1991.

Committee on Infectious Diseases, American Academy of Pediatrics: 1997 red book: report of the committee on infectious diseases, ed 24, Elk Grove Village, Ill., 1997, The Academy.

Coniglio SJ, Stevenson RD, and Rogol AD: Apparent growth hormone deficiency in children with cerebral palsy, Dev Med Child Neurol 38:797-804, 1996.

Craft S et al: Changes in cognitive performance in children with spastic diplegic cerebral palsy following selective dorsal rhizotomy, Pediatr Neurosurg 23:68-75, 1995.

Dabney KW, Lipton GE, and Miller F: Cerebral palsy, Curr Op Pediatr 9:81-88, 1997.

Dallas E, Stevenson J, and McGurk H: Cerebral-palsied children's interactions with siblings—I, influence of severity of disability, age, and birth order, J Child Psychol Psychiat 34:621-647, 1993a.

Dallas E, Stevenson J, and McGurk H: Cerebral-palsied children's interactions with siblings—II, - II. interactional structure, J Child Psychol Psychiatr 34:649-671, 1993b.

Damiano DL and Abel MF: Functional outcomes of strength training in spastic cerebral palsy, Arch Phys Med Rehabil 79:119-125, 1998.

Delfico AJ et al: Intraoperative anaphylaxis due to allergy to latex in children who have cerebral palsy: a report of six cases, Dev Med Child Neurol 39:194-197, 1996.

DeLuca PA: The musculoskeletal management of children with cerebral palsy, PCNA 43:1135-1150, 1996.

de Paz AC Jr, Burnett SM, and Braga LW: Walking prognosis in cerebral palsy: a 22-year retrospective analysis, Dev Med Child Neurol 36:130-134, 1994.

Dormans JP: Orthopedic management of children with cerebral palsy, Pediatr Clin North Am 40:645-657, 1993.

Dorval J: Achieving and maintaining body systems integrity and function: clinical issues. In Lollar DJ, editor: Preventing secondary conditions associated with spina bifida or cerebral palsy: proceedings and recommendations of a symposium, Washington, DC, 1994, Spina Bifida Association of America.

Evans PM and Alberman E: Certified cause of death in children and young adults with cerebral palsy, Arch Dis Child 65:325-329, 1990.

Fletcher NA and Marsden CD: Dyskinetic cerebral palsy: A clinical and genetic study, Dev Med Child Neuro 38:873-880, 1996.

Gersh E: What is cerebral palsy? In Geralis E, editor: Children with cerebral palsy: a parent's guide, ed 2, Bethesda, Md., 1998a, Woodbine House.

Gersh E: Medical concerns and treatment. In Geralis E, editor: Children with cerebral palsy: a parent's guide, ed 2, Bethesda, Md., 1998b, Woodbine House.

Gerszten PC, Albright AL, and Berry MJ: Effect on ambulation of continuous intrathecal baclofen infusion, Pediatr Neurosurg 27:40-44, 1997.

Hirose T and Ueda R: Long-term follow-up study of children with cerebral palsy and coping behaviour of parents. In Smith JP, editor: Research and its application, London, 1994, Blackwell Scientific Publications.

Hirtz DG and Nelson K: Magnesium sulfate and cerebral palsy in premature infants, Curr Op Pediatr 10:131-137, 1998.

Houle AM et al: Bladder function before and after selective dorsal rhizotomy in children with cerebral palsy, J Urol 160:1088-1091, 1998.

Huang Y-C et al: Acyclovir prophylaxis of varicella after household exposure, Pediatr Infect Dis J 14:152-154, 1995.

Im D and McDonald CM: New approaches to managing spasticity in children with cerebral palsy, WJM 166:271, 1997.

Katz N, Cermak S, and Shamir Y: Unilateral neglect in children with hemiplegic cerebral palsy, Percept Mot Skills 86:539-550, 1998.

Kotagal S, Gibbons VP, and Stith JA: Sleep abnormalities in patients with severe cerebral palsy, Dev Med Child Neurol 36:304-311, 1994.

Leibold S: Achieving and maintaining body systems integrity and function: personal care skills. In Lollar DJ, editor: Preventing secondary conditions associated with spina bifida or cerebral palsy: proceedings and recommendations of a symposium, Washington, DC, 1994, Spina Bifida Association of America.

Little WJ: On the influence of abnormal parturition, difficult labors, premature birth, and asphyxia neonatorum, on the mental and physical condition of the child, especially in relation to deformities, Transactions of the Obstetric Society of London 3:293-344, 1861-1862.

Lorenz JM et al: A quantitative review of mortality and developmental disabilities in extremely premature newborns, Arch Pediatr Adolesc 152:425-435, 1998.

Mayo M: Lower urinary tract dysfunction in cerebral palsy, J Urol 147:419-420, 1992.

McLaughlin JF et al: Selective dorsal rhizotomy: Efficacy and safety in an investigator-masked randomized clinical trial, Dev Med Child Neurol 40:220-232, 1998.

Morse J: Personal communication, November 30, 1998.

Minear WL: A classification of cerebral palsy, Pediatrics 18:841-852, 1956.

Mutch L et al: Cerebral palsy epidemiology: where are we now and where are we going? Dev Med Child Neurol 34:547-555, 1992.

Nelson KB: Magnesium sulfate and risk of cerebral palsy in very low-birth-weight infants, JAMA 276:1843-1844, 1996.

Newacheck PW and Halfon N: Prevalence and impact of disabling chronic conditions in childhood, Am J Public Health 88:610-617, 1998.

Newacheck PW and Taylor WR: Childhood chronic illness: prevalence, severity, and impact, Am J Public Health 82:364-371, 1992.

Okumura A et al: MRI findings in patients with spastic cerebral palsy: II, correlation with type of cerebral palsy, Dev Med Child Neurol 39:369-372, 1997.

Palisano R et al: Development and reliability of a system to classify gross motor function in children with cerebral palsy, Dev Med Child Neurol 39:214-223, 1997.

Palmer FB and Hoon AH: Cerebral palsy. In Parker S and Zuckerman B, editors: Behavioral and developmental pediatrics: a handbook for primary care, New York, NY, 1995, Little, Brown, & Co.

Pellegrino L: Cerebral palsy. In Batshaw ML, editor: Children with disabilities, ed 4, Baltimore, Md., 1997, Paul H. Brookes.

Pellegrino L and Dormans JP: Definitions, etiology, and epidemiology of cerebral palsy. In Dormans JP and Pellegrino L, editors: Caring for children with cerebral palsy: a team approach, Baltimore, Md., 1998a, Paul H. Brookes.

Pellegrino L and Dormans JP: Making the diagnosis of cerebral palsy. In Dormans JP and Pellegrino L, editors: Caring for children with cerebral palsy: a team approach, Baltimore, Md., 1998b, Paul H. Brookes.

Pharoah POD and Cooke RWI: A hypothesis for the aetiology of spastic cerebral palsy-the vanishing twin, Dev Med Child Neurol 39:292-296, 1997.

Pinto-Martin JA, Torre C, and Zhao H: Nursing screening of low-birth-weight infants for cerebral palsy using goniometry, Nurs Res 46:284-287, 1997.

Plioplys AV et al: Survival rates among children with severe neurologic disabilities, SMJ 91:161-172, 1998.

Rawlins P: Patient management of cerebral origin spasticity with intrathecal baclofen, J Neurosci Nurs 30:32-46, 1998.

Rogers BT et al: Hypoxemia during oral feeding of children with severe cerebral palsy, Dev Med Child Neurol 35:3-10, 1993.

Rose J and McGill KC: The motor unit in cerebral palsy, Dev Med Child Neurol 40:270-277, 1998.

Schendel DE et al: Prenatal magnesium sulfate exposure and the risk for cerebral palsy or mental retardation among very low-birth-weight children aged 3 to 5 years, JAMA 276:1805-1810, 1996.

Stallings VA et al: Body composition in children with spastic quadriplegic cerebral palsy, J Pediatr 126:5, 1995.

Steinbok P, Reiner A, and Kestle JRW: Therapeutic electrical stimulation following selective posterior rhizotomy in children with spastic diplegic cerebral palsy: a randomized clinical trial, Dev Med Child Neurol 39:515-520, 1997.

Stevenson RD: Measurement of growth in children with developmental disabilities, Dev Med Child Neurol 38:855-860, 1996.

Stevenson RD: North American growth in cerebral palsy project 1998, Website: http://hsc.Virginia.edu/~mon-grow/healthcare/bodyfat.html

Stevenson RD et al: Clinical correlates of linear growth in children with cerebral palsy, Dev Med Child Neurol 36:135-142, 1994.

Strauss D and Shavelle R: Life expectancy of adults with cerebral palsy, Dev Med Child Neurol 40:369-375, 1998.

Thomas SS et al: Does gait continue to improve 2 years after selective dorsal rhizotomy? J Pediatr Orthop 17:387-391, 1997.

United Cerebral Palsy Associations: Cerebral palsy—facts and figures, Washington, DC, 1996, The Associations.

United Cerebral Palsy Research and Educational Foundation: Causes of death of persons with disabilities due to cerebral palsy, Washington, DC, 1995, The Foundation.

Urbano MT: Preschool children with special health care needs, San Diego, Calif., 1992, Singular Publishing Group, Inc.

Wadsworth JS and Harper DC: The social needs of adolescents with cerebral palsy, Dev Med Child Neurol 35:1015-1024, 1993.

Willard-Holt C: Academic and personality characteristics of gifted children with cerebral palsy: a multiple case study, Exceptional Children 65:37-50, 1998.

Winch R et al: Women with cerebral palsy: obstetric experience and neonatal outcome, Dev Med Child Neurol 35:974-982, 1993.

Wilson-Costello D: Perinatal correlates of cerebral palsy and other neurologic impairment among very low birth weight children, Pediatrics 102:315-322, 1998.

Wollack JB and Nichter CA: Static encephalopathies. In Rudolph AM, Hoffman JU, and Rudolph CD, editors: Rudolph's pediatrics, ed 20, Stamford, Conn., 1996, Appleton & Lange.

Wright V et al: Evaluation of selective dorsal rhizotomy for the reduction of spasticity in cerebral palsy: a randomized controlled trial, Dev Med Child Neurol 40:239-247, 1998.

Yokoyama Y, Shimizu T, and Hayakawa K: Prevalence of cerebral palsy in twins, triplets and quadruplets, Int J Epidemiol 24:943-940, 1995.

Young RR: Spasticity: a review, Neurol 44(suppl):512-520, 1994.

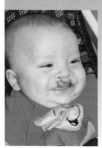

CHAPTER 15

Cleft Lip and Palate

Ginny Curtin

Etiology

Cleft lip and cleft palate result when there is a failure of the median maxillary, premaxillary, and palatine processes to fuse early in gestational age (Gorlin, Cohen, and Levin, 1990). The lip and alveolar ridge or primary palate is fully formed between 5 and 7 weeks' gestation and the secondary palate between 6 and 12 weeks' gestation (Gorlin, Cohen, and Levin, 1990). The specific etiology is usually unknown, although there is evidence to suggest that maternal folic acid deficiency may play a role (Tolarova, 1993). Ingestion of teratogens such as alcohol and some prescriptive anti-seizure medications such as phenytoin (Dilantin) as well as folic acid antagonists and retinoic acid have been implicated (Gorlin, Cohen, and Levin, 1990), but not definitively proven (Kelly, 1984). Occasionally a positive family history of clefting is noted.

All infants with cleft lip and cleft palate need to be examined by a dysmorphologist. There may be associated midline abnormalities, and the clefting may be a component of a recognized syndrome (Gorlin, Cohen, and Levin, 1990; American Cleft Palate-Craniofacial Association, 1993). Isolated cleft palate (i.e., without cleft lip) is more commonly accompanied by other findings than cleft lip and palate together (Gorlin, Cohen, and Levin, 1990). For example, cleft palate with micrognathia (small mandible) and glossoptosis (enlarged tongue) is known as Pierre Robin sequence and has important management implications. In this situation, researchers postulated that in fetal development the micrognathia is the primary problem and the cleft palate is a result of the tongue being placed superiorly, obstructing the movement of the maxillary shelves into the midline (Gorlin, Cohen, and Levin, 1990).

Incidence

The generally accepted incidence rate of clefting is 1/700 births, although some ethnic differences exist. American Indians have an incidence of 3.6/1000 live births followed in descending order by Japanese, Chinese, Caucasian, Hispanic, and African Americans with the lowest reported incidence of 0.3/1000. Incidence rates are based on varied reporting mechanisms, and problems occur with mixing together studies of live births, stillbirths, and spontaneous abortions. No registry or national database exists documenting clefting birth defects. Clefting may or may not be recorded when it is a component of a known syndrome. Submucous cleft palate is frequently undetected until the preschool years when the speech is unintelligible secondary to velopharyngeal insufficiency (Gorlin, Cohen, and Levin, 1990; Tolarova and Cervenka, 1998).

Clinical Manifestations at Time of Diagnosis (Box 15-1)

Cleft lip is an obvious birth defect noted in the delivery room. It is described as unilateral or bilateral and incomplete or complete depending on whether the clefting extends into the nasal cavity (Figure 15-1). A microform cleft lip is characterized by very minor notching or the appearance of a well-healed surgical scar or "seam"; however, microform cleft lip is usually only described by a craniofacial team or plastic and reconstructive surgeon.

Cleft palate may involve the primary palate (lip and alveolus anterior to the incisive foramen) and the secondary palate (hard and soft palate) (Figure 15-2). A submucous cleft palate is characterized by

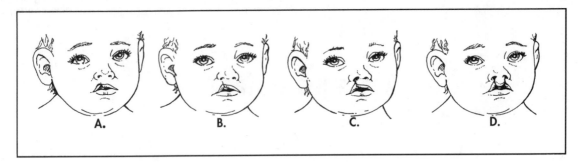

Figure 15-1 Varieties of lip clefts. **A, B,** and **C** show unilateral, or one-sided, clefts in the lip and gum ridge. A bilateral, or two-sided, cleft is seen in **D.** (Redrawn from Moller KT, Starr CD, and Johnson SA: A parent's guide to cleft lip and palate, Minneapolis, 1990, University of Minnesota Press.)

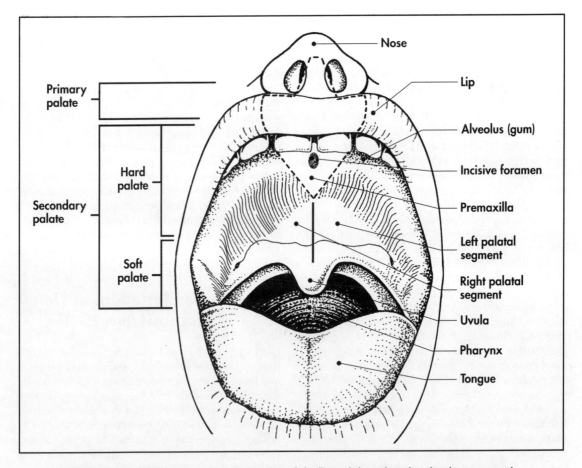

Figure 15-2 The dashes outline the portion of the lip and the palate that develops separately from the hard and soft palate. Unilateral clefts of the lip occur on one side or the other along the dotted line through the lip and possibly the palate. Bilateral clefts of the lip occur on both sides of the incisive foramen and include the prolabium (i.e., the part of the lip attached to the premaxilla). (Redrawn from Berkowitz S: The cleft palate story, Chicago, 1994, Quintessence Publishing Co., Inc.)

Box 15-1

Clinical Manifestations at Time of Diagnosis

Cleft lip and palate—physical findings

Cleft palate—difficulty feeding because of infant's inability to create a seal around the nipple

Pierre Robin sequence—signs and symptoms of upper airway obstruction as a result of tongue repositioning in the airway, micrognathia

Submucous cleft palate—nasal sounding speech

Box 15-2

Findings Apparent in Infants with Pierre Robin Sequence

1. Increasing levels of carbon dioxide when measured serially as a result of carbon dioxide retention from intermittent upper airway obstruction with retropositioning of the tongue.
2. Transient oxygen desaturations measured by pulse oximetry accompanied by increased work of breathing with chest wall retractions and gasping sounds as the tongue blocks the upper airway. These episodes usually self-correct within a short time as the infant repositions the tongue forward; however, the frequency may increase as the infant tires.
3. Difficulty during feedings, especially when the nipple is removed from the mouth and the infant is still swallowing residual milk. The tongue becomes retropositioned easily without the stimulus of the nipple to move it forward. Gagging sounds may be heard and become worse with supine positioning.
4. Deceleration on the growth curve despite adequate intake of formula or expressed breast milk. This should signal a possible worsening respiratory status.

From Sher AE: Mechanisms of airway obstruction in Pierre Robin sequence: implications for treatment, Cleft Palate Craniofac J 29:224-251, 1992.

Singer L and Sidoti EJ: Pediatric management of Pierre Robin sequence, Cleft Palate Craniofac J 29:220-223, 1992.

---

a notch at the posterior spine of the hard palate and translucence at the midline. No standard classification system to describe cleft palate exists (Smith et al, 1998); clinicians draw a diagram or use physical descriptors to define tissue deficiencies (Millard, 1980; Millard, 1993) (Figure 15-3).

Infants with isolated cleft palate should be examined carefully for other anomalies, and as previously mentioned, all infants with clefting need a physical examination by a dysmorphologist (Hofstee, Kors, and Hennekam, 1993). Not all clefts of the palate are noted by the staff in the delivery room. Infants who are unable to successfully breast feed, are unable to "latch on," or exhibit difficulties with bottle feedings such as prolonged (>30 to 45 minutes) feeding times should be reexamined carefully for the presence of clefting. Even a small cleft of the soft palate usually produces ineffective sucking as a result of the infant's inability to create a seal to draw the milk out of the nipple (Curtin, 1990). Infants with cleft palate will present shortly after birth with feeding problems. The mother may initially report that the baby will nurse for 45 minutes yet does not seem satisfied. The mother's breasts may still feel engorged at the end of a feeding and there is never a feeling that the breast is empty of milk. Frequent snacking usually results; however, urine output is inadequate and the baby continues to be fussy. After approximately 4 to 5 days of this feeding behavior, the infant becomes more sleepy, lethargic, and exhibits signs of dehydration including weight loss. For bottle-fed infants, the scenario is the same and parents report that it may take over 1 hour for the infant to

consume 1 oz of formula. It is at this time that a palatal cleft may be noted. Somnolent, dehydrated 4-day-old infants may be hard to examine because they are resistant to opening their mouth. Insertion of a water-moistened gloved finger may be useful in examining palatal integrity (American Cleft Palate-Craniofacial Association, 1993).

Pierre Robin sequence often has a rather benign presentation with the findings of cleft palate, glossoptosis, and micrognathia (Box 15-2). Discovery of airway obstruction may not be present until the infant is 2 weeks of age or until the first upper respiratory tract infection. Therefore it is prudent to

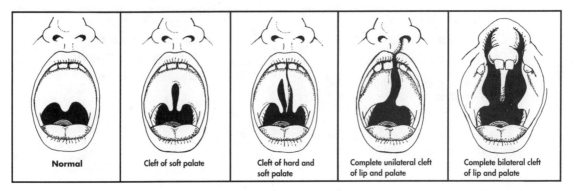

Figure 15-3   Types and examples of clefts. (Redrawn from Lynch JI, Brookshire BL, and Fox DR: A curriculum for infants and toddlers with cleft palate, Austin, 1993, Pro-Ed, Inc.)

Normal

Cleft of soft palate

Cleft of hard and soft palate

Complete unilateral cleft of lip and palate

Complete bilateral cleft of lip and palate

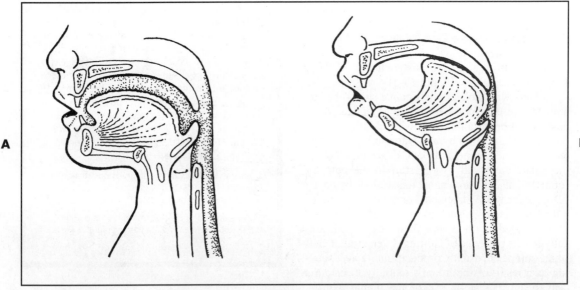

A

B

Figure 15-4   Pierre Robin sequence. Anatomical features of larynx: **A,** Normal. **B,** Mandibular hypoplasia. Note that posterior placement of tongue makes larynx appear more anteriorly situated than normal.

follow these infants closely during the first months of life and consider a baseline pediatric pulmonary evaluation within the first weeks of life. The infants are able to maintain adequate oxygen and carbon dioxide saturations initially after birth, but can tire over time with increased work of breathing. The tongue is retropositioned in the mandible and the infant has difficulty expiring carbon dioxide, which particularly occurs when the baby is placed supine

and also during sleep when the ventilatory effort is diminished (Figure 15-4).

The presentation of a child with a submucous cleft palate is more elusive. The observation of a posterior notch in the nasal spine at the juncture of the hard and soft palates along with a translucence of the soft palate is unusual unless there is clinical symptomatology to warrant closer physical examination of the soft palate. There may or may not be a bifid uvula, which can also be a normal variant, and a short soft palate with muscle separation in the midline.

Children who have nasal-sounding speech for all sounds should have a more detailed examination of their velopharyngeal mechanism. This nasal tone is often not noted until age 3 to 5 years. When the submucous cleft palate is found, then a primary care provider may retrospectively find a predictable history of nasal regurgitation of fluids, inability to breast feed in infancy, initial feeding problems, slow weight gain, and prolonged bottle feeding times. Additionally, a child may have a history of frequent episodes of serous and acute otitis media as a result of eustachian tube dysfunction associated with the cleft palate (Goldman, Martinez, and Ganzel, 1993; Muntz, 1993). Only submucous cleft palates that are symptomatic require intervention (McWilliams, 1991).

Treatment

Goals of Treatment and/or Team Care
(Box 15-3)

Goals of treatment are (1) to achieve optimum function in growth, speech, hearing, dental, and psychosocial development and (2) to achieve optimal aesthetic repair. The American Cleft Palate-Craniofacial Association believes that every individual with cleft lip or cleft palate is best served by the multidisciplinary coordinated approach offered by a cleft palate or craniofacial team (see appendix at the end of this chapter for listings). Parents may either contact the team independently, or contact can be facilitated by their primary health care provider.

Newborns should be referred to a team before discharge from the birthing hospital. Older children can and should be referred for team consultation because management occurs over the first 18 years of life. The team must include a qualified speech pathologist, an orthodontist, and a plastic surgeon. Other specialties on a cleft palate team often include: audiology, otolaryngology, dental specialties (e.g., pediatric dentistry, prosthodontics, oral and maxillofacial surgery), genetics/dysmorphology, genetic counseling, nursing, social work, psychology, and pediatrics. Teams that care for children with more complex craniofacial deformities may

---

Box 15-3

Treatment

- Establishment of adequate feeding
- Airway management for infants with Pierre Robin sequence
- Plastic surgery and oral-maxillofacial reconstruction
- Otolaryngology management
- Speech pathology treatment
- Dental/orthodontic care
- Psychosocial support

---

also include members from anesthesia, neurosurgery, ophthalmology, radiology, and psychiatry.

Initial management of a newborn with a cleft involves diagnosis clarification (i.e., rule out associated syndromes), psychosocial support for the grieving family of the child with a congenital birth defect, feeding issues, and airway management for infants with Pierre Robin sequence.

Establishment of Adequate Feeding

The goal of feeding is to maintain optimum nutrition using a technique that is as normal as possible. Infants with an isolated cleft lip or a cleft lip and alveolus (gum) do not generally experience any feeding difficulties. Infants with cleft palate, on the other hand, require some minor adaptations to establish effective feeding. Establishment of negative intraoral pressure is necessary to draw milk out of a nipple, and an infant with a cleft palate is unable to accomplish this aspect of the sucking process. There is generally no problem with the infant's ability to swallow, and despite "noisy" feeding sounds there is not an increased incidence of aspiration pneumonia in infants with cleft palate. Therefore the feeding technique must deliver the milk into the oral cavity so the baby can swallow it normally.

Although infants with a cleft lip or cleft lip and alveolus may be able to breast feed with minor positioning modifications, infants with cleft palate are not able to breast feed owing to the inability to create a seal and develop adequate suction.

The most common feeding device utilized is the Mead Johnson Cleft Lip and Palate Nurser

(Figure 15-5), which has a soft plastic compressible bottle and a cross-cut nipple that is slightly longer and narrower than regular nipples. The nipple, however, is not the crucial element of this device as evidenced by some infants' preference for an orthodontic type of nipple that is also effective. The orthodontic nipple is useful in large clefts because it can obturate the cleft. This large nipple can provide some tongue stabilization during the sucking process, and its single hole provides a faster flow of milk. The soft plastic bottle allows the parent to control the rate of milk delivered, with rhythmic squeezing of the bottle timed to the infant's cues of swallowing. The nipple should be aimed at the parts of the palate that are intact to take advantage of any possible nipple compression between the tongue and the palate.

Alternatives to the Mead Johnson nurser are available but are more costly and complicated

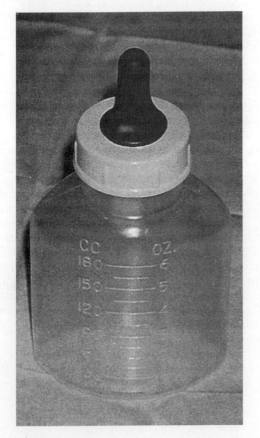

Figure 15-5   The Mead Johnson cleft palate nurser.

without being more effective in establishing feeding. The Medula Company distributes a Haberman feeder, which provides milk flow when the nipple is manually compressed by the feeder or when the infant's gums apply pressure to the plastic nipple. There are varying flow rates and also a one-way valve between the nipple and bottle to decrease the chances of air ingestion with milk. The bottle has several plastic pieces and requires more training to use correctly than the Mead Johnson system. Additionally, the cost is $22.00 vs. approximately $2.00 to $3.00 for each Mead Johnson bottle.

Another feeding device alternative is to cut the hole of a cross-cut nipple larger to ¼″ in length. A 2-oz bottle works well initially with the enlarged cross-cut nipple to provide jaw support more easily with a finger during the feeding. The Ross Cleft Palate nipple is intended for postoperative feeding and is not appropriate for newborns because the flow rate is too fast. Likewise, the Lamb's nipple is an outdated device that is bulky and causes gagging.

Whatever feeding method is chosen, there are principles or guidelines most effective in achieving appropriate weight gain. The family needs personalized teaching within the first week of life regarding assessment, feeding methodology, and evaluation of response to feeding by a practitioner experienced in management of infants with clefts (American Cleft Palate-Craniofacial Association, 1993). Ideally this practitioner should be a member of a cleft palate or craniofacial team. Consistency with a chosen technique for a minimum of 24 hours is important to allow both parent and infant to adapt. Continuous switching of nipples is confusing. Feedings should last no longer than 30 to 45 minutes, and the frequency should not be less than every 2½ to 3 hours. These guidelines promote conservation of energy and decreased caloric expenditure during the feeding process.

Infants who have Pierre Robin sequence require a careful airway assessment, and effective management strategies must be in place before addressing feeding issues. This strategy may vary from placing a tracheostomy for severe, obstructive, upper airway problems to prone positioning at rest and sitting upright during feedings for mild airway symptomatology (Sher, 1992; Singer and Sidoti, 1992).

The use of feeding appliances or acrylic prosthetic devices varies across the country. These devices assist the infant with a cleft in making a seal over the palatal cleft and creating negative intraoral pressure. Additionally, the appliance is used in maintaining or, in the case of an active appliance, manipulating the position of the dental arches and promotes the normal positioning of the tongue in the bottom of the oral cavity. The appliance is custom-made by a dental specialist (i.e., pedodontist, prosthodontist, or orthodontist) and is worn 24 hours a day, only to be removed for cleaning. It is larger than the airway and cannot be swallowed. Sometimes a thin coat of denture adhesive is required to maintain placement in the cleft area. This device may be useful in feeding but does not enable an infant to successfully breast feed, and bottle feeding can be established without it.

Surgical Reconstructive Management

There is a frequent misconception that cleft lip or palate or both are merely surgical problems that are corrected in early childhood when the lip and palatal holes are closed. Parents who are very eager to learn of the timing of surgical repairs soon learn of the multidisciplinary rehabilitative services that must be coordinated with the surgeries. Specific timing of surgery is varied between different teams and individual primary care providers.

Surgical Reconstruction of a Cleft Lip

Surgical repair of cleft lip is generally done between 3 and 5 months of age. Many surgeons use the rule of 10's—10 weeks of age, 10 g/dl hemoglobin level, and 10 pounds in body weight—in planning the repair. Occasionally if the cleft is very wide, especially in a unilateral defect, a surgical cleft lip adhesion is done at about 1 month of age to better approximate the lip tissue in preparation for the definitive procedure at the usual age.

Postoperative management for an infant with cleft lip has changed dramatically in recent years. Unrestricted breast or bottle feeding immediately after surgery has been shown to decrease the length of hospital stay, increase oral intake, and improve parental satisfaction without negatively affecting suture line integrity (Boekelheide et al, 1992). Surgery is now performed on an outpatient basis with the infant discharged with elbow restraints. Parents are instructed to clean the suture line with normal saline for 1 to 2 weeks, and pain management is usually adequate with oral acetaminophen.

Secondary lip revisions may be necessary before beginning school or during the school-age years. A nasal repair during the toddler years to lengthen the columella (soft tissue from nasal tip to nostril sill area) is frequently indicated for children with bilateral clefts.

Surgical Reconstruction of a Cleft Palate

Surgical repair of a cleft palate is usually done between 9 and 18 months of age. This is timed to provide the reconstructed palate needed for speech development (see Figure 15-6). The repair is most commonly done at one time; however, a staged palatal reconstruction of the hard and soft palates is an option. The postoperative management usually dictates a 2-night hospital stay for airway monitoring and adequate enteral hydration. The use of elbow restraints and avoidance of straws and utensils for feeding for 2 weeks are routine. The use of bottles 24 to 48 hours after palatal surgery is variable depending on the center. Cup-feeding is taught for liquids and blenderized solid food. Some centers use mist tents for 1 night to provide humidification for dried bloody nasal and oral secretions. Good pain management usually requires a parenteral narcotic (e.g., morphine sulfate) on the day of surgery followed by an enteral narcotic analgesic (e.g., acetaminophen with codeine elixir) on the first postoperative day followed by an enteral analgesic (e.g., acetaminophen).

Secondary palatal surgery may be recommended by the speech pathologist in order to address persistent nasal speech after a period of speech therapy. The procedures either create a smaller space in all dimensions (i.e., sphincter pharyngoplasty) or create a flap of tissue in the middle (i.e., pharyngeal flap) with two side ports to produce velopharyngeal sufficiency or closure during speech. This second surgery is most commonly done on children of preschool age in order to achieve clear speech before school entry (Witt and D'Antonio, 1993).

Repair of the bony defect along the gum or alveolar ridge is timed according to dental development and eruption of secondary teeth (Berkowitz, 1996; Millard, 1980). Roots of the teeth need to be anchored on bone, and generally iliac crest cancellous bone is harvested and packed into the alveolar cleft defect. This surgical procedure is usually done at 7 to 9 years of age. Dietary restrictions and the use of blenderized food for 2 weeks by cup are indicated.

A

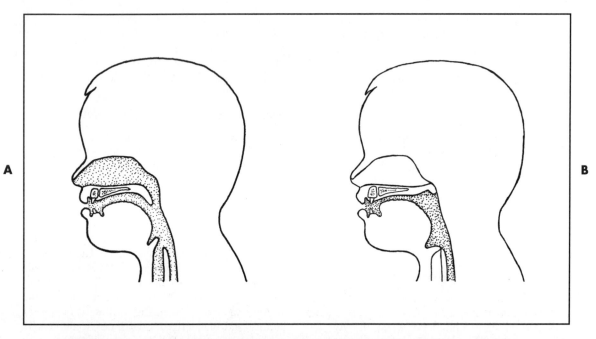

B

Figure 15-6   Anatomy of the roof of the mouth. The hard and soft palates separate the nasal cavity from the mouth. **A,** Soft palate open. Muscles relax for breathing and making certain speech sounds. **B,** Soft palate closed. Muscles in the soft palate and throat seal off the nasal cavity for swallowing foods and liquids and making certain speech sounds. (Redrawn from Looking forward: a guide for parents of the child with cleft lip and palate, Evansville, Ind., 1997, Mead Johnson & Co.)

Final nasal reconstruction surgical repair (i.e., rhinoplasty) is done when full growth has been attained (i.e., after menstruation in females and the growth spurt in males).

Some teens also require midface oral and maxillofacial surgery to address facial imbalances as a result of growth disturbance from the clefting that cannot be completely corrected by orthodontics.

Otolaryngology Treatment

Otolaryngology management involves monitoring persistent serous otitis media and aggressive management with placement of ventilation tubes in the tympanic membranes (Muntz, 1993). Ventilation tubes should be considered if there is fluid in the middle ear space at the time of any other surgical procedures (i.e., cleft lip or palate repair). Because of the high incidence of middle ear problems, some centers favor placement of ventilation tubes at the time of surgical palate repair for all children.

Following placement of the tubes, parents are advised to use silicone ear plugs that work well in the pediatric population and are available in local pharmacies. Children should use plugs while bathing and swimming to prevent water from entering the middle ear cleft.

A small percentage of children have chronic eustachian tube dysfunction after 5 years of age and may require multiple replacements of ventilating tubes to maintain normal hearing through the school-age years. The indication for tubes may be recurrent or persistent serous otitis media or severe retraction of the tympanic membrane in which there is little air present in the middle ear space, resulting in an increased risk for cholesteatoma. The tympanic membranes may be very scarred and a persistent perforation of the tympanic membrane may be present after extrusion of the ventilating tube. This membrane does not need to be patched surgically if the perforation is functioning like a patent ventilating tube. When the child is a teenager, it may be patched if the eustachian tube functioning improves with time (Muntz, 1993).

Dental and/or Orthodontic Treatment

A child with an isolated cleft palate requires regular pediatric dental care and orthodontic services. The palatal growth forward and laterally may be restricted—especially if the cleft extends into the hard bony palate. The surgical palate procedure in infancy creates scarring along areas that normally experience significant growth during childhood. As a result, a palatal expansion appliance may be necessary in order to achieve adequate dental occlusion.

Children with Pierre Robin sequence who have micrognathia in infancy usually experience catch-up mandibular growth during the first year of life. Sometimes, however, children may need orthodontic management to deal with dental crowding as a result of the small mandible.

Children with bilateral or unilateral clefts of the alveolar ridge require considerable orthodontic management. Until the eruption of secondary dentition, these children should be followed by a pediatric dentist.

Recent and Anticipated Advances in Diagnosis and Management

There has been a recent focus on fetal surgery for cleft lip and palate repair (Oberg, Kirsch, and Hardesty, 1993). Proposed advantages of such surgical intervention include: decreased scar formation in fetal wound healing; decreased potential costs as a result of less need for extensive postoperative care, orthodontia, and speech therapy; and minimized psychologic trauma associated with facial deformity. This type of surgical repair has been done in the laboratory in fetal mice, rabbits, sheep, and monkeys.

Obvious limitations to this treatment modality include accurate prenatal diagnosis through ultrasound, which would capture some infants with cleft lip but would not include those with isolated cleft palate. The potential risks to the mother and the early fetus are considerable and probably do not justify the intervention because clefting is not considered a life-threatening problem. Nonetheless, the current research will be beneficial for an increased

---

Box 15-4
Associated Problems

- Feeding difficulty
- Audiology/otolaryngology problems
- Speech pathology
- Dental/orthodontic problems
- Psychosocial adjustment to a physical deformity

---

understanding of craniofacial development and early effects of management upon wound healing.

Potential advances in the management of children with cleft lip and palate include genetic testing to identify the genes that are transformed when an infant has a clefting disorder (Oberg, Kirsch, and Hardesty, 1993). Further research regarding the effects of maternal vitamin deficiencies and environmental factors on gene transformation may provide clues into preventive measures that may be used during pregnancy (Tolarova, 1993).

Associated Problems (Box 15-4)

Audiology and/or Otolaryngology

Infants and children with an isolated cleft lip or cleft lip and alveolus generally do not have abnormal audiologic findings at a rate above the general population. Infants and children with cleft palate, however, have significant audiologic and otolaryngologic problems. Audiologic testing is appropriate in children with cleft palate to monitor the degree of conductive hearing loss in order to guide the clinician in providing appropriate interventions and documenting the effectiveness of management. Newborns can be tested by audiologic screening known as algorithm auditory brain stem response screening, or ALGO (Amer CP-Cranf Assoc, 1993). If an infant does not pass the ALGO screening, the primary care provider may find it appropriate to proceed with more complex testing known as auditory brain stem response testing (ABR), which monitors the sensorineural auditory system.

Children who are at least 6 to 9 months of age may be tested by behavioral audiologic testing. This type of testing requires some degree of cooperation and is given when an infant can sit and respond to sounds. These findings should ideally correlate with the physical examination by the oto-laryngologist so a combined approach to management can then be devised.

The dynamic functioning of the eustachian tube, which serves as the communication link between the middle ear space and the back of the throat, is controlled by the palatal musculature. The child with cleft palate has abnormal placement and under-development of palatal musculature. As a result, the functioning of the eustachian tube is suboptimal. When a child develops an upper respiratory tract infection, fluid normally accumulates in the middle ear space. This fluid usually drains into the oral cavity when the infection and swelling of the eustachian tube subside (Figure 15-7). In a child with cleft palate, however, the eustachian tube may only rarely open, and as a result the fluid remains behind the tympanic membrane on a chronic basis (Goldman, Martinez, and Ganzel, 1993). Infants and children with cleft palate have an 80% incidence of developing chronic serous otitis media associated with eustachian tube dysfunction.

Monitoring children with ear tubes in place is usually done every 6 months and more frequently as necessary for blocked, infected, or prematurely extruded tubes. It is especially important to monitor for the presence of middle ear fluid and resultant conductive hearing loss in children who are rapidly acquiring speech and language skills and are already challenged by the cleft palate, which makes this acquisition more difficult.

Many parents query the primary care provider as to why the eustachian tube dysfunction continues after the surgical repair of the cleft palate. Even though palatal tissue is restored closer to normal, the dynamic mechanisms that control the influence of the palatal musculature on eustachian tube function are not normalized.

Speech Pathology

Children with isolated cleft lip usually do not have significant speech articulation problems. These children may only require short-term therapy that focuses on the anterior and bilabial sounds found in *m* and *b* and *p,* which require competent lip closure. Children with clefts of the alveolus have additional challenges with anterior sounds as well as with managing air leakage from the front of the gums into the anterior nasal cavity before the cleft is surgically repaired with eruption of secondary dentition (Peterson-Falzone, 1986).

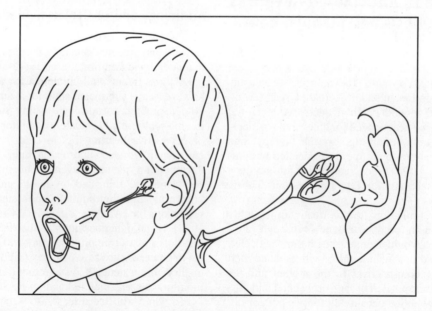

Figure 15-7   Ear-eustachian tube relationship and proximity to the palate. (Redrawn from Ross Laboratories, Columbus, Ohio.)

Children with clefts of the palate have problems with speech articulation (Witt and D'Antonio, 1993). Even before surgical repair of the palate at 9 to 18 months of age, children develop compensatory articulation errors to attempt to correct the nasal air escape caused by a cleft palate. The speech pathologist should meet with the family before the emergence of expressive speech and language development. Parents benefit from knowing how normal communication develops in their child. All families do not appreciate the fact that babies need to receive speech input directed at them and need to reciprocate in a turn-taking fashion with the use of body language and prespeech babbling behavior. Anticipatory guidance is standard practice for such families.

Following surgical closure of the cleft palate, parents can benefit from another visit with the speech pathologist for information about speech sounds and communication styles (e.g., turn-taking and expectations of oral communication). Formal speech therapy can begin with children as young as 2 years of age. Without this intervention, it is common to see toddlers who have developed a complex jargoning system of partially articulated words and gestures to which the people in their environment respond. Their children become frustrated in their inability to expand in expressive speech and language skills and may develop behavioral responses such as temper tantrums in order to communicate. Additionally, the child is unable to communicate even simple desires to strangers because the stranger is unfamiliar with the gestural system.

Ongoing monitoring and parental guidance on a 6-month basis with the speech pathologist is appropriate during the toddler and preschool years. At some point during this time, the speech pathologist usually determines that the child could benefit from regular speech therapy services. For children under 3 years of age, therapy may be provided by an infant development program that has specific speech therapy services or a speech pathologist that is community- or hospital-based. After 3 years of age, the child usually receives speech therapy that is provided by the local school district. An individualized education program (IEP) is necessary for this isolated service because it is a component of special education services. The speech pathologist at the craniofacial or cleft palate center should continue to monitor progress every 6 to 12 months and

provide feedback and suggestions to the speech pathologist providing the therapy.

The desired outcome following cleft palate surgery and speech therapy is clear articulation by 4 years of age. Although many variables have been studied, including type of cleft, age of surgical repair, type of surgical technique used, initiation time and length of speech therapy services, no one factor has been determined to provide the desired outcome (Tatum and Senders, 1993; Witt and D'Antonio, 1993). Rather it is a combination of factors that produce the optimal outcome.

Children who do not have clear speech development by 4 years of age may require secondary surgical palatal management—ideally before school entry. This surgery is particularly helpful if the articulation of sounds is good but there is persistent nasal air emission as a result of a deficiency of palatal tissue or a palate that has inadequate motion. If secondary surgical or prosthetic management is done, follow-up speech therapy is usually needed to obtain maximum benefit from the intervention. It is not unusual for school-age children to receive speech therapy during school, especially because they receive active orthodontic services that may further challenge speech articulation.

Dental and/or Orthodontic

Some children with a cleft alveolus have missing or extra supernumerary teeth. Care should be taken not to remove these teeth because they maintain alveolar bone mass in a dental arch that is deficient in bone at the area of the cleft. Children often develop a crossbite in primary dentition because of the bony deficiency and alveolar and palatal collapse of the arches as a result of the cleft and the growth disturbance of the hard palate from surgical closure. The crossbite does not always need to be corrected in primary dentition, but some pediatric dentists do offer early interceptive orthodontic treatment. Children may also have delayed dental eruption (Pham, 1997).

At 5 to 7 years of age, it is appropriate for a child with an alveolar cleft to have an orthodontic consultation, baseline records (e.g., photographs, dental study models, radiographs, examination), and a treatment plan. Initial management focuses on expansion of the maxillary arch with a removable or fixed active appliance in preparation for surgical grafting with iliac crest donor bone. The orthodontist usually indicates the appropriate time to perform the grafting surgery. Following the grafting procedure, the teeth adjacent to the cleft are mobilized and repositioned into the "new" alveolar bone mass (Millard, 1980).

Orthodontic management is usually done in phases and may have periods of rest when the teeth are held in place by a passive retention type of appliance. The timing and phase of intervention is dependent on the maxillary and mandibular growth that occurs into the teen years. It is not uncommon for orthodontic management to span a period of 10 years. Compliance with the recommended regimen is crucial because active movement of teeth depends on keeping frequent appointments, maintaining appliances, and practicing good oral hygiene (Figueroa, Polley, and Cohen, 1993). Maintaining regular pediatric dental care services during the orthodontic treatment is also important.

Psychosocial Adjustment to a Physical Deformity

Parents of the infant with a cleft are the first clients for the long-term psychosocial management of the child. According to observations, families who positively accommodate to their child's chronic condition have children who appear to cope at a higher level than parents who exhibit negative adaptative behaviors. The degree of clefting is not predictive of the level of psychosocial functioning (Moller, Starr, and Johnson, 1990).

The birth of an infant with a facial deformity is a constant reminder of the physical condition. Any bonding and attachment activities are related to the infant's face, and it takes some time to adjust and positively regard an abnormal face (Moller, Starr, and Johnson, 1990). Most families learn over time to appreciate their infant's own personality and special way of expressing a "wide smile." Some families have a secondary grief reaction once the child's lip is repaired and express that they "miss the cleft" (Curtin, 1990). A second adjustment to the "new" face is necessary and may take 1 to 2 weeks after surgery. Parents do not regret deciding to have the lip repair done, but rather, it is a normal adjustment. Parents are reassured when the team providers give them anticipatory guidance about their feelings. All parents initially experience grief reactions related to the loss of a perfect infant.

These feelings can resurface at times of stress such as hospitalization, initiation of speech, dental eruption, and school entry.

Children in the preschool years gain an increased understanding of their clefting birth defect as they develop a sense of self-awareness and experience teasing from peers. Simple explanations about the cleft can be reviewed and strategies for deflecting the teasing can be suggested. School-age children may need support and strategies to cope with teasing and to promote a positive self-image. Teenagers are able to articulate their wishes and priorities in treatment planning and should participate in the decision-making process. Teenagers also have increased self-image concerns and may benefit from counseling services.

Prognosis

The long-term prognosis for children with cleft lip and palate is excellent. The goals of team management are to achieve good speech articulation, functional dental occlusion, normal hearing acuity, an acceptable appearance, and a positive self-regard. Children with Pierre Robin sequence additionally have a goal of achieving adequate airway function. They are generally cared for in tertiary medical centers with cleft-craniofacial teams that work with pediatric pulmonary or pediatric otolaryngology specialists to achieve adequate airway function.

PRIMARY CARE MANAGEMENT

Health Care Maintenance

Growth and Development

Growth and development in general is not known to be negatively affected in children with a clefting disorder. In the past, infant feeding devices used to provide nutrition for neonates with a cleft palate were suboptimal. With the evolution of the squeeze bottle and the proliferation of team care and trained professionals to provide teaching, this aspect of management has been simplified. Additionally, current postoperative feeding routines are simpler and hospital stays are shorter, which all contribute to a more normalized nutritional status.

Infants with cleft lip and palate are expected to grow along the same parameters as infants without clefting. Once the feeding methodology has been taught by a member of the cleft-craniofacial team, the primary care provider will monitor the child's growth.

All children with craniofacial abnormalities should be referred to a pediatric endocrinologist if short stature (other than constitutional) is identified (Cunningham and Jerome, 1997). A midline pituitary deficiency can result in depressed growth (Rudman et al, 1978). Children who have a known syndrome may have growth and developmental problems related to the syndrome. The primary care provider needs to refer to literature found in medical genetics-dysmorphology texts to determine the usual findings and prognoses for the specific disorder identified.

Diet

Mothers of infants with cleft palate can provide expressed breast milk for their children. Hospital-grade electric pumps work the best and can be rented from a lactation consultant who is trained to provide education and support regarding long-term pumping and storage of breast milk. Most mothers use a double pumping system attachment to decrease the amount of time spent pumping milk. Mothers with a low income may be able to procure an electric pump from their local women, infants, and children (WIC) agency.

Mothers who are pumping breast milk 4 to 6 times a day in addition to bottle-feeding the milk 6 to 8 times per day need support and assistance from others. It is important to balance the needs of the mother and the family with the needs of the infant with a cleft in such a way that the mother not only feels encouraged to continue but also feels support if she decides to discontinue pumping. Mothers who are able to persevere with providing their infant expressed breast milk will be encouraged by a study that linked breast milk intake to a decreased incidence of otitis media specifically in infants with clefts (Paradise, Elster, and Tan, 1994).

Upright positioning of the infant during feeding will decrease the amount of nasal regurgitation. Parents should be reassured that a small amount of nasal regurgitation is expected and should be handled by simply wiping the nose of the infant with a cloth rather than interpreted as a signal of a problem. Cleansing of the nose and mouth with water or a cotton-tipped applicator or bulb syringe is not necessary because the mouth is self-cleaning and the nasal secretions and milk will drain by gravity. The parent may need to be reassured about the anatomy of the cleft palate. The oral and nasal cavity are combined and the parent may have an unspoken fear that the feeding will hurt the infant or that the nasal turbinates and the vomer represent brain tissue that can be injured with feeding.

The primary care provider can provide anticipatory guidance by discouraging the use of bottles—especially when filled with formula, milk, or juice—in bed. The supine position favors accumulation of the fluid into the middle ear space when the eustachian tube is open in a population that is already at risk for recurrent otitis media.

Occasionally infants with clefting do not grow along the expected norms. There may be extenuating psychosocial factors that challenge the parent and/or caretaker in feeding the infant. Initially an observation and review of methodology of feeding should be pursued along with a 24- to 72-hour diet record. Serial weight checks can provide both parental and health care provider reassurance. For the infant with Pierre Robin sequence, deceleration on the growth curve should prompt a careful reassessment of ventilatory status and the probable finding of some degree of upper airway obstruction.

For an infant who is 4 to 6 months old, introduction of solid foods and progression to table foods is sequenced the same as for noncleft infants. There may be some nasal regurgitation as the infant learns this new skill. Varying textures can sometimes alleviate this issue. Some parents require extra encouragement to proceed with the introduction of solid foods by spoon. Delayed initiation of this normal developmental skill can create negative feeding behaviors and may interfere with the normal oral motor development necessary in producing prespeech sounds. Using bottle type of infant feeders or enlarging nipple holes to accommodate solid foods also delays normal development. Messy spoon feedings are expected, and nasal reflux of solids should be handled calmly similar to the milk intake. Infants and children have only minor dietary restrictions. Some tricky foods for a child with an unrepaired cleft palate include peanut butter, soft cheese, and sweets, which are all gummy in texture. Avoiding foods that are a "choking risk," such as peanuts, popcorn, and pellet candy, is advised because these foods can get lodged in the nasal cavity. Parents are very concerned with future speech development in their infant with a cleft palate and therefore may respond to solid food progression as an aid toward a speech goal.

Safety

In addition to routine anticipatory guidance on safety issues, the child may have some restrictions during the first 2 to 4 weeks following reconstructive surgical procedures. Elbow restraints are generally used for 1 to 2 weeks after reconstructive surgery in the infant and toddler. Older preschool children may especially need these restraints, which are referred to as "reminders," at naptime and bedtime.

Dietary restrictions that are recommended postoperatively (e.g., avoidance of utensils, straws, and textured foods) are generally only necessary for about 2 weeks after surgery to allow for nontraumatic healing of the oral tissues. Some families may actually need to be encouraged and reassured to advance to soft foods 2 weeks after the surgery and an unrestricted diet 1 month after the surgery.

Youngsters need to avoid contact sports for 2 to 4 weeks after alveolar bone grafting procedures, nasal reconstruction, and midface jaw procedures to prevent disruption of the surgery before bone healing.

Infants with Pierre Robin sequence who require prone positioning for adequate ventilation may need a car safety bed rather than a car seat when traveling in an automobile; these beds are available commercially (see the list of resources at the end of this chapter).

Immunizations

Infants and children with cleft lip and palate should receive all routine immunizations at the ages recommended by the American Academy of Pediatrics. A planned surgical procedure is not a rationale for deferring routine immunizations; the child is better protected within the hospital setting when immunization status is current.

Administration of immunizations within 24 hours of a planned surgical procedure is not advisable because a low-grade fever following vaccine administration may preclude surgery. Administration of the MMR or varicella vaccine within a week before scheduled surgery is not recommended for similar reasons.

Screening

Vision: Routine vision screening is recommended. Children with isolated cleft palate should have a pediatric ophthalmology dilated examination at approximately 1 year of age and again before school entry at age 4 or 5 years to screen for Stickler syndrome, which is associated with myopia and sometimes leads to retinal detachment.

Hearing: A high index of suspicion and prompt referral to an audiologist and otolaryngologist should be made if audiologic screening in the school-age years is not passed. Detailed audiologic testing (as previously described) is done by the specialty center in the early years of life.

Dental: Routine screening is recommended for a child with an isolated cleft lip. Dental and orthodontic care is indicated for children with clefts of the alveolar ridge or the secondary palate. A pediatric dental provider is strongly advised—even if the family needs to travel some distance to obtain the service. The primary care provider should promote good oral hygiene practices, including initiation of tooth brushing or cleansing with a rough face cloth with eruption of the first tooth. Parents must be counseled on the hazards of baby-bottle tooth decay.

Dental eruption may be slightly delayed in a child with a cleft. Many families believe that once their child starts orthodontic care they no longer need to see the regular pediatric dentist. The dental cleanings and topical fluoride treatment are actually even more important during active orthodontic management.

Blood pressure: Routine screening is recommended.

Hematocrit: Routine screening is recommended.

Urinalysis: Routine screening is recommended.

Tuberculosis: Routine screening is recommended.

Common Illness Management

Differential Diagnosis

Fever

The parents of a child with a cleft are alerted to the increased incidence of middle ear disease. The presence of a fever, increased irritability, tugging at the ears, and asking family members to repeat verbalizations all signal the need to have the ears examined for acute or serous otitis media. Children with cleft palate are defined as an outlying population by the current AAP recommendations regarding middle ear disease favoring ongoing monitoring of serous otitis media rather than aggressive surgical management (Otitis Media Guideline Panel, 1994). Primary care providers are advised to refer these children to the otolaryngologist for a microscopic office examination if they have persistent (i.e., longer than 1 to 2 months) middle ear fluid or recurrent (i.e., every 1 to 2 months) acute otitis media. Management of acute otitis media is with the usual oral antibiotics and possibly prophylactic antibiotics. If the fluid remains throughout the prophylaxis period of about 2 months or longer, or if there are breakthrough infections, more aggressive surgical management is usually indicated.

Drug Interactions

Medications are not required as part of the normal treatment regimen.

Developmental Issues

Sleep Patterns

Infants and children with a unilateral cleft lip usually have a deviated nasal septum that causes noisy breathing during upper respiratory tract infections but does not negatively effect air exchange.

Children who have secondary palatal surgery to address nasal speech have a smaller upper airway space in the velopharyngeal area. These children are particularly at risk for sleep state upper airway obstruction during the first 6 weeks following surgery when local edema is present. Symptoms may include chest wall retractions with or without partial ventilation, irregular snoring with pauses greater than 15 to 20 seconds, diaphoresis, nighttime waking—especially after an apneic episode, daytime somnolence, and enuresis (Sirois et al, 1994). The child's symptomatology should be reported to the specialty center physician, which may be a pediatric pulmonologist or otolaryngologist. The severity of the symptoms will be assessed and medical management (e.g., steroid administration or inpatient observation) may be warranted. The surgical procedure rarely needs to be revised because the symptomatology is usually temporary and the desired outcome is to provide a decreased nasal airflow during speech without negatively affecting the ventilatory capabilities.

An infant with Pierre Robin sequence may have a disrupted sleep experience as a result of sleep state obstructive apnea. Careful history taking, evaluation, and management by the pediatric pulmonologist or otolaryngologist is appropriate.

Sleep patterns are usually disrupted following hospitalizations. Families should be told of this probable change in sleeping pattern at both the pre- and postoperative visits. A required postoperative change in favored sleeping position from stomach to back to prevent rubbing of a facial incision site may also temporarily affect sleep.

Toileting

There is no physiologic effect on toileting. The psychologic impact of stressful surgeries and hospitalization experiences can temporarily delay acquisition of toileting skills or result in regression of recently acquired skills.

Discipline

Parents of children with a congenital birth defect often feel guilty that they "caused" the problem in some way. This feeling can then translate into an altered perception of the child as being special and requiring extra attention to overcompensate for the guilt. Additionally, parents are very saddened to learn of the long-term management, especially the initial surgeries that their child will require. Many parents report that they wish the treatment could be done on them rather than on the child. Because the initial surgeries are done in infancy, the psychologic burden is thrust on the parents.

Parents must be encouraged to return to the infant's or child's normal routine following hospitalizations. A routine is reassuring for the child and promotes normalcy and a quicker return to normal behavior. Parents who focus exclusively on the needs of the infant or child who is sick and cater to every whim soon find that this is not functional or pleasant for the child or the family. Symptoms of this phenomenon include: no structured feeding or meal routine; irregular nap times; nighttime waking; nighttime feedings; co-sleeping in the parental bed (only if this is not the family's usual practice); excessive fussiness, irritability, or clinginess; loss of previously achieved developmental milestones; and inability to get along with others (Elmendorf, D'Antonio, and Hardesty, 1993). These are all normal reactions to a stressful experience such as a hospitalization but usually do not persist beyond 2 to 6 weeks after a 24- to 48-hour hospital stay. Parents can benefit from anticipatory guidance and encouragement to promote normalcy, which initially may appear harsh and unsympathetic. When it is presented as comforting for the child, however, most parents embrace the concept.

Issues of discipline arise again when a child with a cleft lip or palate enters school, especially if the child appears very different from peers and is teased. Overprotectiveness and lack of appropriate limits can actually exacerbate these problems. The child and family can often benefit from short-term counseling regarding self-image concerns and development of skills to cope with teasing from others.

Child Care

Child care in a group daycare setting can be stressful for parents of a child who is at risk for frequent ear infections. For this reason, some parents choose a setting with a more limited number of children—especially during the winter months.

Once children are old enough to attend a Head Start program or structured preschool, they should. Such programs can be helpful as an adjunct to speech therapy because a child's peers will promote expressive language development. Peers usually do not understand the elaborate gesturing system and monosyllabic vocalizations that substitute for expressive language and may encourage children to expand their repertoire by modeling.

Schooling

Children with cleft palate are eligible for special education services, namely speech therapy, under IDEA, PL 101-476 (see Chapter 5). Parents should request in writing a speech evaluation focused on articulation when a child is 2 years 9 months of age. It is helpful if the parents provide medical information and any prior speech evaluations.

Peer teasing can occur as a child progresses through school. Some parents and children use the "class presentation" approach to explain clefting, and teachers can incorporate this into their lesson plans about "differences" between people. A child rarely reports teasing and ridicule so severe that school phobia and frequent absences become an issue. It is important to query parents about these issues at primary care visits and offer supportive services and coordinated efforts between the primary care providers and the school system.

Children with cleft lip and palate are not predisposed to academic difficulties. Children who have an isolated cleft palate that is part of a syndrome may have a lower intellectual potential that is specifically associated with the syndrome (Strauss and Broder, 1993). These children should be evaluated by special education professionals as appropriate.

Sexuality

No special sexual problems are associated with cleft lip and palate. The obvious concerns about self-image may be exaggerated during adolescence.

When discussing reproductive issues, the risks of recurrence for clefting must be addressed. The rates quoted are between 2% and 7% (Gorlin, Cohen, and Levin, 1990; Hofstee, Kors, and Hennekam, 1993), depending on previous family history and the presence of a concurrent syndrome. Clefting is more common in males, so females theoretically have a higher genetic component and therefore a slightly higher risk of recurrence. A bilateral cleft lip is rare and more severe than a unilateral and also has a slightly higher risk of recurrence. As a result, a male with a unilateral cleft lip is at the low end (2%), and a female with a bilateral cleft lip is at the high end (7%). A complete family history and physical examination of an affected individual by a geneticist and genetic counselor is necessary to provide the most accurate information.

Women with increased risk for having a child with a cleft are eligible for a detailed ultrasound that has a better resolution of the facial features than a traditional ultrasound. Women of child-bearing age are counseled to take a multivitamin that contains folic acid on a daily basis in the hope of preventing a clefting condition (Tolarova, 1993).

Transition to Adulthood

State funding for care of children with cleft lips and palates is available to financially eligible children up to age 21 years. Most individuals are able to complete the orthodontic and oral-maxillofacial surgical procedures by this age. Problems are encountered if there were treatment lapses or delays during crucial stages of dental development or orthodontic management that necessitated restarting the treatment. Additionally, orthodontic interventions are effective during active treatment, and then the position of the teeth and the occlusion are often maintained with removable appliances (e.g., a retainer worn at night). Adolescents and their families often do not appreciate the need for these appliances, so relapse occurs. If relapse occurs before the insurance is terminated, some active management can be reinitiated. Otherwise young adults must usually pay for these services as out-of-pocket expenses. It is hard for young adults to gain third-party payment for follow-up lip or nasal surgery because such procedures appear to be cosmetic even if they relate to a congenital birth defect.

Special Family Concerns and Resources

Parents of children with a cleft lip worry about their child's physical attractiveness to others, especially strangers. Parents are sensitive to the reactions and comments of professionals and their family and look at others' facial and emotional reactions when viewing their baby with a facial deformity. Fears of feeding or hurting the face and the mouth and concern that the cleft extends into the brain are common. Demonstrating feeding techniques and pro-moting normal infant care routines provide opportunities for learning and alloying anxieties.

It is beneficial to recommend that parents photograph their infant with a facial cleft, as well as to discuss with parents the usefulness of retaining a photograph that will be available for the child to view when older. If the parents are resistant, stating that they prefer to forget this time of sadness and wish to defer picture taking until after cleft lip repair, it may be prudent for a professional working with the family to take a photograph to keep in the infant's chart.

Families may verbalize oral, auditory, and dental concerns as they become more informed. These concerns and consequent stressors recur over time with rehospitalizations, tooth eruption, initial speech, school entry, and adolescent self-image concerns. Orthodontic services are a crucial component of the rehabilitation process and are covered by the local state CCS program if a family is financially eligible. Families who do not meet the financial eligibility often find this care very expensive.

Special cultural issues that affect families who have a child with a cleft lip and palate are mostly concerned with the etiology of the clefting condition. Superstitions about why clefting occurs often originate in a family's country of origin. Hispanic and Filipino cultural folklore believe that clefting is related to the lunar cycle. A lunar eclipse or a crescent moon during a woman's pregnancy predisposes her unborn child to clefting. Some Asian cultural folklores relate construction, cutting, a fall, or moving the mother's bed during pregnancy with birth defects—especially clefting. In Chinese culture the center of a person's face is very important and central to that person's being (i.e., instead of the heart, which is common in Western culture). This view has implications for a cleft lip and palate deformity in its central location.

Most young parents acknowledge that such beliefs are part of cultural folklores and are explanations that their parents and grandparents provided for the untoward events that happened during a pregnancy. Trying to disprove these theories is unnecessary, especially because the etiology of clefting is unknown. It is more useful to focus on the common feeling of maternal guilt associated with a birth defect and work through the grief process over time.

Some families bring with them extreme fears of surgery and hospitalization, but fear usually seems to be experience-related (i.e., a relative who died after a surgical procedure) rather than related to a specific cultural framework. The concept of health care in general, especially preventive health care (e.g., the routine dental care or anticipatory guidance needed to prevent speech articulation problems), is unfamiliar to some families. The very idea of seeking nonemergent health care services is particularly unknown in families who originate from other countries outside the United States that do not have many health care resources.

Resources

American Cleft Palate-Craniofacial Association (ACPA)
104 South Estes Drive, Suite 204,
Chapel Hill, NC 27514;
(919) 933-9044; (919) 933-9604 (fax);
cleftline@aol.com, www.cleft.com.
CLEFTLINE 1-800-24-CLEFT.
Referral to local cleft-craniofacial team, written pamphlets and fact sheets in English and Spanish; distribution of document; Parameters for Evaluation and Treatment 3/93.

About Face—USA PO
Box 737 Warrington, PA 18976
1-800-225-FACE; abtface@aol.com
Provide newsletter, information, and support.

Cleft lip and palate critical elements of care, ed 1, Seattle, 1997, Children's Hospital and Regional Medical Center.
206-527-5709 ext. 1.

Wide Smiles Newsletter,
PO Box 5153 Stockton, Calif. 95205-0153;
(209) 942-2912
widesmiles@aol.com

Mead, Johnson, & Co Nutritional Division
Evansville, IN 47721-0001;
(812) 429-5000
1-800-BABY123.
Free booklet for cleft lip and palate nursers, "Your cleft lip and palate child: a basic guide for parents."

Medela, Inc
4610 Prime Parkway
McHenry, Ill. 60050-7005;
(800) 435-8316; (816) 362-1166
For breast pump rentals and Haberman feeders. COSCO Columbus, In. (800) 468-0174. Dream Ride infant car bed/car seat: car safety bed for infants with Pierre Robin sequence who require prone positioning.

Books for Parents

Moller KT, Starr CD, and Johnson SA: A parent's guide to cleft lip and palate, Minneapolis, 1990, University of Minnesota Press.
Berkowitz S: The cleft palate story, Chicago, 1994, Quintessence Publishing.

Videocassettes for Parents

Feeding the Newborn with a Cleft Palate
Hospital for Sick Children—Cleft Lip and Palate Program
555 University Avenue
Toronto, Ontario M5G1X8
(416) 813-7490
(416) 813-6637 (Fax)

Teasing and How to Stop It
British Columbia's Children's Hospital
4480 Oak St.
Vancouver, BC V6H 3V4
(604) 875-2345

Summary of Primary Care Needs for the Child with Cleft Lip and Palate

HEALTH CARE MAINTENANCE

Growth and development

Expectations for physical growth and development are the same as those for the noncleft population.

Diet

Use of cleft palate nurser enhances bottle feeding

Cleft palate—provision of expressed breast milk with use of an electric pump.

Introduction of solids by spoon at the same time as noncleft population.

Safety

Elbow restraints following surgical procedures.

Avoidance of utensils, straws, and textured foods approximately 2 weeks after surgical procedures to allow for nontraumatic oral healing.

Avoidance of contact sports for 2 to 4 weeks after surgeries.

Prone positioning for infants with Pierre Robin sequence; may need car safety bed vs. car seat.

Immunizations

All routine immunizations should be given on schedule.

May elect not to administer DaPT within 24 hours of a surgical procedure and MMR/varicella 1 week before a surgery.

Screening

Vision: Routine screening is recommended.

Children with isolated cleft palate or Pierre Robin sequence need a dilated eye examination by a pediatric ophthalmologist at 1 year of age and 4 to 5 years of age to rule out myopia, which is found in Stickler syndrome.

Hearing: Audiology screening for children with cleft lip and alveolus.

Ongoing close monitoring for conductive hearing loss in children with cleft palate.

Dental: Screening for milk bottle caries.

Routine pediatric dental care for children with cleft lip. In addition to routine pediatric dental care children with cleft alveolus and palate need an orthodontic evaluation by age 5 to 7.

Blood pressure: Routine screening is recommended.

Hematocrit: Routine screening is recommended.

Urinalysis: Routine screening is recommended.

Tuberculosis: Routine screening is recommended.

COMMON ILLNESS MANAGEMENT

Differential diagnosis

Fever: Rule out acute otitis media.

Drug interactions: None.

DEVELOPMENTAL ISSUES

Sleep patterns: Unilateral cleft lip and palate—deviated septum, noisy breathing especially with URI.

Increased risk of sleep state obstructive apnea following secondary palatal surgical procedures.

Disruption of sleep patterns following surgical procedures and hospitalization.

Signs of sleep state obstructive apnea requiring careful pulmonary evaluation and management in infants with Pierre Robin sequence.

Toileting: Temporary regression following surgical procedure and hospitalization.

Discipline: Expectations are normal, with allowances during hospitalizations and 1 to 2 weeks after surgery.

Overprotectiveness or lack of limit setting may result if family pities child.

Child care: May need to be in smaller group setting during winter months because of increased risk of otitis media.

Speech therapy sessions need to be coordinated with child care arrangements.

Schooling: Speech therapy to begin at age 3 for children with cleft palate, requires an individualized education program (IEP).

Continued

***Summary of* Primary Care Needs for the Child with Cleft Lip and Palate—cont'd**

Peer teasing may negatively impact performance.

Teasing may occur because of lip, nose, and dentition appearance or speech articulation problems.

Sexuality: Genetic counseling recommended to discuss recurrence risks.

Women of childbearing age recommended to take folic acid to hopefully prevent clefting.

During pregnancy a detailed ultrasound is available to ascertain whether the fetus has a cleft lip.

Transition into adulthood: Treatment plan should be completed by age 21.

There is difficulty in procuring third-party payment for any orthodontic, oral-maxillofacial, or plastic surgical services in adulthood.

Special family concerns and resources

There is heightened awareness of physical appearance

Pre-surgical photographs are important.

Speech, audiology, and dental issues are challenging for families.

Cultural superstitions are common regarding the etiology of clefting.

Multiple surgical procedures during childhood are stressful for families.

References

American Cleft Palate-Craniofacial Association: Parameters for evaluation and treatment of patients with cleft lip and palate or other craniofacial anomalies, Cleft Palate-Cranf J 30:(Suppl 1), 1993.

Berkowitz S: Secondary Alveolar Bone Grafting: After Lip and Palate Closure. In Berkowitz, S: Cleft Lip and Palate vol I and II, San Diego, 1996, Singular Publishing Group. 103-113.

Boekelheide A et al: Comparison of postsurgical feeding techniques following cleft lip repair on suture line integrity, volume of oral fluid intake and length of hospital stay: a multicenter study. Presented at the American Cleft Palate-Craniofacial Association Annual Meeting, Portland, Or., 1992.

Cunningham ML, Jerome JT: Linear Growth Characteristics of Children with Cleft Lip and Palate, J Pediatrics, 131(5):707-711, 1997.

Curtin G: The infant with cleft lip or palate: more than a surgical problem, J Perinat Neonatal Nurs 3:80-89, 1990.

Elmendorf EN, D'Antonio LL, and Hardesty RA: Assessment of the patient with cleft lip and palate—a developmental approach, Clinics in Plastic Surgery 20:607-621, 1993.

Figueroa AA, Polley JW, and Cohen M: Orthodontic management of the cleft lip and palate patient, Clinics in Plastic Surgery 20:733-753, 1993.

Goldman JL, Martinez SA, and Ganzel TM: Eustachian tube dysfunction and its sequelae in patients with cleft palate, Southern Medical Journal 86:1236-1237, 1993.

Gorlin RY, Cohen MM, and Levin LS: Orofacial clefting syndromes: general aspects. In Gorlin RY, Cohen MM, and Levin LS (editors): Syndromes of the head and neck, ed 3, New York, 1990, Oxford University Press, pp 693-714.

Hofstee Y, Kors N, and Hennekam RCM: Genetic survey of a group of children with clefting: implications for genetic counseling, Cleft Palate-Cranf J 30:447-451, 1993.

Kelly TE: Teratogenicity of anticonvulsant drugs. 1: review of the literature, Am J Med Genet 19:413-434, 1984.

McWilliams BJ: Submucous clefts of the palate: how likely are they to be symptomatic?, Cleft Palate-Cranf J 28:247-249, 1991.

Millard DR: Cleft craft: the evolution of its surgery, vol 1: the unilateral deformity; vol 2: bilateral and rare deformities; vol 3: alveolar and palatal deformities, Boston, 1980, Little, Brown, & Co.

Millard DR: Introduction, clefts 1993, past, present and future, Clinics in Plastic Surgery 20:597-598, 1993.

Moller KT, Starr CD, and Johnson SA: A parent's guide to cleft lip and palate, Minneapolis, 1990, Univ. of Minnesota Press.

Muntz HR: An overview of middle ear disease in cleft palate children, Facial Plastic Surgery 9:177-180, 1993.

Oberg KC, Kirsch WM, and Hardesty RA: Prospectives in cleft lip and palate repair, Clinics in Plastic Surgery 20:815-821, 1993.

Otitis Media Guideline Panel: Quick reference guide for clinicians managing otitis media with effusion in young children, J Am Acad Nurse Pract 6(10):493-499, 1994.

Paradise JL, Elster BA, and Tan L: Evidence in infants with cleft palate that breast milk protects against otitis media, Pediatrics 94:853-860, 1994.

Peterson-Falzone S: Speech characteristics: Updating clinical Decisions, Sem Speech Lang 7(3):269-295, 1986.

Pham AN et al: Developmental dental changes in isolated cleft lip and palate, Pediatr Dent 19(2):109-13, 1997.

Rudman D et al: Prevalence of growth hormone deficiency in children with cleft lip or palate, J Pediatr 93:378-382, 1978.

Sher AE: Mechanisms of airway obstruction in Pierre Robin sequence: implications for treatment, Cleft Palate-Cranf J 29:224-231, 1992.

Singer L and Sidoti EJ: Pediatric management of Pierre Robin sequence, Cleft Palate-Cranf J 29:220-223, 1992.

Sirois M et al: Sleep apnea following a pharyngeal flap: a feared complication, Plastic Reconstructive Surgery 93(5):943-947, 1994.

Smith AW et al: A Modification of the Kernahan "Y" classification in cleft lip and palate deformities, Plastic Reconstructive Surgery 102(6):1842-1847, 1998.

Strauss RP and Broder H: Children with cleft lip and palate and mental retardation: a subpopulation of cleft-craniofacial team patients, Cleft Palate-Cranf J 30:548-556, 1993.

Tatum S and Senders C: Perspectives on palatoplasty, Facial Plastic Surgery 9:225-231, 1993.

Tolarova M: Primary prevention of cleft lip with or without cleft palate by vitamins and high folic acid. Presented at the American Cleft Palate-Craniofacial Association Annual Meeting, Pittsburgh, Pa., 1993.

Tolarova MM and Cervenka J: Classification and birth prevalence of orofacial clefts, Am J Med Gen 75:126-137, 1998.

Witt PD and D'Antonio LL: Velopharyngeal insufficiency and secondary palatal management—a new look at an old problem, Clin Plastic Surgery 20:707-721, 1993.

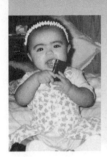

CHAPTER 16

Congenital Adrenal Hyperplasia

Judith A. Ruble and Betty M. Flores

Etiology

The adrenal glands are small triangular organs located at the top of each kidney. They are divided into two major components: the adrenal medulla, which is in the center of the gland, and the adrenal cortex, which surrounds the medulla.

The adrenal cortex synthesizes glucocorticoids (i.e., primarily cortisol), mineralocorticoids (i.e., mainly aldosterone), and androgens through complex metabolic pathways. A simplified diagram of these pathways is shown in Figure 16-1. Cortisol, aldosterone, and adrenal androgens play a crucial role in maintaining homeostasis by helping to regulate the body's blood pressure; glucose, sodium, and water levels; sexual development, and other metabolic processes (Bacon et al, 1990; New, 1995).

Congenital adrenal hyperplasia (CAH) is caused by a deficiency of one of the enzymes used by the adrenal cortex to produce cortisol and aldosterone. Although there are six possible enzyme defects, over 90% of CAH is caused by 21-hydroxylase deficiency (New, 1998; Pang, 1997). The other five enzyme defects are rare and are not discussed here. Each of the enzyme defects causing CAH is inherited as a separate autosomal recessive genetic trait. The gene responsible for CAH is located on the short arm of chromosome 6 and is linked to the loci for HLA-B and DR antigens (New, 1995; Pang, 1997).

Adrenal production of glucocorticoids is regulated by a feedback system to the hypothalamus and pituitary gland (Figure 16-2). The hypothalamus normally secretes corticotropin-releasing factor (CRF), which causes the pituitary gland to produce adrenocorticotropic hormone (ACTH). In turn, ACTH stimulates the adrenal glands to synthesize glucocorticoids (i.e., primarily cortisol). The "switch" that controls this feedback system is corti-

sol. When blood levels of cortisol are low, the system turns on: the hypothalamus releases CRF, which signals the pituitary to release ACTH, stimulating the adrenal glands to synthesize cortisol. When blood levels of cortisol rise, the system turns off, the hypothalamus stops releasing CRF, the pituitary gland stops releasing ACTH, and the adrenal glands stop synthesizing cortisol. Because cortisol production is blocked in CAH, the hypothalamic-pituitary-adrenal system is not turned off, resulting in high ACTH levels that continuously stimulate the adrenal glands (Bacon et al, 1990; New, 1998). The continual stimulation by ACTH leads to hypertrophy of the adrenal glands, a buildup of precursors to cortisol, and an overproduction of adrenal androgens (see Figure 16-1). Aldosterone synthesis is primarily regulated by the renin-angiotensin system of the kidney, so a block in aldosterone synthesis will cause very high activity levels of plasma renin, just as a block in cortisol synthesis will cause high ACTH levels (Bacon et al, 1990).

There are two forms of "classical" 21-hydroxylase deficiency: salt-losing CAH and non–salt-losing (i.e., simple virilizing) CAH. In the salt-losing form both cortisol and aldosterone production are blocked (see Figure 16-1). The absence of aldosterone results in excessive sodium loss through the kidneys and the inability to maintain normal serum electrolyte balance. In the non–salt-losing form, only cortisol production is blocked and aldosterone production meets the body's normal needs. There may be a mild deficit of aldosterone, however, as indicated by elevated plasma renin activity levels or mild hyponatremia during stress (Bacon et al, 1990; Migeon and Donohoue, 1991; New, 1998).

The alterations in adrenal steroid metabolism caused by 21-hydroxylase deficiency lead to the buildup of precursors of cortisol and aldosterone

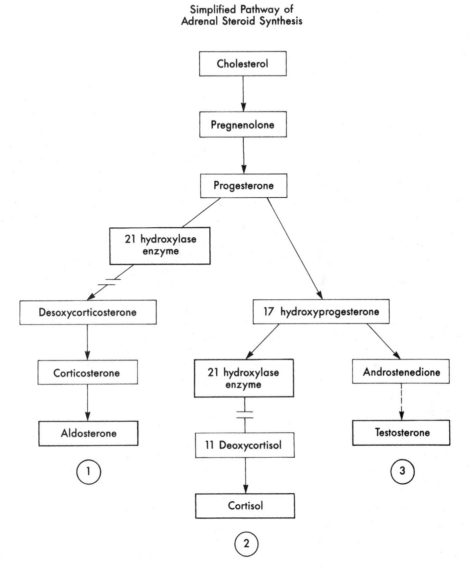

Figure 16-1   In salt-losing CAH, pathways 1 and 2 are blocked, causing aldosterone and cortisol deficiencies. In non–salt-losing CAH, only pathway 2 is blocked, causing cortisol deficiency. In both forms of CAH, there is a buildup of precursors and an overproduction of adrenal androgens.

and overproduction of adrenal androgens, which do not require the 21-hydroxylase enzyme (see Figure 16-1). Laboratory assays for precursors, (e.g., serum 17-hydroxyprogesterone [17-OHP] or urine 17-ketosteroids and pregnanetriol) are used to monitor the adequacy of cortisol replacement ther-

apy for CAH. Laboratory assay of plasma renin activity is used to monitor the mineralocorticoid replacement in the salt-losing form of CAH (New, 1998; Pang, 1997).

Another type of 21-hydroxylase deficiency, which is commonly called the "nonclassic" form, is

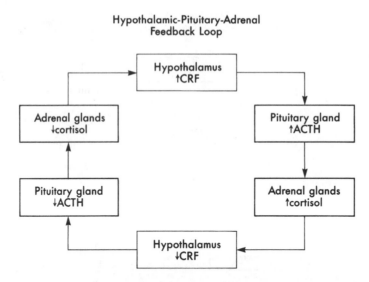

Figure 16-2 Blood levels of cortisol turn the hypothalamic-pituitary-adrenal system "on" and "off". Low cortisol levels cause the hypothalamus to make CRF; CRF causes the pituitary to release ACTH; ACTH stimulates the adrenal cortex to synthesize cortisol; high cortisol levels cause the hypothalamus to stop making CRF; without CRF, the pituitary stops producing ACTH; without ACTH, the adrenal cortex stops synthesizing cortisol; the cycle repeats.

not apparent at birth by physical findings. This form of CAH is more prevalent than the classic form (Brosnan et al, 1998). Its clinical features are similar to those of classical 21-hydroxylase deficiency but occur later in childhood and are much milder (i.e., many are asymptomatic) without salt-losing and acute adrenal insufficiency (New, 1995). Nonclassical 21-hydroxylase deficiency does not present the management difficulties and risks of the classical form.

Incidence

As of 1995, more than 7.5 million newborns worldwide have been screened for 21-hydroxylase deficiency CAH. Screening reports from Brazil, Canada, France, Germany, Israel, Italy, Japan, New Zealand, Portugal, Saudi Arabia, Scotland, Spain, Sweden, Switzerland, and the United States show incidences ranging from 1 : 5,000 live births in Saudi Arabia to 1 : 23,000 live births in New Zealand (Pang and Shook, 1997). The overall incidence of classical 21-hydroxylase deficiency is estimated to be 1 : 15,000 live births worldwide (New, 1998), although some isolated populations (e.g.,

the Yu'pik-speaking Eskimos of Alaska) have an extraordinarily high incidence of CAH (i.e., 1 : 282) (Trautman et al, 1996). Two thirds to three fourths of cases are the salt-losing form (New, 1998). The incidence of 21-hydroxylase deficiency reported by clinical diagnosis is lower than that reported by neonatal screening (Pang and Shook, 1997). This discrepancy may be the result of early deaths of infants with salt-losing CAH before a diagnosis was made. Methods for prenatal diagnosis and neonatal screening of individuals known to have a blood relative with CAH are available. Screening could significantly reduce the number of deaths from undiagnosed CAH, as well as reduce the morbidity associated with nonfatal episodes of acute adrenal insufficiency and excessive virilization (New, 1995).

Clinical Manifestations at Time of Diagnosis

Nearly all female infants with CAH will have virilization apparent on physical examination at birth (Figure 16-3). The findings range from a mildly

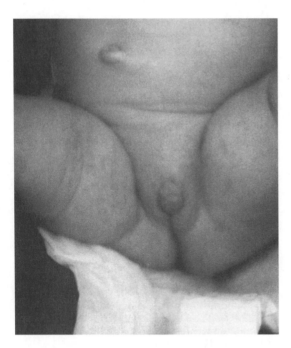

Figure 16-3 An infant girl with CAH-caused clitoromegaly.

enlarged clitoris to complete fusion and rugation of the labia with the urethra opening through a urogenital sinus at the base of the phallus or even on the phallus (Box 16-1) (New, 1995).

Female infants with a mildly enlarged clitoris often go undetected, but an alert primary care provider can identify these infants by paying close attention to clitoral size. When measured at the base with redundant skin retracted, the normal clitoral breadth—not length—in a female infant is 2 to 6 mm; this range applies to all gestational ages of newborns and for infants up to 1 year of age (Riley and Rosenbloom, 1980). The middle range virilization of a female infant looks abnormal enough to prompt an immediate search for the cause. Unfortunately, severely virilized female infants may go undiagnosed because they are mistaken for cryptorchid males with hypospadias or micropenis.

Male newborns with CAH look normal and cannot be reliably identified by physical examination, although the penis may be slightly enlarged and genital pigmentation mildly increased (New, 1995).

The label "ambiguous genitalia" should be applied to any infant with either hypospadias and no palpable gonads or a micropenis and no palpable gonads. Because the most common cause of ambiguous genitalia is CAH, it should be high on the clinician's index of suspicion and part of the diagnostic work-up (New, 1995).

Newborns with salt-losing CAH will have elevated activity levels of plasma renin at birth, although elevated serum potassium levels and decreased serum sodium levels may not be apparent for 1 week (Pang, 1997). Newborns with either form of classical CAH will have significantly elevated 17-OHP levels by 24 to 36 hours of age (the infant's age should be noted on the specimen). False positive results are possible, however, in premature or low birth weight infants (Bacon et al, 1990; Pang and Shook, 1997). If salt-losing CAH is not diagnosed and replacement therapy is not started at birth, both male and female infants will have symptoms of acute adrenal insufficiency and a salt-losing crisis within the first few weeks of life. These symptoms include failure to thrive, weakness, vomiting, and dehydration (Pang, 1997). Unfortunately these symptoms are nonspecific and usually prompt a workup for sepsis, pyloric stenosis, or severe malabsorption. Because the routine evaluation of infants with these symptoms normally includes serum electrolyte values, hyponatremia and hyperkalemia should signal clinicians to suspect acute adrenal insufficiency.

The lack of specific symptoms combined with a low index of suspicion on the part of medical personnel can lead to a high mortality rate for undiagnosed infants—especially boys. The difference in the frequency of salt-losing CAH when based on early case reports vs. when based on newborn screening reinforces the belief that many of these infants die because of a salt-losing crisis before being diagnosed (Zucker, 1996).

Children with non–salt-losing CAH (i.e., who have only cortisol deficiency) may go undiagnosed for years. These children have an impaired ability to withstand stress, so minor illnesses (e.g., acute otitis media, streptococcal pharyngitis, bronchitis) and febrile (i.e., temperature >38.4° C) illnesses may cause excessive weakness, pallor, hypotension, and prolonged convalescence (Burnett, 1980). Severe stressors (e.g., surgery or a fractured bone) can trigger acute adrenal insufficiency with extreme weakness, abdominal pain, vomiting, dehydration, hypotension, and—if not adequately treated—vascular collapse and death (Bacon et al, 1990).

Treatment

It was not until the 1950s that an understanding of the metabolic defect in CAH led to the current concept of replacement therapy, and it was another decade before adequate therapy was routinely used (Bartter, 1977; Migeon and Donohoue, 1991). It is not yet possible to correct the genetic defect that blocks the adrenal metabolic pathways, but the clinical consequences of the defect can be controlled by replacing the blocked end products of cortisol and aldosterone (Box 16-2). The goals of replacement therapy are to prevent acute adrenal insufficiency crises and further virilization and to achieve normal growth and adult stature and normal fertility (Helleday, 1993). In both salt-losing and non–salt-losing CAH, hydrocortisone tablets or liquid (Cortef) are given as a replacement for cortisol; in salt-losing CAH, however, fludrocortisone acetate (Florinef) is added as a replacement for aldosterone (New, 1998).

Basal Hydrocortisone

The basal, nonstress dose of hydrocortisone is intended to suppress ACTH stimulation of the adrenals and the resultant overproduction of adrenal androgens. Determining an optimal replacement dose is crucial to minimize side effects while achieving desired therapeutic effects. Excessive hydrocortisone dosage can lead to obesity, stunted linear growth, and signs of Cushing's syndrome (e.g., truncal obesity, striae, bruising, hirsutism, muscle weakness, and hypertension) (Cornean,

Box 16-2
Treatment

Glucocorticoids; dose increased for stress
Mineralocorticoids (salt-losing)
Sodium chloride supplement (salt-losing infants)
Injectable hydrocortisone for emergencies

1998; New, 1998). Inadequate dosage puts a child at risk for acute adrenal insufficiency and allows excessive androgen production, which causes virilization and accelerates growth and advancement of bone age. A common regimen is 15 to 25 mg/m^2/day divided into three doses and given orally every 8 hours, but there is considerable disagreement on the optimal dosage regimen (Bacon et al, 1990; New, 1998; Sandrini, Jospe, and Migeon, 1993).

Stress Hydrocortisone

The basal hydrocortisone dose is doubled or tripled during the acute phase of an illness (e.g., temperature >38.4° C, significant malaise, or pain) or mild to moderate stress. Stress doses do not require prolonged tapering and should be returned to basal levels as soon as the acute stress is resolved (Bacon et al, 1990). Examples of stresses and dosage guidelines are provided in Box 16-3.

If a child vomits more than once, the stress is severe, or the child does not respond to oral treatment, injectable hydrocortisone (Solu-Cortef) must be given. The typical dose of 50 to 100 mg is based on the size and usual replacement dose of a child and should be prescribed in conjunction with an endocrinologist (Bacon et al, 1990). Parents should have injectable hydrocortisone on hand, know the indications for using it, and learn how to prepare and give an intramuscular (IM) injection. Parents who are unable to give injectable hydrocortisone must have rapid (i.e., 5- to 10-minute) access to a hospital emergency room or health care provider equipped to administer hydrocortisone parenterally.

If the necessity of giving emergency treatment is uncertain, there is no physical harm in treating suspected acute adrenal insufficiency that is not present, and the consequence of not treating acute adrenal insufficiency can be the death of a child (Bacon et al, 1990; Lim, Batch, and Warne, 1995).

Box 16-3

Guidelines on Stress Doses of Hydrocortisone*

1. For a temperature of 38.4° to 38.9° C (orally) or for mild illness, give double the basal dose orally.
2. For a temperature of 38.9° C or higher (orally) or for moderate illness, give triple the basal dose orally.
3. For minor injury (e.g., sprain), give double the basal dose orally.
4. For vomiting once and acting well, wait 20 minutes and give double the basal dose orally.
5. For vomiting once but acting ill, vomiting more than once, or acting ill in spite of increased oral dose, give hydrocortisone intramuscularly.
6. For serious injury (e.g., fracture or concussion), give hydrocortisone intramuscularly.
7. If the child looks severely ill or has symptoms of acute adrenal insufficiency, give hydrocortisone intramuscularly and go to the emergency room.
8. If the child is unconscious for any reason, give injectable hydrocortisone intramuscularly and go to the emergency room.
9. In general, emotional stress does not require increased hydrocortisone doses; for severe, prolonged emotional upheaval, consult with the endocrinologist for advice.
10. Call the endocrinologist or primary care provider for all but mild illnesses.
11. Consult the endocrinologist before all surgical procedures.

NOTE: When in doubt, give stress doses of hydrocortisone. The stress dose should be reduced to basal levels after the acute phase of the illness, injury, or stress; it does not require a prolonged taper.

*From Children's Hospital, Oakland, California.

Box 16-4

Signs and Symptoms of Acute Adrenal Insufficiency

1. Nausea or vomiting
2. Pallor
3. Cold, moist skin
4. Weakness
5. Dizziness or confusion
6. Rapid heart rate
7. Rapid breathing
8. Abdominal, back, or leg pain
9. Dehydration
10. Hypotension

In such situations it is always best to err on the side of prompt, aggressive treatment.

In a medical setting, acute adrenal insufficiency is treated with hydrocortisone (Solu-Cortef) or hydrocortisone 21-phosphate given intravenously in 5 to 10 times the basal dose along with appropriate intravenous (IV) therapy to restore intravascular volume and electrolyte balance (Box 16-4) (New, 1995). If IV access is not available, hydrocortisone should be given intramuscularly instead of waiting until IV therapy can be started.

Fludrocortisone

Salt-losing CAH requires mineralocorticoid replacement with fludrocortisone (Florinef), in addition to hydrocortisone therapy (New, 1998). Children with non–salt-wasting CAH may have mild impairment of aldosterone synthesis, as evidenced by elevated plasma renin activity, even though such impairment is not apparent clinically. Adding fludrocortisone to the treatment regimen will normalize the plasma renin activity levels and may permit a reduction of the hydrocortisone dose and improve linear growth (Lim, Batch, and Warne, 1995; Duck, 1980).

The usual dose of fludrocortisone is 50 to 200 mg daily given orally in a single dose. Newborns may temporarily need doses as high as 200 to 300 mg daily for stabilization, and adolescents may also require up to 250 to 300 mg daily during the rapid growth period (Bacon et al, 1990; Lim, Batch, and Warne, 1995). Excessive amounts of mineralocorticoid will result in hypokalemia, weight gain, edema, hypertension, and headache. Inadequate doses will impair growth and put a child at risk for a salt-losing crisis (Rosler et al, 1977).

The basal mineralocorticoid dose does not need to be increased during illness because the increased amount of hydrocortisone given during stress has enough mineralocorticoid activity to make additional fludrocortisone acetate unnecessary (Stern and Tuck, 1986).

Sodium chloride supplementation may be required in infants if salt loss exceeds salt intake—in spite of mineralocorticoid therapy (Lim, Batch, and Warne, 1995). The usual dose is 3 to 5 mEq/kg/day divided into two to four doses and dissolved in formula or other liquid (Bacon et al, 1990; Mullis, Hindmarsh, and Brook, 1990).

Most girls with CAH have severe enough virilization of the external genitalia to require surgical correction. Corrective surgery often requires more than one procedure (e.g., clitoral reduction, separation of the fused labia, correction of a urogenital sinus, and vaginoplasty), with initial corrections done before 2 years of age (Bailez et al, 1992; Donahoe and Gustafson, 1994; Premawardhana et al, 1997). Although satisfactory cosmetic and functional results are usually achieved, additional surgery may be necessary during adolescence to enlarge the vagina to allow for intercourse and avoid the need for repeated dilatation (New, 1995). Newer surgical techniques may allow even severe virilization of infant girls to be corrected with a single procedure performed before 1 year of age (Donahoe and Gustafson, 1994). Longer term observation is needed, however, because delayed stenosis could develop, requiring additional surgery (Donahoe and Gustafson, 1994).

All surgical procedures are a major stress to the child and require consultation with an endocrinologist for perioperative management.

Recent and Anticipated Advances in Diagnosis and Management

Newborn Screening

Newborn screening efforts for CAH in 13 countries and 17 U.S. states have resulted in early diagnosis with associated reductions in morbidity and mortality. Improvements in assay types and reference ranges for low birth weight and preterm infants have contributed to more accurate newborn screening for CAH. Although false positive results in preterm and low birth weight infants are still problematic, this issue is being addressed through the continued refinements of newborn screening (Pang and Shook, 1997; Therrel et al, 1998).

Prenatal Diagnosis and Treatment

Recent advances have been made in prenatal diagnosis and prenatal treatment of CAH. Prenatal diagnosis can be made in the first trimester by HLA typing or DNA analysis performed by chorionic villus sampling at or after 9 weeks gestation. Second trimester diagnosis can be made by amniocentesis measuring adrenal steroids in amniotic fluid at or after 14 weeks gestation. Virilization of female fetuses with CAH can be prevented or reduced by administering dexamethasone to mothers during pregnancy. Dexamethasone therapy must be started before virilization begins at about 10 weeks' gestation. Because a prenatal diagnosis of CAH may not be available at this time, the treatment decision initially includes unaffected fetuses and their mothers.

Although initial attempts at prenatal dexamethasone treatment have shown some favorable outcomes and appear to have no complications for infants, results have been variable in preventing virilization. Maternal side effects can also be significant, and long-term effects on growth and psychomotor development in treated children are unknown. More experience is warranted to establish a standard of treatment with prenatal dexamethasone. Long-term studies evaluating the effects of prenatal dexamethasone exposure on the growth and psychomotor development of treated children are also necessary (Mercado et al, 1995; New, 1998; Pang, 1997; Trautman et al, 1995). The procedures, potential benefits, risks, and unknown long-term effects in treated children should be fully explained to families seeking genetic counseling who have a first-degree relative with CAH (Levine and Pang, 1994).

Prenatal diagnosis and treatment of CAH are areas of intense interest and rapid progress. These procedures will likely be refined and become readily available in the future.

Other Areas of Research

There is an ongoing search for improved treatment regimens that achieve the therapeutic goals while reducing or eliminating undesirable side effects. Current management of CAH often involves choosing between the effects of excess cortisol and the effects of excess androgen because extraphysiologic doses of hydrocortisone are required to fully suppress adrenal androgen overproduction.

One promising solution to this dilemma is reducing the dose of hydrocortisone to physiologic levels and adding flutamide and testolactone to the treatment regimen (Laue, 1996). Flutamide is an antiandrogen that is able to block the effects of androgen excess. Testolactone blocks the conversion of androgen to estrogen, which may help improve final height because estrogen accelerates advancement of bone age (Laue, 1996). A reduced, physiologic dose of hydrocortisone eliminates the side effects of hypercortisolism. Preliminary results with this regimen showed a normalization of linear growth, weight gain, and bone age. Further studies are needed, however, to evaluate the safety and long-term results. One obvious drawback of this regimen is that it increases the complexity of treatment, which may lead to decreased adherence.

Some clinicians have suggested adrenalectomy as a way of simplifying and improving the management of CAH (Ritzen and Wedell, 1996; VanWyk and Gunther, 1996). The rationale for adrenalectomy is that there is no need to suppress adrenal androgens, so lower doses of hydrocortisone can be used and improved final heights might be achieved. Proponents of adrenalectomy restrict its use to individuals with a complete absence of 21-hydroxylase, because they are the most difficult to manage and have the lowest final heights (Ritzen and Wedell, 1996; VanWyk and Gunther, 1996). Adrenalectomy as a treatment for severe salt-losing CAH is highly controversial, however, and is not widely accepted by endocrinologists.

Other areas of research that may lead to improved therapy in the future include gene therapy and development of an ACTH or CRH antagonist (Cutler, 1996).

Associated Problems

The problems associated with CAH are limited in children receiving appropriate therapy. Primary care providers must be aware, however, of the potential for acute adrenal insufficiency, growth disorders, virilization, and problems surrounding issues of sexuality (Box 16-5).

Box 16-5

Associated Problems

Acute adrenal insufficiency
Accelerated growth and bone age
Virilization
Precocious puberty
Fertility problems

Acute Adrenal Insufficiency

Children with CAH may develop acute adrenal insufficiency with any significant illness or injury because they lack the ability to produce increased amounts of cortisol as part of the body's normal stress response.

Accelerated Growth and Bone Age

Excessive androgen production causes accelerated linear growth and muscle development in children with undiagnosed or inadequately treated CAH (e.g., a 5-year-old child could have the height and build of an 8- or 10-year-old). Another consequence of excessive androgen production is rapidly advancing bone age with early closure of the growth plates (e.g., a 5-year-old with the height and build of a 10-year-old may have the bone age of a 15-year-old). This consequence means that children who were unusually large for their age during the early years will stop growing early because of premature closure of the growth plates and end up a significantly short adolescent and adult (New, 1995).

Virilization

Virilization of the fetus begins at approximately the tenth week of gestation, so virtually all newborn girls with CAH have virilized genitalia requiring surgical correction (Bacon et al, 1990; Donahoe and Gustafson, 1994; New, 1995). By early school age, untreated boys may have an adult-sized penis (although the testes remain normal size for age), and untreated girls will be severely virilized with fused labia and a markedly enlarged clitoris. Both sexes will have adult-appearing pubic and axillary hair and acne. If the condition remains untreated until adolescence, changes from prolonged exposure to very high testosterone levels may no longer be reversible. Boys may have benign testicular tumors and impaired testicular development or spermatogenesis, and girls will not have breast development or menarche (Srikanth et al, 1992).

Puberty

Most children with consistently well-controlled CAH will have normal onset and progression of puberty (Lim, Batch, and Warne, 1995). Some children, however, may enter puberty prematurely. The onset of precocious puberty is believed to be caused by the "priming" of the pubertal timing system by chronically high androgen levels, triggering the complex—and poorly understood—system of pubertal development (Pescovitz et al, 1984). Children who do experience precocious puberty can be successfully treated with gonadotropin-releasing hormone (GnRH) analogs (Dacou-Voutetakis and Karidis, 1993; Pescovitz et al, 1984). GnRH analogs are available as subcutaneous (SQ) injections given daily (e.g., leuprolide acetate [Lupron]), IM injections given every 4 weeks (e.g., leuprolide acetate [Lupron Depot-Ped]), and intranasal spray (e.g., nafarelin [Synarel]) given four times a day.

The occurrence of precocious puberty not only increases the complexity, expense, and burden of a family's medical regimen but also increases psychosocial stresses. Children with precocious puberty are faced with physical sexual development that they are not emotionally ready for, as well as with teasing and sexual harassment. These children are also at increased risk for sexual abuse (Jackson and Ott, 1990). Parents of a child with precocious puberty must meet with school and daycare personnel to ensure that teasing and sexual harassment are not tolerated. Children must be taught how to maintain their "sexual boundaries" (i.e., what kind of remarks, activities, or touching are "OK" and "not OK") and where to go for help (Jackson and Ott, 1990; Ott and Jackson, 1989).

Reduced Fertility

Menstrual irregularities and hirsutism caused by androgen excess are common in adolescent girls with CAH and may contribute to reduced fertility (Kuhnle and Bullinger, 1997). Although most women with CAH are fertile, their fertility rates are somewhat lower than those of unaffected women (Bacon et al, 1990; Helleday, 1993; Premawardhana et al, 1997). Factors that are associated with higher fertility rates for women with CAH are early diagnosis, consistently adequate replacement therapy, and non–salt-wasting status (Premawardhana et al, 1997).

Both a physical and hormonal explanation for the lower fertility rates found in women with CAH, as well as for the difference between women with salt-wasting vs. non–salt-wasting CAH, have been proposed. Women with salt-wasting CAH are more likely than women with non–salt-wasting CAH to have an inadequate vaginal introitus, which could impair sexual activity and conception (Mulaikal, Migeon, and Rock, 1987). Women with CAH also have higher than normal levels of circulating progestational hormones for significant periods of time, even with generally adequate replacement therapy. Women with salt-wasting CAH tend to have higher levels than women with the non–salt-wasting form, which may have the effect of an endogenous "mini pill" that suppresses fertility (Helleday, 1993).

Prolonged exposure to high levels of androgens in undiagnosed or inadequately treated children will eventually result in irreversible infertility and virilization in girls and may cause impaired fertility in boys (Mulaikal, Migeon, and Rock, 1987; New, 1995).

Testicular Masses

Benign testicular masses are an uncommon complication of CAH in males and most often occur in males with chronically inadequate replacement therapy (Berg, 1996; Srikanth, 1992).

Congenital Anomalies

The incidence of congenital anomalies associated with CAH is not thought to be significantly increased over that of the general population. Although there have been reports of an increased incidence of upper urinary tract abnormalities associated with CAH, these have not been clearly established (Bacon et al, 1990).

Prognosis

The major risk for children with CAH is death from an unrecognized salt-losing crisis early in infancy or from inadequately treated acute adrenal insufficiency during stress. Screenings of individuals with a family history of CAH for the carrier state, prenatal screenings, and routine neonatal screenings have the potential to greatly reduce the number of children who die of CAH (New, 1995). CAH screening is now included in the newborn screening programs of 17 U.S. states, and other states are considering adding it to their programs (Brosnan et al, 1998). Nearly all female infants with CAH have morbidity associated with prenatal virilization and the surgical procedures necessary to correct it. If prenatal treatment of female fetuses to prevent virilization becomes available as a standard treatment, it should have a substantial effect on reducing the morbidity in girls with CAH (New, 1995).

PRIMARY CARE MANAGEMENT

Health Care Maintenance

Growth and Development

Because abnormal linear growth is an indication of inappropriate treatment or poor compliance, careful monitoring of growth is essential. Linear growth should be measured every 1 to 4 months for infants and every 3 to 6 months for children over 2 years of age. These measurements should be done carefully, using an infantometer for lengths and a stadiometer for heights. The standard, scale-mounted measuring device is not accurate enough to detect slight variations in growth. Measurements should be plotted on a standardized growth chart and assessed for changes in growth rate (e.g., an increase or decrease in centile).

Poor Growth

Linear growth is acutely sensitive to excessive levels of hydrocortisone, therefore any decrease in height centile on the growth chart should prompt a reassessment of the hydrocortisone dosage. A child's hydrocortisone therapy will occasionally be increased based on a high laboratory 17-OHP result when the result was high because of an acute illness, stress from an unusually traumatic venipunc-ture, or frequently missed hydrocortisone doses before sampling. To avoid unnecessary and possibly harmful increases in hydrocortisone doses, clinicians must rule out these other causes of high 17-OHP values before increasing medication doses. Clinicians can do this by taking a careful history and comparing the prescribed dose of hydrocortisone with the established dose ranges. The primary care provider may be in a position to identify the problem and should contact the endocrinologist with this information.

Another cause of poor linear growth in children with CAH is chronically inadequate mineralocorticoid levels (Duck, 1980). A plasma renin activity level that is abnormally high indicates that a child needs additional mineralocorticoid or dietary sodium. A careful history and comparison with established dose ranges will determine if this problem is one of compliance or inadequately prescribed doses.

A child with poorly controlled CAH, or one who was not diagnosed until preschool or school age, may have early cessation of growth because of premature closure of the epiphyses. If such premature closure is suspected, radiographic studies of bone age should be done to assess skeletal maturity.

Excessive Growth

Inadequate hydrocortisone replacement will cause excessive androgen synthesis by the adrenals, resulting in accelerated linear growth. An elevated serum 17-OHP level or clinical findings of increased virilization (e.g., pubic and axillary hair, oily skin, acne, enlargement of the phallus) confirm the cause of excessive growth. Clinicians must be careful to assess whether the inadequate hydrocortisone replacement is secondary to an inappropriately prescribed dose or to poor adherence.

Excessive Weight Gain

Glucocorticoid replacement therapy—even at doses within the accepted therapeutic range—has been associated with obesity (Cornean, 1998). Clinicians must closely monitor weight gain, avoid overtreatment with glucocorticoids, and encourage good dietary and activity habits to reduce any tendency towards obesity.

Development

Children with CAH who are diagnosed in infancy or very early in childhood and receive consistently adequate treatment should develop normally (Lim,

Bach, and Warne, 1995). If the diagnosis of CAH is not made until late childhood, however, the child will be much taller and more mature looking than peers. Because of their mature physical appearance, people may expect these children to have the emotional maturity and behavior of older children. This expectation may lead to frustration for all concerned, inappropriate demands and punishment, and the creation or exacerbation of behavior problems.

When these children stop growing early because of premature epiphyseal closure, they will go from being the tallest to the shortest children in their peer group. Short stature has an effect on behavior and social relationships and probably has an even greater effect on someone who spent early childhood as the tallest person in any group of peers (Holmes, Karlsson, and Thompson, 1986; Young-Hyman, 1986).

Children with CAH should be regularly evaluated for premature sexual development in order to determine the adequacy of therapy. Clinicians should include appropriate counseling regarding sexual development to the child and family.

Parents, school personnel, child care workers, and others who regularly interact with these children should be given clear, frequently reinforced guidelines on age-appropriate expectations to avoid demanding too much of tall but immature children or too little of short adolescents.

Diet

The main modification to a normal diet is an allowance for adequate sodium intake. Although an appropriate dose of mineralocorticoid prevents significant sodium depletion in children with salt-losing CAH, these children should be offered salty foods and allowed to salt their food to taste. This recommendation also applies to children with non–salt-losing CAH because they may have a mild salt deficit when compared with unaffected children (Rosler et al, 1977). As mentioned previously, good dietary habits are essential to reduce the tendency to gain excessive weight (Cornean, 1998). The advice of a dietician can be helpful in identifying "nutritionally dense" foods that meet a child's dietary needs without excessive calories.

Safety

Children with CAH are not physically impaired or at increased risk for any of the usual physical haz-

ards of childhood, but they are at risk for having their special needs neglected when away from home. Injuries such as a broken bone may not be recognized as potentially life-threatening events. Teachers, child care personnel, coaches, and others in regular contact with the child should have written information describing the condition and the need for prompt treatment in an emergency. The child should wear a Medic-Alert bracelet with this information on it.

The decision of whether or not to keep injectable hydrocortisone at school or daycare depends on the situation and must be made on a case-by-case basis. Factors to consider are as follows: (1) Can the primary care provider or emergency room be reached in 5 to 10 minutes? (2) Is a parent always available at short notice? (3) Are there trained personnel at the site who are willing to give an IM injection? (4) Does the child engage in activities with a high risk of serious injury?

If injectable hydrocortisone is kept at school or daycare, the most convenient preparation is the 100-mg Solu-Cortef Mix-O-Vial (Pharmacia & Upjohn), which is easy to use and store. Written indications for use and dosage should be provided by the endocrinologist.

Participation in sports is a normal part of childhood and should be encouraged; if possible, however, children with CAH should be directed toward activities with a low risk of serious injury (e.g., swimming, track, or tennis). Minor injuries (e.g., bruises, mild or moderate sprains, or abrasions) are not cause for special concern. If these children are involved in high-risk sports (e.g., football), parents should meet with the coach to explain their child's special needs in an emergency, as well as provide appropriate written materials, instructions, and authorization for treatment. A parent or team physician should ideally be present and have hydrocortisone for IM injection on hand during competition. Their presence should be mandatory if the activity takes place more than 15 minutes away from a source of emergency care.

Immunizations

Children with CAH are not immunosuppressed and should receive all standard immunizations at the usual ages. There is currently no recommendation for or against giving additional immunizations (e.g., pneumococcal or influenza), but the benefits of immunity to these diseases must be weighed against the possibility of adverse reactions to the vaccine. In weighing these factors, many clinicians believe that giving additional immunizations is worthwhile to reduce the risk of acute adrenal insufficiency triggered by illness.

It is not necessary to increase the basal dose of hydrocortisone before immunizations are given unless there is a history of adverse reactions to previous immunizations with that vaccine. A common but discretionary recommendation is to give a child acetaminophen a few hours before giving an immunization that is likely to produce a rapid-onset febrile reaction and continue it for 24 to 48 hours afterward.

For new vaccines or new combinations of vaccines, the package insert should be referred to for information on the type and timing of possible reactions and families should be counseled to observe their child closely on the days when reactions are likely to occur (e.g., 5 to 12 days after measles vaccination).

Stress doses of hydrocortisone should be given if a child develops a temperature of more than 38.4° C or is fussy or lethargic after an immunization (see Box 16-3). Any immunization reaction should be documented so that stress doses of hydrocortisone can be given before subsequent immunizations with the same vaccine.

Screening

Vision: Routine screening is recommended.

Hearing: Routine screening is recommended.

Dental: Routine screening is recommended.

Blood pressure: Blood pressure should be checked at each primary care visit, which requires special equipment (e.g., a Dinamap [Critikon]) for infants. Every effort should be made to relax and quiet children so that readings are accurate.

Elevated blood pressure in a quiet child may indicate excessive mineralocorticoid or hydrocortisone dosage, whereas low blood pressure may indicate an inadequate mineralocorticoid or hydrocortisone dosage. Either situation should prompt an evaluation of the replacement therapy regimen and compliance.

Hematocrit: Routine screening is recommended.

Urinalysis: Routine screening is recommended.

Tuberculosis: Routine screening is recommended.

Condition-Specific Screening

Serum 17-OHP: Primary care providers may want to order additional screening tests to more closely monitor the adequacy of replacement therapy in children who have difficulty with compliance. The serum 17-OHP level is widely accepted as a measure of hydrocortisone therapy, even though it has the disadvantage of being influenced by temporary stress (e.g., traumatic venipuncture), the length of time since the last hydrocortisone dose, and diurnal fluctuations. To help evaluate the significance of 17-OHP results, clinicians should note on the specimen the time of day (i.e., preferably morning) and the time of the last dose of hydrocortisone. Androstenedione and testosterone levels can be evaluated along with 17-OHP to monitor adequacy of hydrocortisone therapy. Some clinicians rely on 24-hour urinary 17-ketosteroid and pregnanetriol levels to monitor hydrocortisone therapy because of the lack of short-term fluctuations, despite the difficulty in collecting a 24-hour specimen. Serum 17-OHP levels should be no more than three times above normal (i.e., preferably less than 200 ng/dl). Urinary 17-ketosteroid and pregnanetriol levels should also be in the normal to near-normal range for age, as should plasma renin activity. Specimens ordered by the primary care provider should be coordinated with the endocrinologist and sent to the same laboratory to ensure consistency.

Plasma renin activity: Mineralocorticoid therapy is monitored by measuring plasma renin activity level. The primary care provider who is monitoring 17-OHP levels should include a plasma renin activity assay for individuals with salt-losing CAH.

Bone age: The frequency of radiographic studies of bone age depends on the clinical course. Bone-age evaluations are not helpful in newborns. Initial bone age should be determined early in childhood (i.e., at 2 to 3 years of age or at the time of diagnosis if the diagnosis is delayed) and can be used as a baseline for future studies. If a child is growing normally and has consistently acceptable 17-OHP and plasma renin activity levels, routine screening should not be necessary more than every few years.

If a child has growth acceleration, physical findings of increased virilization, or consistently high 17-OHP laboratory results, bone age should be determined to further assess the effects of androgen excess. If bone age is accelerated, this finding can be used to help impress on the family the serious and permanent consequences of poor adherence. All bone-age studies should ideally be read by the same person to avoid inconsistencies in interpretation.

Common Illness Management

Differential Diagnosis

Children with CAH are not immunosuppressed and their susceptibility to common childhood illnesses is no different from that of their peers; it is their ability to withstand the stress of illness that is impaired (Box 16-6). During periods of illness, these children must be followed closely; consultation with an endocrinologist is necessary if a child shows any signs or symptoms of acute adrenal insufficiency (see Box 16-4).

The primary care provider caring for a child with CAH should keep injectable hydrocortisone in the office for emergencies. The most commonly used preparation is the 100-mg Solu-Cortef Mix-O-Vial (Pharmacia & Upjohn) because of its long shelf life and convenience (e.g., it does not require refrigeration). When reconstituted by rotating and depressing the plunger-stopper, it contains 100 mg of hydrocortisone in 2 ml and can be given intramuscularly or intravenously.

In addition to a Medic-Alert bracelet or necklace, the child and family should carry written materials (e.g., a wallet card) stating the diagnosis, stress dose of hydrocortisone, indications for administering the stress dose, and the name and telephone number of the endocrinologist. This emergency information should be updated regularly.

Box 16-6

Differential Diagnosis

Upper respiratory infections and allergies
Acute illness
Fever
Vomiting
Injury
Acute adrenal insufficiency

Upper respiratory infections and allergies: If the symptoms are mild and the child does not have fever or marked malaise, no specific treatment or increase in basal dose of hydrocortisone is necessary for upper respiratory infections or allergies. Parents should watch for worsening of symptoms, fever, or unusual lethargy; and school-aged children should know to report these symptoms to their teacher and contact their parents. If symptoms worsen or complications develop, children should be promptly treated with a stress dose of hydrocortisone and seen by the primary care provider for assessment and specific therapy for the illness.

Acute illnesses: Any known or suspected bacterial illness (e.g., acute otitis media, urinary tract infection, streptococcal pharyngitis, and cellulitis) should be treated aggressively with the appropriate antibiotic and stress doses of hydrocortisone during the acute phase of the illness if fever, pain, and malaise are present (see Box 16-3). When the diagnosis is uncertain or there is a significant risk for secondary infections or complications (e.g., a suspicious but not clearly inflamed tympanic membrane, viral pneumonia, or prolonged or marked nasal congestion in a child with a history of frequent acute otitis media or sinusitis), it is wise to treat the child with antibiotics rather than wait for the situation to worsen. The child must be followed closely, with an initial office visit for diagnosis and assessment of the child's overall condition and daily telephone progress reports until the acute phase of the illness has passed. Follow-up office visits should be scheduled as for any other child.

Fever: Although fever is a physiologic response to illness, it is also a stress. Therefore fever in a child with CAH should be treated with acetaminophen in the recommended dose for age. Stress doses of hydrocortisone should be given using the guidelines in Box 16-2. It is important to advise families that reducing the fever does not cure the illness and that other treatments (e.g., antibiotics and stress doses of hydrocortisone) should continue to be given as directed. The child must be followed closely (i.e., as described for bacterial and viral illnesses) until the illness has resolved.

Vomiting: If a child with CAH vomits once but otherwise appears well, twice the usual oral dose of hydrocortisone should be given about 20 minutes later, and the child should be closely observed. If a child appears weak or lethargic after vomiting once or vomits more than once, the family should give injectable hydrocortisone intramuscularly and contact the endocrinologist immediately. If family members are not able to give injectable hydrocortisone, they must immediately take the child to the nearest emergency room to receive parenteral hydrocortisone and appropriate fluid and electrolyte therapy because this can be a life-threatening situation. The emergency room staff should contact the endocrinologist but should not delay hydrocortisone therapy while awaiting consultation. A wallet card or other written information on the child's diagnosis, emergency treatment, and endocrinologist can facilitate prompt and appropriate care.

Injury: A child with a significant injury (e.g., a fracture, concussion, or injury from an automobile accident) should immediately be given hydrocortisone intramuscularly and evaluated further for acute adrenal insufficiency at an emergency room. Emergency room personnel should contact the endocrinologist but not delay hydrocortisone therapy while awaiting consultation.

Acute adrenal insufficiency: Acute adrenal insufficiency is a life-threatening situation. Symptoms of acute adrenal insufficiency include weakness, nausea, abdominal discomfort, vomiting, dehydration, and hypotension. Any of these signs or symptoms in a child with CAH should be presumed to indicate acute adrenal insufficiency and be treated with hydrocortisone intravenously or intramuscularly at three to five times the basal dose. This administration should be done at home—or in the primary care setting if the child is there—instead of delaying initial treatment until the child arrives at an emergency room.

The diagnosis of acute adrenal insufficiency can be confirmed by laboratory values showing hyponatremia and hyperkalemia. Although consultation with an endocrinologist should be sought, treatment should not be delayed.

An IM injection of hydrocortisone or IV therapy in an emergency room is a frightening experience that no one wants to go through unnecessarily. In this type of situation, however, it is always best to err on the side of aggressive treatment.

Drug Interactions

Families are often afraid of giving their child steroids because of negative publicity in the popular press. It is important to stress to families that the hydrocortisone and fludrocortisone medications their child takes for CAH are replacing substances normally produced in the body and that the recommended doses are calculated to match normal blood levels as closely as possible. This is very different from taking high doses of glucocorticoids to treat inflammatory diseases. Families may have read stories of athletes having severe side effects from using steroids to increase muscle mass, so they should be told that anabolic steroids are completely different from hydrocortisone in actions and side effects. Replacement therapy for CAH is also an entirely different situation from taking a foreign substance such as an antibiotic. Because the medications for CAH replace hormones normally present in the body, concern about using other medications is limited to their effect on the absorption or rate of metabolism (Box 16-7).

Barbiturates (e.g., phenobarbital [Donnatal], butalbital [Fiorinal, Fioricet], pentobarbital [Nembutal], secobarbital [Seconal], phenytoin [Dilantin], rifampin [Rifadin, Rifamate, Rimactane]) increase the rate of metabolism of glucocorticoids. Therefore children with CAH who are taking any of these medications for more than a few weeks may require a higher than usual dose of hydrocortisone for adequate cortisol replacement (Stern and Tuck, 1986). A serum 17-OHP level done approximately 2 weeks after the start of any of the medications listed here will show if an adjustment in the hydrocortisone dose is necessary. Short-term use of barbiturates perioperatively or prophylactic use of rifampin for *Haemophilus influenzae* meningitis should not require a change in hydrocortisone dose.

Antibiotics, decongestants, antihistamines, cough preparations, analgesics, antipyretics, and topical preparations have no unusual adverse effects.

Box 16-7

Drug Interactions

Barbiturates
Phenytoin
Rifampin

Developmental Issues

Sleep Patterns: Children with CAH do not differ from their peers in their sleep patterns or needs. Unusual fatigue may indicate an illness or inadequate cortisol replacement and should be evaluated.

Toileting: Children who have obvious virilization of their external genitalia should be given privacy when using the toilet to avoid teasing. The initial corrective surgery for girls who are virilized is usually done at an early age to avoid problems related to looking different. Although boys who are excessively virilized may have some regression in pubic hair and penile size once they establish consistently adequate treatment, they will be noticeably different from their peers until adolescence. These children are otherwise no different in toileting readiness or skills than their peers and are not unusually prone to constipation, incontinence, enuresis, polyuria, or other disorders related to toileting.

Discipline: Children with CAH should be expected to behave appropriately for their age. The only special consideration has to do with children who appear older than their actual age. Parents, teachers, and others must be given clear guidelines on appropriate expectations for a child's developmental stage if it is different from his or her appearance.

Another area that raises disciplinary issues is compliance with taking medication, especially during toddlerhood and adolescence when children struggle with issues of dependency and autonomy. Parents should be advised from the beginning to use a matter-of-fact approach and avoid negotiating something that is nonnegotiable. During infancy and early school years, parents have full responsibility for giving medications. As children mature and are able to assume more responsibility, parents should encourage their child's active participation (e.g., by remembering when it is "pill time," marking off the calendar for each dose, or filling a pillbox). Adolescents should have the primary responsibility for taking the medication with the parents offering support. Using a watch with a beeper is helpful for adolescents, as is a pillbox, which also provides an unobtrusive way for a parent to see if the medication disappears on schedule.

Clinicians can help make older children and adolescents aware of the consequences of poor adherence by pointing out signs of virilization to girls and slowed growth to both sexes and emphasizing that it is within their power to "get back to normal." The risks of acute adrenal insufficiency and impaired fertility associated with poor adherence should also be discussed with adolescents, again with emphasis that such things are avoidable.

An adolescent will occasionally choose to make adherence to medications the focus of serious rebellion. Every effort should be made to explain the purpose and necessity of medication, and counseling should promptly be sought if the problem is severe or chronic.

Child Care: Parents should meet with child care personnel before enrollment to explain their child's special needs. Child care personnel do not require detailed knowledge of CAH but should be given a clear explanation that a child has a metabolic disorder that requires simple—but important—treatment. Written information for the child care center should include written authorization to give hydrocortisone orally with instructions on the dose, time, and purpose; instructions on when to call parents and the telephone numbers where they can be reached, what symptoms or events require emergency care; where to take the child for care; authorization for treatment; and the name and telephone number of the primary care provider and endocrinologist. It is neither necessary nor desirable to have special rules or restrictions on activities at school or child care for children with CAH. The usual policies on safety and appropriate play are sufficient to avoid serious injury.

Because hydrocortisone is usually given every 8 hours, many children will need at least one dose while at daycare. Mineralocorticoid is given once daily to children with salt-losing CAH and can be administered at home. Although most child care providers are conscientious, they occasionally miss or delay doses of hydrocortisone because they do not understand its importance and are distracted by other demands on their attention. A routine that ties medication time to a regular activity (e.g., rest period or story time) can be established, or the child can wear a watch programmed to beep at the desired time. A letter from the primary care provider or the endocrinologist is helpful in making this invisible condition real to the people caring for these children.

Schooling: Children with CAH may have more absences than usual because of their need for close observation at home during acute illnesses. Concerns about excessive absences should be brought to the attention of the primary care provider, who can assess their appropriateness. Legitimate absences include any illness that would keep other children at home. In addition, symptoms such as a scratchy throat and malaise that might be ignored in other children should be initially observed at home.

Studies of cognitive abilities and school function in children with CAH have shown inconsistent results. Although earlier studies found normal or above normal cognitive function in individuals with CAH (Ehrhardt and Baker, 1977; Galatzer and Laron, 1989; Nass and Baker, 1991), more recent studies have found an increased prevalence of cognitive impairment or learning disabilities (Helleday, 1994; Plante et al, 1996).

Although it is not possible to identify what influence CAH itself has on cognitive and educational function with the information currently available, it is clear that acute CAH crises have a deleterious effect. Not surprisingly, children who had episodes of acute adrenal insufficiency with hypoglycemia or convulsions have a significantly higher prevalence of learning difficulties than children—with or without CAH—who did not suffer such events (Donaldson et al, 1994; Nass and Baker, 1991). Because hypoglycemia and convulsions are associated with learning difficulties, these findings may represent a complication of poor management rather than the biochemical abnormality inherent in CAH. A child with CAH who has had severe hypoglycemia and convulsions should be assessed for learning difficulties and referred for special education intervention if indicated.

Sexuality: Virilization is nearly always present at birth in infant girls. Because genital surgery is nearly always needed and considerable attention is paid to genital examination during clinic visits, these girls get the message that there is something "wrong" with them and that it has to do with their genitals. It is important to reassure these girls that they have all the normal female organs, hormones, and chromosomes, and that any surgeries are simply to correct a cosmetic mistake that happened before they were born (Mazur, 1983).

Menstrual irregularities due to androgen excess are common in adolescent girls with CAH. Androgen excess can also cause hirsutism and acne in children and adolescents of either sex and may con-

tribute to impaired fertility (Kuhnle and Bullinger, 1997).

Although many observers have noted "tomboyish" behavior (e.g. "rough and tumble play") or "increased activity levels" in girls with CAH, most of the early studies are difficult to interpret because of small sample size, lack of data on adequacy of treatment, and lack of control groups (Ehrhardt and Baker, 1977; Galatzer and Laron, 1989; Hines and Kaufman, 1994; Hochberg, Gardos, and Benderly, 1987; Money, Schwartz, and Lewis, 1984). Stereotyping behavior as "masculine" or "feminine" also remains controversial. Some recent studies using better methodology have shown significant differences in the gender-stereotypic activities and sexual behaviors of girls and women with CAH and those of their unaffected sisters. Investigators attribute these differences to prenatal exposure to high levels of adrenal androgens (Dittmann et al, 1990; Dittmann, Kappes, and Kappes, 1992; Zucker, 1996). The data suggest that, compared with their unaffected sisters, more women with CAH delay or fail to establish intimate heterosexual relationships (Dittmann, Kappes, and Kappes, 1992; Kuhnle, Bullinger, and Schwartz, 1995). The data are conflicting, however, on whether there is an increased prevalence of homosexual orientation among women with CAH (Dittmann, Kappes, and Kappes, 1992; Kuhnle, Bullinger and Schwartz, 1995). Prenatal androgen exposure is considered to be a predisposing—rather than a causative—factor in gender behavior, and all aspects of psychosocial development must be considered in the care of girls with CAH (Dittmann, Kappes, and Kappes, 1992). Primary care providers must use caution when interpreting these data and base discussions of sexuality on an individualized assessment of each child and family.

Women with CAH—particularly those with the salt-losing form—may not have an adequate introitus for comfortable sexual function, in spite of surgical intervention (Helleday, 1993; Mulaikal, Migeon, and Rock, 1987). Additionally, women who become pregnant may require cesarean delivery because of a small birth canal (Mulaikal, Migeon, and Rock, 1987). One study evaluated fertility in eight women with CAH who were diagnosed early, were generally compliant with treatment, had an introitus that was adequate for intercourse, and were sexually active (Premawardhand et al, 1997). Five of the eight women conceived (i.e., three of this five had salt-wasting CAH and two had non–salt-wasting CAH), for an overall fertility rate of slightly greater than 60%. It is important to note that a significant number of women had successful pregnancies in spite of late diagnosis and treatment of CAH, inadequate reconstruction of the introitus, and poor compliance with replacement therapy (Mulaikal, Migeon, and Rock, 1987).

Promising developments that may improve sexual function for women with CAH include better surgical techniques for clitoroplasty and vaginoplasty (Donahoe and Gustafson, 1994), as well as prenatal treatment to prevent virilization of affected female fetuses (Levine and Pang, 1994; Mercado et al, 1995). Males with CAH generally do not have problems with sexual function or fertility, although prolonged androgen excess can eventually result in infertility (New, 1995). When children with CAH reach adolescence, their primary care provider or endocrinologist should discuss with them the availability and purpose of genetic counseling, screening for carriers, and prenatal and neonatal diagnosis. Because CAH is an autosomal recessive trait, children must receive an abnormal gene from each parent to have the disorder; if one parent has CAH and the other is not a carrier, their children will not have CAH. All unaffected children with a parent with CAH will be carriers of the trait.

Transition to Adulthood

As children with CAH approach adulthood, the primary care provider needs to help their families identify an internist or family practice provider to assume primary care responsibilities. If a child has had specialty care through a pediatric endocrinologist, the transition must also be made to adult endocrine care; the pediatric endocrinologist usually has a list of names available. Counseling for early prenatal care (i.e., prenatal screening, diagnosis and potential treatment) should be provided as well.

Unfortunately, insurance may become a problem when children reach an age when they are no longer covered by government-sponsored insurance for children with disabilities or their parents' insurance. Medicaid—for those who meet the criteria—and group insurance through employment—for those with medical benefits—will cover care for CAH. Other possibilities are coverage through the Genetically Handicapped Persons Program (GHPP) and purchasing pools. Information on these and other programs can be sought from county social services agencies, health departments, and state insurance commissions.

Special Family Concerns and Resources

The parents of an infant girl with CAH must cope with the effect of ambiguous genitalia and of possibly a delayed or even incorrect gender assignment. The initial explanations and reassurances that health care personnel give to the family must be both sensitive and accurate to prevent serious misperceptions of the child's condition and prognosis. Discussions with parents should focus on listening to the parents' concerns and reinforcing the normality of their daughter's internal female organs and chromosomes and explaining that the appearance of the external genitals is correctable and the underlying condition treatable.

People tend to blame the occurrence of an abnormality in a baby on something the mother or father did. It is important to discuss this issue with the parents and the extended family and to repeatedly reinforce the lack of fault. Even after the best of explanations and reassurances, these families continue to have much anxiety and guilt about their child's condition, so constant reinforcement and support are necessary.

Families must be taught to be assertive in communicating the urgency of their child's need for hydrocortisone to health care personnel who are not familiar with the child or CAH. Unfortunately, treatment is commonly delayed because of a lack of understanding of the implications of acute illness in children with CAH. Primary care providers can help avoid delays in treatment by alerting other health care personnel (e.g., call group, emergency room staff) to a child's special needs. The endocrinologist should be consulted for any questions about treatment. In addition, the child should wear a Medic-Alert bracelet or necklace, and the family should carry written information on the child's condition (e.g. wallet card) to facilitate prompt treatment.

Parents have initial difficulty believing the seriousness of CAH unless the diagnosis was made during an episode of acute adrenal insufficiency. Once parents experience the rapidity with which their child can change from being robustly healthy to being deathly ill, however, they may be fearful of future episodes. It is difficult for these parents to find a balance between protecting their child from serious harm and allowing the child to have an active, normal life. This balance must be assessed at each primary care visit by asking about the child's social and academic progress, outside interests and activities, and special concerns. Any problem areas should then be discussed.

Children with CAH may experience emotional disturbances related to multiple factors involved in having this chronic condition. Such factors include being concerned about sexuality and fertility, being perceived and treated as different by others—including their parents, receiving mixed or confusing messages from health care personnel, being overprotected by their parents, and dealing with their own fears related to life-threatening crises they may have experienced. Psychotherapy is indicated for significant emotional disturbance and behavioral problems. Newborn siblings should be screened for CAH, and if the screening results are positive, confirming tests should be done. If the diagnosis of CAH is confirmed, treatment can be immediately initiated in order to prevent an adrenal crisis (Brosnan, 1998; Pang, 1997). Because non–salt-wasting CAH can present with virilization or accelerated growth, all older siblings with these findings should be screened.

Although prenatal diagnosis and treatment are still being refined, they should be discussed in detail with parents. Testing for the carrier state is also available and should be explained to unaffected siblings and other first-degree relatives (New, 1995).

The effect of CAH on a family varies with their cultural beliefs about the cause of congenital disorders and their attitudes toward sexuality. Primary care providers must determine what these beliefs are in order to provide sensitive and successful care to the child and family. Families will usually tell providers their beliefs if asked.

Individuals from cultures in which sexual topics are not openly discussed can be expected to have difficulty asking questions about CAH. Primary care providers and endocrinologists are faced with the challenge of presenting information on a sensitive subject without offending a family's values. It may be helpful to have a male health care provider speak to the men in the family and a female provider speak separately to the women in the family.

Resources

There is no national organization for CAH, but individual families can ask to be introduced to one another through their endocrinology clinic. Literature available on the subject of CAH is typically produced by individual medical centers and is available to families and health professionals who request it (i.e., usually for a small charge).

Informational materials:

Burnett J: A boy with CAH, Am J Nurs 80:1306-1308, 1980. This article is easy to read, and families will identify with the description of life with a child with CAH. This is also a good article to give to school and child care personnel because it gives a simple explanation of the disorder and its management without overwhelming readers with technical information.

Congenital Adrenal Hyperplasia, A Pamphlet for Parents that Describes CAH and Its Treatment, is available from The Magic Foundation, 1327 N. Harlem Ave., Oak Park, Ill. 60302; (708) 3830808; (708) 383-0899 (fax); (800)-3-MAGIC 3 (parent help line); http://www.magicfoundation.org. This pamphlet is suitable for families and health care professionals who are unfamiliar with CAH.

Guidelines for the Child Who Is Cortisol Dependent is a leaflet from the Department of Education, University of Wisconsin Hospital, 600 Highland Ave, Madison, Wis. 53792. It provides parents with information on cortisone replacement and illness management. *How to Mix and Inject Injectable Hydrocortisone* is a small pamphlet (also from University of Wisconsin Hospital) for parents with a clear description of this procedure. *Congenital Adrenal Hyperplasia* is an 8-page handout explaining CAH and its management. It is primarily for families but also is of interest to professionals unfamiliar with CAH.

Congenital Adrenal Hyperplasia is a 28-page illustrated booklet from the Patient/Parent Education Department of British Columbia's Children's Hospital, 4480 Oak Street, Vancouver, British Columbia, V6H 3V4, describing the condition and treatment. It is primarily for families but also is of interest to professionals unfamiliar with CAH.

Summary of Primary Care Needs for the Child with Congenital Adrenal Hyperplasia

HEALTH CARE MAINTENANCE

Growth and development

If CAH is diagnosed in infancy and adequately and consistently treated, growth and development are normal.

Accelerated linear growth occurs if CAH is inadequately treated.

Accelerated bone age advancement and early closure of epiphyses with reduced final adult height will occur if CAH is inadequately treated.

Stunted linear growth will occur if CAH is overtreated with hydrocortisone.

Precocious puberty may occur with improved treatment.

Diet: Children should be allowed to salt food to taste and eat salty foods.

Good dietary and activity habits are necessary to counteract the tendency for hydrocortisone therapy to promote excessive weight gain.

Safety: These children have no increased susceptibility to injury.

There is a risk of acute adrenal insufficiency with a serious injury (e.g., fracture, concussion).

A Medic-Alert bracelet or necklace should be worn, and written information should be carried stating the diagnosis, stress dosage of hydrocortisone, and the name and telephone number of the endocrinologist.

Immunizations: Routine immunizations are recommended.

Giving additional vaccines (e.g., pneumococcal, influenza) is discretionary.

Increased stress doses of hydrocortisone are not prophylactically necessary unless the child has a history of previous adverse reaction to the vaccine.

Give increased stress dose of hydrocortisone for immunization reactions involving fever, unusual malaise, and lethargy.

Giving acetaminophen before immunization with likelihood of febrile reaction is discretionary.

Routine screening

Vision: Routine screening is recommended.

Hearing: Routine screening is recommended.

Dental: Routine screening is recommended.

Blood pressure: Blood pressure should be checked at each visit (including infants). Children with abnormal findings should be referred to an endocrinologist.

Hematocrit: Routine screening is recommended.

Urinalysis: Routine screening is recommended.

Tuberculosis: Routine screening is recommended.

Special screening: Screening serum 17-OHP levels or 24-hour urine pregnanetriol values may be indicated and should be coordinated with the endocrinologist.

Checking plasma renin activity levels may be indicated and should be coordinated with the endocrinologist.

Bone age should be checked every 2 to 3 years or more often if there are indications of androgen excess.

COMMON ILLNESS MANAGEMENT

Differential diagnosis

If the child has nausea or vomiting, pallor, cold moist skin, weakness, dizziness or confusion, rapid heart rate, rapid breathing, abdominal, back or leg pain, dehydration, or hypotension, then acute adrenal insufficiency should be ruled out.

A temperature greater than 38.4° C, significant malaise, pain, lethargy, or persistent vomiting (regardless of cause) should be covered by stress doses of hydrocortisone in addition to appropriate specific therapy.

If the child has hypertension, excessive dietary sodium intake and/or overtreatment with mineralocorticoids or glucocorticoids should be ruled out.

Summary of Primary Care Needs for the Child with Congenital Adrenal Hyperplasia—cont'd

COMMON ILLNESS MANAGEMENT—cont'd

Differential diagnosis—cont'd

If the child has hypotension, inadequate mineralocorticoid and/or glucocorticoid dosage should be ruled out.

Drug interactions

Long-term use of barbiturates, phenytoin, or rifampin increases the rate of metabolism of glucocorticoids. Adjustments in dosage may be required.

DEVELOPMENTAL ISSUES

Sleep patterns: Unusual fatigue or lethargy may indicate the need for increased doses of hydrocortisone.

Toileting: There is no impairment in readiness or functioning. Children with obvious virilization should be allowed privacy.

Discipline: Expectations are normal based on age and developmental level.

Physical appearance may differ from age and developmental level, leading to inappropriate expectations.

Child care: Child care providers must be aware of special needs with illness and injury and the importance of routine and stress medication.

Schooling: Children with CAH who have a history of acute adrenal insufficiency and/or hypoglycemic seizures should be assessed for learning difficulties.

School personnel should be aware of special needs of the child's illness and injury.

Sexuality: Virilization of infant girls requires surgical correction.

Inadequate treatment results in continued virilization, acne, hirsutism, menstrual irregularities, infertility in girls, and—eventually—impairment of fertility in boys.

Most children will be fertile.

Transition to adulthood

Transition to providers of adult primary care and endocrine care.

Source of medical insurance must be identified.

Special family concerns

Rapid onset of acute adrenal insufficiency is possible.

Appropriate emergency treatment may be delayed because of health care providers' lack of awareness or knowledge of CAH.

The normality of girls should be stressed.

Others in the family may be affected (e.g., siblings, children of affected child). Genetic counseling, prenatal screening, diagnosis, and treatment are available.

Family members may have difficulty speaking openly about sexuality and genitals.

The *Hydrocortisone/Florinef Handout* is a concise 2-page handout for parents that includes information on illness management. It is available from: Pediatric Endocrinology, CB 7220, Burnett-Womack, University of North Carolina at Chapel Hill, Chapel Hill, NC 27599.

Medication Instructions for Patients with Congenital Adrenal Hyperplasia: Instructions for Families is available from Pediatric Endocrinology Nursing Society, PO Box 2933, Gaithersburg, Md., 20886-2933; www.pens.org. It also describes dosages. *Cortisol Replacement Therapy* is a booklet of instructions on cortisol replacement that is primarily for families but also of interest to professionals unfamiliar with cortisol replacement.

Organization

Pediatric Endocrinology Nursing Society (PENS). This organization has members in many regions who are willing to speak to parent, school, professional, or other groups. PENS, PO Box 2933, Gaithersburg, Md., 20886-2933; www.pens.org

Products

Medic-Alert bracelets and necklaces, which are recommended for all children with CAH, are available from the Medic-Alert Foundation, PO Box 1009, Turlock, Ca. 95381-1009; www.medicalert.org (in the United States) or www.medicalert.ca (in Canada).

References

Bacon G et al: A practical approach to pediatric endocrinology, ed 3, Chicago, 1990, Year Book Medical Publishers.

Bailez M et al: Vaginal reconstruction after initial construction of the external genitalia in girls with salt-wasting adrenal hyperplasia, J Urol 148:680-682, 1992.

Bartter F: Adrenogenital syndromes from physiology to chemistry (1950-1975). In Lee P et al, editors: Congenital adrenal hyperplasia, Baltimore, 1977, University Park Press.

Berg N et al: Testicular masses associated with congenital adrenal hyperplasia: MRI findings, Urology 47(2):252-253, 1996.

Brosnan C et al: A comparative cost analysis of newborn screening for classic congenital adrenal hyperplasia in Texas, Public Health Rep 113(2):170-178. 1998.

Burnett J: A boy with CAH, Am J Nurs 80:1304-1305, 1980.

Cornean R, Hindmarsh P, and Brook C: Obesity in 21-hydroxylase deficient patients, Arch Dis Child 78:261-263, 1998.

Cutler G: Treatment of congenital adrenal hyperplasia: the case for new medical approaches, J Clin Endocrinol Metab 81(9):31853186, 1996.

Dacou-Voutetakis C and Karidis N: Congenital adrenal hyperplasia complicated by central precocious puberty: treatment with LHRH-agonist analog, Ann NY Acad Sci 687:250-254, 1993.

Dittmann R, Kappes M, and Kappes M: Sexual behavior in adolescent and adult females with congenital adrenal hyperplasia, Psychoneuroendocrinology 17:153-170, 1992.

Dittmann R et al: Congenital adrenal hyperplasia I: gender-related behavior and attitudes in female patients and sisters, Psychoneuroendocrinology 15:401-420, 1990.

Donahoe P and Gustafson M: Early one-stage surgical reconstruction of the extremely high vagina in patients with congenital adrenal hyperplasia, J Pediatr Surg 29(2):352-358, 1994.

Donaldson M et al: Presentation, acute illness, and learning difficulties in salt wasting 21-hydroxylase deficiency, Arch Dis Child 70:214-218, 1994.

Duck S: Acceptable linear growth in congenital adrenal hyperplasia, J Pediatr 97:93-96, 1980.

Ehrhardt A and Baker S: Males and females with congenital adrenal hyperplasia: a family study of intelligence and gender-related behavior. In Lee P, Plotnick L, and Kowarski A, editors: Congenital adrenal hyperplasia, Baltimore, 1977, University Park Press.

Galatzer A and Laron Z: The effects of prenatal androgens on behavior and cognitive functions. In M Forest, editor: Androgens in childhood, 1989, Karger & Basel.

Helleday J et al: Subnormal androgen and elevated progesterone levels in women treated for congenital virilizing 21-hydroxylase deficiency, J Clin Endocrinol Metab 76(4):933-936, 1993.

Helleday J et al: General intelligence and cognitive profile in women with congenital adrenal hyperplasis (CAH), Psychoneuroendocrinology 19(4):343-356, 1994.

Hines M and Kaufman F: Androgen and the development of human sex-typical behavior: rough-and-tumble play and sex of preferred playmates in children with congenital adrenal hyperplasia (CAH), Child Dev 65:1042-1053, 1994.

Hochberg Z, Gardos M, and Benderly A: Psychosexual outcome of assigned females and males with 46XX virilizing congenital adrenal hyperplasia, Eur J Pediatr 146:497-499, 1987.

Holmes C, Karlsson J, and Thompson R: Longitudinal evaluation of behavior patterns in children with short stature. In Stabler B and Underwood L, editors: Slow grows the child, Hillsdale, NJ, 1986, Lawrence Erlbaum Assoc.

Jackson P and Ott M: Perceived self-esteem among children diagnosed with precocious puberty, J Ped Nurs 5:190-203, 1990.

Kuhnle U and Bullinger M: Outcome of congenital adrenal hyperplasia, Pediatr Surg Int 12:511-515, 1997.

Kuhnle U, Bullinger M, and Schwarz H: The quality of life in adult female patients with congenital adrenal hyperplasia: a comprehensive study of the impact of genital malformations and chronic disease on female patients life, Eur J Pediatr 154:708-716, 1995.

Laue L et al: A preliminary study of flutamide, testolactone, and reduced hydrocortisone dose in the treatment of congenital adrenal hyperplasia, J Clin Endocrinol Metab 81(10):3535-39, 1996.

Levine L and Pang S: Prenatal diagnosis and treatment of congenital adrenal hyperplasia, J Pediatr Endocrinol 7(3):193-200, 1994.

Lim Y, Batch J, and Warne G: Adrenal 21-hydroxylase deficiency in childhood: 25 years' experience, J Paediatr Child Health 31(3):222-227, 1995.

Mazur T: Ambiguous genitalia: detection and counseling, Pediatr Nurs 9:417-422, 1983.

Mercado A et al: Prenatal treatment and diagnosis of congenital adrenal hyperplasia owing to steroid 21-hydroxylase deficiency, J Clin Endocrinol Metab 80(7):2014-2020, 1995.

Migeon C and Donohoue P: Congenital adrenal hyperplasia caused by 21-hydroxylase deficiency, Endocrinol Metab Clin North Am 20(2):277-296. 1991.

Money J, Schwartz M, and Lewis V: Adult erotosexual status and fetal hormonal masculinization and demasculization: 46XX congenital virilizing adrenal hyperplasia and 46XY androgen-insensitivity syndrome compared, Psychoneuroendocrinology 9:405-414, 1984.

Mulaikal R, Migeon C, and Rock J: Fertility rates in female patients with congenital adrenal hyperplasia as a result of 21-hydroxylase deficiency, N Engl J Med 316:178-182, 1987.

Mullis P, Hindmarsh P, and Brook C: Sodium chloride supplement at diagnosis and during infancy in children with salt-losing 21-hydroxylase deficiency, Eur J Pediatr 150:22-25, 1990.

Nass R and Baker S: Learning disabilities in children with congenital adrenal hyperplasia, J Child Neurol 6:306-312, 1991.

New M: Congenital adrenal hyperplasia. In DeGroot L et al, editors: Endocrinology, ed 3, Philadelphia, 1995, W.B. Saunders.

New M: Diagnosis and management of congenital adrenal hyperplasia, Ann Rev Med 49:311-328, 1998.

Ott M and Jackson P: Precocious puberty, Nurse Pract 14:21-30, 1989.

Pang S: Congenital adrenal hyperplasia, Endocrinol Metab Clin North Am 26(4):853-891, 1997.

Pang S and Shook M: Current status of neonatal screening for congenital adrenal hyperplasia, Curr Opin Pediatr 9(4):419-423, 1997.

Pescovitz H. et al: True precocious puberty complicating congenital adrenal hyperplasia: treatment with a luteinizing hormone-releasing hormone analog, J Clin Endocrinol Metab 58(5):857-861, 1984.

Plante E et al: Elevated androgen, brain development and language/learning disabilities in children with congenital adrenal hyperplasia, Dev Med Child Neurol 38:423-437, 1996.

Premawardhana L et al: Longer term outcome in females with congenital adrenal hyperplasia (CAH): the Cardiff experience, Clin Endocrinol 46(3):327-332, 1997.

Riley W and Rosenbloom A: Clitoral size in infancy, J Pediatr 96:918-919, 1980.

Ritzen E and Wedell A: Adrenals of patients with severe forms of congenital adrenal hyperplasis do more harm than good!, J Clin Endocrinol Metab 81(9):3182-3184, 1996.

Rosler A et al: The interrelationship of sodium balance, plasma renin activity, and ACTH in congenital adrenal hyperplasia, J Clin Endocrinol Metab 45:500-512, 1977.

Sandrini R, Jospe N, and Migeon C: Temporal and individual variations in the dose of glucocorticoid used for the treatment of salt-losing congenital virilizing adrenal hyperplasia as a result of 21-hydroxylase deficiency, Acta Paediatr Suppl 388:56-60, 1993.

Srikanth M et al: Benign testicular tumors in children with congenital adrenal hyperplasia, J Pediatr Surg 27:639-641, 1992.

Stern N and Tuck M: The adrenal cortex and mineralocorticoid hypertension. In Lavin N, editor: Manual of endocrinology and metabolism, Boston, 1986, Little, Brown, & Co.

Therrell B et al: Results of screening 1.9 million Texas newborns for 21-hydroxylase-deficient congenital adrenal hyperplasia, Pediatrics 101(4 Pt 1):583-590, 1998.

Trautman P et al: Effects of early prenatal dexamethasone on the cognitive and behavioral development of young children: results of a pilot study, Psychoneuroendocrinology 20(4):439-449, 1995.

Trautman P et al: Mothers' reactions to prenatal diagnostic procedures and dexamethasone treatment of congenital adrenal hyperplasia, J Psychosom Obstet Gynaecol 17(3):175-181, 1996.

VanWyk J and Gunther D: The use of adrenalectomy as a treatment for congenital adrenal hyperplasia, J Clin Endocrinol Metab 81(9):3180-3182, 1996.

Young-Hyman D: Effects of short stature on social competence. In Stabler B and Underwood L, editors: Slow grows the child, Hillsdale, NJ, 1986, Lawrence Erlbaum Assoc.

Zucker K et al: Psychosexual development of women with congenital adrenal hyperplasia, Horm Behav 30:300-318, 1996.

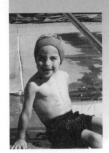

CHAPTER 17

Congenital Heart Disease

Elizabeth H. Cook and Sarah S. Higgins

Etiology

Congenital heart disease (CHD) results from the abnormal development of structures within the heart or those leading to or from the heart. This condition is present—though not always manifested—at birth. Approximately one half of the infants born with CHD are symptomatic within the first year of life and need some form of intervention.

CHD is commonly categorized as acyanotic or cyanotic, depending on the hemodynamic changes that occur as a result of the specific heart anomaly. In acyanotic heart disease, the systemic circulation is not exposed to unoxygenated blood; in cyanotic heart disease, unoxygenated blood mixes in the systemic circulation (see Figure 17-1). A brief description of the intracardiac pressure-flow relationship may clarify this classification of CHD.

Depleted of oxygen, blood returns to the heart from the venous system and enters the right atrium. From the right atrium, blood flows through the tricuspid valve into the right ventricle, where it is pumped through the pulmonary arteries into the lungs to pick up oxygen. Therefore the oxygen saturation in the right side of the heart is low (i.e., approximately 70%). The pressure in the right-sided circulation is also relatively low (i.e., approximately 25/2 mm Hg in the right ventricle and 25/10 mm Hg in the pulmonary arteries).

The blood that enters the left atrium from the lungs is rich in oxygen, with the oxygen saturation reaching 95% to 100%. The blood flows through the mitral valve into the left ventricle, where it is pumped into the systemic circulation via the aorta. Pressure in the left ventricle is under high pressure (e.g., approximately 100/5 mm Hg), as is that in the aorta (i.e., approximately 100/60 mm Hg).

Because the pressure in the left side of the heart is greater than that in the right side, blood flows from the left to the right side of the heart if there is an abnormal connection between the two sides. This flow is called left-to-right shunting. Because of the significant difference in left- and right-sided oxygen saturations, heart defects that cause left-to-right shunting are acyanotic. Left-to-right shunts commonly cause overcirculation of the lungs and may result in congestive heart failure (CHF).

Cyanosis usually results from one or both of the following physiologic problems: (1) right-to-left shunting, which results from obstruction of blood flow to the lungs plus an intracardiac communication; or (2) intracardiac mixing of oxygenated and deoxygenated blood. Figure 17-2 summarizes and illustrates the most common defects. Additional information on cardiovascular disorders in children can be found in the text by Smith and associates (1996).

Most heart defects occur between the fourth and seventh weeks of gestation (Hazinski, 1993). It was widely believed that the majority of congenital heart defects have a multifactorial cause, in which there is an interplay of a genetic predisposition for abnormal cardiac development with an environmental trigger (e.g., a virus or maternal ingestion of certain drugs) at the vulnerable time of cardiac development. The genetic basis of many congenital heart defects and conditions, however, is being increasingly recognized (Clark, 1995).

Many defects are associated with a syndrome in which other systems also are affected (Table 17-1 on page 379). One of the most common genetic associations with CHD is Down syndrome; over 40% of these children have a heart defect (see Chapter 20)(Cousineau and Lauer, 1995). Other syndromes that do not have an identified chromosomal defect (e.g., asplenia syndrome and VACTERL* syndrome) often have CHD as one of many anomalies.

---

*VACTERL syndrome refers to a constellation of abnormalities of the vertebrae, anus, cardiovascular system, trachea, esophagus, renal system, and limb buds.

**CLASSIFICATION OF
CONGENITAL HEART
DEFECTS**

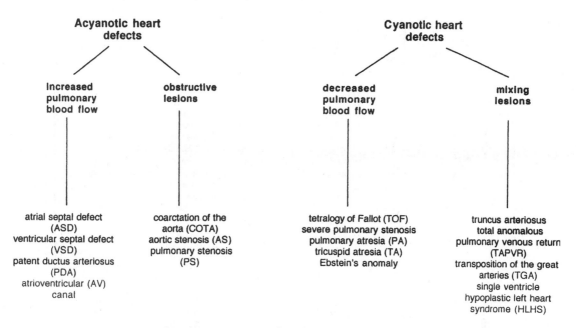

Figure 17-1 Acyanotic and cyanotic heart defects.

Maternal exposure to teratogens during cardiac development of the fetus may result in heart defects. The fetus is vulnerable to cardiac teratogens from 2 to 10 weeks of gestation (Reiss, 1995). This exposure may be from a maternal infection or condition or maternal ingestion of drugs (see Table 17-1).

Incidence

CHD generally occurs in 0.5% to 0.8% of live births (Clark, 1995). The incidence of specific heart defects is shown in Table 17-2. Boys tend to have a higher overall incidence of serious CHD, and certain defects exhibit some sex preference.

The risk of CHD recurring in the same family depends on several factors. The odds for recurrence are greatest if the mother or full sibling—instead of the father or half-sibling—has the heart defect. If the defect is part of a syndrome or chromosomal abnormality, the recurrence risk of the heart lesion is related to the recurrence risk of the syndrome. Additional information indicates that certain left-sided cardiac lesions (i.e., most notably hypoplastic left heart syndrome) have a very high recurrence rate (Clark, 1995).

Clinical Manifestations at the Time of Diagnosis

The clinical presentation of a child with CHD varies depending on the specific defect. Symptoms usually relate to the degree of CHF or cyanosis (Box 17-1).

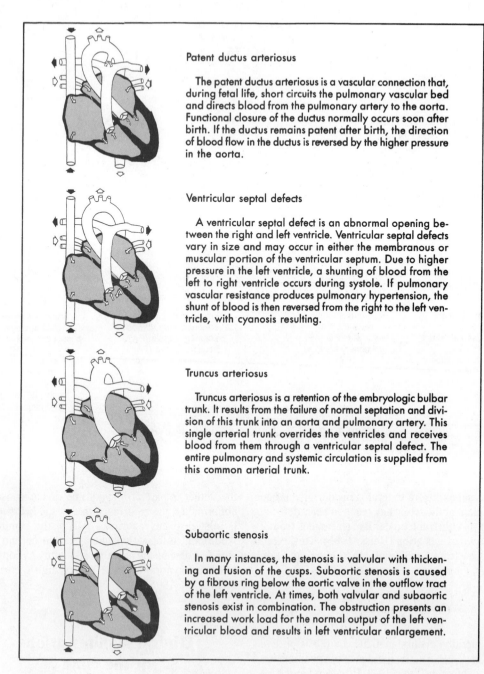

Patent ductus arteriosus

The patent ductus arteriosus is a vascular connection that, during fetal life, short circuits the pulmonary vascular bed and directs blood from the pulmonary artery to the aorta. Functional closure of the ductus normally occurs soon after birth. If the ductus remains patent after birth, the direction of blood flow in the ductus is reversed by the higher pressure in the aorta.

Ventricular septal defects

A ventricular septal defect is an abnormal opening between the right and left ventricle. Ventricular septal defects vary in size and may occur in either the membranous or muscular portion of the ventricular septum. Due to higher pressure in the left ventricle, a shunting of blood from the left to right ventricle occurs during systole. If pulmonary vascular resistance produces pulmonary hypertension, the shunt of blood is then reversed from the right to the left ventricle, with cyanosis resulting.

Truncus arteriosus

Truncus arteriosus is a retention of the embryologic bulbar trunk. It results from the failure of normal septation and division of this trunk into an aorta and pulmonary artery. This single arterial trunk overrides the ventricles and receives blood from them through a ventricular septal defect. The entire pulmonary and systemic circulation is supplied from this common arterial trunk.

Subaortic stenosis

In many instances, the stenosis is valvular with thickening and fusion of the cusps. Subaortic stenosis is caused by a fibrous ring below the aortic valve in the outflow tract of the left ventricle. At times, both valvular and subaortic stenosis exist in combination. The obstruction presents an increased work load for the normal output of the left ventricular blood and results in left ventricular enlargement.

Figure 17-2 Congential heart abnormalities. (Reprinted with permission of Ross Laboratories, Columbus, Ohio; From Clinical Education Aid No. 7, 1970.) *Continued*

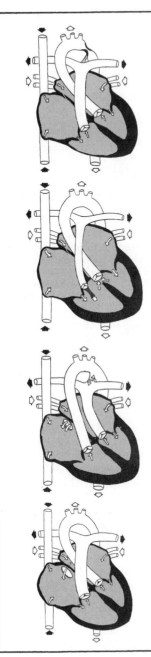

Coarctation of the aorta

Coarctation of the aorta is characterized by a narrowed aortic lumen. It exists as a preductal or postductal obstruction, depending on the position of the obstruction in relation to the ductus arteriosus. Coarctations exist with great variation in anatomic features. The lesion produces an obstruction to the flow of blood through the aorta causing an increased left ventricular pressure and work load.

Tetralogy of Fallot

Tetralogy of Fallot is characterized by the combination of four defects: (1) pulmonary stenosis, (2) ventricular septal defect, (3) overriding aorta, (4) hypertrophy of right ventricle. It is the most common defect causing cyanosis in patients surviving beyond two years of age. The severity of symptoms depends on the degree of pulmonary stenosis, the size of the ventricular septal defect, and the degree to which the aorta overrides the septal defect.

Complete transposition of great vessels

The anomaly is an embryologic defect caused by a straight division of the bulbar trunk without normal spiraling. As a result, the aorta originates from the right ventricle, and the pulmonary artery from the left ventricle. An abnormal communication between the two circulations must be present to sustain life.

Atrial septal defects

An atrial septal defect is an abnormal opening between the right and left atria. Basically, three types of abnormalities result from incorrect development of the atrial septum. An incompetent foramen ovale is the most common defect. The high ostium secundum defect results from abnormal development of the septum secundum. Improper development of the septum primum produces a basal opening known as an ostium primum defect, frequently involving the atrio-ventricular valves. In general, left to right shunting of blood occurs in all atrial septal defects.

Figure 17-2, cont'd For legend see previous page.

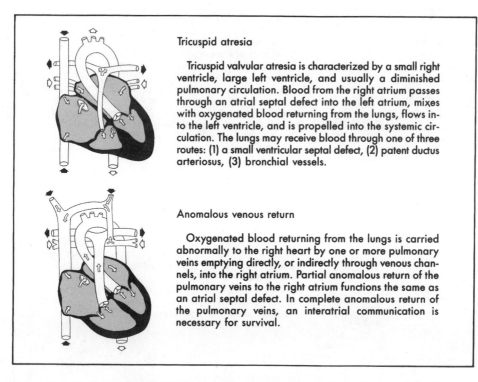

Tricuspid atresia

Tricuspid valvular atresia is characterized by a small right ventricle, large left ventricle, and usually a diminished pulmonary circulation. Blood from the right atrium passes through an atrial septal defect into the left atrium, mixes with oxygenated blood returning from the lungs, flows into the left ventricle, and is propelled into the systemic circulation. The lungs may receive blood through one of three routes: (1) a small ventricular septal defect, (2) patent ductus arteriosus, (3) bronchial vessels.

Anomalous venous return

Oxygenated blood returning from the lungs is carried abnormally to the right heart by one or more pulmonary veins emptying directly, or indirectly through venous channels, into the right atrium. Partial anomalous return of the pulmonary veins to the right atrium functions the same as an atrial septal defect. In complete anomalous return of the pulmonary veins, an interatrial communication is necessary for survival.

Figure 17-2, cont'd   For legend see page 375.

Congestive Heart Failure

The majority of cases of CHF result from CHD, and most occur within the first year of life. CHF occurs when there is a strain on the myocardium from pressure or volume overload that is severe enough to reduce cardiac output to a level insufficient to meet the body's metabolic demands (Talner, 1995). Symptoms of CHF result from the decreased cardiac output and the body's compensatory mechanisms and include cardiac hypertrophy, cardiac dilatation, and stimulation of the sympathetic nervous system. Infants with CHF are tachypneic, dyspneic, tachycardic, pale, cool, diaphoretic, and easily fatigued. Additional symptoms include periorbital edema, hepatomegaly, and a persistent cough. A history of difficult feeding and decreased food intake is a classic sign of CHF. Therefore growth failure is a common consequence of CHF in infancy and childhood (Ackerman et al, 1998).

CHF is manifested in neonates with a severe cardiac defect (e.g., transposition of the great arter-

ies, hypoplastic left heart syndrome, or critical aortic stenosis). Infants with defects causing left-to-right shunts (e.g., ventricular septal defect [VSD]) do not usually develop symptoms until 4 to 8 weeks of age, when the high pulmonary vascular resistance of the fetal period becomes low enough to cause increased pulmonary blood flow. The onset of symptoms is usually gradual; tachypnea, changes in feeding patterns, and poor weight gain are often early clues. Other defects causing left-to-right shunts (e.g., patent ductus arteriosus [PDA] and AV canal) display symptoms dependent upon the degree of shunting. Premature infants with a left-to-right shunt may develop symptoms of CHF earlier than term infants because their pulmonary vascular resistance drops faster than that of term infants.

Hypoxemia and Cyanosis

Hypoxemia is the presence of an arterial oxygen saturation that is below normal. Cyanosis is the

Table 17-1
Conditions Commonly Associated with Cardiac Malformations

Condition	Associated Defect
Infant Syndrome	
Trisomy 13 syndrome	VSD, PDA, dextrocardia
Trisomy 18 syndrome	VSD, PDA, PS
Trisomy 21 syndrome	AV canal, VSD, ASD
Turner's syndrome	COTA, ASD, AS
Marfan syndrome	Great artery aneurysms, aortic insufficiency (AI), mitral regurgitation (MR)
Noonan's syndrome	PS, ASD, idiopathic hypertrophic subaortic stenosis (IHSS)
Cri du chat syndrome	VSD, PDA, ASD
Ellis-van Creveld syndrome	ASD, single atrium
Osteogenesis imperfecta	Aortic valve disease
DiGeorge syndrome	Interrupted aortic arch, TOF, truncus arteriosus, ASD
Holt-Oram syndrome	ASD, VSD, single atrium
Treacher Collins syndrome	VSD, PDA, ASD
Asplenia syndrome	VSD, single ventricle, common AV valve, TGA
VACTERL syndrome	TOF
Maternal Condition	
Rubella	PDA, ASD, VSD, peripheral pulmonary stenosis
Diabetes	TGA, VSD, COTA, cardiomegaly
Lupus erythematosus	Heart block
Phenylketonuria	TOF, VSD, ASD
Maternal Ingestion	
Alcohol	VSD, PDA, ASD
Trimethadione	TGA, TOF, HLHS
Lithium	Ebstein's anomaly, ASD, TA
Retinoic acid	VSD
Amphetamines	VSD, PDA, ASD, TGA
Hydantoin	PS, AS, COTA, PDA
Sex hormones	VSD, TGA, TOF
Thalidomide	TOF, truncus arteriosus, VSD, ASD

AS, aortic stenosis; ASD, atrial septal defect; AV, atrioventricular; COTA, coarctation of the aorta; HLHS, hydroplastic left heart syndrome; PDA, patent ductus arteriosis; PS, pulmonary stenosis; TA, tricuspid atresia; TGA, transposition of the great arteries; TOF, tetralogy of Fallot; VSD, ventricular septal defect.
Adapted from Nora JJ: Etiologic aspects of heart disease. In Adams FH and Emmanouilides GC, editors: Moss's heart disease in infants, children and adolescents, ed 4, Baltimore, 1989, Williams & Wilkins.

blue coloration of the skin and mucous membranes caused by deoxygenated hemoglobin. This coloration is usually seen in the lips, gums, nail beds, and around the eyes and mouth. Cyanosis is difficult to detect in children with dark skin pigmentation and is best perceived by observing mucous membranes and nail beds in natural light. Children with cyanosis often have slowed growth, although they are not usually poor feeders. Polycythemia occurs in children who are chronically hypoxemic, because the body attempts to increase its oxygen-carrying capacity. Toddlers who are cyanotic usually limit their activity but still become easily fatigued and breathless if running, climbing stairs, or playing for long periods of time. Children with symptomatic tetralogy of Fallot (TOF) may assume a squatting position for relief of exertional dyspnea and fatigue. Increasing cyanosis may be subtle and difficult to discern; monitoring increasing hemoglobin may facilitate the determination of progressive hypoxemia (O'Brien and Smith, 1994).

Table 17-2
Incidence of Specific Heart Defects

Defect	CHD (%)
Ventricular septal defect (VSD)	20 to 25
Patent ductus arteriosus (PDA)	10 (excluding premature)
Tetralogy of Fallot (TOF)	10
Coarctation of the aorta (COTA)	8
Atrial septal defect (ASD)	5 to 10
Pulmonary stenosis (PS)	5 to 8
Transposition of the great arteries (TGA)	5
Aortic stenosis (AS)	5
Atrioventricular (AV) canal	3 to 4
Hypoplastic left heart syndrome (HLHS)	1 to 2
Tricuspid atresia (TA)	1 to 2
Total anomalous pulmonary venous return (TAPVR)	1
Pulmonary atresia (PA)	1
Ebstein's anomaly	1
Truncus arteriosus	1
Single ventricle	1

Adapted from Park MK: Pediatric cardiology for practitioners, ed 3, Chicago, 1996, Mosby.

Box 17-1

Clinical Manifestations of CHD

Congestive Heart Failure

- Tachypnea
- Tachycardia
- Hepatomegaly
- Dyspnea
- Pale, cool skin
- Diaphoresis
- Periorbital edema
- Persistent, dry cough
- Poor feeding; failure to thrive
- Easily fatigued

Hypoxemia and Cyanosis

- Blue coloration of lips, gums, nailbeds, around eyes and mouth, skin, and mucous membranes
- Slowed growth
- Decreased activity
- Polycythemia

Treatment

Medical management of the child with CHD is aimed at allowing these infants to grow and their organs to mature so that surgery can be performed at the optimal time (Box 17-2). One goal of primary care management is to control CHF, which is usually achieved with the use of digitalis and diuretics. Because failure to thrive is a common complication of CHF, support with feeding is also a priority in management. Support may include methods of decreasing fatigue during feeding, increasing the caloric concentration of formula, and occasionally providing gavage feeding.

Infants who are cyanotic additionally require monitoring for progressive cyanosis, anemia, and dehydration. Parents of children who are cyanotic must learn to identify increasing blueness and cyanotic spells.

The decision for surgery depends on the severity of the lesion, associated defects, the child's age and size, concurrent medical or surgical problems, and family and cultural factors. The cardiologist follows the progress of a defect through cardiac ultrasound or echocardiography. For most defects, this diagnostic technique provides all of the information needed to perform surgery (Sanders, 1992). For some cardiac defects, however, cardiac catheterization or magnetic resonance imaging (MRI) may also be performed before surgery to determine the precise anatomy and physiology of a child's heart.

The natural history of some defects (e.g., VSD, PDA, and atrial septal defect [ASD]) is such that spontaneous improvement or closure may occur, so that surgery can be avoided. Most lesions, however, require surgery. The timing of surgical intervention varies among cardiac centers. As surgical techniques improve, the nationwide trend is toward earlier corrective surgery (i.e., often by early or middle infancy). Early corrective surgery decreases the negative consequences of longstanding hypoxemia, myocardial strain, and pulmonary overcirculation.

Crucial factors in determining the timing of surgery include preventing irreversible pulmonary hypertension and the development of aortopulmonary collateral vessels, as well as maintaining adequate ventricular function. Large left-to-right shunts rarely cause irreversible changes in the pulmonary vasculature before 12 to 18 months of age. Once these irreversible changes occur, however, surgery is contraindicated and the child becomes progressively cyanotic.

Some neonates with complex defects require an initial palliative surgery at birth and definitive surgery later. These infants have either inadequate pulmonary blood flow or uncontrolled CHF and need close follow-up after surgery to ensure that pulmonary blood flow is maintained (i.e., when cyanotic) and excessive pulmonary blood flow is restricted (i.e., with CHF).

Infants who need surgery are closely followed by a cardiologist to manage CHF or cyanosis and to time surgery. Communication between the cardiologist and the primary care provider is important. Symptoms of increasing tachypnea, decreasing feeding, slowed weight gain, or increased cyanosis should be reported to the cardiologist.

Cardiac defects that may warrant delaying surgery for several years include those that rarely develop early pulmonary hypertension or myocardial strain (e.g., small PDAs, ASDs, VSDs, and mild coarctation of the aorta). Children with these defects are usually asymptomatic. They may have more contact with their primary care provider than their cardiologist after initial diagnosis, so communication with the cardiologist is again important.

For an increasing number of defects, interventional cardiac catheterization has replaced surgery as the treatment of choice. Some forms of aortic and pulmonary valvar or vascular stenosis can be repaired through balloon valvuloplasty and angioplasty. Vascular stents are being placed within the vessel to maintain the patency of stenosed vessels after balloon angioplasty has been performed. Closure of PDAs, septal defects, and unnecessary collateral blood vessels is being performed via placement of various occlusive devices within the defect (Callow, 1994; Radtke, 1994). Clinical results of PDA closure with transcatheter coils are comparable to surgical closure, with no significant long-term complications and a significant decrease in cost (Prieto et al, 1998). In addition, electrophysiologic studies are used in conjunction with

---

> ## Box 17-2
>
> ### Treatment of CHD
>
> - Control CHF
> - Support feeding
> - Monitor for worsening cyanosis
> - Cardiac catheterization—diagnostic or interventional
> - Time surgery based on defect and symptoms

cardiac catheterization to identify cardiac dysrhythmias, evaluate the effectiveness of certain drugs under controlled circumstances, and abolish or ablate the accessory pathway causing the dysrhythmia (Darling, 1994; Finkelmeier, 1994). The field of interventional cardiac catheterization has become a valuable therapy in managing many children with CHD.

Recent and Anticipated Advances in Diagnosis and Management

Further advances in the devices and techniques associated with interventional cardiac catheterization continue to expand treatment options for children with CHD. The use of echocardiography as the primary diagnostic tool in CHD is simultaneously decreasing the need for purely diagnostic cardiac catheterizations. Clinical electrophysiology (i.e., including pacemaker therapy) is another growing field. Rhythm control—whether accomplished via advanced antiarrhythmic drugs, ablative therapy, or implantable devices—continues to evolve as more clinical experience is gained and new technologies are refined. Several mechanical assist devices for children with cardiac failure are used to provide circulatory support until myocardial function recovers or cardiac transplantations occurs. These devices have met with varied success and will continue to evolve. Cardiac transplantation has advanced remarkably in the past decade, which is primarily due to the evolution of immune suppression strategies. Data from the Heart and Lung Transplant Registry reveal that the 1600 newborns to adolescents who have undergone cardiac transplantation since 1980 have a 5-year survival rate of approximately 70% (Registry of the International Society for Heart and Lung Transplantation, 1992). This number will undoubtedly increase as techniques of immune suppression are refined (see Chapter 30).

Associated Problems (Box 17-3)

Hematologic Problems

Children with cyanotic heart disease develop polycythemia to increase the oxygen-carrying capacity of the blood. If the hematocrit reaches 60% or higher, there is a marked increase in the viscosity of the blood, an increase in the tendency for thrombus formation, and a possible decrease in oxygen delivery (Zuberbuhler, 1995). Bleeding disorders are also seen in children with polycythemia, most commonly thrombocytopenia and defective platelet aggregation. These children may bruise easily or develop petechiae, gingival bleeding, or epistaxis (Park, 1996).

Anemia can be a special problem in children with CHD. In children with existing CHF, decreased hemoglobin may exacerbate myocardial strain. In cyanotic infants, iron deficiency anemia has been associated with cerebral vascular accidents and slowed growth (O'Brien and Smith, 1994). Children who are cyanotic with a low hematocrit may exhibit hypoxic spells more readily than if the oxygen-carrying capacity of the blood were normal. Cyanosis will not be as obvious in children with anemia as in children with a normal or elevated hemoglobin. Because of these problems associated with anemia, children with an acyanotic heart defect should have a hemoglobin level within the normal range for their age. Although it is important for children who are cyanotic with a low hematocrit to receive iron therapy, it is equally important to monitor their response to the therapy in order to prevent the hematocrit from rising to undesirably high levels, thus increasing blood viscosity (Fyler and Nadas, 1992).

Adequate hydration must be maintained in children with cyanotic heart disease to avoid increased hemoconcentration. Problems associated with fever and exposure to hot weather can cause excessive perspiration; vomiting and diarrhea can cause dehydration (Miner and Canobbio, 1994).

Box 17-3

Associated Problems in CHD

- Hematologic
  Polycythemia
  Bleeding disorders
  Anemia
- Recurrent respiratory infections
- Infective endocarditis
- CNS complications
  Brain abscess in older children who are cyanotic
  CVA
- Dysrhythmias
- Failure to thrive
- Slowed growth and development
- Vulnerable child syndrome

Infectious Processes

Children with significant heart defects are at high risk for developing a variety of infections. Recurrent respiratory tract infections are especially common in children with lesions causing increased pulmonary blood flow. Other systemic infections (e.g., sinusitis) are common nonspecific infections in older children who are cyanotic. Infections can significantly affect a child's health in the following ways: (1) severe respiratory tract infections can exacerbate hypoxemia in cyanotic children; (2) fever can increase oxygen demands and precipitate myocardial decompensation; (3) dehydration in a child with polycythemia can lead to thrombus formation; and (4) electrolyte imbalances from vomiting, diarrhea, or fever in a child receiving digoxin can lead to digoxin toxicity.

Children with asplenia syndrome (i.e., a condition that includes absence of the spleen and complex cardiac defects) are extremely susceptible to bacteremia with a high mortality. Streptococcus pneumonia and *Haemophilus* influenza type B are the most common pathogens. Daily antimicrobial prophylaxis should be strongly considered for children under 5 years of age with asplenia syndrome. Some experts continue prophylaxis throughout childhood and into adulthood in particularly high-risk clients with asplenia.

Recommended dosage is oral penicillin V (i.e., 125 mg twice a day for children under 5 years, and 250 mg twice a day for children 5 years and older). Some experts recommend amoxicillin 20 mg/kg/day (Committee on Infectious Diseases, 1997).

Infective Endocarditis

Endocarditis may occur because of blood-borne bacteria that lodge on damaged or abnormal heart valves, prosthetic material, or the endocardium near congenital anatomic defects. Endocarditis may occur if prophylaxis precautions are not followed during most dental procedures and surgical or invasive procedures involving mucosal surfaces or contaminated tissues. Most cases of endocarditis, however, are not attributable to an invasive procedure (Box 17-4) (Dajani et al, 1997). The most common organisms are streptococci and staphylococci, which account for 80% to 90% of cases (Park, 1996). The current recommendation for prophylaxis for dental, oral, respiratory tract, or esophageal procedures is amoxicillin (i.e., 50 mg/kg for children; 2.0 g for adults) given orally 1 hour before the procedure. Note that the follow-up dose is no longer recommended (Box 17-5) (Dajani et al, 1997).

Central Nervous System Complications

In children who are cyanotic, bacteria normally filtered out of the blood in the pulmonary circulation may be shunted directly to the systemic circulation. As a result, these children are at increased risk for brain abscess, most commonly after 2 years of age. Infants who are cyanotic with iron deficiency anemia are prone to develop cerebral vascular accidents. A possible explanation for this finding is that relative anemia secondary to cyanosis leads to increased blood viscosity and increased coagulability and thus venous thrombosis (Newberger, 1992).

Dysrhythmias

Rhythm disturbances can occur in children with CHD as a direct result of the cardiac defect or the surgical repair. Atrial dysrhythmias are more common than ventricular rhythm disturbances in children. Infants with Ebstein's anomaly are predisposed to develop supraventricular tachycardia (SVT). Anatomically corrected transposition of the great arteries (L-TGA) is a rare congenital heart de-

fect that may also lead to SVT or varying degrees of heart blockage.

Postoperatively, disturbances in atrial rhythms may be seen in children after surgical manipulation of the atrium (e.g., the Fontan procedure, repair of total anomalous pulmonary venous return [TAPVR], ASD repair, or the Mustard procedure). Postoperative second- or third-degree heart block may occur in surgeries involving the ventricular septum (e.g., repair of VSD, atrioventricular [AV] canal repair, and TOF repair). In addition, children who have had a complete repair of TOF can develop ventricular ectopy, which can infrequently lead to sudden death (Denfield and Garson, 1990).

Digoxin toxicity can cause a wide variety of dysrhythmias, including profound bradycardia, ventricular dysrhythmias, and varying degrees of heart block (Koren and Gorodischer, 1992). A low serum potassium concentration potentiates the effects of digoxin. A child receiving a non–potassium-sparing diuretic (e.g., furosemide [Lasix]) without potassium replacement may be at particular risk of digoxin toxicity. A therapeutic digoxin level is generally 0.5 to 2 ng/ml, although toxicity has been seen at lower levels and may not be seen at higher levels in some infants (Koren and Gorodischer, 1992). A sound rule is to assume that a dysrhythmia noted in a child on digoxin therapy is caused by digoxin until proved otherwise. If extra beats or an abnormal rhythm—including bradycardia and tachycardia—is identified by the primary care provider, an electrocardiogram should be obtained and the child should be referred to the cardiologist for further evaluation as soon as possible.

Failure to Thrive

Growth failure has often been observed in children with CHD (Ackerman et al, 1998; Barton et al, 1994; Cameron, Rosenthal, and Olson, 1995; Gaedeke, Norris, and Hill, 1994). The decreased growth is usually more pronounced in weight than in height. CHF is one of the most potent factors in the development of failure to thrive because of both inadequate caloric intake secondary to tachypnea and the relative hypermetabolism associated with CHF and pulmonary hypertension (Ackerman et al, 1998; Barton et al, 1994) Growth failure is particularly important to recognize because it may suggest significant hemodynamic compromise, necessitating an alteration in

Box 17-4

Infective Endocarditis Prophylaxis*

Cardiac Conditions

Endocarditis prophylaxis recommended for:
- High-risk category
    Prosthetic cardiac valves
    Previous history of bacterial endocarditis
    Complex cyanotic heart defects (e.g., transposition, TOF, single type of ventricle defects)
    Surgically constructed systemic-pulmonary shunts or conduits
- Moderate-risk category
    Most other congenital cardiac defects (i.e., other than those listed here)
    Rheumatic and other acquired valvular dysfunction
    Mitral valve prolapse with valvular regurgitation
    Hypertrophic cardiomyopathy

Endocarditis prophylaxis not recommended for:
- Negligible-risk category (no greater risk than the general population)
    Isolated secundum atrial septal defect
    Surgical repair without residua beyond 6 months of secundum ASD, VSD, or PDA
    Physiologic, functional, or innocent heart murmurs
    Mitral valve prolapse without valvular regurgitation
    Previous Kawasaki disease without valvular dysfunction
    Previous rheumatic fever without valvular dysfunction
    Intravascular and epicardial cardiac pacemakers and implanted defibrillators
    Previous coronary artery bypass graft surgery

Procedures for which Endocarditis Prophylaxis is Recommended:

Dental procedures known to induce gingival or mucosal bleeding, including professional cleaning
Tonsillectomy and/or adenoidectomy
Surgical procedures that involve intestinal or respiratory mucosa

Bronchoscopy with rigid bronchoscope
Sclerotherapy for esophageal varices
Esophageal stricture dilation
Endoscopic retrograde cholangiography with biliary obstruction
Biliary tract surgery
Cystoscopy
Urethral dilatation
Prostatic surgery
Urethral catheterization if urinary tract infection is present

Procedures for which Endocarditis Prophylaxis is not Recommended:

Dental procedures not likely to cause gingival bleeding (e.g., simple adjustment of orthodontic appliances or fillings above the gum line, restorative dentistry)
Shedding of deciduous teeth
Insertion of tympanostomy tubes
Bronchoscopy with flexible bronchoscope, with or without biopsy**
Endotracheal intubation
Transesophageal echocardiography**
Cardiac catheterization
Implanted cardiac pacemakers or defibrillators
Endoscopy with or without gastrointestinal biopsy**
Cesarean section
Uncomplicated vaginal delivery**
Vaginal hysterectomy**
In the absence of infection for urethral catheterization, uterine dilatation and curettage, therapeutic abortion, sterilization procedures, or insertion or removal of intrauterine devices

*This table lists common pediatric conditions and procedures but is not meant to be all-inclusive.

**Prophylaxis is optional for high-risk patients.

Adapted from Dajani AS et al.: Prevention of bacterial endocarditis: recommendations by the American Heart Association, Circulation 96:358-366, 1997.

the drug regimen or surgery. Corrective surgery—particularly in infancy—generally restores a normal growth pattern. Weight usually improves more quickly than height. Palliative surgery generally improves growth, although not to the same degree as corrective surgery.

Development

The majority of children with CHD show development within the normal range (Oates et al, 1995; Wright and Nolan, 1994). Past studies of the effects of cyanosis on IQ have suggested that children who are cyanotic may have a lag in intellec-

---

Box 17-5

Endocarditis Prophylaxis Recommendations

For dental, oral, respiratory tract, or esophageal procedures:

1. For most patients: amoxicillin 50 mg/kg (maximum 2.0 g) orally 1 hour before procedure.
2. For patients unable to take oral medications: ampicillin 50 mg/kg (maximum 2.0 g) IM or IV 30 minutes before procedure.
3. For patients allergic to amoxicillin, ampicillin, and/or penicillin: clindamycin 20 mg/kg (maximum 600 mg) orally 1 hour before procedure;

   or

   cephalexin* or cefadroxil* 50 mg/kg (maximum 2.0 g) orally 1 hour before procedure;

   or

   azithromycin or clarithromycin 15 mg/kg (maximum 500 mg) orally 1 hour before procedure.
4. For patients allergic to amoxicillin, ampicillin, and/or penicillin who are unable to take oral medications: clindamycin 20 mg/kg (maximum 600 mg) IV 30 minutes before the procedure;

   or

   cefazolin 25 mg/kg (maximum 1.0 g) IM or IV 30 minutes before the procedure.

For gastrointestinal and genitourinary tract procedures:

1. For high-risk patients: ampicillin 50 mg/kg (maximum 2.0 g) IM or IV, plus gentamicin 1.5 mg/kg (maximum 120 mg) IM or IV within 30 minutes before procedure, then ampicillin 25 mg/kg (maximum 1 g) IM or IV or amoxicillin 25 mg/kg (maximum 1 g) orally 6 hours after initial dose.
2. For high-risk patients allergic to ampicillin and/or amoxicillin: vancomycin 20 mg/kg (maximum 1.0 g) IV over 1 to 2 hours plus gentamycin 1.5 mg/kg (maximum 120 mg) IM or IV; complete injection and/or infusion within 30 minutes of starting procedure.
3. For moderate risk patients: amoxicillin 50 mg/kg (maximum 2.0 g) orally 1 hour before procedure;

   or

   ampicillin 50 mg/kg (maximum 2.0 g) IM or IV within 30 minutes of starting procedure.
4. For moderate-risk patients allergic to ampicillin and/or amoxicillin: vancomycin 20 mg/kg (maximum 1.0 g) IV over 1 to 2 hours; with the infusion completed within 30 minutes of starting procedure.

*Cephalosporins should not be used in patients with immediate type of hypersensitivity reactions to penicillins.

Adapted from Dajani AS et al.: Prevention of bacterial endocarditis: recommendations by the American Heart Association, Circulation 96:358-366. 1997.

---

tual development (Linde, Rasof, and Dunn, 1970; Wright and Nolan, 1994). It has been felt that early correction of cyanotic lesions results in improved intellectual functioning (Newberger et al, 1984; Newberger, 1992). More recent analysis of children with cyanotic heart disease reveals no significant correlation between intelligence quotient (IQ) or visual motor integration ability and degree of hypoxemia or age of repair (Uzark et al, 1998; Oates et al, 1995). Surgery necessitating hypothermic circulatory arrest, however, has been consistently associated with a higher risk of delayed motor development and neurologic abnormalities (Kern et al, 1998, Uzark et al, 1998; Walsh, Morrow and Jonas, 1995).

CHF and cyanosis may significantly affect gross motor development. Children with CHD may sit, crawl, and walk much later than their peers. Parental overprotection and lack of activity may also contribute to delayed development (Linde et al, 1966; Wright and Nolan, 1994). Although delayed development has been identified in some studies, researchers have emphasized that both cyanotic and acyanotic groups have IQs well within the normal range, and the practical importance of the difference in IQ may be insignificant (O'Brien and Smith, 1994; Wright and Nolan, 1994).

Vulnerable Child Syndrome

Although overprotection may generally be a problem for children with a chronic condition, children with a heart defect are at high risk for overprotection and altered parent-infant attachment (Goldberg et al, 1991). Parental anxiety can occur as a result of the disturbing array of clinical symptoms and feeding problems of a child with CHF or cyanosis, as well as the fear of a sudden catastrophic event (Goldberg et al, 1991; Stinson and McKeever, 1995). The mere presence of the defect unrelated to the severity of the heart disease, however, can produce severe anxiety leading to overprotection and placement of inappropriate limits on a child (Linde et al, 1966; Wright and Nolan, 1994). The dilemma of developing independence vs. dependence is a challenge for adolescents and young adults with CHD (Tong et al, 1998). Because overprotection may delay development in children with existing physical impediments to development, primary care providers should be aware of feelings of vulnerability in parents and children and reinforce the importance of treating these children normally.

Prognosis

The prognosis for children with CHD is good for the majority of lesions. Only the most complex defects require multiple surgeries. Therefore many children have had definitive repair by their first year. The surgical mortality for less-complex defects is generally under 5% (Park, 1996). Children with these defects usually are symptom-free postoperatively and do not require further surgery. The operative risk for most complex lesions is under 15%. The 5-year survival rate for children with hypoplastic left heart syndrome, however, is around 60% (Kern et al, 1998; Mosca et al, 1995). The majority of children after surgery require long-term assessment of potential problems related to myocardial changes, ventricular failure, prosthetic materials, electrophysiologic sequelae, and infective endocarditis (Higgins, 1994).

PRIMARY CARE MANAGEMENT

Health Care Maintenance

Growth and Development

Significant delays in both height and weight are seen in children with symptomatic CHD (Barton et al, 1994; Cameron et al, 1995; Combs and Marino, 1993). Height is generally not affected as much as weight, and head circumference is not affected at

all. If growth is slowed to a point where a child's growth curve flattens, the child should be referred to the cardiologist for an evaluation of worsening CHF. Because growth of a child whose CHF is well-controlled may still be slow, it is important to look at trends of weight gain, as well as make comparisons with the norms.

In assessing the developmental and emotional status of children with CHD, primary care providers must take into account factors such as hypoxemia, CHF, parental overprotection, and physical incapacity. Preoperatively, infants with CHF are often too exhausted to pass all of the developmental tasks in screening tests. If a child is developing at a slower but progressive rate, referral for additional developmental testing is not immediately warranted. If there appear to be significant alterations in the level of alertness or if there is no progress in mastering developmental tasks, further assessment is advised. If CHD is part of a syndrome that involves developmental delay, referral and enrollment in an infant-stimulation program would be important.

Crying is a major developmental concern of most parents of children with CHD, who worry that it will hurt the heart or precipitate a medical crisis. Parents must be informed that short periods of crying will not harm an infant, and that they should treat crying as if the child did not have a heart defect. Parents can be told that prompt attention to crying usually consoles infants faster and reduces crying and irritability in subsequent months (Barnard, 1978). Parents should attend to a child who is crying for these reasons—not because they think that crying is dangerous for the child. Discuss crying issues with both parents because there are often differences in philosophies and subsequent conflicts between parents regarding crying in children.

When discussing developmental concerns with parents, they should be helped to normalize responses to their child with a chronic condition. Primary care providers can guide parents in treating their child normally by reinforcing that children who are symptomatic will limit themselves naturally.

Diet

Feeding is often a major problem for children with CHD, particularly if they are experiencing CHF.

During feeding, infants with CHF often have difficulty coordinating sucking, swallowing, and breathing. The distribution of calories in these infants is similar to the recommended dietary allowances, but the caloric needs of infants with CHF and failure to thrive are about 150 kcal/kg/day (Gaedeke, Norris, and Hill, 1994). If infants are not adequately gaining weight, their caloric intake may need to be increased by concentrating the formula. Concentrating the formula to 24 to 30 calories per ounce will elevate the total calories without increasing the total volume. If formula is concentrated by decreasing the amount of water added to powder or concentrate, the increased renal solute load the infant receives must be considered (Forchelli et al, 1994). An alternative is to add low-osmolarity glucose polymers or oils to standard formulas to increase the caloric density. A diet providing increased carbohydrates and fats may lead to increased retention of nitrogen for growth (Gaedeke, Norris, and Hill, 1994). Two common preparations used are Polycose, which delivers 23 cal/15 cc, and medium chain triglycerides (or MCT oil), which deliver 120 calories/15 cc. Consulting a nutritionist and the cardiologist is advised if nutritional manipulations are used.

Breast feeding children with even a hemodynamically significant heart defect is not contraindicated if growth is adequate. Breast milk is the best source of nutrition for infants with a chronic illness, such as CHD (Committee on Nutrition, 1999). The physiologic stress of breast feeding is actually less than the stress related to bottle feeding (Marino, O'Brien, and LoRe, 1995). Methods to decrease the work of feeding during breast or bottle feeding include holding infants at a 45-degree angle to minimize tachypnea, feeding them for no longer than 40 minutes at a time to minimize fatigue, allowing them to develop their own rhythm of feeding and resting, and following their cues for hunger, satiety, and tiring.

A child rarely will not gain weight despite aggressive feeding and formula concentration. Such children may need gavage feedings to minimize the calories used with feeding. Using a pacifier during gavage feeding helps an infant develop a strong suck, facilitates the transition to oral feeding after surgery, and promotes future language development (Bernbaum et al, 1983).

Parents often need a tremendous amount of support for feeding a child with CHD. Children with CHF and tachypnea have difficulty consuming enough calories to satisfy hunger and may be irritable. Both infants and mothers may contribute to a less than optimal feeding situation. Infants with CHD give fewer feeding cues and respond less to caregivers, and mothers of infants with CHD may exhibit less fostering behavior (e.g., eye contact, smiling, and cuddling) during feeding (Lobo and Michel, 1995). Parents may also feel the pressure of getting a child to gain weight for surgery. In addition, a parent's self-esteem may be tied to the feeding and growth of the child. Primary care providers should stress to parents that feeding can be a positive time for bonding and nurturing. Ongoing support includes teaching the parents to be sensitive to the infant's cues for hunger, satiety, and distress; pointing out the positive aspects of the child; and reinforcing feeding skills. Through feeding, the parent and child are developing their relationship. A primary care provider who understands the potential problems of feeding can be instrumental in fostering a positive feeding relationship by providing support and counseling.

Safety

In addition to standard safety precautions, children with CHD have unique safety needs. For example, digoxin elixir has a pleasant taste and attractive color, which increases the potential for accidental ingestion by the child or siblings. Therefore safe storage and administration of medications is essential. Marking a syringe at the correct dose, giving written instructions on medication administration, and allowing parents to practice drawing the medication will help ensure the safe use of digoxin, which is a valuable but potentially dangerous medication.

Electrical safety is critical for children with permanent pacemakers. An electric shock may irreparably damage the pacemaker requiring immediate surgical replacement. There is no risk of electromagnetic interference between a permanent pacemaker and common household items such as electrical appliances, radios, cellular phones, or electronic equipment. Both microwave ovens and pacemakers have filtering systems that prevent interference with the pacemaker's function. Large magnets placed directly over the pacemaker will temporarily change its function; therefore magnetic resonance imaging (MRI) is contraindicated for children with a permanent pacemaker (Moses et al, 1987). Metal detectors should also be avoided because they have an electromagnetic field that may temporarily alter a pacemaker's function, as well as set off the alarm as a result of the metal in the pacemaker. Small magnet toys, however, will not alter a pacemaker's function. A pacemaker identification card or letter from the primary care provider should be sufficient to allow a child to avoid metal detectors. Older children with pacemakers and children on anticoagulants should wear Medic-Alert bracelets for emergencies.

Children with permanent pacemakers or on anticoagulants for prosthetic valves can maintain most normal activities. They should be counseled to avoid contact sports (e.g., football, boxing, or karate), which could damage the pacemaker or cause excessive bleeding (American College of Cardiology and American College of Sports Medicine, 1994).

Travel may need to be altered for children with CHD. Altitudes of 5000 feet or higher are not recommended for children with moderate to severe pulmonary hypertension, severe CHF, or significant hypoxemia (i.e., PO_2 of 50 mm Hg) (Canobbio, 1987). These children may require precautions to fly on an airplane because cabin pressure is usually equivalent to an altitude of 5000 to 7500 feet. Supplemental oxygen can be supplied by the airlines to increase the inspired oxygen to 20%.

It has been reported that training parents of children with CHD in cardiopulmonary resuscitation (CPR) is effective and particularly warranted for certain problems (Higgins, Hardy, and Higashino, 1989). Suggesting CPR training to parents as a skill that is worthwhile for any parent to know can allay potential concerns about the importance of learning CPR. The American Red Cross or the American Heart Association may offer CPR training to families.

Immunizations

The standard immunization protocol, including the varicella vaccine, is recommended for children with CHD. Standard guidelines for immunization against hepatitis A and B should be followed for children with CHD. A significant percentage of children with CHD, however, are behind in their immunization schedule (Basco, Reckner, Dasden, 1996). Immunizations should not be given before

cardiac catheterization or surgery because a fever would delay the procedure. After surgery, immunizations should be delayed approximately 6 weeks so that a fever from an immunization is not confused with a postoperative infection.

Children with hemodynamically significant CHD may be more susceptible to complications of influenza and should receive the influenza vaccine yearly starting at 6 months of age (Committee on Infectious Diseases, 1997). The recommended dosage is 0.25 cc from 6 to 35 months and 0.5 cc thereafter. Polyvalent pneumococcal vaccine (i.e., as a single intramuscular or subcutaneous 0.5 ml dose) is recommended for children who have asplenia and are at least 2 years old and older (Committee on Infectious Diseases, 1997).

Screening (Box 17-6)

Vision: Routine screening is recommended.
Hearing: Routine screening is recommended.
Dental: Routine dental care should be meticulously followed to prevent caries and gum disease, which may predispose a child to bacteremia if left untreated. Endocarditis prophylaxis is recommended during all dental procedures except simple adjustment of braces and shedding of deciduous teeth (see Boxes 17-4 and 17-5) (Dajani et al, 1997). Because oral procedures (e.g., dental cleaning, drilling at the gum level, or pulling a permanent tooth) produce a higher inoculum of bacteria over a longer period of time than the shedding of deciduous teeth, antibiotic coverage is recommended for these procedures (Danilowicz, 1995). Many chil-

---

Box 17-6

Screening

- Vision, hearing, tuberculosis, and urinalysis—routine recommended
- Dental—endocarditis precautions
- Blood pressure—check upper and lower extremities children with COTA
  check contralateral arm of scar after Blalock-Taussig shunt
- Hematocrit—anemia problematic in CHF and cyanosis
  rising hematocrit levels in cyanotic children may indicate progressive cyanosis

dren with CHD need antibiotic prophylaxis before dental procedures. The specific regimen depends on the type of defect, the procedure being performed, and the child's sensitivity to penicillin. The child's cardiologist should communicate this information to the dentist. Wallet-size cards that outline specific prophylactic regimens are available from the American Heart Association.

Blood pressure: Blood pressure should be obtained in upper and lower extremities for children with pre- or postoperative repair of the aorta to identify discrepancies in pressure readings that may indicate progression of the heart defect. A child who has had a Blalock-Taussig shunt procedure to increase blood flow to the lungs or a subclavian flap repair of coarctation of the aorta will have a diminished or absent pulse in the upper extremity on the side of the surgical scar.

Hematocrit: A rise in hemoglobin and hematocrit may indicate progressive hypoxemia in the child with a cyanotic heart defect. Furthermore, because of the problems associated with anemia in the child with cyanosis or CHF, hemoglobin and hematocrit levels should be checked regularly. Iron supplementation should be prescribed if the hemoglobin level is low for a child's specific condition. Because the child's cardiologist will be checking these values periodically, communication with the cardiologist may save a child the pain and expense of repeated laboratory tests.

Urinalysis: Routine screening is recommended.

Tuberculosis: Routine screening is recommended.

Common Illness Management

Differential Diagnosis

Children with CHD may be susceptible to common pediatric problems that can be more severe than in children with structurally normal hearts. Therefore it is important for primary care providers to know the common problems that can lead to serious complications. It is equally important, however, that they treat these children normally and look for the simple, uncomplicated problems. Families need reinforcement that these children are normal but have special medical needs. Children who have had heart surgery are often scared or hesitant of

---

Box 17-7
Differential Diagnosis

Fever
Focus found: common intercurrent illness unrelated to CHD postoperatively *vs.*

- Wound infection: wound erythema, drainage
- Postpericardiotomy syndrome: pericardial friction rub, malaise, chest pain
- Infective endocarditis: malaise, anorexia, night sweats, new murmur

Respiratory compromise
- URI or LRI: fever, productive cough, infiltrates on chest radiograph *vs.*
- CHF: poor feeding, sweating, dry cough, cardiomegaly

Gastrointestinal symptoms
- Acute gastroenteritis *vs.*
- Digoxin toxicity
- Worsening CHF

Neurologic symptoms
- CVA
- Brain abscess

Chest pain
- Musculoskeletal problems, pulmonary conditions *vs.*
- Cardiac etiology

Syncopes
- Autonomic nervous system, seizures, hyperventilation *vs.*
- Cardiac abnormalities

---

examinations—particularly of their chest. If the child's trust is gained before the examination, visits will be less stressful for the child and more productive for the primary care provider (Box 17-7).

Fever: Although febrile illnesses can have serious consequences in children with CHD, an acute fever may also be caused by a common, uncomplicated childhood illness. Primary care providers should investigate and treat fever the same way they would for any child the same age, while being mindful of the more serious possibilities. The chronic use of antibiotics without a diagnosis just because the child has CHD is not warranted and will put the child at risk of developing infections from resistant organisms (Lieberman, 1994; Woodin and Morrison, 1994).

A fever within a few weeks after heart surgery may be a sign of an operative infection or postpericardiotomy syndrome (i.e., an inflammatory reaction of the pericardial sac after heart surgery). A careful and complete examination is necessary to identify a source of infection. If no focus of infection (e.g., otitis media or pharyngitis) is found, the primary care provider should obtain a complete blood count (CBC) with differential and a blood culture and should consult with or refer the child to the cardiologist or surgeon. In addition, if there are any signs of a superficial wound infection, the child should be referred to the cardiologist or surgeon. Postpericardiotomy syndrome should be suspected by the presence of a fever soon after surgery with a pericardial friction rub, chest pain, malaise, irritability, or enlargement of the cardiac silhouette on a chest radiograph. It is rarely seen in children under 2 years of age and generally appears 7 days to 2 months after surgery (Rheuban, 1995). Referral to the cardiologist is necessary.

A fever will increase the metabolic demands and thus the work of the heart. It is therefore important to evaluate a febrile child with symptomatic CHD for the development or worsening of CHF.

Infants or children with asplenia are at particular risk for infection. These children must be seen by the primary care provider immediately on developing a fever for a complete work-up to identify the cause and initiate antibiotic therapy.

Infective endocarditis: Primary care providers should be alert to signs of endocarditis in children with CHD who have a sustained, unexplained fever because symptomatology may be nonspecific and insidious. Fever may be associated with decreased activity, anorexia, malaise, night sweats, petechiae, splenomegaly, or a new murmur. Children with an unexplained fever and these symptoms should be referred to their cardiologist for evaluation (i.e., including an echocardiogram) to look for vegetation within the heart. Blood cultures should be drawn before initiating antibiotics. Over half of the cases of pediatric infective endocarditis occur in children at least 10 years of age. Children who have palliative systemic to pulmonary shunts, prosthetic valves, and who have had a previous episode of infective endocarditis are at high risk (Dajani et al, 1997).

Parental knowledge of measures to prevent endocarditis is limited (Cetta et al, 1993). Therefore primary care providers must reinforce instructions on endocarditis prophylaxis at each visit.

Respiratory infection: Children with CHD—particularly those with a defect causing left-to-right shunting—may have frequent or significant upper and lower respiratory infections. It is important to evaluate the degree of respiratory compromise compared with the child's baseline respiratory status. If there is an increase in respiratory effort or the presence of adventitious breath sounds, a chest radiograph should be obtained to rule out pneumonia or worsening CHF. Infiltrates evident by radiograph, fever, and productive cough could indicate a lower respiratory infection. Cardiomegaly, poor feeding, sweating, and a dry cough would indicate CHF. The primary care provider should have follow-up contact with a family 24 hours after initial contact to evaluate the child's progress.

Gastrointestinal symptoms: Vomiting or anorexia may occur secondary to gastroenteritis, worsening CHF, or digoxin toxicity. If the history and physical findings are not compatible with more common causes of gastrointestinal (GI) symptoms, a child must be evaluated for other symptoms of CHF and a serum digoxin level obtained.

Excessive fluid losses from vomiting, diarrhea, or anorexia can lead to dehydration and thrombus formation in children who are cyanotic and polycythemic. Replacement fluids or consultation with the cardiologist to hold diuretic therapy may be necessary until the GI disturbance is resolved.

Neurologic symptoms: A child with unexplained fever, headache, focal neurologic signs, or seizures must be immediately referred to a medical center because of the risk of a brain abscess or cerebrovascular accident (CVA).

Chest pain: Only a very small percentage of children complaining of chest pain have symptoms caused by significant cardiovascular abnormality (Hardy, 1994). The majority of these children have pain associated with musculoskeletal problems (e.g., costochondritis or trauma), pulmonary conditions (e.g., reactive airway disease, bronchitis, or pneumonia), hyperventilation, gastrointestinal reflux, or psychogenic chest pain, which is fairly common in adolescents. Cardiac etiologies of chest pain include coronary artery ischemia, tachydysrhythmias (i.e., particularly in toddlers unable to differentiate pain from unusual sensations of dysrhythmias), myocarditis, or pericarditis.

Critical components in a child's history that may clarify the cause can be determined with the following questions: (1) Is the chest pain related to exercise, eating, or breathing? (2) Is there related lightheadedness or syncope? (3) Are there any other serious medical problems? (4) Is there unusual stress at home or school? (5) Is there a family history of sudden death or heart disease? (6) Did the child experience recent physical trauma or new physical activity? (7) Is there a history of illicit drug use? A careful history and physical examination can usually differentiate benign conditions from dangerous ones. An electrocardiogram and referral to a cardiologist should occur if the primary care provider identifies chest pain in conjunction with syncope, dizziness, easy fatigue, palpitations, exertion, drug use, fever, or associated medical problems (e.g., lupus erythematosus, diabetes, Marfan syndrome, or Kawasaki disease) (Cohn, 1993; Hardy, 1994).

Syncope: Syncope is the transient loss of consciousness, usually from decreased cerebral blood flow. Causes of syncope include autonomic nervous system abnormalities, cardiac dysrhythmias, obstructive cardiac lesions, seizures, hyperventilation, vestibular diseases, drug use, or psychogenic causes (Hardy, 1994; Heydemann, 1993). As with chest pain, a thorough history and physical examination are critical. Particular attention should be paid to the head, eyes, ears, nose, and throat for possible vestibular disease. A neurologic examination should be performed if symptoms suggest seizures; and cardiac auscultation should be done to identify a murmur, click, or rub. Worrisome elements of the history include exercise-induced syncope or clonictonic movements suggesting seizures.

The most useful diagnostic test to evaluate for possible cardiac causes of syncope is the electrocardiogram (Hardy, 1994). Referral to a cardiologist for further evaluation (i.e., including an exercise test and tilt-table test) will be needed if the ECG is abnormal.

Drug Interactions

Children with CHF or dysrhythmias often receive combinations of digoxin, diuretics, and other medications. The following issues need to be considered when managing children on these medications: (1) Coadministration of digoxin and quinidine (Cin-Quin), verapamil (Calan, Isoptin), or amiodarone (Cordarone) may elevate digoxin plasma concentrations (Koren and Gorodischer, 1992). (2) Aminoglycosides can affect renal function and alter excretion of digoxin. (3) Children with severe CHF may require medications (e.g., captopril [Capoten] or enalapril [Vasotec]) to decrease resistance to left ventricular ejection (i.e., afterload), thus decreasing the workload on the heart. These drugs may increase serum potassium; therefore if a child is on a potassium-sparing diuretic (e.g., spironolactone [Aldactone]) along with captopril, serum potassium should be checked periodically. (4) Decongestants should be avoided in a child with a rapid heart dysrhythmia (e.g., supraventricular tachycardia or atrial fibrillation) or hypertension because they may exacerbate tachydysrhythmias or increase blood pressure. (5) Aspirin should be avoided for 3 weeks before surgery because of its anticoagulant properties and should be avoided altogether in children receiving warfarin (Coumadin). It is important for the primary care provider to counsel parents to read labels of over-the-counter medications because they may contain aspirin. (6) Some antibiotics may alter the absorption of Coumadin. Any time a child on Coumadin requires antibiotics, the primary care provider should consult with the cardiologist before administering them to prevent possibly altering the prothrombin time.

The primary care provider may be monitoring certain drug levels (digoxin, antidysrhythmics) or response to drugs (prothrombin time in the child taking anticoagulants) in close association with the cardiologist.

Developmental Levels

Sleep Patterns

Infants with CHF who are tachypneic may be unable to satisfy their hunger and thus have a difficult time sleeping through the night. Referral to the cardiologist is advised if a child's respiratory status is deteriorating to the point of interfering with feeding and sleeping. When discussing sleep with parents, primary care providers should ask them where the child sleeps. Primary care providers should reinforce the stability of a child to help parents deal with their anxiety. The transition to the child's bed should not occur when the child's routine or security has been disrupted (e.g., around the time of hospitalization or surgery).

Toileting

Children on diuretic therapy may have difficulty with toilet training. If a child is receiving diuretics for a short period of time, parents may want to delay toilet training until the medication has been discontinued. If a child is on chronic diuretic therapy, the timing of the diuretic may need to be adjusted to facilitate toilet training.

Discipline

Behavioral expectations of children with CHD should be similar to those for children without a heart defect. It is not uncommon for parents to overprotect and pamper children with CHD. Linde and associates (1966) observed that the mere label of CHD effects complex changes in a family's approach and attitudes not only to the child with the disease but also to the normal siblings. Primary care providers can play a key role in reinforcing the importance of setting limits and disciplining children as if there were no heart disease, as well as helping to normalize family dynamics in light of the risk of overprotection.

On the other hand, infants with CHF who are irritable, hard to console, and difficult to feed may present a very stressful situation for parents. Primary care providers must be aware of family stressors and infant characteristics that may lead to abuse of a child with a chronic condition.

Child Care

Some parents choose to stop working when they have a child with a chronic condition, but many do not. Child care is necessary for most families. Several factors that must be balanced when parents are deciding to return to work include the following: (1) the financial and emotional need to return to work; (2) parental anxiety about leaving the child; (3) the increased incidence of infection for children in child care (Takala et al, 1995; Thacker et al, 1992) and the effect of infection on a child's cardiovascular status; and (4) parental confidence in a child care provider's ability to recognize symp-

toms, give medications properly, and respond to emergencies appropriately.

Before surgery or cardiac catheterization, parents may be counseled to take their child out of child care to avoid exposure to infections that would cancel the procedure. Children with asplenia or DiGeorge syndrome are at the highest risk of infection. For these children who are prone to infection, home or small group daycare is advised. For 6 weeks after surgery, parents should limit activities that stress the child's sternum (e.g., climbing, pulling, heavy lifting, rough playing, or lifting the child under the arms). Parents must communicate these restrictions to the child care provider to see if it is realistic or safe for the child to return to daycare before normal activity is allowed. Primary care providers can play a key role in educating child care providers about a child's condition, as well as in reinforcing activity limits—and lack of limits.

Schooling

Most school-age children with CHD can attend school with their peers, although children with cyanotic heart disease are at risk for having difficulties in school (Wright and Nolan, 1994). Missed school is often related to hospitalization, recuperation from surgery, and visits to the cardiologist. Primary care providers can play an important role in assessing the need for home or in-hospital schooling for prolonged absences and facilitating services. Absenteeism may also be associated with parental perception of a child's vulnerability and their lack of control over improving their child's health status.

As children enter junior high and high school, they may have body image concerns related to their scar, small stature, and/or ability to keep up with peers. Parents often underestimate their child's activity tolerance (Casey, Craig, and Mulholland, 1994), and adolescents with heart disease perceive their physical limitations as worse than medically indicated (Koster, 1994). Children should generally be encouraged to participate in physical activity to their tolerance based on discussions that include the child, primary care provider, cardiologist, parents, and school professionals (Committee on Sports Medicine and Fitness, 1994). The twenty-sixth annual Bethesda Conference in January, 1994 outlined detailed recommendations for determining the level of activity related to each congenital car-

RECOMMENDATIONS FOR PHYSICAL ACTIVITY IN SCHOOL
FOR CHILDREN WITH HEART DISEASE

DATE_____

To Whom it May Concern:

_____ is a patient of mine for a congenital heart condition. The following recommendations are guidelines for physical activity in school. The child's cardiac diagnosis is
_____
_____.

____(1) May participate in the entire physical education program, including varsity competitive sports without any restriction.

____(2) May participate in the entire physical education program EXCEPT for varsity competitive sports where there is strenuous training and prolonged physical exertions, such as football, hockey, wrestling, soccer, basketball, etc. Less strenuous sports such as baseball and golf are acceptable at varsity level. All activities during the regular physical education program are acceptable.

____(3) May participate in the physical education program except for restrictions from all varsity sports and from excessively stressful activities such as rope climbing, weight lifting, sustained running (i.e., laps) and fitness testing. MUST be allowed to stop and rest when tired.

____(4) May participate only in mild physical activities such as walking, golf, and circle games.

____(5) Restricted from the entire physical education program.

____(6) Additional remarks: (see other side)

____(7) Duration of recommendations: _____

If there are any additional questions about these recommendations, please contact me.

Sincerely,

_____ (cardiologist signature)

Figure 17-3   Sample letter or recommendation for activity.

diac lesion, dysrhythmia, or acquired heart disease (American College of Cardiology, 1994).

A standard letter of recommendations for activity (Figure 17-3) will clarify expectations and limits so that children can participate in physical activities to their highest potential. The cardiologist may perform stress testing to develop an individualized activity plan. This information should be relayed to the primary care provider. An ongoing discussion with parents and children will reinforce the realistic goals for activity and help prevent overprotection.

Sexuality

Technologic and surgical advances have enabled the majority of young women with CHD to reach childbearing age. Many can successfully carry a pregnancy through delivery. A woman with complex congenital heart defects, however, warrants a careful evaluation of maternal and fetal risk (Canobbio, 1988; Canobbio et al, 1996). The increased risk of CHD in the offspring of individuals with CHD should be discussed with a cardiologist or a genetic counselor before conception if possible.

The issues of contraception and safety of pregnancy must be discussed with parents before their daughter becomes an adolescent, as well as when she is in early adolescence (Uzark, VonBargen-Mazza, and Messiter, 1989). Communication with the cardiologist will give the primary care provider critical information about a girl's risk factors for contraception and pregnancy given her particular physical status.

Oral contraceptives are not advisable for women with pulmonary hypertension, cyanotic CHD, prosthetic valves, and who smoke cigarettes because of the risks associated with increased coagulation and thrombus formation (Gleicher and Elkayam, 1990). Because of the potential for cervicitis and subsequent bacteremia, intrauterine devices (IUD) are contraindicated in women at risk for developing infective endocarditis (Canobbio, 1988; Gleicher and Elkayam, 1990). Barrier methods (e.g., condoms and diaphragms with spermicidal cream) are safe methods of birth control from a cardiac standpoint but are not as effective in preventing pregnancy. The condom is the best method for preventing sexually transmitted diseases; it is an acceptable form of contraception for the young women with CHD, provided that their partners use it reliably (Gleicher and Elkayam, 1990).

For women at very high risk for cardiac compromise with pregnancy, surgical sterilization should be discussed. Tubal ligation in women with longstanding pulmonary hypertension leading to Eisenmenger's syndrome carries with it a high surgical risk and should not be performed unless absolutely necessary (Gleicher and Elkayam, 1990). If tubal ligation is recommended, it is best to wait—if possible—until young adulthood when a woman has gained maturity and can participate in the decision (Canobbio, 1994). Therefore if there is a single sexual partner, vasectomy may be the preferred method of sterilization.

Experts often look at a client's cardiovascular status based on the New York Heart Association (NYHA) Functional Classification to determine the relative risk of pregnancy. Adolescents with mild heart disease that has not been operated upon or those with well-repaired cardiac defects (NYHA Class I or II) are generally at no higher risk from pregnancy than the general population (Canobbio et al, 1996; Gleicher, 1992). Adolescents in class III or above with CHF need special attention during pregnancy. Pregnancy in adolescents with pulmonary vascular disease carries a high risk for morbidity and mortality and may need to be terminated for the safety of the mother (Perloff and Koos, 1998). It is important for primary care providers to discuss the risks of pregnancy with the cardiologist so that the recommendation can be reinforced to the adolescent. A multidisciplinary approach involving the cardiologist, the high-risk obstetrician, and the primary care provider should be used for adolescents with CHD who are pregnant.

Transition to Adulthood

There are approximately 500,000 adults with surgically treated CHD in the United States. An estimated additional 150,000 adults have untreated or unrecognized CHD (Steiner et al, 1995). Adolescents or adults are generally classified according to their postoperative clinical status: Category I—complete repair, asymptomatic; Category II—palliation/complete repair, asymptomatic; Category III—repair with residual defects, minimal; and Category IV—palliation/inoperable, moderate to severe symptoms (Canobbio, 1988). Problems requiring long-term follow-up include electrophysiologic sequelae, myocardial changes, prosthetic materials, ventricular failure, and infective endocarditis (Perloff, 1991).

The occurrence rate of dysrhythmias following intraatrial operations such as atrial septal defects is about 9%. Intraatrial baffling procedures (e.g., the Mustard procedure) for transposing the great arteries have essentially been replaced by arterial switch procedures because of dysrhythmias in over 50% of children and adolescents. The incidence rate of postoperative dysrhythmias in common intraventricular procedures is 30% in TOF and 10% in ventricular septal defect repair (Vetter, 1991).

Additional long-term postoperative concerns include ventricular failure, which is particularly problematic after intraatrial baffling procedures, and systemic-to-pulmonary shunts in functional single ventricles. Myocardial ischemia and fibrosis in open-heart repairs can affect the long-term performance of the myocardium (Somerville, 1991).

Synthetic valves can be associated with infective endocarditis and thromboembolism. These complications have been reduced with the use of human cadaver homograft valves, which do not require anticoagulation and have a lower incidence of endocarditis (Tong and Sparacino, 1994).

Long-term surveillance of adolescents and adults with repaired or unrepaired CHD for infective endocarditis is of central importance. Individuals with the following conditions constitute the greatest risk: (1) rigid prosthetic—especially left-sided—valves; (2) prosthetic conduits, such as the Fontan type of operations; (3) cyanotic defects; (4) defects with high turbulence flow areas, such as VSDs; and (5) palliative shunts, such as the Blalock-Taussig anastomosis (Child and Perloff, 1991; Newberger, 1992). Inadequate knowledge of endocarditis prophylaxis in many adults with CHD underscores the importance of repetitive patient education in this area at every follow-up clinic visit (Cetta and Warnes, 1995; Kantoch et al, 1997).

Evaluating clients' late postoperative concerns, as well as psychologic and social well-being, is central as they progress to adulthood. The goal for individuals who have survived CHD is to provide them with the best possible quality of life throughout adulthood (Higgins and Reid, 1994).

Special Family Concerns and Resources

The family of a child with CHD may have ongoing concerns about symptoms, feeding problems, sudden death, finances, and the long-term physical and emotional effects of multiple surgeries. When parents are counseled about symptoms, it is important that primary care providers convey that the parents will be watching for trends over time rather than minute-by-minute. Reinforcing the fact that parents become the experts in observing their child for changes decreases their feelings that only health care providers can adequately monitor their child.

Young, Shyr, and Schork (1994) found that a substantial number of parents of children with CHD believe that their primary care provider is un-able to meet many of their child's illness needs. Parental information needs related to caring for their infant after cardiac surgery are significant, and their level of understanding may be limited (Stinson and McKeever, 1995). A review of postoperative instructions by the primary care provider and ongoing, careful evaluation of the child will help solidify the parents' knowledge base and reinforce the health provider's position as a valuable asset to the child's care.

The insurability of a child with heart disease depends on the particular defect and repair. As children become older, they often lose their parents' coverage and have difficulty obtaining insurance as adults (Canobbio, 1988; Hellstedt, 1994). Parents must investigate the options for extended coverage of the child on their health insurance plan well before the policy's coverage expires for the child. Depending on their parents' income, children with CHD may qualify for the supplemental insurance of Crippled Children's Services.

Parents may also be concerned about the occurrence of CHD in subsequent children. The cardiologist or genetic counselor should advise a family about specific risks to future children; and the primary care provider should reinforce this information and support the family in their decision making. Early prenatal diagnosis of CHD is possible through ultrasound of the fetal heart (i.e., fetal echocardiogram).

Parent support groups are valuable resources and provide an important network for families who are coping with anxieties related to caring for a child with CHD. Newsletters and special interest groups often develop from parent networking (see section on organizations at the end of this chapter). The primary care provider should contact the local American Heart Association (AHA) or the pediatric cardiology department to see if such groups exist. Written information on many aspects of CHD is also available through the AHA. Public health or home health nursing may be an additional source of support, especially for families learning to identify symptoms, give multiple medications, provide adequate nutrition to a newly diagnosed infant with CHD, or care for a child with complex home care needs.

The Internet has a wealth of information about heart defects, surgical procedures, and support for families of children with heart defects. Parents should be warned to always take the information received on these web pages with a grain of salt. Information changes rapidly, and if individuals reading the information do not have a medical background, they can misunderstand some of the information. The AHA has a website (see the following section of informational materials for the address), which is a good starting place for families to collect information on the web.

Informational Materials

The following resource booklets and pamphlets are available for families through the local or national chapter of the AHA (this is not a complete listing of resources):

> *If Your Child Has a Heart Defect—A Guide for Parents*
> *Feeding Infants with Heart Disease—A Guide for Parents*
> *Dental Care for Children with Heart Disease*
> *Abnormalities of Heart Rhythm—A Guide for Parents*
> *Caring for a Child with a Heart Condition—A Guide for Parents [San Francisco Chapter]*
> *Marfan's Syndrome*
> *Kawasaki's Disease*
> *AHA Scientific Statement: Guidelines for Parent Support Groups (1998)*

Organizations

American Heart Association
National Center
7272 Greenville Ave
Dallas, Texas 75231
www.americanheart.org

Various parent support groups exist across the nation. Check with the local AHA for listings.

Summary of Primary Care Needs for the Child with Congenital Heart Disease

HEALTH CARE MAINTENANCE

Growth and development

Significant delays in weight and height are common in children with symptomatic CHD preoperatively; corrective surgery improves growth.

Intellectual development is not significantly impaired by CHD; cyanosis, parental overprotection, and CHF may contribute to delayed development.

Neurologic abnormalities may occur in children with CHD.

Infant crying is a major—but unnecessary—concern for parents.

Diet

Feeding is a major problem for children with CHD—especially for a child in CHF; required daily allowances are normal, but formula may need to be concentrated for adequate caloric intake.

Breast feeding is encouraged if growth is adequate.

Parents should be taught methods to decrease work of feeding.

Feeding is a major source of stress for parents, who will need much support.

Safety

Safe storage of digoxin is critical.

For the child with a pacemaker, electrical safety is critical. There is no risk of damage with usual household appliances, including microwaves. Children with pacemakers should not have MRIs and should avoid metal detectors and wear a Medic-Alert bracelet.

Air travel and altitude may need to be limited depending on the defect.

Cardiopulmonary resuscitation training for parents is warranted for certain defects.

Immunizations

Standard immunization protocol is recommended; delay should occur only around cardiac catheterization or surgery.

With significant CHD, influenza vaccine is recommended.

With asplenia syndrome, daily antimicrobial prophylaxis and pneumococcal vaccine is recommended for children at least 2 years of age.

Screening

Vision: Routine screening is recommended.

Hearing: Routine screening is recommended.

Dental: Dental care is important to prevent caries, which predispose a child to bacteremia and endocarditis. Endocarditis prophylaxis is recommended for all dental procedures except routine adjustment of braces and shedding of deciduous teeth (see Boxes 17-4 and 17-5).

Blood pressure: Check blood pressure in all four extremities for children with coarctation of the aorta pre- and postoperatively. Children with a Blalock-Taussig shunt will have low or absent blood pressure values in the arm on the side of the shunt.

Hematocrit: A rise in hematocrit may indicate worsening cyanosis. Anemia is problematic in children with CHF or cyanosis. Monitor hemoglobin levels closely in coordination with the cardiologist.

Urinalysis: Routine screening is recommended.

Tuberculosis: Routine screening is recommended.

COMMON ILLNESS MANAGEMENT

Differential diagnosis

Fever: Postoperatively rule out (1) wound infection and (2) postpericardiotomy syndrome. If no focus is found, obtain CBC and blood culture. The child with asplenia with fever must be seen immediately.

Infective endocarditis: Symptoms are often vague; a high level of suspicion is needed for diagnosis. It is rarely seen in children under 2 years of age.

Refer to the cardiologist if fever, malaise, anorexia, splenomegaly, or night sweats are present.

Respiratory infection: Frequent or significant upper and lower respiratory infections may occur; rule out CHF or pneumonia.

Continued

Summary of Primary Care Needs for the Child with Congenital Heart Disease

Gastrointestinal symptoms: Rule out digoxin toxicity and CHF; excessive fluid losses are dangerous in children who are cyanotic or taking diuretics and digoxin.

Neurologic symptoms: Cyanotic children are at increased risk for brain abscess (if <2 years) or CVA (if >2 years); unexplained fever, headaches, seizures, or focal neurologic signs require immediate referral to a medical center.

Children with CHD are at increased risk of neurologic abnormalities (e.g., seizures, muscle tone abnormalities, and motor asymmetry).

Chest pain: Most chest pain is caused by noncardiac problems.

Careful history and physical examination usually differentiate benign from dangerous conditions.

Syncope: There are many cardiac and noncardiac causes.

Close attention should be paid to head, eyes, ears, nose, and throat to rule out vestibular disease.

An electrocardiogram is useful to rule out cardiac causes.

Drug interactions: Accurate administration of digoxin is critical.

Phenobarbital may lower the plasma level of digoxin.

Aminoglycosides may decrease renal function and increase the digoxin level.

Decongestants are not recommended for children with rapid heart dysrhythmias or hypertension.

Digoxin or anticoagulant dosages may need to be monitored.

DEVELOPMENTAL ISSUES

Sleep patterns: Children may have difficulty sleeping through the night if they are tachypneic and unable to satisfy their hunger.

Toileting: Toilet training children receiving diuretics may be difficult.

Discipline: Normal behavior should be expected from children regardless of CHD. Parents often overprotect and pamper children with CHD.

Child care: The provider must understand medications, be able to recognize symptoms, and know emergency procedures.

Infants with DiGeorge syndrome or asplenia syndrome are prone to infection, so home daycare or small-group daycare is recommended.

Vigorous activity should be limited for 6 weeks after surgery.

Schooling: Children may need home tutoring around hospitalization and surgery time.

Children may develop self-image concerns about their scar, ability to keep up with peers, and small stature.

The AHA publishes guidelines for activity limits based on each defect. Generally, children limit themselves. Children who have a pacemaker or are taking anticoagulants should avoid rough contact sports.

Parents frequently underestimate their child's activity tolerance.

Sexuality: Oral contraceptives are not recommended for individuals with pulmonary hypertension, cyanotic CHD, or prosthetic valves.

An intrauterine device is not recommended for individuals at risk for developing endocarditis.

An individual's heart defect and functional ability (i.e., as assessed by the cardiologist) determine risks associated with pregnancy; teens need early and thorough counseling.

Transition to adulthood: Late postoperative concerns include dysrhythmias, ventricular failure, myocardial ischemia, prosthetic failure, thromboembolism, and infective endocarditis.

SPECIAL FAMILY CONCERNS AND RESOURCES

Families have ongoing concern about symptoms, multiple surgeries, and sudden death.

Children with CHD have difficulty finding insurance coverage.

Parents may be concerned that CHD will occur in subsequent children and may want genetic counseling; prenatal diagnosis of CHD is possible through fetal echocardiography.

References

Ackerman IL et al: Total but not resting energy expenditure is increased in infants with ventricular septal defects, Pediatrics 102:1172-1177, 1998.

American College of Cardiology and American College of Sports Medicine: 26th Bethesda conference recommendations for determining eligibility for competition in athletes with cardiovascular abnormalities, J Am Coll Cardiol 24:845-899, 1994.

Barnard K, editor: The nursing child assessment satellite training series: learning resources manual, Seattle, 1978, University of Washington School of Nursing Publications.

Barton JS et al: Energy expenditure in CHD, Arch Dis Child 70:5-9, 1994.

Basco W Jr, Reckner JC, and Darden PM: Who needs an immunization in a pediatric subspecialty clinic?, Arch Pediatr Adolesc Med 150:508-511, 1996.

Bernbaum JC et al: Nonnutritive sucking during gavage feeding enhances growth and maturation in premature infants, Pediatrics 71:41-45, 1983.

Callow LB: Nursing implications of interventional device placement in pediatric cardiology and pediatric cardiac surgery, Crit Care Nurs Clin North Am 6(1):133-151, 1994.

Cameron JW, Rosenthal A, and Olson AD. Malnutrition in hospitalized children with CHD, Arch Pediatr Adolesc Med 149:1098-1102, 1995.

Canobbio MM: Counseling the adult with CHD. In Roberts WC, editor: Adult CHD, Philadelphia, 1987, F.A. Davis.

Canobbio MM: Postoperative follow-up and counseling of adults with CHD. In Jillings CR, editor: Cardiac rehabilitation nursing, Baltimore, 1988, Aspen Publishers.

Canobbio MM: Reproductive issues for the woman with CHD, Nurs Clin North Am 29(2):285-298, 1994.

Canobbio MM et al: Pregnancy outcomes after Fontan repair, J Am Coll Cardiol 28:763-767, 1996.

Casey FA, Craig BG, and Mulholland HC: Quality of life in surgically palliated complex CHD, Arch Dis Child 70:382-386, 1994.

Cetta F et al: Parental knowledge of bacterial endocarditis prophylaxis, Pediatr Cardiol 14:220-222, 1993.

Cetta F and Warnes CA: Adults with CHD: patient knowledge of endocarditis prophylaxis: Mayo Clin Proc 70(1):50-54,1995.

Child JS and Perloff JK: Infective endocarditis. In Perloff JK and Child JS, editors: Congenital heart disease in adults, Philadelphia, 1991, W.B. Saunders.

Clark EB: Epidemiology of congenital cardiovascular malformations. In Emmanouilides GC et al, editors: Moss and Adams heart disease in infants, children and adolescents, ed 5, Baltimore, 1995, Williams & Wilkins.

Cohn HE: Chest pain. In Dershewitz RA, editor: Ambulatory pediatric care, ed 2, Philadelphia, 1993, J.B. Lippincott.

Combs V and Marino BL: A comparison of growth patterns in breast and bottle fed infants with CHD: Pediatr Nurs 19:175-179, 1993.

Committee on Infectious Diseases: Report of the committee on infectious diseases, ed 24, Elk Grove Village, Ill., 1997, The American Academy of Pediatrics.

Committee on Nutrition: Pediatric nutrition handbook, ed 4, Elk Grove Village, Ill, 1998, The American Academy of Pediatrics.

Committee on Sports Medicine and Fitness: Medical conditions affecting sports participation, Pediatrics 94:757-760, 1994.

Cousineau AI and Lauer RM: Heart disease and children with Down syndrome. In Van Dyke DC et al, editors: Medical and surgical care for children with Down syndrome: a guide for parents, Bethesda, Md., 1995, Woodbine House.

Dajani AS et al: Prevention of bacterial endocarditis: recommendations by the American Heart Association; Circulation 96:358-366, 1997.

Danilowicz D: Infective endocarditis, Pediatrics in Review 16:148-154, 1995.

Darling EJ: Overview of cardiac electrophysiologic testing. Crit Care Nurs Clin North Am 6(1):1-14, 1994.

Denfield SW, Garson A Jr: Sudden death in children and young adults, Pediatr Clin North Am 37:215-231, 1990.

Finkelmeier BA: Ablative therapy in the treatment of tachyarrhythmias, Crit Care Nurs Clin North Am 6(1):103-110, 1994.

Forchelli LM et al: Children with heart disease: A nutritional challenge. Nutrition Reviews, 52, 348-353, 1994.

Fyler DC, Nadas AS: Trends. In DC Flyer, (editor): Nadas' pediatric cardiology, Philadelphia, 1992, Hanley and Belfus, Inc, pp 273-280.

Gaedeke-Norris MK, Hill CS: Nutritional issues in infants and children with CHD, Crit Care Nurs Clin North Am 6(1):153-163, 1994.

Gleicher N: Principles and practices of medical therapy in pregnancy, ed 4, Connecticut, Appleton and Lange, 1992.

Gleicher N and Elkayam U: Fertility control in the cardiac patient. In U Elkayam and N Gleicher, (editors): Cardiac problems in pregnancy: Diagnosis and management of maternal and fetal disease, ed 2, New York, 1990, Alan R Liss, pp 453-460.

Goldberg S et al: CHD, parental stress, and infant-mother relationships, J Pediatr 119:661-666, 1991.

Hardy CE: Syncope and chest pain: to worry, or not?, Contemp Pediatr 11:19-42, 1994.

Hazinski MF: Cardiovascular disorders. In MF Hazinsli, (editor): Nursing care of the critically ill child, ed 2, St Louis, 1993, Mosby, pp 117-394.

Hellstedt LF: Insurability issues facing the adolescent and adult with CHD, Nurs Clin North Am 29(2):331-343, 1994.

Heydemann PT: Syncope. In RA Dershewitz, (editor): Ambulatory pediatric care, ed 2, Philadelphia, 1993, JB Lippincott Co, pp 694-697.

Higgins SS: Long-term follow-up of the postoperative patient with CHD, Nurs Clin North Am 29(2):221-231, 1994.

Higgins SS, Hardy CE, and Higashino SM: Should parents of children with CHD and life-threatening dysrhythmias be taught cardiopulmonary resuscitation?, Pediatrics 84:1102-1104, 1989.

Higgins SS and Reid AR: Common congenital heart defects: long-term follow-up, Nurs Clin North Am 29(2):233-248, 1994.

Kantoch MJ et al: Adult patients' knowledge about their CHD, Can J Cardiol 13(7):641-645, 1997.

Kern JH et al: Early developmental outcome after the Norwood procedure for hypoplastic left heart syndrome, Pediatrics 102:1148-1152, 1998.

Koren G and Gorodischer R: Digoxin. In Yaffe SJ and Aranda JV, editors: Pediatric pharmacology: therapeutic principles in practice, ed 2, Philadelphia, 1992, W.B. Saunders.

Koster NK: Physical activity and CHD, Nurs Clin North Am 29(2):345-356, 1994.

Lieberman JM: Bacterial resistance in the 90s, Contemp Pediatr 11:72-99, 1994.

Linde LM et al: Attitudinal factors in CHD, Pediatrics 38:92-101, 1966.

Linde LM, Rasof B, and Dunn OJ: Longitudinal studies of intellectual and behavioral development in children with CHD, Acta Paediatr Scand 59:169-176, 1970.

Lobo ML and Michel Y: Behavioral and physiological response during feeding infants with CHD: a naturalistic study, Prog Cardiovasc Nurs 10(3): 26-34, 1995.

Marino BL, O'Brien P, and LoRe H: Oxygen saturations during breast and bottle feedings in infants with CHD, J Pediatr Nurs 10:360-364, 1995.

Miner PD and Canobbio MM: Care of the adult with cyanotic heart disease, Nurs Clin North Am 29(2):249-267, 1994.

Mosca ES et al: Hemodynamic characteristics of neonates following the first stage palliation for hypoplastic left heart syndrome, Circulation 92:II-267-271, 1995.

Moses HW et al: A practical guide to cardiac pacing, ed 2, Boston, 1987, Little, Brown.

Newberger JW: Central nervous system sequelae of CHD. In Fyler DC, editor: Nadas' pediatric cardiology, Philadelphia, 1992, Hanley & Belfus, Inc.

Newberger JW et al: Cognitive function and age at repair of transposition of the great arteries in children, N Engl J Med 310:1495-1499, 1984.

Oates RK et al: Intellectual function and age of repair in cyanotic CHD, Arch Dis Child 72:298-301, 1995.

O'Brien P and Smith PA: Chronic hypoxemia in children with cyanotic heart defects, Crit Care Nurs Clin North Am 6(1):215-226, 1994.

Park MK: Pediatric cardiology for practitioners, ed 3, St Louis, 1996, Mosby.

Perloff SK: CHD in adults: a new cardiovascular subspecialty, Circulation 84:1881, 1991.

Perloff JK and Koos B: Pregnancy and CHD. In Perloff JK, editor: CHD in adults, ed 2, Philadelphia, 1998, W.B. Saunders.

Prieto LR et al: Comparison of cost and clinical outcome between transcatheter coil occlusion and surgical closure of isolated paten ductus arteriosus, Pediatrics 101:1020-1024, 1998.

Radtke WAK: Interventional pediatric cardiology: state of the art and future perspective, Eur J Pediatr 153:542-547, 1994.

Registry of the International Society for Heart and Lung Transplantation: Ninth annual report, J Heart Lung Transplant 11:599-606, 1992.

Reiss RE: Maternal diseases and therapies affecting the fetal cardiovascular system. In Emmanouilides GC et al, editors: Moss and Adams heart disease in infants, children and adolescents, ed 5, Baltimore, 1995, Williams & Wilkins.

Rheuban KS: Diseases of the pericardium. In Emmanouilides GC et al, editors: Moss and Adams heart disease in infants, children and adolescents, ed 5, Baltimore, 1995, Williams & Wilkins.

Sanders SP: Echocardiography. In Fyler DC, editor: Nadas' pediatric cardiology, Philadelphia, 1992, Hanley & Belfus, Inc.

Smith JB et al: Cardiovascular critical care problems. In Curley MAQ, Smith JB, and Moloney-Harmon PA, editors: Critical care nursing of infants and children, Philadelphia, 1996, W.B. Saunders.

Somerville J: The physician's responsibility: residua and sequelae, J Am Coll Cardiol 18:325, 1991.

Steiner RM et al: CHD in the adult patient: the value of plane film chest radiography, Journal of Thoracic Imaging 10:1-25, 1995.

Stinson J and McKeever P: Mothers' information needs related to caring for infants at home following cardiac surgery, J Pediatr Nurs 10(1):48-57, 1995.

Takala AK et al: Risk factors for primary invasive pneumococcal disease among children in Finland, JAMA 273:859-864, 1995.

Talner NS: Heart failure. In Emmanouilides GC et al editors: Moss and Adams heart disease in infants, children and adolescents, ed 5, Baltimore, 1995, Williams & Wilkins.

Thacker SB et al: Infectious diseases and injuries in child day care, JAMA 268:1720-1726, 1992.

Tong E and Sparacino PS: Special management issues for adolescents and young adults with congenital heart defects, Crit Care Nurs Clin North Am 6:199-214, 1994.

Tong EM et al: Growing up with CHD: the dilemmas of adolescents and young adults, Cardiology in the Young 8:303-309, 1998.

Uzark K et al: Neurodevelopmental outcomes in children with Fontan repair of functional single ventricle, Pediatrics 101:630-633, 1998.

Uzark K, VonBargen-Mazza P, and Messiter E: Health education needs of adolescents with congenital heart disease, J Pediatr Health Care, 3:137-143, 1989.

Vetter VL: Electrophysiologic residua and sequelae, J Am Coll Cardiol, 18:331, 1991.

Walsh, AZ, Morrow, DF, & Jonas, RA: Neurologic and developmental outcomes following pediatric cardiac surgery, Nurs Clin North Am 30:347-364, 1995.

Woodin KA and Morrison SH: Antibiotics: mechanisms of action, Pediatr Rev 15:440-447, 1994.

Wright M and Nolan T: Impact of cyanotic heart disease on school performance, Arch Dis Child 71:64-70, 1994.

Young PC, Shyr Y, and Schork A: The role of the primary care physician in the care of children with serious heart disease, Pediatrics 94(3):284-290, 1994.

Zuberbuhler JR: Tetralogy of Fallot. In Emmanouilides GC et al, editors: Moss and Adams heart disease in infants, children and adolescents, ed 5, Baltimore, 1995, Williams & Wilkins.

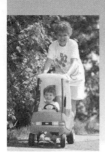

CHAPTER 18

Cystic Fibrosis

Ann Hix McMullen

Etiology

Cystic fibrosis (CF), a condition characterized by complex multisystem involvement, is the most common life-shortening genetic illness among white children, adolescents, and young adults. Significant advances in genetic and biomedical research have been made over the past 15 years that have influenced health professionals' understanding of the condition and its cause, clinical management, and approaches to detection. Although still without cure, CF is no longer considered a terminal childhood disease but a chronic illness with a median life expectancy of more than 30 years of age (National Patient Registry data, CF Foundation, 1997).

After a succession of scientific breakthroughs in genetics, in 1989 the CF gene was isolated on the long arm of chromosome 7, which encodes a protein product (i.e., cystic fibrosis transmembrane conductance regulator [CFTR]) (Rommens et al, 1989). More than 700 unique mutations in the CFTR gene have been reported, the most common of which is the delta F508 mutation, which accounts for 70% of CF alleles (Fernbach and Thomson, 1992; Zeitlin, 1998). Scientists continue to pursue a relationship between specific mutations, defects in CFTR functioning, and subsequent clinical manifestations of the disease. Those genotype-phenotype relationships are complex and probably complicated by factors such as multiple person-environment interactions and the presence of other gene modifiers (Cutting, 1994; Tsui and Durie, 1997). This area of scientific study should be closely followed by primary care providers because findings will have specific implications for the genetic counseling of carriers and parents considering prenatal diagnosis, as well as for the development of novel therapeutic approaches for individuals with the illness.

Breakthroughs in genetics have been accompanied by advances in biomedical research, which are leading to an improved understanding of the pathophysiology of CF. At least one function of CFTR appears to be as a chloride ion channel regulated by cyclic AMP (Quinton, 1990; Ramsey, 1996). This impermeability to chloride ions leads to decreased water movement across cell membranes, which causes secretions to become viscous and less well-hydrated and lumen of airways and ducts to be obstructed (Cutting, 1994). The pathogenesis of an ion-transport defect leads to pathologic sequelae of mucus-obstructing ducts in various body organs. Progressive pathologic changes are produced in nearly every organ of the body. The most consistent changes occur in the exocrine glands (e.g., pancreatic acini, bile ducts and gallbladder, prostatic glands, salivary and lacrimal glands, mucous glands of the tracheobronchial tree, upper respiratory tract and intestinal wall, and the sweat glands) (Abrons, 1993). Table 18-1 is an overview of cystic fibrosis that delineates organ system pathogenesis, clinical manifestations, and treatment.

Incidence

The transmission of CF follows an autosomal recessive mode of inheritance in whites and occurs in approximately 1 in 3200 live births. The incidence in other races, however, is lower. In blacks, it is about 1 in 15,000; in Asians, it is about 1 in 31,000; in Native Americans, it is about 1 in 11,000; and in Hispanics, it is about 1 in 9,000. Occurrence is possible in any race, however. With a gene frequency in whites of 1 in 28, it is estimated that 1 in 400 to 500 couples are both carriers of this recessive trait, with a subsequent 1 in 4 risk of bearing an affected child with each pregnancy (Fitzsimmons, 1993; Hamosh et al, 1998).

Table 18-1
Overview of Cystic Fibrosis

System	Pathogenesis	Clinical Manifestations	Complications	Management
Sweat glands	Abnormal electrolytes	High rate of salt loss; salt depletion	Heat prostration	Dietary salt replacement, sweat test
Lungs	Thick, tenacious mucus	Cough; decreased exercise tolerance	Infection	Chest physiotherapy: postural drainage, cupping/vibration; alternative methods of CPT
	Mucus plugging	Air trapping: increased anteroposterior chest diameter	Fibrosis, bronchiectasis	Antibiotics: oral, intravenous, aerosolized
	Obstruction; Decreased mucociliary clearance	Hyperresonance; Wheezing, fine and coarse crackles, clubbing	Atelectasis; Hypoxia, respiratory failure; Pneumothorax; Hemoptysis; Cor pulmonale; Allergic bronchopulmonary aspergillosis;	Bronchodilators; DNase; Antiinflammatories; Ibuprofen; Cromolyn sodium; Inhaled steroids; Oral corticosteroids;
			Failure to thrive (increased energy expenditure); Hypertrophic osteoarthropathy	High calorie diet
Upper airway	Viscous mucus	Chronic sinusitis; Nasal polyposis	Obstruction, mouth breathing	Decongestants (intermittent use) Nasal cromolyn sodium or corticosteroids; Antibiotics; Surgery

Clinical Manifestations at Time of Diagnosis

The pathophysiologic hallmarks of CF are as follows: (1) pancreatic enzyme deficiency from duct blockage by viscous mucus; (2) progressive chronic obstructive lung disease associated with viscous infected mucus and subsequent interstitial destruction; and (3) sweat gland dysfunction, resulting in abnormally high sodium and chloride concentrations in the sweat (Welsh and Smith, 1995).

There are three common clinical presentations (Box 18-1). The first is meconium ileus in neonates, which occurs in 7% to 10% of newly diagnosed

Box 18-1

Common Clinical Manifestations at Time of Diagnosis

Meconium ileus in the neonate
Malabsorption with failure to thrive
Chronic or recurrent upper and/or lower respiratory infections

Table 18-1
Overview of Cystic Fibrosis—cont'd

System	Pathogenesis	Clinical Manifestations	Complications	Management
Gastrointestinal (GI tract)	Inspissated tenacious meconium; Maldigested food and viscous mucus in gut;	No passage of meconium; Abdominal distension; Cramping abdominal pain	Obstruction: meconium ileus, Distal ileal obstruction syndrome (DIOS); Fecal mass in colon; Volvulus, intussusception	Enema, surgery; Pancreatic enzyme; Dietary changes to avoid constipation; Laxatives Gastrografin with Tween 80 enema or Go-LYTELY;
Pancreas	Viscous secretions obstructions, fibrosis; Abnormal electrolytes; Suboptimal enzyme function	Maldigestion; bulky, foul-smelling stools; Fat malabsorption (including fat-soluble vitamins)	Pancreatitis; Fibrosis; Failure to thrive; Delayed maturation; Rectal prolapse	Enzyme replacement; Antacids; H_2 antonists; High-energy diet; Normal fat intake; Concentrated dietary supplements; Aggressive nutritional supplementation;
			Vitamin deficiency; Glucose intolerance	Vitamin supplements Insulin or oral hypoglycemics
Biliary	Obstruction; Fibrosis	Subclinical cirrhosis	Cirrhosis; Portal hypertension; Cholelithiasis	Urosodiol (Actigall); Cholecystectomy
Salivary glands	Abnormal electrolyte concentrations	Probably not clinically significant		
Reproductive tract	Abnormal viscous secretions	Male: obliteration of vas deferens, sterility Female: thick vaginal and decreased cervical secretions		Genetic and reproductive counseling

infants. The occurrence of meconium ileus should be presumed to be CF until testing confirms or rules out the diagnosis. Meconium plug syndrome—although less frequently associated with the diagnosis of CF—should also raise the primary care provider's suspicion.

The second common clinical presentation is failure to thrive with malabsorption as a result of lost or diminished exocrine pancreatic function, which occurs in 80% to 90% of children with CF. These children exhibit varying degrees of weight loss or poor growth patterns usually in the presence of a normal to voracious appetite; frequent foul-smelling, greasy, bulky stools; rectal pro-

lapse (i.e., in 25% of children); and a protuberant belly with decreased subcutaneous tissue of the extremities.

The third common clinical presentation is the occurrence of chronic or recurrent upper and lower respiratory infections. Manifestations include the following: nasal polyps, chronic sinusitis, recurrent pneumonia and bronchitis, bronchiectasis, or atelectasis. Children with these manifestations have a chronic cough that persists after a respiratory infection and may become paroxysmal and productive, provoking choking and vomiting. Auscultatory findings may include fine crackles and expiratory wheezes—particularly in the upper lobes and right middle lobe, however, some children have no findings on auscultation. Infants may have recurrent episodes of wheezing and tachypnea. *Staphylococcus aureus,* which is often seen initially, and subsequently *Pseudomonas aeruginosa* and *Haemophilus influenzae* are frequent isolates in a respiratory tract culture. Fungi—including *Candida albicans* and *Aspergillus fumigatus* are also often cultured from the respiratory tract (Colin and Wohl, 1994). Early roentgenographic changes include air trapping and peribronchial thickening, followed by atelectasis, infiltrates, and hilar adenopathy (Rosenstein and Langbaum, 1984; Schwartz, 1987). Without treatment, these early signs and symptoms progress and complications occur. Box 18-2 and Figure 18-1 summarize the clinical picture of CF lung disease.

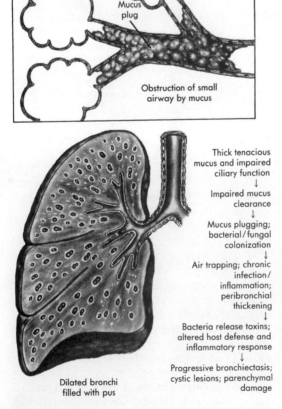

Figure 18-1 Pathophysiology of CF lung disease.

Box 18-2

Progressive Changes in the Clinical Picture of Cystic Fibrosis

I. Early
  A. Dry, hacking, nonproductive cough
  B. Increased respiratory rate
  C. Decreased activity
II. Moderate
  A. Increased cough, increased sputum production
  B. Rales, musical rhonchi, scattered or localized wheezes
  C. Repeated episodes of respiratory tract infection
  D. Signs of obstructive lung disease
    1. Increased anteroposterior diameter
    2. Depressed diaphragm
    3. Palpable liver border
  E. Decreased appetite
  F. Failure to gain weight or grow, or weight loss
  G. Decreased exercise tolerance
III. Advanced
  A. Chronic, paroxysmal, productive cough
  B. Increased respiratory rate, shortness of breath on exertion, orthopnea, dyspnea
  C. Diffuse and localized fine and coarse crackles
  D. Signs of severe obstructive lung disease
    1. Marked increase in anteroposterior diameter (barrel chest, pigeon breast)
    2. Limited respiratory excursion of thoracic cage
    3. Depressed diaphragm
    4. Hyperresonance over entire chest
    5. Decreased ventilation, persistent hypoxemia
  E. Noisy respirations
  F. Marked decrease in appetite
  G. Muscular weakness
  H. Cyanosis
  I. Digital clubbing
  J. Rounded shoulders
  K. Fever, tachycardia, toxicity
  L. Hemoptysis
  M. Pneumothorax
  N. Lung abscess
  O. Signs of cardiac failure (cor pulmonale, edema, enlarged tender liver)
  P. Bone pain and osteoarthropathy

Although these presentations are most common, CF's multisystem involvement (see Table 18-1) may lead to the presentation of variable and subtle symptoms, possibly leading to diagnostic delays and creating an anxious and difficult period for the family and the primary care provider. Manifestations may be minimal or absent during childhood. In 1997, 8% of new diagnoses were made in individuals over 10 years of age (National Patient Registry data, CF Foundation, 1997a). Diagnostic delays may be decreased if primary care providers maintain a high level of suspicion of the various symptoms associated with CF. See Box 18-3 for indications for sweat testing, which is the gold standard test for diagnosing CF.

Diagnosis of CF requires a positive sweat test in the presence of either (1) clinical symptoms consistent with CF or (2) a family history of CF. Sweat testing is done by pilocarpine iontophoresis with quantitative analysis of sweat sodium and chloride. Sweat should only be collected and assayed through a qualified laboratory. All of the 115 regional CF centers certified by the CF Foundation have clinical chemistry laboratories that meet specifications for the accuracy and reliability of sweat tests. Sweat sodium and chloride concentrations above 60 mEq/L are consistent with a diagnosis of CF. A value of 40 to 60 mEq/l is considered borderline and should be repeated. These values should only be considered reliable if an adequate quantity of sweat (i.e., minimally 75 mg) has been collected (National Committee for Clinical Laboratory Standards, 1993). Adequate quantities of sweat may be difficult to obtain from infants under 4 weeks of age, so CF centers may elect to obtain DNA analysis to facilitate early diagnosis in these children. Once the diagnosis has been established in a child, all siblings should be sweat tested. In a small number of individuals with clinical symptoms suggestive of CF, the sweat test may be borderline or even high normal. In these situations, the primary care provider should consult with CF specialty providers who can use expanded laboratory criteria and methods (e.g., identifying CF mutations by DNA analysis and abnormal bioelectric properties of nasal epithelium) to diagnose CF (Rosenstein and Cutting, 1998; Stern, 1997; Wilmott, 1998).

Treatment

Pancreatic Enzyme Deficiency

The principal treatment for the resulting malabsorption in cystic fibrosis is oral pancreatic enzyme replacement (Box 18-4). Enteric coating of enzyme preparations decreases the likelihood of inactivation by gastric acid, and doses may be adjusted to achieve weight gain and one to two formed stools per day. Concerns have been raised,

---

Box 18-3

Indications for Sweat Testing

Pulmonary

Chronic cough
Recurrent or chronic pneumonia
Staphylococcal pneumonia
Recurrent bronchiolitis
Atelectasis
Hemoptysis
Mucoid *Pseudomonas* infection

Gastrointestinal

Meconium ileus, steatorrhea, malabsorption
Rectal prolapse
Childhood cirrhosis (portal hypertension or bleeding esophageal varices)
Hypoprothrombinemia beyond newborn period

Other

Family history of CF
Failure to thrive
Salty sweat, salty taste when kissed, salt frosting of skin
Nasal polyps
Heat prostration, hyponatremia, and hypochloremia, especially in infants
Pansinusitis
Azoospermia
Digital clubbing
Recurrent pancreatitis

Modified from Ewig JM: Cystic fibrosis. In Hoekelman RA, editor: Primary pediatric care, ed 3. St Louis, 1997, Mosby.

<table>
<tr><td colspan="2" style="text-align:center">Box 18-4</td></tr>
<tr><td colspan="2" style="text-align:center">Treatment</td></tr>
</table>

Box 18-4

Treatment

Nutrition
Enzyme and vitamin supplementation
Salt replacement
High-calorie diet

Respiratory
Chest physical therapy
Antibiotics
Antiinflammatory therapy
Bronchodilators
Antifungal therapy
rhDNAse
Lung transplantation

Table 18-2
Factors Contributing to a Poor Response to Pancreatic Enzyme Therapy

Enzyme factors	Outdated prescription
	Enzymes not stored in cool place
Dietary factors	Excessive juice intake
	Parental perception that enzymes are not needed with milk or snacks
	"Grazing" eating behavior
	High-fat "fast foods"
Poor adherence to the prescribed enzyme regimen	Toddler willful refusal
	Chaotic household, multiple meal givers
	Anger or desire to be "normal"
	Teenage girls' desire to be slim
Acid intestinal environment	Poor dissolution of enteric coating
	Microcapsule contents released all at once
Concurrent gastro-intestinal disorder	Biliary disease, cholestasis, Crohn's disease and others

From Drucy S et al: Use of pancreatic enzyme supplements for patients with cystic fibrosis in the context of fibrosing colonopathy, J Pediatr 127:681-684, 1995.

however, by reports of colonic strictures in children with CF (Borowitz et al, 1995). These strictures have occurred in children under 12 years of age receiving enzyme doses of more than 6,000 lipase units/kg/meal. Current recommendations are that pancreatic enzyme doses should be reduced to the lowest effective dose without altering a child's diet. Dosing guidelines of 1000 to 2000 lipase units/kg/meal are now used by most CF centers as a safe range. The safety of doses between 2500 and 6000 lipase units/kg/meal is not known, so such doses should be used with caution (Borowitz et al, 1995; FitzSimmons, Burkhart, and Borowitz, 1997).

Children often experience continued problems with malabsorption despite reasonable coverage with enzymes. Table 18-2 lists factors that contribute to a poor response to pancreatic enzyme therapy. Initial assessment and intervention should address adherence, enzyme storage, and a child's eating habits (e.g., small frequent snacks without taking enzymes). Neutralizing gastric acid with antacids or inhibiting its production with histamine-receptor antagonists may improve the efficacy of the enzyme preparation. If the problem persists, consultation with the CF center may be helpful.

Because fat malabsorption is particularly problematic in CF and deficiencies in fat-soluble vitamins have been reported, CF centers recommend doubling the recommended daily allowance of multivitamins and adding a water-miscible form of vitamin E supplement. Vitamin K may also be supplemented during infancy, in the presence of hemoptysis, or when clotting studies are prolonged.

Newer water-miscible preparations combining the fat-soluble vitamins A, D, E, and K have recently been marketed, providing the convenience of supplementation with a single vitamin preparation for most children (CF Clinical Practice Guidelines, CF Foundation, 1997b; Erdman, 1999).

Caloric and protein requirements are increased in children with CF because of malabsorption related to pancreatic insufficiency, inadequate enzyme supplementation, and progressive pulmonary disease. Most authorities agree that these children have a basal energy requirement that is 25% to 50% greater than the usual recommended daily allowance for energy intake (Erdman, 1999; MacDonald, 1996). With progression of pulmonary disease, children usually have chronic weight and nutrition problems as a result of their increased pulmonary energy requirements. The goal is for children with CF to maintain a weight-height index greater than or equal to 90%. Evidence is growing that children maintained at more than 96% of their ideal weight for height have much better long-term outcomes (CF Clinical Practice Guidelines, CF Foundation, 1997; Nutrition in CF Consensus Report, 1992).

Box 18-5

Tips to Boost Energy Intake

- Include snacks regularly, especially before bedtime. Serve snacks at least 2 hours before the next meal.
- Serve vegetables with cheese or cream sauces.
- Serve meats, potatoes, and other foods with sauces and gravies.
- When preparing fruit juice from concentrate, reduce water added by one fourth.
- Use whole milk fortified with powdered milk as a beverage, in cooking, and on food (e.g., cereal).

Make the following additions to foods served:

Amount	Food	Adds (calories)	Use in or on
1 tsp	Butter or margarine	40	Hot cereal, vegetables, sandwiches, soups, casseroles, breads
1 tbs	Sour cream	26	Vegetables, salads
1 tbs	Mayonnaise	100	Salads, sandwiches, vegetables, deviled eggs
1 oz	Light cream	60	Cereal, hot chocolate, in cooking
1 oz	Evaporated milk*	50	Hot cereal, hot chocolate; substitute for water or milk in cooking
1 tbs	Powdered milk*	23	Whole milk, milkshakes, mashed potatoes, scrambled eggs, meatloaf, or hamburgers
1	Hard boiled egg*	80	Casseroles, meatloaf
1	Egg yolk, chopped*	60	Sandwich spreads
1 tbs	Peanut butter*	100	Bread, crackers, toast, apples or celery, hot cereal, baked goods, milk shakes
1 oz	Cheese*	100	Vegetables, casseroles, meats, sandwiches, salads, pasta, soup, dips
1 oz	Cream cheese	100	Toast, sandwiches, raw vegetables, scrambled eggs, jello salads
1 tbs	Chopped nuts*	49	Puddings, ice cream, salads, casseroles, cereal, baked goods, fruit cup

*These foods add protein in addition to calories.

From Adams EA: Nutrition care in cystic fibrosis: nutrition news, Seattle, 1988, University of Washington Child Development and Mental Retardation Center.

Calories are encouraged in both complex carbohydrates and fats. Dietary fat is the highest density source of calories and also improves the palatability of foods and maintains normal essential fatty acid status. Whenever possible, children with CF should follow a normal diet pattern with no specific restrictions (Nutrition in CF Consensus Report, 1992). Energy-boosting tips are found in Box 18-5. An individual may have difficulty with certain high-fat foods, which may be limited; but children should generally be encouraged to cover high fat intake with additional enzymes. Aggressive nutritional supplementation (i.e., oral, enteral, and parenteral) has been used for children with weight loss problems and growth delay despite a reasonable intake. Early short-term studies documented improved weight gain and stabilization of pulmonary function with this approach (Levy et al, 1985; Soutter et al, 1986). More recent long-term studies have documented decreased mortality, improved growth, and—for some individuals—a decreased rate of pulmonary decline (Steinkamp and von der Hardt, 1994).

Pulmonary Disease

Progressive lung disease is the major cause of morbidity and mortality in CF. The pathophysiologic basis of CF lung disease is impaired mucociliary clearance of dehydrated mucus followed by endobronchial infection. Children with CF become chronically colonized with gram-negative organisms, which may be quantitatively decreased with antimicrobial therapy but cannot be eradicated. A child's susceptibility to this bacterial growth is not fully understood, and there is widespread controversy over the optimal approach to its long-term treatment. General agreement exists, however, that bacterial infection—especially *Pseudomonas aeruginosa* with its virulence factors—and the intense host inflammatory response to infection (i.e., antibody response and neutrophil influx) lead to chronic bronchiectasis and progressive damage to lung tissue (see Figure 18-1). CF centers recognize that antimicrobial therapy is of primary importance in decreasing the rate of this deterioration and has played a significant role in the increased survival of individuals with CF (Denton and Wilcox, 1997; Marshall and Samuelson, 1998).

Pulmonary exacerbations often follow mild viral illnesses, particularly upper respiratory infections. It has been hypothesized that viruses may suppress host defenses, although this mechanism has not been clearly defined (Prober, 1991; Rosenfeld and Ramsey, 1992). It can be argued that an early course of oral antibiotic therapy should be used with viral illness symptoms to prevent exacerbation of the bacterial pulmonary infection during the viral illness. Continuous oral antibiotic coverage to reduce the frequency of exacerbations in young children, however, has come under question. In a multicenter trial of continuous *Staphylococcus* prophylaxis with cephalexin vs. with a placebo for 5 to 7 years, there were no differences in the pulmonary and nutritional outcomes of each group; but the group treated with antibiotics had a higher rate of *Pseudomonas aeruginosa* colonization (Ramsey, 1996).

Traditional concerns about the development of resistant organisms with overuse of antibiotics must be balanced against the greater concern for progressively deteriorating bronchiectasis. The initial choice of antibiotic and dose should consider broad-spectrum coverage (i.e., specifically for *Staphylococcus aureus, Streptococcus pneumoniae,* and *Hemophilus influenza*). Further considerations in children whose pulmonary infections do not respond to initial therapy include antibiotic susceptibility or resistance, lack of compliance, or abnormal pharmacokinetics (MacLuskey, 1993; Ramsey, 1996).

Other ongoing pulmonary therapeutic interventions are aimed at relief of bronchial obstruction through clearance of pulmonary secretions. Chest physical therapy (e.g., postural drainage and cup-

ping and/or clapping and/or vibration two to four times a day) has been effective and has been standard therapy for years. Other techniques of airway clearance have been developed for school-age children and adolescents; such techniques include active cycle of breathing (ACB) and forced expiration technique (FET), autogenic drainage (AD), positive expiratory pressure (PEP), and airway oscillation (e.g., Flutter device, mechanical percussor, vest). The common advantage of these techniques is that they allow the child independence in clearing the airway of mucus. Although more definitive studies are needed, these techniques have been effective (Davidson and McIlwaine, 1995).

Routine chest therapy is recommended for all children with pulmonary involvement; the specific regimen recommended for an individual with CF should be made by the CF center's physician and respiratory or physical therapist. Exercise (i.e., particularly an aerobic conditioning program) is also encouraged because it positively influences general health, cardiopulmonary and musculoskeletal function, and airway clearance (DeJong et al, 1994; Loutzenhiser and Clark, 1993). Reactive airways disease (RAD) may result from chronic inflammation and infection. Bronchodilators are often used if a clinical response can be observed or if a beneficial response of a more than 10% increase in forced vital capacity 1 second after bronchodilator use is shown by pulmonary function testing (Pattishall, 1990; Ramsey, 1996). Many children with CF use an aerosolized bronchodilator before chest physical therapy, and some may also be on a theophylline preparation.

Children with CF mount an intense inflammatory response to chronic bronchial infection, which contributes to parenchymal destruction and disease progression. Konstan and associates (1994) reported that adolescents and adults with mild CF lung disease who appeared clinically healthy were found to have evidence of bacterial infection and significant local inflammatory response on bronchoalveolar lavage. Even bronchoalveolar lavage fluid from infants has been shown to have increased DNA levels, which is an early marker for inflammation (Kirchner et al, 1993). Clinicians have long recognized the clinical efficacy of antiinflammatory therapy and have used short courses of oral and inhaled corticosteroids, as well as cromolyn sodium, in reactive airway disease associated with CF. Findings of small studies have supported these practices; but large, long-term trials are needed to determine the specific use of both short courses of oral corticosteroids, as well the use of inhaled steroids (Konstan, 1998). Although participants in a study of the chronic use of systemic corticosteroids had improved lung function, they developed significant side effects (i.e., cataracts, growth retardation, and glucose abnormalities) (Rosenstein and Eigen, 1991). More recently, long-term use of high-dose ibuprofen by preadolescents with mild lung disease has been reported to decrease the progression of lung disease over a 4-year period (Konstan et al, 1995). Ibuprofen use is expected to increase in the future and requires serum drug levels to be monitored so that therapeutic doses can be established (Konstan, 1998). Individuals most likely to benefit should be selected by the CF center team.

Pharmacotherapies that clear airways of thick, tenacious secretions indirectly improve inflammation. In 1994, the FDA released aerosolized recombinant human DNAse (rhDNAse), which was a breakthrough in new CF pharmacotherapy. rhDNAse cleaves extracellular DNA, which is present in high concentrations in purulent CF airway mucus, and reduces its viscosity to a more liquid form (Hubbard et al, 1992). Studies have shown its efficacy in improving pulmonary function as well as decreasing the frequency of hospitalizations, school or work absenteeism, and CF-related symptoms in individuals with mild to moderate pulmonary disease (i.e., FVC >40% predicted). Side effects were limited to upper airway irritation (i.e., resulting in hoarseness, rash, chest pain and conjunctivitis) and were usually mild and transient (Accurso, 1995; Hodson, 1995; Shak, 1995). Children started on rhDNAse should be monitored by serial pulmonary function testing and clinical markers of morbidity. The selection of children to be started on DNAse should be based on data on the effectiveness and long-term outcomes of pulmonary function, which continue to emerge. Initial studies document that ongoing efficacy is based on daily use (Ramsey, 1993).

Recent evidence that actin, which is released by polymorphonuclear leukocytes in the airway, may inhibit mucus clearance. Gelsolin is a naturally occurring protein that depolymerizes actin and may reduce the viscosity of CF secretions; studies are underway to determine its potential efficacy in CF (Vasconcellos et al, 1994). Acetylcysteine (Mucomist), which is a mucolytic agent, and expectorants

have no clear effectiveness; in fact, acetylcysteine may irritate the respiratory tract (Rosenstein, 1990).

Aerosolized antibiotics have been increasingly effective by delivering high concentrations of antibiotics to the site of infection while decreasing the risk of systemic absorption and toxicity. These antibiotics have been used most effectively as suppressive therapy in individuals chronically colonized with *Pseudomonas aeruginosa*. Aminoglycosides and colistin (Coly-Mycin M Parenteral) have been the most consistent choices; and tobramycin has been the most extensively studied aminoglycoside. Aerosolized aminoglycosides may reduce the frequency of intravenous antibiotic therapy, but the potential for developing resistant strains of *Pseudomonas* spp. concerns primary care practitioners. Therefore clinical expertise in CF management is recommended when appropriate individuals, the specific drug and dosage, and the length of therapy are selected (Marshall and Samuelson, 1998).

When pulmonary exacerbations are not controlled by oral and aerosolized antibiotics, intravenous antibiotics may be necessary. A pulmonary and nutritional "tune-up" or "clean-out" may be initiated in the hospital or home. These 2-week—or longer—courses of therapy allow the CF-center team to employ more aggressive strategies to contain infection and supplement nutrition. Such strategies include using intravenous antibiotics (i.e., often an aminoglycoside with either a synthetic penicillin or third generation cephalosporin), as well as increased pulmonary toilet, physical therapy, exercise, and nutritional support measures. Intravenous antibiotics are chosen for their effectiveness in treating *Pseudomonas aeruginosa*, which is less responsive to oral therapy. Quinolone antibiotics are currently the only available oral preparations that effectively treat *Pseudomonas* spp; and of these, ciprofloxacin (Cipro) has been the most extensively studied in CF. Because of the lack of data on side effects in children, quinolones have not been approved by the FDA for use in individuals under 18 years of age. In clinical trials of Cipro, however, children with CF generally tolerated it well, so many CF centers use it judiciously in children. Clinicians should be aware that *Pseudomonas* spp. rapidly develops resistance to oral quinolones; frequent use and use in more severely affected individuals is often associated with a suboptimal response (Marshall and Samuelson, 1998).

Recent and Anticipated Advances in Diagnosis and Management

Genetic Testing

The effect of genetic discoveries on understanding etiology and pathophysiology is only beginning to unfold while approaches to detection are changing and reflect the new technologic advances. Carrier screening is available and reliable for siblings and family members of a child with CF whose deletions have been identified. Appropriate studies of DNA deletion and linkage analysis are highly complex, and any family member contemplating such a screening should be referred to a regional CF center with a pediatric genetics center for counseling.

Prenatal diagnosis is now available to parents of a child affected with CF and other at-risk couples. As a result, increasing numbers of at-risk families are using these diagnostic resources and confronting the ethical dilemma of having a therapeutic abortion vs. continuing the pregnancy. Such decision making occurs while the science of treatment is advancing and clinicians observe the variability of the phenotypic expression of CF in an individual child. Chorionic villus sampling (CVS) at 8 to 10 weeks' gestation or amniocentesis at 12 to 16 weeks' gestation may provide information on CF mutations in the fetus. Wertz and associates (1992) surveyed parents of childbearing age who had a child with CF about their attitudes on prenatal diagnosis. Almost half of the couples surveyed desired more children and intended to use prenatal diagnosis. Of those who expected to use prenatal diagnosis, 44% would carry a fetus found to have CF to term, 28% would abort, and 28% were undecided. Prenatal diagnosis services, along with related counseling, is an area of specialization and should be coordinated by the regional CF center (Fernbach and Thomson, 1992; Shapiro and Seilheimer, 1994).

Heterozygote (carrier) detection of the general population is technically possible. Specialized genetic laboratories now offer screening for up to 70 of the most common CF mutations, which account for about 85% to 90% of mutant CF genes in North America. In 1990 a National Institutes of Health (NIH) workshop report recommended that carrier screening should only be offered to the general population if a 90% to 95% level of carrier detection could be achieved. The report also noted that a number of mass population screening issues were unstudied (i.e., public and professional education, the system's ability to provide genetic counseling services, and the effects of information on legislative and health insurance systems). Before mass screening becomes a feasible and responsible endeavor, data from pilot screening programs, which are currently underway in several areas of the country, should be analyzed (NIH Workshop on Population Screening for the CF Gene, 1990).

Neonatal screening of immunoreactive trypsinogen (IRT)—although possible—is controversial because of the high number of false positives. The test accuracy is increased, however, when coupled with DNA testing for gene mutations. Statewide screening programs in Colorado and Wisconsin are addressing the dilemma of the benefits of early diagnosis vs. the cost of testing newborns and educating and counseling the family (Shapiro and Seilheimer, 1994). There is growing evidence that early diagnosis of CF is medically beneficial. As more targeted therapies are developed, early diagnosis may become even more beneficial to a child. No national consensus on screening, however, has yet been achieved (Rock, 1997).

Pharmacologic and other Advances

New breakthroughs in pharmacologic interventions that focus on the treatment of CF lung disease, which is the major determinant of morbidity and mortality in CF, are currently being tested. Interventions are designed to interrupt the cascade of pathophysiologic phenomena by either preventing the development of abnormal airway secretions and lung infections or treating the existing infection and inflammation (Figure 18-2). Four of the most promising areas of research are as follows:

1. Modulation of salt and water transport in CF airway epithelium—Initial studies of aerosolized amiloride and uridine triphosphate (UTP) showed success in stimulating chloride secretion and inhibiting sodium absorption in the airway epithelium of children with CF, leading to more hydrated airway mucus. Multicenter trials are underway (Knowles et al, 1995).

Use of **standard*** and *experimental*+ therapy

To alter the pathologic sequence of CF lung disease

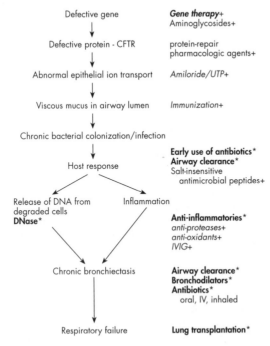

Figure 18-2 Pathologic sequence of CF lung disease and the therapies used.

2. Interruption of the neutrophil-mediated inflammatory cascade with agents such as antiproteases, pentoxifylline, and intravenous immune globulin (Davis, 1994, Moss et al, 1994).

3. Novel therapeutic approaches directed at the common defects of CFTR (e.g., protein-repair therapy)—These approaches include the use of aminoglycosides, phenylbutyrate, CPX, genistein, melrinone, and gene therapy. Gene therapy, however, has received the most attention by the lay CF community. The first human trial of gene therapy for CF was initiated at the NIH in April of 1993 (Wilson, 1994). The goal of this therapy is to insert coding for normal CFTR protein in airway epithelial cells. For all of these therapies, clinical studies of safety, efficacy, and methodology are in progress in research centers across America. Individuals with CF, their families, and their health care providers ultimately hope that gene therapy and other therapeutic approaches will eventually be collectively realized in a cure for CF (Wilson, 1994; Zeitlin, 1998).

4. Bilateral lung transplantation—This has emerged as a viable therapeutic option for individuals with end-stage CF lung disease. As of 1998, estimates of 3-year survival with CF are 56% for individuals transplanted since 1992 as compared with 46% for those transplanted before 1992. The current overall 5-year survival rate is 48%. Improved surgical techniques and anti-rejection drugs have had—and will continue to have—a marked impact on survival statistics. The biggest impediment to more widespread use of this intervention is the critical shortage of suitable organ donors (Yankaskas et al, 1998). Although this procedure offers hope to individuals with end-stage disease and their families, it also presents them with significant psychosocial and financial challenges. Because the waiting time prior to transplant is increasing, referral should be made when the clinical course predicts length of survival to be about 2 years. Because such complex decisions are involved, consideration of transplantation, individual and family counseling, and referral for evaluation should be coordinated through the CF center.

Associated Problems (Box 18-6)

Salt Depletion: Hyponatremia and Dehydration

Children with CF have abnormal sodium and chloride loss in their sweat and are therefore at risk for dehydration secondary to electrolyte imbalance. Risk factors include hot weather, febrile illnesses with or without vomiting and diarrhea, and strenuous physical activity. Excessive salt loss may lead to listlessness, vomiting, heat prostration, and dehydration. Infants are at particular risk because of the low salt content of breast milk, commercial infant formulas, and infant foods. Prevention includes supplementing salt in infant formulas (e.g., ¼ tsp/day) and adding salt to an older child's diet (Adams, 1988).

Rectal Prolapse

Rectal prolapse, which can occur in as many as 20% to 25% of individuals with CF (Littlewood, 1992), may be the presenting symptom and may occur only once or be a recurrent problem. Initiation of appropriate enzyme replacement or adjustment of enzyme dosage often prevents its reoccurrence. Persistent or recurrent prolapse may rarely require surgical intervention (Borowitz, 1994). The first episode of rectal prolapse is frightening for both parents and child, and its reduction usually requires both immediate guidance (i.e., via phone) and assistance in the primary care provider's office or emergency room.

If a child experiences recurrent episodes of rectal prolapse, parents may learn to manually reduce a prolapse. With the child lying on his or her side, a parent (i.e., using a glove and lubricant jelly) is usually able to gently invert the mucosa through the rectal opening.

Nasal Polyps and Pansinusitis

Nasal polyps occur in 10% of children with CF and, if found on physical examination of a child, should raise the suspicion of CF if not already diagnosed. The upper respiratory tract (i.e., including sinuses) is lined with respiratory epithelial cells similar to the lining in the lungs and is therefore also affected by CF pathology. Sinuses are often chronically infected, producing symptoms such as frontal headaches, tenderness on palpation, purulent nasal discharge, and postnasal discharge, which further contributes to the chronic cough. Treatment includes extended use of antibiotics and nasal cromolyn sodium and steroids, as well as intermittent use of nasal decongestants. Children

may also find warm mist and saline nasal rinses to be comfort measures; some CF clinicians and otolaryngologists recommend sinus irrigations with saline. Surgical interventions for polyposis and sinusitis are sometimes necessary and are usually followed by stringent postsurgical nasal and/or sinus hygiene regimens (Stern, 1998).

Distal Ileal Obstruction Syndrome and/or Constipation

Although the prevalence of distal ileal obstruction syndrome (DIOS) is higher in adolescents and young adults, young children with CF are also at risk for developing total or partial intestinal obstruction. Constipation is often the result of a combination of malabsorption (i.e., from inadequate pancreatic enzyme doses or failure to take enzymes), decreased intestinal motility, and abnormally viscous intestinal secretions. DIOS is seen when intestinal contents build up at the ileocecum. Abdominal cramping with either diarrhea or the absence of stool and anorexia occurs. A stool mass may be palpable in the right lower quadrant. If the obstruction becomes complete, vomiting and increased pain and distention occur. Appendicitis, intussusception, and volvulus occur more frequently in children with CF and must be considered. A plain abdominal film may help to confirm the diagnosis of DIOS. Contrast enemas (e.g., gastrograffin with Tween 80) may be both diagnostic and therapeutic and are the treatment of choice for children with complete obstruction. Children with partial obstruction may be treated with polyethylene-glycol solutions (Golytely, Colyte) or gastrograffin given orally or by nasogastric tube (Borowitz, 1994). Follow-up should include long-term use of some combination of stool softener, mild stimulant, and bulk laxative, as well as the addition of bulk to the diet, consistent enzyme use, and exercise (MacLusky, 1993).

Hemoptysis

It is not uncommon in CF for blood-streaked sputum and small quantities of bright red blood to be expectorated from the lungs. Although initially alarming to the child and family, this bleeding is usually self-limiting. Bleeding reflects increased bronchial infection, inflammation, and irritation,

---

Box 18-6

Associated Problems

Hyponatremia
Rectal prolapse
Nasal polyps
Sinusitis
DIOS
Hemoptysis
Gastroesophageal reflux

which require more aggressive treatment. Initiation or change of antibiotic therapy should be considered in addition to increasing routine pulmonary toilet. Massive hemoptysis (i.e., usually >240 ml/24 hrs), however, requires immediate referral to the CF center team for management.

Gastroesophageal Reflux

Heartburn and regurgitation may be reported by more than 20% of individuals with CF, although the frequency with which reflux exacerbates pulmonary disease is unknown. Symptoms of reflux should be evaluated and treated if documented (Orenstein and Orenstein, 1988). In addition to pharmacologic management with a histamine-receptor antagonist and motility agent, dietary measures and an upright position after feedings and/or meals should be instituted. Postural drainage should always be done before feedings and/or meals.

Other Associated Problems

CF is a multisystem condition with an increased rate of complications and morbidity with age and disease progression. The complications listed in Box 18-7 are more serious and usually require the expertise of the CF center team. Primary care providers must recognize the early signs and symptoms of these complications so that timely referral for evaluation and treatment is possible.

Of note, colonization with *Burkholderia cepacia* has emerged as a perplexing problem in some CF centers. This organism is highly resistant to an-

tibiotic therapy and has been implicated in the rapid progression of lung disease. *Cepacia* and other resistant organisms are known to be transmitted between children with CF, and appropriate infection-control measures for patients are the subject of ongoing debate within the CF community (MacLusky, 1993).

Prognosis

Despite 40 years of remarkable progress and a recent surge of new approaches to treatment, CF remains a progressive disease without cure. The median survival age is over 30 years of age (Figures 18-3 and 18-4), and survival has markedly

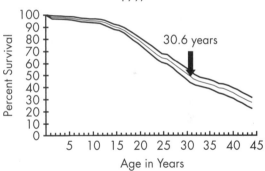

Figure 18-3 Survival curve for all CF patients for the year 1997. (Courtesy Cystic Fibrosis Foundation, National CF Patient Registry, 1997.)

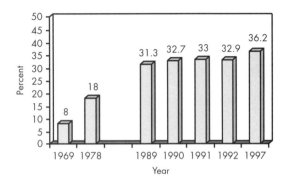

Figure 18-4 Aging of the CF population: percent of CF patients ≥18 years, 1969-1997. (Courtesy Cystic Fibrosis Foundation, National CF Patient Registry, 1997.)

Box 18-7

Serious Complications
of Cystic Fibrosis

Cor pulmonale
Massive hemoptysis
Pneumothorax
Hypertrophic pulmonary osteoarthropathy
Liver disease including portal hypertension
Gallbladder disease
Glucose intolerance, including insulin dependent diabetes
Allergic bronchopulmonary aspergillosis (ABPA)
Pancreatitis

increased over the past 20 years. This change is likely a result of not only an improved understanding of pathophysiology and treatment but also an appreciation and detection of the milder phenotypic expressions of the disease. With continued improvement in survival, CF is becoming a chronic illness of children, adolescents, and a growing population of adults (Fitzsimmons, 1993).

PRIMARY CARE MANAGEMENT

Health Care Maintenance

Growth and Development

Growth delay and difficulty maintaining an adequate weight:height ratio are common problems in CF. Weight loss and linear growth retardation may be presenting clinical signs both in infancy and early adolescence. Catch-up growth is often observed after diagnosis and initiation of pulmonary and nutritional therapy.

Growth and developmental failure may be seen in children with CF who have significant progression of pulmonary disease. Such failure may be more evident as children approach puberty and during adolescence when a growth spurt is normally expected. These delays involve not only height and weight but also skeletal and sexual maturation and are explained by a complex interrelationship of the degree and severity of pulmonary disease, maturational delay, and caloric intake (MacDonald, 1996; Pencharz and Durie, 1993). Aggressive nutritional supplementation has been associated with long-term improvement in growth velocity and well being, as well as with slowed decline in pulmonary function (Dalzell et al, 1992; Erdman, 1999; Steinkamp and von der Hardt, 1994). A metaanalysis of the literature on behavioral, oral, enteral, and parenteral treatment approaches to malnutrition in CF was conducted (Jelalian et al, 1998). All interventions effectively produced weight gain, although the selection of appropriate individuals for specific therapies remains unclear and supports continued research. Primary care providers should be alert to weight loss or a flattened growth curve associated with loss of appetite because these may indicate a pulmonary exacerbation. The presence of either should prompt further investigation with the child and family for an increase in pulmonary symptoms.

Growth retardation should also prompt a review of gastrointestinal status (i.e., specifically stool pattern and consistency), as well as symptoms of abdominal cramping or gastric "burning." Primary care providers may adjust the enzyme dosage if stools are frequent and greasy, but consultation with the CF center team about further interventions may be necessary.

The mean age of the onset of puberty in children with CF is 14.9 years; this delay may be an acute source of concern for adolescents. Primary care providers may be able to help teenagers understand that this delay is not unusual or unexpected and that sexual development—though delayed—will occur. Menarchal age has been associated with severity of illness, and adolescent girls who are underweight because of advancing disease—despite rigorous efforts in nutritional supplementation—need support and reassurance (Johannesson et al, 1997).

CF is not associated with intellectual deficits or delays in cognitive development. Problems in school performance are more likely related to either absenteeism as a result of physical illness or fatigue associated with an impending exacerbation.

Diet

Children with CF require high-calorie, high-protein diets. In infancy, breast feeding should be continued whenever possible with enzyme supplementation and—when necessary—supplementation of a higher calorie/ounce formula. Formula-fed infants and breast-fed infants requiring supplemental formula are often given a hydrolysate formula with medium-chain triglycerides (e.g., Pregestimil, Alimentum). Even though these formulas are predigested, enzyme supplementation is often necessary. Enzymes are given to infants by mixing the beads in the capsule into pureed fruit (e.g., applesauce) and feeding this by mouth.

Parents often have questions about enzyme supplementation doses. Requirements depend on the degree of pancreatic insufficiency, the fat content of the food ingested, the quantity eaten, and the type of enzymes used. Doses are adjusted by trial until the stool pattern is acceptable (e.g., one to two stools per day in older children, and more in infancy) and the child demonstrates reasonable growth. Enzymes should be taken within 30 minutes of eating, and the beads should not be chewed or crushed; destroying the enteric coating inactivates the enzymes and may excoriate the oral mucosa. Children should be encouraged to add extra enzymes when high-fat foods are eaten.

As toddlers and preschoolers experience developmentally appropriate changes in eating patterns, parents are often anxious about providing adequate food intake to maintain the child's well-being and growth. In a study of eating behaviors of preschool children with CF, Stark and associates (1997) found that children with CF consumed at least as much as their peers but did not achieve dietary recommendations. The parents of these children also perceived more eating problems in them. Parents need help in understanding that abnormal emphasis on food, force feeding, and mealtime battles should be avoided. They should instead provide appropriate foods, set limits for mealtimes, and suggest their child try some of each food offered. Multiple small servings and nutritious snacks may also boost a child's nutritional intake.

In preschool-age and older children, high-calorie, high-protein supplementation may be orally achieved with commonly purchased foods (see Box 18-5). The nutritionist at the CF center can provide many suggestions for fortifying a child's diet, and printed educational material is also available to families.

Taking enzymes in front of classmates may be difficult for school-age children. The parents, teacher, school nurse, and child can devise the best plan for enzyme administration. As children grow older and have more control in selecting their diets, parents must pay particular attention to the quality of snack foods available at home. Parents often find that an adolescent's intake is better if a structured mealtime is maintained, despite individual schedules.

Safety

In addition to routine anticipatory guidance about safety issues, primary care providers should emphasize safe storage and handling of the large quantities of medications often used by children with CF. The issue of accidental ingestion of pancreatic enzymes by another child may arise because ample supplies of these enzymes are often available at mealtimes in the home and carried by the child for use. Medications are not likely to be harmful if small quantities are ingested; they are activated in the small intestine and excreted in stool without major absorption in the bloodstream.

Immunizations

Infants and children with CF should receive all routine immunizations at the ages recommended by the American Academy of Pediatrics (AAP). In a few instances the CF team may recommend a brief delay in order to stabilize an acute pulmonary or nutritional problem, but there is no evidence to support delay of routine immunizations.

Following AAP guidelines, a single dose of the FDA-approved (April 1995) varicella vaccine should be given to children with CF between 12 and 18 months of age who do not have a history of chicken pox. Older children with CF and no history of varicella may be immunized at the earliest opportunity. Two doses of vaccine 4 to 8 weeks apart are recommended for adolescents. Children who are steroid dependent should be immunized with caution, and the CF center should be consulted (American Academy of Pediatrics, 1997).

Immunization with an annual influenza vaccine is also recommended, following CDC guidelines, which include the use of split-virus vaccine in children under 13 years of age. Use of amantadine or rimantadine chemoprophylaxis may be indicated in children and adolescents with more significant lung disease. Consultation with the CF center team about selection of appropriate individuals is recommended. A pneumococcal vaccine is also routinely recommended for children over 2 years of age in an effort to prevent pneumococcal pneumonia and a CF pulmonary exacerbation (Committee on Infectious Diseases, 1997).

Screening

Vision: Routine screening is recommended. Steroid-dependent children should be monitored annually by a pediatric ophthalmologist for early detection of cataracts or glaucoma.

Hearing: Routine screening is recommended. Children should be monitored by an audiologist for occurrence of high-frequency hearing loss with each course of intravenous aminoglycoside therapy.

Dental: Routine screening is recommended. Precautions for the use of tetracycline before permanent tooth formation are advised.

Hematocrit: Routine screening is recommended. The roles of pancreatic insufficiency and pancreatic enzyme replacement therapy in iron absorption in CF is unclear. If anemia is present, iron status should be periodically evaluated and appropriate supplementation provided (Nutrition Assessment and Management in Cystic Fibrosis: A Consensus Report, 1992).

Tuberculosis: CF centers routinely perform skin tests with the Mantoux test. Although active disease caused by *Mycobacterium tuberculosis* is probably no more prevalent in individuals with CF than in the general population, recent reports have documented the presence of atypical mycobacteria in individuals with CF. The general prevalence and clinical pathogenesis, however, have not yet been determined (Kilby et al, 1992).

Condition-Specific Screening

Pulmonary function testing: Pulmonary function testing (PFT) is routinely performed in children over 6 years of age during CF-center visits every 6 months and more often as indicated. PFTs and chest roentgenography monitor the progression of pulmonary disease and identify acute problems.

Multisystem screens: Other screening routinely performed at CF-center visits include sputum cultures with antibiotic sensitivities; blood and urine assays of liver and renal function; blood cell counts; and serum and anthropometric measures of nutritional status. The CF-center team routinely shares the results of these screens and PFTs and their management of abnormalities with primary care providers.

Common Illness Management

Differential Diagnosis

Symptoms associated with common pediatric illnesses may also be symptoms specific to CF, and questions about their cause and management often arise. Parents may often need to hear that their child will develop common, minor childhood illnesses and will usually respond to routine management. Parents may be reassured that the CF-center team is available to the primary care provider whenever questions about the cause and treatment of an acute illness arise. Thorough history taking and examina-

---

Box 18-8
Differential Diagnosis

Constipation: Common vs. DIOS
Abdominal pain: Rule out appendicitis, volvulus, intussusception, gallstones, pancreatitis
Fever: Viral illness with exacerbation of chronic infection
Chest pain: Pneumothorax vs. muscle pull vs. GER
Cough: Sinusitis vs. lower respiratory tract exacerbation
Wheezing: Heightened bronchial reactivity due to chronic infection and inflammation

---

tion are not only necessary for primary care providers to make a differential diagnosis but are also reassuring to parents and the child (Box 18-8).

Gastrointestinal symptoms: Diarrhea, constipation, and abdominal cramping may be presenting complaints of a partial or complete intestinal obstruction. A history of cramping pain and changes in stool pattern in the absence of other acute gastrointestinal and systemic symptoms is suggestive of distal ileal obstruction syndrome (DIOS). Abdominal pain may also be suggestive of gallstones or pancreatitis, and a careful pain history is essential. Appendicitis, intussusception, and volvulus should always be in the differential diagnosis (Borowitz, 1994).

Fever and viral illness: Fever associated with a CF pulmonary exacerbation is a relatively uncommon presentation, and evaluation of fever in children with CF should elicit the same broad-based approach used with other children. An initial brief febrile period with a viral illness should be anticipated in children with CF and symptomatically treated per usual practice protocols. When a viral illness exacerbates lower respiratory tract symptoms—as often occurs with upper respiratory tract infections, an increase in chest physical therapy and prompt, sustained (i.e., 2 to 3 weeks) oral antibiotic coverage are usually recommended. Prevention of hyponatremia and dehydration during febrile illness includes adding salt to a child's intake and reviewing warning signs of dehydration with parents. When a rehydration solution is indicated, electrolyte-balanced clear liquids (e.g., Pedialyte [Ross Laboratories]) may be used.

Chest pain: Children with CF often complain of chest pain. These complaints should always be evaluated because of the potential occurrence of pneumothorax. Complaints associated with pneumothorax are typically a sudden onset of sharp pain unilaterally followed by dull aching and accompanied by profound shortness of breath and activity intolerance. This complication, confirmed by physical examination and chest roentgenogram, is best managed at the regional CF center following local emergency stabilization as indicated.

Bilateral musculoskeletal pain from coughing paroxysms is usually diffuse and occurs with a pulmonary exacerbation. Such pain may also be localized, however, and a child will have pain on palpation at the site. Both diffuse and localized pain usually respond to the use of nonsteroidal antiinflammatory and pain therapy. Some children and adolescents with CF experience midline chest and epigastric burning related to gastroesophageal reflux (GER) and esophagitis (Schidlow, Taussig, and Knowles, 1993). If antacids are not effective, the CF-center team should be consulted, specifically regarding the use of histamine-receptor antagonists.

Varicella: There has been no report in the CF literature of higher rates of complications from chicken pox in children with CF; however, there have been reports of exacerbation of pulmonary symptoms (MacDonald, Morris, and Beaudry, 1987). Varicella immunization is strongly recommended. If a child with CF develops chicken pox, management of coryzal symptoms is no different from that for other children. The same approach to antibiotic use with increased pulmonary symptoms should also apply to this viral illness. Use of antipruritic medications is not contraindicated, but they may suppress a child's cough, so parents should increase chest physical therapy as soon as lesions permit. In some children with severe CF lung disease, the CF center may recommend varicella-zoster globulin (VZIG) with exposure to chicken pox. If recommended, it should be administered within 48 hours of exposure. The CF center may recommend that acyclovir be given within 24 hours of onset of the rash of chicken pox to attenuate the clinical course in children with moderate to severe lung disease (American Academy of Pediatrics, 1997).

Cough: A chronic cough that may vary in intensity is a hallmark of CF lung disease. At baseline, it may be present in the early morning and with exercise. An increase in cough is always of significance and requires intervention. Nighttime coughing may develop and be associated with reactive airway disease, increased pulmonary infection and inflammation, or postnasal discharge from sinusitis or rhinitis. Delineating a clear cause can be challenging. Both antibiotic therapy and initiation of or increase in the use of aerosolized bronchodilators and antiinflammatory agents may be helpful. Cough suppressants are generally contraindicated and should only be used after consultation with the CF center team. A trial of decongestants may be useful. Antihistamines may be used when allergy plays a role in symptomatology, but primary care providers should be aware that antihistamines may increase the viscosity of mucus, inhibiting its mobilization.

Wheezing: Wheezing is a common manifestation of CF—particularly in infancy—that is most often attributed to heightened bronchial reactivity from chronic infection and inflammation (Schidlow et al, 1993). Aerosolized bronchodilators and antiinflammatory agents may be effective, as will a course of an antibiotic. Wheezing in infancy may be difficult to alleviate but often diminishes with age (Stern, 1989).

Drug Interactions

Primary care providers routinely include anticipatory guidance about substance abuse to children, adolescents, and parents. The effect of tobacco smoke—both active and passive—is an obvious burden for children with CF. Evidence of an increased incidence of viral respiratory illness in all children exposed to passive smoke was documented in the 1980s (Wall, 1987), making caregiver smoking an added risk for children with CF. Even more alarming are Campbell and associates' findings (1992) of a significant association between heavy exposure to tobacco smoke and lower clinical scores, poorer pulmonary function results, and higher rates of hospitalization in children with CF. Smoke also increases airway reactivity (Stern, 1987).

In addition to the overall effect of alcohol, smoke, and psychoactive drugs on the organ systems of children and adolescents with CF, specific interactions have been reported. Alcohol use in individuals on chloramphenicol or cephalosporins has been associated with episodes of nausea, vomiting, and headache. Alcohol has also been associated with increased pulmonary symptoms—perhaps from suppression of the cough reflex—with episodes of hemoptysis.

Primary care providers should also be cognizant of certain interactions of drugs commonly used to manage CF lung disease. Erythromycin and ciprofloxacin alter the metabolism and excretion of theophylline, requiring a reduction in the theophylline dose when either of these drugs is used. With use of these antibiotics, primary care providers should review signs of theophylline toxicity with children and parents and discuss a plan for dose reduction if indicated. Increased ultraviolet light sensitivity may occur in some children on tetracyclines and sulfonamides, so their use should be avoided when sun exposure is anticipated.

Use of antifungals and macrolide antibiotics (e.g., erythromycin, azithromycin) is contraindicated in children with gastroesophageal reflux being treated with cisapride. Primary care providers should consult with the CF center about cardiac screening if cisapride use is contemplated (Levine et al, 1998).

Developmental Issues

Sleep Patterns

Children with CF have a busy early morning routine, which requires early rising for school-age children and adolescents. They are also often more vulnerable to fatigue because of their increased basal metabolic rate. Although sleep requirements are not necessarily greater in these children, sleep should not be reduced. Nighttime coughing may also interfere with rest and contribute to general fatigue. Nighttime symptoms are usually relieved by an added treatment with a bronchodilator and a chest physical therapy session, but these symptoms should be reported to the primary care provider and consideration should be given to initiating or changing antibiotic and antiinflammatory therapy.

Toileting

As in other children, toilet training should proceed as cues of developmental readiness are noted in a child. Many children with CF, however, continue to

have stools more than once a day and may have some abdominal cramping before producing stool—even with adequate enzyme therapy. These problems may impede the child's interest in toileting, and parents should allow for this delay.

Even though enzymes improve digestion of nutrients, some maldigested food passes through the intestine. As a result, stools may be malodorous and embarrassing for children and adolescents. Parents, teachers, and friend's parents should be aware of the need for privacy during toileting and help a child manage bathroom odor.

Discipline

From the time of diagnosis, parents of children with CF not only grieve the loss of a healthy child but also feel guilty about their genetic contribution. Parents struggle to redefine a future for their child and family. The primary care provider can provide ongoing support and counseling during this difficult adjustment period. Helping parents to set limits and encourage similar responsibilities for the child with CF and siblings makes it easier for them to maintain consistency in family life.

The time commitment of daily therapy may not only create periodic conflicts between parents and children but may also be viewed by siblings as an inequity in parental attention. Conscious efforts by parents to give individual attention to each child may prevent feelings of jealousy and guilt. Coyne (1997) identified effective parental coping strategies, including assigning meaning to the illness, sharing the burden, and incorporating therapy in a schedule. Extended family and community support is an important ingredient in daily therapy because parents need respite and the opportunity to develop individual interests (Quittner et al, 1992).

Parents of adolescents with CF are often frustrated and anxious about disease progression when they have difficulty maintaining their child's adherence to the treatment program. Factors influencing compliance with CF regimens are numerous and complex (Gudas, Koocher, and Wypij, 1991). Normal adolescent behavior (e.g., testing limits, perceiving themselves as invincible, and taking risks) is complicated by the chronicity and morbidity of CF. Experimentation with medications—both over- and underuse—and refusal of chest physical therapy often occurs. Teenagers with CF often experience no immediate consequences of such experimentation, further reinforcing their behavior. Although the relative risk of not doing therapy is difficult to quantify, documentation of the efficacy of chest physical therapy cannot be ignored. Parents who begin to transfer responsibility for illness management to their child during early school years often report fewer problems in adolescence. Even children 5 to 6 years of age are old enough to understand the need for treatment such as enzymes and vitamins. Adolescents with CF may also be more compliant if allowed to control parts of their illness management (e.g., using a mechanical percussor, flutter device, or independent drainage technique, or substituting an exercise program for a therapy session). Encouraging school-age children and adolescents to actively participate in clinic visits and involving them in decision making is essential to their development of accountability. Behavioral contracts may be useful tools for families and health care providers who are experiencing more problems with an adolescent (Parcel et al, 1994).

Child Care

Parents of children with CF often struggle with daycare issues. Parents need reassurance that a child with CF is not immunocompromised and will mount an adequate response to communicable diseases. Choosing a daycare setting with fewer children (i.e., and potentially lower viral illness exposure), however, may be a more appropriate decision for parents of infants or toddlers. When a daycare program has been selected, daycare providers should be specifically educated on issues such as: (1) the child's individual nutritional and pulmonary treatment program; (2) the child's chronic cough and lack of contagion; and (3) methods to prevent the spread of viral illness in the setting. (See the list of educational materials at the end of this chapter.)

Schooling

A number of issues may surface for children with CF in the school environment, and it may be helpful for a CF-center provider to make a school visit and meet with the school nurse, classroom teacher(s), physical education teacher, principal, and—when appropriate—the director of special education. School personnel commonly have questions about the child's cough, bowel and pul-

monary toilet needs, exercise tolerance, nutrition and medication requirements during the school day, and absenteeism for illness and hospitalization. Advice in handling these issues greatly depends on the severity of a child's illness. Specific educational materials for school personnel are also available (see the list of education materials at the end of this chapter).

The degree to which short stature, difficulty in gaining and maintaining weight, and delayed pubertal development are present varies. When significant, these affect the development of a positive body image and self-esteem, particularly in adolescence. These delays are often associated with increasing pulmonary involvement and alter a child's ability to fully participate in academics, social life, and sports and exercise programs. The primary care provider may be able to suggest recreational activities and skills that are more likely to be tolerated and in which the child may be able to excel (e.g., swimming, diving, baseball, archery, gymnastics, certain track and field events, playing a musical instrument, and art) (Committee on Sports Medicine and Fitness, 1994).

Sexuality

Of the men with CF, 98% are sterile because of blockage or absence of the vas deferens; a sperm count is recommended to confirm the expected aspermia (Kotloff, 1994). Male adolescents need reassurance that this condition does not indicate impotency and will not diminish their ability to have normal sexual relations. Women with CF may have more difficulty becoming pregnant because of thick cervical mucus. A woman should also be carefully evaluated and counseled about the degree of risk of pregnancy in her individual condition. This counseling is complex and includes considerations of the woman's level of pulmonary function and overall health status, the statistical genetic risk of having a child with CF, and the woman's shortened life expectancy (Hillman et al, 1996).

Contraception alternatives for adolescent and young adult women with CF have been controversial. Oral contraceptives have been reported to increase the viscosity of cervical mucus and therefore theoretically carry the increased risk of having a similar effect on pulmonary mucus viscosity, although this has not been documented. Because of the comparative risk of pregnancy, many CF-center providers recommend oral contraceptives after fully discussing these issues with a young woman. Reproductive issues in CF should be managed in consultation with the CF-center team and its high-risk obstetrician/gynecologist consultant.

Transition to Adulthood

Adolescents with CF whose parents were given a less-than-optimistic picture of survival at diagnosis are being challenged to set goals for a future that may include college and/or vocational education, a career, and social relationships (e.g., marriage). At the same time, these adolescents struggle with increasing morbidity and higher rates of CF complications as they grow older.

Primary care providers and CF-center providers are faced with meeting the needs of a growing population of young adults. In most regional CF centers, 35 to 40% of the client population is over 18 years of age. Transition programs that move adolescents into the care of adult providers have been developed in many of these centers, and adult programs are planned to be in place at most centers within the next 2 to 3 years. These programs feature a committed team of adult providers who have developed expertise in CF care and become jointly involved with pediatric providers in delivering care during adolescence. Although their implementation has not been without problems, these programs have innovatively addressed clients' developmental needs for independence and identity and acknowledged the need for age appropriate care in a growing population of adults with CF (Clinical Practice Guidelines, CF Foundation, 1997).

Special Family Concerns and Resources

Families who deal with CF have myriad special concerns, including the stress of its prognosis, the added financial burden of medical care, and the maintenance of family life despite the uncertainty of exacerbations, hospitalizations, and disease progression. It has been demonstrated that families—though stressed—generally cope successfully (Buchanan and Morrison, 1992; Ievers and Drotar, 1996). Circumstances that place a family dealing

with CF at high risk for dysfunction and maladaptation have been identified (Walker, Van Slyke and Newbrough, 1992) and include single-parent families, families with an adult with CF, and families with a limited income.

Parents often need guidance in presenting information to and answering questions about CF for their child and other family members. In addition to the help of the CF-center team, written material (e.g., including books for school-age children [see list of education materials at the end of this chapter]) is available. By age 10 to 12 years, the cognitive development of most children is reaching formal operational thinking. Information on morbidity and mortality should be presented honestly and within a framework of hope for continued breakthroughs in treatment research.

The financial burden of this condition is formidable, and families often need additional assistance with health care costs. The diagnosis of CF is covered in most states by programs for physically handicapped children or children with special needs. Eligibility requirements, as well as benefits, are highly variable; the CF center staff can help to coordinate these efforts for a family.

CF is commonly seen in whites of European origin. In the population of a CF center, it is not unusual to find few—if any—black, Asian, or Indian children. When these children are diagnosed, they and their families face the additional problem of limited support networks within the community. One-to-one contact between families may be helpful and can be facilitated by the CF center.

In Amish and Mennonite families, as well as in a growing number of families in general, use of herbal medicine (e.g., garlic and pleurisy root) to treat the pulmonary and nutritional problems of CF is common. Remedies are often shared among families by mail. Coverage of health care costs can be a significant issue for families in many of the Anabaptist communities. Neither private insurance nor government programs are often acceptable to these communities because of their religious beliefs. In addition, homes may not have electricity. Providers of health care to these children should be both sensitive and creative as they address issues in care delivery with these families.

When considering genetic testing of cultural, ethnic, and racial subpopulations, it is important to identify differences in the prevalence of various CF mutations and their potential phenotypic expressions within and among these groups (e.g., Amish, Mennonite, and Hutterite communities; blacks, Ashkenazi Jews). Cultural differences in beliefs, attitudes, and feelings, as well as in behavior during testing and intervention, should also be identified and understood by the counselor (Miller and Schwartz, 1992).

Community Resources

The CF Foundation is a national organization committed to supporting research for the treatment and cure of CF. Local chapters are found in many larger cities in the United States. The CF Foundation also develops and distributes excellent informational material for public and the professional community (see the list of educational materials at the end of this chapter). The Foundation has also supported the development of CF Clinical Practice Guidelines (CF Foundation, 1997b), which are a distillation of the standards of care for individuals with CF. These guidelines have helped to ensure a uniform level of care and service at all CF centers in the United States. The 115 regional CF care centers in the United States offer expertise in the care and management of CF-related issues. Parents should be encouraged to keep in regular contact with the center because this ongoing and regular specialist care has been shown to correlate with improved survival statistics (Wood, 1984). CF centers offer a specialty team approach with physicians, nurses or nurse practitioners, nutritionists, social workers, respiratory or physical therapists, and clinical psychologists. These centers have a family focus in programming, which often includes parent, adolescent, and young adult support groups, education programs, education and support for newly diagnosed families, genetic counseling and testing services, and medical specialty consultation for multiple organ system involvement in CF.

Educational Materials

This is a brief partial listing of helpful information for children and families. Contact a regional CF center for help with additional resources, particularly in specific content areas.
Cystic Fibrosis Foundation
6931 Arlington Road
Bethesda, Md. 20814
1-800-FIGHT CF
   Publications include: *Chest Physical Therapy: Segmental Bronchial Drainage; An Introduction*

to Cystic Fibrosis; and *The Genetics of Cystic Fibrosis.*

   Farmer G and Wilcox S: Fat and loving it. This is a book on nutrition written in 1990 for individuals with CF and is available from Gail Farmer, PO Box 5127, Belmont, Calif. 94002.

   Orenstein DM: Cystic fibrosis: a guide for patient and family, ed 2, New York, 1997, Raven Press.

   Ribando C and Langbaum T: I have cystic fibrosis, Baltimore, Md., 1985, The Johns Hopkins Medical Institutes. This is a story for school-aged children.

   Nakielna B, O'Loane M, and Durbach E: For adults with cystic fibrosis, Vancouver, BC, 1986, Shaughnessy Hospital CF Clinic.

   Sondel S and Hartman L: A way of life: cystic fibrosis nutrition handbook and cookbook, 1988. Available for $5.00/copy from Karen Luther, F4/120 Food and Nutrition Services, University of Wisconsin Hospital and Clinics, Madison, Wis. 53792

   Storey M and Adams E: Snacks and more, Rochester, New York, 1988, Pediatric Pulmonary Center, University of Rochester Medical Center.

Available through pharmaceutical representatives:

   A guide to cystic fibrosis for parents and children is a manual and video available from McNeil Pharmaceuticals.

   Ryan LL: Cystic fibrosis in the classroom: a handbook for teachers, Marietta, Ga., 1996, Solvay Pharmaceuticals, Inc.

   Luder E: Living with cystic fibrosis: family guide to nutrition, Spring House, Penn., 1987, McNeil Pharmaceuticals.

   Mandolfo A: Cystic fibrosis, Marietta, Ga., 1988, Solvay Pharmaceuticals, Inc. This is a booklet for young children.

   Stanzone A and Godwin SL: Let's look at me, Marietta, Ga., 1989, Solvay Pharmaceuticals, Inc. This is a workbook for young children.

   Websites:
   CF Foundation—http://www.cff.org
   CF Research, Inc.—http://www.cfri.org
   Cystic fibrosis index of online resources—http://vmsb.csd.mu.edu/~5418lukasr/cystic.html
   CF-WEB—http://www.cf-web.mit.edu
   There are many other websites and online resources. Each source should be evaluated for accuracy and reliability of information.

Summary of Special Primary Care Needs of Children with Cystic Fibrosis

HEALTH CARE MAINTENANCE

Growth and development

Growth and developmental delay reported and variable; associated with severity of pulmonary disease and maturational delay.

Degree of malabsorption and presence of pulmonary exacerbation are also factors affecting growth delay.

Pubertal delay may be anticipated in most adolescents.

Diet

High-calorie, high-protein diet recommended.

Fat intake not restricted; target of 35% to 40% of daily intake in fat sources.

Pancreatic enzyme replacement and vitamin supplementation necessary in children with malabsorption.

Safety

Safe storage of multiple medications emphasized.

Immunizations

All routine immunizations should generally be given on schedule.

Influenza vaccine should be given annually per CDC guidelines.

Pneumococcal vaccine is recommended for all children over 2 years of age.

Screening

Vision: Routine screening is recommended.

Hearing: Routine screening is recommended. An audiology screen for high-frequency hearing loss should be done with aminoglycoside therapy.

Dental: Routine care.

Hematocrit: Routine screening recommended with full review of iron status as indicated.

Tuberculosis: Routine testing with PPD at CF center.

Condition-specific screening: PFTs, chest roentgenography, sputum culture with drug sensitivities and blood and urine assays of liver and renal function, cell counts and differential, glucose and nutritional status are usually monitored at routine CF center visits.

Drug Interactions

Erythromycin and ciprofloxacin may increase serum theophylline levels.

Alcohol use with cephalosporins or chloramphenicol may cause headaches, nausea, and vomiting.

Cisapride should not be used with macrolides and antifungals. The CF center should be consulted before cisapride is started.

COMMON ILLNESS MANAGEMENT

Differential diagnosis

Constipation or diarrhea: Rule out DIOS.

Abdominal pain: Rule out DIOS, appendicitis, volvulus, intussusception.

Chest pain: Rule out pneumothorax.

Cough: Further differentiation of componens of reactive airways disease (RAD), lower respiratory tract infection and/or inflammation, rhinitis and/or sinusitis may be helpful in selecting treatment choices.

DEVELOPMENTAL ISSUES

Sleep patterns: Early morning routines require adjustment of bedtime. Nighttime coughing may interfere with rest and require prompt attention.

Toileting: Delayed bowel training may occur secondary to increased frequency of stools and associated abdominal cramping.

Discipline: Expectations should be normal, with allowances during periods of illness exacerbation. Lack of compliance with treatment programs may affect disease progression in adolescence.

Child care: Home care and small daycare programs are recommended during first year of life to reduce viral exposure. Daycare workers need information on CF.

Summary of Special Primary Care Needs of Children with Cystic Fibrosis—cont'd

Schooling: Multiple school questions may be best addressed in a school visit.

Adjustment problems related to altered body image and self-esteem are possible during adolescence.

School performance may be affected by fatigue and lethargy with an impending pulmonary exacerbation.

School absenteeism for hospitalizations requires coordination for ongoing academic services.

Sexuality: Male sterility should be confirmed.

Female reproductive issues are complex and require specialty consultation and counseling.

Transition to adulthood: Developmentally appropriate, specialty health care should begin in adolescence.

Special family concerns

Uncertainty of illness progression and predicted lethality.

Family functioning during illness exacerbations requiring hospitalizations.

Effect of treatment program—particularly chest physical therapy—on family life.

Cultural issues of minority and subpopulations include isolation, use of alternative therapies, sensitive counseling for genetic screening, and insurance coverage for health care.

Available through the CF Center:

The *Cystic fibrosis family education program* is a comprehensive program developed by DK Seilheimer and associates at Baylor College of Medicine, Texas Children's Hospital. Distribution was underwritten by Genentech.

References

Abrons HL: Cystic fibrosis: current concepts, W V Med J 89(6):236-240, 1993.

Accurso FJ: Aerosolized dornase alfa in cystic fibrosis patients with clinically mild lung disease, Dornase Alfa Clinical Series 2(1):1-6, 1995.

Adams EA: Nutrition care in cystic fibrosis: nutrition news Seattle, 1988, University of Washington Child Development and Mental Retardation Center.

American Academy of Pediatrics Committee on Sports Medicine and Fitness: Medical conditions affecting sports participation, Pediatrics 94(5):757-760, 1994.

American Academy of Pediatrics: Report of the committee on infectious diseases, Elk Grove Village, Ill., 1997, The Academy.

Borowitz D: Pathophysiology of gastrointestinal complications of cystic fibrosis, Semin Respir Crit Care Med 15(5):391-401, 1994.

Borowitz D et al: Use of pancreatic enzyme supplements for patients with cystic fibrosis in the context of fibrosing colonopathy, J Pediatr 127:681-684, 1995.

Buchanan E and Morrison LM: Cystic fibrosis: a full-time occupation or more of a way of life?, Eur J Clin Nutr 46(suppl 1):S41-S46, 1992.

Campbell PW et al: Association of poor clinical status and heavy exposure to tobacco smoke in patients with cystic fibrosis who are homozygous for the delta F 508 deletion, J Pediatr 120(2):261-264, 1992.

Colin AA and Wohl MEB: Cystic fibrosis, Pediatr Rev 15(5):192-200, 1994.

Coyne IT: Chronic illness: the importance of support for families caring for a child with cystic fibrosis, J Clin Nurs 6(2):121-129, 1997.

Cutting GR: Genotype defect: its effect on cellular function and phenotypic expression, Semin Respir Crit Care Med 15(5):356-363, 1994.

Cystic Fibrosis Foundation: National Patient Registry data, Bethesda, Md., 1997, The Foundation.

Cystic Fibrosis Foundation: Clinical Practice Guidelines, Bethesda, Md., 1997, The Foundation.

Dalzell AM et al: Nutritional rehabilitation in cystic fibrosis: a 5-year follow-up study, J Pediatr Gastroenterol Nutr 15(2):141-145, 1992.

Davidson AGF and McIlwaine M: Airway clearance techniques in cystic fibrosis, New Insights into Cystic Fibrosis 3(1):6-11, 1995.

Davis PB: Advances in treatment of cystic fibrosis, plenary session presented at the 8th Annual North American Cystic Fibrosis Conference, Pediatr Pulmonol (suppl 10):69-70, 1994.

deJong W et al: Effect of a home exercise training program in patients with cystic fibrosis, Chest 105(2):463-468, 1994.

Denton M and Wilcox MH: Antimicrobial treatment of pulmonary colonization and infection by Pseudomonas aeruginosa in cystic fibrosis patients, J Antimicrob Chemother 40:468-474, 1997.

Erdman SH: Nutritional imperatives in cystic fibrosis therapy, Pediatr Ann 28(2):129-136, 1999.

Fernbach SD and Thomson EJ: Molecular genetic technology in cystic fibrosis: implications for nursing practice, J Pediatr Nurs 7(1):20-25, 1992.

FitzSimmons SC: The changing epidemiology of cystic fibrosis, J Pediatr 122:1-9, 1993.

Fitzsimmons SC, Burkhart GA, and Borowitz D: High-dose pancreatic enzyme supplements and fibrosing colonopathy in children with cystic fibrosis, N Engl J Med 336:1283-1289, 1997.

Gudas LJ, Koocher GP, and Wypij D: Perceptions of medical compliance in children and adolescents with cystic fibrosis, J Dev Behav Pediatr 12:236-242, 1991.

Hamosh A et al: Comparison of the clinical manifestations of cystic fibrosis in African Americans and Caucasians, J Pediatr 132:255-259, 1998.

Hilman BC, Aitken ML, and Constantinescu M: Pregnancy in patients with cystic fibrosis, Clin Obstet Gynecol 39(1):70-86, 1996.

Hodson ME: Aerosolized dornase alfa (rhDNase) for therapy of cystic fibrosis, Am J Respir Crit Care Med 151:S70-S74, 1995.

Hubbard RC et al: A preliminary study of aerosolized recombinant human deoxyribonuclease I in the treatment of cystic fibrosis, New Engl J Med 326(12):812-815, 1992.

Ievers CE and Drotar D: Family and parental functioning in cystic fibrosis, J Dev Behav Pediatr 17(1):48-55, 1996.

Jelalian E et al: Nutrition intervention for weight gain in cystic fibrosis: a metaanalysis, J Pediatr 132(3):486-492, 1998.

Johannesson M, Gottlieb C, and Hjelte L: Delayed puberty in girls with cystic fibrosis despite good clinical status, Pediatrics 99(1):20-34, 1997.

Kilby JM et al: Nontuberculous mycobacteria in adult patients with cystic fibrosis, Chest 201(1):70-75, 1992.

Kirchner KK et al: Increased DNA levels in bronchoalveolar lavage fluid obtained from infants with cystic fibrosis, Pediatr Pulmonol (suppl 9):288, 1993.

Knowles MR et al: Pharmacologic modulation of salt and water in the airway epithelium in cystic fibrosis, Am J Respir Crit Care Med 151:S65-S69, 1995.

Konstan MW: Therapies aimed at airway inflammation in cystic fibrosis, Clin Chest Med 19(3):505-513, 1998.

Konstan MW et al: Bronchoalveolar lavage findings in cystic fibrosis patients with stable, clinically mild lung disease suggest ongoing infection and inflammation, Am J Respir Crit Care Med 150:448-454, 1994.

Konstan MW et al: Effect of high dose ibuprofen in patients with cystic fibrosis, New Engl J Med 332(13):848-854, 1995.

Kotloff RM: Reproductive issues in patients with cystic fibrosis, Sem Respir Crit Care Med 15(5):402-413, 1994.

Levine A et al: QT interval in children and infants receiving cisapride, Pediatrics 101(3):464, 1998.

Levy LD et al: Effects of long-term nutritional rehabilitation on body composition and clinical status in malnourished children and adolescents with cystic fibrosis, J Pediatr 107:225-230, 1985

Littlewood JM: Gastrointestinal complication, Br Med Bull 48:847-859, 1992.

Loutzenhiser JK and Clark R: Physical activity and exercise in children with cystic fibrosis. J Pediatr Nurs 8:112-119, 1993.

MacDonald A: Nutritional management of cystic fibrosis, Arch Dis Child 74(1):81-87, 1996.

MacDonald N, Morris R, and Beaudrey P: Varicella in children with cystic fibrosis, Pediatr Infect Dis J 6:414-416, 1987.

MacLusky I: Cystic fibrosis for the primary care pediatrician, Pediatr Ann 22(9):541-549, 1993.

Marshall BC and Samuelson WM: Basic therapies in cystic fibrosis: does standard therapy work?, Clin Chest Med 19(3):487-504, 1998.

Miller SR and Schwartz RH: Attitudes toward genetic testing of Amish, Mennonite, and Hutterite families with cystic fibrosis, Am J Public Health 82(2):236-242, 1992.

Moss R et al: Safety and pharmacokinetics of a mucoid Pseudomonas aeruginosa immune globulin, intravenous (human) in patients with cystic fibrosis. Preliminary results of a phase I/II trial, Abstract presented at the 8th Annual North American Cystic Fibrosis Conference, Orlando, Fla., October 1994.

National Committee for Clinical Laboratory Standards: Sweat testing: sample collection and quantitative analysis, proposed guideline, NCCLS document C34-P, Villanova, Pa., 1993, The Committee.

National Institutes of Health Workshop on Population Screening for the CF Gene: New Engl J Med 323:70-71, 1990.

Nutrition assessment and management in cystic fibrosis: a consensus report, Am J Clin Nutr 55:108-116, 1992.

Orenstein SR and Orenstein DM: Gastroesophageal reflux and respiratory disease in children, J Pediatr 112:847-858, 1988.

Parcel GS et al: Self management of cystic fibrosis: a structural model for education and behavioral variables, Soc Sci Med 38(9):1307-1315, 1994.

Pattishall EN: Longitudinal response of pulmonary function to bronchodilators in cystic fibrosis, Pediatr Pulmonol 9:80-85, 1990.

Pencharz PP and Durie PR: Nutrition management of cystic fibrosis, Ann Rev Nutr 13:111-136, 1993.

Prober CG: The impact of respiratory viral infections in patients with cystic fibrosis, Clin Rev Allergy Immunol 9(1):87-102, 1991.

Quinton PM: Cystic fibrosis: a disease of electrolyte transport, FASEB J 4:2709-2717, 1990.

Quittner AL et al: The impact of caregiving and role strain on family life: comparisons between mothers of children with cystic fibrosis and matched controls, Rehab Psychol 37:275-290, 1992.

Ramsey B, Fartell P, and Pencharz P: Nutritional assessment and management in cystic fibrosis: consensus conference, Am J Clin Nutr 55:108-116, 1992.

Ramsey BW: A summary of the results of the phase III multicenter clinical trial: aerosol administration of recombinant human DNase reduces the risk of respiratory tract infection and improves pulmonary function in patients with cystic fibrosis, Pediatr Pulmonol (suppl 9):152-153, 1993.

Ramsey BW: Management of pulmonary disease in patients with cystic fibrosis, New Engl J Med 335(3):179-188, 1996.

Rock MJ: Controversies in newborn screening: the Wisconsin experience, New Insights into Cystic Fibrosis 5(2):1-6, 1997.

Rommens JM et al: Identification of the cystic fibrosis gene: chromosome walking and jumping, Science 245:1059-1065, 1989.

Rosenfeld M and Ramsey B: Evolution of airway microbiology in the infant with cystic fibrosis: role of nonpseudomonal and pseudomonal pathogens, Sem Respir Infect 7:158-167, 1992.

Rosenstein BJ: Cystic fibrosis. In Oski FA, editor: Principles and practice of pediatrics, Philadelphia, 1990, J. B. Lippincott.

Rosenstein BJ and Cutting GR: The diagnosis of cystic fibrosis: a consensus statement, J Pediatrics 132:589-595, 1998.

Rosenstein BJ et al: The diagnosis of cystic fibrosis: a consensus statement, J Pediatr 132:589-595, 1998.

Rosenstein BJ and Eigen H: Risks of alternate-day prednisone in patients with cystic fibrosis, Pediatrics 87:245-246, 1991.

Rosenstein BJ and Langbaum TS: Diagnosis. In Taussig LM, editor: Cystic fibrosis, New York, 1984, Theime Stratton, Inc.

Schidlow DV et al: Cystic Fibrosis Foundation consensus conference report on pulmonary complications of cystic fibrosis, Pediatr Pulmonol 15(3):187-198, 1993.

Schidlow DV, Taussig LM, and Knowles MR: Cystic fibrosis foundation consensus conference report on pulmonary complications of cystic fibrosis, Pediatr Pulmonol 15(3):187-198, 1993.

Schwartz RH: Cystic fibrosis. In Hoekelman RH, editor: Primary pediatric care, ed 3, St Louis, 1997, Mosby.

Shak S: Aerosolized recombinant human DNAse I for the treatment of cystic fibrosis, Chest 107(2):65S-70S, 1995.

Shapiro SK and Seilheimer DK: Screening for cystic fibrosis: clinical issues and genetic counseling implications, New Insights into Cystic Fibrosis 2(1):6-11, 1994.

Soutter VA et al: Chronic undernutrition/growth retardation in cystic fibrosis, Clin Gastroenterol 15(1):137-155, 1986.

Stark LF et al: Descriptive analysis of eating behavior in school-age children with cystic fibrosis and health control children, Pediatrics 99(5):665-671, 1997.

Steinkamp G and von der Hardt H: Improvement of nutritional status and lung function after long-term nocturnal gastrostomy feeding in cystic fibrosis, J Pediatr 124:244-249, 1994.

Stern RC: Sinus disease in CF: current concepts, New Insights into Cystic Fibrosis 6(1)1-5, 1998.

Stern RC: The diagnosis of cystic fibrosis: current concepts, New Engl J Med 336(7):487-491, 1997.

Stern RC et al: Recreational use of psychoactive drugs by patients with cystic fibrosis, J Pediatr 111:293-299, 1987.

Stern RC: The primary care physician and the patient with cystic fibrosis, J Pediatrics 114(1):31-36, 1989.

Tsui LC and Durie PR: What is a CF diagnosis?—genetic heterogeneity, New Insights into Cystic Fibrosis 5(1):1-5, 1997.

Vasconcellos CA et al: Reduction in viscosity of cystic fibrosis sputum in vitro by gelsolin, Science 263: 969-971, 1994.

Walker LS, Van Slyke DA, and Newbrough JR: Family resources and stress: a comparison of families of children with cystic fibrosis, diabetes, and mental retardation, J Pediatr Psychol 17:327-343, 1992.

Wall M: Update on the effects of passive smoking in children, J Respir Dis 8(7):31-36, 1987.

Welsh MJ and Smith AE: Cystic fibrosis, Scientific American, December 1995, pp. 52-59.

Wertz DC et al: Attitudes toward abortion among parents of children with cystic fibrosis, Am J Public Health 81:992-996, 1992.

Wilmott RW: Making the diagnosis of cystic fibrosis, J Pediatr 132:563-565, 1998.

Wilson JM: Cystic fibrosis: strategies for gene therapy, Sem Respir Crit Care Med 15(5):439-445, 1994.

Wood RE: Prognosis. In Taussig LM, editor: Cystic fibrosis, New York, 1984, Thieme-Stratton, Inc.

Yankaskas JR et al: Lung transplantation in cystic fibrosis: consensus conference statement, Chest 113(1) 217-226, 1998.

Zeitlin PL: Therapies directed at the basic defect in cystic fibrosis, Clin Chest Med 19(3):515-525, 1998.

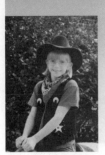

CHAPTER 19

Diabetes Mellitus (Type 1)

Elizabeth A. Boland and Margaret Grey

Etiology

Diabetes mellitus was first described in the Egyptian *Ebers Papyrus* in 1500 BC. Type 1, or insulin-dependent diabetes mellitus, most commonly occurs in young people and is characterized by beta-cell failure. In type 2, or non–insulin-dependent diabetes mellitus, individuals are often overweight and usually more than 30 years of age, overproduce insulin, and have a receptor-site defect. Therefore individuals with type 2 diabetes can often be treated orally with hypoglycemic agents, but those with type 1 diabetes must be treated with insulin.

The cause of type 1 diabetes is unknown, but many factors have been hypothesized to contribute to the cause of the disease. It is clear that type 1 diabetes is an autoimmune disease. In autoimmunity, "self" antigens are no longer recognized as such, so a self-destructive process occurs. Islet cell antibodies can be detected in a majority of individuals newly diagnosed with type 1 diabetes, and evidence of an autoimmune response may be present up to 9 years before the onset of clinical symptoms (Bingley, Bonifacio, and Gale, 1993). Genetic susceptibility is a necessary precursor to the development of type 1 diabetes. Certain histocompatibility leukocyte antigen (HLA) genes are thought to play a role in the genetic inheritance of the tendency to develop type 1 diabetes. Individuals with type 1 diabetes have an increased frequency of HLA genes B8, B15, DR3, and DR4. The HLA-DR genes are known to be associated with autoimmunity. Evidence of autoimmunity is necessary but not sufficient for the development of type 1 diabetes. It is hypothesized that without genetic susceptibility, other factors will not initiate the autoimmune process. Other factors (e.g., host and environmental factors) may influence the development of the illness because the concordance rate is only 50% in identical twins. Such factors include age, race, stress, and infectious agents (Leslie and Elliott, 1994).

Incidence

Type 1 diabetes mellitus is the most common metabolic disorder of childhood, affecting 1.7 people per every 1000 younger than 20 years of age, as well as approximately 127,000 children (American Diabetes Association [ADA], 1996). Overall, the annual incidence of type 1 diabetes in the United States is approximately 18 new cases per 100,000 people under the age of 20, with a peak incidence at about 10 to 12 years of age in girls and 12 to 14 years in boys (ADA, 1996).

Clinical Manifestations at Time of Diagnosis

Despite the fact that the autoimmune process may be longstanding before the diagnosis of diabetes is made, the signs and symptoms of type 1 diabetes are usually present for a short period of time (Box 19-1). Once the autoimmune process has destroyed enough of the pancreatic beta, or islet, cells to produce clinical evidence of illness, the classic symptoms (i.e., polydipsia, polyuria, polyphagia) of diabetes occur. As can be seen in Figure 19-1, the lack of insulin production leads to disturbances in metabolism of carbohydrate, protein, and fat.

The hormone insulin, produced by the pancreatic beta cells (i.e., islets of Langerhans), is responsible for the use of glucose in the cell. In the absence of insulin, there are three general alterations, as follow: (1) reduced entry of glucose into the cell; (2) unavailability of carbohydrate as a substrate for energy needs; and (3) the cell's use of alternate substrates (i.e., fatty acids derived from adipose stores and amino acids from body protein). Thus when there is lack of insulin, glucose cannot be used in the cell for energy, and hyperglycemia results. The extraordinary concentration of glucose in the blood promotes an osmotic diuresis, so that large amounts of urine are produced. This osmotic diuresis is responsible for the symptom of polyuria, and as the body struggles to maintain homeostasis, polydipsia ensues.

If glucose is not available as a source of energy, alternative sources must be used. The body relies upon lipolysis, as well as proteolysis. When this occurs, polyphagia becomes prominent as the body tries to avoid starvation. If these symptoms go uncorrected, the hyperglycemia and ketonemia secondary to increased lipolysis will progress to severe levels, and diabetic ketoacidosis will occur.

The diagnosis of diabetes is easily established. Any children with the classic symptoms should have their levels of blood and urinary glucose and urine ketone levels determined. If the blood glucose level is more than 200 mg/dl and symptoms of diabetes are present, the diagnosis is established. Alternatively, if fasting blood glucose (i.e., no calories in 8 hours prior to the test) is greater than or equal to 126 mg/dl or the 2-hour plasma glucose level is greater than or equal to 200 mg/dl on a glucose tolerance test, then the diagnosis is established (ADA, 1999).

Treatment

Management of type 1 diabetes has changed dramatically since the release of the Diabetes Control and Complications Trial (DCCT) results in 1993. Before these results were published, a convincing benefit of intensive therapy had not been demonstrated, despite suggestions from animal and epidemiologic studies (DCCT Research Group, 1986). The DCCT was a multicenter, randomized clinical trial designed to compare intensive diabetes therapy with conventional therapy to determine its effects on the development and progression of early vascular and neurologic complications of type 1 diabetes (DCCT Research Group, 1993b). A total of 1441 people aged 13 to 39 years with type 1 diabetes—726 of whom had no retinopathy at baseline and 715 of whom had mild retinopathy—were randomly assigned to intensive or conventional therapy.

Intensive therapy comprised three or more injections per day of insulin with frequent blood glucose monitoring; conventional therapy comprised one or two insulin injections per day. The goals of intensive therapy were to reduce glucose to the normal range and keep glycosylated hemoglobin in the normal range. Subjects in the intensive therapy group had monthly visits and were often followed via telephone (Santiago, 1993). After 6.5 years, the study was terminated because the results were so impressive; in the group without retinopathy, the risk for developing it decreased 76% with intensive therapy, and in the secondary prevention group, the progression of retinopathy was slowed by 54%. Further, microalbuminuria was reduced by 39%, albuminuria by 54%, and clinical neuropathy by 60%. Intensive therapy, however, was associated with a two- to threefold increase in severe hypoglycemia and clinically significant weight gain. There were no differences between the mean total scores on a quality of life measure of the individuals in the intensive treatment group and those of the individuals in the conventional group. Based on these findings, the researchers and the ADA recommended that for individuals with type 1 diabetes, "a primary treatment goal should be blood glucose control at least equal to that achieved in the intensively treated cohort" (ADA, 1993).

Among the 1441 clients in the DCCT were 195 adolescents (i.e., 13 to 17 years of age at entry), 125 with no retinopathy and 70 with mild retinopa-

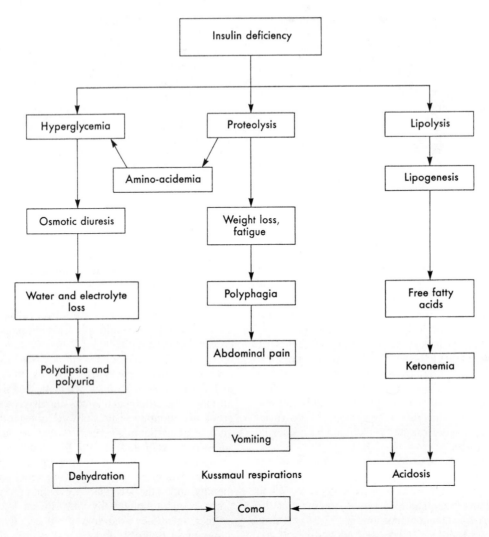

Figure 19-1 Signs and symptoms of type 1 diabetes mellitus.

thy. Because adolescents face unique issues compared with adult subjects with regard to diabetes, data on these subjects were analyzed separately (DCCT Research Group, 1994). In contrast with the larger study group, the adolescents took longer to attain near-normal glycosylated hemoglobin (i.e., 6 to 12 months vs. 6 months at nadir). Nevertheless, similar positive results of intensive treatment were also found within this group: the risk of retinopathy, retinopathy progression, microalbuminuria, and clinical neuropathy decreased by 53% to 70%. In terms of quality of life, none of the sub-

jects voluntarily withdrew from the study, and adolescents in the intensively treated group did not differ from the conventional treatment group on a measure of quality of life. Thus the DCCT Research Group (1994) recommends that most teens with diabetes be treated with intensive therapy because the potential for reduction of long-term complications was substantial. The research group also noted that the adolescents in the DCCT were the most difficult to manage and required the most time of the treatment team, but that the potential savings in suffering and long-term costs to young people

Box 19-2

Treatment

- Insulin to achieve near-normal blood glucose
- Diet sufficient for growth
- Monitoring of blood sugars at least 4 times daily
- Glycosylated hemoglobin to assess overall control

Table 19-1
Types and Actions of Insulin Preparations

Class/name	Approximate Action Curves (hr)		
	Onset	Peak	Duration
Quick Acting			
Insulin lispro	0.25	1	2 to 4
Rapid Acting			
Regular	0.5 to 1	2 to 4	4 to 6
Intermediate Acting			
NPH	1.5 to 2	6 to 12	18 to 24
Lente	1.5 to 2	6 to 12	16 to 24
Long Acting			
Ultralente	4 to 8	10 to 20	16 to 24

with type 1 diabetes are worth the investment of treatment resources.

Since the release of the results of the DCCT, many diabetes providers recommend intensive therapy regimens to achieve the goals of treatment (i.e., to return the blood glucose levels to near normal and to prevent complications for most young people with diabetes) (Box 19-2) (ADA, 1999; Tamborlane, et al, 1994). The ADA (1998) guidelines recommend the blood glucose level be normalized using intensive treatment regimens as the goal of treatment for children and adolescents. Intensive therapy involves three or more insulin injections per day or insulin delivered by continuous subcutaneous insulin infusion (CSII). Although many providers are reluctant to use pumps in adolescents, a recent report suggests that adolescents on pumps have improved metabolic control and less hypoglycemia than those taking multiple injections (Oesterle et al, 1998). Insulin doses are often adjusted according to frequent blood glucose monitoring (i.e., at least four times per day, and once per week at 3 AM), strict dietary intake, and anticipated exercise. Treatment goals may be more relaxed in children under 7 years of age because of the risk of severe hypoglycemia. The concern with severe hypoglycemia in young children is the effect of lowered blood sugar on brain development and functioning. These regimens require frequent and careful monitoring by the diabetes team (i.e., physician, nurse, dietitian, behaviorist), and are difficult to accomplish in a primary care setting (Drash, 1993).

There are multiple approaches to providing insulin to children and adolescents with type 1 diabetes. The appropriate regimen should be determined by the child and the family. The available types of insulin shown in Table 19-1 can be combined to create a regimen that fits the child's lifestyle and the provider's and family's goals.

Most children use genetically engineered human insulin preparations.

Insulin replacement results in a dramatic reversal of the disease symptoms. At diagnosis, most children are hospitalized—in part for correction of the metabolic derangement but also for education in the management of the condition. Once any acidosis is corrected, subcutaneous treatment with insulin is the mainstay of therapy. Most children are adequately controlled on an initial regimen of two injections of insulin per day: one before breakfast, and one before the evening meal. These injections usually consist of rapid-acting and intermediate-acting insulin. Based on the blood glucose response, the dose is titrated to achieve blood glucose levels as close to normal as possible.

Shortly after the diagnosis is made, many children experience a sharp reduction in the insulin requirement. In some cases, no insulin is necessary for a period of time, which may last up to 6 months, but some health care providers continue a small dose to maintain the injection schedule. The insulin requirement eventually returns, and children should be cautioned that this "honeymoon period" does not indicate that the diabetes has gone away. Once destruction of the beta cells is complete—usually within 2 years of diagnosis—most children will require insulin replacement of approximately 1 unit/kg of body weight/day, although 2 or more units/per kg of body weight may be necessary.

Once the honeymoon is over, it is difficult to achieve optimal metabolic control without using intensive insulin regimens. Intensive regimens consist of three or more daily injections or the use of an insulin pump. Multiple daily injection (MDI) regimens usually consist of rapid or quick-acting insulins before meals with NPH or Ultralente insulin twice per day. Such regimens more closely mimic the body's normal response to a carbohydrate meal. Insulin pumps (Figure 19-2) even more closely mimic the normal moment-to-moment response and are increasingly being used with young people on intensive regimens.

Because replacement of insulin is not perfect, regulation of both diet and exercise help to minimize variation in blood glucose levels. Children with diabetes—unlike individuals with type 2 diabetes—are often slender. Therefore the goal of dietary therapy is to provide sufficient calories for normal growth and development. A meal plan based on an individual's usual intake pattern is used to integrate insulin therapy into typical eating and exercise patterns. Such a meal plan helps avoid hyperglycemia, prevent hypoglycemia, and maintain metabolic balance. Consistent with the current recommendations of the American Academy of Pediatrics, American and Canadian Diabetes Associations, and the American Dietetic Association, a meal plan should comprise 55% to 60% carbohydrate, 10% to 20% protein, and 10% to 20% fats, with less than 10% saturated fats (ADA, 1998). As discussed in the section below on diet, carbohydrate counting is an approach that allows for more flexibility in dietary management.

Daily caloric requirements can be estimated to be 1000 calories for the first year of life with approximately 100 calories added each year until age 10 to 12 years. Thereafter, unless they are exceptionally active on a regular basis, females may need their total calories reduced to the common adult level of 1400 to 1600 calories daily. Males, however, will continue to need approximately 2000 calories daily. Shortly after diagnosis, children may need an additional 200 to 700 kcal per day to make up the negative energy balance at diagnosis.

Maintenance of near-normal or normal blood glucose levels requires constant self-monitoring. Self-monitored blood glucose (SMBG) levels allow people with diabetes to have more precision in monitoring than with urine testing. Glucose is not found in the urine until the blood glucose level rises above the renal threshold (i.e., usually about 180 mg/dl). The goal of therapy is to maintain blood glucose levels from 80 to 120 mg/dl before meals and 100 to 140 mg/dl at bedtime (ADA, 1998). Therefore self-monitoring of blood glucose levels lets children know exactly what the blood glucose level is at any moment and adjust the dose of insulin in response to their actual blood glucose level.

Most children are advised to test their blood at least four times daily, at various times throughout the day, and when symptoms are present. The results of SMBG testing are used to identify asymptomatic hypoglycemia, determine patterns in insulin action, and appropriately alter the insulin dose. For example, if a child consistently has high blood glucose levels before lunch, the morning intermediate-acting insulin (i.e., NPH or Lente) is increased to prevent this effect.

Children and adolescents with diabetes are evaluated every 3 months by the diabetes treatment team. Quarterly visits correspond to the rate at which the glycosylated hemoglobin levels can be expected to change. Glycosylated hemoglobin, or Hemoglobin A1c, is a measure of the attachment of glucose to the circulating hemoglobin molecule. In individuals without diabetes, glycosylated hemoglobin comprises 3% to 6% of the total hemoglobin; those with diabetes, however, have levels in excess of 6% that vary in proportion to the blood glucose levels. The glycosylated hemoglobin level reflects the average blood glucose level over the most recent 3 months because the lifespan of the hemoglobin molecule is approximately 120 days. This level is not affected by short-term fluctuations and is considered to be an objective and accurate

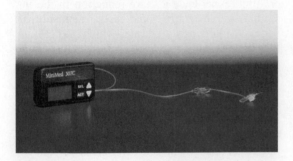

Figure 19-2 Example of an insulin pump used for continuous subcutaneous insulin infusion. (Courtesy MiniMed, Sylmar, Calif.)

measure of long-term diabetes control (ADA, 1998; Goldstein et al, 1995).

Recent and Anticipated Advances in Diagnosis and Management

The Diabetes Prevention Trial-Type 1 (DPT-1) is currently being conducted in the United States. All consenting first-degree relatives of people with type 1 diabetes are being screened to see if they are at risk for developing the disease in the next 5 years. Any relatives who test positively will be asked to have more specific testing, including glucose tolerance testing and HLA typing. If these tests show a relative to be at significant risk, the relative will be asked to participate in a randomized clinical trial to determine if small doses of insulin will prevent onset of the disease. The trial is based on animal and human studies with small samples that suggest that small doses of insulin may protect the pancreatic beta cells from the destruction associated with type 1 diabetes by preventing the autoimmune process from proceeding (Keller, Eisenbarth, and Jackson, 1993).

In addition, researchers are developing artificial insulin delivery systems and transplantation of beta cells (Lacy, 1994) as new methods of treatment. The artificial insulin delivery systems will improve on the CSII by incorporating a feedback loop that will alter the insulin delivered according to the blood glucose level. Transplantation of beta cells or the whole pancreas results in a cure for people with diabetes who are already on immunosuppression for previous organ transplants (Sutherland and Gruessner, 1997). The remaining challenge is to prevent autoimmune destruction of these cells in individuals who are not immunosuppressed. Techniques have been developed to encapsulate the islets, and studies are underway to determine if these techniques will be effective early in the course of the disease.

New insulin delivery systems are also being tested. Data from a recent trial of inhaled insulin were presented at the ADA meeting in 1998 and suggested that adults can achieve control similar to conventional therapy with a regimen of inhaled insulin with meals and long-acting insulin at night (Skyler et al, 1998). Studies are underway to determine the effects of these new insulin delivery systems in adolescents. Implantable insulin pumps that deliver insulin intraperitoneally have also been used in adults, but not yet in children (Dunn et al, 1997).

Research advances are also being made in home blood glucose monitoring. With future technology, blood glucose levels will be able to be measured on an almost continuous basis. Near-infrared and indwelling continuous monitoring devices may either decrease or eliminate the pain and inconvenience of home blood glucose monitoring (Mastrototaro et al, 1998). This increased monitoring is likely to improve metabolic control and decrease the risk of hypoglycemic episodes.

Associated Problems

Diabetic Ketoacidosis and Hypoglycemia

Figure 19-1 shows the physiologic process that results in diabetic ketoacidosis (DKA) when there is a lack of insulin. Any potential stressor (e.g., illness, fever, injury, and psychosocial stress) can increase the risk of metabolic derangement caused by disturbances in counterregulatory hormones and lead to DKA. Thus any stressor in a child with diabetes must be managed with care (Box 19-3).

Children with well-controlled diabetes will occasionally experience episodes of hypoglycemia. Because the symptoms of DKA and hypoglycemia can sometimes be confused, they are compared in Box 19-4. Hypoglycemia may be caused by too much insulin, too little food, too much exercise, or a combination of these. Although hypoglycemia is easily treated, prevention is the best approach.

Box 19-3

Associated Problems

- Diabetic ketoacidosis
- Hypoglycemia
- Monilial vaginitis
- Complications associated with:
  Cardiovascular disease
  Renal failure
  Eye degeneration
  Neuropathies

Again, SMBG determination is helpful. With SMBG testing, children can identify patterns of lower blood glucose levels that may indicate periods of increased risk. During these periods, the insulin dose can be altered to prevent the hypoglycemia. If a child anticipates unusual physical activity, both insulin and diet can be adjusted to prevent low glucose levels.

Hypoglycemia presents particular problems at different ages. Infants are unable to express the feelings associated with hypoglycemia, so they must be observed for listlessness, sleepiness, or irritability. Parents should be instructed that unusual behavior at any time is an indication for blood glucose levels to be measured. If the result is less than 60 mg/dl, a conscious infant should be given 2 to 4 oz of sweet liquids or a small amount of cake frosting and an unconscious or convulsing infant should be given ¼ to ½ cc of glucagon by injection. Older children can be taught the symptoms of hypoglycemia and how to prevent its occurrence. They should also be instructed to carry high-sugar foods with them at all times. All children with type 1 diabetes should wear medical identification so that they can be diagnosed and treated appropriately if they lose consciousness while away from home. In the DCCT, intensive regimens were associated with a threefold increase in the incidence of severe hypoglycemia (DCCT Research Group, 1995), so extra care must be taken by children on intensive regimens.

Some substances can increase the likelihood of hypoglycemia. Adolescents need to know that alcohol augments the glucose-lowering effects of insulin and that the symptoms of alcohol intoxication and hypoglycemia are similar. Low blood glucose levels can increase the body's sensitivity to alcohol, and many experimenting teenagers have found themselves in the emergency room with profound hypoglycemia. Stimulants such as amphetamines and cocaine may increase metabolism and decrease appetite, so hypoglycemia may occur.

Candidial Infections

Once healthy girls are toilet trained, monilial infections of the perineum are rare until adolescence, when the estrogenation of the vagina provides a potential environment for growth of *Candida* spp. Hyperglycemia also leads to increased glucose levels in vaginal secretions, which provides an ideal medium for *Candida* spp. Thus girls with poorly controlled diabetes are at increased risk for monilial vaginitis; any complaint of vaginal discharge and itching should be investigated with a potassium hydroxide preparation and treated appropriately.

Prognosis

Diabetes is the sixth leading cause of death in the United States (National Center for Health Statistics, 1996). Children with diabetes at the age of 10 can be expected to live until the age of 54 years, but their peers without diabetes can be expected to live

---

Box 19-4
Comparison of Diabetic Ketoacidosis and Hypoglycemia

Diabetic ketoacidosis (hyperglycemia)	Hypoglycemia
• Slow onset	• Rapid onset
• Increased thirst and urination	• Excessive sweating
• High blood and urine glucose levels	• Fainting
• Urinary ketones	• Headache
• Weakness and abdominal pain	• Trembling and shaking
• Heavy, labored breathing	• Hunger
• Anorexia	• Unable to wake
• Nausea and vomiting	• Irritability
• Candidial infections	• Personality change

to the age of 72 years (ADA, 1996). For the most part, this early mortality is a result of the long-term complications of the illness.

Complications can range from asymptomatic mild proteinuria to blindness, renal failure, painful neuropathies, cardiovascular disease, and death. Hyperglycemia is a necessary—but not sufficient—factor for the development of complications. In addition to hyperglycemia, genetic factors seem to influence the development of complications. Epidemiologic evidence suggests that the prevalence of microvascular complications is relatively high in the general diabetic population, with approximately 40% of affected individuals experiencing renal failure and 50% having diabetic retinopathy after 15 years (ADA, 1996). Although the DCCT showed that improvement in metabolic control to near normal levels delays the onset or progression of complications, complications were not eliminated. It is clear, however, that the better the metabolic control, the better the chance of avoiding complications.

PRIMARY CARE MANAGEMENT

Health Care Maintenance

Growth and Development

Because type 1 diabetes is a metabolic disorder affecting carbohydrate metabolism, growth and sexual development may be slowed. Children and adolescents whose diabetes is less well-controlled may fail to grow normally. Therefore accurate measurement of height and weight and comparison with growth norms are imperative.

Even when children have normal linear growth, there may be delays in the onset and progression of puberty if glycemic control is inadequate. At each visit, Tanner stages should be assessed and recorded. Any deviation from the normal pattern should be investigated. In girls, menarche may be delayed. Loss of regular menses once cycling has been established may indicate a further degeneration in diabetic control and should be investigated.

Obesity can occur in children and adolescents with type 1 diabetes, especially in those on intensive regimens. In the DCCT, intensive therapy was associated with a 73% higher risk of becoming overweight (DCCT Research Group, 1995).

Management of this obesity should be done carefully, with attention to the need to maintain self-monitoring, because glucose levels may change dramatically when a weight loss diet is followed.

Adolescents who manipulate weight by overeating or reducing or omitting insulin are another concern. Some adolescent girls with type 1 diabetes engage in insulin withholding to maintain body shape or lose weight (Pollack et al, 1995). Researchers have studied the incidence of eating disorders in adolescents with type 1 diabetes with conflicting results. Some have found that adolescents with diabetes are at higher risk for eating disorders than those without diabetes (Polonsky et al, 1994), but others have not found differences between the two groups of adolescents (Striegel-Moore, Nicholson, and Tamborlane, 1992). Nevertheless, alterations in insulin dosage may affect an adolescent's ability to grow and develop normally and should be considered in evaluation of children with growth difficulties.

Diet

Although insulin therapy is the cornerstone of treatment, a dietary plan is important in maintaining near-normoglycemia without wide swings in blood glucose levels. Long-term adherence to the dietary plan is probably the most difficult aspect of management for families.

Many meal plans are based on the exchange system. Current exchange lists can be obtained from the ADA (see the list of resources at the end of this chapter), but the basic components are listed in Table 19-2. There are six food groups, including a "free" group. Within the groups, the nutritional composition of a serving of different foods is relatively constant. For example, in the starch category, one exchange is one slice of bread, one-half cup of white rice, or one medium, baked potato. This system helps families learn portion sizes and healthy childhood nutrition.

All dietary management plans have the goal of providing adequate calories and nutrients for normal growth and maintaining blood glucose as normal as possible. The consistency of daily intake with regular meals and snacks is important. Families, in consultation with the diabetes team, should select the appropriate meal plan because they are in the best position to judge the approach that will work. Imposing a rigid approach on an unwilling

Table 19-2
Dietary Exchange System

| Food Exchange | Calories | Approximate Content gm/Serving | | |
		Carbohydrate	Protein	Fat
Fruit	60	12	0	0
Starch	68	15	2	0
Milk				
Whole	170	12	8	10
Skim	90	12	8	Trace
Meat				
Lean	55	0	7	3
Medium fat	75	0	7	5
High fat	95	0	7	8
Fat	45	0	0	5
Free	0	negligible	0	0

family only leads them to not adhere to the diet. In addition, most children will not adhere without question to a diet perceived as different from that of peers. Thus primary care providers must be understanding in their approach and work with families to ensure as much dietary consistency as possible.

The two approaches to dietary management most commonly used with children are the ADA Exchange Lists (see Table 19-2) and carbohydrate counting. With the ADA Exchange Lists, the goal is for children to have adequate calories for growth that are distributed appropriately over the day and through the food groups. This dietary plan should be developed with the child and parents so that usual routines and favorite foods can be incorporated.

Carbohydrate counting is used most frequently by those on intensive regimens (DCCT Research Group, 1993a). This method provides more flexibility in the diet by providing for varying amounts of carbohydrates at meals and snacks with appropriate coverage with rapid-acting insulin. Protein and fat intake are not controlled, but efforts to stay within low-fat guidelines are encouraged. For example, adolescents who choose to eat a second sandwich at lunch (i.e., 30 g extra carbohydrate in the bread) may need to take 5 to 10 units of rapid-acting insulin before the meal, depending on their regimen.

The wide availability of artificially sweetened foods and drinks has eased some of the difficulties children with diabetes faced in following the meal plan. Parents sometimes express concern, however, that extensive use of artificial sweeteners will be problematic for their children. There are three non-nutritive sweeteners approved for use by the FDA in the United States: saccharine, aspartame, and acesulfame K. For these and all other additives, the FDA determines an acceptable daily intake (ADI) (i.e., the amount that can be safely consumed on a daily basis over a person's lifetime without any adverse effects), which includes a 100-fold safety factor. Average intake is actually much less than the acceptable daily intake. For example, the average aspartame consumption in the general population (i.e., including children) is 2 to 3 mg/kg/day or approximately 4% of the US ADI of 50 mg/kg (ADA, 1998).

Safety

The safety issues faced by families with a child or adolescent with diabetes are twofold. As discussed earlier, hypoglycemia is a significant risk for all affected children, so families and others in a child's social sphere should be prepared to respond appropriately. Older children need to know how to prevent severe hypoglycemia, especially when exercising. Children should be taught to eat a snack of complex carbohydrate and protein before exercise, not to inject insulin into an exercising muscle, and to carry glucose with them at all times. When traveling or on school day trips, children or their parents should carry the supplies with them—not in checked baggage—and always have food available in case a meal is delayed. Some airlines require a letter from a health care provider explaining the need for syringes to be carried on board an airplane.

Parents or caretakers must learn to treat episodes of severe hypoglycemia with glucagon. Glucagon is the antagonist hormone to insulin and releases glycogen from the liver. When a child or adolescent cannot take sugar by mouth, glucagon is administered by intramuscular injection to rapidly raise the blood glucose. The dose for infants or toddlers is 0.5 mg (0.5 cc), and the dose for older children is 1 mg (1.0 cc).

The other important safety issue is the proper disposal of syringes. Children and parents must be taught the importance of proper disposal of syringes to reduce the risk of injury to themselves and others.

Immunizations

Children and adolescents with diabetes should follow the immunization schedule—including vaccines for hepatitis A and B and varicella—recommended by the American Academy of Pediatrics. Children with diabetes are potentially at an increased risk for developing complicated influenza illness; therefore they may benefit from yearly influenza vaccination after the age of 6 months (American Academy of Pediatrics, 1998). Some providers also recommend that youths with diabetes receive the pneumococcal vaccine, but with improved metabolic control, there is less risk for infection.

Screening

Vision: Vision screening is particularly important in children with diabetes because visual problems are common. A small number of children develop cataracts early in the course of the illness; therefore observing the normalcy of the red reflex during the ophthalmic examination is very important. Fluctuations in blood glucose levels can also affect visual acuity. Children experiencing hypoglycemia may complain of visual disturbances, and those with hyperglycemia may also complain of blurred vision. Thus it is important to relate the results of routine visual screening to the level of metabolic control,

because improvement in metabolic control may improve the results of the visual testing.

Parents and children are often most concerned about the risk of diabetic retinopathy. Retinopathy of diabetes is the leading cause of blindness. Therefore the ADA (1998) recommends that funduscopic examination be performed in individuals with diabetes at each primary care visit. Furthermore, an annual examination with dilation by a pediatric ophthalmologist is recommended for children over 12 years of age who have had diabetes for at least 5 years.

Hearing: Routine screening is recommended.

Dental: Routine screening is recommended. If metabolic control is poor, children may experience increased dental caries and gingivitis due to increased glucose in saliva. Thus, those with poorer control should have frequent dental screening and appropriate treatment.

Blood pressure: Screening should be performed at each visit. Hypertension has been reported in up to 45% of all individuals with diabetes. Thus the ADA (1999) recommends that orthostatic measurements be performed and recorded routinely.

Hematocrit: Routine screening is recommended.

Urinalysis: Screening is performed yearly, with examination for levels of ketones, glucose, and protein. After 5 years of diabetes or after puberty, total urinary protein excretion should be measured yearly by the microalbuminuria method to screen for renal complications. If proteinuria is detected, serum creatinine clearance or blood urea nitrogen concentration should be measured and glomerular filtration assessed.

Tuberculosis: Routine screening is recommended.

Condition-Specific Screening

Lipids: Individuals with type 1 diabetes are at risk for disorders of lipid metabolism, and these disorders may increase the risk of macrovascular complications. Children with type 1 diabetes should be screened with blood lipid profiles yearly after puberty. If a child has other risk factors, lipid screening should begin earlier, as is true for children without diabetes.

Thyroid: Because diabetes is an autoimmune disease, it is associated with other autoimmune diseases—especially Hashimoto's thyroiditis

(Eisenbarth, 1986). Children and adolescents who show any change in growth pattern or develop signs and symptoms of hypothyroidism (e.g., fatigue, dry skin, constipation) or hyperthyroidism (e.g., heat intolerance, tremor, diarrhea) should be tested with thyroid function studies (i.e., triiodothyronine, thyroxine, and thyroid-stimulating hormone levels).

Common Illness Management

Differential Diagnosis (Box 19-5)

Management of Vomiting and Diarrhea and Prevention of Diabetic Ketoacidosis

Provided that their diabetes is under reasonable metabolic control, children and adolescents with diabetes are not at higher risk than their peers for most common infectious diseases of childhood. Because any stressor may lead to DKA in a child with diabetes, infections and other stressors must be managed with care.

Regardless of the insult, there are several important principles for management. A child's need to continue to take insulin even when unable to eat a normal diet is of utmost importance because the excess of counterregulatory hormones released in response to the stressor will more than offset the decreased oral intake. Thus even though dietary intake may be decreased, insulin requirement may be increased.

The principles of management include monitoring parameters of control, maintaining hydration, preventing hypoglycemia, and preventing DKA. For these principles to work effectively, it is imperative that the child and family know that any illness or insult involving fever, gastrointestinal symptoms, congestion in the head or chest, or urinary symptoms should be managed as a sick day. Once a day is identified as a sick day, the usual rules for self-monitoring are altered to reflect the need for closer monitoring. Blood glucose levels should be tested every 1 to 4 hours, and individuals with blood glucose levels greater than 200 mg/dl should test their urine for ketones. Blood glucose levels of more than 400 mg/dl on two determinations and moderate or high ketone levels in the urine that do not decrease with additional insulin should be viewed as an indication that the child should be seen and evaluated by either the primary care provider or the specialist.

Maintaining hydration is important to help clear extra glucose and ketones, and hydration must be carefully monitored if vomiting or diarrhea is present. If children cannot eat their usual diet, a large fluid intake should be maintained. In adolescents, this amount should be more than 8 oz of fluid hourly. Such fluids should contain adequate amounts of carbohydrate (i.e., 50 to 75 gm in 6 to 8 hr) to maintain the usual caloric intake. Children often drink regular (i.e., not diet) sodas, flavored gelatin water, or suck on ice pops when ill. If a child is vomiting or has diarrhea, broth or electrolyte solutions help replace sodium losses.

A child may need additional insulin to prevent DKA. If the blood glucose level is greater than 300 mg/dl, the family should generally administer the usual dose of insulin and add up to 20% of the total daily dose as rapid-acting insulin every 4 hours. Such management should be undertaken in careful consultation with the child's diabetes team. Recent studies have shown that treatment with insulin lispro during ketosis and hyperglycemia may result in quicker correction than with conventional rapid-acting insulin (Attia et al, 1998).

Box 19-6 lists the indications for which children or adolescents should be seen and evaluated. Most important is the need for children with any alteration in mental status to be evaluated. Primary care providers should never assume that sleepiness in children with diabetes is merely the result of the fatigue associated with an illness.

Other Conditions

Vaginal discharge: Young women with diabetes are prone to Candidial infections when glucose

---

Box 19-5

Differential Diagnosis

- Stressors, including illness, can lead to DKA.
- Illness requires "sick day" management.
- Important to maintain hydration during illness.
- Vaginal discharge may be candidial infection.
- Skin manifestations may require referral.
- Weight loss may indicate poor metabolic control.
- Gastroparesis may be the cause of prolonged vomiting.

control is inadequate. Treatment with an antifungal agent is warranted in young girls if vaginal discharge with itching exists without evidence of other sexual activity. If there has been sexual contact of any kind, the vagina should be examined, and testing for other infections (e.g., Chlamydia) should be performed.

Other skin manifestations: Children and adolescents with diabetes may develop skin lesions associated with diabetes (e.g., necrobiosis diabeticorum). If these scaly lesions develop—usually on extensor surfaces—treatment by a dermatologist is warranted.

Weight loss: The most common cause of weight loss in youth with diabetes is worsening metabolic control. Therefore evaluation of weight loss should include assessment of overall glucose control. If control is inadequate and attempts to improve control are not successful, then deliberate withholding of insulin for weight control should be investigated. Individuals with diabetes may also develop bulimic characteristics as a method of weight control, but vomiting and abdominal distress in youth with long-standing diabetes may also be a symptom of diabetic gastroparesis. Evaluation for gastroparesis includes radiographic gastric emptying studies that should be done under the direction of a specialist.

Drug Interactions

Many over-the-counter medications and antibiotics contain glucose, and some contain alcohol or traces of gluconeogenic substances, such as sorbitol or glycerine (Kumar, Weatherly, and Beaman, 1991). In the amounts usually ingested, these compounds may raise blood glucose levels slightly but should not markedly impair metabolic control. Pseudoephedrine has the potential to increase blood glucose levels because of its stimulant effect. This effect is minimal at usual doses, but all such products contain warnings that individuals with diabetes should consult their provider before taking the product, so primary care providers should be aware of the potential effect.

Developmental Issues

Sleep Patterns: Children with diabetes who are in good control should have no problems sleeping. Those who are hyperglycemic overnight, however, will have difficulty sleeping because of the recurrent need to urinate. This problem can be managed by improving metabolic control.

Nighttime hypoglycemia is a concern of parents. A child may not wake with the usual early signs and symptoms, and the first sign may be a severe event with nightmares or seizures. Therefore it is important to prevent nighttime hypoglycemia by appropriately adjusting the evening insulin dose and offering a bedtime snack with carbohydrate and protein or fat. Parents should also be instructed in the use of the counterregulatory hormone glucagon in case the child is not able to be aroused.

Nightmares are common in young children and may be caused by hypoglycemia. Parents should determine the blood glucose level before assuming the cause of a nightmare. If the cause is hypoglycemia, treatment includes administration of glucose. If the nightmares are not related to hypoglycemia, appropriate comfort measures should be instituted. Prevention is the key, however, and significant nighttime hypoglycemia is to be avoided as much as possible by careful adjustment of diet and insulin.

Toileting: Several issues related to toileting are important in the management of diabetes in children. Many children have secondary enuresis at the time of diagnosis. It is important to tell children who were previously dry that diabetes is the cause of their enuresis and that the enuresis should remit when the diabetes is adequately controlled. Enuresis can occur, however, with well-controlled

---

Box 19-6

Indications for Evaluation by a Health Care Provider

Vomiting for more than 6 hours or more than five diarrheal stools in 1 day.

Any change in mental status.

Syncope.

Temperature greater than 38.9° C for 12 hours.

Blood glucose levels more than 400 mg/dl twice.

Moderate or high ketone levels that do not decrease with extra insulin intake.

Dysuria or other symptoms of urinary tract infection.

Decreased urinary output.

diabetes. Other methods of diagnostic confirmation and treatment should be explored with these families.

Although testing urine for glucose is not as critical to management as it was before SMBG testing was available, urinary ketone levels are important indicators of status when a child is ill. Parents should know how to obtain such samples from infants and toddlers. Cotton balls tucked into a diaper can provide an adequate sample for use on a dipstick to determine ketone levels in children who are not yet toilet-trained. Urine is readily obtainable when a child uses a potty chair during toilet training. When children move onto the bathroom commode, parents needs to teach them to urinate into a paper cup so that the urine can be tested. If taught when a child is feeling well, this task can be made into a game so that, when necessary, the behavior has been learned (Lipman et al, 1989).

Discipline: Although the issues related to discipline of a child with diabetes are not different from those of all children with a chronic condition, parents of children with diabetes report that their second most common concern in raising the child is discipline (Hodges and Parker, 1987). Parents most often worry that a hypoglycemic episode will be missed by attributing the unruly behavior to lack of discipline. It is appropriate for parents to test the blood glucose level at any time hypoglycemia is suspected. Then if the result is within the normal range, the child can be appropriately disciplined. Blood testing should be performed matter-of-factly, so that children do not misinterpret the test as a punishment. Some parents also worry that the stress of imposed discipline will raise the blood glucose level because of the presence of counter-regulatory hormones. Although severe stressors may increase blood glucose levels (Aikens et al, 1992), no evidence suggests that usual disciplinary measures increase blood glucose levels or worsen diabetic control. Indeed, some authors (Betschart, 1993; Lipman et al, 1989) have suggested that parents who set reasonable limits for their children are more likely to have children in good metabolic control.

Child care: Toddlers and preschoolers with diabetes benefit from the socialization of preschool programs. They do not need specialized medical daycare. Preschool teachers should be informed of parental expectations, such as blood glucose testing and insulin administration. Snack and lunch intake

are very important, so preschool teachers must be aware of the child's need to eat and what should be served at each mealtime. They should be aware of appropriate food substitutions when food is refused. All caregivers should be told how to manage symptoms of hypoglycemia. Emergency telephone numbers should always be available and should include telephone numbers of the parents, another emergency contact, the primary care provider, and the diabetes specialists.

Parents of children with diabetes often express concerns about the abilities of baby-sitters or day-care workers to manage a young child's diabetes. Parents of young children can begin by leaving the child for only short periods of time, thus reassuring themselves that the sitter can successfully care for the child. Clear instructions on the child's diet and management of hypoglycemia should be provided in writing. Parents should be encouraged to train sitters in blood glucose monitoring and recognition of hypoglycemic symptoms. Emergency telephone numbers should always be available.

Schooling: Children whose diabetes is adequately controlled should attend school regularly and participate in any activities for which they are otherwise suited. Parents should be encouraged to inform the school nurse and the child's teachers when the diabetes is diagnosed. It is important that school personnel are knowledgeable about the child's care so that hypoglycemia or illness can be appropriately managed. The need for other involvement (e.g., SMBG testing or injections) depends on the child's usual regimen.

With older children, providers need to work with the child, family, and school personnel to arrange a school schedule that fits the child's diabetes regimen (Jornsay and Carney, 1992). For example, a child who has had regular and NPH insulin at 7:00 AM should probably have a snack before a gym class that precedes a late lunch period. Arrangements must be made so that the child can always have access to glucose-containing foods or tablets in case of a hypoglycemic episode. The child should always have food available on field trips. A sack lunch with all food groups serves nicely as a substitute if a meal is unexpectedly delayed.

Sports are also encouraged. Coaches should be aware of the diabetes and keep foods containing glucose on hand. Depending on the degree of exercise on extra-activity days, the insulin dose may be lowered or the diet increased or both in an attempt to prevent hypoglycemia. Hypoglycemia following exercise may occur up to 12 hours after the event, so children should be carefully monitored when any new activity is undertaken. Children should be advised that insulin is absorbed more rapidly from exercising muscle; therefore if a muscle is to be exercised, insulin should be injected in another site. For example, if a child will run track, the insulin could be administered in the arm or the abdomen instead of the leg.

Children whose diabetes is in poor control may experience difficulties in school performance. Because hypoglycemia can cause a child to lose the ability to concentrate when the blood glucose level is low, learning can be a problem. When the blood glucose level is consistently too high, many children experience difficulties in concentration and grades may suffer. Thus any child with diabetes whose school performance changes should be carefully assessed for alterations in metabolic control.

As with all children with chronic conditions, emphasis should be on the normality of the child—not the diabetes. Such an approach helps to minimize the sense of being different that is experienced by all affected children.

Because children and adolescents with diabetes are encouraged to participate fully in sports and other activities, they may be encouraged to go to camp as well. There are specialized camps for children with diabetes, which may help young people to learn about their diabetes and meet peers who also have diabetes. Children and adolescents with diabetes may also safely attend regular camps. Whether the camp is diabetes-specific or not, care should be taken to adjust the insulin dose and food intake to account for the markedly increased physical activity at camp. Extra blood glucose monitoring may be necessary.

Sexuality: Achievement of normal growth and development is a goal of therapy. If the diabetes is adequately controlled, sexual development should be normal. If sexual development is delayed, however, normal concerns about self- and physical adequacy may be amplified. Primary care providers need to monitor secondary sexual development carefully in children with diabetes, and any deviation from normal should be investigated. Tightening the metabolic control often improves growth. If not, the cause should be investigated.

All sexually active teenagers need information about birth control. Such information is especially important for those with diabetes because the risks for complications of pregnancy are at least 5 times greater than the already high risk for adolescents. Because of the risk for acquired immunodeficiency syndrome (AIDS), many providers are encouraging condoms over all other birth control methods. Unfortunately, as with all teenagers, proper and consistent use of condoms is variable. Other barrier methods (e.g., diaphragms, foams, and creams) may also be used by those with diabetes but share the same disadvantages as condoms and do not prevent sexually transmitted diseases.

Teenagers who are willing to use contraceptives often find using the birth control pill acceptable. Earlier versions of the combination pill (i.e., containing both estrogen and progesterone) carried risks for cerebral ischemia, myocardial infarction, and rapid progression of retinopathy and were not recommended for adolescents with diabetes. Newer low-dose estrogen combination pills, however, seem to be reasonably well-tolerated and are the oral contraceptive of choice.

Although avoidance of adolescent pregnancy is clearly preferred, some teenagers express the desire to become pregnant. It has been clearly demonstrated (Aucott et al, 1994), however, that pregnancy outcomes can be dramatically improved if euglycemia is maintained both in the months preceding conception and throughout the pregnancy. Therefore female adolescents at risk for pregnancy or contemplating pregnancy should be counseled about pregnancy outcomes and helped to achieve better metabolic control.

Male adolescents often express concern about the well-known complication of impotence in adult men. Impotence is thought to be a result of both vascular and neurologic compromise in those with long-standing diabetes. Fortunately, impotence caused by diabetes is very rare in adolescence, so most of these individuals can be reassured.

Transition to Adulthood

The challenges of making the transition into adulthood may be more complex for adolescents with type 1 diabetes because of the extraordinary demands of disease self-management on the client and the family. Wysocki and associates (1992) found that older adolescents had worse adjustment to diabetes and metabolic control than younger children, as well as that difficulties in adjustment in early adolescence tended to persist into young adulthood. Further, other studies have suggested that young adults with type 1 diabetes have more difficulty with vocational adjustment and marital relationships (Karlsson, Holmes, and Lang, 1988) than other young adults. Thus the care provided during this crucial time may be important for long-term quality of life.

Wysocki and associates (1992) also found that adolescents who were better adjusted had better metabolic control in early adulthood. This finding suggests that the care provided in early adolescence with attention to improving psychosocial adjustment is just as important as providing quality transitional care. Little empirical work on the provision of care in the transition from adolescence to adulthood has been accomplished, but Court (1993) surveyed adolescents on their views about the transfer process from pediatric to adult care. Court found that adolescents value continuity of care by a provider they trust, as well as expect confidentiality and privacy, informality, and waiting rooms tailored to their needs. In addition, young adults and late adolescents may be less capable of insulin self-regulation than providers assume (Pless et al, 1988). Therefore transition to adult care must be designed to respect the wishes of these young people and to support their assumption of self-care and development in their vocational and social roles.

Another concern of young adults is the increasing risk of complications. A recent study (Dunning, 1995) found that concerns about complications were common among young adults with type 1 diabetes and included concerns about eye disease, pregnancy and childbirth, hypoglycemia, and loss of independence. It is clear that these young people need help implementing intensive insulin regimens and self-care management styles that will help to delay complications.

Compliance is a behavioral coping strategy (Grey and Thurber, 1991) that is an issue in many chronic conditions and therefore is not discussed in depth here. Any child or adolescent with repeated problems in management (e.g., poor control with or without repeated hospitalization), however, should be carefully questioned about adherence to the diabetes treatment regimen.

Special Family Concerns and Resources

Families worry about the appropriate assumption of self-care because of its importance in preventing long-term complications. Recommendations for understanding the levels at which children should assume various self-care activities are available (Daneman, 1991). There is, however, broad disagreement among professionals as to the appropriate age for management of skills (Wysocki et al, 1990), and some authors (Ingersoll et al, 1986) have suggested that a too-early assumption of self-management is associated with poorer psychologic and metabolic outcomes. Therefore decisions about the assumption of self-care activities should be made with the family, child, and providers working together. Adolescents whose families maintain more involvement with their child's diabetes care have better metabolic control than those who are less involved (Grey et al, 1998). Until more data on the effect of assuming self-care at different ages are available, providers' strict regulation of such activities may be unwarranted.

In studies of parental concerns (Hauenstein et al, 1989; Hodges and Parker, 1987), several issues are prominent. First is the adherence to the diabetes regimen—especially diet and the assumption of self-care. Second is the question of genetics and inheritance. In addition, psychosomatic issues may be of particular importance to families dealing with diabetes because poorly functioning families have been shown to be associated with poorer diabetic control (Kovacs et al, 1989). Parents frequently also express concerns about long-term complications and the risk of hypoglycemia. As noted earlier, the risk of severe hypoglycemia is 3 to 4 times greater in children on intensive treatment regimens. Parents may be more concerned about their child participating in sports, going on field trips, or spending the night at a friend's house if he or she is on an intensive treatment regimen.

Guilt is often of concern to parents of children with diabetes, particularly because the disease is inherited. Families must be provided with appropriate genetic counseling so that they are aware of the risks to other family members and to offspring of the individual with diabetes. Such information often helps to assuage the guilt present at diagnosis because the risk for first-degree relatives is low. The sibling of a child with type 1 diabetes has about a 5% to 10% risk, and an offspring of one parent with diabetes has about a 1% to 2% risk as compared with a 0.05% risk for the general population. The current DPT-1 trial has introduced the concern that testing at-risk siblings may lead to labeling a child as having diabetes before the disease actually occurs. In addition, because treatment of high-risk relatives in the DPT-1 involves daily insulin injections, parents may be concerned about the ethics of this treatment for someone who does not yet have diabetes.

Considerable attention has been paid to family problems and their effect on metabolic control in children with diabetes. Studies of the influence of family life on diabetes control have been inconclusive (Kovacs et al, 1989). Some families, however, exhibit psychosomatic characteristics that clearly have an adverse effect on the child with diabetes. Such families should be referred for family therapy.

Social issues (e.g., cultural differences) may also influence adaptation to diabetes in youth, but little work on these questions has been done with adolescents with type 1 diabetes. Auslander and associates (1990) demonstrated that black children and children from single-parent families were at higher risk for poor control. Hanson, Henggeler, and Burghen (1987) and Delameter and associates (1991) found that black children and adolescents had worse metabolic control than white children. Hanson and associates (1987) did not find differences in psychosocial status and family functioning between white and black families. Differences in metabolic control between these families may be because of cultural dietary factors (e.g., eating more foods that affect blood glucose swings or participating in less exercise). Because eating behaviors and participation in sports may be influenced by cultural values, families should be assessed for their beliefs and values about food and exercise.

Resources

Two national organizations provide help for families coping with diabetes in a child: the American Diabetes Association (ADA) and the Juvenile Diabetes Foundation (JDF) (see the list of organizations that follows). The ADA is the largest such organization, composed of both lay individuals and professionals. The ADA supports research, education, fund raising, and camps, as well as provides lobbying efforts related to diabetes. It publishes several pamphlets and books for families to use in understanding diabetes. At the local level, many affiliates provide support and educational programs for families and children. The ADA deals with all types of diabetes, not only type 1 diabetes.

Research toward a cure for type 1 diabetes is the primary focus of the JDF. The organization does provide some support for families, but its major effort is devoted to fund raising for research to find a cure for type 1 diabetes. Some families find that working toward the cure helps deal with the illness in their family.

Organizations

American Diabetes Association
1660 Duke Street
Alexandria, Va. 22314
(800) ADA-DISC
www.diabetes.org

Juvenile Diabetes Foundation
23 E 26th Street
New York, NY 10010
(212) 689-7868
www.jdfcure.org
   Relevant websites:
CDC Diabetes Home Page: www.cdc.gov
National Institute of Diabetes and Digestive and Kidney Disease (NIDDK): www.nih/niddk.gov
Children with Diabetes: www.childrenwithdiabetes.com
Diabetes Book Store: www.members.aol.com/healthbook/diabetes/
Diabetes Monitor: www.mdcc.com
KidsRPumping: www.members.aol.com/CamelsR-Fun/index.html/
Insulin pumpers: www.insulin-pumpers.org/index.html/
Health: Diseases and Conditions: Diabetes: www.yahoo.com/Health/Diseases_and_Conditions/Diabetes/
   News and chat groups:
misc.health.diabetes: This is the place to find people to talk with about diabetes.
alt.support.diabetes.kids: A support group for parents with children with diabetes.

Summary of Primary Care Needs for the Child with Diabetes Mellitus (Type 1)

HEALTH CARE MAINTENANCE
Growth and development
Height and weight are normal unless diabetes control is less than adequate.

Secondary sexual development may be delayed.

Rapid weight gain may require intervention.

Weight loss usually indicates poor control.

Diet
Maintenance of normoglycemia is critical.

Stress the importance of regular distribution of meals and snacks.

Safety
Prevent hypoglycemia with careful monitoring; be sure a glucose source is always available.

Dispose of syringes properly.

Use glucagon for severe hypoglycemic episodes.

Immunizations
Routine immunizations are recommended.

Yearly influenza vaccine recommended.

Screening
Vision: Check red reflex and perform funduscopic examination at each visit.

A thorough pediatric ophthalmologic examination every 5 years is advised.

Cataracts are possible at diagnosis.

Hearing: Routine screening is recommended.

Dental: Routine screening is recommended.

Blood pressure: Blood pressure and orthostatic variation should be checked at each visit.

Hematocrit: Routine screening is recommended.

Urinalysis: Perform urinalysis yearly for ketones, glucose, and protein determinations; after 5 years screen for microalbuminuria yearly.

Tuberculosis: Routine screening is recommended.

Condition-specific screening: Check hemoglobin A_{1c} every 3 months.

Perform thyroid function studies if a change in growth patterns occurs.

Perform other studies as indicated.

COMMON ILLNESS MANAGEMENT
Differential Diagnosis
Illness requires "sick day" management.

It is important to maintain hydration during illness.

It is most important to evaluate for hypoglycemia with changes in mental status.

Candidial vaginal infections are more common in adolescent females. Skin lesions must be evaluated. Weight loss may indicate poor diabetic control.

Drug Interactions
Beware that many OTC medications and antibiotics contain glucogenic substances or alcohol.

Pseudoephedrine may increase blood glucose as a result of stimulant effect.

DEVELOPMENTAL ISSUES
Sleep patterns: Prevention of nighttime hypoglycemia is important.

Nightmares may be the result of hypoglycemia.

Toileting: Enuresis may be present when control is poor.

Measurement of urinary ketones is important when blood glucose levels are high or when the child is ill.

Discipline: Unruly behavior may be caused by hypoglycemia.

The potential for conflict over diet, blood testing, and insulin administration should be recognized.

Child care: Teachers and baby-sitters need training in management of dietary needs and hypoglycemia.

Summary of Primary Care Needs for the Child with Diabetes Mellitus (Type 1)—cont'd

Schooling: Full attendance and participation are expected.

School personnel must be aware of the child's special needs.

If diabetic control is poor, performance may be affected.

Sexuality: If diabetes is adequately controlled, sexual development should be normal.

Pregnancy prevention is very important because of combined risks of diabetes and adolescent pregnancy.

Low-dose estrogen combination oral contraceptives are recommended because of the risk for complications with BCP or oral contraceptives containing estrogen.

Pregnancy outcomes are dramatically improved if euglycemia is maintained preceding and during pregnancy.

Impotency caused by long-term vascular and neurologic compromise is a rare problem during adolescence.

Transition to adulthood: Challenges in the transition to adulthood may be more complex for adolescents with type 1 diabetes because of the extraordinary demands of the disease self-management.

Vocational adjustment and marital relationships may be more difficult for some young adults with type 1 diabetes than others.

If adjustment is better in early adolescence, young adults are more likely to have better adjustment and metabolic control.

SPECIAL FAMILY CONCERNS

Assumption of self-care activities and adherence to the regimen are prime concerns.

Parents often experience guilt about the inheritance of type 1 diabetes.

Psychosomatic families may have more problems with diabetic management.

Black children and children from single-parent homes are at highest risk for poor metabolic control.

Black children and adolescents tend to have worse metabolic control than white children and adolescents. Differences in metabolic control may be from cultural dietary factors or participation in less exercise, both of which may be influenced by cultural values.

References

Aikens JE et al: Daily stress variability, learned resourcefulness, regimen adherence, and metabolic control in type I diabetes mellitus: evaluation of a path model, J Consult Clin Psychol 60:113-118, 1992.

American Academy of Pediatrics: Summaries of infectious diseases. In Peter G, editor: 1998 red book: report of the committee on infectious diseases, ed 25, Elk Grove Village, Ill., 1998, The Academy.

American Diabetes Association: Diabetes: 1996 vital statistics, Alexandria, Va., 1996, The Academy.

American Diabetes Association: Position statement: implications of the Diabetes Control and Complications Trial, Diabetes 42:1555-1558, 1993.

American Diabetes Association: Clinical practice recommendations 1999, Diabetes Care 22(suppl 1): S1-S114, 1999.

Attia N et al: Comparison of human regular and lispro insulins after interruption of continuous subcutaneous insulin infusion and the treatment of acutely decompensated IDDM, Diabetes Care 21:817-821, 1998.

Aucott SW et al: Rigorous management of insulin-dependent diabetes mellitus during pregnancy, Acta Diabetologica 31:126-129, 1994.

Auslander W et al: Risk factors to health in diabetic children: a prospective study from diagnosis, Health Soc Work 15:133-142, 1990.

Betschart J: Children and adolescents with diabetes, Nurs Clin North Am 28:35-44, 1993.

Bingley PJ, Bonfacio E, and Gale EAM: Can we really predict IDDM? Diabetes 42:213-220, 1993.

Court JM: Issues of transition to adult care, J Pediatr Child Health 29(suppl 1):S53-S55, 1993.

Daneman D: When should your child take charge? . . . diabetes care, Diabetes Forecast 44:60-66, 1991.

Delamater AM et al: Racial differences in metabolic control of children and adolescents with type I diabetes mellitus, Diabetes Care 14:20-25, 1991.

DCCT Research Group: The Diabetes Control and Complications Trial (DCCT): design and methodologic implications for the feasibility phase, Diabetes 35:530-545, 1986.

DCCT Research Group: Expanded role of the dietitian in the DCCT: implications for clinical practice, J Am Diet Assoc 93:758-767, 1993a.

DCCT Research Group: The effect of intensive treatment of diabetes on the development and progression of long-term complications in insulin-dependent diabetes mellitus, New Engl J Med 329:435-459, 1993b.

DCCT Research Group: Effect of intensive diabetes treatment on the development and progression of long-term complications in adolescents with insulin-dependent diabetes mellitus: DCCT, J Pediatr 125:177-188, 1994.

DCCT Research Group: Adverse events and their association with treatment regimens in the diabetes control and complications trial, Diabetes Care 18:1415-1427, 1995.

Drash AL: The child, the adolescent, and the DCCT, Diabetes Care 16:1515-1516, 1993.

Dunn FL et al: The implantable insulin pump trial study group, Diabetes Care 20:59-63, 1997.

Dunning PL: Young-adult perspectives of insulin-dependent diabetes, Diabetes Education 21:58-65, 1995.

Eisenbarth GS: Type I diabetes mellitus: a chronic autoimmune disease, N Engl J Med 314:1360-1368, 1986.

Franz MJ et al: Nutritional principles for the management of diabetes and related complications, Diabetes Care 17:490-518, 1994.

Goldstein DE et al: Tests of glycemia in diabetes (technical review), Diabetes Care 18:896-909, 1995.

Grey M et al: Personal and family factors associated with quality of life in adolescents with diabetes, Diabetes Care 21:909-914, 1998.

Grey M and Thurber FW: Adaptation to chronic illness in childhood: diabetes mellitus, J Pediatr Nurs, 1991.

Hanson CL, Henggeler SW, and Burghen GA: Race and sex differences in metabolic control of adolescents with type 1 diabetes: a function of psychosocial variables, Diabetes Care 10:313-318, 1987.

Hauenstein EJ et al: Stress in parents of children with diabetes mellitus, Diabetes Care 12:18-23, 1989.

Hodges LC and Parker J: Concerns of parents with diabetic children, Pediatr Nurs 13:22-24, 1987.

Jornsay DL and Carney TM: Diabetes care in schools, Diabetes Spectrum 5:260-265, 1992.

Ingersoll GM et al: Cognitive maturity and self-management among adolescents with insulin-dependent diabetes mellitus, J Pediatrics 108(4):620-623, 1986.

Karlsson JA, Holmes CS, and Lang R: Psychosocial aspects of disease duration and control in young adults with type I diabetes, J Clin Epidemiol 41:435-440, 1988.

Keller RJ, Eisenbarth GS, and Jackson RA: Insulin prophylaxis in individuals at high risk of type I diabetes, Lancet 341:927-928, 1993.

Kovacs M et al: Family functioning and metabolic control of school-aged children with type 1 diabetes, Diabetes Care 12:409-414, 1989.

Kumar A, Weatherly M, and Beaman DC: Sweeteners, flavorings, and dyes in antibiotic preparations. Pediatrics 87:352-360, 1991.

Lacy PE: Pancreatic islet cell transplant, Mt Sinai J Med 61:23-31, 1994.

Leslie DG and Elliot RG: Early environmental events as a cause of IDDM: evidence and implications, Diabetes 43:843-850, 1994.

Lipman TH et al: A developmental approach to diabetes in children: birth through preschool, Moll Cell Neurosci 14:225-259, 1989.

Mastrototaro J et al: Clinical results from a continuous glucose sensor multi-center study, Diabetes 47(suppl 1):A61, 1998.

National Center for Health Statistics: Advance report of final mortality statistics, MVSR Monthly Vital Stat Rep 45(6), 1996.

Oesterle A. et al: CSII: A "new" way to achieve strict metabolic control and lower the risk of severe hypoglycemia in adolescents, Diabetes 47(suppl 1):A342, 1998.

Pless IB et al: Expected diabetic control in childhood and psychosocial functioning in early adult life, Diabetes Care 11:387-392, 1988.

Pollock M et al: Eating disorders and maladaptive dietary/-insulin management among youths with childhood-onset insulin dependent diabetes mellitus, Am Acad Child Adolesc Psychiatr 34:291-296, 1995.

Polonsky WH et al: Insulin omission in women with IDDM, Diabetes Care 17:1178-1185, 1994.

Santiago JV: Lessons from the Diabetes Control and Complications Trial, Diabetes 42:1549-1554, 1993.

Skyler JS, Gelfand RA, and Kourides IA for the Inhaled insulin phase II study group: Treatment of type 1 diabetes mellitus with inhaled human insulin: a 3-month multicenter trial, Diabetes 47(suppl 1):A61, 1998.

Striegel-Moore RH, Nicholson TJ, and Tamborlane WV: Prevalence of eating disorder symptoms in preadolescent and adolescent girls with type 1 diabetes, Diabetes Care 15:1361-1368, 1992.

Sutherland DER and Gruessner RWG: Current status of pancreas transplantation for the treatment of type 1 diabetes mellitus, Clin Diabetes 152-156, July-August 1997.

Tamborlane WV et al: Implications of the DCCT in treating children and adolescents with diabetes, Clin Diabetes, 115-116, 1994.

Torlone F et al: Pharmacokinetics, pharmacodynamics, and glucose counter-regulation following subcutaneous injection of the monomenic insulin analogue (Lys(B28)Pro(B29), Diabetologia 37:713-720, 1995.

Wysocki T et al: Survey of diabetes professionals regarding developmental changes in diabetes self-care, Diabetes Care 13:65-68, 1990.

Wysocki T et al: Diabetes mellitus in the transition to adulthood: adjustment, self-care, and health status, Dev Behav Pediatr 13:194-201, 1992.

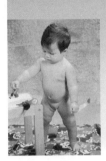

CHAPTER 20

Down Syndrome

Wendy M. Nehring and Judith A. Vessey

Etiology

Down syndrome, which was first described by Jean Etienne Esquirol in 1838 and promulgated by John Langdon Down in 1866, is a condition that is associated with a recognizable phenotype and limited intellectual endowment because of extra chromosome 21 material. It is the most frequent autosomal chromosomal anomaly. The exact band of chromosomal material implicated in Down syndrome has been isolated, which indicates that an entire replication of chromosome 21 is not necessary for expression.

Nondisjunction

Nondisjunction of chromosome 21 is responsible for the majority of cases of Down syndrome and is not inherited. Nondisjunction (i.e., the uneven division of chromosomes) can occur during anaphase 1 or 2 in meiosis (i.e., reduction and division of germ cells) or in anaphase of mitosis (i.e., somatic cell division). Although the exact mechanism is unconfirmed, the pair of chromosomes fail to separate and migrate properly during cell division. When this occurs in meiosis, the haploid number for the respective daughter cells is unequal. If the cell receiving 24 rather than 23 chromosomes is fertilized, a trisomic zygote results (Figure 20-1).

Nondisjunction may also occur early in mitosis. The resulting zygote will possess two or more cell lines with varying chromosomal constitutions. The earlier that nondisjunction occurs, the greater the percentage of affected cells. This inheritance pattern (i.e., mosaicism) is associated with fewer phenotypic features (Figure 20-2).

Translocation

In Down syndrome caused by translocation, there are also three copies of chromosome 21. The third copy does not occur independently, however, but is attached to another chromosome—usually to one of the D or G group. Robertsonian translocations, where the long arms of chromosome 21 attach to the long arms of chromosome 14, 21, or 22, are the most common translocations, although other forms can occur (Roizen, 1997).

The total chromosome count in Down syndrome is 46, even though material for 47 chromosomes is present. Although the phenotype for Down syndrome caused by translocation is the same as that for nondisjunction, the inheritance pattern is quite different. With translocation, the disorder may reoccur in future pregnancies. If one parent has 45 chromosomes—including a translocation of chromosome 21, the gametes produced could result in a trisomic zygote. Although six combinations are theoretically possible, three are nonviable. Of the three that are viable, one is normal (i.e., N = 46), one results in a balanced translocation (i.e., N = 45), and one is an unbalanced translocation resulting in Down syndrome (i.e., N = 46) (Figure 20-3). Although this would translate to a 33% chance of having a child with Down syndrome with each pregnancy, in clinical practice the actual distribution differs from the theoretical distribution. If the mother is the carrier, the risk of recurrence is 10% to 15%; if the father is the carrier, the risk is 5% to 8%.

A variety of hypotheses as to the cause of Down syndrome have been offered over the years, including the following: (1) a genetic predisposition to nondisjunction; (2) autoimmunity; (3) hormonal alterations in aging women; (4) viral disease; (5) environmental factors such as abdominal radiation before conception and drug exposure; and (6) frequency of coitus (Pueschel, 1992). No one factor has been confirmed, although new genetic findings suggest that the cause is probably multifactorial.

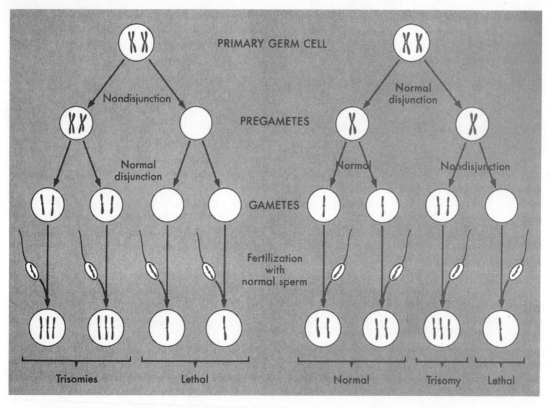

Figure 20-1   The mechanisms of maldistribution of chromosomes during first and second meiotic divisions caused by nondisjunction.

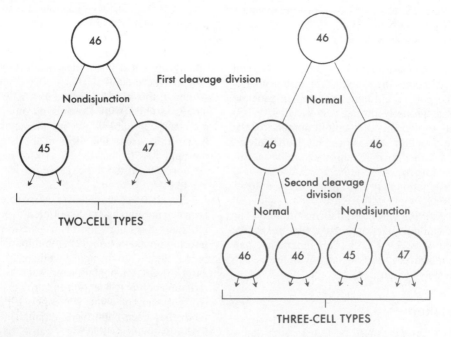

Figure 20-2   Nondisjunction during the first and second mitotic division of the zygote, resulting in a mosaic phenotype. (From Whaley L and Wong D: Nursing care of infants and children, ed 4, St Louis, 1991, Mosby.)

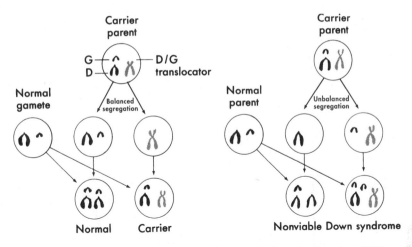

Figure 20-3 Possible zygotes from the union of a somatically normal carrier of D/G translocation and with a genetically and somatically normal individual. (From Wong D et al: Whaley and Wong's nursing care of infants and children, ed 6, St Louis, 1999, Mosby.)

Incidence

The prevalence rate for Down syndrome is 1 in 650 to 1000 live births, with the incidence rate dropping to approximately 1 in 800 live births (Lashley, 1998). Prenatal diagnosis of women of advanced maternal age explains this difference. Prevalence rates vary by inheritance pattern. Nondisjunction is found in 93% to 95% of cases; mosaicism in 1% to 2% of cases; and translocation in 4% to 5% of cases (Rogers, Roizen, and Capone, 1996; Roizen, 1997).

Down syndrome caused by translocation is independent of parental age, and the incidence is stable across age cohorts, although one third of the cases of translocation Down syndrome are inherited from parents (Jones, 1997). Advanced parental age, however, is implicated in nondisjunction. For women in their early 20s, the incidence is approximately 1 in every 2000 births. The incidence rises gradually until maternal age surpasses 35 and then climbs to approximately 42 in every 1000 live births for 45-year-old women (Hecht and Hook, 1996). Advanced paternal age (i.e., age 55 years and older) has also been shown to affect the incidence of nondisjunction Down syndrome in approximately 5% of the cases (Lashley, 1998). Although the extra chromosome is paternal in origin, nondisjunction still occurs after fertilization. Be-

cause the overwhelming percentage of cases of Down syndrome are caused by nondisjunction, parental age directly affects the overall incidence (Figure 20-4).

Trisomic Down syndrome occurs more frequently in males (Sharav, 1991), and translocation Down syndrome occurs more often in females (Staples et al, 1991). Down syndrome is found in all races and ethnic groups. Although the incidence rates of Down syndrome vary little among whites, blacks, and Hispanic infants born to mothers under 35 years of age, rates are significantly higher in Hispanic infants born to mothers over 35 years of age. Differences in these rates may reflect differences in early prenatal care, prenatal diagnosis, and views on abortion (Centers for Disease Control and Prevention [CDC], 1994).

Clinical Manifestations at Time of Diagnosis

Down syndrome is most often diagnosed immediately after birth as a result of its distinctive phenotype. In infants of color or those born very prematurely, diagnosis may be delayed because the clinical features may not be as clearly recognized. Although more than 50 physical characteristics can

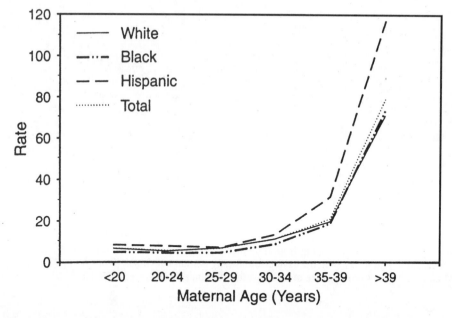

Figure 20-4   Rate* of Down syndrome at birth, by race/ethnicity of mother and maternal age group—17 state-based birth defects surveillance programs,† United States, 1983-1990.§

be identified at birth (Box 20-1), no one feature is considered diagnostic. Features vary in their expression and are not always present. Some of the most commonly associated features, however, include generalized hypotonia, epicanthal folds, single transverse palmar creases, neck skinfold, and widely spaced first and second toes.

A variety of congenital anomalies are commonly associated with Down syndrome. Congenital cardiac disease is seen in approximately 40% to 66% of children with Down syndrome, with endocardial cushion defects accounting for about 29% and septal defects comprising another 39% to 44% of cardiac malformations (Marino and Pueschel, 1996; Rogers, Roizen, and Capone, 1996; Wells et al., 1994). Gastrointestinal (GI) malformations are

seen in 5% of children with Down syndrome; among the most common problems are duodenal or esophageal atresia, congenital megacolon (Hirschsprung's disease), imperforate anus, tracheoesophageal fistula, and pyloric stenosis (Pueschel and Pueschel, 1992; Rogers, Roizen, and Capone, 1996). An increase in urogenital conditions (e.g., micropenis, hypospadias, and cryptorchidism) in males has also been documented, although no rise in the incidence of anatomic abnormalities of the kidneys or ureters was noted (Lang et al, 1987). Anomalies can usually be surgically corrected in the neonatal period. Although many children experience total correction of the anomaly, others will suffer from untoward sequelae throughout their lives.

Treatment

No treatment can eliminate the chromosomal defect that causes Down syndrome. Extensive interdisciplinary services and research over the last 20 years has, however, transformed society's view of children with Down syndrome and accepted treatment protocols. Accepted approaches include

---

*Per 10,000 live-born infants (US Department of Health and Human Services: Down syndrome prevalence at birth—United States, 1983-1990, MMWR Morbid Mortal Wkly Rep 43:617-622, 1994).

†Arizona, Arkansas, California, Colorado, Georgia, Hawaii, Illinois, Iowa, Kansas, Maryland, Missouri, Nebraska, New Jersey, New York, North Carolina, Virginia, and Washington.

§Because of the variability in surveillance periods (e.g., 1983-1987 or 1986-1989) and the low number of annual cases in some states, rates are presented as period prevalence rates. Includes infants from all racial/ethnic groups and infants for whom race/ethnicity was unknown.

Box 20-1

Clinical Manifestations in Down Syndrome

Skull

False fontanel
Flat occipital area
Brachycephaly
Separated sagittal suture
Hypoplasia of midfacial bones
Reduced interorbital distance
Underdeveloped maxilla
Obtuse mandibular angle

Eyes

Oblique narrow palpebral fissures
Epicanthal folds
Brushfield spots
Strabismus
Nystagmus
Myopia
Hypoplasia of the iris

Ears

Small, shortened ears
Low and oblique implantation
Overlapping helices
Prominent antihelix
Absent or attached earlobes
Narrow ear canals
External auditory meatus
Structural aberrations of the ossicles
Stenotic external auditory meatus

Nose

Hypoplastic
Flat nasal bridge
Anteverted, narrow nares
Deviated nasal septum

Mouth

Prominent, thickened and fissured lips
Corners of the mouth turned downward
High arched, narrow palate
Shortened palatal length
Protruding enlarged tongue
Papillary hypertrophy (early preschool)
Fissured tongue (later school years)
Periodontal disease
Partial anodontia
Microdontia
Abnormally aligned teeth
Anterior open bite
Mouth held open

Neck

Short broad neck
Loose skin at nape

Chest

Shortened rib cage
Twelfth rib anomalies
Pectus excavation or carinatum
Congenital heart disease

Abdomen

Distended and enlarged abdomen
Diastasis recti
Umbilical hernia
Muscle tone and musculature
Hyperflexibility
Muscular hypotonia
Generalized weakness
Integument
Skin appears large for the skeleton
Dry and rough
Fine, poorly pigmented hair

Extremities

Short extremities
Partial or complete syndactyly
Clinodactyly
Brachyclinodactyly

Upper extremities

Short, broad hands
Brachyoclinodactyly
Single palmar transverse crease
Incurved short fifth finger
Abnormal dermatoglyphics

Lower extremities

Short and stubby feet
Gap between first and second toes
Plantar crease between first and second toe
Second and third toes grouped in a forklike position
Radial deviation of the third to the fifth toe
Physical growth and development
Short stature
Increased weight in later life
Other findings seen in newborns
Enlarged anterior fontanel
Delayed closing of sutures and fontanels
Open sagittal suture
Nasal bone not ossified, underdeveloped
Reduced birth weight

genetic counseling, prompt referral for surgical correction of congenital anomalies, and enrollment in an early intervention program (Box 20-2).

Genetic Counseling

Validation of Down syndrome and its genotype by chromosomal analysis via karyotype should be considered for all affected children during the neonatal period (Haddow, 1998). Although this validation will not affect a child's treatment or prognosis, it has significant implications for the genetic counseling of family members. Because translocation is the cause of 4% to 5% of cases, parents and siblings must be tested to determine their carrier status, as well as have the risk of recurrence in future pregnancies carefully explained to them.

Surgery

Surgical corrections of most major cardiac, GI, and genitourinary anomalies are now performed routinely, but this was not the standard practice in some settings. Amidst moral and ethical controversy, however, the federal judiciary decreed in 1984 that treatment of life-threatening congenital anomalies could not be refused only because a child was developmentally disabled (Mahon, 1990) (see Chapter 6).

Surgery is not without risk. The risk for upper airway compromise during and after surgery is increased in Down syndrome because of clinical features such as subglottic stenosis, tracheal stenosis, hypotonia, and a narrow nasopharyngeal inlet. Atlantoaxial instability also poses a surgical risk, although if cervical spine radiographs are normal, any neck flexion or extension during the surgical

period does not pose a problem (Abramson et al, 1995). Furthermore, postextubation stridor (deJong et al, 1997; Goldstein et al, 1998) and apnea (Bower and Richmond, 1995) are common, and a longer hospital stay is recommended for children with Down syndrome. Specifically, perioperative and late cardiac mortality are only associated with complete atrioventricular septal defect (Reller and Morris, 1998).

In addition to life-saving surgeries, some children with Down syndrome also undergo plastic surgery to alter their phenotypic appearance. As these children continue to become more integrated into society, they may be stigmatized because of their physiognomy. Some parents, concerned about their child's social acceptance, seek plastic surgery for the child (e.g., partial glossectomies, neck resections, Silastic implants for the chin and nose, and reconstruction of dysplastic helices). Better articulation of speech, less mouth breathing, fewer and less severe upper respiratory tract infections, and improved mastication and swallowing may be realized. The degree of success, however, may be small or nonexistent. There are surgical risks, surgery is expensive, and it is most often not covered by insurance. Any parents and/or children with Down syndrome wanting to undergo plastic surgery should talk at length with their primary care provider and surgeon before the procedure so that they understand the risks (Van Dyke, 1995).

Early Intervention

Infant stimulation programs and continued early childhood education are designed to optimize a child's rate of development and minimize the amount of developmental lag that will occur between children with Down syndrome and their developmentally normal peers. Specific therapeutic exercises are devised to stimulate an infant's cognitive, social, motor, and language domains. Researchers have found motor and cognitive improvement in infants after their participation in an early intervention program (Hines and Bennett, 1996). Parents are usually taught these skills by special education teachers, physical therapists, occupational therapists, and speech pathologists so that therapy can be conducted at home. Timing seems to be a critical factor, however, with earlier interventions correlated with greater developmental

---

Box 20-2

Treatment

- Genetic counseling
- Medical and pharmacologic treatment of deficiencies and/or disorders
- Surgical correction of abnormalities
- Early intervention programs
- Choosing appropriate educational settings (e.g., inclusion)

gains. These children will later be referred to a specialized program designed to continue these intervention strategies and then integrated into generic child care or school.

Numerous other approaches (e.g., patterning, cell therapy, megavitamin therapy, and the administration of butoctamide hydrogen succinate) designed to improve the developmental outcomes of these children have also been tried. Unfortunately, the results of these interventions have been disappointing. The drug, piracetam, which some consider to be a cognitive enhancer, has received the most attention of late. Funding for a double blind study is being sought, but until such a study is completed, use of piracetam should be cautioned against (Van Dyke, 1995).

Recent and Anticipated Advances in Diagnosis and Management

Maternal age has been the traditional screening risk factor for Down syndrome. Researchers and physicians are calling for a screening policy based on statistical modeling and decision analysis (i.e., using financial and human factors) (Cuckle, 1998; Serra-Prat et al, 1998). Pregnant women must be aware of the screening options available to them (i.e., biochemical screening, ultrasound, and/or amniocentesis) based on maternal age. Moreover, a fourth serum marker, inhibin, has been added, increasing the detection rate. Ultrasound measurement of nuchal translucency has not been consistently developed, and its technique has not been standardized for consistent results in all settings. Research on the use of polymerase chain reaction (PCR) amplification with three DNA markers on the 21st chromosome is being done and may be the screening technique of the near future (Haddow, 1998).

Human growth hormone (hGH) therapy for children with Down syndrome is investigational and controversial. Children with Down syndrome should be treated with hGH only if they are deficient in this hormone because an increase in brain growth stimulated by hGH has not been found to increase cognitive function. Many ethical issues about its usage exist, such as: What are the goals of treatment? How are the children being evaluated? What are the parents' roles in treatment decisions?

When is such treatment appropriate when its scientific efficacy is unfounded? How will this child benefit from being taller? Is the discomfort associated with the therapy warranted? Who will pay for the therapy? Moreover, hGh therapy has been associated with leukemia. The risks vs. the benefits of this therapy have not yet been clearly evaluated (Foley, 1995; Kodish and Cutler, 1996).

Associated Problems (Box 20-3)

Mental Retardation

The intellectual capabilities of children with Down syndrome vary dramatically. Most of these children are moderately retarded (i.e., intelligence quotient [IQ] of 40 to 55, standard deviation [SD] of 15), but a small percentage are either mildly affected (i.e., IQ of 56 to 69, SD of 15) or severely impaired (i.e., IQ of 39, SD of 15). For a few children, their IQs are not consistent with a diagnosis of mental retardation (Pueschel, 1992). Known correlates to the intelligence and adaptive behavior skills of children are their physical condition, home environment, and individualized early intervention

---

Box 20-3

Associated Problems

- Mental retardation
- Cardiac defects
- Celiac disease
- Gastrointestinal tract anomalies
- Malignancies
  —Testicular germ cell
  —Leukemia
- Growth retardation
- Musculoskeletal and motor disabilities
- Vision problems
- Hearing loss
- Immune system deficiency
- Dental changes
- Altered respiratory function
- Thyroid dysfunction
- Sleep disordered breathing
- Seizure disorders
- Skin conditions

(Mattheis, 1995). Unfortunately, cognitive function often deteriorates with age, and significant losses in intelligence, memory, and social skills are seen earlier (i.e., often by age 40 years) than in persons without Down syndrome (Carlesimo, Marotta, and Vicari, 1997).

Mental retardation may also be accompanied with behavior disorders. Depression, autistic-like behavior, and psychotic episodes have been reported. Neurologic deterioration, institutionalization, disturbed family life, stress associated with inclusion, and normal childhood stressors may affect the mental health of children with Down syndrome.

Cardiac Defects

Approximately 40% to 66% of children with Down syndrome have congenital heart defects. In order of decreasing frequency, the most common heart anomalies include atrioventricular septal defect (i.e., endocardial cushion defect and atrioventricular canal defect), ventricular septal defect, patent ductus arteriosus, and atrial septal defect (see Chapter 17). Other heart or cardiac-associated conditions that may also occur in Down syndrome include tetralogy of Fallot, polycythemia, pulmonary artery hypertension (Cousineau and Lauer, 1995), and pulmonary vascular obstructive disease, which can progress to congestive heart failure and death (Roizen, 1997). Children with Down syndrome and cardiac defects requiring surgery also are at risk for developing subacute bacterial endocarditis (Cousineau and Lauer, 1995). In addition, children with Down syndrome who do not have congenital heart disease are at risk for developing mitral valve prolapse with age; by the end of adolescence, mitral valve prolapse has been detected in over 50% of the individuals tested (Geggel, O'Brien, and Feingold, 1993).

Celiac Disease

The frequency of celiac disease in children with Down syndrome is 1% to 4%; in the general population, celiac disease generally occurs in 1 in 2000 live births (Amil Dias and Walker-Smith, 1990; Zubillaga et al, 1993). Screening has been successfully done with the antiendomysium antibody of the IgA class. Researchers recommend screening all individuals with Down syndrome (Carlsson et al, 1998; George et al, 1996) because a gluten free diet can be started to relieve symptoms and protect against future malignancy (George et al, 1996).

Gastrointestinal Tract Anomalies

Common congenital gastrointestinal tract anomalies include tracheoesophageal fistula, pyloric stenosis, duodenal atresia, annular pancreas, aganglionic megacolon, and imperforate anus (Pueschel and Pueschel, 1992). Most of these anomalies require immediate surgical correction and careful follow-up throughout life.

Malignancies

Leukemia

Children with Down syndrome are 10 to 30 times more likely to acquire leukemia than children without Down syndrome (Shen et al, 1995; Zipursky, 1996). One form of leukemia, transient leukemia (TL), occurs most often in infants with Down syndrome. This form of leukemia occurs during the newborn period and disappears within the first 3 months. In approximately one fifth of these cases, the child develops acute megakaryoblastic leukemia (AMKL) before age 4 years (Doyle and Zipursky, 1994). Researchers and health care professionals do not know if this is a reoccurrence of transient leukemia or onset of a new and different type of leukemia for which children with Down syndrome are at high risk (Zipursky, 1996).

The overall incidence of AMKL in children with Down syndrome is approximately 500 times greater than in children without Down syndrome, but children with Down syndrome who acquire AMKL have a better prognosis and respond to treatment better than other children (Lange et al, 1998). AMKL primarily occurs in children with Down syndrome before the age of 4 years (Zipursky, 1996; Zipursky, Poon and Doyle, 1992).

Acute lymphatic leukemia (ALL) also occurs at a higher rate (i.e., almost 10 times greater than that in the general population) in children with Down syndrome. ALL occurs most often after the age of 4 years (Lange et al, 1998; Zipursky, 1996).

Germ Cell Tumors

The incidence of testicular germ cell tumors may be increased in males with Down syndrome. More study is needed, however, to understand this trend (Satge et al, 1997).

Growth Retardation

At birth, infants with Down syndrome weigh less, are typically shorter, and have smaller occipital-frontal circumferences than unaffected children (Palmer et al, 1992). The velocity of linear growth is also reduced, with the most marked reductions between 6 and 24 months of age. This reduction in velocity reoccurs during adolescence, when the growth spurt—which is less vigorous than would normally be expected—occurs earlier in adolescents with Down syndrome (Arnell et al, 1996). This reduction in linear growth is not unexpected because children with Down syndrome have hypothalamic dysfunctions that affect the secretion of growth hormone (Pueschel, 1993). Other causes for the reduction in linear growth may be congenital heart disease, thyroid disorders, and/or nutrition problems, and each should be evaluated if suspected (Earl and Blackwelder, 1998).

Children with Down syndrome tend to be overweight. Beginning around 2 years of age, these children often have untoward weight gain that persists throughout their lives. For virtually every age, more than 30% of children with Down syndrome are above the 85th percentile for weight-height ratios, but some researchers have found this percentage to be as high as 50%. Children of school age show the greatest propensity for weight-height percentile gain (Cronk et al, 1988; Foley, 1995; Luke et al, 1994; Troiano et al, 1995). Yet when Luke and associates (1994) compared children with Down syndrome with those of similar height and weight, they found the children with Down syndrome consumed fewer calories and had similar activity levels. Significant differences have been seen between the growth parameters of children with Down syndrome—with and without congenital heart defects, with the severity of growth delay correlating to the severity of disease (i.e., especially during infancy prior to cardiac surgery) (Cousineau and Lauer, 1995).

Musculoskeletal and Motor Abilities

Orthopedic problems are second only to cardiac defects as a cause of morbidity in Down syndrome. Flaccid muscle tone and ligamentous laxity occur to some extent in all children with Down syndrome, possibly because of an intrinsic defect in their connective tissue. Among these conditions are pes planus, patellar subluxation, scoliosis, dislocated hips, atlantoaxial subluxation, joint and muscle pain, and rapid muscle fatigue. These problems may occur throughout a child's life, and the primary care provider should carefully screen for them at each visit.

Surgical correction may be indicated for patellar hypermobility with subluxation, scoliosis, or dislocated hips. Although the incidence of congenital dislocated hip in children with Down syndrome is similar to that of unaffected peers, approximately 1 in 20 will acquire dislocated hips between the time they learn to walk and the end of their school-aged period.

Another significant disorder associated with Down syndrome is atlantoaxial instability. Atlantoaxial instability results from a "loose joint" between C1 and C2 and increased space between the atlas and odontoid process and affects approximately 15% of children with Down syndrome (Committee on Sports Medicine and Fitness, 1995; Lawhon, 1995; Pueschel, 1998). At least 98% to 99% of affected children are asymptomatic. Subluxation or dislocation may result; and early manifestations may include neck pain, torticollis, deteriorating gait, or changes in bowel or bladder function. If left untreated, symptoms may progress to frank neurologic findings associated with spinal cord compression. The atlantodens interval may change over time in a small percentage of children (i.e., generally narrowing but occasionally widening) (Pueschel, Scola, and Pezzullo, 1992). Secondary to the numerous studies done on atlantoaxial instability, other cervical spinal abnormalities (e.g., degenerative disk diseases including premature arthritis and spondylosis) have been noted (Lawhon, 1995).

Vision

The increased prevalence of numerous ocular deviations is associated with Down syndrome. The most commonly occurring abnormalities are—in order of decreasing frequency: slanted palpebral fissures, spotted irises, refractive errors, strabismus, nystagmus, cataracts, blepharitis, pseudopapilledema, and keratoconus (Roizen, Mets, and Blondis, 1994). A significant loss in visual acuity will result if many of these conditions are not diagnosed and treated in early childhood. Moreover, visual problems—especially refractive errors—increase with age (Wong and Ho, 1997).

Hearing

The incidence of hearing loss in children with Down syndrome is approximately 67%. Structural deviations of the skull, foreface, external auditory canal, middle and inner ears, and throat accompanied by eustachian tube dysfunction are associated with congenital and acquired hearing loss that can be sensorineural or conductive or both and occur unilaterally or bilaterally (Roizen et al, 1993). The immune deficiency present in children with Down syndrome also effects recurrent ear infections (Roizen, 1997).

Immune System

Children with Down syndrome have altered immune function. Immune system deficits directly contribute to the increased incidence and severity of numerous other conditions, including—but not limited to—periodontal disease, respiratory problems, thyroid disorders, lymphocytic thyroiditis, leukemia, diabetes mellitus, alopecia areata, adrenal dysfunction, vitiligo, and joint problems (Smith, CS, 1995). Specifically, diabetes occurs in 1 in 250 in children with Down syndrome, which is more than twice the rate in the general population (Roizen, 1997).

Dental Changes

Children with Down syndrome seem to develop caries less often than unaffected children. Numerous other dental problems (e.g., bruxism, malocclusion, defective dentition, microdontia, and periodontal disease), however, are more prevalent in these children because of anatomic anomalies of the oral cavity and immunologic dysfunction. The average age of the first tooth eruption in children with Down syndrome is 13 months (Roizen, 1997). Of particular significance is juvenile periodontitis, which occurs in approximately 100% of children with Down syndrome. This disease progresses rapidly and may even be noted in deciduous dentition (Cichon, Crawford, and Grimm, 1998). Poor dental care alone does not account for juvenile periodontitis; the altered immune function in conjunction with the extensive gingival inflammation of children with Down syndrome are thought to also be responsible (Morinushi, Lopatin, and Van Poperin, 1997). Mouth breathing and consumption of a diet high in soft foods—two common occurrences in children with Down syndrome—also contribute to their dental problems.

Respiratory Functioning

Combined with a compromised immune system, pulmonary hypertension and hyperplasia, fewer alveoli, a decreased alveolar blood capillary surface area, and associated upper airway obstruction (e.g., lymphatic hypertrophy in the Waldeyer ring) predispose children with Down syndrome to respiratory tract infections. If recurrent severe respiratory tract infections occur, they will have a significant effect on a child's development.

Thyroid Dysfunction

Thyroid dysfunction in Down syndrome is commonly associated with autoimmune dysfunction (Foley, 1995; Ivarsson et al, 1997) and is usually an acquired rather than a congenital condition. The prevalence of thyroid dysfunction may reach 20% in adults. Specifically, congenital hypothyroidism has an incidence of 1 in 141 infants with Down syndrome, which is 28% higher than that of the general population. Subclinical hypothyroidism is seen in 30% to 50% of school-age children with Down syndrome (Roizen, 1997). Graves' disease, goiter, chronic lymphocytic thyroiditis, and hypothyroidism occur most often. Although thyroid dysfunction may remain subclinical for an extended period, alterations in thyroid-stimulating hormone and thyroid-binding globulin may be seen (Foley, 1995).

Sleep-Disorder Breathing

Anatomic and physiologic differences (e.g., midfacial hypoplasia, glossoptosis) predispose children with Down syndrome to obstructive sleep apnea and other sleep-disorder breathing problems (Kavanaugh, 1995). A study by Marcus and associates (1991) showed that overnight polysomnograms were abnormal in 100% of the children tested. Problems frequently diagnosed included hypoventilation (81%), obstructive sleep apnea (63%), desaturation (56%), and multiple abnormalities (63%). Age, obesity, and cardiac disease did not affect the incidence of these problems.

Seizure Disorders

Children with Down syndrome have an increased frequency of seizure disorders, with approximately 6% of these children being diagnosed with epilepsy. Structural differences and biochemical changes associated with Down syndrome have been implicated, although this has not been confirmed. The distribution of the onset of seizures is bimodal, occurring before age 3 years and after 13 years. Of the affected children, 40% begin to have seizures (i.e., generally infantile spasms and generalized tonic-clonic seizures) before 1 year of age. The prognosis of infantile spasms in children with Down syndrome is better than in the general population (Roizen, 1997; Stafstrom and Konkol, 1994). The onset of seizures again peaks in adults in their 30s, with tonic-clonic seizures and partial simple and partial complex seizures being the most common. Seizures in adulthood can be indicative of Alzheimer's disease (Mattheis, 1995) (see Chapter 21).

Skin Conditions

Several skin conditions—most of an immune origin—are common in individuals with Down syndrome. These conditions include atopic dermatitis, cheilitis, seborrheic dermatitis, ichthyosis, and vitiligo (Pueschel and Pueschel, 1992; Roizen, 1997).

Prognosis

Because Down syndrome is associated with numerous anatomic and physiologic aberrations, life expectancy is reduced, with approximately a 10% mortality rate in the first year of life that rises to 14% by 10 years of age (Carr, 1994). The number and severity of congenital anomalies significantly decrease life expectancy for some of these children. Premature aging and a high incidence of Alzheimer's disease are also seen in Down syndrome and may reduce life expectancy for adults. With correct medical, educational, and social interventions, most individuals live well into adulthood and have satisfying, productive lives (Carr,

1994). Successful outcomes seem to depend heavily on the early interventions children and their families receive. If children with Down syndrome are to reach their full potential, aggressive, interdisciplinary management is paramount.

PRIMARY CARE MANAGEMENT
Health Care Maintenance

Primary care providers are encouraged to consult the *Health Care Guidelines for Individuals with Down Syndrome* (Cohen, 1996) and the *Health Supervision Guidelines for Individuals with Down Syndrome* (Committee on Genetics, 1994). Both sets of guidelines cover the lifespan and are under review for revision in 1999.

Growth and Development

Evaluating the growth of children with Down syndrome is a detailed process. When linear growth is assessed, primary care providers must take into account the variations in velocity. Whereas growth adequacy is often determined by maintaining a particular percentile rank, variations in growth velocity affect the growth curves of these children during early childhood. Growth velocities for children with and without Down syndrome are similar during the school-aged period, however, and stability is then seen in percentile curves.

Measurements should be plotted on both the National Center for Health Statistics (NCHS) growth charts and growth charts specifically normed for children with Down syndrome (Figures 20-5 to 20-10). The NCHS growth charts allow children with Down syndrome to be compared with their chronologic-age peers and also provide a frame of reference for parents. The weight-height percentiles on the NCHS growth charts are independent of a child's age and are also useful in determining appropriate weight in children before adolescence. The specialty charts, where all percentiles for stature are less than their analogous percentiles on the NCHS charts, provide an excellent reference point for comparing growth among children with Down syndrome and determining those at risk for failure to thrive or obesity. The methodology used in obtaining the growth charts for children with Down syndrome has been questioned, but it is recommended that these charts

Text continued on p. 460.

Boys with Down Syndrome:
Physical Growth: 1 to 36 Months

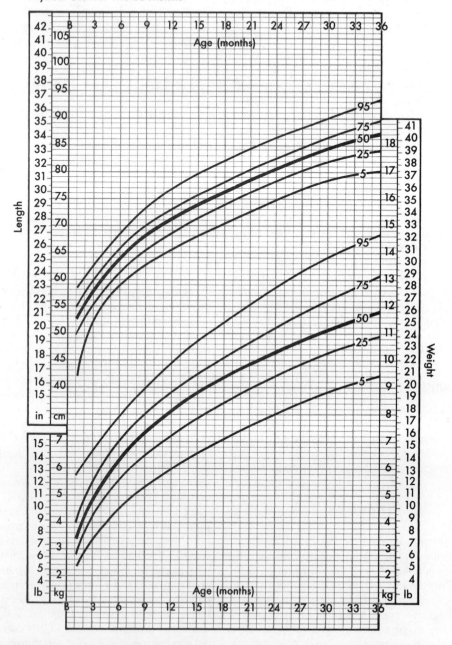

Figure 20-5 This graph is based on data from the Developmental Evaluation Clinic of the Children's Hospital, Boston, The Child Development Center of Rhode Island Hospital, and the Clinical Genetics Service of the Children's Hospital of Philadelphia. (Supported by March of Dimes grant 6-449.)

Girls with Down Syndrome:
Physical Growth: 1 to 36 Months

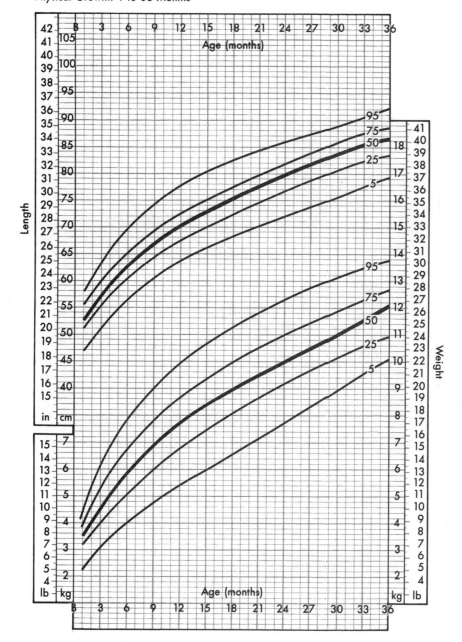

Figure 20-6   This graph is based on data from the Developmental Evaluation Clinic of the Children's Hospital, Boston, The Child Development Center of Rhode Island Hospital, and the Clinical Genetics Service of the Children's Hospital of Philadelphia. (Supported by March of Dimes grant 6-449.)

Boys with Down Syndrome:
Physical Growth: 2 to 18 Years

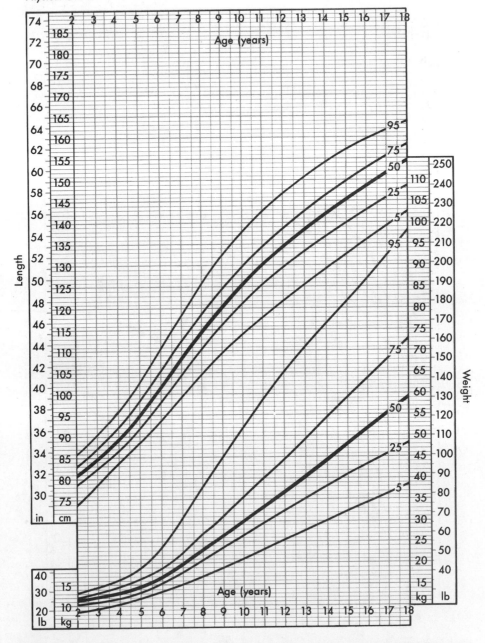

Figure 20-7 This graph is based on data from the Developmental Evaluation Clinic of the Children's Hospital, Boston, The Child Development Center of Rhode Island Hospital, and the Clinical Genetics Service of the Children's Hospital of Philadelphia. (Supported by March of Dimes grant 6-449.)

Girls with Down Syndrome:
Physical Growth: 2 to 18 Years

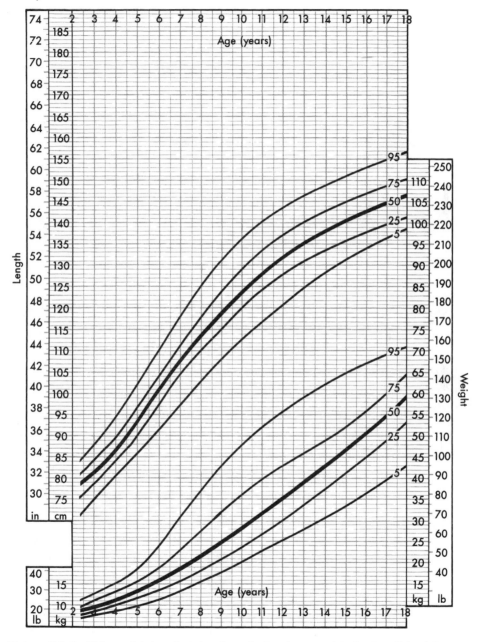

Figure 20-8   This graph is based on data from the Developmental Evaluation Clinic of the Children's Hospital, Boston, The Child Development Center of Rhode Island Hospital, and the Clinical Genetics Service of the Children's Hospital of Philadelphia. (Supported by March of Dimes grant 6-449.)

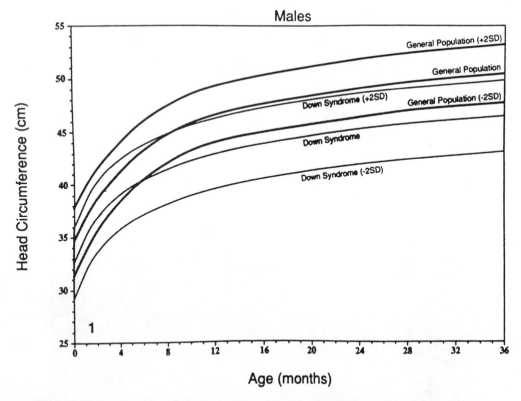

Figure 20-9   Head circumference growth curves for males with Down syndrome compared with those for males in the general population. (From Palmer CGS et al: Head circumference of children with Down syndrome (0 to 36 months), Am J Med Genetics 42:61-67, 1992.)

be consulted until future charts are available (Cohen and Patterson, 1998). Because inappropriate growth and excessive weight gain have ramifications for motor performance and social acceptance for children with Down syndrome, yearly assessments are required. Interventions for weight management may be introduced as necessary. Caloric reduction and increased exercise incorporated into a behavior management program are likely to be the most effective approach.

Because Down syndrome is associated with global development delay, virtually all children with Down syndrome will have IQs below the second standard deviation on standardized tests such as the Weschler Intelligence Scale for Children—Revised or the Stanford-Binet Intelligence Test. Performance on other language, motor, and social aptitude tests will also be below normal for almost all children.

Children with Down syndrome have the most difficulty with language development, especially with expressive language. They often do not speak their first word until 24 months of age (Kumin, 1996). Encouragement of nonverbal communication skills (e.g., turn-taking with toys and social interaction between parents and the child) facilitates the development of verbal language development (Mundy et al, 1995). The MacArthur Communicative Development Inventory is an appropriate parent report tool for measuring vocabulary development (Miller, Sedley, and Miolo, 1995).

Children with Down syndrome will pass through the normal developmental milestones but at a much slower rate than expected. The primary care provider can assist in a child's development by referring the family to an early intervention program as soon as possible after the child's birth. As

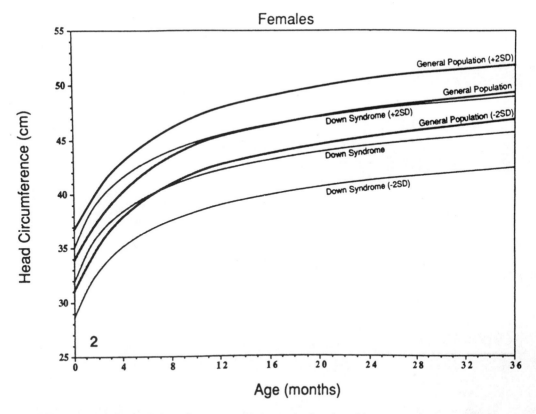

Figure 20-10 Head circumference growth curves for females with Down syndrome compared with those for females in the general population. (From Palmer CGS et al: Head circumference of children with Down syndrome (0 to 36 months), Am J Med Genetics 42:61-67, 1992.)

the child grows older, a variety of activities that are known to assist in development (e.g., Special Olympics and summer camp) can be encouraged. If a child has significant congenital anomalies, program personnel will need guidance as to the intensity of activity the child is allowed. A child's progress should be carefully documented on standardized developmental schedules (Figure 20-11) at each primary care visit. Sharing the results of the child's developmental gains with the parents will objectively demonstrate the child's improvement, thus reinforcing the parents' efforts.

Diet

Among the most significant concerns are feeding difficulties in young children and obesity in older children. Feeding problems may be encountered because of the disproportionately large tongues, muscle flaccidity, poor coordination, significantly delayed social maturation, thyroid or pituitary disorders, and congenital heart disease found in children with Down syndrome.

For infants, breast feeding should be encouraged. The immunogenic qualities of breast milk offer additional protection against upper respiratory tract infections and other illnesses. The extra effort required of infants who are breast feeding also helps them to develop orofacial muscles and tongue control and promotes greater jaw stability. Breast feeding may take longer at first, and mothers will need to be encouraged in their efforts. In addition to the standard guidance for breast feeding, primary care providers may also suggest other helpful tips, including the following: (1) waking the infant for feeding as necessary; (2) initially

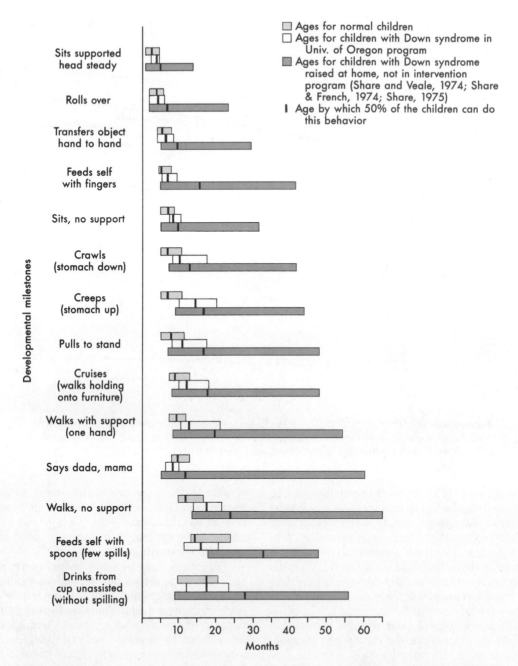

Figure 20-11.   Stray-Gunderson K: Babies with Down syndrome: a new parents' guide, ed 2, Bethesda, Md., 1995, Woodbine House.

expressing some milk to encourage the infant to latch onto the breast; (3) ensuring that the infant's nose and mouth are free of mucus; (4) checking that the infant's lip is turned out during feeding; and (5) holding the infant in an upright position during feeding. The LaLeche League of America has material on breast feeding infants with Down syndrome. Using soft, large-hole nipples may be helpful for infants who are not breast feeding.

Blended and chopped foods and shallow-bowl, latex-covered spoons may help children who are learning to eat solids. If significant problems (e.g., aspiration) occur, an occupational therapist or other developmental therapist should be consulted in designing an individualized feeding program (Frazier and Friedman, 1996).

There are no routine dietary restrictions for older children. Care should be taken to avoid excessive caloric intake if inappropriate weight gain is a problem. A balanced diet, a program of physical exercise, and vitamin and mineral supplementation are recommended as necessary (Luke et al, 1996).

Safety

Safety issues for children with Down syndrome are the same as for their developmental—not chronologic—peers. Primary care providers must adjust their normal schedule for providing anticipatory guidance to the development of children with Down syndrome. If information is given too far in advance of a child's developmental progression, parents may forget or find the information to be a painful reminder that their child is progressing more slowly than unaffected children.

Children with Down syndrome are more likely to sustain joint injuries as a result of their musculoskeletal problems. For children with atlantoaxial instability or those who have not yet been adequately evaluated, contact sports, somersaults, or other activities that may result in cervical injury should be restricted. Documentation that the child is not in danger of subluxation may be required for children participating in the Special Olympics.

Immunizations

Children with Down syndrome tend to develop autoantibodies at a higher frequency than the general population, which is possibly due to accelerated aging of their immune system. More research is needed on this topic to further understand how and why this development occurs. As a result of the development of autoantibodies, additional immunizations may be necessary because these children are at high risk for infection. In areas endemic for specific diseases, antibody titer levels may be assessed to determine a child's immune status. Researchers believe that immunoglobulin A (IgA) and immunoglobulin G (IgG) deficiencies are increased in children with Down syndrome, but the incidence is unknown. There is some evidence that deficiencies in IgG subclasses 2 and 4 occur more often in children with Down syndrome. If diagnosed, human immune globulin can be given (Smith CS, 1995).

There are, however, no contraindications for immunizations for children with Down syndrome, unless they have a cell-mediated disorder. If so, live viral vaccines are contraindicated (Smith CS, 1995). In most cases, the national immunization schedule—including the immunizations for varicella—should be followed (Committee on Infectious Diseases, 1999).

Pneumococcal polysaccharide vaccine (Pneumovax) is indicated for this population and is given at 2 years of age. Yearly immunoprophylaxis for influenza should also be considered for all children over 6 months of age. In cases of recurrent infections, antiviral medications (e.g. amantadine) may be considered to prevent the occurrence of influenza (Smith CS, 1995).

Screening

Vision: Because of the large number of ocular defects associated with Down syndrome, all children should be evaluated by an ophthalmologist by 6 months of age to assess for strabismus and cataracts. Early referral is critical considering the synergistic effects that diminished vision and hearing have on development. Significant visual impairment is usually preventable because the conditions common in Down syndrome (e.g., strabismus and myopia) are treatable (Roizen, 1997). Future screening recommendations should be determined in conjunction with the ophthalmologist according to the status of the child's eyes. At minimum, the primary care provider should screen for visual problems at each well child visit. Such screening should include testing acuity, examining the red reflex and optic fundi, and checking alignment and oculo-motor functions. Because children with Down syndrome may have difficulty using a Snellen or lazy E chart, acuity screening performed with the Titmus picture test, Teller acuity cards, or Allen picture cards will yield more valid results.

Many children with Down syndrome have difficulty keeping their glasses in place, so parents should be counseled that purchasing glasses with lightweight plastic lenses and using an elastic strap around the child's occiput to secure them will help correct this problem. Contact lenses are not routinely recommended but may be appropriate for children with keratoconus.

Hearing: Because good hearing is a requisite for cognitive, social, and language development and because these children are at high risk for conductive hearing loss, careful assessment is necessary. It is recommended that all infants be evaluated for auditory brainstem responses (ABR) during the first 6 months of life (Roizen et al, 1993). If the external ear orifice is so stenotic or there are other difficulties that preclude adequate pneumootoscopic examination, alternate methods of evaluation must be used. Tympanometry provides one useful adjunct to assessment but is not reliable in children under 1 year of age. Because of the importance of early intervention, infants between 9 and 12 months of age should be referred for microotoscopy if examination is difficult. The accumulation of cerumen leading to impacted canals is common; removal of cerumen every 6 months is recommended for children with this problem. When middle ear disease occurs, it deserves aggressive intervention and close follow-up if further developmental insult is to be prevented. Therefore a hearing evaluation should take place every 6 months until the child is 3 years old and on an annual basis thereafter (American Academy of Pediatrics, Joint Committee on Infant Hearing, 1995).

If hearing aids are required, those that fasten onto the earpiece of eyeglasses may be better than ear molds. Hearing aids dependent on ear molds are hard to fit for children who are just beginning to wear them. These children often do not like the increased sound. Parents may need help finding methods (e.g., behavior management) to help improve their child's compliance for leaving the hearing aid in place. Parents must also be cautioned to devise mnemonic cues for remembering to change the batteries routinely because it is unlikely that their child will be able to realize that the hearing aid is malfunctioning.

Dental: Because of the extremely high prevalence of dental problems in young children, aggressive dental care is necessary. Primary care providers must document and carefully follow the dental problems of these children. All children with Down syndrome should be evaluated before the age of 18 months by a dentist or pedodontist skilled in caring for children with developmental disabilities. Locating such dentists is often difficult for parents, and specific referrals to professionals may be warranted.

Good dental hygiene—including frequent brushing and flossing—is indicated to reduce the amount of periodontal disease. If good dental hygiene is difficult to achieve, using a Water Pik should be considered. Effective toothbrushing techniques may be difficult to achieve because of the child's limited manual dexterity, enlarged tongue, and small mouth. Close supervision is required, and independent toothbrushing and mouth care may not be feasible until the child is at least of preschool age.

Weaning children from a bottle by 18 months and diets that contain low-sugar, crunchy foods (e.g., fresh vegetables) also help deter dental deterioration and should be encouraged. In areas where the water supply is nonfluoridated, fluoride supplementation should be initiated. Sealants may also be necessary (Nowak, 1995). If periodontal disease is severe, chemical plaque control may be necessary. For children with congenital heart disease, prophylactic antibiotics should accompany all dental interventions (Cousineau and Lauer, 1995; Earl and Blackwelder, 1998) (see Chapter 17).

Blood pressure: Routine screening is recommended. If there is a history of cardiac disease or a positive family history of cardiac disease or hypertension, more careful assessment is required. A cardiac evaluation—including an echocardiogram, however, is warranted during infancy to rule out congenital heart disease and/or cardiac defects (Roizen, 1997).

Hematocrit: Routine screening is recommended.

Urinalysis: Routine screening is recommended.

Tuberculosis: Routine screening is recommended. No special precautions must be taken unless the child is or has been institutionalized.

Condition-Specific Screening (Box 20-4)

Thyroid dysfunction: Because the abnormalities seen in Down syndrome are similar to some seen in thyroid dysfunction, it is difficult to diagnose thyroid problems by clinical examination. Thyroid-stimulating hormone levels should be assessed at 4 to 6 months of age, again at 12 months, and annually thereafter (Committee on Genetics, 1994). If there are any signs or symptoms suggestive of thyroid dysfunction, a complete thyroid panel should be drawn.

Atlantoaxial instability: Primary care providers must appraise the risk of atlantoaxial subluxation for all children with Down syndrome who are planning to engage in physically active exercise and/or the Special Olympics or who are to undergo surgical or rehabilitative procedures (Morton et al, 1995). In general, cervical spine radiographic studies and a neurologic examination should be considered after age 2½ years (Pueschel, 1998; Roizen, 1997), as well as at 12 years and 18 years (Earl and Blackwelder, 1998).

Hip dislocation: Assessing hip stability through age 10 years is indicated because early detection (i.e., before the dislocation is fixed and acetabular dysplasia occurs) allows for optimal surgical correction. Early presenting signs of habitual dislocation are an increasing limp, decreasing activity, and an audible click. Pain does not usually occur unless the dislocation is acute. In older children, radiographic studies may be necessary for assessment.

Mitral valve prolapse: Screening should begin in adolescence. Echocardiographic evaluations are recommended before surgical or dental procedures (Roizen, 1997; Wiet et al, 1997).

Celiac Disease: Although screening is not mandatory for individuals with Down syndrome, increased attention has been brought to the incidence of celiac disease in persons with Down syndrome. IgA-antiendomysium antibodies (EMA) have been found to be a good immunologic marker in screening for this disease (Carlsson et al, 1998; George et al, 1996).

Common Illness Management

Differential Diagnosis (Box 20-5)

Immune dysfunction: The significant changes in the immune systems of children with Down syndrome have significant implications for primary care providers. Specifically, all infections must be treated aggressively because negative sequelae are more likely to develop. The incidence of many autoimmune diseases (i.e., including diabetes mellitus and juvenile rheumatoid arthritis) is also much greater in this population. If a child exhibits signs and symptoms compatible with a diagnosis of any of these diseases, a thorough evaluation is indicated. Parents must be educated about the signs and symptoms of conditions and the need to seek medical advice promptly (see Chapters 19 and 27).

Upper respiratory tract infections: Children with Down syndrome are prone to upper respiratory tract infections. These infections should be managed aggressively because untoward sequelae—including

---

Box 20-4

Screening

Karyotype

- Thyroid dysfunction
- Atlantoaxial instability
- Hip dislocations
- Congenital heart disease and defects, including mitral valve prolapse

Refractive errors and other ophthalmic disorders

- Hearing loss
- Sleep apnea
- Periodontal disease
- Celiac disease
- Behavioral and mental health issues
- Signs and symptoms of leukemia and diabetes

Box 20-5

Differential Diagnosis

- Immune dysfunction requires aggressive treatment.
- Upper respiratory tract infections are common.
- Behavioral changes may have physical cause.
- Gastrointestinal symptoms in infants may be due to congenital anomalies.
- Leukemia is 10 to 30% more likely to be acquired than in general population.

otitis media and pneumonia—are apt to develop. Children with congenital heart disease should be examined at the first signs of illness because these children are more likely to develop secondary problems and parents may confuse an upper respiratory tract infection with early congestive heart failure. These children may also need to be given subacute bacterial endocarditis prophylaxis (see Chapter 17).

Behavioral changes: Behavioral changes may be caused by a variety of physiologic and psychologic problems, including the following: (1) thyroid dysfunction, (2) obstructive sleep apnea, (3) neurodegeneration (primarily in older individuals), (4) declining physical competence (e.g., congestive heart failure), (5) disturbed home environment, and (6) overstimulation. Attention has been given to attention deficit hyperactivity disorder (ADHD) and aggressive behavior (Myers and Pueschel, 1991) (see Chapter 28). Interventions must be cause-specific. Trials with stimulants, antidepressants, or antipsychotic drugs may be indicated in some cases after a thorough evaluation.

Gastrointestinal symptoms: Because pyloric stenosis and Hirschsprung's disease are more common in children with Down syndrome, primary care providers should carefully pursue reports of persistent vomiting, constipation, or chronic diarrhea in infants. Constipation, which is a common problem, may also be related to inadequate peristalsis, poor diet, lack of exercise, or thyroid dysfunction. The cause of constipation must clearly be assessed so that the correct interventions are initiated.

Leukemia: Children with Down syndrome acquire leukemia 10 to 30 times as often as other children. Easy bruising, unusual pallor, or listlessness must be fully evaluated. Parents must be alerted to immediately seek health care for their child if any of these signs or symptoms develop.

Drug Interactions

Because children with Down syndrome are at risk for health problems affecting any organ or system of their body, they may often be taking medications. It is important that family members understand how to administer the medications, what the side effects are, and to report any allergic reactions to the primary care provider. Primary care providers should know what drug interactions could occur. For example, if a child has hyperthyroidism and is taking methimazole (Tapazole) or propylthiouracil and develops a bacterial infection, bloodwork for white blood cell and neutrophil counts must be drawn (Foley, 1995). Over-the-counter medications are often ineffective (e.g., with skin problems), and prescription medications are needed.

Developmental Issues

Sleep patterns: Sleep disorders are uncommon in children with Down syndrome, with the exception of obstructive sleep apnea and related conditions. Anatomic and immunologic differences predispose school-aged children in particular to this condition. The primary care provider should have a high index of suspicion if the child has a history of snoring, restless sleep, being awake for hours during the night, night terrors, or daytime somnolence, as well as if failure to thrive, pulmonary hypertension, or behavioral problems are present. Referral to a sleep laboratory for periodic overnight polysomnography is warranted (Carskadon, Pueschel, and Millman, 1993; Lefaivre et al, 1997). Surgical treatment can range from tonsillectomy and adenoidectomy to a combination of skeletal and soft tissue alterations (Lefaivre et al, 1997).

Toileting: The median age for toilet training children with Down syndrome is approximately 36 months. Parents must be advised of this to reduce frustrations associated with unrealistic expectations. Routine toilet training techniques are effective. It takes longer, however, to train a child with Down syndrome, and additional positive reinforcement is necessary.

Children with Down syndrome may suffer from constipation secondary to their generalized muscle flaccidity and low activity levels. Dietary corrections, occasional use of bulk laxatives, and increases in exercise can alleviate this problem.

Discipline: Children with Down syndrome are usually not more difficult to discipline than other children. Parents must be encouraged to remember that discipline needs to be appropriate for the child's developmental—not chronologic—age. Children with Down syndrome should not receive special compensation just because they have Down syndrome. Parental expectations should be consistent, and limits should be set for all children in the family. Behavior management programs can be developed for specific discipline problems when a child has not been responsive to the parents' usual methods.

Child care: Daycare should provide appropriate social, cognitive, and physical stimulation for a child with Down syndrome. When selecting the type of daycare setting, parents should be encouraged to consider the child's personality and medical needs as well as their own philosophy about inclusion. Many generic daycare centers include children with Down syndrome into their programs and are sufficiently staffed to provide an excellent experience for these children. If a child has significant medical problems, specialized daycare, which is often available through the school system, may be a better option. Primary care providers should be aware of resources in their community to assist parents with daycare placement. Local parent groups for children with Down syndrome, as well as the local affiliates of the Arc of the United States, the Association for the Care of Children's Health, and other specialty agencies may also help with placement.

If a child is highly susceptible to infections, a home care setting (i.e., with less than six children) is recommended. As with all individuals who are immunocompromised, immunizations are an important component in prevention.

Schooling: A variety of options—from total inclusion to residential placement—for academic placement exist. If circumstances permit, children with Down syndrome do best in an environment fully integrated with nondisabled peers. Children with Down syndrome, however, need support from their families while they deal with being exceptional and with social pressures from peers. Parents and teachers working together to create a supportive environment can ensure that a child has some social and academic successes. Otherwise, the child may become frustrated and demoralized, which can lead to disruptive behavior and poor self-esteem.

Families may need assistance in choosing the school setting they deem most appropriate for their child. Primary care providers can be instrumental in helping families locate appropriate community services (e.g., mental health and/or mental retardation base service units) to assist in educational placement. All children with Down syndrome are eligible for educational provisions under Public Law 105-17 (IDEA) (see Chapter 5). Parents should be encouraged to contact their social worker or local office of mental retardation shortly after the child's birth so that they can receive the educational, vocational, and supportive services for which the child is eligible.

Sexuality: Pubertal changes in adolescents with Down syndrome occur at approximately the same time as in their unaffected peers (Scola and Pueschel, 1992). Accompanying these physical changes, adolescents will have social interests and biologic drives similar to those of their chronologic-age peers and must be given the opportunity to participate in social activities with their peers. For parents who are highly protective, the social and sexual education that must accompany their child's increasing independence are often difficult and sensitive issues (Smith K, 1995). Primary care providers need to help parents recognize their responsibility in ensuring that children can handle themselves in a socially and sexually appropriate manner.

Individualized instruction about self-care skills, biologic changes, social implications, and contraception is paramount to minimizing both the appearance of sexual impropriety and the risk of being sexually exploited. Routine pelvic examination is not recommended for females who are not sexually active, and the young woman, her parents, and the primary care provider should discuss the frequency of this examination (Earl and Blackwelder, 1998). Genetic counseling for both the parents and the child is necessary. Although men are virtually always sterile, women are capable of reproducing. Planned Parenthood, the Arc of the United States, and parent support groups offer printed and audiovisual materials specifically designed for use with these families.

The age at onset of menses for females is similar to that of their mothers (Arnell et al, 1996). Handling pubertal changes is difficult for some female adolescents. Family members must be helped to recognize the behavior changes that may be related to normal hormonal cycles. For those women who are menstruating and are unable to manage their own hygienic care, parents and other caregivers must also take precautions in assisting if she is positive for hepatitis B.

Primary gonadal insufficiency may be present in males and is evidenced by small testes, a concentration of serum follicle-stimulating hormone, and a negative correlation between testicular volume and luteinizing hormone level (Arnell et al,

1996). Some parents may request that their daughter with Down syndrome be sterilized. The right to procreative choice is protected by law, and statutes regarding sterilization vary dramatically from state to state. Primary care providers are strongly suggested to consult with the state office of mental retardation for current guidelines because sterilization is illegal in some jurisdictions. Professional practice standards from the American College of Obstetricians and Gynecologists and the American Academy of Pediatrics provide ethical guidelines for this difficult issue (Committee on Bioethics, 1990). If sterilization is to be pursued, the adolescent must participate in the decision to the extent possible and state and local laws must be strictly followed.

Transition to Adulthood

The life expectancy for individuals with Down syndrome has increased dramatically. Most of these individuals are now reaching adulthood, raising many specific issues that were unaddressed, such as independent living, sexuality, vocational choices, and health maintenance.

Individuals with Down syndrome range in their abilities to live independently; some require ongoing, consistent supervision, and others merely need minimal guidance with complex tasks. Most individuals remain at home until a crisis forces different arrangements. Because individuals with Down syndrome often have aged parents, families can help plan for a smooth transition to a different living situation within the context of normal development. For example, some parents may help their son or daughter move to a group home at about the same age as their other children left for college. Recreation activities such as bowling, swimming, and dancing are encouraged because they promote social relationships and physical fitness. Registering to vote is also an important function of adulthood.

Vocational choices are directed by an individual's cognitive abilities, social skills, and adaptive abilities. Many can seek competitive employment in custodial work, offices, housekeeping, restaurants, landscaping, or other occupations where the required skills are not too difficult, fairly repetitive, and there is ongoing supervision. The skills necessary to survive in the work force (e.g., basic money management, telling time, or using public

transportation) must be mastered before such positions are sought. For others, working in sheltered workshops is a better option because this type of job requires fewer adaptive abilities.

Generally, the overall health of most individuals with Down syndrome is good, although premature aging occurs as early as age 20 with dental changes. Dermatologic, thyroid, cardiac, and sensory problems are the most troublesome and worsen with age. Changes in mental health are also a concern after children complete formal schooling at 21 years of age. The overall prevalence of psychiatric disorders is 22%, with depression and dementia being the most common (Carr, 1994). This prevalence may be a result of decreased social opportunities and lack of readily available transportation. Perhaps of greatest concern is Alzheimer's disease, which occurs in 15% to 20% of adults with Down syndrome over 40 years of age (Holland and Oliver, 1995). IQ levels also decline over time. These changes do not bode well for maintaining the self-help skills and independence that individuals with Down syndrome worked so hard to achieve during their childhood. Further longitudinal study of adults with Down syndrome—especially documentation of health status changes—is warranted.

Special Family Concerns and Resources

Parenting a child with Down syndrome can be difficult. Although Down syndrome is associated with numerous health and developmental needs, most parents meet these challenges with resilience and adaptive functioning (Cahill and Glidden, 1996). For some parents, however, raising these children can become overwhelming. Locating and coordinating acceptable medical, educational, and ancillary personnel may produce stress. Parents may spend more time providing child care and less time working and participating in social activities (Barnett and Boyce, 1995). Primary care providers may be of tremendous assistance to the families in identifying appropriate resources (e.g., respite care) and helping parents become their child's lifelong case manager. Mothers in particular may find it difficult to balance their time and responsibilities among their children and spouse. Although many concerns are similar for all families who have a child with special needs, one notable issue for families of children with Down syndrome is the need for long-range planning. Most children with Down syndrome may never become totally self-sufficient, and families must plan for a child's lifetime through, for example, estate planning and custody arrangements. They must also enroll an adult child to receive social security income (SSI). Other children with Down syndrome, however, may marry and live semiindependent lives. The severity of the child's difficulty, the internal strengths of the family, and the support from extended family and community networks all affect a family's adjustment.

Parents of children with Down syndrome will experience joy and pride in their child. They may also experience chronic sorrow. A natural response to an abnormal event, chronic sorrow is the prolonged sadness that parents may periodically experience at points throughout their child's life (Olshansky, 1962). This sorrow most commonly occurs when developmental milestones (e.g., graduating from high school) are missed (Wikler, Wascow, and Hatfield, 1981). This continued grief work is discomfiting for some parents, particularly if it is misinterpreted by professionals as pathologic grieving. Primary care providers have the unique opportunity to assist families in recognizing that chronic sorrow is a normal extension of the grieving process and that their reactions are normal and healthy.

Resources

Caring for a child with Down syndrome is a complex task because of the physical, cognitive, and social concerns that must be addressed. Additional resources for professionals and parents of children with Down syndrome are as follows:

Informational materials

Bruni M: Fine motor skills in children with Down syndrome: a guide for parents and professionals, Bethesda, Md., 1998, Woodbine House. Available from Woodbine House, 6510 Bells Mill Rd., Bethesda, Md. 20817.

Hassold TJ: Down syndrome: a promising future, together, New York, 1998, Wiley-Liss. Available from Wiley-Liss, Inc., 605 Third Ave., New York, NY 10158-0012.

Kumin L: Communication skills in children with Down syndrome: a guide for parents, Bethesda, Md., 1994, Woodbine House. Available from Woodbine House, 6510 Bells Mill Rd., Bethesda, Md. 20817.

Martino B and Pueschel SM, editors: Heart disease in persons with Down syndrome, Baltimore, Md., 1996, Paul H. Brookes. Available from Paul H. Brookes Publishing Co., PO Box 10624, Baltimore, Md. 21285-0624.

Nadel L and Rosenthal D, editors: Down syndrome: living and learning in the community, New York, 1995, Wiley-Liss. Available from Wiley-Liss, Inc., 605 Third Ave., New York, NY 10158-0012.

Oelwein PL: Teaching reading to children with Down syndrome: a guide for parents and teachers, Bethesda, Md., 1995, Woodbine House. Available from Woodbine House, 6510 Bells Mill Rd., Bethesda, Md. 20817.

Pueschel SM, editor: Parents guide to Down syndrome: toward a brighter future, Baltimore, Md., 1995, Paul H. Brookes. Available from Paul H. Brookes Publishing Co., PO Box 10624, Baltimore, Md. 21285-0624.

Pueschel SM and Sustrova M, editors: Adolescents with Down syndrome: toward a more fulfilling life, Baltimore, Md., 1997, Paul H. Brookes. Available from Paul H. Brookes Publishing Co., PO Box 10624, Baltimore, Md. 21285-0624.

Stray-Gundersen K, editor: Babies with Down syndrome: a new parents guide, ed 3, Bethesda, Md., 1995, Woodbine House. Available from Woodbine House, Inc, 6510 Bells Mill Rd., Bethesda, Md. 20817.

Van Dyke DC et al, editors: Medical and surgical care for children with Down syndrome: a guide for parents, Bethesda, Md., 1995, Woodbine House. Available from Woodbine House, 6510 Bells Mill Rd., Bethesda, Md. 20817.

Winders PC: Gross motor skills in children with Down syndrome: a guide for parents and professionals, Bethesda, Md., 1997, Woodbine House. Available from Woodbine House, 6510 Bells Mill Rd., Bethesda, Md. 20817.

Organizations

The Arc of the United States (formerly the Association for Retarded Citizens of the United States)
500 E Border Street, Suite 300
Arlington, Texas 76010
(817) 261-6003; (817) 277-3491 (fax)
thearc@metronet.com; http://TheArc.org/welcome.html

Canadian Down Syndrome Society
811-14 Street NW
Calgary, Alberta, Canada T2N 2A4
(403) 270-8500; (403) 270-8291 (fax)
Cdss@ican.net; http://home.ican.net/~cdss/

The Commission on Mental and Physical Disability Law
American Bar Association
750 N. Lake Shore Drive
Chicago, Ill. 60611
(312) 988-5000
Info@abanet.org;
http://www.abanet.org/publicserv/mental.html

National Down Syndrome Congress
7000 Peachtree-Dunwoody Road, NE
Building #5B, Suite 100
Atlanta, Ga. 30328
(800) 232-6372 (NDSC); (770) 604-9898 (fax)
ndsccenter@aol.com;
http://members.carol.net/ndsc/

National Down Syndrome Society
666 Broadway, 8th Floor
New York, NY 10012-2317
(800) 221-4602; (212) 979-2873 (fax)
Info@ndss.org; http://www.ndss.org/

Association for Children with Down Syndrome, Inc.
2616 Martin Avenue
Bellemore, NY 11710-3196
(516) 221-4700; (516) 221-5867 (fax)
info@acds.org; http://www.acds.org/

Summary of Primary Care Needs for the Child with Down Syndrome

HEALTH CARE MAINTENANCE

Growth and development

Children usually have a shorter stature and increased weight (after infancy).

Occipitofrontal circumference may be decreased.

Children should have height and weight measured at each visit and plotted on NCHS growth charts and growth charts for children with Down syndrome. Caloric reduction and increased exercise are recommended.

Virtually all children will have mentally retardation and global developmental delay.

Expressive language problems are common.

Normal progression of developmental milestones occurs but at slower rate.

Early intervention programs are recommended for older children.

Virtually all children will have hypotonia and joint laxity. Obesity compounds these complications.

Cognitive function often deteriorates with age.

Diet: Breastfeeding is encouraged in infancy. Feeding support is needed in infancy to ensure adequate weight gain.

Diets may need to be tailored to help correct constipation or obesity.

Vitamins and mineral supplementation is often recommended.

Potential for aspiration is a concern.

Safety: Anticipatory guidance needs to be based on a child's developmental—not chronologic—age.

There is increased incidence of musculoskeletal and/or joint injuries from laxity.

Atlantoaxial instability is a hazard and must be ruled out before active sports programs or surgery. Spine radiographs are usually done after 2½ years of age.

Summary of Primary Care Needs for the Child with Down Syndrome—cont'd

Immunizations: Routine immunizations are recommended.

Immunity may not be conferred from immunizations because of a compromised immune system. Titer analysis during outbreaks of communicable diseases is recommended.

Pneumococcal polysaccharide and influenza immunoprophylaxis should be considered.

Screening

Vision: The incidence of ocular defects is high. All infants should be evaluated by an ophthalmologist during infancy.

Acuity and alignment testing and examination of the red reflex and optic fundi should be done at each visit.

Hearing: Anatomical abnormalities of ears are common. Auditory brainstem response recommended in infancy. Evaluation by specialist recommended every 6 months until age 3 and then annually.

Otoscopy and tympanometry should be performed at each visit.

Cerumen impaction and otitis media are common.

50% to 76% of these children have hearing loss. Many will require hearing aids.

Dental: Dental screening should be done a minimum of every 6 months from age 18 months because of the high incidence of periodontal disease.

Good dental hygiene is important. If not in water, fluoride is recommended.

Children with CHD may require antibiotic prophylaxis to prevent endocarditis.

Blood pressure: Routine screening is recommended.

A full cardiac evaluation with echocardiogram should be done in infancy.

Hematocrit: Routine screening is recommended.

Urinalysis: Routine screening is recommended.

Tuberculosis: Routine screening is recommended.

Condition-specific screening: Use MacArthur Communicative Development Inventory to measure vocabulary development.

Obtain karyotype in neonatal period

Thyroid-stimulating hormone levels should be checked at 4 to 6 months of age and then at 12 months and yearly.

Cervical spine radiograph studies to determine atlantoaxial stability should be done after age 2½ years or before first surgery or athletic involvement. Reevaluation at 8 years, 12 years, and 18 years may be warranted.

Screening for hip dislocation is necessary through age 10 years or whenever a gait abnormality occurs.

Screening for mitral valve prolapse should start in adolescence.

Screening for celiac disease with IgA-antiendomysium antibodies should be done in symptomatic individuals.

Assess for signs and symptoms of sleep apnea, diabetes, and leukemia.

COMMON ILLNESS MANAGEMENT

Differential diagnosis

Immune dysfunction: Children with Down syndrome are more susceptible to infections and autoimmune disorders.

Upper respiratory tract infections: Upper respiratory tract infections are often associated with otitis media and pneumonia and should be managed aggressively, especially when a child has CHD.

Behavioral changes: Thyroid dysfunction, obstructive sleep apnea, neurodegeneration, declining physical competence, disturbed home environment, overstimulation, and ADHD should be ruled out.

Gastrointestinal symptoms: Pyloric stenosis, Hirschsprung's disease, inadequate peristalsis, and thyroid dysfunction should be ruled out.

Constipation is a common problem and may be due to decreased peristalsis, poor diet, lack of exercise, or thyroid dysfunction.

Continued

Summary of Primary Care Needs for the Child with Down Syndrome—cont'd

Leukemia: Unusual pallor, easy bruising, and listlessness should be fully evaluated.

Drug interactions

Children may be on different medications for different conditions, so primary care providers should be aware of drug interactions and side effects.

Developmental issues

Sleep patterns: Obstructive sleep apnea may occur; it is a problem of primarily school-aged children. Surgical intervention may be necessary. Refer for periodic overnight polysomnography if history warrants further assessment.

Toileting: Delayed bowel and bladder training may occur as a result of developmental lag; constipation is common because of low activity level, decreased peristalsis, and poor diet.

Discipline: Discipline must be developmentally appropriate; behavior management programs are often successful.

Child care: Small group daycare lessens the risk of repeated infections.

Children may be eligible for special programs through Public Law 105-17 (IDEA); infants up to 3 years of age may be eligible for early intervention programs.

Schooling: Children and youth eligible for special education services under programs most commonly used.

Sexuality: Sex education must be taught so that children with Down syndrome are not abused and do not display inappropriate sexual behaviors.

Girls may need assistance with menstrual hygiene.

Boys are usually infertile, but girls may be fertile.

Transition to adulthood: Emphasis should be on independent living, vocational skills, and health maintenance.

Mental health problems (e.g., depression and Alzheimer's disease) may be problematic.

Special family concerns

Special family concerns include long-term care and chronic sorrow.

References

Abramson PJ et al: Neck flexion and extension in children with Down syndrome: a somatosensory study, Laryngoscope 105:1209-1212, 1995.

American Academy of Pediatrics, Joint Commission on Infant Hearing: 1994 position statement, Pediatrics 95:152-156, 1995.

Amil Dias J and Walker-Smith J: Down syndrome and celiac disease, J Pediatr Gastroenterol Nutr 10:41-43, 1990.

Arnell H et al: Growth and pubertal development in Down syndrome, Acta Paediatr 85:1102-1106, 1996.

Bower CM and Richmond D: Tonsillectomy and adenoidectomy in patients with Down syndrome, Int J Pediatr Otorhinolaryngol 33:141-148, 1995.

Barnett WS and Boyce GC: Effects of children with Down syndrome on parent's activities, Am J Ment Retard 100:115-127, 1995.

Cahill BM and Glidden LM: Influence of chronic disease on family and parental functioning: Down syndrome versus other disabilities, Amer J Ment Retard 101:149-160, 1996.

Carlesimo GA, Marotta L, and Vicari S: Long-term memory in mental retardation: evidence for a specific impairment in subjects with Down's syndrome, Neuropsychologia 1: 71-79, 1997.

Carlsson A et al: Prevalence of IgA-antigliadin antibodies and IgA-antiendomysium antibodies related to celiac disease in children with Down syndrome, Pediatrics 101:272-275, 1998.

Carr J: Annotation: long-term outcome for people with Down's syndrome, J Child Psychol Psychiatr 35:425-439, 1994.

Carskadon MA, Pueschel SM, and Millman RP: Sleep-disordered breathing and behavior in three risk groups: preliminary findings from parental reports, Child's Nervous System 9:452-457, 1993.

Centers for Disease Control and Prevention: Down syndrome prevalence at birth—United States, 1983-1990, MMWR Morb Mortal Wkly Rep 43:617-622, 1994.

Cichon P, Crawford L, and Grimm W-D: Early-onset periodontitis associated with Down's syndrome: a clinical interventional study, Ann Periodontal 3:370-380, 1998.

Cohen WI, editor: Health care guidelines for individuals with Down syndrome (Down syndrome preventive medical check list), Down Syndrome Quarterly 1:1-10, 1996.

Cohen WI and Patterson B: News from the Down syndrome medical interest group, Down Syndrome Quarterly 3(3):15, 1998.

Committee on Bioethics: Sterilization of women who are mentally handicapped, Pediatrics 85:868-871, 1990.

Committee on Genetics: Health supervision for children with Down syndrome, Pediatrics 93:855-859, 1994.

Committee on Infectious Diseases: Recommended childhood immunization schedule—United States, January-December 1999, Pediatrics 103:182-185, 1999.

Committee on Sports Medicine and Fitness: Atlantoaxial instability in Down syndrome: subject review, Pediatrics 96:151-154, 1995.

Cousineau AI and Lauer RM: Heart disease and children with Down syndrome. In Van Dyke DC et al, editors: Medical and surgical care for children with Down syndrome: a guide for parents, Bethesda, Md., 1995, Woodbine House.

Cronk C et al: Growth charts for children with Down syndrome: 1 month to 18 years of age, Pediatrics 81:102-110, 1988.

Cuckle H: Rational Down syndrome screening policy, Am J Public Health 88:558-559, 1998.

deJong AL et al: Tenuous airway in children with trisomy 21, Laryngoscope 107:345-350, 1997.

Doyle JJ and Zipursky A: Down syndrome children with neonatal transient leukemia: survival and risk of subsequent myelodysplasia and leukemia, Blood 84:316a, 1994.

Earl DT and Blackwelder RB: Management of chronic medical conditions in children and adolescents, Primary Care 25:253-268, 1998.

Foley TP Jr: Thyroid conditions and other endocrine concerns in children with Down syndrome. In Van Dyke DC et al, editors: Medical and surgical care for children with Down syndrome: a guide for parents, Bethesda, Md., 1995, Woodbine House.

Frazier JB and Friedman B: Swallow function in children with Down syndrome: a retrospective study, Dev Med Child Neurol 38:695-703, 1996.

Geggel RL, O'Brien JE, and Feingold M: Development of valve dysfunction in adolescents and young adults with Down syndrome and no known congenital heart disease, J Pediatr 122:821-823, 1993.

George EK et al: High frequency of celiac disease in Down syndrome, J Pediatr 128:555-557, 1996.

Goldstein NA et al: Postoperative complications after tonsillectomy and adenoidectomy in children with Down syndrome, Arch Otolaryngol Head Neck Surg 124:171-176, 1998.

Haddow JE: Antenatal screening for Down's syndrome: where are we and where next?, Lancet 352:336-337, 1998.

Hecht CA and Hook EB: Rates of Down syndrome at livebirth at one-year maternal age intervals in studies with apparent close to complete ascertainment in populations of European origin: a proposed revised rate schedule for use in genetic and prenatal screening, Am J Med Gen 62:376-385, 1996.

Hines S and Bennett F: Effectiveness of early intervention for children with Down syndrome, Ment Retard Dev Disab Res Rev 2:96-101, 1996.

Holland AJ and Oliver C: Down's syndrome and the links with Alzheimer's disease, J Neurol Neurosurg Psychiatr 59:111-114, 1995.

Ivarsson S-A et al: The impact of thyroid autoimmunity in children and adolescents with Down syndrome, Acta Paediatr 86:1065-1067, 1997.

Jones KL: Smith's recognizable patterns of human malformation, ed 5, Philadelphia, 1997, Saunders.

Kavanaugh KT: Ear, nose, and sinus conditions of children with Down syndrome. In Van Dyke DC et al, editors: Medical and surgical care for children with Down syndrome: a guide for parents, Bethesda, Md., 1995, Woodbine House.

Kodish E and Cutler L: Ethical issues in emerging new treatments such as growth hormone therapy for children with Down syndrome and Prader-Willi syndrome, Curr Op Pediatr 8:401-405, 1996.

Kumin L: Speech and language skills in children with Down syndrome, Ment Retard Dev Disab Res Rev 2:109-115, 1996.

Lang DJ et al: Hypospadias and urethral abnormalities in Down syndrome, Clin Pediatr 26:40-42, 1987.

Lange BJ et al: Distinctive demography, biology, and outcome of acute myeloid leukemia and myelodysplastic syndrome in children with Down syndrome: children's cancer group studies 2861 and 2891, Blood 91:608-615, 1998.

Lashley FR: Clinical genetics in nursing practice, ed 2, New York, 1998, Springer.

Lawhon SM: Orthopedic issues affecting children with Down syndrome. In Van Dyke DC et al, editors: Medical and surgical care for children with Down syndrome: a guide for parents, Bethesda, Md., 1995, Woodbine House.

Lefaivre J-F et al: Down syndrome: identification and surgical management of obstructive sleep apnea, Plast Reconstr Surg 99:629-637, 1997.

Luke A et al: Nutrient intake and obesity in prepubescent children with Down syndrome, J Am Diet Assoc 96:1262-1267, 1996.

Luke AH et al: Energy expenditure in Down syndrome, J Pediatr 125:829-836, 1994.

Mahon M: The nurse's role in treatment decision making for the child with disabilities, Issues Law Med 6:247-268, 1990.

Marcus CL et al: Obstructive sleep apnea in children with Down syndrome, Pediatrics 88:132-139, 1991.

Marino B and Pueschel SM, editors: Heart diseases in persons with Down syndrome, Baltimore, Md., 1996, Paul H. Brookes.

Mattheis P: Neurology of children with Down syndrome. In Van Dyke DC et al, editors: Medical and surgical care for children with Down syndrome: a guide for parents, Bethesda, Md., 1995, Woodbine House.

Miller JF, Sedley AL, and Miolo G: Validity of parent report measures of vocabulary development for children with Down syndrome, J Speech Hear Res 38:1037-1044, 1995.

Morinushi T, Lopatin DE, and Van Poperin N: The relationship between gingivitis and the serum antibodies to the microbiota associated with peridontal disease in children with Down's syndrome, J Peridontal 68:626-631, 1997.

Morton RE et al: Atlantoaxial instability in Down's syndrome: a 5-year follow up study, Arch Dis Child 72:115-119, 1995.

Mundy P et al: Nonverbal communication and early language acquisition in children with Down syndrome and in normally development children, J Speech Hear Res 38:157-167, 1995.

Myers BA and Pueschel SM: Psychiatric disorders in persons with Down syndrome, J Nerv Ment Dis 179:609-613, 1991.

Nowak AJ: Dental concerns of children with Down syndrome. In Van Dyke DC et al, editors: Medical and surgical care for children with Down syndrome: a guide for parents, Bethesda, Md., 1995, Woodbine House.

Olshansky S: Chronic sorrow: a response to having a mentally defective child, Soc Casework 43:190-193, 1962.

Palmer CGS et al: Head circumference of children with Down syndrome (0 to 36 months), Am J Med Genet 42:61-67, 1992.

Pueschel SM: Growth hormone response after administration of L-dopa, clonidine, and growth hormone releasing hormone in children with Down syndrome, Res Devel Disabil 14:291-298, 1993.

Pueschel SM: The child with Down syndrome. In Levine MD, Carey WB, and Crocker AC, editors: Developmental-behavioral pediatrics, ed 2, Philadelphia, 1992, Saunders.

Pueschel SM: Should children with Down syndrome be screened for atlantoaxial instability?, Arch Pediatr Adolesc Med 152:123-125, 1998.

Pueschel SM and Pueschel JK, editors: Biomedical concerns in persons with Down syndrome, Baltimore, Md., 1992, Paul H. Brookes.

Pueschel SM, Scola FH, and Pezzullo JC: A longitudinal study of atlanto-dens relationships in asymptomatic individuals with Down syndrome, Pediatrics 89:1194-1198, 1992.

Reller MD and Morris CD: Is Down syndrome a risk factor for poor outcome after repair of congenital heart defects?, J Pediatr 132:738-741, 1998.

Rogers PT, Roizen NJ, and Capone GT: Down syndrome. In Capute AJ and Accardo PJ, editors: Developmental disabilities in infancy and childhood, vol. II: the spectrum of developmental disabilities, ed 2, Baltimore, Md., 1996, Paul H. Brookes.

Roizen NJ: Down syndrome. In Batshaw ML, editor: Children with disabilities, ed 4, Baltimore, Md., 1997, Paul H. Brookes.

Roizen NJ, Mets MB, and Blondis TA: Ophthalmic disorders in children with Down syndrome, Dev Med Child Neurol 36:594-600, 1994.

Roizen NJ et al: Hearing loss in children with Down syndrome, J Pediatr 123:S9-S12, 1993.

Satge D et al: An excess of testicular germ cell tumors in Down's syndrome: three case reports and a review of the literature, Cancer 80:929-935, 1997.

Scola PS and Pueschel SM: Menstrual cycles and basal body temperature curves in women with Down syndrome, Obstet Gynecol 79:91-94, 1992.

Serra-Prat M et al: Trade-offs in prenatal detection of Down syndrome, Am J Public Health 88:558-559, 1998.

Sharav T: Aging gametes in relation to incidence, gender, and twinning in Down syndrome, Am J Med Genetics 39:116-118, 1991.

Shen JJ et al: Cytogenic and molecular studies of Down syndrome individuals with leukemia, Am J Hum Genet 56:915-925, 1995.

Smith CS: Immune system concerns for children with Down syndrome. In Van Dyke DC et al, editors: Medical and surgical care for children with Down syndrome: a guide for parents, Bethesda, Md., 1995, Woodbine House.

Smith K et al: The role of the pediatric nurse practitioner in educating teens with mental retardation about sex, J Pediatr Health 9:59-66, 1995.

Stafstrom CE and Konkol RJ: Infantile spasms in children with Down syndrome, Dev Med Child Neurol 36:576-585, 1994.

Staples AJ et al: Epidemiology of Down syndrome in South Australia, 1960-1989, Am J Hum Genet 49:1014-1024, 1991.

Troiano RP et al: Overweight prevalence and trends for children and adolescents, Arch Pediatr Adolesc Med 149:1085-1091, 1995.

Van Dyke DC: Alternative and unconventional therapies in children with Down syndrome. In Van Dyke DC et al, editors: Medical and surgical care for children with Down syndrome: a guide for parents, Bethesda, Md., 1995, Woodbine House.

Wells GL et al: Congenital heart disease in infants with Down's syndrome, South Med J 87:724-727, 1994.

Wiet GJ et al: Surgical correction of obstructive sleep apnea in the complicated pediatric patient documented by polysomnography, Int J Pediatr Otorhinolaryngol 41:133-143, 1997.

Wikler L, Wascow M, and Hatfield E: Chronic sorrow revisited: parent and professional depiction of adjustment of parents of mentally retarded children, Am J Orthopsychiatry 51:63-67, 1981.

Wong V and Ho D: Ocular abnormalities in Down syndrome: an analysis of 140 Chinese children, Pediatr Neurol 16:311-314, 1997.

Zipursky A: The treatment of children with acute megakaryoblastic leukemia who have Down syndrome, J Pediatr Hematol Oncol 18:10-12, 1996.

Zipursky A, Poon A, and Doyle J: Leukemia in Down syndrome: a review, Pediatr Hematol Oncol 9:139-149, 1992.

Zubillaga P et al: Down syndrome and celiac disease, J Pediatr Gastroenterol Nutr 16:168-171, 1993.

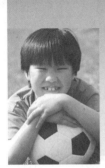

CHAPTER 21

Epilepsy

Judith A. Farley and Marion McEwan

Etiology

Epilepsy is a chronic condition defined by the *repeated* occurrence of seizure activity. Seizures are the abnormal discharge of electric activity within the brain. When a sufficient number of neurons become overexcited, they discharge abnormally. This activity may or may not display clinical manifestations. If clinical manifestations occur, the specific physical activity displayed depends on the origin of the electric activity and its expanse within the brain. Epilepsy may be the result of either an underlying disorder of the central nervous system (CNS) or a disorder that directly or indirectly affects the normal function of the central nervous system. The true cause of epilepsy often remains unknown.

Certain types of epilepsy have a familial predisposition and/or a genetic component. Congenital structural anomalies of the CNS may also cause epilepsy. In the prenatal period, fetal infections, trauma, and maternal diseases have also been identified as precipitating factors of epilepsy (American Association of Neuroscience Nurses, [AANN], 1996; Wolf, Ochoa, and Conway, 1998).

During the first month of life, asphyxia, intracranial hemorrhage, trauma, electrolyte imbalances, and inborn metabolic errors are all thought to be potential causes of epilepsy. Primary infections of the CNS—including encephalitis and meningitis—or systemic infections resulting in persistent high fever have also been implicated as causative factors. Infants born to drug-addicted mothers may withdraw during the neonatal period resulting in frequent reoccurring seizure activity (AANN, 1996; Stafstrom, 1998; Wolf, Ochoa, and Conway, 1998).

The etiology of epilepsy in children over a year old is generally the same as in infants during the first month of life. In addition to the conditions already discussed, this population may present with acute neurologic disorders or chronic conditions that have continued from earlier in life. These conditions may include infections, trauma, intracranial neoplasms, and degenerative disorders, all of which are associated with epilepsy (AANN, 1996; Stafstrom, 1998).

Incidence

The incidence of epilepsy varies greatly with age. The incidence is greatest in children up to 1 year of age, averaging approximately 1 per 1000 in the United States (Epilepsy Foundation of America, 1998). Infants are particularly susceptible to developing epilepsy during the first 12 months of life, but this incidence decreases with age. Of all epilepsy cases, 50% initially occur before 25 years of age with 20% of the cases initially occurring within the first 5 years of life. Approximately 125,000 individuals in the United States are newly affected each year (Epilepsy Foundation of America, 1998; Hauser, 1994).

Clinical Manifestations at Time of Diagnosis

Clinical manifestations at diagnosis depend on the primary cause and the extent and involvement of abnormal electric discharges within neuronal tissue (Box 21-1). Because of the diversities and complexities displayed in seizure activity, the International Seizure Classification System was adopted in 1970 and later revised in 1981 (Table 21-1). This classification system groups seizures that have similar clinical presentations. The general purposes of the classification system are to assist the health care provider with the assessment of the clinical course, to institute appropriate treatment, and to

---

Box 21-1

Clinical Manifestations

- International Seizure Classification System
  - Partial seizures
    - Simple partial seizures
    - Complex partial seizures
  - Generalized seizures
  - Unclassified epileptic seizures
  - Status epilepticus

- Epileptic Syndromes
  - Infantile spasms
  - Lennox-Gestaut syndrome
  - Juvenile myoclonic epilepsy

---

evaluate the individual's response to therapy (Gastaut, 1970; Stafstrom, 1998; Wolf, Ochoa, and Conway, 1998).

Three major classifications within the international system of epilepsy are as follows: (1) partial seizures, (2) generalized seizures, and (3) unclassified epileptic seizures. Each major grouping is divided into subsets based on clinical manifestations and electroencephalographic (EEG) findings.

Partial seizures are characterized by seizure activity that begins in and is usually limited to one part of either the left or right cerebral hemisphere. A *simple partial seizure* refers to seizure activity that occurs without loss of consciousness. A *complex partial seizure* refers to seizure activity that occurs with impairment or alteration in level of consciousness. The clinical activity is contingent on which part of the cortex generates the activity. For example, partial seizures may result in either abnormal activity (e.g., focal muscle-twitching and loss of tone) or sensory changes (e.g., tingling and numbness) (Stafstrom, 1998).

In general, a simple partial seizure is confined to one cerebral hemisphere, whereas a complex partial seizure involves both hemispheres. A partial seizure (i.e., either simple or complex) may evolve into a generalized tonic-clonic, tonic, or clonic convulsion (see Table 21-1) (Stafstrom, 1998; Wolf, Ochoa, and Conway, 1998).

Generalized seizures are those in which the first clinical manifestations indicate that the seizure activity starts or involves both cerebral hemi-

spheres. In this type of seizure, consciousness is impaired. The clinical manifestations may present as convulsive activity, although others (e.g., absence seizures, which are typically characterized by staring) have nonconvulsive activity. Because both hemispheres are involved, the clinical manifestations are almost always bilateral (see Table 21-1).

Not all seizure disorders fit neatly into a classified grouping. Such seizures are referred to as **unclassified epileptic seizures** and characteristically have a wide variety of abnormal clinical activity (e.g., rhythmic eye movements, chewing, and swimming movements). These activities are commonly seen in neonatal seizures (Pellock, 1998).

Status epilepticus is defined as the state of continuing or recurring seizure activity in which recovery between seizures is incomplete. The seizure activity is unrelenting and usually lasts for 30 minutes or more. Any classified seizure activity can evolve into status epilepticus. The state of status epilepticus is considered a medical emergency and requires immediate intervention (AANN, 1996; Scott, 1998; Tasker, 1998; Wolf, Ochoa, and Conway, 1998).

In addition to the seizures classified by the international system, several types of **epileptic syndromes** also exist. These are seizure disorders that display a *group* of signs and symptoms that collectively characterize or indicate a particular condition. An additional classification system of these syndromes has been proposed by the International League Against Epilepsy. This classification system was revised in 1989 (Box 21-2) (Dreifuss et al, 1985; International League Against Epilepsy, 1989). Several syndromes that are associated with epilepsy occur in infants and children. Three syndromes that occur most often are infantile spasms, Lennox-Gastaut syndrome, and juvenile myoclonic epilepsy.

Infantile spasms are a form of epilepsy characterized by a variety of clinical manifestations. Infants may present with episodes of sudden flexion or extension movements involving the neck, trunk, and extremities. The resulting spasms may range in presentation from subtle head nods to violent body contractions (i.e., jackknife seizures). The onset of infantile spasms is usually between 3 and 12 months of age. These spasms may be idiopathic or occur in response to a CNS insult. An EEG will display a classic hypsarrhythmia pattern of epileptic spike and wave discharges on a slow, disorga-

Table 21-1
International Classification System

I. Partial (Focal, Local) Seizures

Partial seizures are those in which the first clinical and electroencephalographic (EEG) changes generally indicate initial activation of a system of neurons limited to part of one cerebral hemisphere. A partial seizure is classified primarily on the basis of whether or not consciousness is impaired during the attack. When consciousness is not impaired, the seizure is classified as a simple partial seizure. When consciousness is impaired, the seizure is classified as a complex partial seizure. Impairment of consciousness may be the first clinical sign, or simple partial seizures may evolve into complex partial seizures. In patients with impaired consciousness, aberrations of behavior (i.e., automatisms) may occur. A partial seizure may not terminate but instead progress to a generalized motor seizure. Impaired consciousness is defined as the inability to respond normally to exogenous stimuli by virtue of altered awareness and/or responsiveness.

There is considerable evidence that simple partial seizures usually have unilateral hemispheric involvement and rarely have bilateral hemispheric involvement; complex partial seizures, however, often have bilateral hemispheric involvement.

Partial seizures can be classified into one of the following three fundamental groups:
- Simple partial seizures.
- Complex partial seizures:
  With impairment of consciousness at onset.
  Simple partial onset followed by impairment of consciousness.
- Partial seizures evolving to generalized tonic-clonic convulsions:
  Simple evolving to generalized tonic-clonic convulsions.
  Complex evolving to generalized tonic-clonic convulsions (including those with simple partial onset).

Clinical Seizure Type	EEG Seizure Type

A. Simple partial seizures (consciousness not impaired)
  1. With motor signs
    (a) Focal motor without march
    (b) Focal motor with march (jacksonian)
    (c) Versive
    (d) Postural
    (e) Phonatory (vocalization or arrest of speech)
  2. With somatosensory or special-sensory symptoms (e.g., simple hallucinations: tingling, light flashes, buzzing)
    (a) Somatosensory
    (b) Visual
    (c) Auditory
    (d) Olfactory
    (e) Gustatory
    (f) Vertiginous
  3. With autonomic symptoms or signs (including epigastric sensation, pallor, sweating, flushing, piloerection, and pupillary dilation)
  4. With psychic symptoms (i.e., disturbance of higher cerebral function); these symptoms rarely occur without impairment of consciousness and are much more commonly experienced as complex partial seizures
    (a) Dysphasic
    (b) Dysmnesic (e.g., déjà vu)
	Local contralateral discharge starting over the corresponding area of cortical representation (not always recorded on the scalp)

Continued

Table 21-1
International Classification System—cont'd

Clinical Seizure Type	EEG Seizure Type
(c) Cognitive (e.g., dreamy states, distortions of time sense) (d) Affective (e.g., fear, anger, etc.) (e) Illusions (e.g., macropsia) (f) Structured hallucinations (e.g., music, scenes)	
B. Complex partial seizures (with impairment of consciousness; may sometimes begin with simple symptoms) 1. Simple partial onset followed by impairment of consciousness (a) With simple partial features, followed by impaired consciousness (b) With automatisms 2. With impairment of consciousness at onset (a) With impairment of consciousness only (b) With automatisms	Unilateral or, frequently, bilateral discharge; diffuse or focal in temporal or frontotemporal regions
C. Partial seizures evolving to secondarily generalized seizures (may be generalized tonic-clonic, tonic, or clonic) 1. Simple partial seizures *(A)* evolving to generalized seizures 2. Complex partial seizures *(B)* evolving to generalized seizures 3. Simple partial seizures evolving to complex seizures evolving to generalized seizures	Discharges listed earlier become secondarily and rapidly generalized

II. Generalized Seizures (Convulsive or Nonconvulsive)

Generalized seizures are those in which the first clinical changes indicate initial involvement of both hemispheres. Consciousness may be impaired, which may be the initial manifestation. Motor manifestations are bilateral. The ictal EEG patterns are initially bilateral and presumably reflect neuronal discharge that is widespread in both hemispheres.

Clinical Seizure Type	EEG Seizure Type
A. Absence seizures 1. Typical absence seizures (a) Impairment of consciousness only (b) With mild clonic components (c) With atonic components	Usually regular and symmetric 3-Hz, but may be 2 to 4-Hz, spike-and-slow-wave complexes; may have multiple spike-and-slow-wave complexes; abnormalities bilateral

nized background (Lombroso, 1983; Pellock, 1998). Infantile spasms manifest a typical clinical course. The spasms usually occur in clusters as frequent as 5 to 150 times a day and are usually worse when waking or falling asleep. Once the spasms begin, the seizure activity increases in intensity and severity over time. There is invariably a loss of developmental milestones with infantile spasms (Pellock, 1998).

Lennox-Gastaut syndrome is characterized by an onset of seizures early in childhood, usually around 1 to 5 years of age. This epileptic syndrome presents with a variety of generalized seizures, in which predominantly tonic-clonic, atonic (i.e., drop attacks), akinetic, absent, and myoclonic activity are seen. Mental retardation and delayed psychomotor development are often associated with Lennox-Gastaut syndrome (Pellock, 1998).

Table 21-1
International Classification System—cont'd

Clinical Seizure Type	EEG Seizure Type

(d) With tonic components
(e) With automatisms
(f) With autonomic components (*b-f* may be used alone or in combination)
2. Atypical absence seizures, which may have:
  (a) Changes in tone that are more pronounced
  (b) Onset and/or cessation that is not abrupt
	EEG more heterogeneous; may include irregular spike-and-slow-wave complexes, fast activity or other paroxysmal activity; abnormalities bilateral but often irregular and asymmetric

B. Myoclonic seizures (single or multiple myoclonic jerks)	Polyspike and wave or sometimes spike and wave or sharp and slow waves
C. Clonic seizures	Fast activity (e.g., ≥10 c/sec) and slow waves; occasional spike-and-wave patterns
D. Tonic seizures	Low voltage fast activity, a fast rhythm of 9 to 10 c/sec, or more decreasing in frequency and increasing in amplitude
E. Tonic-clonic seizures	Rhythm at ≥10 c/sec, decreasing in frequency and increasing in amplitude during tonic phase, interrupted by slow waves during clonic phase
F. Atonic seizures (astatic) (combinations of the above may occur, e.g., *B* and *F, B* and *D*)	Polyspikes and waves or flattening or low-voltage fast activity

III. Unclassified Epileptic Seizures

These include all seizures that cannot be classified because of inadequate or incomplete data and some that defy classification in hitherto described categories. They include some neonatal seizures (e.g., rhythmic eye movements, chewing, and swimming movements).

IV. Addendum

Repeated epileptic seizures occur under a variety of circumstances:
1. As fortuitous attacks, coming unexpectedly and without any apparent provocation.
2. As cyclic attacks, at more or less regular intervals (e.g., in relation to the menstrual cycle, or the sleep-waking cycle).
3. As attacks provoked by nonsensory factors (e.g., fatigue, alcohol, emotion, etc.) or sensory factors, (i.e., sometimes referred to as "reflex seizures").

The term status epilepticus is used whenever a seizure persists for a sufficient length of time or is repeated often enough that recovery between attacks does not occur. Status epilepticus may be divided into partial (e.g., jacksonian) or generalized (e.g., absence status or tonic-clonic status). When very localized motor status occurs, it is referred to as "epilepsia partialis continua."

Adapted from Bancaud J et al: Proposal for revising clinical electroencephalographic classification of epileptic seizures, Epilepsia 22:489-501, 1981.

Juvenile myoclonic epilepsy is a primary generalized epilepsy that usually affects adolescents and young adults. This form of epilepsy is relatively benign, involving myoclonic jerks of neck, shoulders, and arms. The seizures may occur singularly or repetitively. Juvenile myoclonic epilepsy is usually associated with a normal neurologic exam, normal intelligence, and a positive family history of seizures (Pellock, 1998).

Treatment (Box 21-3)

Specific treatment for epilepsy is directed at particular clinical manifestations or the syndrome of seizure activity and its underlying causes. Several other factors must be considered in addition to the clinical manifestations presented at the time of diagnosis. The history and examination, which covers the child's physical and developmental activities, provide invaluable in-

---

Box 21-2

International League Against Epilepsy Classification of Epilepsies and Epileptic Syndromes

1. Localization-related (i.e., focal, local, partial) epilepsies and syndromes
1.1 Idiopathic (with age-related onset)
The following syndromes are established, but more may be identified in the future:
Benign childhood epilepsy with centrotemporal spike
Childhood epilepsy with occipital paroxysms
Primary reading epilepsy
1.2 Symptomatic
Chronic progressive epilepsia partialis continua of childhood (i.e., Kojewnikow's syndrome)
Syndromes characterized by seizures with specific modes of precipitation
1.3 Cryptogenic
Presumed to be symptomatic; etiology unknown
2. Generalized epilepsies and syndromes
2.1 Idiopathic (with age-related onset; listed in order of age)
Benign neonatal familial convulsions
Benign neonatal convulsions
Benign myoclonic epilepsy in infancy
Childhood absence epilepsy (i.e., pyknolepsy)
Juvenile absence epilepsy
Juvenile myoclonic epilepsy (i.e., impulsive petit mal)
Epilepsy with grand mal seizures on wakening
Other generalized idiopathic epilepsies not already defined
Epilepsies with seizures precipitated by specific modes of activation
2.2 Cryptogenic or symptomatic (in order of age)
West's syndrome (e.g., infantile spasms, Blitz-Nick-Salaam Krämpfe)
Lennox-Gastaut syndrome
Epilepsy with myoclonic-astatic seizures
Epilepsy with myoclonic absences
2.3 Symptomatic
2.3.1 Nonspecific etiology

Early myoclonic encephalopathy
Early infantile epileptic encephalopathy with suppression burst
Other symptomatic generalized epilepsies not already defined
2.3.2 Specific syndromes
Epileptic seizures may complicate many disease states; under this heading are diseases in which seizures are the presenting or predominant feature
3. Epilepsies and syndromes undetermined—whether focal or generalized
3.1 With both generalized and focal seizures
Neonatal seizures
Severe myoclonic epilepsy in infancy
Epilepsy with continuous spike-waves during slow-wave sleep
Acquired epileptic aphasia (i.e., Landau-Kleffner syndrome)
Other undetermined epilepsies not already defined
3.2 Without unequivocal generalized or focal features; all cases with generalized tonic-clonic seizures in which clinical EEG findings do not permit classification as clearly generalized or localization related (e.g., in many cases of sleep-grand mal) are considered not to have unequivocal generalized or focal features
4. Special syndromes
4.1 Situations-related seizures (e.g., Gelegenheitsanfälle)
Febrile convulsions
Isolated seizures or isolated status epilepticus
Seizures occurring only when there is an acute metabolic or toxic event caused by such factors as alcohol, drugs, eclampsia, nonketotic, hyperglycemia

Adapted from Commission on Classification and Terminology of the International League Against Epilepsy: Epilepsia 30:389-399, 1989.

---

formation necessary to combine the multitude of pieces that contribute to the diagnosis. The child's birth history and record of milestone achievements must be explored along with a family history of seizures. Reports of presenting signs and symptoms (e.g., associated factors: fever or head trauma) are important considerations for primary care providers. Evaluation and testing include an EEG to isolate the focus or origin and involvement of seizure activity in the brain, and a computerized tomography (CT) scan and a magnetic resonance imaging (MRI) of the brain to investigate the presence of a lesion or abnor-

---

Box 21-3

Treatment

- Need for thorough assessment
- Complete data base
- Evaluation may include:
  - EEG
  - CT scan
  - MRI scan
  - PET scan
  - SPECT scan
  - Metabolic workup
- Therapies
  - Pharmacologic therapy (see Table 21-2)
    - Focal resective surgery
    - Hemispherectomy
    - Considered for intractable hemispheric disease
    - Corpus callosotomy
    - Vagal nerve stimulation
  - Ketogenic diet

---

mal tissue. Finally, a complete metabolic workup must be reviewed to explore the possibility of a deficiency or malabsorption (Pellock, 1998).

Treatment usually begins with anticonvulsant medications (Table 21-2). The epileptic pattern and clinical course often require more than one drug to control the abnormal discharges. The child's age, classification of seizures, medication side effects, and compliance must all be considered when deciding on a medication regimen (Pellock, 1998; Wolf, Ochoa, and Conway, 1998).

Surgery is also a treatment for some forms of epilepsy. As with medical interventions, surgery for epilepsy is directed at the particular clinical manifestations of seizure activity, the EEG findings, and the underlying causes. If a site of origin or a seizure focus is identified, it may be possible to remove this area of the brain, thus eliminating seizure activity with little or no neurologic impairment. Certain forms of partial seizure disorders can be treated successfully with focal resective surgery (Pellock, 1998; Reynolds, 1998).

The surgical removal or disconnection of a cerebral hemisphere is a treatment for children with unilateral hemispheric disease and medically intractable epilepsy. Total or partial hemispherectomy may be performed to control localized epileptic conditions that are extremely complex and have a profound effect on a child's activities and life

span (Pellock, 1998; Reynolds 1998; Wyllie et al, 1998).

Corpus callosotomy is another neurosurgical treatment used to help control generalized seizures (i.e., involving both hemispheres) that are medically intractable. The corpus callosum is basically the connecting bridge between the right and left hemisphere. In this classification of epilepsy, the abnormal electric discharge begins in one hemisphere and then crosses over the corpus callosum to the opposite hemisphere, thereby creating a generalized response. Corpus callosotomy partially or completely severs this connecting bridge. The main objective of this treatment is to stop or decrease generalized seizure activity. A palliative procedure, it is done in an effort to minimize physical injury that may occur during seizure activity and decrease the need for anticonvulsant medications (Spencer and Spencer, 1989).

Vagal nerve stimulation is a recently approved treatment for controlling intractable seizures. This treatment is indicated for individuals with partial or generalized seizures who are not responding to medication or are not candidates for epilepsy surgery. It is used in conjunction with antiepileptic medications (Snively, 1998).

An impulse generator is implanted under the skin of the left upper chest. Tunneled electrode wires are attached to the left vagus nerve in the neck. The generator is programmed to deliver intermittent stimulation to the nerve. The device may also be activated by the child or caregiver when an aura is experienced.

Adverse effects include coughing, hoarseness, tingling, shortness of breath, nausea, and dysphagia. The device has been used in children as young as 4 years of age (McLachlan, 1997).

The ketogenic diet is a form of treatment for certain types of medically intractable epilepsies. This diet consists of foods high in fat and low in carbohydrate and protein. The exact therapeutic mechanism is not completely known. It is thought, however, that the ketone bodies produced by this diet may have an antiepileptic effect. The ketogenic diet has been shown to improve seizure management for children with seizures that are difficult to control. In some cases it is more effective than many of the new antiepileptic drugs (AEDs). Both surgical and nutritional interventions almost always require concurrent medical treatment with antiepileptic drugs.

Table 21-2
Commonly Used Antiepileptic Drugs*

Drug	Dosage/Interval	Therapeutic Plasma Level	Seizure Type	Common Side Effects	Adverse Side Effects
ACTH	Begin 40 units IM qd (taper gradually) Treatment course 2-4 mo		Infantile spasm	Hypertension Gastrointestinal distress Weight gain Electrolyte disturbance	Infection Gastrointestinal bleeding Sodium retention
Clonazapam (Klonopin)	0.1-0.2 mg/kg tid	0.01-0.08	Absence Generalized tonic-clonic Myoclonic Simple partial Complex partial	Drowsiness Ataxia Gastrointestinal distress	Behavioral changes Hyperactivity Cognitive dysfunction
Valproic acid (Depakote)	30-60 mg/kg qid	40-150	Absence Generalized tonic-clonic Myoclonic Simple partial Complex partial	Nausea and/or vomiting Fatigue with initiation of treatment Hair loss	Thrombocytopenia Pancreatitis Hepatic dysfunction Liver toxicity
Primidone (Mysoline)	10-25 mg/kg/day 3-4 times/day	5-12†	Tonic-clonic Complex partial Simple partial	Drowsiness Hyperactivity Ataxia Behavior changes	Oversedation Behavioral disturbances Gastrointestinal dysfunction
Phenytoin (Dilantin)	4-8 mg/kg bid	10-20	Generalized tonic-clonic Simple partial Complex partial	Gingival hyperplasia	Lethargy; ataxia; dizziness Skin reaction (rash) Hepatic dysfunction Rash
Phenobarbitol	2-4 mg/kg qd; bid	15-40	Generalized tonic-clonic Myoclonic Simple partial Complex partial	Fatigue with initiation of treatment Hyperactivity Mood changes Irritability	Lethargy Learning difficulties Behavioral changes Hepatic dysfunction Leukopenia

Drug	Dosage	Therapeutic level	Indications	Side effects	Serious side effects
Carbamazepine (Tegretol)	10-30 mg/kg tid; qid	6-12	Generalized tonic-clonic Simple partial Complex partial	Drowsiness Ataxia; dizziness Gastrointestinal distress Irritability	Movement disorders Rashes Hepatic dysfunction Bone marrow suppression
Felbamate (Felbatol)	15-45 mg/kg bid-tid	37-54	Refractory epilepsy Lennox-Gastaut	Anorexia/weight loss Insomnia	Aplastic anemia Hepatic toxicity Mood/behavior changes
Gabapentin (Neurontin)	10-40 mg/kg/day tid		Partial Secondary generalized Benign rolandic epilepsy	Somnolence Fatigue Dizziness Ataxia	
Lamotrigine (Lamictal)	2-15 mg/kg/day‡ bid		Partial Lennox-Gastaut Infantile spasms Encephalopathic epilepsy	Rash Headache Dizziness Nausea	Hypersensitivity
Topiramate (Topamax)	1 mg/kg/day initial‡ 5-9 mg/kg/day ÷ bid§		Partial Generalized Lennox-Gastaut	Dizziness Fatigue Diplopia Anorexia/weight loss	Word finding difficulty Renal stones
Tiagabine (Gabatril)	4-32 mg/kg‡§ bid		Partial	Dizziness Ataxia Somnolence	
Vigabatrin (Sabril)	40-100 mg/kg/day‖ bid		Partial Infantile spasms Generalized	Sedation Increased appetite	Behavior changes Psychosis Visual field constriction

Modified from Physicians desk reference, ed 52, Montvale, NJ, 1998, Medical Economics Co.
Drug information modified from Appleton 1996, Barron and Hunt 1997, Bourgeois 1996, Holmes 1997, Pellock 1997.
*ACTH, adrenocorticotropic hormone; IM, intramuscular; qd, every day; tid, 3 times daily; qid, 4 times daily; bid, twice daily.
†When testing mysoline levels, always check phenobarbital levels as well.
‡Dose is gradually increased to evaluate for side effects.
§Unpublished data.
‖Not currently approved for use in United States

Recent and Anticipated Advances in Diagnosis and Management

There have been significant advances in the diagnosis and subsequent management of pediatric epilepsy. In general, diagnosis and treatment are directed at the underlying cause. Recent advances in medical technology with EEG studies and neuroimaging support this primary objective. Surgical placement of electrodes directly on the cortex helps obtain diagnostic information to localize the seizure origin. The continued development and refinement of high-resolution magnetic resonance imagery (MRI), positron emission tomography (PET), and single photon emission computed tomography (SPECT) have led to the early identification of underlying pathologies that may have previously gone undetected. Major advances in genetics have allowed researchers to examine the genetic basis for several epilepsies.

Results from diagnostic studies and data lead to the enhancement of treatment options and opportunities for individuals with epilepsy. Genetic counseling, advances in surgical procedures and interventions, and development and introduction of new and challenging antiepileptic medications are all additional considerations for future developments and outcomes.

Associated Problems (Box 21-4)

The etiology, age of onset, type of seizures, frequency of occurrence, and success of treatment influence problems related to epilepsy.

Injury During Seizures

Injury during seizure activity is always possible. A child may sustain direct trauma or may fall or aspirate during a seizure. It is therefore vital for parents, primary care providers, and teachers to be knowledgeable about the appropriate first aid to minimize injury during a seizure (Box 21-5).

Cognitive Dysfunction

Children with epilepsy may also present with various cognitive dysfunctions. In general, the intelli-

---

Box 21-4

Associated Problems

- Vary according to etiology
- Injury secondary to seizures
- Cognitive dysfunction
- Psychiatric problems

Box 21-5

First Aid for Seizure Management

The following is a guide for first aid in the event of a generalized seizure. Parents, teachers, and caretakers must know these steps to follow in the event of such an occurrence:

- It is important to lower the child to the floor or leave the child where he or she is when the seizure begins.
- Be careful to move any objects in the area away from the child to prevent injury. Cushion the child's head from the floor with a pillow or soft barrier.
- Turn and keep the child on his or her side to prevent aspiration. It is very important NOT to attempt to put anything in the child's mouth because this can actually cause injury or further damage (e.g., a broken tooth or a bite to the individual providing aid).
- Loosen tight, restrictive clothing on the child that may be too confining and cause further injury (e.g., a buttoned shirt collar or tie). Clear the location of objects that may cause further injury to flailing extremities.
- Stay with the child and do not restrain movements.
- Try to remain calm.
- When the seizure clears, the child may be sleepy or confused. Allow for adequate rest after the seizure finishes.
- If there are breathing difficulties or the seizure does not stop for an extended period of time, the local Emergency Medical Services (EMS) should be called for further assistance.
- Never hesitate to call EMS for help if concern is present.

gence quotients (IQs) of children with epilepsy are slightly lower than average (Wossum, 1994). Children with seizures emanating from the temporal lobe region may have difficulty with language and memory functions (Wossum, 1994). Children with partial seizures manifested as staring spells may have an impaired attention span. Specific antiepileptic drugs may further alter or impair selected facets of cognition, including memory and attention span (Drane Meador, 1996).

Psychiatric Problems

A greater incidence of psychiatric problems, emotional disturbances, and psychosocial and behavioral problems exist in children with epilepsy in combination with other neurological impairments (Dunn, Austin, and Husker, 1997; Kokkonen et al, 1997).

Prognosis

Prognosis for epilepsy primarily depends on the type and severity of the disorder, the age of onset, the coexisting disorders, and the type and success of medical, surgical, and nutritional therapy. If a child's brain is active with abnormal electric activity, the opportunity for normal growth, development, and learning is limited. The convulsive disorders do not in themselves cause irreversible brain damage, but they detract from the potential of normal brain and intellectual development.

As with the classification of epilepsy and its clinical manifestations and treatment, the prognosis of epilepsy depends on many factors. Some seizure disorders cease or improve with age, some persist at the same level, and some worsen. The type of seizure and the age of onset help to determine a child's responsiveness to treatment and therefore the effect on the child's general prognosis.

Impaired neurologic functioning and altered growth and development occur more frequently in the forms of epilepsies that are more difficult to treat. The functional outcomes in these seizure disorders are more difficult to predict and generally have a poorer prognosis.

PRIMARY CARE MANAGEMENT
Health Care Maintenance
Growth and Development

Primary care provider must monitor body growth and total development in all children. Obtaining body heights and weights regularly on children with epilepsy is particularly important—especially if there have been significant losses, gains, or dramatic growth spurts such as occur with adolescents. This information must be kept current because antiepileptic drug dosages are calculated and usually prescribed for children according to their body weight and maintenance of therapeutic levels.

Primary care management and interventions related to the child's social, cognitive, and motor development depend on the severity of the seizure disorder and the underlying neurologic complications. Accompanied by regular neuropsychologic evaluations, screening and assessment tools (e.g., the Denver Developmental Screening Tool II and Wechsler Intelligence Scale for Children) help to identify the particular strengths and weaknesses (or potential for weaknesses) as a child matures.

If developmental delays are detected, these infants, children, and families may benefit from early intervention programs or infant stimulation programs. These programs are usually community-based and provide therapy for the child and education for the parents, focusing on developmental needs and appropriate child-centered interventions.

Diet

Infants with epilepsy may have difficulty with feeding because of the frequency of their seizure activity or increased lethargy from anticonvulsant therapy or the post-ictal state. In addition, seizure activity may produce a temporary state of increased metabolism. This increase, in combination with poor intake, may result in an inadequate nutritional balance for growth and development. Assessment of growth curves over time in combination with the parents' reports of intake help to determine if interventions such as increased calories per feeding and supplemental feedings are necessary. Temporary assistance and supplementation can be supported with use of a nasogastric tube. Children with persistent weight loss, poor oral feeding abilities, and failure to thrive may require a gastric tube for caloric, fluid, and medication intake.

Conversely, excessive weight gain may occur in infants and children with epilepsy. Neurologic impairments that accompany epilepsy may result in poor motor function leading to decreased physical activity, which requires less caloric intake for normal body growth. Again, assessment of growth curves over time in addition to parental reports of intake help to determine if interventions such as decreased calories per feeding are necessary.

Weight gain is a significant issue in infants with infantile spasms. Infants with this epileptic syndrome commonly present with *extreme* irritability. This irritability is frequently quieted with feeding, and therefore—in an effort to soothe their distressed baby—parents may overfeed their infant. In addition, the treatment of choice for this seizure disorder is administration of adrenocorticotropic hormone (ACTH). A major side effect of this drug is weight gain. The child's weight and growth must be monitored closely while on this medication; they will usually return to normal after the ACTH treatment is discontinued.

The ketogenic diet is an accepted form of therapy to control intractable seizures in children with certain forms of epilepsy with the objective of producing ketosis. An extremely difficult diet for a child to maintain, the ketogenic diet is often associated with weight loss and hypoglycemia. Careful monitoring of the nutritional status of these children is necessary.

Safety

Being aware of the many safety issues particular to infants and children with epilepsy is important. Parents must be educated on any changes that occur and threaten their child's safety (i.e., including instruction on how to intervene safely and appropriately during frequent or prolonged seizure activity). In the event of such an occurrence, parents, teachers, and caretakers must know the following steps: (1) maintain an adequate airway, (2) lower the child to the ground, (3) turn and keep the child on his or her side to prevent aspiration, (4) protect the child from injury to the head and limbs by loosening tight, restrictive clothing and clearing away

objects, and (5) remain with the child and call for help. EMS should be called in situations of prolonged seizure activity (e.g., when dramatically different seizures occur other than baseline or when there is respiratory distress) a call should be made whenever any concern is present. The primary care provider should emphasize to the parents that they should *never* place anything in the child's mouth. In addition, a child's tonic-clonic movements should not be restrained during the seizure activity, unless the child is in danger of greater injury. Parents and child care providers of children with life-threatening seizures should also be certified to perform cardiopulmonary resuscitation (CPR) in the event of a respiratory and cardiac arrest. After a seizure episode, the child may experience a postictal period of confusion, disorientation, or sleepiness. The child should be allowed to rest during this time of recovery following a seizure.

Certain types of seizures—including complex partial seizures, atonic seizures, and Lennox-Gastaut syndrome—often result in a sudden loss of consciousness and a change in body muscle tone. These types of seizures may exhibit loss of muscle tone (i.e., atonic) or extreme tension of muscle groups (i.e., tonic). These changes may occur independently or just before a generalized body convulsion. Because the onset of this seizure activity is unpredictable, the actual clinical manifestation is a sudden body drop to the floor, resulting in a great potential for injury—especially to the head. If the child has ever had these symptoms, the primary care provider should advise the parents to have the child wear a helmet in effort to protect the child's head in case of such seizure activity. A hockey or bicycle helmet provides adequate protection to the areas (e.g., forehead, back of head) most commonly hit during these drop attacks. These helmets are lightweight, come in various colors and sizes, and are available wherever sports equipment is sold. The child's individuality and cooperation may be fostered by placing creative designs, stickers, and labels on the helmet.

For similar reasons, consideration must be given to the child's participation in certain activities that may increase the risk of injury if a seizure occurs. Participation in activities such as swimming and gymnastics is commonly questioned by parents and school teachers. Restricting the child from taking part in these exercises, however, is not necessary provided there is adequate supervision by a responsible adult who is able to intervene appropriately if an emergency arises.

Many safety issues related to the use of various machinery (i.e., lawn mowers, equipment in machine shop classes) exist for adolescents with epilepsy. If adequate adult supervision is possible, participation in such activities supports the child's normal growth and development and peer relationships. Each state has laws pertaining to an individual with epilepsy securing a license to operate a motor vehicle.

Compliance with antiepileptic drugs presents another safety issue for adolescents. Adolescence is a time of tremendous peer pressure and personal challenges. Alcohol use and experimentation with other drugs are common. Intake of these substances often lowers the anticonvulsant's therapeutic effects, therefore lowering the seizure threshold. Education on the individual's personal responsibility for health maintenance may minimize these complications.

As discussed in the previous section, a potential for limited cognitive ability and altered judgment exists in children with epilepsy. This potential is an important concept to discuss with parents when they are considering independence issues.

Immunizations

Much has been written about the controversial opinions and data surrounding immunizations (e.g., with the immunization schedule and the potential interaction in children with neurologic disorders). Infants and children with underlying seizure disorders or a family history of seizures are at increased risk of having a seizure after receiving either the DTP (diphtheria, tetanus, and pertussis) or the measles vaccine (American Academy of Pediatrics [AAP], 1997). These seizures are usually brief, generalized, and associated with a fever. Such characteristics typically classify this type of seizure as a febrile convulsion (AAP, 1997). No evidence suggests that these seizures (1) cause permanent brain damage or epilepsy, (2) increase or advance underlying neurologic disorders, or (3) affect the prognosis of children with underlying disorders (AAP, 1997).

The recommendations from the AAP regarding the DTP immunization in infants and children with neurologic disorders are as follows: (1) administration of the pertussis vaccine may be, and in many cases should be, deferred in children with a progressive neurologic disorder (i.e., infantile spasm, uncontrolled epilepsy). (2) Infants and children with a history of seizures should have the pertussis vaccine deferred until the progress of the neurologic condition is determined. Children with well-controlled seizures who are neurologically stable should receive the pertussis vaccine. (3) Children who are suspected or predisposed to developing a progressive neurologic condition with seizures should have the pertussis vaccine deferred until the diagnosis can be determined. (4) A family history of seizures is not a contraindication for the child to receive the pertussis vaccine (AAP, 1997).

If deferment of the pertussis vaccine is necessary, the AAP recommends that the DTP vaccine be held completely until the child is 1 year of age. At this time a decision to administer either the complete DTP or just the DT vaccine can be made based on the criteria listed here. Receipt of the DTP immunization often results in fever; therefore the AAP also recommends that children who are predisposed to seizures *and receive the DTP vaccine* be given acetaminophen (15 mg/kg/dose) every 4 to 6 hours after the vaccine for as long as 24 hours to prevent a fever that may lower the child's seizure threshold (AAP, 1997). As with all difficult health care questions, primary care providers must view each infant and child in question individually and involve the family in the decision-making process.

Receipt of the measles vaccine frequently results in fever approximately 1 week later. The AAP recommends that the measles vaccine be administered to children who are predisposed to *develop* seizures or have a positive history of seizures. Therefore the same prophylactic therapy of acetaminophen (15mg/kg/dose) for 24 hours after receipt of the vaccine is advised (AAP, 1997).

All other immunizations should be given according to routine schedule.

Screening

Vision: Routine vision screening is recommended.

Hearing: Routine screening is recommended.

Dental care: Routine dental care is recommended. In severe seizure disorders, routine dental care may be difficult with resulting dental caries or gum disease. Gingival hyperplasia is a common occurrence in children on phenytoin (Dilantin) (Physicians' Desk Reference, 1998) therefore children on phenytoin require more frequent brushing and flossing with particular attention given to gums. The dentist should be informed if an individual is taking phenytoin and more frequent dental cleaning should be scheduled.

Blood pressure: Infants treated with ACTH therapy require daily blood pressure monitoring for potential hypertension. Parents should be taught how to take and monitor the infant's blood pressure while the infant is on ACTH therapy. If the parents are unable to do this, the visiting nurse or health care provider should check the blood pressure at least twice a week during therapy.

Hematocrit: Routine screening is recommended.

Urinalysis: Routine screening is recommended.

Tuberculosis: Routine screening is recommended.

Condition-Specific Screening

Drug toxicity screening: Decreased hematocrit with increased bruising or bleeding in a child taking valproic acid (Depakene), carbamazepine (Tegretol), and phenytoin (Dilantin) may indicate thrombocytopenia, blood dyscrasia, and liver dysfunction. Complete blood counts with platelets, SGOT, and SGPT should be obtained every 2 weeks when Depakene or Tegretol is initiated and then monthly for at least the first 6 months of treatment (Physicians' Desk Reference, 1998).

Common Illness Management

Differential Diagnosis (Box 21-6)

Seizurelike episodes: The primary care provider will evaluate children with epilepsy who present with common childhood illnesses that may or may not be related to this underlying disorder. The following presenting signs and symptoms must be evaluated in order to provide appropriate treatment for the illness or change the treatment regimen for the diagnosed seizure disorder.

Gastroesophageal reflux is a condition that produces vomiting. In this condition, the reflux of the stomach contents may enter only the lower esophagus, producing pain and symptoms of choking, laryngospasm, apnea, arching, and occasionally

---

> ### Box 21-6
> ### Differential Diagnosis
>
> - Seizurelike episodes
>   - Gastroesophageal reflex
>   - Breath-holding spells
>   - Migraine headaches
>   - Cardiac dysfunction
>   - Pseudoseizures
>   - Unusual body movements
> - Fever

---

loss of body tone (Pellock, 1993). This event is dramatic and frightening for parents to witness. Parents commonly report that the child has had a seizure or convulsion. Pathophysiologic cause and response may be more common when infants are laid supine after feeding. Diagnosis of gastroesophageal reflux can be confirmed through a barium swallow and esophagram, an esophageal manometry, or a nuclear medicine test called a "scintiscan." Treatment may include thickening feedings, maintaining the child in an upright position for approximately 30 minutes after feeds, using agents to alter sphincter tone, and—as a last resort—performing surgery for fundoplication (Pellock, 1993).

Breath-holding spells are common in infants and young children and present much like seizure activity. Such events usually begin with and are provoked by the child crying. The crying worsens, and the child may hold his or her breath and actually stop breathing. This breath holding leads to cyanosis, the child loses consciousness, and becomes limp. Once the child loses consciousness, normal breathing returns. If persistent apnea occurs, the child may actually have seizure activity (Pellock, 1993). The key to accurate diagnosis of breath-holding spells vs. seizure activity depends on meticulous history taking on the part of the primary care provider. Reliable reporting of a witnessed event by the parents is essential. These attacks are always associated with crying, and the apnea and cyanosis occur *before* loss of consciousness (Pellock, 1993). EEG findings demonstrate no abnormal electric activity. Treatment of breath-holding spells may include use of behavior modification (Pellock, 1993).

Migraine headaches are often difficult to differentiate from seizure activity. Migraine headaches are often associated with clinical manifestations similar to those seen with simple partial seizures (e.g., visual changes, weaknesses, nausea, and flushing). A complete history of presenting signs and symptoms, family history, and EEG findings may help to confirm the differential diagnosis (Buchholz and Reich, 1996).

Treatment of migraine headaches may include use of antiepileptic drugs; 60% of children with migraine headaches report relief with antiepileptic medications (Pellock, 1993).

Cardiac dysfunction, such as arrhythmias and syncopal episodes, may be mistaken for seizure activity. A child may have a loss of consciousness that presents much like drop attacks or an atonic seizure. Cardiac dysfunction is different from seizure activity because it usually presents with a gradual change in consciousness accompanied by dizziness, decreased or irregular pulse, pale clammy appearance, and mild neurologic impairment after the event (i.e., confusion, lethargy). An EEG performed during an event is usually normal. In addition, there may be a positive family history of cardiac anomalies and syncopal attacks (O'Donohoe, 1994).

Pseudoseizures are behavioral manifestations that closely resemble seizures but do not correlate with epileptic activity on an EEG. Pseudoseizures may occur in children and adolescents with a diagnosed seizure disorder. These spells are sometimes quite convincing and are not necessarily intentional. A psychiatric referral in combination with medical therapy is appropriate to evaluate, differentiate, and treat this diagnosis separate from electrically discharged seizures (Nash, 1995).

Unusual body movements in infants and children, such as a hyperstartle response to stimuli, muscle tics, muscle spasticity, and altered gait pattern, are conditions that may be confused with epileptic patterns. Diagnosis can usually be differentiated by careful testing, assessment, precise history taking, and accurate reporting of signs and symptoms experienced by the child and witnessed by the parents.

Differential diagnosis of common pediatric problems are sometimes very difficult and may require additional testing to rule out seizure activity. Referral to other specialists, such as a pediatric neurologist, cardiologist, gastroenterologist, and

---

Box 21-7

Drug Interactions

- Combination drug therapy for epilepsy
- Altered seizure threshold may occur with:
  - Antihistamines
  - Antidepressants
- Aspirin
  - Decreases phenatoin's effectiveness
  - Increases plasma levels of valproic acid
- Anticonvulsants may lessen therapeutic effect of oral contraceptives
- Erythromycin increases plasma level of carbamazepine (Tegretol)

---

psychologist, may also be necessary for supportive consultation and diagnostic confirmation.

Fever: The presence of infection and fever in a child with epilepsy may alter the serum levels and therapeutic effects of antiepileptic drugs. Moreover, the fever may lower a child's seizure threshold. The primary care provider should advise parents of methods of fever management (i.e., increasing fluid intake, controlling environmental factors, and using antipyretics appropriately). Parents should be advised not to increase antiepileptic drugs without consulting the primary care provider.

Drug Interactions (Box 21-7)

Many antiepileptic drugs are available for use today. Control of seizure activity is often enhanced with the use of more than one antiepileptic drug. Primary care providers must know the particular regimen and combination of drug therapy, serum levels, and common side effects (see Table 21-2). Several of these antiepileptic drugs have altered therapeutic effects when combined with common drugs used in pediatric care. Caution should be used in recommending or prescribing antihistamines, antidepressants, aspirin, oral contraceptives, and erythromycin.

Drugs such as antidepressants and antihistamines may alter the threshold of seizure activity and interact with the therapeutic effects of antiepileptic medications. Because of the wide variety of antihistamines and antidepressants available, it is beyond the scope of this chapter to address each interaction specifically. The primary care provider should further explore the individual medication regimen and the potential complications that may arise from combining these drugs.

The use of aspirin may decrease therapeutic plasma levels of phenytoin (Dilantin) by displacing the Dilantin from binding sites. This displacement causes an increase level of free Dilantin, which may result in toxic effects despite a decreased plasma level. The use of aspirin may increase therapeutic plasma levels of valproic acid (Depakote) by displacing the valproate from the protein-binding sites. This displacement would potentiate the drug's toxic side effect (Physicians' Desk Reference, 1998; Wolf, Ochoa, and Conway, 1998).

The therapeutic effect of oral contraceptives may be altered when used in combination with antiepileptics. Failure rates have been reported to be higher in women taking certain antiepileptic drugs. As a result, a higher dose of oral contraceptive may be necessary in some women to achieve a full contraceptive effect.

The use of the erythromycin results in an increased plasma level of carbamazepine (Tegretol). Erythromycin decreases the metabolism or breakdown of Tegretol, potentiating toxic effects (Physicians' Desk Reference, 1998; Wolf, Ochoa, and Conway, 1998).

Developmental Issues

Sleep Patterns

Sleep patterns may be altered if seizure activity occurs at night. Infants and children with seizures are at increased risk for apnea or respiratory difficulties because the seizure activity may be unwitnessed. It is recommended that these children wear a cardiac-apnea monitor during sleep. If a child does not have a history of respiratory difficulties during sleep, a room intercom monitor may be used to alert parents to seizure activity. Early recognition of seizure activity helps limit complications. Pillows should also be used with caution. A firm pillow and mattress are advised.

Seizure activity during the day may result in prolonged post-ictal states, interfering with the child's sleep pattern at night. Parents should be instructed not to allow their child to sleep for extended periods during the day. The post-ictal state often cannot be interrupted, however, and even the greatest effort to keep a child awake may not be successful.

Toileting

There are usually no particular concerns related to toileting the child with epilepsy. Toilet training should be appropriate for the child's developmental level.

Discipline

Children with epilepsy have an increased risk of psychosocial adjustment problems (Mims, 1997). In fact, these children have a greater incidence of psychiatric problems, emotional disturbances, and psychosocial and behavioral problems than children with other chronic conditions (Dunn, Austin, and Husker, 1997; Kokkonen et al, 1997). This invariably influences the parents' and family members' response to discipline. Parents may be hesitant to set limits for their child for fear that this will upset the child and cause a seizure. Parental guidance on discipline should be provided early in a child's life and should always reflect a child's cognitive ability. Need for discipline, direction, and encouragement toward the child's independence should be ongoing. Referral for parent and family counseling may be necessary to assist with the particular needs and challenges that may arise (Mims, 1997).

Child Care

Finding appropriate daycare often presents a challenge for parents. This challenge is even greater for parents of children with a chronic condition such as epilepsy. Primary care providers can assist the family in this endeavor by helping to identify local agencies familiar with the care involved with a child with epilepsy or by providing the necessary education about epilepsy to the child care agencies willing to support these children's special needs.

Specific needs of a child in daycare are dependent on the individual seizure disorder. The child care providers must be educated in the same manner as the parents regarding emergency aid and interventions during seizures (see Box 21-5). They must have an understanding of the clinical manifestations and what type of seizure activity to expect and monitor.

Medications must often be administered to child while they are at daycare. It is therefore necessary for the daycare providers to have information regarding the following: (1) the rationale for the anticonvulsant, (2) the potential side effects, and (3) the proper administration of the prescribed drugs. All medications should be stored in a safe, locked location to prevent accidental ingestion.

Schooling

Children with epilepsy may have social, intellectual, and cognitive difficulties. These difficulties must be assessed and identified so that interventions for a child's particular learning needs can be individualized and addressed. Staff from early intervention or infant stimulation programs should be consulted if the seizure disorder begins during infancy or early childhood. These children are at risk for developmental delay. Early assessment allows appropriate interventions to begin, maximizing learning potentials.

If needed, this preschool plan can be carried into the formal educational program as a child ages. Core evaluations by the individual school systems are necessary and appropriate for children at risk (see Chapter 5).

Establishing a supportive, well-informed environment for a child is important. School staff should be informed of a child's medical diagnosis, even if the child progresses well and does not require special educational classes. This information allows teachers to be helpful in assessing behavioral side effects of anticonvulsant therapy. A teacher who is informed of the potential for seizure occurrence and who has been instructed by the parents and the primary care provider on proper interventions is more apt to be calm and intervene appropriately if necessary.

A tremendous social stigma accompanies a diagnosis of epilepsy. The primary care provider must recognize the stress this diagnosis places on a child and its effect on the child's self-concept and relationships with peers, as well as on the educational system. The unpredictability and lack of control of seizure activity are part of this stress. Misconceptions, fears, apprehensions, and judgments of the peer group commonly have a negative effect on a child's self-esteem (Hanai, 1996; Mims, 1997). Primary care providers should explore opportunities to educate the community and increase knowledge and understanding of this condition. Greater understanding of epilepsy may yield compassion and acceptance rather than ridicule and fear of children with epilepsy.

The primary care provider should inquire about school performance and peer interactions at each well-child visit. It may be appropriate to refer a child for additional counseling and professional support to help manage with these ongoing stresses (Kokkonen et al, 1997; Mims, 1997).

Sexuality

In female adolescents with epilepsy, the seizure threshold may fall with cyclic changes induced by the menstrual cycle. This decline is presumably related to water retention, electrolyte imbalances, and decreased levels of progesterone. Cyclic adjustments of the antiepileptic medications should be considered. Regulation of the menstrual cycle may also help control seizure activity.

As with all women, oral contraceptives should be considered on an individual basis. The therapeutic effect of oral contraceptives may be altered when used in combination with antiepileptics. Therefore a higher dose of oral contraceptive may be necessary in some women to achieve a full contraceptive effect (PDR, 1998). Caution should be taken if a woman with epilepsy becomes pregnant because certain antiepileptic drugs are potentially teratogenic. Antiepileptic drugs such as valproic acid, carbamazepine, primidone, and phenobarbital have been associated with birth defects and fetal loss. The use of particular antiepileptic drugs—especially in combinations—may need to be altered during pregnancy (PDR, 1998).

Transition into Adulthood

The etiology and neurologic status of individuals with epilepsy are significant issues when considering the concept of transition into adulthood. Young adults who have epilepsy that develops as a result of inborn metabolic disease (e.g., congenital malformations, brain trauma, or brain tumors) are less likely to achieve complete seizure control than those with idiopathic epilepsy. As such, the diagnosis of epilepsy and associated complications follow them into adulthood and their life span. Primary care and clinical management of specific issues should be directed by internists in consultation with epileptologists. Consultation and advisement on educational training programs and careers must take into account both an individual's cognitive and physical abilities and the safety concerns regarding environments with significant hazards (e.g., construction work or fire fighting) in case of a seizure.

Special Family Concerns and Resources

Families of children with epilepsy experience some sense of grief as parents mourn for the "loss of the normal" child they once had. Societal stigmas and misconceptions about epilepsy are particularly stressful to the family. The diagnosis has implications through all aspects of growth and development (child care, health care, recreation, education, transportation, employment, and insurance coverage [life and health]).

Epilepsy presents a chronic and intense stress on the family system. This, in addition to the unpredictability of seizure occurrence, often results in overprotective parents and dependent children (Hanai, 1996; Mims, 1997).

Community Resources

The health care system must be empathic to the many needs of these children and their families. Health care workers provide the physical, emotional, and social care that individuals with epilepsy need. Nevertheless, no one understands or feels the problems these children and families face in their day-to-day lives as well as another child or family with the same disorder. For this reason, parent and peer support groups are available to provide this network of support within the community. These resources are not only necessary but also have proven to be a major factor in coping and adaptation for these families.

Epilepsy Foundation of America
National Epilepsy Library and Resource Center
4351 Garden City Drive
Landover, MD 20785-2267
(301) 459-3700
(800) EFA-1000
www.efa.org
National Easter Seal Society
2030 W Monroe St Suite 1800
Chicago, IL 60606-4802
(312) 726-6200; (800) 221-6827
www.seals.com

Summary of Primary Care Needs for Children with Epilepsy

HEALTH CARE MAINTENANCE

Growth and development

Obtain heights and weights at each visit. Medications must be based on current accurate measurements.

Provide regular screening and assessment of cognitive and motor skills.

Provide regular neuropsychologic screening.

If developmental delays present, recommend early intervention with infant stimulation program.

Diet

Diets may be tailored to meet child's caloric needs.

Ketogenic diet is difficult to maintain.

Safety

Provide instructions regarding emergency interventions for seizure activity.

Use helmet for certain seizure types.

Use caution with certain sports and activities.

Use caution with use of machinery, including motor vehicles.

Immunizations

Increased risk for children with underlying seizure disorders of having a seizure after DTP or measles vaccine. May defer pertussis and use DT. Measles vaccine continues to be recommended.

Screening

Vision: Routine screening is recommended.
Hearing: Routine screening is recommended.

Summary of Primary Care Needs for Children with Epilepsy—cont'd

Dental: Routine screening is recommended.

Phenytoin (Dilantin) may cause gingival hyperplasia. Children on Dilantin require more frequent cleaning by the dental hygienist.

Blood pressure: Routine screening is recommended. Infants on ACTH therapy may require daily monitoring of blood pressure.

Hematocrit: Routine screening is recommended.

Urinalysis: Routine screening is recommended.

Tuberculosis: Routine screening is recommended.

Condition-specific screening

Drug toxicity screening: Necessary first 6 months of therapy for valproate/valproic acid (Depakote), carbamazepine (Tegretol), and phenytoin (Dilantin).

COMMON ILLNESS MANAGEMENT

Differential diagnosis

Need to rule out seizurelike symptoms.

Gastrointestinal symptoms: Rule out gastroesophageal reflux.

Respiratory symptoms: Rule out breathholding spells and apnea.

Severe headaches and migraines may occur.

Cardiac symptoms: Arrhythmias, and syncopal episodes may occur.

Pseudoseizures may occur.

Movement disorders, hyperstartle, muscle tics, muscle spasticity, altered gait patterns may occur.

Management of illness with fever: increased risk of seizures. Close observation needed and antipyretic therapy.

Drug interactions

Several antiepileptic drugs have altered therapeutic effects when combined with antihistamines, aspirin, antidepressants, oral contraceptives, and certain antibiotics. Careful monitoring is required.

DEVELOPMENTAL ISSUES

Sleep patterns: May require use of cardiacapnea monitor.

May be altered with prolonged or frequent seizure activity.

Toileting: Reflective of child's cognitive and developmental ability.

Discipline: Developmentally appropriate.

Child care: Instructions to agency on emergency interventions for seizure activity. Instructions on medication given at daycare.

Schooling: Learning needs must be individualized and addressed.

Teachers should be informed of seizure history and instructed on emergency interventions for seizure activity.

Social stigmas of epilepsy may adversely affect a child's self-concept.

Sexuality: Cyclic changes induced by menstrual cycle may alter antiepileptic effects. Some antiepileptic drugs are teratogenic. Counseling may be necessary.

Transition into adulthood: Issues are dependent on complexity of disorder.

Career counseling and recognizing potential safety concerns with seizures are of particular importance.

SPECIAL FAMILY CONCERNS

Chronic sorrow and stress are present.

Social stigmas are present.

Unpredictability of seizure activity is a major concern.

References

American Academy of Pediatrics: Red book report of the Committee on Infectious Diseases, ed 24, Am Acad Pediatr, 1997.

American Association of Neuroscience Nurses: Core curriculum for neuroscience nursing, ed 3 update, Chicago, 1996, The Association.

Appleton R: The new antiepileptic drugs, Arch Dis Child 75:256-262, 1996.

Barron TF and Hunt SL: A review of the newer antiepileptic drugs and the Ketogenic diet, Clin Pediatr 36(9):513-521, 1997.

Bourgeois B: New antiepileptic drugs, Curr Opin Pediatr 8(6):543-548, 1996.

Buchholz DW and Reich SG: The menagerie of migraine, Sem Neurol 16(1):83-93, 1996.

Drane DL and Meador KJ: Epilepsy, anticonvulsant drugs and cognition, Baillieres Clin Neurol 5(4):877-885, 1996.

Dreifuss FE et al: Proposal for classification of epilepsies and epileptic syndromes, Epilepsia 26:268-278, 1985.

Dunn DW, Austin JK, and Huster GA: Behavior problems in children with new onset epilepsy, Seizure, 6(4):283-287, 1997.

Epilepsy Foundation of America, Epilepsy facts and figures, website: http://www.efa.org, 1998.

Freeman JM et al: The efficacy of the Ketogenic diet—1998: a prospective evaluation of intervention in 150 children, Pediatrics 102(6):1358-1363, 1998.

Gastaut H: Clinical and electroencephalographic classification of epileptic seizures, Epilepsia 11:102, 1970.

Hauser WA: The prevalence and incidence of convulsive disorders in children, Epilepsia 35(suppl 2):S1-6, 1994.

Hanai T: Quality of life in children with epilepsy, Epilepsia, 37(suppl 3):28-32, 1996.

Holmes G: Gabapentin for treatment of epilepsy in children, Sem Pediatr Neurol 4(3):244-250, 1997.

International League Against Epilepsy: Proposal for revised classification of epilepsies and epileptic syndromes, Epilepsia 30:389-399, 1989.

Kokkonen J et al: Psychosocial outcomes of young adults with epilepsy in childhood, J Neurol Neurosurg Psychiatry 62(3):265-268, 1997.

Lombroso CT: A prospective study of infantile spasms: clinical and therapeutic correlations, Epilepsia 24:135, 1983.

McLachlan R: Vagus nerve stimulation for intractable epilepsy, a review, J Clin Neurophysiol 14(5):358-368, 1997.

Mims J: Self-esteem, behavior, and concerns surrounding epilepsy in siblings of children with epilepsy, J Child Neurol 12(3):187-192, 1997.

Nash JL: Pseudoseizures: an update, Compr Ther 21(9):486-491, 1995.

O'Donohoe NV: Epilepsies of childhood, ed 3, Oxford, 1994, Butterworth-Heinemann, Ltd.

Pellock JM: Overview of lamotrigine and the new antiepileptic drugs: the challenge, J Child Neurol 12(suppl 1):S48-52, 1997.

Pellock JM: The differential diagnosis of epilepsy: nonepileptic paroxysmal disorders. In Wyllie E, editor: The treatment of epilepsy: principles and practice, Philadelphia, 1993, Lea & Febiger.

Pellock JM: Treatment of seizures and epilepsy in children and adolescents, Neurol 51(5 suppl 4):S8-14, 1998.

Physician's Desk Reference, ed 52, New York, 1988, Medical Economics Company.

Reynolds T: Epilepsy treatment enters a new era, Ann Int Med 128(8):702-704, 1998.

Tasker RC: Emergency treatment of acute seizures and status epilepticus, Arch Dis Child 79(1):78-83, 1998.

Scott RC et al: Status epilepticus: pathophysiology, epidemiology, and outcomes, Arch Dis Child 79(1):73-77, 1998.

Snively C, Counsell C, and Lilly D: Vagus nerve stimulator as a treatment for intractable epilepsy, J Neurosci Nurs 30(5):286-289, 1998.

Spencer DD and Spencer SS: Corpus callosotomy in the treatment of medically intractable secondarily generalized seizures of children, Cleveland Clin J Med 56:69-78, 1989.

Stafstrom CE: The pathophysiology of epileptic seizures: a primer for pediatricians, Pediatr Rev 19(10):342-350, 1998.

Wolf SM, Ochoa JG, and Conway EE: Seizure management in pediatric patients for the nineties, Pediatr Ann 27(10):653-664, 1998

Wossum DJ: Neuropsychologic issues in children with disabilities, Compr Ther 20(2):79-83, 1994.

Wyllie E et al: Seizure outcome after epilepsy surgery in children and adolescents, Ann Neurol 44(5):740-748, 1998.

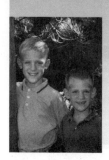

CHAPTER 22

Fragile X Syndrome

Randi J. Hagerman

Etiology

Fragile X syndrome is a relatively newly recognized condition that causes cognitive impairment ranging from mild learning disabilities to severe mental retardation. This condition derives its name from the presence of a fragile site or break in the X chromosome at Xq27.3 (Figure 22-1), which is identifiable by chromosome analysis. Because of the phenotypic variability among children with fragile X syndrome and because this condition was only recently discovered, most individuals with fragile X syndrome remain undiagnosed.

Fragile X syndrome is caused by a mutation in the gene called the Fragile X Mental Retardation 1 gene (FMR1), which is located at Xq27.3. The FMR1 gene was discovered and sequenced in 1991 by an international collaborative effort (Oberle et al, 1991; Verkerk et al, 1991; Yu et al, 1991). The FMR1 gene has a unique trinucleotide expansion located within the gene. This expansion is the source of the mutation that causes fragile X syndrome. All individuals have the FMR1 gene, but when the trinucleotide repeat expansion $(CGG)_n$ increases in size dramatically, this expansion causes dysfunction and lack of protein production from the FMR1 gene. Normal individuals in the general population have between 6 and 54 CGG repeats within their FMR1 gene. Individuals who are carriers for fragile X syndrome have an expansion of the CGG repetitive sequence that goes beyond 54 repeats up to 200. This change in the DNA is called a "premutation" and causes an increase in the instability of this region so that further expansion can take place when this mutation is passed on to the next generation through a female carrier. Individuals who are significantly affected by fragile X syndrome have over 200 repeats (i.e., "full mutation"). This full mutation is usually associated with methylation, which is a process of silencing the gene so that no FMR1 protein is produced from a full mutation. The absence of protein production actually causes the physical, behavioral, and cognitive problems that compose fragile X syndrome.

Incidence

Fragile X syndrome is the most common cause of inherited mental retardation known. Down syndrome, which rarely is inherited, has an incidence of approximately 1 per 1000. In comparison, fragile X syndrome causes mental retardation in approximately 1 per 4000 individuals in the general population (Turner et al, 1996). Studies by Rousseau et al (1995) have shown that approximately 1 in 259 females in the general population is a carrier of the premutation. Screenings of individuals with mental retardation in institutional and other residential settings have shown that 2% to 10% (Hagerman et al, 1988) of this high-risk population have fragile X syndrome as the cause of their mental impairment.

Population studies of such diverse groups as the Aborigines in Australia, the Zulus of Africa, and individuals screened in Sweden, Finland, New South Wales, England, and France suggest that fragile X is equally common among all racial and ethnic groups (Sherman, 1996). As mentioned earlier, however, the majority of families affected by this syndrome are still undiagnosed and therefore remain unaware of available treatment and intervention.

Clinical Manifestations at Time of Diagnosis

When most health care providers hear the word syndrome, they think of an individual who appears phenotypically abnormal. Similarly, most syndromes

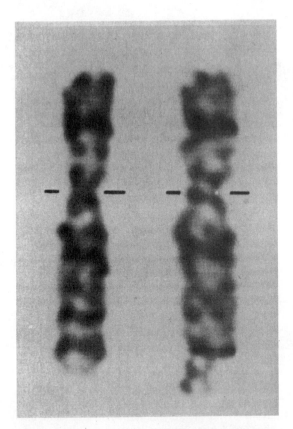

Figure 22-1   A normal X chromosome and a fragile X chromosome demonstrating the fragile X site at Xq27.3.

have consistent cognitive and physical features that succinctly describe the clinical manifestations (Box 22-1). Although most individuals with fragile X syndrome share certain clinical findings, there is much variability. Health care providers should note that children with this syndrome may not be immediately recognizable by their phenotype.

Males

Most males with fragile X syndrome have intelligence quotients (IQs) in the mild to moderate range of mental retardation. A significantly smaller percentage are severely to profoundly retarded. Approximately 13% of males with fragile X syndrome have an IQ above 70 and are therefore not mentally retarded (Hagerman 1996a). Most of these males have a variant pattern on DNA testing, including a

---

Box 22-1

Clinical Manifestations

Males

Severe learning disabilities or mental retardation

Delayed onset of language

Long or narrow face

Prominent or cupped ears

Enlarged testicles

Hyperextensible finger joints

Hyperactivity or Attention Deficit Hyperactivity Disorder

Perseveration in speech

Females

Shyness, social anxiety

Prominent ears

Long, narrow face or high palate

Hyperextensible finger joints

Attentional problems but less prominent hyperactivity

---

lack of complete methylation of the full mutation or a mosaic pattern, some cells with the premutation, and some cells with the full mutation. This is not a rare occurrence but instead a continuum of the cognitive spectrum of involvement. The cognitive profile of males with fragile X includes difficulty with abstract reasoning, math, and attention.

Delayed onset of language is present in nearly all males with fragile X syndrome. In some children, difficulties are only evidenced by language problems related to weaknesses in abstract reasoning. Other children as young as 18 months of age have delayed speech and significant deficits in receptive and expressive language. Perseveration and echolalia (i.e., repetitive speech) are common speech characteristics of individuals with fragile X. A fast rate of speech, cluttering, mumbling, rambling, and poor topic maintenance are also frequent findings (Madison, George, and Moeschler, 1986; Newell, Sanborn, and Hagerman, 1983; Scharfenaker and Schreiner, 1989).

The three classic physical features associated with the fragile X syndrome phenotype are a long narrow face, prominent or large ears, and, in males, enlarged testicles. Approximately 80% of males with fragile X will exhibit one or more of these fea-

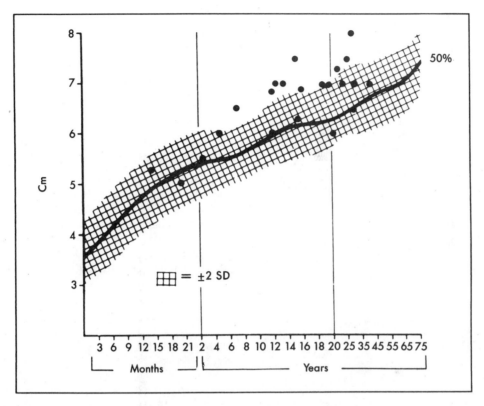

Figure 22-2 Mean ear length. (From Hagerman R, Smith ACM, and Manner R: Clinical features of the fragile X syndrome. In Hagerman R and McBogg P, editors: The fragile X syndrome: diagnosis, biochemistry and intervention, Dillon Colo., 983, Spectra).

tures (Hagerman, 1996a). A long, narrow face is a more subjective measurement, although Butler and associates (1991) and Loesch, Lafranchi, and Scott (1988) have described anthropometric methods that may lead to better characterization of facial features.

Large ears (i.e., >2 SD above the norm) are seen in 50% of boys with fragile X (Figure 22-2). Prominent or cupped ears are often a more useful discriminating feature among this younger group. This finding is observed in 60% to 70% of boys and is often the only obvious physical feature associated with fragile X syndrome (Hagerman, 1996a; Simko et al, 1989).

Enlarged testicles are often seen in the mentally retarded population; 70% to 90% of men with fragile X have a testicular volume greater than 30 ml (Hagerman, 1996a). An orchidometer (Figure 22-3) consisting of ellipsoid shapes of varying size is a useful instrument to measure testicular volume,

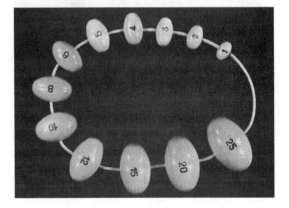

Figure 22-3 Prader orchidometer used to measure testicular volume.

especially in prepubescent boys whose testicular volume may be less obvious (e.g., 4 ml or greater in approximately 30% of boys with fragile X compared with a normal testicular volume of 2 ml in those up to 8 years of age).

Other more subtle physical features noted in the fragile X population include a prominent jaw, prominent forehead, and long palpebral fissures (Butler et al, 1991; Hagerman, 1996a). A high-arched palate, mitral valve prolapse, hypotonia, hyperextensible finger joints, and flat feet suggest that these individuals may have an underlying connective tissue disorder (Hagerman, 1996a).

It is very important to recognize that the majority of males with fragile X—especially the younger boys—appear physically normal (Figure 22-4). What is often more concerning to the parents are the behavioral characteristics. Hyperactivity is observed in more than 70% of boys with fragile X syndrome yet

frequently disappears after puberty. Poor attention span, often combined with impulsivity, is also problematic for all boys with fragile X—regardless of the level of cognitive functioning (Hagerman, 1996a). Approximately 90% have poor eye contact (Hagerman, 1996a; Pueschel and Finelli, 1984), and 60% to 70% display unusual hand mannerisms, including hand flapping and hand biting (Hagerman, 1996a).

Females

Overall, females affected by fragile X syndrome display milder phenotypic features than males, although some have been described with moderate and severe retardation (Figure 22-5).

Females who carry the premutation (i.e., CGG repeat number between 54 and 200) are usually unaffected intellectually by fragile X. Females who carry the full mutation, however, are often affected

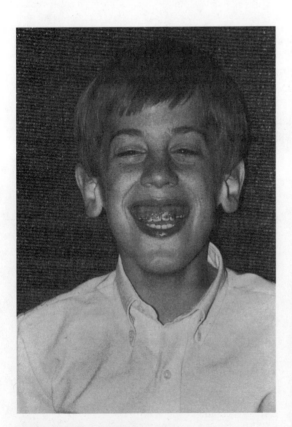

Figure 22-4   Prepubertal fragile X male.

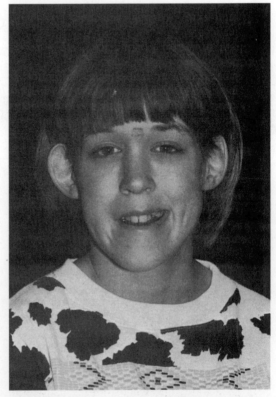

Figure 22-5   Young heterozygous fragile X female who is affected physically and cognitively by fragile X syndrome.

to a mild or severe degree. Approximately 70% of females with the full mutation have cognitive deficits including a borderline IQ or mild to moderate mental retardation (deVries et al, 1996). Executive function deficits—including attention and organizational difficulties—are common in most females with the full mutation but with an overall normal IQ. In addition, math difficulties, shyness, and poor eye contact are also common in females with the full mutation (Freund, Reiss, and Abrams, 1993; Hagerman, 1996a; Mazzocco, Pennington, and Hagerman, 1993; Sobesky et al, 1994).

Speech and language difficulties are noted in children with a heterozygote gene pattern. Although more work is needed in this area, receptive and expressive language deficits (i.e., including difficulties with auditory processing, inappropriate and tangential speech, poor topic maintenance, and written language difficulties) have been reported (Hagerman, 1996a; Madison, George, and Moeschler, 1986; Scharfenaker and Schreiner, 1989).

The physical characteristics in females are less obvious than those described for males with fragile X. Prominent ears, a long narrow face, a prominent forehead and jaw, and hyperextensible finger joints

have been described by some authors (Cronister et al, 1991; Hagerman 1996a). Phenotypic expression is more frequently observed in the mentally impaired population, but penetrance of the fragile X gene or genes is also seen in normal functioning heterozygous females (Cronister and Schreiner, 1991; Loesch and Hay, 1988).

To improve diagnosis in fragile X syndrome, primary care providers must be familiar with the characteristic gestalt that defines this very common condition. None of the physical, behavioral, or psychologic characteristics looked at individually are diagnostic of fragile X syndrome. The finding of one or more of these features in combination with developmental delay or mental retardation of unknown cause, however, should alert the clinician to order DNA studies for the FMR1 mutation. The fragile X checklist (Table 22-1) was designed to assist primary care providers with screening children who have developmental delays or mental retardation. A child receives a zero for each feature not present, one point for those present in the past or questionably present, and two points for those definitely present. The higher the score, the greater the risk for fragile X syndrome (Hagerman, Amiri, and Cronister, 1991).

Table 22-1
Fragile X Checklist

	Score		
	0 (Not Present)	1 (Borderline or Present in the Past)	2 (Definitely Present)
Mental retardation	_____	_____	_____
Perseverative speech	_____	_____	_____
Hyperactivity	_____	_____	_____
Short attention span	_____	_____	_____
Tactile defensiveness	_____	_____	_____
Hand flapping	_____	_____	_____
Hand biting	_____	_____	_____
Poor eye contact	_____	_____	_____
Hyperextensible finger joints	_____	_____	_____
Large or prominent ears	_____	_____	_____
Large testicles	_____	_____	_____
Simian crease or Sydney line	_____	_____	_____
Family history of mental retardation	_____	_____	_____
TOTAL SCORE: _____			

Adapted from Hagerman RJ: Fragile X syndrome, Curr Probl Pediatr 17:621-674, 1987.

Treatment

Few health care professionals are knowledgeable about the diagnosis and treatment of individuals with fragile X syndrome. It is not uncommon, however, for an undiagnosed child with fragile X to be seen by the primary care provider for one of several associated medical problems including repeated ear infections, strabismus, hyperactivity, delayed language, tantrums, violent outbursts, seizures, or hypotonia. Although much of the medical intervention is approached as it would be with any child, certain treatment options specific to the fragile X diagnosis can significantly improve the developmental outcome for these children.

Any signs that indicate developmental delay, sensory integration dysfunction, or language delays deserve immediate and aggressive treatment in a child with fragile X. All areas of a child's presenting signs and symptoms should be addressed, and thus a multidisciplinary approach to evaluation and therapy is essential (Box 22-2).

Medication

Medical management of hyperactivity and attentional problems can augment learning and behavioral management at home and in school. Central nervous system (CNS) stimulant medication has

---

Box 22-2

Treatment

Medications for hyperactivity
  Methylphenidate (Ritalin), dextroamphetamine (Dexedrine), or delroamphetamine/amphetamine (Adderall)
  Folic acid
  Catapres (clonidine) or Tenex (guanfacine)
Medications for aggression or severe mood lability
  Anticonvulsants (carbamazipine [Tegetrol], valproic acid [Depakote], or gabapentin [Neurotonin])
  Selective serotonin reuptake inhibitors (SSRIs)
Special education support including speech and/or language therapy and occupational therapy
Genetic counseling for all extended family members at risk

---

proved the most reliable, with improvements in as many as two thirds of affected children (Hagerman, Murphy, Wittenberger, 1988). No one drug is effective for all children. Children are most commonly prescribed methylphenidate (Ritalin), but dextroamphetamine or detraamphetamine/amphetamine (Dexedrine, Adderall) are also beneficial (Hagerman, 1996b) (see Chapter 28).

Folic acid therapy appears to be helpful for approximately 50% of prepubertal boys with fragile X (Hagerman, 1996b). Its use is controversial, however, and several studies have shown a lack of efficacy. Other studies have shown noticeable improvements in activity level, attention span, unusual mannerisms, and coping skills. The mechanism of action of folate is unclear, but it does not appear to be specific to fragile X syndrome. Because harmful side effects are rare, many families request that their child be given folic acid as a trial. A prepubescent child can be placed on a regimen of 10 mg/day (i.e., divided twice daily) for 3 to 6 months. Regardless of the dosage, careful follow-up is warranted to monitor vitamin B_6 and zinc serum levels, which may become deficient. If improvements are not noticeable within the trial period, however, the clinician should consider an alternative treatment.

Clonidine (Catapres) has been beneficial in approximately 80% of children with fragile X syndrome who have significant hyperactivity. Clonidine is a high blood pressure medication that lowers plasma and CNS norepinephrine levels. This medication is particularly helpful for children with severe hyperactivity, overexcitability, and aggression. It has an overall calming effect on hyperactivity and can be used in conjunction with stimulants (Hagerman et al, 1995).

Individuals who suffer from significant mood lability, mood instability, or aggression may benefit significantly from the use of anticonvulsants (e.g., carbamazepine [Tegretol] valproic acid [Depakote] or gabapentin [Neurontin]), which stabilize moods (Hagerman, 1996b; Hagerman, 1999).

In adolescence, aggression can be a significant difficulty, and serotonin agents (e.g., fluoxetine [Prozac]) have been helpful in fragile X syndrome (Hagerman et al, 1994a). A survey of fluoxetine's efficacy in fragile X reported that 70% of the individuals had a beneficial response, including a decrease in aggression, improvement in anxiety, and improvement in moodiness or outburst behavior. Fluoxetine is widely known as an antidepressant medication but may also be helpful in decreasing obsessive or compulsive behavior. The side effects of fluoxetine can include gastrointestinal upset or nausea and an activation effect, which can sometimes exacerbate hyperactivity. A rare child may experience an increase in obsessive or compulsive behavior, aggression, or suicidal ideation while taking fluoxetine. For this reason, children should be followed in therapy on a weekly basis while taking this medication.

Educational Intervention

Several studies have indicated that IQ declines with age (Borghgraef et al, 1987; Dykens et al, 1989; Lachiewicz et al, 1987). Some males, however, whose IQs have remained stable over time have been followed (Hagerman et al, 1989), and an occasional individual may maintain an IQ within the normal range (Hagerman et al, 1994b). This finding has been associated with a novel pattern on DNA testing: an unmethylated or partially unmethylated full mutation (i.e., CGG expansion >200). This finding is unusual because the full mutation is typically completely methylated. The lack of methylation in these high-functioning males has been associated with a limited level of FMR1 protein production, leading to a less severe degree of involvement intellectually and behaviorally than typical fragile X males (Hagerman et al, 1994b; Merenstein et al, 1994; Tassone et al, 1999). There is a tendency for individuals with fragile X to perform better on some academic tests than their IQ score would predict. Children with fragile X syndrome are typically better visual than auditory learners. Significant memory abilities and well-developed skills in recognizing visual gestalts make reading, spelling, and vocabulary obvious areas of strength for many (Kemper, Hagerman, and Altshul-Stark, 1987; Scharfenaker et al, 1996; Wilson et al, 1994).

When developing an educational program, a child's overall intellectual abilities must be considered. Mainstreaming is a realistic goal for some children, but others may need a more structured and specialized program. Children with fragile X will improve most significantly if they are shown appropriate role models. Educational intervention strategies should emphasize a child's strengths (e.g., imitating abilities, memory, visual skills, and vocabulary). The curriculum should focus on areas of a child's interest (Scharfenaker and Schreiner, 1989; Scharfenaker et al, 1996). Logo reading is an example of a learning tool developed to capitalize on a child's interesting sense of incidentally acquired knowledge (Braden, 1996). The idea is to use logos from popular television commercials and advertisements as the basis for a sight word vocabulary. The logos are gradually faded away so that only the word, phrase, or number remains.

Another learning tool that has proved successful is the use of computers for learning enhancement. This medium may be used to enhance language ability and academic progress in reading, spelling, and math. It can use visual matching skills and can help focus attention with colorful programs (Hagerman, 1999).

Speech and language and occupational therapy intervention are critical components of the education program and are recommended for all children with fragile X syndrome. Therapy is most effective when it incorporates a child's primary areas of interest. When possible, speech and language therapy sessions should include one or two other children who function at a higher level. Again, early intervention and vigorous treatment can optimize a child's speech and language abilities (Scharfenaker and Schreiner, 1989; Scharfenaker et al, 1996). Occupational therapy can be combined with speech and language therapy so that attention is maintained and the child is provided with an experimental approach to language (Scharfenacker et al, 1996; Windeck and Laurel, 1989).

Because children with fragile X are easily overstimulated, occupational therapy should be geared toward helping them reorganize, interpret, and adjust to sensory stimulation. For this reason, sensory integration therapy is the method of choice when working with these children. With this form of treatment, improvements should be noticeable in motor skills, balance, coordination, movement, sequencing, and attention (Scharfenaker et al, 1996).

Genetic Counseling

Fragile X syndrome is known to affect generation after generation, and many families have two or more children affected by this condition (Figure 22-6). Early diagnosis can provide relatives with important information about fragile X inheritance,

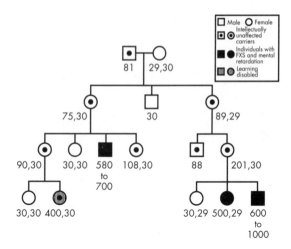

Figure 22-6 A family tree with individuals affected by fragile X syndrome (FXS). The numbers underneath the circles and squares represent the CGG repeat number in the FMR1 gene.

recurrence risks, carrier testing, and family planning options (Cronister, 1996).

Fragile X syndrome is inherited in an X-linked fashion. Males are typically affected by any deleterious gene that they carry on the X chromosome. Females, on the other hand, are usually normal because the abnormal gene on one X chromosome is compensated for by the normal gene on the other X chromosome. Heterozygous females have a 50% chance of passing the abnormal gene to their children. Males who carry the fragile X gene, however, will pass the premutation to all of their daughters but none of their sons.

Males who are carriers have the premutation, which is a CGG repeat between 54 and 200. When males pass on this premutation to all of their daughters, only minimal changes occur in the CGG repeat number and it never increases to the full mutation. When the premutation is passed on by a female, however, there is a high probability that the premutation will increase to a full mutation in the offspring who inherit the fragile X chromosome. The larger the size of the premutation in the carrier mother, the greater the chance that expansion will occur to a full mutation. In women with a premutation of 100 CGG repeats, the expansion to the full mutation will occur 100% of the time when the fragile X chromosome is passed on to the next generation. All family members who are at risk to

carry either the premutation or the full mutation should be studied by DNA testing, which is done on a blood sample. DNA testing is available throughout the United States and at large genetic centers internationally. For a list of laboratories that can carry out DNA testing for fragile X syndrome, contact the National Fragile X Foundation.

Because fragile X syndrome is inherited, it is essential that a thorough family history or pedigree be taken. Questions about intellectual deficits, learning disabilities, emotional problems, and physical features associated with fragile X syndrome should be asked. Any relative with positive findings should be suspected as either a carrier or an affected individual.

Prenatal diagnosis is available to all families with a confirmed diagnosis of fragile X syndrome or those with a history of mental retardation. This testing includes amniocentesis (performed at 14 to 18 weeks' gestation), chorionic villi sampling (performed at 9½ to 12 weeks' gestation) and percutaneous umbilical blood sampling (18 to 22 weeks' gestation). Each procedure has specific benefits and drawbacks that should be carefully discussed with a genetic counselor before pregnancy or testing is pursued (Cronister, 1996). The accuracy of prenatal diagnostic testing has improved significantly (i.e., >98% accurate) with DNA-FMR1 studies.

Recent and Anticipated Advances in Diagnosis and Management

A recent, significant advance is the use of antibodies to the FMR1 protein to identify individuals who have fragile X syndrome (Tassone et al, 1999; Willemsen et al, 1997). Because unaffected individuals produce a normal level of FMR1 protein, the antibody test will light up the protein within the lymphocytes of individuals who are normal. An antibody test, however, usually detects little or no protein in males with the full mutation (Tassone et al, 1999). Females, on the other hand, produce some level of FMR1 protein because their other normal X chromosome is producing FMR1 protein to a level dependent on the pattern of X-inactivation in the female. Therefore this diagnostic test does not clearly differentiate females with the full mutation compared with controls because of the variable FMR1 protein expression in females. This antibody test should be considered as a screening for individuals who may be affected by fragile X syndrome, and then the diagnosis should be confirmed by DNA testing.

In the future, new medications will be developed that will help with the behavior problems, including hyperactivity and aggression, in children with fragile X syndrome. Within the next 10 years the technology to either replace the FMR1 protein or replace a normal FMR1 gene in individuals who are affected by this syndrome will probably be developed. This very important advance could mean a cure or significant alleviation of this disorder. Extensive animal studies will be needed over the next decade to improve methods for inserting a gene or normal FMR1 protein inside of neurons. It is unclear at this time how significant the improvements will be in children or adults who receive a new gene or normal levels of FMR1 protein (Rattazzi and Ioannou, 1996).

Associated Problems (Box 22-3)

Otitis Media

Recurrent otitis media has been reported in 45% to 60% of all children with fragile X syndrome. Approximately 40% of these children will require myringotomy tube insertions (Hagerman, Altshul-Stark, and McBogg, 1987; Simko et al, 1989). There has been some speculation that this may be caused by an unusual angle or collapsibility of the eustachian tube (Hagerman, 1996a). Appropriate intervention is critical to avoid conductive hearing loss and a compounding of language deficits typical for fragile X (Rapin, 1979).

Connective Tissue Problems

Of all individuals with fragile X syndrome, 50% will have pes planus (Davids, Hagerman, and Eilert, 1990). Clubfoot has also been reported and may be related to hypotonia in utero. In the study by Davids and associates (1990), joint laxity was documented in approximately 70% of children 10 years or younger. For reasons not clearly understood, hypotonia tends to disappear with age. Sco-

> **Box 22-3**
> ## Associated Problems
> Otitis media
> Connective tissue problems
>   Pes planus
>   Scoliosis
>   Mitral valve prolapse
> Vision problems
>   Strabismus
>   Nystagmus
> Seizures
> Oral problems
> Autistic-like features (e.g., hand flapping, hand biting)
> Psychiatric manifestations
> Surgery integration difficulties

liosis may be present, and hernias appear to be more common in children with fragile X than in the general population. These problems may also be related to an underlying connective tissue disorder. Routine intervention is recommended.

Cardiac problems have also been noted in individuals with fragile X syndrome and may be secondary to a connective tissue disorder. Mitral valve prolapse has been diagnosed in 22% to 55% of affected individuals (Loehr et al, 1986; Sreeran et al, 1989). Although usually benign, mitral valve prolapse can predispose a person to arrhythmias. This has not yet been noted in males with fragile X, but 30% of heterozygous females complain of heart palpitations (Cronister et al, 1991). Mild dilation of the base of the aorta has also been observed with ultrasound studies in as many as 50% of this population but does not appear to be progressive (Loehr et al, 1986; Sreeran et al, 1989).

Vision Problems

Strabismus (i.e., either esotropia or exotropia) appears to be present in approximately 30% to 56% of those with fragile X syndrome (King, Hagerman, and Houghton, 1995; Maino et al, 1990). Other eye problems, such as myopia, nystagmus, and ptosis, have been observed with and without strabismus (Schnizel and Largo, 1985; Storm, DeBenito, and Ferretti, 1987).

Seizures

Seizures have been documented in approximately 20% of individuals with fragile X. Generalized seizures and partial complex seizures have been reported (Musumeci et al, 1988a, b; Wisniewski et al, 1991). A careful history should be taken and if clinical seizures are present, treatment with an anticonvulsant such as carbamazepine (Tegretol) is warranted (Hagerman, 1996b).

Oral Problems

A high-arched palate is seen with greater frequency among the fragile X population and can explain the increased incidence of dental malocclusion (Partington, 1984). Several reports of Pierre Robin syndrome (micrognathia and cleft palate) have also been noted in combination with fragile X syndrome.

Autistic-like Tendencies

Much has been written to suggest an association between autism and fragile X syndrome. Studies have estimated that approximately 15% of individuals with fragile X meet the *Diagnostic and Statistical Manual of Mental Disorders DSM-IV* criteria for autism (Brown et al, 1982, 1986; Hagerman 1996a; Partington, 1984). Most individuals, however, are more appropriately described as autistic-like. In addition to poor eye contact and unusual hand mannerisms, many children have fascinations with certain objects such as vacuum cleaners and record players. What differentiates most individuals with fragile X from those with autism is that those who are autistic characteristically lack an ability to relate. Although social anxiety is obvious at times, many children with fragile X can be intermittently quite sociable, demonstrating a spontaneous and natural sense of humor (Hagerman, 1987; Scharfenaker et al, 1996).

Psychiatric Manifestations

Researchers have only recently investigated the psychiatric manifestations of the fragile X gene in females. As with males with fragile X, social anxiety is a common complaint. Many of the affected girls appear shy, are withdrawn, and have poor eye contact (Freund, Reiss, and Abrams,

1993; Hagerman et al, 1992). Cognitively normal women occasionally recall that their childhood was burdened by similar types of problems. Poor self-image and depression have also been described (Hagerman and Sobesky, 1989; Reiss et al, 1988). Reiss and colleagues (1988) have reported an increased incidence of schizotypal features, including emotional withdrawal and odd communication patterns. The schizotypal features appear to be related to the executive function or frontal deficits that are seen in most females with the full mutation (Mazzocco, Pennington, and Hagerman, 1993; Sobesky et al, 1994).

Sensory Integration Difficulties

Other behavioral concerns include a child's inability to calm when overstimulated or overwhelmed. New stimuli or novel situations can be frightening. Many parents describe their child as being hypersensitive to touch or tactilely defensive. Sensory integration difficulties are evidenced by an inability to screen out noises, lights, or confusion. Common responses to this overloading can include tantrums or outburst behavior, aggressive behavior, emotional instability, and—rarely—psychotic behavior (Hagerman, 1996a, b; Scharfenaker and Schreiner, 1989; Scharfenaker et al, 1996).

Prognosis

Individuals with fragile X syndrome are expected to live a normal life span regardless of intellectual functioning.

PRIMARY CARE MANAGEMENT
Health Care Maintenance

Growth and Development

Increased head circumference (i.e., greater than the 75th percentile) at birth and throughout childhood has been reported by several authors (Borghgraef, Fryns, and Van den Berghe, 1990) and may lead to a possible misdiagnosis of Sotos' syndrome (i.e., cerebral gigantism). Others, however, have concluded that this deviance of head circumference into the upper range of normal occurs only occasionally and therefore is not a consistent finding (Partington, 1984). No special intervention is necessary for a large head circumference.

Controversy also exists about birth weights and growth. Prouty and associates (1988) found growth to be normal and noted only a mild increase in growth percentiles from childhood into adult life. Partington (1984) reported similar findings. Sutherland and Hecht (1985), on the other hand, reported that 9 of 29 (31%) boys studied were above the 95th percentile.

In addition to deficits in cognitive functioning and speech, children with fragile X may be delayed in meeting other age-appropriate developmental milestones. Developmental delay will be evident with early developmental testing, such as the Bayley Scales of Infant Development (see Chapter 2). Other early warning signs are clumsiness and poor balance. Toe walking, unusual gait, lack of flow of movement, and trouble with motor planning may also occur secondary to hypotonia, joint laxity, and sensory integration difficulties (Scharfenaker, et al 1996).

Diet

Obsessive-compulsive behavior can be seen in children with fragile X syndrome and may involve food cravings. Obesity has been a problem for a small subgroup of children with fragile X (Fryns et al, 1987), which may be secondary to perseverative eating or hypothalamic dysfunction (Fryns et al, 1987). A subgroup of patients with fragile X may have a Praderwilli-like phenotype or general overgrowth (deVries et al, 1995). Parents of obese children should be encouraged to place their children on appropriate diets. Exercise programs for older children may also be beneficial, as well as exercise videos, which encourage children to use their visual and mimicking abilities. Failure to thrive is not uncommon in infants with fragile X syndrome but may be the result of aversion to some food textures, frequent infections, or problematic mothering skills (i.e., if the mother herself is affected by the syndrome).

Safety

Families and educators should not expect every child with fragile X to be able to learn age-appropriate safety. It will depend on each child's individual strengths and weaknesses. With strong visual and mimicking abilities and through the use of repetition, many children can be taught to follow safety tips.

Hyperactivity may lead to more accidents, so these children should be monitored closely. Because children with fragile X can be overstimulated by their environment, the home setting—particularly the child's playroom and bedroom—should be a calm and uncluttered environment. The use of bean bag chairs, vibrating pillows, musical tapes, and appropriate environmental changes can be discussed with an occupational therapist.

Parents also may be concerned about the safety of their child if self-injurious behavior is displayed. Head banging is rare but can be harmful to the child. Hand biting, despite its frequency, does not commonly cause scarring. Nevertheless, parents may wish to pursue behavior management therapies to decrease the frequency of these behaviors. Parents and professionals should also be advised of possible seizure activity and taught appropriate intervention.

Immunizations

Vaccination regimen is the same as it would be for any infant or child. If a child has a seizure disorder, the American Academy of Pediatrics guidelines for administering pertussis and measles vaccinations to those with seizures should be followed (see Chapter 21) (Committee on Infectious Diseases, 1994).

Screening (Box 22-4)

Vision: An eye examination is recommended as early as possible after fragile X is diagnosed to rule out strabismus and the less frequent findings of myopia, hyperopia, astigmatism, nystagmus, and ptosis. The evaluation should include a complete case history, visual acuity evaluation, refractive error determination, oculomotor assessment, and fundoscopy. Other testing may include an assessment of focusing function and visual developmental-perceptual skills. Yearly screening is sufficient unless visual difficulty is suspected. Early intervention is encouraged to avoid the development of blurred vision, amblyopia, or diplopia as a result of an uncorrected refractive error or strabismus.

Box 22-4

Screening

Vision
Hearing
Dental
Cardiac examination
Speech and/or language delays
Connective tissue problems
Seizures

Treatment for many of the ophthalmologic problems includes corrective lenses or patching or both (i.e., treatment that is relatively inexpensive and noninvasive). For some cases of strabismus, however, surgery may be the treatment of choice. Although early intervention may not dramatically influence cognitive functioning, corrected vision will maximize a child's learning potential.

Hearing: Because of the increased risk for recurrent ear infections, hearing evaluations are strongly recommended in newly diagnosed children. Audiometry testing is usually sufficient to assess hearing. Any child with a history of recurrent ear infections is best referred to an ear, nose, and throat (ENT) specialist to determine whether pressure equalizing (PE) tubes are warranted.

Dental: A routine dental screening by the practitioner may reveal a high-arched palate, cleft palate, or dental malocclusion, all of which compound speech problems. Any child requiring dental work should be evaluated for mitral valve prolapse. If it is present, prophylactic antibiotic treatment to avoid subacute bacterial endocarditis is warranted (see Chapter 17). Although not always possible, families should be referred to a pedodontist experienced in working with developmentally delayed and hyperactive children.

Blood pressure: Routine screening is recommended.

Hematocrit: Routine screening is recommended.

Urinalysis: Routine screening is recommended.

Tuberculosis: Routine screening is recommended.

Condition-Specific Screening

Mitral valve prolapse: Children with fragile X syndrome are at increased risk of mitral valve prolapse. Careful screening to detect a click or murmur is essential to detect this problem or any other cardiac involvement. Any child with an abnormal cardiac examination should be referred to a cardiologist for formal evaluation.

Speech and language: Some children will have early speech delays that may be so subtle that they go undetected by parents or teachers. An early and annual speech and language evaluation should be performed to detect any speech or language deficits that can be improved through early intervention. Because of the diversity of speech and language difficulties in children with fragile X, no one screening tool is recommended. Each child should be approached on an individual basis. Routine screening tools (e.g., the Denver II) will identify developmental delays, but subsequent DNA testing is necessary to identify fragile X syndrome as the cause of the delays. Children identified with fragile X syndrome should have a formal evaluation by a licensed speech and language pathologist who is preferably experienced with fragile X syndrome.

Connective tissue problems: Early detection of scoliosis can often prevent further sequelae. Screening should also include a careful examination for excessive joint laxity and other complications of loose connective tissue (e.g., hernias).

Seizures: When the clinical history suggests seizures, an electroencephalogram (EEG) is indicated. Unusual findings can include a slow background rhythm and spike-wave discharges that are often similar to rolandic spikes (Musumeci et al, 1988a, 1988b). Any child who appears to be having seizures should be treated with anticonvulsant medication and followed closely by a pediatric neurologist. If a child is taking medication to control seizures, anticonvulsant serum levels should be followed (see Chapter 21).

Common Illness Management

Differential Diagnosis (Box 22-5)

Recurrent otitis media: As mentioned earlier, a frequent pediatric health problem in children with fragile X is ear infections. These children must be vigorously monitored and treated for recurrent otitis media to avoid sequelae that could further compromise language development and learning.

Parents of young children may not recognize otitis as the cause of their child's irritability. It may be helpful to inform parents of children with fragile X that recurrent otitis media is a common problem and review which signs or symptoms are indicators of infection.

To best determine a child's individualized medical management, newly diagnosed families should be referred to a health care team with expertise in fragile X syndrome for a thorough evaluation and consultation.

Drug Interactions

Carbamazepine is a commonly prescribed anticonvulsant that is also used to control behavior problems (e.g., violent outbursts, aggression, and self-injurious behavior). Concurrent treatment with macrolide antibiotics, cimetidine (Tagamet), propoxyphene (Darvon), and isoniazid (INH) can interfere with the breakdown of carbamazepine, causing nausea, vomiting, and lethargy. Folic acid therapy may worsen the seizure frequency in children with epilepsy.

Developmental Issues

Sleep Patterns

Frequent wakefulness in early childhood is a common problem in children with fragile X. Overstimulation can often interfere with sleeping, and calming techniques (e.g., music) are useful in quieting the child in preparation for bedtime.

Toileting

Parents of children with fragile X often need help setting realistic expectations about toilet training. Some children achieve this milestone on time, but delayed training is more common. Parents should not be discouraged if a child takes longer to learn. The establishment of a predictable routine and consistent positive reinforcement are general principles that are helpful for children with fragile X. As with parents of any child having toilet-training difficulties, parents are discouraged from being overly critical or reprimanding.

Discipline

Children with fragile X syndrome are especially noncompliant in response to an unexpected event or change in routine and therefore need a highly structured environment. Sending the child to school the same way each day, having meals on a scheduled basis, and using the same nightly routines are encouraged. Behavior problems should be anticipated if a child is faced with an unexpected event. The prevention of unpredictable events in the home or at school is obviously an unrealistic expectation and should not be overemphasized. On the other hand, change and transitions should be gradually programmed into the child's learning and home environment. Setting limits, giving the child timeouts, and being consistent are appropriate responses when disciplinary action is required.

Child Care

Issues related to child care are common concerns for parents of a child with fragile X. Because of the short attention span and hyperactivity of children with fragile X, child care providers should be knowledgeable about behavior modification techniques. The environment in which a child is placed is also important. Colors, noise level, and the amount of light can be altered to avoid overstimulation. Slowly but gradually new events can be programmed into a child's day. Setting a common time each week to introduce a new game, playing in a new space, or meeting a new daycare provider can help a child anticipate and deal more effectively with change. If these aspects of daycare are well managed, there is no reason why a child with fragile X cannot be placed in full-day or half-day programs. Placement with nonaffected children is very helpful for modeling appropriate behavior.

Schooling

Most children with fragile X syndrome that has been identified are receiving special education. Mainstreaming is a potential goal as described under the treatment section in this chapter. Children can be mainstreamed in preschool programs as well, but child care providers should be experienced in specialized education. A program that provides for individualized attention and a high teacher-student ratio is best. The success of any approach depends on a number of factors specific to each child, including the child's level of cognitive functioning, distractibility, impulsivity, the structure of the class, classroom environment, and appropriate role models.

Because few educators are knowledgeable about fragile X syndrome, the health care professional can play an active role in helping families educate the teachers and therapists about the specialized needs of their child and why an integrative approach that emphasizes a child's overall strengths and weaknesses is essential for effective learning.

Parents should be encouraged to become actively involved in their child's program. Frequent visits to the classroom and observing therapy sessions helps establish open communication among parents, teachers, and support personnel.

Sexuality

Masturbation and other forms of self-stimulatory behavior are common among the mentally retarded population and are occasionally problematic for adolescents with fragile X. Families can be supportive by providing appropriate sex education and talking openly about sexuality issues. This need can also be met through family or individual counseling (Brown, Braden, and Sobesky, 1991). Counseling or therapy can also train new behaviors that can replace socially inappropriate behavior (e.g., masturbation in public). Most important, counseling can provide an environment in which the adolescent can discuss and deal with issues of sexuality in a supportive environment.

Fertility is usually normal in men with fragile X, although reproduction is rare because of cognitive deficits (Cantú et al, 1976). All female children of males with fragile X will have the premutation because only the premutation—not the full mutation—is carried in the sperm. Ovarian problems and premature menopause have been reported in women with the premutation (Cronister et al, 1991; Hagerman, 1996a). Individuals with mild redardation will require support in parenting. Sex education and genetic counseling should therefore be available to them.

Transition to Adulthood

The transition to adulthood is usually difficult for adolescents with fragile X syndrome because living independently is a problem as a result of mental retardation. It is important for adolescents to have adequate vocational training. Most individuals affected by fragile X syndrome can carry out jobs in the community that are consistent with their level of mental functioning. Many individuals require a job trainer who can work with them for the first several days or first few weeks when a new job is started. If they are to be successful in living independently or semi-independently, a focus on daily living skills is also critical for young adults with fragile X syndrome. Individuals with mild or moderate mental retardation can learn how to use public transportation and carry out activities in the home, including laundry, self-care, and cooking. Most adults affected by fragile X syndrome do well with limited supervision in an apartment living situation. Females affected with fragile X syndrome have most difficulty when trying to raise their children who are affected by fragile X syndrome. This role can be extremely stressful and may overwhelm their limited resources, particularly if the mother is mildly retarded. Additional help from family or from social services agencies is usually necessary.

The connective tissue problems usually improve in adulthood and medical complications are uncommon. Hernia and mitral valve prolapse are more common in adulthood than childhood. Follow-up with a cardiologist and the use of antibiotic prophylaxis for subacute bacterial endocarditis (SBE) prevention are necessary for mitral valve prolapse.

Approximately 30% of young adults—particularly males—with fragile X syndrome may have difficulty with episodic outburst behavior. This behavior should be treated with medications such as the serotonin agents, fluoxetine or sertraline, in addition to counseling. Counseling can help with development of calming techniques and recognition of environmental situations that can lead to outburst behavior.

Special Family Concerns and Resources

Perhaps the most frustrating aspect of having a child with fragile X syndrome is realizing that few professionals have a good understanding of this disorder and how it can affect a child and other family members. As a consequence many parents become the main advocate for their child in both the educational and medical settings. Health care professionals who are unfamiliar with fragile X syndrome should make every effort to listen carefully to families. It is also the parents' responsibility to educate themselves about this unique disorder so that they too appreciate the specialized needs of these children, as well as to recognize their own needs if they require additional support because they may also be affected by the syndrome.

Fragile X syndrome occurs in all ethnic and racial groups that have been studied. There is no evidence of increased prevalence in any individual group. In some cultural groups, such as certain Asian populations, it is sometimes difficult to do genetic counseling in extended family members because of the negative cultural implications of knowing about a genetic disorder that affects large numbers within the family tree. When these cultural concerns exist, often permission will not be given to inform extended family members about this genetic disorder. In these cases it is helpful to write an explanatory letter about fragile X syndrome that the immediate family can pass out to other family members who may be affected or be carriers for fragile X syndrome.

The National Fragile X Foundation was established to educate parents, professionals, and the public on the diagnosis and treatment of fragile X syndrome and other forms of X-linked mental retardation. In addition, the National Fragile X Foundation promotes research pertaining to fragile X syndrome in the areas of biochemistry, genetics, and clinical applications. All parents who have a child diagnosed with fragile X syndrome and professionals interested in working with the developmentally delayed population are encouraged to write or call the foundation so that they may receive the newsletter and other services available to them.

Resources

Foundations:
National Fragile X Foundation
  PO Box 190488
  San Francisco, Calif. 94119
  (510) 763-6030; (800) 763-6030
  http://www.frax.org
FRAXA Research Foundation
  PO Box 935
  West Newbury, Mass. 01985-0935
  (978) 462-1866; (978) 463-9985 (fax)
  http://www.fraxa.org; info@fraxa.org
  Fragile X syndrome listserv sponsored by FRAXA: to be added to the listserv, email "SUBSCRIBE FRAGILEX-L" to listserv@listserv.cc.emory. edu
Fragile X Research Foundation of Canada
  167 Queen Street West
  Brampton, Ontario
  Canada, L6Y 1M5
  (905) 453-9366
  FXRFC@ibm.net;
    http://dante.med.utoronto.ca/Fragile-X/linksto.htm
The Fragile X Society (England)
  53 Winchelsea Lane
  Hastings, East Sussex
  TN35 4LG
  011-424-813147
The International Fragile X Alliance (Australia)
  263 Glen Elra Rd.
  Nth Caulfield 3161
  Melbourne, Australia
  (03) 9528-1910; (03) 9532-9555 (fax)
  jcohen@netspace.net.au
Fragile X Association of Australia, Inc.
  15 Bowen Close
  Cherrybrook, NSW
  Australia
  (019) 987012
  fragilex@ozemail.com.au
Newsletters:
National Fragile X Foundation Newsletter—Call the National Fragile X Foundation at (800) 688-8765.

FRAXA Research Foundation Newsletter—Subscriptions through FRAXA, PO Box 935, West Newbury, Mass. 01985

National Fragile X Advocate—Quarterly magazine for parents and professionals. (800) 434-0322. Avanta Media Corporation, PO Box 17023, Chapel Hill, NC 27516-1702.

Reading for children:

O'Connor R: Boys with fragile X syndrome, 1995. Can be obtained from the National Fragile X Foundation: (800) 688-8765

Steiger C: My brother has fragile X syndrome, Chapel Hill, NC, 1998, Avanta Publishing. (800) 434-0322

General family support—internet:

The Family Village
http://www.familyvillage.wisc.edu
This site was organized by the Waisman Center of the University of Wisconsin-Madison and integrates resources and communication opportunities on the Internet for people with disabilities, their families, and those that support and serve them. Selections include: Library (information about disabilities), Coffee Shop (connections with other families), Hospital (links for: health care concerns), Shopping Mall (assistive technology suppliers), and others.

Family Voices
http://www.ichp.edu/mchb/fv
Family Voices is a national grassroots network of families and friends speaking on behalf of children with special health care needs. Selections include: About Family Voices, ACCESS-MCH/Family Voices, PIC Project, To Join Family Voices, Voices Newsletter, Español, Search.

National Parent Network on Disabilities (NPND)
http://www.npnd.org
NPND was established to provide a presence and national voice for parents of children, youth, and adults with special needs. NPND shares information and resources in order to promote and support the power of parents to influence and affect policy issues concerning the needs of people with disabilities and their families. Selections include: News Releases, the Friday Fax (i.e., weekly newsletter from the Department of Health and Human Services), Conferences, Federal Issues, links to Federal Government sites, and information on IDEA.

PACER Center
http://www.pacer.org
PACER stands for Parent Advocacy Coalition for Educational Rights. Selections include: Publications (including order forms), Who We Are, PACER Center Articles, Events, Legislative Information (including alerts), Frequently Asked Questions, Projects, National Information (links to other organizations).

PEP: Parents, Educators, and Publishers
http://www.microweb.com/pepsite/index.html
The PEP site is intended as an informational resource for parents, educators, and children's software publishers. The creators of this site have developed it in response to the interests and needs of these three audiences. Selections include: Children's Software Revue, Educational Software Publishers, Computer Camps, Shopper Resources, and Cool School Sites.

Summary of Primary Care Needs for the Child with Fragile X Syndrome

HEALTH CARE MAINTENANCE

Growth and development

Physical growth is usually within normal limits. Some children are reported to have large heads for body size.

Deficits in cognitive function and speech are common.

Developmental delays in gross motor skills are common.

Diet

Obsessive eating may result in obesity in older children.

Infants may have failure to thrive.

Summary of Primary Care Needs for the Child with Fragile X Syndrome—cont'd

Safety

Cognitive dysfunction may limit these children's awareness of safety issues.

Hyperactivity may make these children more accident prone.

Self-injurious behavior may occur, and parents can be taught behavior management therapies.

If seizures are present, seizure precautions are necessary.

Immunizations

Routine immunizations are recommended.

AAP guidelines for immunizations in children with seizures should be followed where indicated.

Screening

Vision: Eye examination for strabismus, refractive errors, and visual perceptual skills is recommended at the time of diagnosis. If no problems are found, annual vision screening is recommended.

Hearing: An increased risk of otitis media warrants audiometric testing. A child may need referral to an ENT specialist for PE tubes.

Dental: Screening for palate and dental abnormalities is recommended. If mitral valve prolapse is present, prophylactic antibiotics will be needed for dental work.

Blood pressure: Routine screening is recommended.

Hematocrit: Routine screening is recommended.

Urinalysis: Routine screening is recommended.

Tuberculosis: Routine screening is recommended.

Condition-specific screening

Mitral valve prolapse: In the presence of an abnormal cardiac examination, mitral valve prolapse must be evaluated by a cardiologist.

Speech and language: Speech and language evaluation should be done annually, with early intervention if a problem is detected.

Connective tissue problems: Children should be screened for flat feet, scoliosis, and excessive joint laxity.

Seizures: A clinical history suggestive of seizures should be evaluated by electroencephalography. If a child is taking anticonvulsants, blood levels must be monitored.

COMMON ILLNESS MANAGEMENT

Differential diagnosis

Recurrent otitis media is common.

Drug interactions

Carbamazepine is altered by macrolide antibiotics, cimetidine, propoxyphene, and isoniazid.

See Chapter 19 for drug interactions with seizure medications.

DEVELOPMENTAL ISSUES

Sleep patterns: Frequent wakefulness in early childhood is not uncommon.

Overstimulation should be avoided.

Toileting: Delayed continence is not uncommon.

Discipline: Children behave better in highly structured environments.

Consistent limit setting is beneficial.

Positive reinforcement is essential.

Child care: Short attention span and hyperactivity may be modified by subdued environments.

New activities must be introduced slowly.

Schooling: Most children receive special education services. The provider can help educate the school system personnel on condition and treatment.

Sexuality: Self-stimulatory behaviors are common. Counseling may help decrease inappropriate behavior.

Fertility is normal in men; carrier females may experience premature menopause.

Sex education, birth control, and genetic counseling are necessary.

Continued

Summary of Primary Care Needs for the Child with Fragile X Syndrome—cont'd

Transition to adulthood: Living independently is difficult, individuals will likely need support from others.
Connective tissue problems will improve.
Outburst behavior may be a problem.

SPECIAL FAMILY CONCERNS

Families may have difficulty adjusting to the diagnosis; parents may also be affected.
Genetic counseling is warranted.
Because the condition is not well known, care may be nonspecific.

References

Borghgraef M et al: Fragile X syndrome: a study of the psychological profile in 23 patients, Clin Genet 32:179-186, 1987.

Borghgraef M, Fryns JP, and Van den Berghe H: The female and the fragile X syndrome: data on clinical and psychological findings in fragile X carriers, Clin Genet 37:341-346, 1990.

Braden ML: Fragile, handle with care: understanding fragile X syndrome, ed 2, Chapel Hill, NC, 1997, Avanta Publishing.

Brown J, Braden M, and Sobesky W: Treatment of behavioral and emotional problems. In RJ Hagerman and AC Silverman, editors: The fragile X syndrome: diagnosis, treatment, and research, Baltimore, 1991, Johns Hopkins University Press.

Brown WT et al: Fragile X and autism, Am J Med Genet 23:341-352, 1986.

Brown WT et al: Autism is associated with the fragile X syndrome, J Autism Dev Disord 12:303-307, 1982.

Butler MG et al: Anthropomorphic comparisons in mentally retarded males with and without the fragile X syndrome, Am J Med Genet 38:260-268, 1991.

Cantú JM et al: Inherited congenital normofunctional testicular hyperplasia and mental deficiency, Hum Genet 33:23-33, 1976.

Committee on Infectious Diseases: Report of the Committee on Infectious Diseases, ed 23, Elk Grove Village, Ill., The American Academy of Pediatrics, 1994.

Cronister A et al: The heterozygous fragile X female: historical, physical, cognitive, and cytogenetic features, Am J Med Genet 38:269-274, 1991.

Cronister AJ: Genetic counseling. In Hagerman RJ and Cronister A, editors: Fragile X syndrome: diagnosis, treatment, and research, ed 2, Baltimore, 1996, Johns Hopkins University Press.

Davids JR, Hagerman RJ, and Eilert RE: The orthopaedic aspects of the fragile X syndrome, J Bone Joint Surg BR 72:889-896, 1990.

de Vries BB et al: General overgrowth in the fragile X syndrome: variability in the phenotypic expression of the FMR1 gene mutation, J Med Genet 32(10):764-9, 1995.

de Vries BB et al: Mental status of females with an FMR1 gene full mutation, Am J Med Genet 58(5):1025-32, 1996.

Dykens E et al: The trajectory of cognitive development in males with the fragile X syndrome, J Am Acad Child Adolesc Psychiatry 28:422-426, 1989.

Freund LS, Reiss AL, and Abrams M, Psychiatric disorders associated with fragile X in the young female, Pediatrics 91:321-329, 1993.

Fryns JP et al: A peculiar subphenotype in the fragile X syndrome: extreme obesity, short stature, stubby hands and feet, diffuse hyperpigmentation. Further evidence of disturbed hypothalamic function in the fragile X syndrome? Clin Genet 32:388-392, 1987.

Hagerman RJ: Medical follow-up and pharmacotherapy. In Hagerman RJ and Cronister A, editors: Fragile X syndrome: diagnosis, treatment, and research, ed 2, Baltimore, 1996a, Johns Hopkins University Press.

Hagerman RJ: Physical and behavioral phenotype. In Hagerman RJ and Cronister A, editors: Fragile X syndrome: diagnosis, treatment and research, ed 2, Baltimore, 1996b, Johns Hopkins University Press.

Hagerman RJ: Fragile X syndrome, Curr Probl Pediatr 17:621-674, 1987.

Hagerman RJ: Selected neurodevelopmental disorders: diagnosis and treatment, New York, 1999, Oxford University Press.

Hagerman RJ, Amiri K, and Cronister A: The fragile X checklist, Am J Med Genet 38:283-287, 1991.

Hagerman RJ et al: Institutional screening for the fragile X syndrome, Am J Dis Child 142:1216-1221, 1988.

Hagerman RJ et al: Fluoxetine therapy in fragile X syndrome, Developmental Brain Dysfunction 7:155-164, 1994a.

Hagerman RJ et al: High functioning fragile X males: demonstration of an unmethylated fully expanded FMR1 mutation associated with protein expression, Am J Med Genet 51:298-308, 1994b.

Hagerman RJ et al: A survey of the efficacy of clonidine in fragile X syndrome. Developmental Brain Dysfunction, 8:336-344, 1995.

Hagerman RJ, Murphy M, and Wittenberger M: A controlled trial of stimulant medication in children with fragile X syndrome, Am J Med Genet 30:377-392, 1988.

Hagerman RJ et al: Longitudinal IQ changes in fragile X males. Am J Med Genet 33:513-518, 1989.

Hagerman RJ, Altshul-Stark D, and McBogg P: Recurrent otitis media in boys with the fragile X syndrome, Am J Dis Child 142:1216-1221, 1987.

Hagerman RJ, Smith ACM, and Mariner R: Clinical features of the fragile X syndrome. In RJ Hagerman and PM McBogg, editors: The fragile X syndrome: diagnosis, biochemistry and intervention, Dillon, Colo., 1983, Spectra Publishing, pp 83-94.

Hagerman RJ and Sobesky WE: Psychopathology in fragile X syndrome, Am J Orthopsychiatry 59:142-152, 1989.

Hagerman RJ et al: Consideration of connective tissue dysfunction in the fragile X syndrome, Am J Med Genet 17:111-121, 1984.

Kemper MB, Hagerman RJ, and Altshul-Stark D: Cognitive profiles of boys with the fragile X syndrome, Am J Med Genet 30:191-200, 1987.

King RA, Hagerman RJ, and Houghton M: Ocular findings in fragile X syndrome. In press Developmental Brain Dysfunction, 1995.

Lachiewicz AM et al: Declining IQ scores of young males with fragile X syndrome, Am J Med Genet 30:272-278, 1987.

Loehr JP et al: Aortic root dilatation and mitral valve prolapse in the fragile X syndrome, Am J Med Genet 23:189-194, 1986.

Loesch DZ and Hay DA: Clinical features and reproductive patterns in fragile X female heterozygotes, J Med Genet 25:407-414, 1988.

Loesch DZ, Lafranchi M, and Scott D: Anthropometry in Martin-Bell syndrome, Am J Med Genetics 30:149-164, 1988.

Madison LS, George C, and Moeschler JB: Cognitive functioning in the fragile X syndrome: a study of intellectual, memory and communication skills, J Ment Defic Res 30:129-148, 1986.

Maino DM et al: Ocular anomalies in fragile X syndrome. J Am Optom Assoc 61:316-323, 1990.

Mazzocco MM, Pennington BF, and Hagerman RJ: The neurocognitive phenotype of female carriers of fragile X: additional evidence for specificity, J Dev Beh Ped 14:328-335, 1993.

Merenstein SA et al: Fragile X syndrome in a normal IQ male with learning and emotional problems, J Am Acad Child Adoles Psychiat 33:1316-1321, 1994.

Musumeci SA et al: Prevalence of a novel epileptogenic EEG pattern in the Martin-Bell syndrome, Am J Med Genet 30:207-212, 1988a.

Musumeci SA et al: Fragile X syndrome: a particular epileptogenic EEG pattern, Epilepsia 29:41-47, 1988b.

Newell K, Sanborn B, and Hagerman RJ: Speech and language dysfunction in the fragile X syndrome. In RJ Hagerman and P McBogg, editors: The fragile X syndrome: diagnosis, biochemistry and intervention, Dillon, CO, 1983, Spectra Publishing, pp 175-200.

Oberle I et al: Instability of a 550-base pair DNA segment and abnormal methylation in fragile X syndrome, Science 252:1097-1102, 1991.

Partington MW: The fragile X syndrome: preliminary data on growth and development in males, Am J Med Genet 17:175-194, 1984.

Prouty LA et al: Fragile X syndrome: growth development and intellectual function, Am J Med Genet 30:123-142, 1988.

Pueschel SM and Finelli PV: Neurologic investigations in patients with fragile X syndrome. Proceedings of the American Academy of Cerebral Palsy and Developmental Medicine, Washington, DC, April 1984 (abstract).

Rapin I: Conductive hearing loss effects on children's language and scholastic skills: a review of the literature, Ann Otol Rhinol Laryngol 88:3-12, 1979.

Rattazzi MC and Ioannou YA: Molecular approaches to therapy. In Hagerman RJ and Cronisten A. (eds.) Fragile X syndrome. Diagnosis, treatment, and research. 2nd ed. Johns Hopkins University Press, Baltimore, 1996.

Reiss AL et al: Psychiatric disability in female carriers of fragile X chromosome, Arch Gen Psychiatry 45:25-30, 1988.

Rousseau F et al: Prevalence of carriers of premutation—size alleles of the FMRI gene—and implications for the population genetics of the fragile X syndrome, Am J Hum Genet 57:1006-1018:1995.

Rousseau F et al: Surprisingly low prevalence of FMR1 premutation among males from the general population, Am J Hum Genet 59(suppl):A188-1069, 1996.

Scharfenaker S et al: An integrated approach to intervention. In Hagerman RJ and Cronister A, editors: Fragile X syndrome: diagnosis, treatment, and research, ed 2, Baltimore, 1996, Johns Hopkins University Press.

Scharfenaker S and Schreiner R: Cognitive and speech language characteristics of the fragile X syndrome, Rocky Mountain J Commun Disorders, 1989.

Sherman S: Epidemiology. In Hagerman RJ and Cronister A, editors: Fragile X syndrome: diagnosis, treatment, and research, ed 2, Baltimore, 1996, Johns Hopkins University Press.

Schnizel A and Largo RH: The fragile X syndrome (Martin-Bell syndrome) clinical and cytogenetic findings in 16 prepubertal boys and in 4 of their 5 families, Helv Paediatr Acta 40:133-152, 1985.

Simko A et al: Fragile X syndrome: recognition in young children, Pediatrics 83:547-552, 1989.

Sobesky WE et al: Emotional and neurocognitive deficits in fragile X, Am J Med Genet 51:378-384, 1994.

Sreeran N et al: Cardiac abnormalities in the fragile X syndrome, Br Heart J 61:289-291, 1989.

Storm RL, De Benito R, and Ferretti C: Ophthalmologic findings in the fragile syndrome, Arch Ophthalmol 105:1099-1102, 1987.

Sutherland GR, Hecht F: Fragile sites on human chromosomes, New York, 1985, Oxford University Press.

Tassone F et al: FMRP expression as a potential prognostic indicator in fragile X syndrome, Am J Med Gen 4:250-261, 1999.

Turner G et al: Prevalence of fragile X syndrome, Am J Med Gen 64(1):196-7, 1996.

Verkerk AJMH et al: Identification of a gene (FMR-1) containing a CGG repeat coincident with a breakpoint cluster region exhibiting length variation in fragile X syndrome, Cell 65(5):905-914, 1991.

Willemsen R et al: Rapid antibody test for prenatal diagnosis of fragile X syndrome on amniotic fluid cells: a new appraisal, J Med Genet 34(3):250-1, 1997.

Wilson P et al: Issues and strategies for educating children with fragile X syndrome: a monograph, Dillon, CO, 1994, Spectra Publishing Co, Inc.

Windeck SL and Laurel M: A theoretical framework combining speech-language therapy with sensory integration treatment, Am Occup Ther Assoc Sensory Integration Spec Interest Sect Newslett 12:1-5, 1989.

Wisniewski KE et al: The fragile X syndrome: neurological, electrophysiological, and neuropathological abnormalities, Am J Med Genet 38:476-480, 1991.

Yu S et al: Fragile X genotype characterized by an unstable region of DNA, Science 252:1179-1181, 1991.

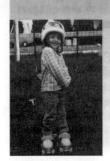

CHAPTER 23

Head Injury

Carole Low* and Patricia A. Murphy

Etiology

In children, the head is often involved in traumatic injuries because it is proportionally the largest part of a child's body. Therefore when a child falls or is thrown, the most energy from the impact is transmitted to the head. The major concern about a head injury is whether there has been damage to the brain. Traumatic brain injury (TBI) is defined as physical damage to or functional impairment of the brain from acute mechanical energy exchange (Michaud, Duhaime, and Batshaw, 1993).

Craniocerebral trauma is the most common cause of acquired disability in the pediatric population, with nearly one fourth of head injuries being inflicted in children under 2 years of age (Reynolds, 1992; Michaud, Duhaime, and Batshaw, 1993). Due to a child's immature brain, the pattern of injury and response to injury varies from that of adults. Of the children that are hospitalized with a head injury, approximately 15% will be categorized as having severe head injury with mortality rates approaching 50% (Adelson and Kochanek, 1998; Tullous, 1992). The majority of head injuries are preventable.

The *primary injury* to the brain occurs at the moment of impact from a direct traumatic force. Concussions, contusions, lacerations, skull injuries, and diffuse axonal injuries are examples of primary injuries. The brain damage that occurs from the primary injury is irreversible.

The primary injury elicits a secondary response from the brain, which includes a cascade of biochemical and physiologic events that—if not controlled or prevented—contribute to further brain injury (Adelson and Kochanek, 1998; Adelson et al,

1996). Secondary injuries include the development of intracranial hypertension, cerebral edema, cerebral hemorrhage, seizures, systemic hypotension, hypercapnia, infection, or hypoxemia, and significantly increase the morbidity and mortality in children with TBI. Unlike the primary injury, secondary responses and the resulting injury to the brain are amenable to medical and pharmacologic intervention.

The mechanisms of the primary injury associated with TBI are a result of direct traumatic forces and include the forces of *deceleration,* which occur when the head strikes an immovable object, (e.g., the ground or the dashboard of a car) and *acceleration* forces, which occur when the head is struck by an object (e.g., a baseball bat or forceful hand slap). Coup-contrecoup, or acceleration-deceleration injuries, occur in combination (Figure 23-1). The first injury occurs when the brain strikes the cranium on the side of impact; the second occurs when the brain rebounds and strikes the cranium on the contralateral side (Chipps, Clanin, and Campbell, 1992; Woestman et al, 1998). Contrecoup injuries are considered more severe and the size of the impact area also affects the injury severity; the smaller the area of impact, the greater the severity of the injury as a result of the concentration of force in the smaller area (Walleck and Mooney, 1994).

Rotational trauma is characterized by a twisting of the brain during deceleration or acceleration, which frequently occurs in combination with coup-contrecoup injuries, resulting in shearing of the tissues. Blunt trauma or gunshot wounds to the brain are examples of *deformation* injuries, which are the result of direct blows to the head that change the skull contour and symmetry; the higher the velocity of impact, the greater the explosive effect within the cranium (Chipps, Clanin, and Campbell, 1992; Woestman et al, 1998).

*The authors gratefully acknowledge the contributions of the late Carole Low.

Head Injury Classification

Severity of Head Injury

Head injuries are classified by severity of response during the immediate postinjury period (Table 23-1). Mild head injuries are associated with high Glasgow Coma Scale (GCS) scores (Table 23-2) and usually full recovery, and severe head injuries are associated with low GCS scores and potential long-term morbidity or mortality.

Open or Closed Head Injuries

Head injuries are classified as either open or closed. Open head injuries are the result of penetrating wounds to the skull. Closed or blunt head trauma can result in cerebral concussion, contusion, or hematoma.

Focal or Diffuse Injuries

Head injuries are further classified as focal (i.e., when brain damage is localized to one area due to an expanding mass), tissue or vascular lacerations or contusions, or diffuse (i.e., when brain damage

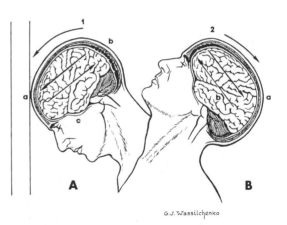

G.J. Wassilchenko

Figure 23-1 Coup and contrecoup head injury following blunt trauma. **A,** Coup injury: impact against object. Site of impact and direct trauma to brain *(a)*. Shearing of subdural veins *(b)*. Trauma to base of brain *(c)*. **B,** Contrecoup injury: impact within skull. Site of impact from brain hitting opposite side of skull *(a)*. Shearing forces through brain *(b)*. These injuries occur in one continuous motion—the head strikes the wall (coup), then rebounds (contrecoup). (From Rudy E: Advanced neurological and neurosurgical nursing, St Louis, 1984, Mosby.)

Table 23-1
Severity of Head Injury

Mild	Moderate	Severe
Asymptomatic or Minimal loss of consciousness with rapid clearing of mental status or Headache or Vomitinge or Irritability GCS 13-15	>10 min posttraumatic unconsciousness or Posttraumatic seizures or Focal neurologic deficits or Retrograde amnesia lasting >30 min or Evidence of depressed skull fracture, basilar skull fracture, or CSF leak or Severe headache or Persistent vomiting or Irritability GCS 9-12	Respiratory distress or Circulatory instability or Altered mental status (unresponsiveness, coma) or Marked irritability or Signs of increased intracranial pressure GCS ≤8

Adapted from Fox J: Primary healthcare of children, St Louis, 1997, Mosby.
Berman S: Pediatric decision making, St Louis, 1997, Mosby.
GCS, Glascow Coma Score.

Table 23-2
Glasgow Coma Scale

	Child >2 Years Old or Adult		Child <2 Years Old or Developmentally Delayed	
Best eye-opening response	Spontaneously	4	Spontaneously	4
	To verbal command	3	To verbal command	3
	To pain	2	To pain	2
	No response	1	No response	1
Best verbal response	Oriented, converses	5	Coos, babbles	5
	Disoriented, converses	4	Irritable cry	4
	Inappropriate words	3	Cries to pain	3
	Incomprehensible sounds	2	Moans to pain	2
	No response	1	None	1
Best motor response				
To verbal command	Obeys	6	Spontaneous	6
To painful stimulus	Localizes pain	5	Withdraws to touch	5
	Flexion-withdrawal	4	Withdraws to pain	4
	Flexion-decorticate	3	Abnormal flexion	3
	Extension-decerebrate	2	Abnormal extension	2
	No response	1	None	1
Total		(3-15)		(3-15)

Adapted from Chipps EM, Clanin NJ, and Campbell VG: Neurologic disorders, St Louis, 1992, Mosby.
Hazinski MF: Neurologic disorders. In Hazinski MF, editor: Nursing care of the critically ill child, St Louis, 1992, Mosby.

is widespread due to generalized brain edema or ischemia, systemic hypoxia, or hypotension). Brain injuries in children are most commonly diffuse closed head injuries.

Skull Fracture

Skull fractures occur less commonly in children than adults because their skulls are more pliable. When fractures do occur, they are most often linear and reflect a significant impact and potential for brain injury. Fractures that cross underlying blood vessels increase the risk of intracranial hemorrhage (Goldstein and Powers, 1994).

Concussion

The least serious type of traumatic brain injury is a concussion, which is a transient neurologic dysfunction involving immediate and transitory alterations in consciousness, equilibrium, and vision (Bruce, 1995). Although these injuries may be considered minor, they can be deceiving and may lead to complications and a prolonged course of recovery. The duration of unconscious-

ness can indicate the severity of the concussion (i.e., the longer the coma, the worse the injury). Long-term sequelae or postconcussive syndrome can include fatigue, dizziness, headache, irritability, poor concentration, memory difficulties, emotional lability, decreased attention span, and cognitive changes lasting from a week to years after the injury (Walleck and Mooney, 1994; Woestman et al, 1998).

Contusion and Laceration

Cerebral contusions result in bruising of neuronal tissue due to hemorrhage into cortical tissue. Contusions are the most frequently seen lesions in older children after a head injury. Common locations for contusions include the frontal, occipital, and parietal areas. Lacerations are more serious than contusions and occur due to a penetrating injury. Lacerations involve tearing of the cortical surface with damage to the surrounding tissues. As a result, lacerations tend to bleed profusely because of the poor vasoconstrictive ability of the cortical vasculature (Walleck and Mooney, 1994).

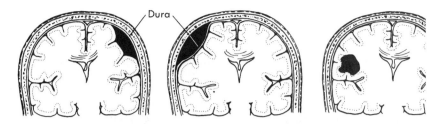

Figure 23-2   Different types of hematomas. **A,** Subdural. **B,** Epidural. **C,** Intracerebral. (From Thelan LA et al: Critical care nursing: diagnosis and management, ed 2, St Louis, 1994, Mosby.)

Diffuse Axonal Injury

Diffuse axonal injury (DAI) is a term used to describe widespread cerebral damage that results from shearing, tearing, or stretching of axons within the white matter of the brain. This lesion is the most common cause of prolonged coma following a traumatic brain injury (Michaud, Duhaime, and Batshaw, 1993). The symptoms of DAI include prolonged unresponsiveness, pupillary changes, and decerebrate posture (Slazinski and Johnson, 1994). DAI results from damage to nerve fibers produced by linear and rotational sheer strains following high-speed deceleration injuries (i.e., a significant fall or hitting a windshield in a car accident (Alexander, 1995). The severity of injury corresponds with the amount of shearing force applied. The resulting injury to the brain tissue leads to widespread cerebral edema and neuronal dysfunction. The prognosis ranges from severe disabilities, persistent vegetative state, to death.

Cerebral Hemorrhage or Hematoma

Cerebral hemorrhage, or hematoma, results in a mass lesion effect that causes elevated intracranial pressure (Figure 23-2). Of individuals with skull fractures, 25% develop a surgically significant hematoma. Epidural hematomas occur between the dura and the skull and are often arterial. Subdural hematomas occur 5 to 10 times more frequently than epidural hematomas and occur between the dura and the arachnoid. They are frequently venous and slower in formation (Chipps, Clanin, and Campbell, 1992; Coburn, 1992). Subdural hematomas occur in approximately 10% to 20% of all traumatic brain injuries (Walleck and Mooney, 1994; Woestman et al,

1998). Intracerebral hemorrhages occur within the cortical tissue and vary significantly in size and effect on brain function. Surgical evacuation of an intracerebral hematoma only occurs when medical therapies to decrease intracranial pressure fail.

Cerebral Edema

Cerebral edema, either focal or generalized, is the result of an increase in tissue fluid from intracellular or extracellular sources. It may be caused by either the initial injury to the neuronal tissue or secondarily in response to hypoxia, hypercapnia, or cerebral ischemia. Signs and symptoms of increased intracranial pressure include irritability, lethargy, nausea and vomiting, headache, photophobia, pupillary changes, abnormal reflexes, seizures, widening pulse pressure, bradycardia, and apnea.

Peak response for cerebral edema usually occurs up to 72 hours after the neurologic insult, and gradually resolves over a 2- to 3-week period (Walleck and Mooney, 1994). If left untreated or poorly controlled, cerebral edema can have a devastating effect, resulting in intracranial hypertension and altered cerebral perfusion. These results can lead to neuronal tissue hypoxia, ischemia, cerebral herniation and death.

Brain herniation can occur after a traumatic brain injury if the increased intracranial pressure fails to adequately respond to aggressive management. Downward displacement of the cerebellar tonsils of the lower brainstem through the foramen magnum can lead to irreversible loss of brain function. The prognosis associated with brainstem injuries is poor as a result of the brainstem's control of vital functions (Aldrich et al, 1992; Chipps, Clanin, and Campbell, 1992).

Incidence

Trauma is the leading cause of death and disability in the pediatric population of the United States, with head injuries significantly contributing to both mortality and morbidity (Adelson and Kochane, 1998). The annual incidence of hospital admitted traumatic brain injury is approximately 200 to 400 per 100,000 children in the United States with over 4,000 children dying due to head injury and up to 45 per 100,000 becoming disabled (Jennett, 1998). For every child who dies of a head injury, 40 children will require hospitalization and 1,000 children will be seen in the emergency room (Stylianos, 1998). Head injuries in children commonly result from falls, motor vehicle accidents, sports, and assaults. Of traumatic head injuries in children, 82% are considered mild, 14% are moderate or severe, and 5% are fatal. Factors influencing traumatic head injury in children include gender (i.e., males are affected more often than females at a ratio as high as 4 : 1 during adolescence), socioeconomic factors (i.e., increased incidence in low socioeconomic classes), and time of the year (i.e., increased incidence in spring and summer) (Adelson and Kochanek, 1998). Peak occurrence is during evenings, nights, weekends, and holidays when children are outside playing, swimming, riding bicycles, traveling in cars, or victims of gunshot wounds.

Clinical Manifestations at Time of Diagnosis

The clinical manifestations at the time of diagnosis vary depending on the primary brain injury and the extent and involvement of secondary responses (Box 23-1). Children with head injuries can present with varying levels of alertness and responsiveness, depending on the degree of increased intracranial pressure. Children with significant brain injury can initially present awake and alert and become confused, lethargic, and unresponsive within minutes to hours (Woestman et al, 1998). Alterations in level of consciousness after head injury can result in irritability, agitation, restlessness, and

confusion to coma. Acute pain can be manifested by verbalization of a headache, irritability, or crying. Skull fractures may or may not show bony displacement or swelling.

Children with closed head injuries may have a transient period of unconsciousness with recovery in minutes to hours with residual amnesia and memory loss. Hemorrhage from a hematoma may first present with a transient loss of consciousness followed by a lucid period and then suddenly deteriorate with signs of rapidly increasing intracranial pressure. Seizures, unilateral pupillary changes, and hemiplegia may be present. As cerebral edema and increased intracranial pressure rise, the following may be evident: changes in level of consciousness, abnormal respiratory patterns, loss of protective reflexes (e.g., cough, gag, or corneal), changes in blood pressure and pulse pressure with bradycardia, pupillary dysfunction, papilledema, changes in motor function or posturing, nausea and projectile vomiting, positive Babinski's sign, and visual disturbances (Adelson and Kochanek, 1998; Chipps, Clanin, and Campbell, 1992).

The GCS has become the most widely used tool to measure a child's level of consciousness and severity of head injury (Altimier, 1992; Vernon-Levett, 1991). The GCS objectively scores the child's best responses to motor, verbal, and eye opening stimulation (see Table 23-2). The highest combined score is 15 and the lowest is 3. Any score less than a maximum of 15 is considered an alteration in the level of consciousness. GCS scores of 13 to 15 reflect a minor injury; scores of 9 to 12 reflect moderate brain injury; and scores of 8 or less are considered a severe brain injury.

Despite its limitations for use in infants and preverbal children, individuals with a preinjury

---

Box 23-1

Clinical Manifestations

Physical findings determined by severity and type of injury
Assessment tools for TBI
   Glascow Coma Scale (GCS)
   Children's Coma Scale (CCS)
   Rancho Los Amigos Scale of Cognitive Functioning

deficit (i.e., hemiparesis), or individuals who are intubated, this scoring method is routinely used as an assessment tool because it is universally understood and provides for a rapid assessment of the child's level of consciousness. The modified GCS has proven to be more useful for assessing children with a head injuries who are under 2 years of age, nonverbal, or developmentally delayed. The GCS, along with the clinician's physical assessment, should be used in evaluating children with a head injury during the acute care period.

A Children's Coma Score (CCS) was developed as a method of assessing infants and toddlers who are preverbal or unable to follow commands appropriately (Table 23-3) (Ghajar and Hariri, 1992). The maximum score of the CCS is 11 compared with 15 on the adult GCS. Although gaining in popularity, many clinicians continue to use the GCS because it is familiar and universally accepted.

The Rancho Los Amigos Scale of Cognitive Functioning is useful in assessing the level of recovery from head injury and is primarily used during the rehabilitation phase (Table 23-4). This table categorizes the cognitive functioning and behaviors of individuals with brain injuries in more descriptive terms. The scale is divided into eight cognitive levels that range from purposeful

and appropriate responses to no response to any stimulus. This table is useful in tracking the sequence of recovery from coma (Walleck and Mooney, 1994).

Treatment (Box 23-2)

Treatment of children with TBI is dependent on the severity of the injury. Initial treatment begins with control and support of the airway, breathing, and circulation. The goal of treatment is to stabilize the effects of the primary injury and prevent the secondary injuries due to hypoxia, hypercarbia, cerebral edema, seizures, infection, and aspiration.

Medical management begins in the prehospital setting where the goal is rapid, accurate assessment of the primary injury and the prevention or management of associated secondary responses or injuries (Altimier, 1992). Standard treatment consists of elevating the head of the bed and keeping the head in a midline position to facilitate cerebral venous drainage. Frequent clinical assessments are part of the treatment plan and are necessary in caring for children because of the rapid and often unanticipated changes they make in their clinical presentation. Children with head injuries should be treated for cervical spine injuries until definitive neurodiagnostic studies demonstrate otherwise (Cox, 1994). Children who are considered to be high risk for hypoxia, hypercarbia, or aspiration and are unable to protect their airway should have an artificial airway placed. Children with a GCS of

---

Table 23-3
Children's Coma Scale

Maximum score = 11
Minimum score = 3
Motor response: maximum score = 4
  4 flexes and extends
  3 withdraws from painful stimulus
  2 hypertonic
  1 flaccid
Verbal response: maximum score = 3
  3 cries
  2 spontaneous respirations
  1 apneic
Ocular response: maximum score = 4
  4 pursuit
  3 extraocular muscles (EOM) intact, reactive pupils
  2 fixed pupils of EOM impaired
  1 fixed pupil and EOM paralyzed

Adapted from Ghajar J and Hariri R: Management of pediatric head injury, Pediatric Clinics of North America 39:1093-1125, 1992.

Box 23-2

Treatment

- Prehospital stabilization
- Early treatment determined by severity of TBI
- Need to control hypoxia, increased cerebral CO_2, and brain edema
- Surgical intervention for bleeding, trauma, or cerebral edema may be necessary
- Recovery from coma follows predictable patterns but with varied time sequence
- Rehabilitation program key to long-term recovery

Table 23-4
Rancho Los Amigos Scale of Cognitive Functioning

Level	Response	Description
1	None	Completely unresponsive to any stimulus
2	Generalized	Reacts inconsistently and nonpurposefully to stimuli; may respond with physiologic changes, gross body movements, or utterances
3	Localized	Reacts specifically but inconsistently to stimuli; responds directly to a stimulus; shows vague awareness of self and body; may pull at tubes and react to discomfort
4	Confused Agitated	Heightened state of activity but unable to process information correctly; reacts to internal confusion; nonpurposeful behavior with confabulation present; cries, screams, and manifests aggressive behavior; cannot discriminate among people; performs gross motor activities but not self-care activities
5	Confused Inappropriate	Follows simple commands; may show agitated behavior from inability to cope with external demands; gross inattention to environment, easily distracted; impaired memory and inappropriate verbalization; cannot initiate tasks; often uses things incorrectly
6	Confused Appropriate	Displays goal-directed behavior but requires direction from others; follows simple commands; shows carryover of information from previously learned tasks; memory problems persist; inconsistently oriented to time and place; increased awareness of self and others
7	Automatic Appropriate	Oriented in hospital and home settings but performs tasks in robotlike manner; superficial awareness of own condition but lacks good problem-solving abilities; carryover for new learning; independent in self-care activities; needs structure but can initiate tasks of interest
8	Purposeful Appropriate	Alert and oriented; few memory problems; can begin vocational rehabilitation; carryover for new learning; social, emotional, and intellectual capacities may be decreased from pretrauma level

Modified from original scale developed by Los Amigos Research and Education Institute, Inc. of Rancho Los Amigos Medical Center, Downey, California. From Walleck CA and Mooney KF: Neurotrauma: head injury. In Barkin E, editor: Neuroscience Nursing, St Louis, 1994, Mosby.

8 or less should be provided with intubation and hyperventilation immediately. Hypoxia and hypercarbia exacerbate secondary injury by producing vasodilation and subsequently an increase in intracranial pressure (Adelson and Kochanek, 1998; Walleck and Mooney, 1994). Even moderate reductions in PaO_2 (<60 mm Hg) can contribute to neuronal injury by causing vasodilatation and increased cerebral edema (Forbes et al, 1995; Pigula et al, 1993)

Artificial hyperventilation is used to decrease intracranial pressure by lowering the $PaCO_2$ to 30 and 35 mm Hg, leading to vasoconstriction of cerebral vasculature and decreased intracranial pressure (AANA, 1995; Cox, 1994). The goal is to avoid systemic hypotension and maintain adequate cerebral perfusion. A single episode of systolic blood pressure below 90 mmHg decreases survival fourfold and increases morbidity in survivors (Kokoska et al, 1998). Because neuronal tissue lacks metabolic reserves, it depends on arterial blood flow to meet its metabolic needs (Walleck and Mooney, 1994). Injuries to the cerebral contents cause edema and loss of autoregulation, increase intracranial pressure, decrease cerebral perfusion pressure, and ultimately decrease cerebral blood flow. Vasopressors may be used to maintain adequate cerebral perfusion pressure.

Fluid restrictions and osmotic diuretics are used to decrease cerebral edema. Anticonvulsants are often given to prevent early posttraumatic seizures (Adelson and Kochanek, 1998; Paolin et al, 1998). In addition, decreasing the cerebral metabolic rate by use of mild hypothermia, sedation, paralytic agents, and barbiturate coma can be effective in lowering cerebral metabolism, ultimately leading to further decreases in intracranial pressure (Reynolds, 1992).

Surgical management to lower intracranial pressure includes removal of mass lesions, drainage of CSF, placement of burr holes to relieve internal pressure on the brain, and placement of devices to measure intracranial pressure.

Recovery from Coma

Most children who lapse into a coma as a result of a traumatic brain injury eventually regain consciousness (Adelson and Kochanek, 1998; Michaud, Duhaime, and Batshaw, 1993). Recovery from a coma can be lengthy and painful for family members to witness. Families are often relieved and elated that their child has survived the initial critical care phase but become frustrated and agitated with the slowness of the recovery phase and the uncertainty that their child will regain consciousness. Despite individual variations in recovery due to the mechanism and severity of injury, there are certain patterns of behavior commonly seen in children (Michaud, Duhaime, and Batshaw, 1993). A child's initial response to external stimuli may include unresponsiveness; generalized, purposeless motor response; or an inability to localize. Autonomic dysfunction (i.e., central fever, systemic hypertension, agitation, restlessness, teeth grinding, or diffuse intermittent diaphoresis) may also be seen. Spontaneous eye opening may occur, but there is no tracking or fixation on objects, little recognition of familiar objects or family members, and the visual gaze is often dysconjugate (Michaud, Duhaime, and Batshaw, 1993). As children are emerging from a coma, they typically demonstrate frequent alterations in their level of consciousness.

There is rarely a sudden or smooth rise to being alert and oriented. Periods of intermittent agitation, which include pulling at restraints, entanglement in bed linens, nonpurposeful crying, moaning or movement, using vulgarity or repetitive movements, are frequent. The agitation periods begin to subside as the child shows an increased awareness of surroundings. The child may begin to verbalize a familiar phrase or word, follow a simple command, show a common gesture, or visually focus on a familiar face or object. This heightened level of awareness will initially come

and go and be brief, but as the child progresses through the coma, he or she will become more aware of the environment and respond appropriately. The return of consciousness is functionally defined as the child's ability to reliably and consistently follow commands (Michaud, Duhaime, and Batshaw, 1993).

In aphasic or preverbal children, however, a more general assessment must be used in observing the child's behaviors or purposeful actions. Passive interventions such as range-of-motion exercises can then be modified to include those movements that encourage more active participation by the child. During this period of rehabilitation, assessment of the child's abnormal physical, behavioral, and cognitive problems is necessary in order to establish long-term goals (Michaud, Duhaime, and Batshaw, 1993). Behavioral problems for the child with a head injury can include altered attention span and memory, poor impulse control and emotional outbursts, and frustration at the lengthy process of rehabilitation and adaptation.

Long-Term Management and Rehabilitation

The goals of rehabilitation in children with a head injury are to maximize abilities and functions in physical, cognitive, communicative, emotional, and social areas (Michaud, Duhaime, and Batshaw, 1993). Rehabilitation can hasten and maximize restoration of lost functions, promote adaptation to disabilities, and aid in age-appropriate independence and reintegration into family and school life. Rehabilitation can enhance the quality of life of these children and reduce future health care expenditures.

Once a child is able to show some awareness of the environment and some ability to respond to it, he or she can be transferred to a rehabilitation program suitable for the care of children. Rehabilitation provides the services necessary for children to maximally recover and adequately compensate for lost or impaired function while continuing to develop physically, cognitively, and socially to their fullest potential (Chorazy et al, 1998). Rehabilitation helps to prevent problems that are secondary in nature. Passive range-of-motion exercises, limb splinting, and proper support and positioning are methods aimed at preventing physical deformities (e.g., extremity contractures) that result from prolonged immobilization and increased tone.

Due to the complexity of caring for a child and family after a head injury and the promotion of recovery, rehabilitation often uses a multidisciplinary approach of team experts. The team of specialists is often directed by a pediatric physiatrist (i.e., a physician specializing in the care of children recovering from a significant injury or illness). A pediatric physiatrist is familiar with all aspects of a child's development, as well as with the pathologic sequelae related to brain injury and their effects on a dynamically changing nervous system (Chorazy et al, 1998). Within the team of experts, physical and occupational therapists attend to a child's physical limitations by promoting normal locomotion and adaptation to hindering physical disabilities. Emotional, social, and behavioral aspects of a child's recovery are guided by the team's psychologists, psychiatrists, social workers, and life therapists. Cognition and school reentry are directed by the team's speech and language pathologists and special education teachers. A child's medical problems during the recovery period are managed by a physiatrist, nursing staff, and other subspecialists when appropriate.

During rehabilitation, significant emphasis is placed on the return of function and avoidance of additional medical and physical problems. This phase of care may continue throughout a lifetime for some children and their families (Ylvisaker, Hartwick, and Stevens, 1991).

The role of the primary care provider is often incorporated into the final stages of inpatient rehabilitation. The provider is updated on the child's medical conditions and functional limitations, the team of subspecialists providing services, and the types of therapy and equipment necessary after discharge. Together the primary care provider and the rehabilitation staff evaluate the community resources and services and implement the support that will be necessary to the child and family upon returning home.

The decision to be discharged to home is often difficult and traumatic—both physically and emotionally—for the child and family (Nash et al, 1998). Extensive discharge planning is needed to provide a smooth transition from the inpatient setting to the home and community setting.

The process of recovery does not stop when a child is discharged from the inpatient unit. Continued emotional, physical, medical, nursing, and cognitive support for the child and family is needed until the quality of life is acceptable to the child, family, and care providers. In addition, respite opportunities for the family and other providers are important and should be arranged. The decision to discharge the child from a rehabilitation program should be considered when reasonable treatment goals have been achieved or no further progress is demonstrated.

Reliable predictions of outcome in the child with a severe head injury can be provided between 6 and 12 months after injury, at which point children have regained 90% of their probable neurologic function (Ghajar and Hariri, 1992).

Recent and Anticipated Advances in Diagnosis and Management

Current advances in the management and treatment of children with head injuries center around monitoring and preventing or treating secondary responses and injuries. Maintaining adequate cerebral perfusion pressure is essential to avoid cerebral ischemia, but the ideal value is unknown. Therefore future research using measurements of cerebral blow flow and metabolism may help determine adequate cerebral perfusion pressure. Intracranial monitoring has been the gold standard when treating severe head injuries; however, the shift is now to obtain more information about intracerebral dynamics to more effectively manage intracranial pressure and maintain adequate cerebral perfusion pressure. Assessment of cerebral blood flow by xenon-CT scan, transcranial doppler, or radioactive Xe is used to determine regional cerebral blood flow (Forbes, Kochanek, and Adelson, 1999). Near-infrared spectroscopy tracks the oxidative state of cytochromes in the brain and provides an indication of reduced cerebral oxygenation flow (Forbes, Kochanek, and Adelson, 1999). This modality has just begun to be evaluated in children with head injuries (Adelson et al, in press).

Magnetic resonance imaging (MRI) is currently not used in the initial evaluation of head injuries but is being used more during the critical and acute care phase as a tool for evaluating the evolution of cerebral edema, quantification of cerebral blood flow, aging of various intracranial bleeds, and documentation of brain stem and spinal cord abnormalities (Barzo et al, 1996; Forbes et al, 1997)

Associated Problems (Box 23-3)

Neurologic Dysfunction

Posttraumatic hydrocephalus occurs in a small number of individuals after head trauma, most commonly in those who have suffered a subarachnoid hemorrhage. Cerebral ventriculomegaly may arise weeks or months after head injury. In children with severe head injury, the ventriculomegaly may be due to cerebral atrophy. If a diagnosis of hydrocephalus is made, treatment consists of placement of a valve-regulating shunt (see Chapter 25) (Humphreys, 1991). Surgical management via a shunt relieves the acute symptoms (see Chapter 25).

Posttraumatic meningitis may be associated with a basilar skull fracture. Indications of cerebrospinal fluid (CSF) leakage from the nares or ear canal, periorbital ecchymosis, Battle's sign, scleral hemorrhage, fever, irritability, or an altered level of consciousness indicates the need for further assessment and CSF sampling. Once meningitis has been treated successfully, surgical intervention is necessary to repair the dural opening or close the CSF fistula.

The incidence of posttraumatic seizures varies from 0.7% to 10%, depending on the severity of the head injury (Annegers et al, 1998). Children who experience an open head injury have a much higher incidence than children with a closed head injury (Altimier, 1992; Walleck and Mooney, 1994). Posttraumatic seizures show no correlation with age, location of skull fracture, parenchymal injury, fixed neurologic deficits, or type of cranial operation (Humphreys, 1991). Posttraumatic seizures are classified as early (i.e., occurring within 7 days of injury) or late (i.e., occurring >7 days after injury) (Yablon, 1993). Studies have indicated that prophylactic administration of anticonvulsants during the first week reduces the incidence of early seizures; extended use of anticonvulsants, however, does not reduce the incidence of late seizures (Manaka, 1992; Temkin, Dikmen, Wilensky, 1990). Anticon-

> ### Box 23-3
> ### Associated Problems
>
> - Neurologic dysfunction
>   - Posttraumatic hydrocephalus
>   - Posttraumatic meningitis
>   - Seizures
>   - Postconcussion syndrome
> - Abnormal motor and sensory function
> - Feeding problems
> - Endocrine dysfunction
> - Altered cognitive and neuropsychologic functions
> - Psychosocial and psychiatric deficits
> - Additional physiologic problems (see Box 23-4)

vulsants should therefore only be given prophylactically for 1 week and then discontinued unless chronic seizures develop.

Chronic seizures are usually well controlled with anticonvulsant medications. The onset of these seizures varies greatly, from soon after the initial injury to 2 years following the injury. (See Chapter 21 on epilepsy.)

Postconcussion syndrome can occur after a mild head injury. The most common symptoms include headaches, irritability, anxiety, behavioral disturbances, dizziness, fatigue, impaired concentration, forgetfulness, blurred vision, nausea, and sleep disturbances (Ingebrigtsen, Waterloo, Marup-Jensen, 1998). This syndrome usually appears days to weeks after the initial injury and can persist up to a year postinjury.

Abnormal Motor and Sensory Function

Common motor disabilities for children following a head injury include incoordination, quadriparesis, hemiparesis, spasticity, rigidity, tremors, decreased motor speed, and ataxia (Michaud, Duhaime, and Batshaw, 1993). For children with any impairment at all after craniotrauma, difficulty in walking is the single most frequently impaired function (DiScala et al, 1991). Tics have also been shown to occur after CNS insult (e.g., anoxia secondary to trauma). As many as 10% of new onset tic disorders arise following head trauma (Moskowitz, 1994). In addition, audiologic problems and visual deficits may develop. Occupational and physical therapies are provided at regular intervals to maximize balance, coordination, and strength, as well as to retrain individuals in assisted (followed by independent) ambulation and other functional activities leading to developmentally appropriate self-care. Adaptive equipment (i.e., crutches, walkers, wheelchairs, lifts, and mechanical seats) may be used as needed. Pharmacologic management of spasticity with baclofen, dantrolene, or benzodiazepines may have variable levels of success (Michaud, Duhaime, and Batshaw, 1993).

Feeding Problems

Many children cannot eat on their own because of physical limitations or inability to coordinate chewing and swallowing. Children often have nasogastric tubes or gastrostomies to facilitate nutrition. A child's ability to feed is often an area of focus for a family due to the emotional, social, and cultural beliefs surrounding feeding and nutrition. Use of a registered dietitian to maintain fluid balance, appropriate caloric intake, and nutrition status for growth is highly recommended. These children often go on to develop weight problems due to inactivity and therefore need to decrease caloric intake.

Endocrine Dysfunction

After a severe head injury, children may initially show signs of antidiuretic dysfunction. Diabetes insipidus (i.e., a deficiency of antidiuretic hormone secretion) presents as hypernatremia, polydipsia, and polyuria. Current treatment consists of fluid boluses to maintain hydration and administration of intranasal vasopressin. Syndrome of inappropriate secretion of antidiuretic hormone (SIADH) consists of hyponatremia and decreased urinary output. Treatment of SIADH consists of fluid restriction and sodium administration. Either dysfunction resolves in most children but is a life-long issue for some.

Precocious puberty may present after a severe head injury with early signs of secondary sexual characteristics. If unrecognized or untreated, precocious puberty can result in accelerated skeletal growth and fusion of the skeletal epiphyses, leading to short stature.

Altered Cognitive and Neuropsychologic Function

In children who have developed verbal skills, alterations in speech and language capability can be either expressive, receptive, or mixed. In preverbal children, delays in expressive and receptive language can be present. Deficits may be noted in the areas of memory, word retrieval, naming, verbal organization, comprehension of verbal information, comprehension of verbal abstractions, efficient verbal learning, and effective conversation and discourse. Difficulties in attention and concentration, poor judgment, and impulsivity may persist (Michaud, Duhaime, and Batshaw, 1993). There may also be perceptual impairment, poor motor planning, tactile sensory dysfunction, and spatial disorientation. Improvement of speech is consistent with gains in motor function. Improvement in language ability (predominantly a cognitive function) may lag in severe cases despite aggressive therapy by speech and language specialists.

Psychosocial and Psychiatric Deficits

Postconcussion syndrome may be seen after a mild head injury or any form of head trauma. Personality changes—which can be the most difficult to manage—mood lability, loss of self-confidence, impaired short-term memory, headaches, and subtle cognitive impairments can be present (Walker, 1993; Walleck and Mooney, 1994). There is no specific treatment. Reassurance and support for the child and family are key factors in management.

Deficits noted include lack of goal direction and initiative, social withdrawal, depression, denial of disabilities, immature behavior, apathy, reduced self-image, self-centeredness, disinhibition, and aggression. Peer acceptance is extremely important because without it social isolation may persevere.

Additional Problems Associated with Traumatic Brain Injury

Box 23-4 lists additional physiologic problems found in children with TBI.

Box 23-4

Traumatic Brain Injury Sequelae and Complications

Focal neurologic deficits
Neurogenic pulmonary edema
Pneumonia
Gastrointestinal hemorrhage
Cardiac dysrhythmias
Disseminated intravascular coagulation
Pulmonary emboli
Heterotopic ossifications
Increased muscle tone
Contractures
Aspiration
Hypertension
Disturbances of respiratory control
Hypopituitarism
Impaired nutritional status
Bladder incontinence
Bowel incontinence
Hyperphagia

Adapted from Chipps EM, Clanin NJ, and Campbell VG: Neurologic disorders, St Louis, 1992, Mosby.

Table 23-5
Staging Prognosis in the Child with a Neurotrauma Injury

Time	Examination	Prognosis
Within 24 hours following resuscitation	Absent ocular brainstem reflexes	Poor
	GCS ≤8	Significant probability of death or major neurologic deficits
	GSC ≥8	Low probability of death but with high risk of temporary or permanent neurologic deficits
Within first week after neurotrauma with GCS <8	Patient meets brain death criteria	Follow institutional protocol
	Intracranial pressure (ICP) consistently >40 mm Hg	Significant probability of death or major neurologic deficit including persistent vegetative state
	ICP generally <20 mm Hg	Low probability of death; high probability of long-term neurologic deficits

Adapted from Walker C: The young pediatric patient: Predicting outcome after cerebral insult, Headlines 4:4-11, 1993.

Prognosis

The key factor associated with overall outcome is the severity and type of traumatic brain injury. Of the children who sustain traumatic brain injury, 95% survive; of the children who sustain a severe head injury, however, only 65% survive (Jennett, 1998; Michaud, Duhaime, and Batshaw, 1993). Children with diffuse injury have better outcomes than those with focal lesions in addition to a diffuse injury. Secondary brain injuries have a significant effect on both the survival and quality of cognitive and physical outcome. In addition, significant extracranial injuries—most notably those involving the chest or abdomen and related problems of hypoxia and hypotension—are also associated with a poorer survival rate and outcome (Michaud, Duhaime, and Batshaw, 1993).

Neurologic assessment protocols have been developed and may provide some insight into the child's likely course of management and outcome (Table 23-5) (Ghajar and Hariri, 1992). Children in a coma will either meet the preestablished criteria for brain death or will respond to external stimulation within the first 2 weeks post injury. A child's eventual outcome after eye opening can range from a persistent vegetative state to the preinjury state. It should be recognized that in even the best of situations, other behavioral and personality changes may occur.

Despite improvements in imaging techniques and aggressive management for infants, toddlers, and young children with traumatic brain injuries,

Box 23-5

Glascow Outcome Scale

Vegetative state:
No cerebral cortical function that can be judged by behavior
Severe disability:
Conscious but dependent
Moderate disability:
Independent but disabled
Good recovery:
Able to participate in normal social life and can return to daily activities

From Chipps EM, Clanin NJ, and Campbell VG: Neurologic disorders, St Louis, 1992, Mosby.

Table 23-6
Glasgow Coma Scale Scores vs. Glasgow Outcomes Scale

GCS at 24 Hrs	Good Recovery or Moderate Disability %	Vegetative or Dead %
11-15	91	6
8-10	59	27
5-7	28	54
3-4	13	80

From Chipps EM, Clanin NJ, and Campbell VG: Neurologic disorders, St Louis, 1992, Mosby.

initial appearance, level of consciousness, and recovery time are still the best tools for primary care providers in determining long-term prognosis (Walker, 1993). Potential outcomes range from coma and permanent neurologic damage to a brief loss of consciousness followed by the resumption of full neurologic functioning. Of survivors with traumatic brain injury, 20% have a residual disability: 10% in mild injuries, and 90% to 100% for severe injuries (Michaud, Duhaime, and Batshaw, 1993) (Box 23-5 and Table 23-6). The initial GCS scores can be helpful in providing a gross predictor of outcome. In addition, other factors (i.e., pupillary response to light and intracranial pressure measurements) can improve the accuracy in predicting mortality and morbidity (Walker, 1993).

The highest mortality rate occurs in children under 2 years of age, reflecting the increased risk of physical abuse and resultant subdural hematomas. A second rise in mortality occurs during midadolescence related to increased motor vehicle accidents and resultant diffuse axonal injury (Michaud, Duhaime, and Batshaw, 1993). The duration of coma is also an important factor associated with severity of the underlying brain injury—longer duration is associated with a less favorable outcome (Michaud, Duhaime, and Batshaw, 1993). The speed at which a child recovers from coma provides a good predictive scale of how well the child will recover long-term (Walker, 1993).

The effect of age at the time of injury on neuro-

logic outcome is complex. Cerebral water content, extent of normal myelination, level of brain development, developmental stage, amount of cortical function, and neurochemical content vary in children at different ages. Each of these factors may have an effect on brain plasticity and the potential level of functional recovery (Michaud, Duhaime, and Batshaw, 1993).

Long-term prognosis is more difficult to evaluate. Although being realistic is important, the primary care provider should not convey an overly pessimistic outlook in counseling families because there have been many stories of children who have defied the odds and made remarkable recoveries. The reasons for higher percentages of good neurologic outcome in the pediatric population are unclear but could be attributed to the resilient properties of the immature brain.

PRIMARY CARE MANAGEMENT

Health Care Maintenance

Growth and Development

Body growth and total development must be monitored in children with a head injury. Head circumference measurements should be taken at each visit and recorded on a head circumference chart from birth to late adolescence (see Chapter 25 on hydrocephalus). For children with seizures, doses of antiepileptic drugs are calculated based on body weight for therapeutic effectiveness. Alterations in growth for weight and height may be present because of altered nutritional intake (see the following section on diet), therefore weight and height measurements should be taken and plotted on each visit.

Precocious puberty may occur in association with CNS lesions, including head trauma. As a result of this insult and potential disruption of the normal hypothalamus and pituitary function, children with a traumatic brain injury are at risk and should be monitored for clinical features of puberty before age 8 years in girls or age 9 years in boys. Premature sexual characteristics can take the form of isolated breast or pubic hair development. The most significant long-term complication is early epiphyseal fusion, resulting in short stature as an adult. If these sexual changes arise, referral to a pediatric endocrinologist is recommended for more in-depth management.

Children who have suffered a severe head injury often demonstrate signs of regression and may take on infantlike behavior. These children are completely dependent on supportive nursing care by health professionals and family members (Appleton, 1994). Major motor milestones are often delayed in young infants. Developmental progress should be monitored, as well as progress in therapy programs. Contractures and impaired motor function may persist as a result of alterations in muscle tone, decreased range of motion, and immobility.

Diet

Feeding difficulties often affect children who have sustained a traumatic brain injury. These difficulties include poor manual dexterity in handling utensils, dysphagia, inability to communicate when hungry, vomiting, insufficient caloric intake to meet metabolic demands, and gastroesophageal reflux. A decreased level of arousal interferes with adequate nutrition, and a negative nitrogen balance develops. Difficulty with immobility may lead to increased bone calcium loss as a result of inadequate weight bearing (Boss, 1994). Management of these nutritional difficulties usually begins with hyperalimentation during the acute phase and then transition to high-calorie, gastric tube feedings when bowel function is stabilized. At this point, tube feedings may continue indefinitely. Placement of a gastrostomy tube and fundoplication may be

considered for long-term management. Potential aspiration or gastroesophageal reflux concerns may be addressed by placing the child in a side-lying position during and after meals.

Once the level of consciousness has improved along with an intact cough and gag reflex, occupational and speech therapy can assist in optimizing feeding positions, evaluating swallowing function, facilitating coordinated tongue-lip-jaw control, and promoting oral desensitization. Alterations in smell and taste may also be associated with feeding difficulties (Michaud, Duhaime, and Batshaw, 1993). Disability in the dominant hand requires new spatial and motor learning for effective self-feeding.

Oral hygiene, mucosal and tongue lesions, and poor dentition may affect appetite, as well as depression, overstimulation, fatigue, and frustration with trying to relearn how to self-feed. Cognitive or behavioral deficits can cause poor intake through problems with confusion, inability to concentrate, attentional deficits, and distractibility.

Children who must learn new eating skills may be unable to eat without repeated cueing and supervision (Whitney, 1994). Soft foods that are easy to swallow should be offered with assistance in feeding. Inadequate oral intake of a high-calorie, balanced diet consisting of three small meals with three snacks during the daytime may be supplemented by tube feedings at nighttime. Weight should be monitored at regular intervals and more often if there is evidence of inadequate weight gain or the presence of excessive weight gain as a result of poor motor function and decreased physical activity. In addition, supplementation of vitamins and minerals may be considered to address the amount of calcium loss.

Safety

Safety practices and injury prevention are important in children who have sustained a traumatic brain injury. These children are at an increased risk for future injury as a result of neuropsychologic and neurobehavioral deficits resulting in overactivity, poor judgment, impulsivity, and perceptual deficits (Michaud, Duhaime, and Batshaw, 1993). Keeping an environment free of clutter, sharp-angled objects, steps, or uneven surfaces is recommended along with adequate anticipatory supervision as independence increases (see Chapter 28 on learning disabilities). Assistive devices (e.g., wheelchairs and walkers) should be assessed for safety and kept repaired (Whitney, 1994). Consideration of appropriate emergency exit routes from the home and other locations should be evaluated. Family members and care providers should be knowledgeable of seizure precautions and seizure first aid (see Chapter 21 on epilepsy).

Use of appropriate motor vehicle passenger seat restraints, helmets, and home child-proofing should be reinforced. Normal childhood activities (i.e., bike riding, swimming, gymnastics, and softball) should be considered for each individual child with regard to the benefits gained from active participation vs. the possible risks. Adolescents with post-TBI may have increased safety risks as a result of neuropsychiatric sequelae impairing judgment and motor-coordination. Parents may need help determining appropriate adolescent responsibilities and activities.

Immunization

Infants and children with head injuries and post-traumatic seizures are at a slightly increased risk of having a seizure after receiving either the diphtheria, tetanus, and acellular pertussis (DTaP) vaccine or the measles vaccine (Committee on Infectious Diseases, 1997). Withholding these immunizations during the acute phase should be considered. The immunizations can be given when the neurologic situation is stabilized. Postimmunization fever management with acetaminophen is recommended for children with seizures.

The risk of contracting these diseases vs. the risk of the vaccine's side effects should be discussed with the family. Consulting the child's neurologist is recommended during the acute and rehabilitation period. Known exposure to a vaccine-preventable illness can be managed with disease-specific immunoglobulin therapy.

Screening

Vision and hearing: A thorough evaluation is recommended 6 to 8 weeks postinjury during the recovery period (Humphreys, 1991). Both vision and hearing can be adversely affected in children

after a traumatic brain injury. Formal evaluation including brainstem auditory or visual evoked potentials should be considered in assessing function. Mild deficits of either disorder should be corrected if possible to facilitate recovery (Michaud, Duhaime, and Batshaw, 1993). Continued routine periodic screening is recommended if deficits are not determined in the immediate postinjury period.

Dental: Routine dental care is recommended. Children with head injuries may have fractured or missing teeth secondary to facial trauma. Sedation may be necessary for dental work if voluntary cooperation is difficult because of spasticity. Assessment of gingival hyperplasia is recommended with more frequent dental examinations at 3-month intervals for children on phenytoin (Dilantin) therapy. For persistent bruxism, a mouth guard should be considered.

Blood pressure: Routine screening and evaluation during episodic visits are recommended. Persistently elevated blood pressure should be evaluated, including assessment of the blood pressure on all four extremities—particularly in the presence of an intracranial shunt.

Hematocrit: Routine screening is recommended.

Urinalysis: Bimonthly screening is recommended for the first 6 months after head injury to rule out indications of trauma or diabetes insipidus. Then routine screening is recommended.

Tuberculosis: Routine screening is recommended. If prophylactic medications are needed, evaluate potential drug interactions in children on anticonvulsant therapy. Consultation with the child's neurologist and pharmacist are recommended.

Condition-Specific Screening

Posttraumatic seizure therapy: CBC counts and chemistry panels to assess for blood dyscrasias and liver dysfunction are recommended. This screening should be done biweekly and then monthly for 6 months postinjury, then periodically thereafter. Anticonvulsant medications must be titrated for therapeutic effect and management of adverse side effects. Repeat drug levels should be done within 2 weeks of adjustments in dosage (see Chapter 21 on epilepsy).

Common Illness Management

Differential Diagnosis (Box 23-6)

Alterations in cognition or level of consciousness: A thorough knowledge of the child's baseline health and neurological status, level of consciousness, and behavior is the key to accurate assessment. Children with neurologic system impairment are more at risk for developing an acute illness. A significant change in cognitive function should be viewed as pathologic and assessed (Boss, 1994). Many different etiologies may produce decreases in arousal or cognition. Various types of trauma, infections, tumors, and metabolic imbalances may cause such alterations. The severity and the site of the pathology can often help to determine if it is an acute exacerbation of the child's chronic condition or a new focus. The onset may be sudden, subacute over a period of several days, or progressive over several weeks to months. Fevers should be assessed early, especially in children with seizures (see Chapter 21).

Respiratory tract infections: Upper respiratory tract illnesses are common in children and adolescents. Acute illnesses (i.e., fever, otitis media and other respiratory infections) may exacerbate the manifestations of post-TBI (e.g., worsening posttraumatic seizure pattern or level of consciousness) and should be appropriately monitored and treated (Martinez, Schreiber, and Hartman, 1991). Children with severe motor or neurologic sequelae need to be closely evaluated for respiratory complications (i.e., pneumonia and aspiration). Any adjustments to antiepileptic medications should be withheld until the acute phase of the respiratory illness has passed.

Common infectious diseases (i.e., varicella, rubella, or rubeola) can cause potentially serious complications such as pneumonia or worsening encephalopathy in children with a serious head injury. Any signs of acute deterioration should be urgently evaluated and further treatment initiated.

Nausea and vomiting: Symptoms of nausea and vomiting are of concern, particularly in children with an intracranial shunt. Mild gastrointestinal symptoms should be evaluated and then reevaluated in 24 to 48 hours by telephone or a return appointment with close follow-up by the family or primary care provider. Fluid rehydration either orally or via gastroesophageal or gastrostomy tube

---

> ### Box 23-6
> ## Differential Diagnosis
>
> - Need to know child's current baseline neurologic status.
> - Respiratory tract infections—children with severe neurologic or motor deficits are more prone to complications such as pneumonia or aspiration.
> - Nausea and vomiting—may be indicative of shunt malfunction in children with posttraumatic hydrocephalus. Prolonged or severe vomiting may require aggressive rehydration in children with poor nutritional intake.
> - Skin rashes—evaluate for possible allergic reaction to medication, especially anticonvulsant drugs.
> - Headaches—post-TBI often associated with frequent headaches. Headache diaries may help determine frequency, intensity, and effectiveness of mild analgesics.

---

may be necessary in children with severe vomiting or difficulty feeding. Persistent vomiting or development of lethargy should be evaluated urgently.

Skin rashes: The onset of skin rashes should be evaluated for early signs of a possible allergic reaction, particularly when a new anticonvulsant has been initiated for seizure management. Potentially serious complications may require consideration of alternate anticonvulsant therapies.

Headaches: Posttraumatic headaches can be a frequent concern, especially in older children. Use of a 2-week log by the family or primary care provider can be extremely valuable in recording patterns of onset, frequency, and relief-producing actions. Symptom management with mild analgesics is usually adequate. If the headaches persist in frequency to a chronic pattern, as indicated by continuation of the headache log book, further evaluation is recommended.

Drug Interactions

Drug interactions between multiple medications—especially multiple anticonvulsants—should be evaluated. Antihistamines should be used with caution in combination with anticonvulsants. The use of erythromycin-based antibiotics should be avoided with carbamazepine (Tegretol). Aspirin can alter therapeutic effects of anticonvulsants and should be used with caution. Acetaminophen is recommended instead of aspirin (see Chapter 21). The use of stimulant medications (e.g., methylphenidate [Ritalin], dextroamphetamine [Dexedrine], pemoline [Cylert]) can result in a prolonged half-life of many anticonvulsants (e.g., phenytoin [Dilantin], primidone [Mysoline], phenobarbital) (see Chapter 21). Consultation with a pharmacist and the child's neurologist may be indicated.

Developmental Issues

Sleep Patterns

Alterations in a child's sleep-wake cycle may result from the irregular pattern experienced during the acute phase of management. Children may experience excessive wakefulness or insomnia and irregular sleep patterns, or they may be fearful and experience nightmares as a result of the recent head injury. Alterations in a child's sleep routine may lead to difficulties in the family's or care provider's sleeping routine because of the need for adequate supervision. A 2-week sleep log may help in identifying specific patterns.

Irregular sleep-wake patterns are generally managed with behavioral therapy. A schedule of daily activities may be necessary to develop a consistent pattern. A regular bedtime that allows a sleep period of 8 to 10 hours should be established with a short daytime nap if needed. A regular arousal time in the morning can strengthen circadian rhythms and lead to regular times of sleep onset. Regular daily exercise can deepen existing sleep patterns. A soothing evening bath or shower can increase relaxation. A light snack may enhance sleep. Caffeinated beverages (e.g., tea, soda, cocoa) may need to be withheld. The number and duration of daytime naps may need to be limited (Boss, 1994). Timing of medication doses may need to be adjusted if a correlation with sleep patterns is identified. Encouraging verbalization of fears and concerns and the use of relaxation techniques may be helpful. Appropriate pain management also should be addressed.

Transient insomnia is treated symptomatically with short-term use of antihistamines (for their sedative effect) or intermediate-acting hypnotics

(e.g., chloral hydrate). Long-acting hypnotics are contraindicated because of impairment in daytime functioning (Boss, 1994).

Toileting

Bowel and bladder continence may be disrupted in older children who had voluntary control before the head injury. Establishing a progressive training program with positive reinforcement as cognition increases will help them regain control. This routine may also be helpful for younger children when ready for toilet training.

Routine toileting every 2 hours can reduce the incidence of incontinence. Longer interval periods are introduced as continence is achieved. The goal should be to obtain bowel and bladder control during the waking hours and then progress to nighttime hours. Children should be monitored for adequate fluid intake during the daytime hours with limitation of fluid intake near bedtime. Caffeinated beverages (e.g., tea, soda) may need to be withheld during the training schedule (Whitney, 1994). Appropriately sized disposable diapers, easy to manipulate clothing, and adaptive equipment can facilitate the training program. In addition, labeling bathroom doors with large pictures and using a night light in the room at night may be helpful (Bunting and Fitzsimmons, 1994).

Children with a head injury who are immobile can be prone to constipation. These children may require the use of natural or medicated stool softeners, glycerin suppositories, additional fluid intake, dietary bulk expanders, or manual rectal stimulation for assisted elimination (Coffman, 1992).

Discipline

Alterations in behavior and personality should be anticipated, even following mild brain injury. The most common behavioral changes are social withdrawal, decreased attention span, hyperactivity, aggression, and poor anger control. If deficits secondary to traumatic brain injury persist, they may lead to behavior and learning problems. Children may have changes in temperament including apathy, poor motivation, and social withdrawal or may be hyperactive, irritable, impulsive, aggressive, or inattentive (Michaud, Duhaime, and Batshaw, 1993).

Parents and primary care providers must be encouraged to be consistent with discipline and reinforce normal household rules as much as possible (Diamond, 1994). Persistent behavior difficulties at home, altered family and peer relationships, disruption in the school setting, or issues in the use of leisure time can lead to interruption in learning situations.

Difficulties with behavior and discipline are generally managed with behavioral therapy. Clear, simple expectations should be established and explained at an appropriate cognitive level for the child. Consistency in the style of discipline and behavior management of care providers is important to avoid giving mixed messages of appropriate and acceptable behavior. Regular unrestricted physical activities can help in releasing excessive energy. Role modeling of acceptable behavior should be done by the parents, care providers, and other family members. Acceptable behaviors should be positively reinforced. Unacceptable behaviors should have an appropriate consequence.

Referral and evaluation by a behavior specialist should be considered for persistent behavior suggestive of attention deficit hyperactivity disorder syndrome. These problems are often more easily recognized in the school setting, where the group situation may provide distractions that magnify the child's attentional difficulties. The primary care provider helps coordinate and collect data from the parents, school teachers, the child, and significant others in a child's life for a comprehensive evaluation. Several standardized behavior rating scales can be used for assessment (Kelly and Aylward, 1992).

Appropriate assessment and management in a multidimensional, interdisciplinary, and adaptive behavior modification program should do the following: (1) reflect a developmental base, (2) survey multiple developmental and behavioral dimensions, (3) use several norm-based, curriculum-based, and clinical judgment scales, (4) blend the assessments of several team members and parents or care providers, (5) link assessment and curriculum goals, (6) adapt tasks for various disabilities, and (7) monitor the child's program (Bagnato et al, 1988).

Pharmacologic management with the use of stimulants (e.g., Ritalin, Dexedrine, Cylert) or other psychotropic medications (e.g., clonidine) may be considered (see Chapter 28). These medications should never be used as an isolated treatment program and should be initiated on a trial basis.

Child Care

Short-term child care or longer periods of respite care are often priority needs of families (Coffman, 1992). Household members provide most of the care to meet the needs of these children's activities of daily living (Folden and Coffman, 1993). Mildly disabled children may be appropriately cared for in a daycare or home care setting. Severely disabled children often require assisted nursing care in the home.

Respite care can provide an important gift of time and potential peace of mind. This time can be used to go on errands, provide a needed vacation from the day-to-day activities of providing care, spend extra time with other family members, or become involved in new activities. Respite providers must be aware that although their assistance is very supportive, their presence can also be disruptive to the family dynamics and relationships (Coffman, 1992). Federal funds from Title XX of the Social Security Act are available for respite services, homemaker services, and foster home care (Folden and Coffman, 1993).

For children in a daycare or preschool setting, an individualized health program (IHP) can be useful in communicating medical information with early childhood educators and individual curriculum goals.

Schooling

Discharge from an acute care or rehabilitation facility marks a return to normalcy for children and families. Discharge can also be a time of confrontation with the realities of the physical, cognitive, psychiatric, or neuropsychologic impairments, however, as a result of the brain injury.

A critical phase in recovery for children with a head injury is the return to school. Successful school reentry is determined by intellect and cognitive ability, social skills, and peer relationships. Home schooling, tutoring, or part-time attendance may initially be appropriate on return to a school program, especially if limited endurance or fatigue problems are present.

Cognitive recovery ranges from a return to preinjury ability to severely impaired intellectual function and is often not as complete as motor function recovery (Michaud, Duhaime, and Batshaw, 1993). Unlike other special education students who have a stable neurologic status, children who have experienced a traumatic brain injury continue to change neurologically for weeks, months, and even years after resuming their school program. In young children with a head injury—particularly in the preschool age—many of the school difficulties may not occur until 2 or 3 years later when they are expected to develop math and reading skills.

Behavior and cognitive difficulties after a head injury may be sufficient to interfere with learning in a mainstream classroom setting and warrant referral for special education evaluation and services. Public Law 101-476, the Individuals with Disabilities Education Act of 1990, identifies traumatic brain injury as a specific disability category within special education (Michaud, Duhaime, and Batshaw, 1993). Parents and family members should be introduced early to advocacy skills that will assist in developing an IEP.

Neuropsychologic deficits can include information processing, impaired attention and memory, problem-solving skills, processing of abstract information, judgment, and organizational skills. Performance IQ can be more adversely affected than verbal IQ (Michaud, Duhaime, and Batshaw, 1993). Recent research indicates that psychostimulants can be very effective in treating attention disorders secondary to brain injury in children (Mahalick et al, 1998). Neurobehavioral and neuropsychologic problems may not be recognized as resulting from a previous traumatic brain injury, especially if there has been much time between the injury and the detection of deficits. Formal neuropsychologic and school performance testing can help identify problems and develop an IEP.

Depending on the depth of persistent deficits, children with traumatic brain injury can receive services ranging from regular classes with help in a resource room to special education classes, speech-language therapy, occupational or physical therapies, special services for hearing or visual impairments, behavior management, and counseling as components of their IEP (Michaud, Duhaime, and Batshaw, 1993). Flexibility in educational programming is of utmost importance because the children's changing profile may at no point resemble that of other children classified under existing special education categories. The child's strengths and weaknesses should be identified and used in the IEP assessment and planning process. Family counseling in regard to realistic performance expectations and anticipatory guidance for the parents and primary care providers in their role as the child's advocate in the school reentry process are important and should be emphasized.

Sexuality

Individuals who have sustained a head injury may have altered inhibitions or may make socially inappropriate sexual comments and gestures. Impairment in motor and sensory function or impaired communication may alter sexual functioning. Concerns about sexuality expressed by the child or adolescent, family, and significant others should be addressed early (Chipps, Clanin, and Campbell, 1992; Miller, 1991). For adolescents, educational programs or counseling sessions should include the topics of sexuality, substance abuse, and other risk-taking behaviors. For female adolescents on long-term antiepileptic medication, teratogenic effects should be considered when prescribing or altering medications (see Chapter 21).

Transition to Adulthood

Traumatic brain injury may have a major effect on the subsequent education, vocational development, independent living skills, and future productivity of affected individuals. Supported living programs, supervised housing, shared services, or foster care should be evaluated with respect to the level of assistance provided for the activities of daily living (Jackson, 1994). School guidance and vocational counselors should be aware of the importance of appropriate work experiences for children and adolescents with a head injury offered in adult rehabilitation programs (Goldberg and Sachs, 1992). Supervised work experiences may be necessary to develop appropriate skills, work habits, and attitudes in order to succeed in gainful employment and contribute to the community. Health care insurance coverage and financial assistance programs should also be addressed as adolescents enter adulthood.

Special Family Concerns and Resources

Severe stresses on the family arise after the sudden occurrence of a head injury. Families want to know exactly how their child is going to be at the end of the recovery period, even though this is difficult to predict. They want to know whether their child will have the same intelligence, personality, and sensory motor functions that were present before the head injury. The need to deal with the physical, social, cognitive, and communicative changes is emotionally draining—especially if there is a likelihood of permanent disability (Michaud, Duhaime, and Batshaw, 1993; Miller, 1991; Wade et al, 1998). An uncertain outcome followed by numerous weeks and months of medical treatment further contributes to the family's stress. Parents, family members, and primary care providers should be encouraged to become actively involved in the day-to-day care of the child because this will reduce their sense of helplessness and result in confidence building (Appleton, 1994). They should be actively involved in any recommendations or decision. Support groups or family counseling for both parents and siblings may help them express and discuss any concerns or anxieties during the rehabilitation and recovery period (Miller, 1991; Appleton, 1994).

The primary caretaker, usually the mother, may have difficulty meeting the care needs of the injured child along with those of the spouse and siblings. The noncaretaker parent, usually the father, may feel neglected by the exhausted mother who is coping with the child for the majority of the daytime hours. There are often unresolved feelings of denial, guilt, and remorse. It is not uncommon for marriages to dissolve within 1 to 2 years following the onset of a significant brain impairment in a child (Miller, 1991).

Siblings of the child who had the head injury also suffer from a loss of parental attention and may demonstrate guilt feelings. Many siblings may initially experience a sense of relief that the injury happened to their brother or sister and not to them, which is followed by a sense of guilt over having been spared. Younger siblings may fear that the same thing or worse may happen to them (Miller, 1991).

Significant financial issues and conflict related to the parents' return to work may arise, adding to the family's stress. Long-term family support and counseling should be advocated.

Use of a home health record would help parents and primary care providers organize health care information about the child's disabilities and ongoing health condition. As an adjunct to formal medical records, this health summary could be used during respite care or travel. Components of a home health record include emergency medical information, birth history, hospitalizations, medications used, information about primary health care, growth and nutrition, use of special equipment or supportive devices, daily schedule and special care routines, therapy and communication needs, and toileting regimen (Smigielski and Parton, 1992).

Head trauma in the pediatric population does not discriminate and can occur in all walks of life. Despite the tremendous benefits of family-centered care, cultural differences may become a barrier to adequate services. Differences in English-speaking capability, level of literacy, knowledge of the sophisticated level of care required, coordination of health services, compliance in the treatment regimen, and adequacy of health care resources based on legal residency status are all issues to be addressed by these families. Primary health care providers are in a key position to help provide comprehensive care services that are congruent with and respectful toward the child's and family's cultural background (Folden and Coffman, 1993).

Caring for a child with a head injury is a complex task because of the physical, cognitive, and psychosocial concerns that must be addressed. The following is a list of additional resources for professionals as well as for parents and primary care providers of these children.

Neurologic Organizations

American Brain Tumor Association
2720 River Rd. Suite 146
Des Plaines, Ill. 60018
(800) 886-2282
www.abta.org

American Speech, Language, Hearing Association
10801 Rockville Pike
Rockville, Md. 20852
(800) 638-8255
www.asha.org

Brain Injury Association
105 N. Alfred Street
Alexandria, Va. 22314
(800) 444-6443 (Family Helpline 9 to 5 EST);
(703) 236-6000 (Administration office)
www.biausa.org

National Rehabilitation Information Center
8455 Colesville Rd, Suite 935
Silver Spring, Md. 20910
(301) 588-9284

Rehabilitation Services Administration
Department of Human Services, Rm 101M
605 G Street NW
Washington, DC 20001
(202) 727-3211

Neurologic Organizations for Professionals:

American Congress of Rehabilitative Medicine
4700 West Lake Ave.
Glenview, Ill. 60025
(847) 375-4725
www.acrm.org

Association of Rehabilitation Nurses
5700 Old Orchard Rd, 1st Floor
Skokie, Ill. 60077-1024
(800) 299-7530; (708) 966-3433
www.rehabnurse.org

National Stroke Association
96 Inverness Dr. East, Suite 1
Englewood, Co. 80112
www.stroke.org

Summary of Primary Care Needs for the Child with a Head Injury

HEALTH CARE MAINTENANCE
Growth and development
Height, weight, and head circumference should be assessed to monitor growth. Medications (e.g., anticonvulsants) are based on current accurate weight measurements for therapeutic effectiveness.

Delayed development may be present. Cognitive and motor skills should be regularly screened and assessed. Interventional therapy programs are recommended.

Signs of precocious puberty and short stature should be monitored.

Diet
Eating and feeding problems contribute to poor growth patterns. Decreased physical activity and immobility may lead to excessive weight gain. Dietary intake should be tailored to meet the child's caloric needs.

Protective reflexes should be regularly monitored to prevent potential of aspiration and determine need for fundoplication with feeding tube placement.

Occupational and speech therapy can assist with optimal feeding programs.

Safety
Increased risk of injury is present as a result of instability, incoordination, potential seizures, and delays in motor skill acquisition.

Ongoing anticipatory guidance on general safety precautions should be provided.

Emergency seizure procedures and helmet use for certain seizure types should be reviewed.

Caution should be taken with risk-taking sports and activities.

Emergency exit routines should be evaluated.

Immunization
Routine immunizations should be avoided until a child is well into the postinjury recovery stage.

Children with posttraumatic seizures are at increased risk for having a seizure after a DPT or measles vaccine. Pertussis vaccine may be deferred and DT used instead. Benefit of measles immunization should be evaluated vs. risk of contracting disease with potentially serious complications in endemic areas.

Fever prophylaxis with acetaminophen is recommended.

Other immunizations are given as recommended.

Summary of Primary Care Needs for the Child with a Head Injury—cont'd

Screening

Vision: A complete evaluation is recommended 6 to 8 weeks post-injury during the recovery period, with correction of minor deficits.

Hearing: A complete evaluation is recommended 6 to 8 weeks post-injury during the recovery period, with correction of minor deficits.

Dental: Routine screening is recommended. Possible dental trauma should be evaluated after a head injury.

More frequent evaluations may be necessary for children on phenytoin.

Blood pressure: Monitor blood pressure with each visit. Assess elevations from baseline.

Hematocrit: Routine screening is recommended.

Hematologic monitoring for chronic medication therapy may be warranted.

Urinalysis: A child should be monitored periodically for the first 6 months postinjury. Routine screening is then recommended.

Tuberculosis: Routine screening is recommended. If prophylactic medications are needed, potential drug interactions should be evaluated in children on anticonvulsant therapy.

Condition-specific screening

Posttraumatic seizure therapy: Monitor CBC counts and chemistry panels along with anticonvulsant levels for the first 6 months postinjury and periodically thereafter.

COMMON ILLNESS MANAGEMENT

Differential diagnosis

A thorough knowledge of the baseline level of health and neurologic status, level of consciousness, and behavior is key in assessing significant pathologic deviations.

Risk of seizures is increased with acute illness and fever. Closely observe, maintain hydration, and provide antipyretic therapy. Children with severe motor or neurologic sequelae must be monitored for respiratory complications.

Common communicable diseases may result in high incidence of pulmonary or neurologic complications.

The potential for increased intracranial pressure should be monitored in the presence of an intracranial shunt with signs of nausea and vomiting.

Skin rashes must be evaluated for possible indication of allergic reactions to chronic medication therapy.

Evaluation of headaches will require careful history and symptom management.

Drug interactions

Altered therapeutic effects have been seen between several antiepileptic medications and certain antibiotics, antihistamines, behavior stimulants, and aspirin. Careful monitoring is required.

Developmental issues

Sleep patterns: Disruption in sleep patterns may be evident. A structured behavioral program is recommended.

Toileting: Bowel and bladder continence may be delayed in younger children or disrupted in older children who previously had voluntary control. Establishment of a progressive training program with positive reinforcement as cognition increases will help them regain control.

Discipline: Alterations in behavior and personality should be anticipated with early guidance counseling instituted. Standard developmentally appropriate discipline is recommended with reinforcement of normal household rules.

Persistent difficulties with behavior and discipline are managed with behavioral therapy. Referral and evaluation by a behavior specialist may be warranted.

Child care: Child care and respite care have been identified as priority needs by the primary caretakers. Assistance in this area is priority.

Continued

Summary of Primary Care Needs for the Child with a Head Injury—cont'd

Schooling: Cognitive changes continue to occur from weeks to months following the recovery from head trauma.

Assessment of learning needs must be fully individualized and addressed as soon as feasible postinjury. Public Law 99-457 and 101-476 outline mandated educational programs.

Families may require assistance with IEP process.

Toddlers and preschoolers need close monitoring because of increasing cognitive demands with age.

Formal neuropsychologic and school performance testing may be necessary.

Sexuality: Impairment in the motor and sensory function or impaired communication may alter sexual functioning. Anticipatory guidance in counseling is advised.

Transition to adulthood: Traumatic brain injury can have a major effect on the future education, vocational development, and independent living skills of the affected adolescent. School guidance and vocational counseling are recommended.

SPECIAL FAMILY CONCERNS

Severe stresses on the family unit arise following the sudden occurrence of a head injury. Support groups or family counseling for parents and siblings may be helpful.

Cultural differences can be considered a barrier to adequate services despite the benefits of family-centered care. Comprehensive care that is congruent with and respectful toward the child's and family's cultural background is a key element.

References

Adelson PD et al: Cerebral blood flow and CO_2 vasoresponsivity following severe traumatic brain injury in children, Neurosurg 84:357a, 1996.

Adelson PD and Kochanek PM: Head injury in children, J Child Neurol 13(1):2-15, 1998.

Aldrich EF et al: Diffuse brain swelling in severely head-injured children: a report from the NIH Traumatic Coma Data Bank, J Neurosurg 76:450-454, 1992.

Altimier LB: Pediatric central neurologic trauma: issues for special patients, AACN Clin Issues 3:31-41, 1992.

Alexander MP: Mild traumatic brain injury: pathophysiology, natural history and clinical management, Neurol 45:1253-1260.

Annegers JF et al: A population based study of seizures after traumatic brain injuries, New Engl J Med 338(1):20-24, 1998.

Appleton R: Head injury rehabilitation for children, Nurs Times 90:29-31, 1994.

Bagnato SJ et al: An interdisciplinary neurodevelopmental assessment model for brain-injured infants and preschool children, J Head Trauma Rehabil 3:75-86, 1988.

Boss BJ: Coma and cognitive deficits. In Barker E, editor: Neuroscience nursing, St Louis, 1994, Mosby.

Bullock R et al: Guidelines for the management of severe head injury, J Neurotrauma, 13:639-737, 1996.

Bunting L and Fitzsimmons F: Degenerative disorders. In Barker E, editor: Neuroscience nursing, St Louis, 1994, Mosby.

Chipps EM, Clanin NJ, and Campbell VG: Neurologic disorders, St Louis, 1992, Mosby.

Coburn D: Traumatic brain injury: the silent epidemic, AACN Clin Issues 3:9-18, 1992.

Coffman SP: Home care of the child and family after near drowning, J Pediatr Health Care 6:18-24, 1992.

Committee on Infectious Diseases: Report of the committee on infectious diseases, ed 24, Elk Grove Village, Ill., 1997, American Academy of Pediatrics.

Cox SA: Pediatric trauma: special patients/special needs, Crit Care Nurs Q 17:51-61, 1994.

Dandrinos-Smith S: The epidemiology of pediatric trauma, Crit Care Nurs Clin North Am 3:387-389, 1991.

Davies R L et al: The use of cranial CT scans in the triage of pediatric patients with mild head injury, Pediatrics 95:345-349, 1995.

Diamond J: Family-centered care for children with chronic illness, J Pediatr Health Care 8:196-197, 1994.

DiScala C et al: Children with traumatic head injury: morbidity and postacute treatment, Arch Phys Med Rehabil 72:662-666, 1991.

Folden SL and Coffman S: Respite care for families of children with disabilities, J Pediatr Health Care 7:103-110, 1993.

Ghajar J and Hariri R: Management of pediatric head injury, Pediatr Clin North Am 39:1093-1125, 1992.

Goldberg AL and Sachs PR: A guide to evaluating residential post-acute programs for children and adolescents with brain injury, J Cognit Rehabil 10:28-32, 1992.

Goldstein B and Powers K: Head trauma in children, Pediatr Rev 15(6):213-219, 1994.

Hazinski MF: Neurologic disorders. In Hazinski MF, editor: Nursing care of the critically ill child, St Louis, 1992, Mosby.

Humphreys RP: Complications of pediatric head injury, Pediatr Neurosurg 17:274-278, 1991.

Ingebrigtsen T et al: Quantification of post concussion symptoms 3 months after minor head injury in 100 consecutive patients, J Neurol 245 (9):609-612, 1998.

Jackson JD: After rehabilitation: meeting the long-term needs of persons with traumatic brain injury, Am J Occup Ther 48:251-255, 1994.

Jennett B: Epidemiology of head injury, Arch Dis Child 78(5):403-413, 1998.

Kelly DP and Aylward GP: Attention deficits in school-aged children and adolescents: current issues and practice, Pediatr Clin North Am 39:487-512, 1992.

Kirchner KM, and Sammons J: Transdisciplinary approach to a brain injured child, Rehabil Nurs 8:22-23, 26-27, 1983.

Kokoska ER et al: Early hypotension worsens neurological outcome in pediatric patients with moderately severe head trauma, J Pediatr Surg 33(2):333-338, 1998.

Luerssen TG: Acute traumatic cerebral injuries. In Check WR, editor: Pediatric neurosurgery: surgery of the developing nervous system, ed 3, Philadelphia, 1994, W.B. Saunders.

Mahalick DM et al: Psychopharmacologic treatment of acquired attentional disorders in children with brain injuries, Pediatr Neurosurg 29:121-126, 1998.

Manaks S: Cooperative prospective study on posttraumatic epilepsy: risk factos and the effect of prophylactic anticonvulsant, Jpn J Psychiatry Neurol 46:311-315, 1992.

Martinez NH, Schreiber ML, and Hartman EW: Pediatric nurse practitioners: primary care providers and case managers for chronically ill children at home, J Pediatr Health Care 5:291-298, 1991.

Michaud LJ, Duhaime AC, and Batshaw ML: Traumatic brain injury in children, Pediatr Clin North Am 40:553-565, 1993.

Miller L: Significant others: treating brain injury in the family context, J Cognit Rehabil 9:16-25, 1991.

Moskowitz C: Movement disorders. In Barker E, editor: Neuroscience nursing, St Louis, 1994, Mosby, pp 536-558.

Paolin A et al: Cerebral hemodynamic response to CO_2 after severe head injury: clinical and prognostic implications, J Trauma 44(3):495-500, 1998.

Reynolds EA: Controversies in caring for the child with a head injury, MCN 17:246-251, 1992.

Slazinski T and Johnson MC: Severe diffuse axonal injury in adults and children, J Neurosci Nurs 26:151-154, 1994.

Smigielski PA and Parton E: A home health record for children with chronic health conditions, J Pediatr Health Care 6:121-126, 1992.

Stylianos S: Late sequelae of major trauma in children, Pediatr Clin North Am 45(4):853-859, 1998.

Temkin NR et al: A randomized double blind study of phenytoin for the prevention of posttraumatic seizures, N Engl J Med 323:497-502, 1990.

Vernon-Levett P: Head injuries in children, Crit Care Nurs Clin North Am 3:411-421, 1991.

Walker C: The young pediatric patient: predicting outcome after cerebral insult, Headlines 4:4-11, 1993.

Walleck CA and Mooney KF: Neurotrauma: head injury. In Barker E, editor: Neuroscience nursing, St Louis, 1994, Mosby.

Whitney F: Stroke. In Barker E, editor: Neuroscience nursing, St Louis, 1994, Mosby.

Wade Sl et al: Family burden and adaptation during the initial year after traumatic brain injury in children, Pediatrics 102:110-116, 1998.

Woestman R et al: Mild head injury in children: identified clinical evaluating, neuroimaging and disposition, J Pediatr Health Care 12:288-298.

Yablon SA: Post traumatic seizures, Arch Phys Med Rehabil 74:983-1001, 1993.

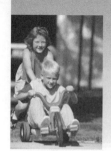

CHAPTER 24

HIV Infection and AIDS

Rita Fahrner and Estrella Manio

Etiology

The human immunodeficiency virus (HIV) causes a continuum of infection to occur, the end stage of which is acquired immune deficiency syndrome (AIDS). HIV type 1 (HIV-1) is a member of the lentivirus genus of the Retroviridae family, which means that its viral RNA is copied into DNA using reverse transcriptase. This virus selectively infects the T-helper (i.e., T4 or CD4) subset of T-cell lymphocytes. Other cells that express CD4 (e.g., monocytes, macrophages, and glial cells) and some cells without detectable cell surface CD4 can become infected. Through a process of replication, HIV perpetuates and integrates itself into the genetic material of the organism it infects. Full intracellular viral life cycling requires the generation of a DNA copy of the HIV-1 RNA genome; integration of this proviral DNA into the host genomic DNA permits viral persistence and impedes the eradication of virus from infected individuals (Luzuriaga and Sullivan, 1998). The primary pathologic condition of HIV causes specific immunodeficiency that destroys the host's ability to withstand infection. In addition, the HIV directly invades other major organ systems, including the peripheral and central nervous system (CNS), lungs, heart, kidneys, and gastrointestinal (GI) tract.

Although HIV infections in children and adults have common pathologic conditions, infants with perinatally acquired HIV infections represent a distinctive immunologic host with a developing, immature immune system (Kamani, 1991). The fetus and neonate have a well-developed T cell, or cell-mediated, immune system, whereas their B cell, or humoral, immune system is physiologically immature (CDC, 1998c). Although the function of both B and T cells is altered in HIV-infected children, the consequences of B-cell dysfunction, including hypergammaglobulinemia and failure to form functional antibodies, are often problematic early in the course of disease. For this reason, children with HIV are more susceptible to bacterial infections than their adult counterparts. T-cell defects, allowing for opportunistic infections (OIs), such as *Pneumocystis carinii* pneumonia (PCP), are also often seen in young infants. In addition, the degree of lymphopenia, percentage of T4 (CD4) cells, absolute T4 (CD4) count, and degree of reversal of the helper-suppressor (T4-T8) ratio are more variable in infants. Depletion of T-cell numbers and inversion of the helper-suppressor ratio generally occurs at a later stage of disease in children than in adults. Another major difference between adults and children with HIV is that the time period from infection to development of signs and symptoms seems to be shorter in children.

HIV is transmitted to children by a variety of modes (Table 24-1). Perinatal transmission is the most common (91%) mode of transmission and may occur transplacentally in utero (vertically from mother to fetus), during delivery by exposure to infected maternal blood and vaginal secretions, and by postpartum ingestion of infected breast milk. Many factors (i.e., maternal, fetal, viral, placental, obstetrical, and neonatal factors) seem to influence mother-to-infant transmission of the virus. The success of the Pediatric AIDS Clinical Trials Group (PACTG) 076 study demonstrated that when zidovudine (AZT) was administered during pregnancy and labor, as well as to the newborn, the risk for perinatal HIV transmission was reduced by two-thirds; infection rates were 25% in the placebo group compared with 8% in the treatment group (Steim et al, 1999) (Boxes 24-1 and 24-2).

Children have become infected with HIV from contaminated blood and blood products, tissues, and factor concentrates received between the years of 1978 and 1985. The risk for infection, however, was extremely high during these years,

---

Box 24-1

AZT to Reduce Vertical Transmission
(From ACTG 076 Protocol)

Maternal:

Antepartum
- Begin after 14 weeks' gestation
- Zidovudine 100 mg PO 5 times daily

Intrapartum
- Zidovudine loading dose 2 mg/kg IV over 1 hr then 1 mg/kg/hr continuous IV infusion until delivery
- Zidovudine 1000 mg should be diluted with 250 mg D$_5$W to prepare a final concentration of 4 mg Zidovudine/ml D$_5$W.

Infant
Begin as soon as possible within the first 12 hours of life

For PO Infant
Zidovudine 2 mg/kg PO q6h 3 to 6 weeks plus extra week supply

For NPO Infant
Zidovudine 1.5 mg/kg IV q6h infuse over 30 to 60 minutes
Zidovudine should be diluted with D$_5$W to prepare a final concentration of 0.5 mg Zidovudine/ml D$_5$W.

Table 22-1
U.S. Pediatric AIDS Cases by Route of Transmission*

Mode of Transmission	%
Mother has or is at risk for HIV infection	91
Recipient of blood, blood product, or tissue	5
Hemophilia or coagulation disorder	2
Undetermined	2
TOTAL	100

Adapted from Centers for Disease Control: HIV/AIDS surveillance report, June 1998.
*N = 8280

Box 24-2

Results of ACTG 076:

A randomized, double-blind, placebo-controlled clinical trial of the efficacy and safety of zidovudine (AZT) in reducing the risk of maternal-infant HIV transmission

- The mothers and infants who took zidovudine had an 8.3% risk of transmission.
- The mothers and infants who took the placebo had a 25.5% risk of transmission.

Data from Connor EM et al: Reduction of maternal-infant transmission of human immunodeficiency virus type I with zidovudine treatment, N Engl J Med 331:1173-80, 1994.

---

with infection estimated to occur in up to 95% of those receiving contaminated products. Because of the safeguards instituted in blood and tissue collection and heat treatment of factor concentrates during the mid-1980s, few new cases of infection from blood and blood products, tissues, and factor concentrates have been reported.

A small number of children have become infected with HIV as a result of sexual abuse. Practitioners caring for children who have experienced abuse must include HIV infection in their differential diagnosis of sexually transmitted diseases. HIV has also rarely been transmitted through blood exposure within household settings, but no cases of transmission within daycare or school settings have been reported (Courville et al, 1998).

Adolescents and young adults aged 13 through 24 years comprise approximately 4% of the AIDS cases in the United States (CDC, 1998a). Of the HIV infection cases reported by the states who track HIV infection, however, adolescents and young adults aged 13 through 24 years comprise

Table 24-2
Pediatric AIDS Cases (*N* = 5095) by Maternal Exposure Category and Race*

Maternal Exposure Category	White (%)	Black (%)	Asian/ Latino (%)	Am Ind/ Pac Is (%)	Alaskan (%)	Total (%)
Injection drug use (IDU)	42	39	41	14	46	40
Sex with IDU	19	15	27	14	27	18
Sex with another at-risk person	19	17	16	37	12	17
Recipient of blood, blood products, or tissue	4	2	2	1	0	2
Risk unspecified	16	27	14	34	15	23
Total						100

Adapted from Centers for Disease Control: HIV/AIDS surveillance report, June 1998.
*Pac Is, Pacific Islander; *Am Ind,* American Indian; *IDU,* injection drug user.

14% (CDC, 1998a). The average time from HIV infection to the development of AIDS is about 11 years, so most young adults with AIDS were infected as teenagers. Teenagers are especially at risk for HIV because many of the behaviors that put a person at risk for HIV begin during adolescence (i.e., sexuality, drug use). In addition, as the management and therapeutic treatments for children with perinatally acquired HIV infection improve, more of these children will reach adolescence.

Incidence

Although pediatric and adolescent AIDS is a reportable condition, the actual incidence and/or prevalence is unknown because AIDS cases are significantly underreported in the United States and worldwide. The actual incidence and/or prevalence of HIV infection in children, however, is becoming better known because national confidential HIV infection reporting now occurs in 28 states. The occurrence of AIDS in children was established as early as 1982; 20 children under 13 years of age were diagnosed by the end of 1981. By mid-1998, more than 8280 cases of AIDS in children (i.e., 1.2% of the total number of reported AIDS cases in the United States) were reported to the CDC (CDC, 1998a). Estimates from the CDC suggest that there are 18,000 to 23,000 infants and children infected with HIV in the United States. The incidence of pediatric HIV is increasing as HIV infection in-

creases in the injection drug-using and heterosexual communities. All states in the United States have reported at least one case of pediatric AIDS.

Because most children with AIDS have been perinatally infected, the demographics of this group closely parallel that of women with AIDS (Table 24-2). In this population, HIV is a disease primarily associated with poverty and drug use and is clustered in inner cities and ethnic minority communities. On the other hand, parenteral cases have a broader geographic distribution and a wider ethnic apportionment.

Clinical Manifestations at Time of Diagnosis

Developing a clinical definition of HIV infection and AIDS in children is a complex task (Box 24-3). The initial pediatric AIDS definition directed surveillance but did not describe the spectrum of infection. Therefore in 1987 the CDC developed a classification system for HIV infection in children; as more information about pediatric HIV became available, however, the 1987 classification system was inadequate. In 1994 the CDC again revised the classification system for children under 13 years of age. The current classification system places perinatally exposed and infected children into mutually exclusive categories according to infection and clinical and immunologic status (Box 24-4). Al-

Box 24-3

Clinical Manifestations Associated with Early HIV Infection in Infancy and Childhood

Failure to thrive
Chronic or recurrent diarrhea
Fever of unknown origin
Atopic dermatitis
Persistent or recurrent fungal infections (e.g., thrush or diaper dermatitis)

Thrombocytopenia
Hepatosplenomegaly
Parotitis
Frequent infections
Developmental delay; loss of milestones

Box 24-4

Diagnosis of HIV Infection in Children*

Diagnosis: HIV Infected

A. A child <18 months of age who is known to be HIV seropositive or born to an HIV-infected mother **and:**

- Has positive results on two separate specimens (excluding cord blood) from any of the following HIV detection tests:
  —HIV culture
  —HIV polymerase chain reaction
  —HIV antigen (p24)
      or
- Meets criteria for AIDS diagnosis based on the 1987 AIDS surveillance case definition

B. A child >18 months of age born to an HIV-infected mother or any child infected by blood, blood products, or other known modes of transmission (e.g., sexual contact) who:

- Is HIV-antibody positive by confirming Western blot or immunofluorescence assay (IFA)
      or
- Meets any of the criteria in *A*

Diagnosis: Perinatally Exposed (Prefix E)

A child who does not meet the previously listed criteria who:

- Is HIV seropositive by ELISA and confirming Western blot or IFA and is ≤18 months of age at the time of test
      or
- Has unknown antibody status but was born to a mother known to be infected with HIV

Diagnosis: Seroreverter (SR)

A child who is born to an HIV-infected mother and who:

- Has been documented as HIV-antibody negative (i.e., two or more negative ELISA tests performed at 6 to 18 months of age or one negative ELISA test after 18 months of age)
      and
- Has had no other laboratory evidence of infection (i.e., has not had two positive viral detection tests, if performed)
      and
- Has not had an AIDS-defining condition

*Adapted from Centers for Disease Control MMWR 43: 2-3, 1994.

though HIV infection is most accurately identified by viral culture from blood or tissue, it is generally diagnosed in adults by the presence of specific antibodies to the virus. The presence of passively acquired maternal antibodies, however, limits the use of HIV antibody testing in infants up to 18 months of age suspected of perinatal infection. For this reason, two definitions of infection in children are necessary: one for infants up to 18 months of age and one for older children (see Box 24-4).

Table 24-3
Pediatric HIV Classification*

	Clinical Categories			
Immunologic Categories	**N: No Signs/ Symptoms**	**A: Mild Signs/ Symptoms**	**B: Moderate Signs/Symptoms**	**C: Severe Signs/Symptoms**
1: No evidence of immune suppression	N1	A1	B1	C1
2: Evidence of moderate immune suppression	N2	A2	B2	C2
3: Severe immune suppression	N3	A3	B3	C3

*Children whose HIV infection status is not confirmed are classified by using the above grid with a letter *E* (for perinatally exposed) placed before the appropriate classification code (e.g., EN2).
Adapted from Centers for Disease Control: MMWR 43: 2-3, 1994.

Children who meet the definition of HIV exposure or infection may be further grouped into one of six mutually exclusive classes based on clinical signs and symptoms and immunologic status (Table 24-3). This classification system is helpful for health care planning and for epidemiologic purposes.

Pediatric HIV/AIDS centers can use more specific laboratory tests to determine infection in perinatally exposed infants. HIV blood culturing is considered the gold standard in virologic testing of infants. Blood culturing is very expensive and labor intensive, however, and results are not usually available for 4 to 6 weeks after specimen processing. The p24 antigen assay is another virologic test that is rather inexpensive and has been available for many years. In the presence of HIV antibodies, however, an immune complex is formed with the p24 antigen, making detection of the antigen itself impossible. This test becomes more accurate in children at 6 months of age, when maternal antibody titers in infants begin to drop. A third test, the polymerase chain reaction (PCR), has proved to be superior to viral culture and p24 antigen assay. PCR is a method of gene amplification that directly detects proviral sequences of HIV within DNA using small amounts of blood. PCR is less expensive than viral culture and more sensitive than p24 antigen assays. In addition, PCR results are usually available within 1 week of processing the specimen.

Using HIV culture or PCR or both, an infant's infection status can be determined with 90% to 100% certainty by 3 to 6 months of age (CDC, 1998c). Because these tests are still not yet widely available, community clinicians caring for these children may not have direct access to them but will need to refer children to the closest pediatric HIV specialty center or contact the National Institute of Allergy and Infectious Diseases or the Maternal-Child Health Bureau for the nearest participating research group.

Because HIV infection is clearly a multisystem disease process, infected infants and children may have a wide range of signs and symptoms. The clinical manifestations that occur early in infection are often nonspecific and may be seen in healthy children and children with other conditions. Children with HIV infection, however, generally experience more chronic and severe signs and symptoms and often fail to respond to appropriate therapy. Some children have acute opportunistic infections (OIs) with the same protozoal, viral, fungal, and bacterial pathogens as adults, which are indicator diseases for an AIDS diagnosis. Others may have nephropathy, hepatitis, cardiomyopathy, and hematologic abnormalities (Pizzo and Wilfert, 1998).

Most children are diagnosed with HIV infection before they exhibit any signs or symptoms of illness. Infants and children born to mothers who are infected with HIV should be tested to determine if they are also infected. Retrospective transfusion programs have identified many children who are infected. Children with hemophilia or other hematologic conditions who received factor concentrates or other blood products before 1985 should be counseled about HIV testing (see Chapter 11).

Treatment

HIV infection has become a chronic, treatable, life-threatening disease. The most significant treatments are those aimed at killing HIV in an attempt to eradicate the virus (Box 24-5). Combination antiretroviral therapy using a variety of agents has become standard therapy (Pizzo and Wilfert, 1998).

Although the pathogenesis of HIV infection and the general virologic and immunologic principles for the use of antiretroviral therapy are similar for all individuals with HIV, there are unique considerations for their use in infants, children, and adolescents. These considerations include the following: (1) perinatal transmission; (2) in utero exposure to antiretrovirals; (3) differences in diagnostic evaluations in perinatal infection; (4) differences in immunologic markers in young children; (5) changes in pharmacokinetics with age caused by the continuing development and maturation of organ systems involved in drug metabolism and clearance; (6) differences in the clinical and virologic manifestations of perinatal HIV infection in relation to the occurrence of primary infection in growing, immunologically immature bodies; and (7) special issues associated with treatment adherence for children and adolescents (CDC, 1998c).

Many questions about the use of antiretrovirals in children are being answered because there are a growing number of investigational treatment protocols for children that address issues such as the optimal time to start treatment, when and how to modify dosage, and how to determine disease progression. Rather than having to prove their efficacy in adults before children are allowed access to them, new drugs are now simultaneously tested in adults and children. This process parallels the approval process for new chemotherapeutic agents used in cancer therapy.

Combination therapy has proved to be superior to monotherapy and is the hallmark of HIV treatment (McKinney et al, 1998). A variety of agents including nucleoside reverse transcriptase inhibitors (i.e. zidovudine [AZT], lamivudine [Epivir], stavudine [Zerit], didanosine [Videx]), non-nucleoside reverse transcriptase inhibitors (i.e.

> ### Box 24-5
> #### Treatment
>
> - Antiretroviral drugs
> - Intravenous immune globulin
> - Therapies for concurrent infectious and other clinical manifestations

nevirapine [Viramune], delavirdine [Rescripton]) and protease inhibitors (i.e. ritonavir [Norvir], nelfinavir [Viracept], indinavir [Crixivan]) are currently used.

Intravenous immune globulin (IVIG) is still used in some centers to reconstitute the immune systems of children with HIV infection. IVIG has been shown to reduce serious bacterial infections in children with HIV but has not increased survival time (Wood, 1998). This benefit, however, did not hold true in children receiving zidovudine in addition to trimethoprim-sulfamethoxazole as *Pneumocystis carinii* pneumonia (PCP) prophylaxis (Spector, 1994).

Without a definitive cure, children with HIV infection are treated with comprehensive, multidisciplinary care with prompt diagnosis and aggressive therapy of concurrent infections and other clinical manifestations of disease. Recurrent and severe systemic bacterial infection, which can progress to pneumonia, meningitis, and sepsis, is one of the most frequent problems in children with HIV infection. Although this type of infection contributes greatly to morbidity, it is potentially preventable and treatable. The major bacterial pathogens encountered are those seen in pediatric practice with children who are immunocompetent. Reducing the frequency and intensity of bacterial infection may potentially modify HIV replication and primary disease progression (Krasinski, 1994).

Most children with HIV infection, even those with symptomatic disease, are active, playful, functional children who see themselves as healthy. They may take medications and spend time in the hospital but also attend daycare and school. It is important for primary care providers to remember that these children will develop common childhood illnesses and that all symptoms are not related to their underlying immunodeficiency. Children with HIV, however, must be quickly assessed and aggressively managed when the possibility of intercurrent illness occurs (Luzuriaga, 1997). A wait-and-see attitude is rarely appropriate. These children and their families must develop a strong partnership with their primary care provider to ensure prompt evaluation and treatment (Teriff, 1998). Children infected with HIV must be linked with a comprehensive pediatric HIV-AIDS treatment center whenever possible. Centers ensure access to clinical trials and the most up-to-date information and expertise, as well as to other children and families living with this condition. Clear lines of access to and responsibility of the primary care provider and the center team must be developed for each family.

Recent and Anticipated Advances in Diagnosis and Management

The CDC published an update to the 1994 PHS guidelines for the use of antiretroviral drugs—both for maternal health and for reducing perinatal transmission of HIV—in pregnant women with HIV (CDC, 1998d). These guidelines are based on the ACTG 076 protocol and confirmation of the efficacy of AZT for reducing perinatal transmission. Along with the substantial advances in the understanding of the pathogenesis of HIV infection and in the treatment and monitoring of HIV disease, standard antiretroviral therapy for adults with HIV now comprises more aggressive combination drug regimens that maximally suppress viral replication. Pregnancy is not a reason to defer standard therapy, therefore offering antiretroviral to infected pregnant women—whether to primarily treat the disease or to reduce the risk of perinatal transmission or both—is recommended. Treatment discussions should include the known and unknown short- and long-term benefits and risks of such therapy for infected women and their infants.

Advances in the early diagnosis of infants at risk for HIV have been dramatic. One of the reasons that the ACTG 076 efficacy results were available earlier than anticipated is because when the study was first drafted in 1990, it was thought that infection could only be ruled out when maternal antibody levels in the infant dissipate (i.e., at 15 to 18 months of age). More recently, however, the use of repeated PCR testing has made diagnosis of HIV possible by 3 to 6 months of age.

The advances in combination antiretroviral therapy have provided substantial clinical benefit to children with HIV with immunologic and/or clinical symptoms of disease (Luzuriaga, 1997). Studies have previously shown concrete improvements in neurodevelopment, growth, and immunologic and/or virologic status with initiation of monotherapy. Recent trials have shown that combination therapy is clinically, immunologically, and virologically superior to monotherapy in previously untreated symptomatic children, as well as that combination therapy including a protease inhibitor is superior to dual nucleoside combination therapy in children who were previously treated (CDC, 1998c).

Adult treatment guidelines are appropriate for post-pubertal adolescents who have been infected by sexual activity or needle-sharing behaviors because their clinical course is more similar to that of adults than to that of perinatally infected children (CDC, 1998b). Adolescents who are long-term survivors of perinatal HIV infection or transfusion-related infection as young children, however, may have a unique clinical course. Doses of medications for HIV infection and opportunistic infection should be based on Tanner staging of puberty rather than age; adolescents in early puberty should be given doses based on pediatric schedules, and those in late puberty should follow adult dosing schedules (CDC, 1998c).

Associated Problems (Box 24-6)

Failure to Thrive

Nutrition can be a significant problem for children with HIV, particularly for those with chronic diarrhea and *Candida* esophagitis. Many infants and children with symptomatic disease demonstrate poor weight gain and often fall below the 5th percentile on the National Center for Health Statistics growth curves for weight. Because most children with HIV and/or AIDS also experience nutritional deficits, malnutrition is thought to be a cofactor of immune dysfunction (Miller and Garg, 1998).

Specific causes of chronic diarrheas (e.g., *Cryptosporidium* spp., *Giardia* spp., and Mycobacterium avium-intracellular [MAI] spp.) are rarely found, even after exhaustive gastrointestinal (GI) and stool examinations. Some children thrive better

---

Box 24-6

Associated Problems

Failure to thrive
  Chronic diarrhea
  Candida sp. esophagitis
  Malnutrition
Neurologic manifestations
  HIV encephalopathy
    Developmental delay
    Deterioration of motor skills and/or cognitive
      functions
  Acquired microcephaly
    Impaired brain growth
    Cortical atrophy
    Calcifications
  Gait disturbances
  Deficits in expressive language
Opportunistic infections
  Major cause of death
  PCP most common OI

Pulmonary disease
  Noninfections
    PLH/LIP
    Nonspecific pulmonary fibrosis
    Pulmonary hypertension
    Aspiration pneumonia
  Infectious
    PCP
    CMV
    RSV
    MTB
Pancytopenia
  Thrombocytopenia
  Anemias
  Leukopenia
    Neutropenia
    Lymphopenia
Fungal infections
  Candidiasis
Drug exposure
  Delayed development
  Learning/behavioral difficulties

---

on lactose-free diets, whereas others experience cyclical diarrhea unresponsive to dietary manipulations. The GI tract is a major target for HIV because it constitutes 60% of all the lymphocytes in the body. Therefore these problems are thought to be caused by changes in the GI tract secondary to direct invasion by HIV (Miller and Garg, 1998).

HIV-associated malnutrition is no different from malnutrition of other causes. Children with chronic conditions who are experiencing malabsorption may also have malnutrition-induced immunodeficiency, which creates an atmosphere where enteric pathogens are likely to thrive. Therefore malabsorption, malnutrition, immunodeficiency, and enteric infections appear to be interrelated (Miller and Garg, 1998). Figure 24-1 shows the obvious necessity of good nutrition in supporting the immune system of children with HIV-infection.

Neurologic Manifestations

The brain is a target site for HIV infection in infants and children, and a variety of clinical patterns of neurodevelopmental involvement emerge. In most children, the neurologic dysfunction appears to be a result of direct infection of the CNS by HIV (Browers, Wolters, and Civitello, 1998). HIV encephalopathy may result in developmental delay, deterioration of motor skills and cognitive functioning, and behavioral abnormalities. This course may be static, progressive, or episodic with plateaus of relative stability that last months alternating with intervals of marked deterioration that last weeks. The degree of neurologic deficit is variable and related to an individual's age at first symptom, stage of disease, rate of disease progression, and the current age (Browers, Wolters, and Civitello, 1998). Some degree of neurologic impairment is usually found in all symptomatic children, but CNS involvement may be the first and only sign of HIV disease in a child.

Acquired microcephaly is often observed in infants and young children with HIV disease. Computerized tomographic (CT) scanning and magnetic resonance imaging (MRI) often show impaired brain growth with diffuse cortical atrophy

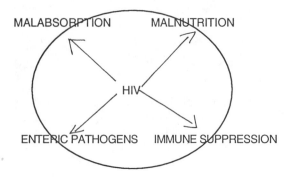

Figure 24-1 Link between malabsorption, malnutrition, and HIV infection. (From Winter HS and Miller TL: Gastrointestinal and nutritional problems in HIV disease. In Pizzo PA and Wilfert CM, editors: Pediatric AIDS: the challenge of HIV infection in infants, children, and adolescents, ed 2, Baltimore, 1994, Williams & Wilkins.)

and basal ganglia calcifications in severely affected infants. Cerebrospinal fluid (CSF)—even if positive for HIV culture—usually shows normal glucose, protein levels, and cell count.

Children with acquired microcephaly may demonstrate gradual apathy, progressive motor deficits resulting in generalized weakness and gait disturbances, and difficulties with expressive language. It is often perplexing to differentiate the effect of HIV infection from the effects of prenatal and perinatal drug exposure, prematurity, chronic disease, and chaotic social environments (Browers, Belman, and Epstein, 1994).

Opportunistic Infections

Opportunistic infections (OIs), including bacterial, mycobacterial, fungal, protozoal, and viral infections, are the major cause of death for children with HIV infection. Serious bacterial infections often occur in children with HIV, and the risk of infection continues throughout childhood (Wilfert, 1998). *Pneumocystis carinii* sp. pneumonia (PCP) is the most frequent AIDS-defining illness in children with HIV, and most cases occur between the third and sixth month of life. The initial episode of PCP is most often fatal, even with appropriate treatment (Cvetkovich and Frenkel, 1993). The high rate of recurrence makes prophylaxis imperative.

Pulmonary Disease

Pulmonary disease and resultant respiratory failure profoundly contribute to the morbidity and mortality of pediatric HIV infection. Over 80% of HIV-infected children develop lung disease during the course of their illness (Andiman and Shearer, 1998). Pulmonary complications of pediatric HIV infection may be divided by noninfectious and infectious etiologies. The lymphoid infiltrates represent a continuum from focal lymphocytic hyperplasia in lung parenchyma (PLH) to more diffuse infiltration of alveolar septa and interstitial tissue (LIP) and then to neoplastic lymphoproliferative disease (Andiman and Shearer, 1998). Symptoms may be subtle and include tachypnea, dyspnea, cough, and exercise intolerance. Treatment is generally symptomatic and supportive but also depends upon antiretroviral therapy aimed at the underlying HIV infection, as well as corticosteroids. PLH/LIP may be complicated by superinfection with viral, bacterial, or other pathogens.

PCP, which is a diffuse, desquamative alveolopathy that results in hypoxia, is the OI seen most often in pediatric AIDS. The clinical manifestations of children with PCP are age- and immune status-dependent. Symptoms are likely to be acute with fever, dyspnea, dry cough, cyanosis, and hypoxemia. Treatment of acute infection usually begins with trimethoprim-sulfamethoxazole (Bactrim, Septra) and corticosteroids. Prophylaxis, both primary and secondary, with oral Bactrim or Septra is extremely effective.

Other pathogens causing pulmonary infection include cytomegalovirus (CMV); respiratory syncytial virus (RSV); *Mycobacterium* spp. tuberculosis; MAI; rubeola; varicella; and other viral, fungal, and bacterial sources. Reactive airway disease is common and considered to be chronic airway inflammation associated with frequent and persistent infection.

Pancytopenia

Hematologic abnormalities, occurring as a result of HIV infection or as an adverse effect of treatment, are common in children with HIV. Some children have thrombocytopenia, which is usually an immune response to circulating platelets, because their bone marrow produces megakaryocytes, which break down into platelets in the peripheral blood. Intravenous immunoglobulin (IVIG) is sometimes effective in raising the platelet count, and platelet transfusions are rarely required. Anemias of chronic disease or iron deficiency are common in this population and often require iron supplementation. Red blood cell (RBC) transfusions are sometimes indicated—especially in AZT-induced anemia. Cytomegalovirus-negative, washed, and irradiated RBCs and platelets are used to avoid introducing new infection and to protect against graft vs. host disease. Abnormalities of the white blood cell (WBC) line (i.e., neutropenia, lymphopenia, and leukopenia) are also often seen.

Fungal Infections

Candidiasis occurs frequently and may be manifested as either oral thrush or diaper dermatitis. Mucosal Candida sp. is the most prevalent opportunistic infection in all individuals with HIV (Walsh et al, 1998). First-line treatments for oral thrush usually include topical nystatin (Mycostatin) and clotrimazole (Mycelex) oral troches. Clotrimazole vaginal suppositories (100 mg) used orally are often more effective because they are 10 times more potent than oral suspensions or troches. Infants can be treated either by placing the suppository into the nipple of a bottle, allowing the infant to suck formula through it, or by dissolving the suppository in warm water and swabbing the mouth. Older children can suck the suppositories. Both nystatin and clotrimazole creams are available for skin infections. Refractory cases of mucous membrane and dermatologic infections may be treated systemically with oral ketoconazole (Nizoral) or the newer fluconazole (Diflucan); IV amphotericin B may be necessary for refractory cases of mucosal Candidiasis.

Prenatal and Perinatal Drug Exposure

Children with HIV who were born to mothers who have HIV and have had drugs and/or alcohol are often premature and small for gestational age and have very immature immune systems. Their development is often delayed, and learning and behavioral difficulties are common (see Chapters 28 and 32).

Prognosis

HIV infection is now the seventh leading cause of death in U.S. children 1 to 14 years of age and is the leading cause of death in children 2 to 5 years old in many U.S. cities (Butz et al, 1998). Over 50% of the children diagnosed with AIDS have died, but the actual mortality rate may be changing along with treatment advances. Two distinct courses of disease of perinatally infected children seem to exist. Infants who have a shorter median survival time seem to develop symptoms by 4 to 6 months of age, qualify for an AIDS diagnosis by 1 year of age, and often die by 2 years of age; and infants with a longer median survival time usually develop mild symptoms during the first year that resolve over the second and third years, may not have an AIDS diagnosis for many years, and may live to be teenagers (Dickover, 1994).

Data now exist to support the well-accepted hypothesis that children who have a rapidly progressive HIV course were infected early in gestation and those with a more indolent course were infected late in gestation or during the delivery process (Pizzo and Wilfert, 1998).

PRIMARY CARE MANAGEMENT
Health Care Maintenance

All children followed by HIV centers must also have a primary care provider. The HIV specialty provider and primary care provider work together to provide the highest level of care.

Growth and Development

The poor growth of children with symptomatic HIV disease appears to be more related to the general failure to thrive associated with the underlying HIV infection than to specific problems with caloric intake or GI losses. Height and weight should be carefully measured by a practitioner or a skilled assistant and plotted on the child's individual National Center for Health Statistics growth chart at least monthly. The same scale should be used at each visit if possible.

As previously noted, cortical atrophy and acquired microcephaly are common findings in severely affected infants. All children up to 3 years of age require serial head circumference measurements at least every 3 months, with results plotted on their growth charts and carefully evaluated.

Standard developmental screening tests used by primary care providers (e.g., the Denver Developmental Screening Test II) are of little value in assessing children with HIV disease. Developmental delay is a hallmark of pediatric HIV infection, and early intervention seems to produce significant results; therefore children must be regularly assessed by a skilled clinical psychologist as part of the comprehensive team approach. It is important for the primary care provider and the psychologist to discuss their developmental assessments and formulate a plan of action together.

Intervention strategies must begin as early as possible in an attempt to maximize a child's capabilities. Infant stimulation programs that focus on motor and language skills and additional specialties (e.g., physical, occupational and speech therapy) can be provided at home, in the hospital, or in clinic or group settings. Preschool and school-aged children with the necessary physical stamina can best be mainstreamed into regular programs with special services added (Abramowitz et al, 1998).

Diet

Children with HIV need a well-balanced diet with emphasis on adequate calories to maintain and increase their weight with growth. Nutritionists must be part of the multidisciplinary primary care team, taking dietary histories and performing nutritional assessments to guide clinical decisions. There are no special dietary recommendations or restrictions based on HIV infection. Because failure to thrive is common in these individuals, however, early nutritional intervention before wasting occurs is important (Deatrick, 1998). Dietary supplementation and special formulas (e.g., Scandi-shakes [Scandipharm] and Instant Breakfast [Carnation] for those who can tolerate dairy products; Pediasure [Ross] for infants and younger children; and Ensure [Ross] for older children and adolescents who are lactose-intolerant) are often beneficial for weight stabilization and potential gain. Enteral feedings and IV alimentation may be used acutely, intermittently, or chronically for children with severe anorexia, vomiting, diarrhea, and other GI prob-

lems. Families should regularly consult the primary care provider regarding the child's particular needs. Oral megestrol (Megace) has proved to increase appetite in some children.

Safety

Primary care providers must teach the families safety precautions for children with neutropenia and thrombocytopenia, as well as how to evaluate a child with neutropenia for signs and symptoms of infection (see Chapter 13).

Caretakers may benefit from education on infectious disease transmission and control (e.g., the need for frequent handwashing and avoiding crowds). Children with HIV and their household contacts must learn universal blood and body substance precautions. Because there is such concern about casual contagion in the community, families must be well-educated and able to withstand the apprehension of others. Several prospective studies of family and school contacts have found no evidence of the spread of HIV within these settings (Courville et al, 1998). Although HIV has been isolated in a variety of body fluids (including blood, CSF, pleural fluid, breast milk, semen, cervical secretions, saliva, and urine), only blood, semen, cervical secretions, and human milk have been implicated in its transmission.

It is important to counsel the child's caretaker about the safe storage of medications and equipment in the home (Maloney, 1998). Parents who are infected with HIV may also have many potentially hazardous medications at home. Children with HIV may be developmentally delayed or exhibit neurologic regression as the infection progresses, and safety precautions must be adjusted accordingly. If a parent with HIV cares for the child, the parent's ability to provide safe care must be frequently assessed because of the dementia often associated with HIV infection in adults (Nehring et al, 1997).

Immunizations

There is much controversy about immunization practices in children with HIV. Live-virus vaccines have not been recommended for children with congenital or drug-induced immunodeficiencies because of the concern that live, attenuated vaccine viruses can produce infection in an immunocompromised host. Prospective studies, however, failed to reveal such problems (AAP, 1999).

In addition, the dysfunction of the B-cell system typical of infants with HIV disease, which includes markedly elevated immunoglobulins, reflects nonspecific stimulation that is suggestive of a poor immune response to antigens and therefore to vaccines. Because of this immunologic dysfunction, immunogenicity and efficacy of vaccines may be lower in these children than in children who are immunocompetent. In general, children with symptomatic HIV infections have poor immunologic responses to vaccines and therefore should be considered susceptible regardless of history of vaccination, as well as receive passive immunoprophylaxis if indicated, when exposed to a vaccine-preventable disease such as measles or tetanus (Committee on Infectious Disease, 1997).

Because live-virus, attenuated immunizations may be ineffective in children who have received IVIG within the last 3 months, the general practice is to administer these vaccinations at the midpoint between monthly IVIG infusions.

Hepatitis B virus (HBV): Hepatitis B vaccine is now recommended as part of the regular schedule of immunizations for all children, including those who are symptomatic with HIV-infection.

Tetanus: Children with HIV should receive human tetanus immune globulin (TIG) regardless of vaccine status following an injury that places them at risk for tetanus infection (Committee on Infectious Disease, 1997).

Polio: Although oral polio vaccine (OPV) has been administered to children with HIV without adverse effects, the injectable enhanced, inactivated poliomyelitis vaccine (EIPV) is recommended because both the child and the HIV-infected family members may be immunosuppressed as a result of HIV infection and therefore may be at risk for vaccine-associated paralytic poliomyelitis caused by vaccine virus infection (Committee on Infectious Disease, 1997). All children in the household—even those not infected with HIV—should receive EIPV (AAP, 1999b).

Measles, mumps, and rubella: The measles, mumps, and rubella (MMR) vaccination should be administered at the standard age of 12 to 15 months unless the risk for measles or rubeola exposure is increased. Monovalent measles vaccine can be used for infants 6 to 11 months old, with revaccination with MMR at 12 months of age or older (Committee on Infectious Disease, 1997).

Regardless of vaccination status, children with both asymptomatic and symptomatic HIV infection should receive prophylaxis with immune globulin (IG) after exposure (Committee on Infectious Disease, 1997). Immune globulin may help prevent or minimize measles if administered within 6 days of exposure and is also indicated for household contacts of children with asymptomatic HIV disease who are measles-susceptible, especially for infants under 12 months of age. IG may be unnecessary if a child is receiving regular IVIG infusions and the last dose was within 3 weeks of exposure (Committee on Infectious Diseases, 1997).

***Haemophilus influenzae* type b (HIB):** Conjugated polysaccharide-diphtheria HIB vaccine is recommended for all children at 2 months of age (Committee on Infectious Diseases, 1997). As previously noted, *H. influenzae* organisms are a common and serious pathogen in children with HIV, increasing the importance of immunization. Even children who have had one or more episodes of documented infection with *H. influenzae* before 2 years of age may not produce enough antibody to prevent subsequent infections, making vaccination imperative. Prophylaxis with rifampin (Rifadin) is required even after vaccination if there is a known contact with HIB (Committee on Infectious Diseases, 1997).

Pneumococcus: Polyvalent pneumococcal vaccine (Pneumovax) should be administered to children with HIV at 2 years of age because of their underlying immunosuppression and because pneumococci are a prevalent pathogen in this population (Committee on Infectious Diseases, 1997).

Influenza: Yearly influenza vaccination with the subvirion (i.e., split-virus) bivalent vaccine is recommended for children over 6 months of age with HIV exposure or infection and their household contacts (Committee on Infectious Diseases, 1997).

Varicella: Varicella (HZV) poses significant risks for dissemination, encephalitis, and pneumonia in children who are immunosuppressed. Although the vaccine is now approved and released for use in healthy children, the efficacy of the vaccine in children with HIV infection is unknown and may vary depending on a child's degree of immune suppression. A study of the use of the varicella vaccine in children with HIV is in progress.

Children with HIV who are susceptible to varicella need to receive varicella-zoster immune globulin (VZIG) intramuscularly within 72 hours of exposure if they have not received IVIG within the past 3 weeks (Committee on Infectious Disease, 1997).

Screening

Vision: Because of the incidence of CMV retinitis in adults with HIV disease and therefore the theoretical risk of a similar process affecting children, primary care providers must elicit a thorough visual history and provide a careful visual and funduscopic examination. Comprehensive pediatric HIV centers may recommend that all children with HIV be referred to a knowledgeable pediatric ophthalmologist for baseline screening. If the findings are normal, the primary care provider can then continue to provide regular follow-up.

Hearing: Because of the frequent acute suppurative otitis media (OM) in children with HIV infection and the possibility of hearing loss, periodic audiometry and tympanometry should be performed. Children who require myringotomy tube placement require special precautions for swimming and showers (e.g., regular use of well-fitting earplugs).

Children with severe neurologic disease, some children with chronic OM, and those on maintenance aminoglycoside therapy need baseline brainstem, auditory evoked-response hearing testing if routine acuity testing cannot be done or is abnormal

Dental: Early screening (i.e., starting at 2 to 3 years of age) is strongly recommended because dental caries can create a focus of infection. Fluoride treatments are recommended if the community water supply does not contain adequate amounts to protect enamel. Severe dental caries and gingivitis, as well as dental abscesses, are reported in some infected children (Ramos-Gomez, 1997). Clinicians must educate families on appropriate oral hygiene and encourage regular dental care. Liquid medications contain sweeteners to increase drug palatability, which also increases the risk of caries.

Blood pressure: Blood pressure measurements should be taken every 3 to 6 months unless changes warrant more frequent measurements. Increased blood pressure can indicate renal disease.

Hematocrit: Screening is deferred because of the need for frequent assessment of CBCs.

Urinalysis: Children with HIV require urinalysis with microscopic examination at least every 3 months because urine abnormalities can be the first sign of illness. Findings can include hematuria and proteinuria and can result in azotemia and nephrotic syndrome. Children taking the protease inhibitor indinavir (Crixivan) need frequent (i.e., at least monthly) urinalysis with microscopic examination for crystals because this drug is known to cause renal stones.

Tuberculosis: Yearly screening is strongly advised. As tuberculosis is being diagnosed more often in adults with HIV, more children in infected households are at risk. Because many individuals infected with HIV demonstrate anergy to skin testing, close surveillance of families may include regular chest radiographic studies. MAI is a common bacterium of the same family as *Mycobacterium tuberculosis,* which is prevalent in individuals with HIV. Unlike *M. tuberculosis,* MAI is not contagious by the respiratory route but may be transmitted through infected GI secretions. Because it can invade many organ systems, including the bone marrow and the GI system, MAI may be responsible for much morbidity.

Condition-Specific Screening

Vital signs: Vital signs should be assessed and documented at each visit. Children can be asymptomatic yet febrile, needing a work-up. Elevations in heart and respiratory rates can indicate pulmonary or cardiac dysfunction.

Complete blood count: Because of bone marrow suppression caused by HIV and some OIs, as well as by many of the drugs used in treatment, children with HIV require that CBCs—with differential and platelet counts—be regularly determined. Asymptomatic children should have a CBC done every 3 to 6 months; symptomatic children usually need them done at least monthly. This blood work can be performed by the primary care provider or at the pediatric HIV center.

If anemia is present, its cause should be investigated because children with iron deficiency anemia usually benefit from oral iron supplementation. A specific cause, however, is not often discovered. Children taking antiretrovirals need their CBCs and reticulocyte counts assessed frequently because anemia is a common adverse effect. CBCs are usually completed every 2 weeks for the first 2 months and then done monthly as long as they are stable. Some children taking antiretrovirals require RBC transfusions. Neutropenia and thrombocytopenia are also common side effects of antiretroviral treatment. Doses of antiretrovirals may be modified based on the degree of bone marrow suppression. Bone marrow-stimulating drugs such as filgrastim (Neupogen) and granulocyte colony stimulating factor (GCSF) may be used.

Immunologic markers: Baseline T- and B-cell counts and quantitative immunoglobulin (QUIG) determinations are necessary to assess immunologic status. T-cell subset values and T4/T8 ratios are usually checked every 3 to 6 months. T4 counts below 500/mm^3 generally indicate that antiretrovirals should be prescribed. Children receiving monthly IVIG infusions do not have serial QUIG assessments because the infused—rather than endogenous—immunoglobulins would be represented.

Clinicians interpreting immunologic markers for children must consider age as a variable. These markers are used in conjunction with other markers to guide antiretroviral treatment decisions and primary prophylaxis for PCP after 1 year of age.

HIV markers: Viral burden can be determined by using quantitative HIV RNA viral load assays of peripheral blood. During primary infection in adults and adolescents, the HIV RNA viral load rises to high peak levels and then—coinciding with the body's humoral and cell-mediated immune response—declines by 2 to 3 logs to a stable lower level some 6 to 12 months later. This leveling off reflects the balance between ongoing viral production and immune elimination (CDC, 1998c). This pattern differs in perinatally infected infants in that high HIV RNA levels usually persist during the first year of life and then gradually decline over the next few years. This pattern may reflect an immature but developing immune system's lower efficiency in containing viral replication and more HIV-susceptible cells.

Trends in HIV RNA levels can be helpful in determining antiretroviral therapy and when the agents should be changed. Because of the complexities of testing and the age-related changes in values, however, interpretation of HIV RNA levels for clinical decision-making should be done by or in consultation with pediatric HIV experts.

Chemistry panel: Routine serum chemistry panels should be obtained every 3 to 6 months and more often for symptomatic children or those taking medications (i.e., AZT, didanosine [ddI]) that might affect liver or kidney function. Children taking ddI and/or 3TC must also be monitored for pancreatitis by having their amylase levels checked. Children taking protease inhibitors need regular lipid panels (including lipase, cholesterol, triglyceride, and glucose levels). Many children with HIV have elevated baseline liver function test results, often with both aspartate aminotransferase (AST) and alanine aminotransferase (ALT) enzyme levels 2 to 3 times that of normal.

Pulmonary function: Children with chronic lung disease need baseline pulmonary function testing with oxygen saturation and regular serial testing based on disease severity. When available, pulse oximetry—a noninvasive technique—is used in place of arterial blood gas sampling. A baseline radiograph is useful as a comparison study for pulmonary complaints. Children with either acute infection or chronic pneumonitis often have no adventitious sounds. Pulmonary consultation is a useful adjunct for the primary care provider in following these children.

Common Illness Management

Differential Diagnosis (Box 24-7)

Fever: Fever is often a sign in children with HIV disease and can be caused by the HIV itself or can indicate a separate infectious process. Practitioners must ensure that families have a thermometer that they can use accurately, as well as clear guidelines about when to contact their primary care provider. Whenever a child's temperature measures at least 38.5° C, the child generally needs to be examined and a treatment plan initiated based on the objective and subjective findings.

A thorough interval history and complete physical examination are the most important part of the work-up of a febrile child with HIV. Some of these children will have otitis media, sinusitis, pneumonia, or sepsis; others will have common colds and other viral infections that can be traced to school or household contacts.

In consultation with the infectious disease specialist or the HIV center, the primary care provider can order cultures of blood and other body fluid as indicated for aerobic, anaerobic, and fungal organisms. Cultures are essential to identifying the infectious process. Cultures are often negative—even in seriously ill children, but positive cultures will determine specific antibiotic therapy. Chest radiographic studies may be an important part of the work-up of a febrile child with HIV.

Respiratory distress: A variety of respiratory complaints may plague children with HIV. History and physical examination are paramount to the differential diagnosis. A dry, hacking cough is a common complaint of children with LIP but can also be a sign of PCP. Children with acute onset of respiratory distress require quick evaluation because the condition can progress extremely rapidly—sometimes within hours. Pulmonary consultation is often necessary. Children with cardiac disease occasionally have respiratory complaints and need cardiologic consultation and diagnosis.

Children with known reactive airway disease may benefit from having equipment and medications for aerosol delivery at home. The primary care provider must evaluate the family's ability to provide such sophisticated assessment and treatment; if parents are capable, they can be taught the necessary skills.

Otitis media: Otitis media (OM) is one of the most common infectious diseases in children with HIV and is often diagnosed on routine physical examination when no pain or fever is present, even when the tympanic membrane may be ruptured with pus filling the external canal. Follow-up must be done after treatment is completed because the OM may not resolve and complications may occur. Children who have persistent and refractory OM should be referred to an ear, nose, and throat (ENT) specialist for evaluation for placement of myringotomy tubes.

Sinusitis: Although sinusitis is uncommon in children, it is seen commonly in children with HIV disease and often occurs after a viral respiratory tract infection. Primary care providers can teach families to report changes in nasal mucus from clear or white to yellow or green, which may indicate infection. If not appropriately treated, sinusitis can lead to mastoiditis and directly extend into the brain, causing meningitis.

Varicella: Because of the risk of dissemination as a result of immunocompromise, varicella is potentially life threatening in children with HIV. Because these children may not respond adequately to vaccines and the general herd immunity to varicella will not be high until the vaccine has been widely distributed for many years, herpes zoster virus (HZV) will continue to cause chickenpox as a primary manifestation and zoster as a secondary manifestation of infection in most children with HIV. If primary prevention with VZIG fails or if a child was not known to be exposed until the rash occurs, the usual practice at most centers is to hospitalize these children and treat them with acyclovir IV as soon as the disease is diagnosed. With this treatment, few children progress to disseminated disease, and most go home within 5 days of starting therapy, continuing with oral therapy to complete a 7-day to 10-day course.

Drug Interactions

Antiretrovirals: The following three groups of agents are used to treat HIV infection: (1) nucleoside reverse transcriptase inhibitors (e.g., AZT, 3TC, ddI, zalcitabine [ddC], d4T); (2) nonnucleoside reverse transcriptase inhibitors (e.g., nevirapine, delavirdine, sustiva); and (3) protease inhibitors (e.g., saquinavir, ritonavir, indinavir, nelfinavir). There are variations in whether each drug may be given on an empty or full stomach, and some must be given separately from other drugs. Many of these drugs have significant drug interactions. It is best to identify the specific considerations of each and every drug that a child with HIV is taking.

Trimethoprim-Sulfamethoxazole (TMP-SMX): Two of the major toxicities of this sulfa combination are hematologic: neutropenia and thrombocytopenia. Children on PCP prophylaxis or treatment regimens who develop persistent neutropenia secondary to TMP-SMX either alone or with AZT must often discontinue TMP-SMX. Intravenous or aerosolized pentamidine can be used as an alternative in older children. Allergic reactions to sulfa are not uncommon, and primary care providers must teach families how to recognize the symptoms of skin rash and hives as part of the reaction complex. Several studies have shown successful treatment using TMP-SMX with a history of previous adverse reactions (Simonds and Orejas, 1998).

IVIG: There are no specific drug interactions noted with IVIG. Allergic reactions have been documented but appear to be rare.

Developmental Issues

Sleep Patterns

Children taking AZT or other medications that interrupt normal sleeping hours may experience difficulty in returning to sleep. Findings from a study on sleep disturbances in children with HIV suggest that sleep disturbances occur frequently (Franck et al, 1998). Therefore parents may need to try a variety of schedules to find one that works best for them and their child to minimize interruptions in their child's sleeping hours. For example, primary care providers must ensure that families have access to a reliable alarm clock so that medication doses are not missed.

Toileting

Children with HIV who are in diapers may experience diaper dermatitis, which is often associated with Candidiasis, as well as with chronic and cyclical diarrhea. Impeccable perineal care—including frequent diaper changes, exposure of the perineum to air, and the use of topical medications—can significantly reduce morbidity. When the perineum is bloody or the child has hematuria or diarrhea, care-

takers should wear gloves to protect themselves during diapering. Neurologic deterioration can lead to incontinence in children who have previously been out of diapers.

Discipline

Discipline is often difficult for the family of a child with a life-threatening illness. Some parents are unable to set developmentally appropriate and necessary limits and need guidance and information from their primary care provider. Discipline needs and appropriate expectations will vary as the illness progresses and neurologic and motor deterioration occurs, so caretakers must be given anticipatory guidance in these areas. Other factors (e.g., homelessness, chaotic lifestyle, and parental illness) can make consistent discipline difficult. Practitioners may help families and caregivers to understand the child's needs for safety and limits.

Child Care

Child care, respite care, and preschool placement are difficult issues for families of children with HIV. Primary care providers must advise parents that children in group settings are at increased risk for exposure to infectious diseases and common childhood illnesses compared with children who stay at home (Takala et al, 1995). The particular setting must be individualized for each child based on the child and family's needs and resources. Practitioners can provide education on universal infection control and infectious disease guidelines for these agencies.

Child care and respite care are important resources for families caring for children with chronic conditions. Some foster families have access to respite hours through their social services division, but others do not. In some areas there are few, if any, child care or respite workers willing to care for infants and children with HIV, which is an enormous problem for families who need time to care for their own HIV, as well as for their infected and uninfected children. The regular availability of respite care and other support services may allow many infected mothers to continue to care for their children.

Public Laws 101-476 and 99-457 may offer valuable services for children with HIV (see Chapter 5). Head Start, a federal preschool program that provides preschool for economically deprived children, is specifically mandated to enroll children with HIV.

Because daycare and preschool are not a legal requirement for children, individual daycare providers may develop their own policies in accordance with local, state, and federal regulations. Many private daycare centers and preschools do not accept children with HIV, probably because of their fears of casual contagion, litigation, and unenrollment if other families discover the diagnosis. Some areas of the country with a high prevalence of pediatric HIV have developed daycare programs specifically for these children. Such services are directed toward children who are too ill to attend regular daycare programs.

Daycare and preschool personnel and families should be educated before a child with HIV is enrolled. It may be useful for the primary care provider to call the preschool, stating that a family is interested in enrolling their child with HIV. The school is notified that there is no "duty to inform" and that the child will not be identified. Feelings about children with HIV infection are explored, and an offer is made to provide in-service training about pediatric HIV and control of general infection.

Some families choose to conceal the HIV in their family, but other families openly discuss it (Wiener, 1998). As more children take antiviral medications such as AZT that must be administered frequently, it is becoming harder to conceal HIV infection from daycare providers. Many families, however, schedule dosing around school hours and create unusual stories about why they need to immediately know about chickenpox or other contagious illnesses in the classroom. Clinicians have an important role to play in helping families decide how, when, and to whom information about HIV disease should be disclosed (AAP, 1999c).

Schooling

The major school issues faced by young children with HIV have little to do with their educational needs and much to do with concerns about confidentiality, information sharing, and infection control. These issues have created strife in many communities nationwide. As children with HIV age, however, their needs for special education programs will undoubtedly increase. Primary care providers can help the families secure the appropriate services (see Chapter 5).

Because AIDS is recognized as a handicap, attendance in public schools is supported by Public Law 101-476. In some areas of the country, public school attendance is decided by committees of educators and public health officials and the child's primary care provider. If the decision to ban the child from attending school is made, the school district must provide home teaching. Children benefit greatly from attending school, so this option should be strongly encouraged. When children are too ill to attend, home teaching is a viable alternative for that time period only. As a child's condition progresses, particularly with neurologic deterioration, frequent meetings of school resource personnel, health care providers, and family members will be needed to ensure that appropriate services are provided.

The legal duty to inform school officials about a child's HIV diagnosis varies from state to state (Cohen, 1997). As more children become aware of their own HIV infection, however, there will be more discussion among these children, which will make more of the school and larger community aware that a child with HIV is in attendance. Providers should be available to the school (i.e., students, faculty, and parents) for educational discussion sessions.

Teenagers with HIV often have difficulty in school. Rumors that circulate about HIV infection and the students thought to be infected can cause tremendous anxiety for an infected adolescent— regardless of the route of infection (Chabon, 1999). Primary care providers can support their teen-aged clients, helping them gain more knowledge and determine whom they might trust with this sensitive information. Referral to the school nurse or counselor may be appropriate (Rogers, 1998).

Sexuality

Children and adolescents with HIV need to learn about sexual and perinatal transmission of this condition. Adolescence is the time for sexual experimentation and the emergence of sexual identity, and sexual activity increases steadily throughout these years. Teens with HIV face much difficulty in attaining a healthy, integrated sexual identity because of the risks of oral and genital sexual transmission. Some teens deny the reality of their HIV, refusing to practice safer sex. Primary care providers must be comfortable discussing transmission and sexual risk reduction strategies, as well as demonstrating the proper use of condoms and dental dams.

Transition to Adulthood

The advent of new and more effective HIV therapies has transformed HIV infection from a terminal illness to a chronic but manageable condition. Survival times have continued to increase; there are now long-term survivors among children who were perinatally infected. These individuals will continue to need a vast array of medical and psychosocial services throughout their childhood and transition to adulthood. Because these children were born to mothers with HIV, many infected family members are often at risk for death from HIV while these children are young. As they reach sexual maturity, these children must be educated about and helped to deal with the fact that they can transmit HIV to their sexual partners.

Children and teenagers who have been infected as a result of nonperinatal transmission (i.e., sexual activity, injection drug use, transfusion, or transplantation) have many other concerns to face. Some of these issues include the risk for sexual transmission, intimacy, and stigma. As HIV infection becomes a more chronic, life-threatening disease integrated into the mainstream of health care, these special issues may gradually decline.

Special Family Concerns and Resources

HIV infection is a family disease, and when a child is diagnosed, a family crisis results. Most children with HIV have infected mothers who are ill, dying, or deceased and may have an infected father and siblings in the family, as well. Most mothers who transmit HIV to their children experience tremendous guilt. The physical and emotional burden of caring for a child who requires frequent medical and supportive treatments, may have developmental delay, and will probably die as a result of the illness is enormous.

The most significant psychosocial issue facing children with HIV and their families is the social stigmatization associated with the disease. Many families initially feel isolated and unable to call on their normal support systems for fear of rejection and retaliation. These families may also lack other resources; they are primarily poor, of minority heritage, undereducated, and burdened by the social ills of inner-city life. With support, these families may reach out to extended family, friends, and community agencies (AAP, 1999d).

Most children who were perinatally infected with the HIV disease are children of color. Some children are placed in foster or adoptive care after birth if their mother is unable to care for them. Others are placed out of the home later when resources cannot support their parents' ability to care for them. Foster and adoptive parents need considerable support (i.e., ongoing education, financial support, respite care, emotional support and counseling, and social and legal counseling) to provide optimal care for these children. Because children in foster care are wards of the juvenile court, decisions about consent for investigational drugs and experimental protocols, as well as do-not-resuscitate orders, must be court-ordered. Working relationships between the primary care provider, HIV center, and social services must be developed to ensure that children with HIV receive optimal care in the child welfare system.

Helping children and families face a chronic, life-threatening illness that may ultimately lead to death is a pivotal role for primary care providers. Counseling about the physical and emotional issues of death and the dying process, options for hospital or home death, hospice services, funeral plans, and bereavement is an integral part of the clinician's role. Support groups are invaluable resources for networking, keeping current, and decreasing social isolation. Most pediatric HIV-AIDS comprehensive treatment centers offer such groups on an ongoing basis. Primary care providers should become familiar with the local, national, and international organizations (see the list of organizations that follows).

Organizations

Camp Heartland
http://www.campheartland.org

Camp Pacific Heartland
3663 Wilshire Blvd.
Los Angeles, Calif. 90010-2798
(213) 464-1235
http://www.camppacificheartland.org

Camp Sunburst National AIDS Project
5350 Commerce Blvd, Suite I
Rohnert Park, Calif. 94928
(707) 588-9477
http://www.sunburstprojects.org

CDC National AIDS Clearinghouse
PO Box 6003
Rockville, Md. 20849-6003
(800) 458-5231
http://www.cdcnpin.org

HIV and AIDS Malignancy Branch (HAMB),
    National Cancer Institute
(301) 496-0328
http://www-dcs.nci.nih.gov/aidstrials

National AIDS Hotline
(800) 342-AIDS

National Center for Youth Law
114 Sansome Street, Suite 900
San Francisco, Calif. 94104-3820
(415) 543-3307
http://www.youthlaw.org

National Foundation for Children with AIDS
3505 South Ocean Drive
Hollywood, Fla. 33019
http://www.childrenwithaids.org

National Pediatric and Family HIV Resource
    Center
15 S 9th Street
Newark, NJ 07107
(800) 362-0071
http://www.pedhivaids.org

NIAID Intramural Trials for HIV Infection
    and AIDS
(800) AIDS-NIH or (800)243-7644

Safe Haven
PO Box 24
Vineyard Haven, Mass. 02568
(508) 693-1767
http://www.charityweb.net/SafeHaven

Sunshine for HIV Kids, Inc
c/o Richard Merck
PO Box 3537
Kingston, NY 12402
(888) SUN-4-KIDS
http://www.songshine.com

The Elizabeth Glaser Pediatric AIDS Foundation
1311 Colorado Avenue
Santa Monica, Calif. 90404
(310) 395-9051
http://www.pedaids.org

Local and State Resources

County health department
State health department
AIDS task forces
AIDS hotlines

Summary of Primary Care Needs for the Child with HIV

HEALTH CARE MAINTENANCE

Growth and development

Growth in both weight and height may be poor and should be measured and plotted monthly.

Cortical atrophy and acquired microcephaly are common in severely affected infants.

Measure and plot head circumference monthly until a child is 3 years of age.

Standard developmental screening tests are not useful; if available, serial screening by a psychologist is recommended.

Early intervention programs are recommended.

Diet

A balanced, high-calorie diet should be emphasized.

Nutritional supplements should be used.

Safety

The risk of infection because of immunocompromise is increased.

Summary of Primary Care Needs for the Child with HIV—cont'd

The risk of bleeding because of thrombocytopenia is increased.

Universal blood and body substance precautions should be taught to the family and community.

Safe storage of medication in the home is important.

Developmental delay or regression may alter safety requirements.

Parents with HIV must be evaluated for safe care practices because of symptoms of dementia.

Immunizations

Hepatitis B Vaccine should be given to all children with HIV.

Tetanus immunoglobulin (TIG) should be given to children at risk for infection due to injury.

Use EIPV for exposed or infected children, all household members, and close contacts.

Give immune globulin within 6 days of measles exposure to prevent or modify course unless a child received IVIG in the previous 3 weeks.

Haemophilus influenzae type b and polyvalent pneumococcal vaccines are recommended.

Pneumovax should be given to children >2 years of age with HIV.

Yearly influenza vaccine is recommended.

Varicella-zoster immune globulin is recommended within 72 hours of varicella exposure.

Screening

Vision: An ophthalmologist should do a baseline funduscopic examination with practitioner follow-up every 3 to 6 months.

Hearing: Periodic audiometry and tympanometry screenings are recommended.

A brain stem evoked-response (BSER) hearing test should be given to children with chronic OM or abnormal screening.

Dental: Early screening is recommended to prevent dental infections and should be followed-up regularly to prevent and/or treat dental caries.

Blood pressure: Measurements should be taken every 3 to 6 months.

Hematocrit: Routine screening is deferred because of the need for frequent CBC tests.

Urinalysis: Urinalysis with microscopic examination should be done at least every 3 months and monthly for children taking indinavir.

Tuberculosis: Yearly screening is recommended. Chest radiographic studies may be needed if a child is anergic.

Condition-specific screening

Vital signs: Temperature, heart rate, and respiratory rate should be checked at each visit.

Complete blood count: A CBC should be assessed every 3 to 6 months if a child is asymptomatic and every 2 to 4 weeks if a child is taking antiretrovirals or other myelosuppressive agents.

Immunologic markers: Baseline T- and B-cell counts, QUIG values, repeat T-cell subset levels, and T4/T8 ratios should be checked every 3 to 6 months.

Chemistry panel: Serum chemistry panels should be obtained every 3 to 6 months if a child is asymptomatic and more often if a child is symptomatic or taking liver or kidney toxic agents. Serum amylase should be obtained for children taking 3TC/ddI. Lipid panel and glucose should be obtained for children taking protease inhibitors.

Pulmonary function: Baseline pulmonary function testing, including pulse oximetry if available, is recommended for children with lung disease.

COMMON ILLNESS MANAGEMENT
Differential diagnosis

Fever: Rule out bacterial infection and OI.

Respiratory distress: Rule out LIP, PCP, and cardiac disease.

Otitis media: Rule out tympanic membrane perforation.

Sinusitis: Rule out bacterial sinusitis, mastoiditis, and meningitis.

Varicella: Use VZIG as primary prevention and acyclovir as secondary prevention.

Continued

Summary of Primary Care Needs for the Child with HIV—cont'd

Drug interactions

Zidovudine: Bone marrow suppression may occur.

Didanosine (ddI): Check amylase for pancreatitis.

Trimethoprim/sulfamethoxazole: Bone marrow suppression (neutropenia, thrombocytopenia) and allergic reactions may occur.

Developmental issues

Sleep patterns: Sleep patterns may be disturbed because of medications needed around the clock.

Toileting: Impeccable perineal care is necessary to reduce morbidity of diaper dermatitis. Caretakers should use gloves for blood or diarrhea.

Discipline: Discipline is often difficult for the family; lifestyle issues can exacerbate problems.

Child care: The child care program should be individualized to meet the child and family's needs.

Public Laws 99-457 and 101-476 cover early intervention services.

Schooling: Public school attendance is aided by Public Law 101-476.

There is no duty to inform school officials of a child's HIV status.

The school community may benefit from education.

Teens may need extra support from the school nurse or counselor.

Sexuality: Sexual and perinatal transmission should be discussed.

Safer sex techniques and the use of condoms and dental dams should be demonstrated.

Transition to adulthood

With improved treatment, HIV may become a chronic condition.

Parents may have died from condition years before.

Individuals must be educated about the possible transmission of HIV to others.

Special family concerns

HIV is a family disease.

Many families lack resources.

HIV is an enormous physical and emotional burden.

Stigmatization is a major issue.

Many children with HIV are placed in foster or adoptive homes.

Counseling on death and dying and during bereavement is helpful.

Many of children with HIV are of color. Primary care providers must be sensitive to specific cultural issues.

References

Abramowitz S, Obten N, and Cohen H: Measuring case management for families with HIV, Soc Work Health Care 27:29-41, 1998.

American Academy of Pediatrics, Committee on Pediatric AIDS: Recommended childhood immunizations schedule—United States, January-December 1999, Pediatrics 103:182-5, 1999a.

American Academy of Pediatrics, Committee on Infectious Diseases: Poliomyelitis prevention: revised recommendations for use of inactivated and live oral poliovirus vaccines, Pediatrics 103:171-2, 1999b.

American Academy of Pediatrics, Committee on Pediatric AIDS: Disclosure of illness status to children and adolescents with HIV infection, Pediatrics 103:164-6, 1999c.

American Academy of Pediatrics, Committee on Pediatric AIDS: Planning for children whose parents are dying of HIV/AIDS, Pediatrics 103:509-11, 1999d.

Andiman WA and Shearer WT: Lymphoid interstitial pneumonitis. In Pizzo PA and Wilfert CM, editors: Pediatric AIDS: the challenge of HIV infection in infants, children and adolescents, ed 3, Baltimore, 1998, Williams & Wilkins.

Browers P, Wolters P, and Civitello L: Central nervous system manifestations and assessment. In Pizzo PA and Wilfert CM, editors: Pediatric AIDS: the challenge of HIV infection in infants, children and adolescents, ed 3, Baltimore, 1998, Williams & Wilkins.

Butz AM et al: Primary care for children with human immunodeficiency virus infection, J Pediatr Health Care 12:10-19, 1998.

Centers for Disease Control and Prevention: 1994 revised classification system for human immunodeficiency virus infection in children less than 13 years of age, MMWR 43(RR-12):1-10, 1994.

Centers for Disease Control and Prevention: HIV/AIDS surveillance report 10:1998a, The Centers.

Centers for Disease Control and Prevention: Guidelines for the use of antiretroviral agents in HIV-infected adults and adolescents, MMWR 47(RR-5):42-82, 1998b.

Centers for Disease Control and Prevention: Guidelines for the use of antiretroviral agents in pediatric HIV infection, MMWR 47(RR-4):1-43, 1998c.

Centers for Disease Control and Prevention: Public Health Service Task Force recommendations for the use of antiretroviral drugs to pregnant women infected with HIV-1 for maternal health and for reducing perinatal HIV-1 transmission in the United States, MMWR 47(RR-2):1-28, 1998d.

Centers for Disease Control and Prevention: Rotavirus vaccine for the prevention of rotavirus gastroenteritis among children: recommendations of the advisory committee on immunization practices (ACIP), MMWR 48(RR-2):1-23, 1999.

Chabon B and Futterman D: Adolescents and HIV, AIDS Clin Care 11:1, 1999.

Cohen J et al: School-related issues among HIV-infected children, Pediatrics 100:E8, 1997.

Committee on Infectious Disease: Report of the Committee on Infectious Disease, ed 24, Elk Grove Village, Ill., 1997, The American Academy of Pediatrics.

Courville TM, Caldwell B, and Brunell PA. Lack of evidence of transmission of HIV-1 to family contacts of HIV-1 infected children. Clin Pediatr 37:175-8, 1998.

Cvetkovich TA and Frenkel LM: Current management of HIV infections in children, Pediatr Ann 22:428-434, 1993.

Deatrick JA et al: Nutritional assessment for children who are HIV-infected, Pediatr Nurs 24:137-41, 1998.

Dickover RE et al: Rapid increases in load of human immunodeficiency virus correlate with early disease progression and loss of CD4 cells in vertically infected infants, J Infect Dis 170:1279-1284, 1994.

Franck LS et al: Sleep disturbances in children with HIV infection, Pediatrics, In Press.

Kamani NR and Douglas SD: Structure and development of the immune system. In Sites DP and Terr AF, editors: Basic and clinical immunology, ed 7, Norfolk, Conn., 1991, Appleton & Lange.

Krasinski K: Bacterial infections. In Pizzo PA and Wilfert CM, editors: Pediatric AIDS: the challenge of HIV infection in infants, children, and adolescents, ed 2, Baltimore, 1994, Williams & Wilkins.

Luzuriaga K and Sullivan JL: Prevention and treatment of pediatric HIV infection, JAMA 280:17-18, 1998.

Luzuriaga K and Sullivan JL: Viral and immunopathogenesis of vertical HIV-1 infection. In Pizzo PA and Wilfert CM, editors: Pediatric AIDS: the challenge of HIV infection in infants, children and adolescents, ed 3, Baltimore, 1998, Williams & Wilkins.

Luzuriaga K et al: Combination treatment with zidovudine, didanosine, and nevirapine in infants with human immunodeficiency virus type 1 infection, NEJM 336:1343-9, 1997.

McKinney RE et al: A randomized study of combined zidovudine-lamivudine versus didanosine monotherapy in children with symptomatic therapy-naïve HIV-1 infection: the pediatric AIDS clinical trials group protocol 300 study team, J Pediatr 133:500-8, 1998.

Maloney C, Damon B, and Regan AM. Pediatric compliance in combination HIV therapy: getting it right the first time, Adv Nurse Pract 6:35-8, 1998.

Miller TL and Garg S: Gastrointestinal and nutritional problems in pediatric HIV disease. In Pizzo PA and Wilfert CM, editors: Pediatric AIDS: the challenge of HIV infection in infants, children and adolescents, ed 3, Baltimore, 1998, Williams & Wilkins.

Nehring WM, Larson B, and Boyer SG: Caring for the child with HIV infection or AIDS: key points for community care, Adv Nurse Pract 5:37-42, 1997.

Pizzo PA and Wilfert CM, editors: Pediatric AIDS: the challenge of HIV infection in infants, children and adolescents, ed 3, Baltimore, 1998, Williams & Wilkins.

Ramos-Gomez FJ: Oral aspects of HIV infection in children, Oral Dis Suppl 1:S31-5, 1997.

Rogers AS et al: The REACH project of the adolescent medicine HIV/AIDS research network: design, methods, and selected characteristics of participants, J Adolesc Health 22:300-11, 1998.

Simonds RJ and Orejas G: Pneumocystis carinii pneumonia and toxoplasmosis. In Pizzo PA and Wilfert CM, editors: Pediatric AIDS: the challenge of HIV infection in infants, children and adolescents, ed 3, Baltimore, 1998, Williams & Wilkins.

Spector SA et al: A controlled trial of intravenous immune globulin for the prevention of serious bacterial infections in children receiving zidovudine for advanced human immunodeficiency virus infection, N Engl J Med 331:1181-1187, 1994.

Steim RE et al: Efficacy of zidovudine and human immunodeficiency virus (HIV) hyperimmune immunoglobulin for reducing perinatal HIV transmission from HIV-infected women with advanced disease: results of pediatric AIDS clinical trials group protocol 185, J Infect Dis 179:567-75, 1999.

Takala AK et al: Risk factors for primary invasive pneumococcal disease among children in Finland, JAMA 273(11):859-864, 1995.

Walsh TJ et al: Fungal infections in children with HIV. In Pizzo PA and Wilfert CM, editors: Pediatric AIDS: the challenge of HIV infection in infants, children and adolescents, ed 3, Baltimore, 1998, Williams & Wilkins.

Wiener LS, Battles HB, and Heilman NE: Factors associated with parents' decision to disclose their HIV diagnosis to their children, Child Welfare 77:115-35, 1998.

Wilfert CM: Invasive bacterial infections in children with HIV infection. In Pizzo PA and Wilfert CM, editors: Pediatric AIDS: the challenge of HIV infection in infants, children and adolescents, ed 3, Baltimore, 1998, Williams & Wilkins.

Wood LV: Immunomodulation and immune reconstitution. In Pizzo PA and Wilfert CM, editors: Pediatric AIDS: the challenge of HIV infection in infants, children and adolescents, ed 3, Baltimore, 1998, Williams & Wilkins.

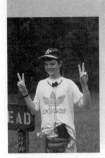

CHAPTER *25*

Hydrocephalus

Patricia Ludder Jackson and Joyce Harvey

Etiology

Hydrocephalus is a condition that results from an imbalance between the production and absorption of cerebrospinal fluid (CSF), leading to an increase in the volume of intracranial CSF, enlargement of the ventricular system, and increased intracranial pressure (ICP) (Raimondi, 1998; Rekate, 1997). Hydrocephalus is most commonly caused by an obstruction in the normal circulation and absorption of CSF (Figure 25-1) Although rare, hydrocephalus may occur when excessive CSF is produced by an intraventricular tumor of the choroid plexus.

CSF is continuously produced by the choroid plexus within the lateral, third, and fourth ventricles and as a by-product of cerebral and spinal cord metabolism. CSF formation occurs at a rate of .3 ml/min (Rekate, 1997). An equal amount of CSF is absorbed from the subarachnoid space into the venous system by projections (i.e., arachnoid villi) in the arachnoid. To reach the subarachnoid space and villi, CSF passes through a series of channels and pathways (see Figure 25-1). Pulsations of the choroid plexus propel CSF through the ventricular system. From the lateral ventricles, CSF flows into the third ventricle via the foramen of Monro. It passes from the third ventricle into the fourth ventricle through the aqueduct of Sylvius and out of the fourth ventricle through either the lateral foramina of Luschka or the foramen of Magendie. CSF exits the ventricular system and travels around the brainstem and spinal cord and over the surface of the brain, where it is absorbed by the arachnoid villi (Raimondi, 1998; Rekate, 1997). Alternate pathways for CSF absorption may come into play when ICP is increased. CSF may travel into the paranasal sinuses, conjunctiva of the eye, and lymphatics, as well as along the cranial or spinal nerves to be absorbed into the systemic circulation (Rekate, 1997).

Hydrocephalus may be classified as congenital or acquired, communicating or noncommunicating, and intra- or extraventricular (Box 25-1). The description of communicating vs. noncommunicating hydrocephalus may be most helpful in understanding the etiology and treatment options for a particular child. Noncommunicating hydrocephalus can result from blockage of any part of the ventricular system, obstructing the passage of CSF from one ventricle into another or from the ventricular system into the subarachnoid cisterns (Barkovich, 1995) and resulting in enlargement of the ventricular system proximal to the site of obstruction. For example, when the aqueduct of Sylvius is obstructed, the lateral and third ventricles enlarge but the fourth ventricle remains normal in size.

The most common obstruction is congenital aqueductal stenosis at the aqueduct of Sylvius. This obstruction may occur as the result of a perinatal infection (e.g., toxoplasmosis, cytomegalovirus, mumps, syphilis, meningitis) or compression and obstruction of the aqueduct by a mass (e.g., congenital aneurysm, arachnoid cyst, subdural hematoma, intraventricular or subarachnoid hemorrhage, or early neonatal brain tumors) (Barkovich, 1995; Raimondi, 1998). Congenital malformations of the brain such as Chiari II malformations, which are commonly associated with myelomeningocele, and Dandy-Walker malformations also result in noncommunication or obstructive hydrocephalus with both intra- and extraventricular blockage of CSF. Noncommunicating hydrocephalus may occur as a result of CNS infections, tumors, trauma, arteriovenous malformations, or systemic bleeding disorders in older children (Barkovich, 1995; Raimondi, 1998).

Communicating hydrocephalus occurs when CSF flow or absorption is blocked in the subarachnoid spaces, basilar cisterns, and the arachnoid villi. CSF may circulate freely throughout the entire ventricular system and cisterns but not be adequately

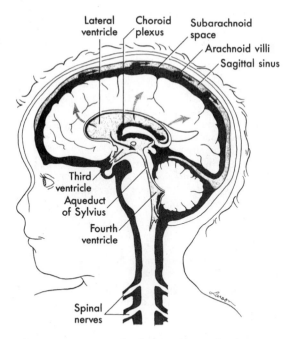

Lateral ventricle
Choroid plexus
Subarachnoid space
Arachnoid villi
Sagittal sinus
Third ventricle
Aqueduct of Sylvius
Fourth ventricle
Spinal nerves

Figure 25-1 CSF circulatory pathway showing a view of the center of the brain. Solid arrows show the major pathway of CSF flow; broken arrows show additional pathways. (From Edwards MS and Derechin M, editors: About hydrocephalus: a book for parents. Drawings by Lynne Larson. San Francisco, 1986, University of California. Reprinted with permission.)

absorbed. Communicating hydrocephalus may be associated with meningitis (bacterial or viral), intraventricular hemorrhage, trauma, or a congenital malformation of the subarachnoid spaces. In communicating hydrocephalus, the lateral, third, and fourth ventricles enlarge (Barkovich, 1995).

Hydrocephalus may also be a component of numerous syndromes (Raimondi, 1998). The cause of hydrocephalus associated with achondroplasia and various cranial facial syndromes is thought to be a result of venous hypertension, leading to a decreased pressure gradient across the arachnoid villi and impaired CSF absorption (Barkovich, 1995). Similarly, infants with a Vein of Galen malformation have a large arteriovenous shunt, which leads to retrograde flow of blood from the high-pressure arterial side to the low-pressure venous side, causing an elevation of the cerebral venous pressure

that will affect absorption of CSF into the venous system (Raimondi, 1998).

Incidence

The overall incidence of hydrocephalus is unknown. The incidence of infantile hydrocephalus is approximately 3 to 4 per 1000 live births (Carey, Tullous, and Walker, 1994), and aqueductal stenosis is responsible for approximately one third of these cases. The incidence of myelomeningocele varies dramatically from region to region. In the United States the incidence is approximately 1 per 1000 births (Carey, Tullous, and Walker, 1994). Of these children, 80% will develop hydrocephalus that requires shunting during the first year of life as a result of either a Chiari II malformation or associated aqueductal stenosis.

Clinical Manifestations at Time of Diagnosis

Although the signs and symptoms of hydrocephalus may vary depending on its cause, there are common clinical manifestations associated with increased CSF volume and ICP (Box 25-2). The presence or absence of an expandable cranium and the volume and compliance of cerebral tissue determine the severity of symptoms (Carey, Tullous, and Walker, 1994). If the accumulation of excessive CSF occurs slowly, an infant or young child may be asymptomatic until the hydrocephalus is advanced. Infants are less likely to be acutely ill because their skull and sutures can expand to accommodate increasing ventricular size, thereby minimizing an elevation in ICP. Full or distended fontanels, frontal bossing, prominent scalp veins, split sutures, and abnormally rapid head growth are common presenting signs in infancy. Poor feeding, vomiting, and irritability may later occur. A loss or delay of developmental milestones may become evident. Increased tone or hyperreflexia may be apparent, particularly in the lower extremities. Late signs include lethargy, sixth nerve palsy, and paralysis of upward gaze (i.e., "sunsetting") (Dias and Li, 1998).

Specific signs and symptoms of increased ICP are evident in children over 18 to 24 months of age with fused cranial sutures. Such symptoms include

---

Box 25-1

Classification of Hydrocephalus

I. Noncommunicating
   A. Congenital
      1. Chiari malformation (usually associated with myelomeningocele)
      2. Aqueductal stenosis
      3. Aqueductal gliosis (postperinatal hemorrhage or infection)
      4. Obstruction from congenital lesions (neoplasms, vascular malformation, vein of Galen)
      5. Arachnoid cyst, benign intracranial cyst
   B. Acquired
      1. Infectious ventriculitis
      2. Obstruction from lesions (neoplasms, vascular malformation)
      3. Chemical ventriculitis
      4. Intraventricular hemorrhage
II. Communicating
   A. Congenital
      1. Arachnoid cyst

   2. Encephalocele
   3. Associated with congenital malformation: craniofacial syndromes, achondroplasia
   4. Dandy-Walker malformation
   B. Acquired
      1. Chemical arachnoiditis
      2. Infections (postmeningitis)
      3. Posthemorrhagic (postsubarachnoid hemorrhage, intraventricular hemorrhage)
      4. Associated with spinal tumors and seeding from CNS tumors

Adapted from Carey CM, Tullous MW, and Walker ML: Hydrocephalus: etiology, pathologic effects, diagnosis, and natural history. In Cheek WR, editor: Pediatric neurosurgery: surgery of the developing nervous system, ed 3, Philadelphia, 1994, W.B. Saunders.

Barkovich AJ: Hydrocephalus. In Barkovich AJ: Pediatric neuroimaging, New York, 1995, Raven Press.

Box 25-2

Clinical Manifestations

Manifestations are determined by degree of hydrocephalus, degree of increased ICP, and etiology.

Associated Symptoms

Associated symptoms in infants:
- Abnormal head growth
- Distended fontanels
- Frontal bossing
- Vomiting
- Irritability or lethargy
- Opisthotonic posturing
- Sixth nerve palsy

Associated symptoms in children >18 months:
- Headache
- Nausea
- Vomiting
- Irritability and/or lethargy
- Alterations in motor development
- Ocular changes

headache, nausea, vomiting, and personality changes (i.e., irritability, lethargy, and loss of interest in normal daily activities). Headaches, especially those that awaken the child from sleep or occur immediately upon awakening, strongly suggest an elevated ICP (Dias and Li, 1998). Depending on the cause of the hydrocephalus and the degree of increased ICP, these symptoms can be either acute in onset or chronic and intermittent (Carey, Tullous, and Walker, 1994). Spasticity or ataxia of the lower extremities, as well as urinary incontinence, may occur. These children often complain of vision problems because increased ICP on the second, third, or sixth cranial nerves results in extraocular muscular paresis and papilledema (Gaston, 1991). Alterations in growth, sexual development, and fluid and electrolyte imbalance may occur if there is increased pressure at the site of the hypothalamus.

Treatment

Surgical treatment for hydrocephalus is directed at restoring CSF flow by either removing the obstruction to CSF flow or creating a new CSF pathway (Box 25-3). The latter usually involves placement of a ventricular catheter or shunt to divert CSF flow to the peritoneal cavity for absorption (Drake and Sainte-Rose, 1995; Rekate, 1994). If the peritoneal cavity is not appropriate for placement of the distal tubing—either due to abdominal malformation, surgery, infection or inadequate absorption—the shunt may be placed in the atrium of the heart (i.e., ventriculoatrial [VA] shunt) or pleural space (i.e., ventriculopleural shunt) (Piatt, 1994; Punt, 1993; Rekate 1994). The distal portion is tunneled under the child's skin to the designated location, where a small incision is made and the shunt is inserted either through the peritoneum into the peritoneal cavity (i.e., VP shunt) or through the neck into the superior vena cava and into the right atrium (i.e., VA shunt) (Figure 25-2). The distal end of the ventriculopleural shunt is guided subcutaneously to an area just below the nipple, where an incision is made and the tube is inserted into the pleural space (Rekate, 1994).

A variety of shunt designs exist, with most consisting of a soft silastic tube with a 1/8-inch diameter, a dome-shaped reservoir, and a one-way valve (Drake and Sainte-Rose, 1995; Shiminski-Maher and Disabato, 1994). The reservoir and tubing are palpable from the burr hole in the skull to the tube's insertion at either the abdomen or chest. Identification of and access to the shunt reservoir are important in evaluating shunt infection and malfunction. The reservoir should be easy to depress and should

rebound readily when released. A small 25-gauge needle can be inserted into the reservoir to collect CSF for culture, obtain ICP readings, or inject radioisotopes for shunt-flow studies (Piatt, 1992; Rekate, 1994).

Although CSF shunting has dramatically improved the prognosis for children with hydrocephalus, shunts still have inherent problems. Shunt revisions are necessary at some time in almost all children who have been treated for hydrocephalus. Most individuals require two to five revisions during childhood and adolescence (Drake and Sainte-Rose, 1995; Lazareff et al, 1998; Lumenta and Skotarczak, 1995; Vernet, Campiche, and de Tribolet, 1995). Shunts in children with tumors and intraventricular hemorrhage were found to have the highest rate of complications requiring revision (Lazareff et al, 1998). The most common complications associated with shunts include blockage (49%), infection (19%), and disconnection (13%) (Casey et al, 1997). Shunt obstruction may occur as a result of chronic or acute inflammation, overgrowth of choroid plexus, accumulation of cellular debris or blood, or occlusion of either the distal or proximal end of the shunt as a result of growth (Drake and Sainte-Rose, 1995; Kast et al, 1994). Repeat shunt failure requiring multiple revisions is a problem for some children. One study found that the interval between revisions became progressively shorter as the number of surgeries increased, so it seems that the primary pathology that resulted in hydrocephalus in these children elicits a reactive inflammatory process that is perpetuated by repeat shunt procedures (Lazareff et al, 1998). Multiple shunt revisions are traumatic for the child and family and pose physical risk because of surgery and increased ICP; the number of revisions alone, however, has not been correlated with poor neurodevelopmental outcome (Lumenta and Skotarczak, 1995; Riva et al, 1994).

The incidence of shunt infection has significantly decreased in the past decade but continues to be a major source of shunt malfunction and potential morbidity. As a foreign body, the implanted shunt creates a medium in the host where normal phagocytosis is impaired, allowing a child to be susceptible to infection of the shunt and cerebrospinal fluid (Drake and Sainte-Rose, 1995; Madikians and Conway, 1997; Marlin and Gaskill, 1994). Irregularities in the wall of the shunt and the glycoproteinaceous film that forms along the shunt tubing

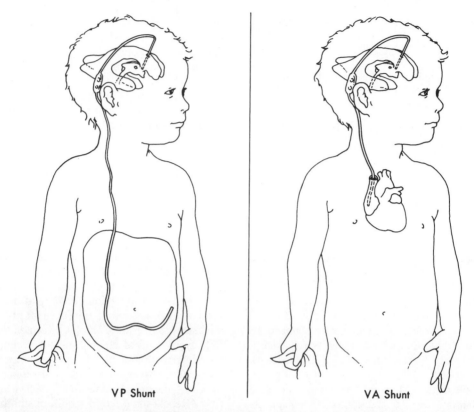

VP Shunt   VA Shunt

Figure 25-2 Pathway used for **A,** ventriculoperitoneal shunt and, **B,** ventriculoatrial shunt. (From Edwards MS and Derechin M, editors: About hydrocephalus: a book for parents. Drawings by Lynne Larson. San Francisco, 1986, University of California. Reprinted with permission.)

increase the risk of infection by providing a niche for adherence and growth of bacteria (Madikians and Conway, 1997). A shunt infection is identified when a bacterial pathogen or pathogens are isolated from ventricular CSF. Reported rates of infection range from 4% to 12% (Casey et al, 1997; Drake et al, 1998; Hoppe-Hirsch et al, 1998; Mancao et al, 1998; Piatt and Carlson, 1993), with infants under 6 months of age having a higher incidence than older children. Other factors associated with infection include premature birth, poor condition of the skin or concurrent foci of infection at the time of surgery, shunt placement following external ventricular drainage, distal end shunt revision, and postoperative wound dehiscence (Drake and Sainte-Rose, 1995; Mancao et al, 1998).

Gram-positive organisms are responsible for most shunt infections with *Staphylococcus epidermidis* identified in 45% to 48% of infections and *Staphylococcus aureus* in 25% (Casey et al, 1997; Lazareff et al, 1998). Infection from Gram-negative organisms, including *Escherichia coli, Pseudomonas aeruginosa, Propionibacterium acne, Haemophilus influenzae,* and *Klebsiella pneumoniae,* are less common. Streptococci and yeast have also been identified in CSF shunt infections (Madikians and Conway, 1997, Mancao et al, 1998). Over 50% of staphylococcal infections occur within 2 weeks of a shunt operation, and 70% of all infections occur within 2 months of surgery, probably due to bacterial colonization at the time of shunt insertion (Mancao et al, 1998). In addition to colonization, the pathogenesis of shunt infections includes possible retrograde spread of organisms from the distal end of the shunt tubing, as well as hematogenous spread (Madikians and Conway, 1997). Although shunt malfunction has not been associated with cognitive deficits, shunt infections—especially resulting from Gram-negative organisms—have a significant detrimental effect (Drake and Sainte-Rose, 1995; Hendrick, 1993).

There is conflicting evidence about the effectiveness of antibiotic prophylaxis in preventing shunt infection. An extensive review of the literature showed a 50% reduction in infection risk when antibiotic prophylaxis was used during CSF shunt procedures at centers where baseline infection rates were higher than 5% (Haines and Walters, 1994). Even with prophylaxis and meticulous surgical technique, it is difficult to achieve an infection rate below 5% (Drake and Sainte-Rose, 1995; Haines and Walters, 1994; Rotim et al, 1997). The incidence of shunt infections following dental or surgical procedures other than shunt placement is relatively low or absent (Graham et al, 1993; Helpin et al, 1998; Pumberger, Lobl and Geissler, 1998). Although antibiotics are administered in nearly all surgical procedures involving the shunt, neurosurgeons do not always recommend prophylaxis before dental or other surgical procedures unless a child has a VA shunt (Helpin et al, 1998). For children with ventriculoatrial shunts, the possibility of bacterial endocarditis as a complication must not be overlooked. Peritoneal shunts are preferred over atrial shunts because the latter often result in cardiac complications.

In light of the multiple problems with ventricular shunts, surgeons continue to look for ways to restore CSF flow without placement of a permanent shunt. The removal of intracranial mass lesions may restore normal CSF flow and cure the associated hydrocephalus. Unfortunately, as many as 25% to 30% of children with brain tumors and hydrocephalus require shunting subsequent to tumor resection (Rekate, McCormick, and Yamada, 1991; Warnick and Edwards, 1991). Clinical and experimental data suggest that the cause of hydrocephalus in these children is more complex than simply obstruction of flow by the lesion (Rekate, McCormick, and Yamada, 1991). These children, as well as others with obstructive hydrocephalus, may benefit from recent advances in neuroendoscopy (Brockmeyer et al, 1998; Rekate, 1997). Using a fiber optic ventriculoscope, neurosurgeons can navigate through the ventricular system and create a new pathway of communication for CSF between the third ventricle and the prepontine subarachnoid cistern. This pathway allows the CSF to circulate in the subarachnoid space and be absorbed normally via the arachnoid villi. Current literature on the success of endoscopic third ventriculostomy in preventing permanent shunt placement in certain individuals with noncommunicating hydrocephalus is promising (Brockmeyer et al, 1998; Rekate, 1997). Neuroendoscopy also helps in guiding shunt placement and creating communication between trapped ventricles or cysts and other CSF spaces (Rekate, 1997).

Investigation of the use of drug therapy to prevent the need for permanent shunting continues (Hack and Cohen, 1998; Hudgins et al, 1994; International PHVD Drug Trial Group, 1998). Acetazolamide (Diamox) and furosemide have been given to reduce the production of CSF in individuals with slowly progressing hydrocephalus (Frim, Scott, and Madsen, 1998). Diamox is often used (either by serial lumbar punctures or tapping of a ventricular access device in combination with CSF drainage) to prevent progressive ventricular enlargement in preterm infants with intraventricular hemorrhage (Frim, Scott, and Madsen, 1998; Rekate, 1994). Follow up of preterm infants has shown that shunt complications, including infection and obstruction, are higher when shunts are placed in extremely premature neonates; therefore prolonging placement of a permanent shunt may improve long-term outcome. Unfortunately, a recent study comparing the use of acetazolamide and furosemide in posthemorrhagic ventricular dilation in infancy with standard treatment (i.e., with serial tapping) revealed a higher rate of permanent shunt placement and increased neurological morbidity in the infants receiving drug therapy (International PHVD Drug Trial Group, 1998). If prescribed, acetazolamide and furosemide may have severe side effects and require close monitoring.

Children with communicating hydrocephalus occasionally outgrow the need for a shunt. Alternative pathways for absorption are thought to be established as a result of persistent increased ICP, therefore compensating for the diminished absorption from the arachnoid villi in communicating hydrocephalus (Barkovich, 1995). This compensated or resolved hydrocephalus usually occurs during the first year of life, although it may not be identified until later when lengthening of the shunt appears necessary as a result of growth. Compensated hydrocephalus is accompanied by stable ventricular size despite documented shunt obstruction. Shunt failure may be verified by the absence of flow after injection of a radioisotope into the shunt reservoir (i.e., shunt function study) or by radiologic confirmation of shunt disconnection (i.e., radiographic shunt series) (Drake and Sainte-Rose, 1995). In this situation, the shunt is left in place unless the risk of infection is high. The child is monitored by periodic brain scans and neuropsychologic examinations. Annual neuropsychologic testing is recommended because intellectual deterioration has been associated with arrested hydrocephalus (Epstein, 1994).

Neuroimaging of the brain is essential for the diagnosis and management of hydrocephalus. The three major imaging modalities include ultrasonography, computed tomography (CT) scan, and magnetic resonance imaging (MRI). Ultrasound is only possible in infants while the anterior fontanel is open. CT scans are most commonly obtained if acute hydrocephalus or shunt malfunction is suspected. Although all techniques are reasonable for follow-up of ventricular size and shunt placement, MRI is superior in defining the cause of hydrocephalus. MRI scans illustrate the central nervous CNS anatomy in multiple planes and allow for detailed imaging of the cerebrum and posterior fossa (Barkovich, 1995). One study compared findings on MRI with those previously identified on CT scans and noted that a different cause for hydrocephalus was discovered in 11% of the subjects and additional information on the effects of hydrocephalus was obtained in 55% (Paakko et al, 1994). Advances in MRI technology can also be used to study the flow dynamics of CSF (Barkovich, 1995; Carey, Tullous, and Walker, 1994). MRI is also useful in determining the success of third ventriculostomy in restoring CSF circulation.

CT and MRI studies are used to evaluate shunt failure and the need for shunt revision. These scans must be compared with prior imaging studies and reviewed in conjunction with clinical findings of probable shunt failure, as assessed by an experienced clinician. In a recent study, initial radiologic reports did not support the diagnosis of shunt malfunction in as many as one third of children presenting with shunt failure (Iskandar et al, 1998). In some cases, ventricular size did not change despite shunt malfunction. In other cases, ventricular enlargement was only noted when compared with

previous scans. Primary care providers must remember that a negative or stable CT scan does not rule out shunt malfunction.

Other diagnostic tools to evaluate shunt function include radionuclide CSF shunt studies, a shunt series (i.e., a lateral radiograph of the skull, neck, chest, and abdomen to ascertain the location and continuity of the shunt apparatus), shunt tap and CSF culture for infection, and ICP monitoring. A measurement of ICP can be obtained either intermittently via the shunt reservoir or by placement of an ICP monitor (Madikians and Conway, 1997). Keeping in mind the morbidity associated with a delay in the diagnosis of a shunt malfunction, primary care providers must have a low threshold for ordering a brain scan or referring a child to the neurosurgeon when symptoms of increased ICP or shunt infection are apparent (Iskandar et al, 1998; Madikians and Conway, 1997).

Recent and Anticipated Advances in Diagnosis and Management

Advances in obstetric and neonatal intensive care have decreased the incidence of hydrocephalus as a result of intraventricular hemorrhage and meningitis (Abdel-Rahman and Rosenberg, 1994; duPlessis and Volpe, 1998; Hack and Cohen, 1998). In addition, nutritional guidelines recommending supplementation of folic acid in women of childbearing age has lowered the incidence of hydrocephalus by decreasing the number of children born with myelomeningocele and other neural tube defects (Canadian Task Force on the Periodic Health Examination, 1994; Rieder, 1994).

Prenatal evaluation (i.e., including high resolution ultrasound and measures of maternal alphafetoprotein [AFP]) has increased the number of fetal anomalies identified. Neural tube defects may be identified by fetal ultrasound and elevated levels of maternal AFP. Assessment for other congenital anomalies and follow-up ultrasounds to detect progressive ventricular enlargement are essential when counseling families (Crombleholme, 1994; Fudge, in press). If severe brain dysfunction or other congenital anomalies are suspected, parents may decide to terminate the pregnancy; otherwise pregnancy can be continued as close to term as possible and a shunt or ventricular access device placed soon after birth (Frim, Scott, and Madsen, 1998).

Prenatal treatment of hydrocephalus has been attempted with placement of a ventriculoamniotic shunt, but the risks for both the fetus and the mother are high (Crombleholme, 1994). More recently, limited success was reported with in utero closure of the myelomeningocele defects in three infants (Tulipan and Bruner, 1998). Each of these babies had a short stent tube placed in the lumbar region to drain CSF into the amniotic sac. There is no current evidence that the long-term outcome for these babies will significantly improve with in utero treatment; so fetal surgery for hydrocephalus remains experimental (duPlessis and Volpe, 1998; Tulipan and Bruner, 1998).

Shunt materials and systems are continually being modified to meet individual needs. Special anti-siphon devices treat symptoms of low pressure or slit ventricle syndrome, and unified systems have decreased complications related to shunt disconnection (Rekate, 1997). Unfortunately, new valve designs may not significantly affect shunt failure rates (Drake et al, 1998). A variable pressure programmable valve (i.e., the Medos-Hakim valve) is currently in clinical trials. This valve allows CSF drainage to be adjusted incrementally and noninvasively and could reduce the number of surgeries caused by valve failure and prevent problems associated with overdrainage (Reinprecht et al, 1997; Rekate, 1997). The valve pressure settings can be altered by exposure to a MRI machine and require adjustment from the neurosurgery staff. The primary provider should consult the neurosurgeon if an MRI is scheduled.

Shunt placement can be guided by endoscope, allowing the ventricular system and shunt placement to be seen (Sainte-Rose and Chumas, 1996). This guidance is particularly helpful when treating individuals with complex hydrocephalus. Posthemorrhagic or postinfectious hydrocephalus may be complicated by the presence of septations or cystic areas within the ventricular system. Adequate CSF drainage may not be possible with one shunt, so these individuals may require multiple shunts with complex connecting systems, thus increasing the likelihood of shunt malfunction. Introducing the ventricular endoscope to fenestrate (i.e., make holes) between these multiple compartments has helped to reduce the number of ventricular catheters used and simplify the shunt system (Brockmeyer et al, 1998; Rekate, 1997). As improvements are made in the handling and visual capabilities of the endoscope, indications for its use will probably increase (Brockmeyer et al, 1998; Buxton et al, 1998; Rekate, 1997).

Associated Problems (Box 25-4)

Intellectual Problems

Intellectual function is difficult to predict early after diagnosis. The cause of the hydrocephalus seems to be the most important determining factor, with uncomplicated hydrocephalus having a better cognitive prognosis than hydrocephalus associated with brain injury, infection, or intraventricular hemorrhage (Casey et al, 1997). In long-term studies, approximately 30% of the children with hydrocephalus had intelligence quotients (IQs) in the normal range above 90; 30% to 60% had mild-to-moderate mental retardation; and 7% to 20% had severe retardation (Hoppe-Hirsch et al, 1998; Lumenta and Skotarczak, 1995; Villani et al, 1995). In children with IQs above 70, performance IQs were lower than full-scale and verbal IQs, and there was evidence of speech impairment, visual motor integration deficits, memory deficits, and decreased performance in school (Blum and Pfaffinger, 1994; Lumenta and Skotarczak, 1995). Integration into the normal school system was possible for 60% of these children, although many required some special education services (Casey et al, 1997; Hoppe-Hirsch et al, 1998). Difficulty with reading comprehension, writing, mathematical skills, and attention span are common areas of concern.

Box 25-4
Associated Problems

- Intellectual deficits
- Ocular abnormalities
- Motor disabilities
- Seizures

As with most developmental measures, social risk factors also affect cognitive outcomes. A recent study found that socioeconomic status was the factor most strongly associated with verbal scores in children with hydrocephalus (Bier et al, 1997). The importance of both social and biologic factors in developmental outcomes must be remembered in counseling families and planning intervention strategies. Preschool and school counseling with neuropsychologic evaluations must be completed early to identify areas of learning disability and resources for intervention.

Ocular Problems

As mentioned earlier, ocular abnormalities are often found at the time of diagnosis or during episodes of shunt malfunction. Increased ICP results in optic nerve pressure, limited upward gaze, extraocular muscle paresis, and papilledema (Gaston, 1991; Neville, 1993). Without prompt treatment for acute hydrocephalus or shunt malfunction, permanent visual damage is a definite risk. Before the era of successful CSF shunting, optic atrophy secondary to hydrocephalus was the leading cause of blindness from congenital malformations (Simpson and Hemmer, 1993). Even with a functioning shunt and controlled hydrocephalus, however, visual problems are common. Gaze and movement problems (e.g., strabismus, astigmatism, nystagmus, and amblyopia) are found in approximately 25% to 33% of children with hydrocephalus (Gaston, 1991; Rosen, 1998). Refractive and accommodative errors are found in about the same percentage of children but not necessarily in the same children. The optic disk is often found to be abnormally light or pale, but papilledema is not normally found (Gaston, 1991). These children may require the use of large print and increased contrast in work materials, as well as placement of work items within their visual field. Abnormalities in vision are associated with lower intelligence scores and may help identify children at risk for mental retardation. Close follow-up and referral to infant stimulation programs for the visually impaired may be necessary (Donders, Canady, and Rourke, 1990; Riva et al, 1994; Rosen, 1998). Correctable visual problems should be attended to as soon as possible so that poor vision does not interfere with learning potential.

Motor Disabilities

Unfortunately, as many as 60% of the children with hydrocephalus will have some form of motor disability (Hoppe-Hirsch et al, 1998). These disabilities vary from severe paraplegia to mild imbalance or weakness. The severity of the motor deficit is most often related to the diagnosis, with conditions such as porencephaly, Dandy-Walker malformation, and myelomeningocele having more serious motor defects than simple congenital hydrocephalus. Hydrocephalus also affects fine motor control. The kinesthetic-proprioceptive abilities of the hands are often negatively affected and—coupled with the impaired bimanual manipulation and frequent visual deficits—make it difficult for children with hydrocephalus to perform well on time-limited, nonverbal intelligence tests (Blum and Pfaffinger, 1994; Riva et al, 1994).

Seizures

Because of increased ICP, seizures are common at the time of initial diagnosis in infancy. Fortunately, only 13% to 33% of children with hydrocephalus continue to have seizures after the first year of life (Hoppe-Hirsch et al, 1998; Kokkonen et al, 1994; Villani et al, 1995). These seizures may be simple or complex, partial or generalized, and usually can be well-managed with standard anticonvulsant therapy. Acquired hydrocephalus is more often associated with seizure activity because of the underlying reason for development of the hydrocephalus (e.g., brain tumor, CNS trauma, or infection). These seizures may be more focal in origin and difficult to control. (See Chapter 21 for further discussion on seizure disorders.)

Prognosis

The outlook for children with hydrocephalus continues to improve with advances in shunt and surgical technology. Morbidity and mortality rates are variable and determined by the cause of hydrocephalus, the number and type of shunt infections, the surgical complications, and the environmental and social factors (Hoppe-Hirsch et al, 1998; Kokkonen et al, 1994; Lumenta and Skotarczak, 1995; Marlin and Gaskill, 1994; Vernet, Campiche, and de Tribolet, 1995). The neurologic prognosis for newborns with hydrocephalus with variable etiologies has been reviewed by du Plessis and Volpe (1998), who report that recent studies indicate a more favorable prognosis for newborns with hydrocephalus. An overall mortality rate of 4% to 11% over a 10-year period for children with hydrocephalus not associated with a brain tumor was reported in recent studies (Hoppe-Hirsch et al, 1998; Iskandar et al, 1998). Primary care providers should remember that children with hydrocephalus are still at risk for increased morbidity and early mortality after years of excellent progress and shunt function. Early detection and treatment of shunt malfunction and complications can reduce morbidity and mortality.

PRIMARY CARE MANAGEMENT

Health Care Maintenance

Growth and Development

Measurements of children seen in a primary care practice are typically done by minimally trained office or clinic personnel. If a child is suspected of having hydrocephalus or known to have hydrocephalus, the primary care provider should measure the head circumference. Until the cranial sutures are completely fused, which is often delayed in these children, head circumference is a major diagnostic tool in evaluating a child's condition. Normal head circumference at birth is 33 to 36 cm. During the first year, head circumference increases 2 cm/month during the first 3 months, 1 cm/month from 4 to 6 months, and 0.5 cm/month from 7 to 12 months. A diagnosis of hydrocephalus is indicated more by increases across growth percentiles than by a normal rate of growth paralleling the 95th percentile (Albright, 1994). Increasing head circumference from hydrocephalus is usually associated with a full fontanel, splayed sutures, and frontal bossing.

Once the diagnosis of hydrocephalus has been made and a shunt inserted, head circumference may decrease 1 to 2 cm as the pressure is relieved. The sutures may become overriding, and the fontanel sunken. After this initial decrease, the head should only grow in proportion to the child's body. Therefore a newborn whose weight and height are in the 50th percentile for age and who has a head size of

40 cm when a shunt is placed shortly after birth may not resume head growth for 2 to 4 months (Figure 25-3). Resumption of growth before that time might indicate shunt malfunction. The significance of head size measurements in a child with a shunt cannot be overestimated, and daily measurements may be necessary during evaluation of shunt-dependent infants for possible shunt malfunction. Weight gain must be assessed carefully because the increasing weight of the heads of infants with hydrocephalus may mask failure to thrive (Neville, 1993).

Endocrine dysfunction resulting in precocious puberty, slow growth velocity, short stature, and amenorrhea have been reported in as many as 40% of children with hydrocephalus (Elias and Sadeghi-Nejad, 1994; Klauschie and Rose, 1996; Proos et al, 1996; Villani et al, 1995). Sexual development before the age of 8 years in girls and 10 years in boys is considered precocious and warrants further diagnostic study. If not compatible with family stature, heights below the 5th percentile indicate growth retardation. Treatment is available for both of these conditions, and children should be referred to an endocrinologist if these signs occur.

The standard early infant developmental assessment tools used in primary care practice (e.g., Denver Developmental Screening Test II) are of little help in assessing infants with hydrocephalus. Tasks that require head control (e.g., elevating the head while in the prone position, rolling over, pulling to a sitting position without head lag, and even sitting unassisted) will be delayed in infants with macrocephaly. It is important for primary care providers to interpret developmental findings in light of other clinical observations to help parents set reasonable expectations for their infant.

Other motor delays can be expected during infancy and childhood given that approximately 60% of children with hydrocephalus have some form of motor disability. Primary care providers must carefully document motor skill acquisition (i.e., even in infants and older school-aged children) because a loss of skill may indicate shunt malfunction or progression of the primary cause. Ataxia, slurred speech, lack of progression in school, incontinence, or other regression in developmental ability may indicate a deterioration in neurologic status and need for further evaluation.

Children with hydrocephalus usually have verbal skills commensurate with their intellectual abil-

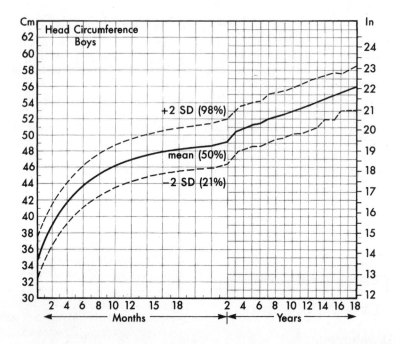

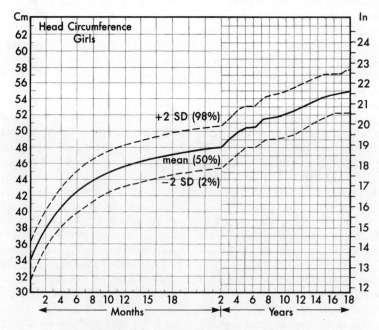

Figure 25-3 Head circumference charts from birth to age 18 years. (From Neilhaus G: Head circumference from birth to eighteen years, Pediatrics 41:106-114, 1968.)

ities and perform better on verbal tests than on fine motor-visual perception tests. For unknown reasons, children with shunted hydrocephalus perform worse than children with arrested hydrocephalus (Brookshire et al, 1995). Primary care providers must assess speech carefully, however, because 25% to 35% of individuals with hydrocephalus develop a hyperverbal pattern of communication with good vocabulary and articulation but shallow intellect, poor social skills, and low academic attainment (Blum and Pfaffinger, 1994; Hendrick, 1993). This speech pattern is called cocktail party chatter and may disguise a lower intelligence than is first apparent. These children often benefit from infant stimulation programs or speech therapy, and primary care providers must be familiar with the program offerings in the family's community to help them identify services that would be most beneficial for their child.

Diet

There are no special dietary requirements for children with hydrocephalus. Many parents become overly concerned about the episodes of regurgitation or vomiting that are common in all infants, and clarification as to what is normal and what is pathologic vomiting should be made soon after the diagnosis of hydrocephalus. Parents may be hesitant to burp their infant because of poor head control or concern over dislodging the shunt. Alternate positions for burping can be demonstrated. If repeated regurgitation does occur, parents should be advised on how to use an infant seat for post-feeding positioning and introduction of solids (if age-appropriate).

Safety

Primary care providers play a major role in educating parents and children about safety. Families may be so overwhelmed with the task of parenting a child with a chronic condition that routine safety measures are overlooked.

The prolonged lack of head control in children with hydrocephalus predisposes them to accidental head injury. In addition, car seat safety studies indicate that infants should be positioned facing the rear in a semireclined position until they are able to sit upright, fully supporting their head. Infants with hydrocephalus may not be able to attain head con-

trol or sit upright until late in their first year of life. This must be reviewed, and parents encouraged to use the infant car seats properly to decrease the risk of head, neck, and abdominal injury. Transportation to and from daycare or school must also be provided with appropriate safety restraints to support the trunk and head of children with severe disabilities (Paley, 1993). Car seats that completely recline and vest restraints for older children are available but may require special fitting. A referral to a pediatric physical therapist may be helpful in determining the appropriate equipment.

As a child grows, activities should be limited as little as possible to encourage normal development and peer relationships. Helmets should be required for all activities that have the potential for falls (e.g., bike and skateboard riding). A child's neurologic disabilities and visual perceptual integration may make competitive sports difficult and operation of motor vehicles hazardous. Few sports are absolutely contraindicated in children with hydrocephalus. Gymnastics, wrestling, tackle football, and hockey might increase the risk of shunt damage or head trauma, so participation in these sports may be restricted (Sheiner, 1996). Each individual's ability must be regularly assessed so that the risks and benefits of activities can be determined (Committee on Sports Medicine and Fitness, 1994).

Immunizations

Diphtheria, tetanus, and pertussis: Pertussis poses a special problem for infants with hydrocephalus. Infants and children with a history of seizures are at increased risk of seizures after receipt of pertussis vaccine (Committee on Infectious Diseases, 1997). As stated previously, seizures at the time of diagnosis during the newborn period may be present in infants with hydrocephalus, but it is difficult to determine which of these infants will continue to have recurrent seizures. An infant's neurologic status should be evaluated at each primary care visit to determine if the pertussis vaccine is contraindicated. Use of acellular pertussis is associated with fewer neurologic side effects and is recommended for children with hydrocephalus (Committee on Infectious Diseases, 1997). Because outbreaks of pertussis still occur in the United States, deferral of the vaccine must be weighed against the potential for disease and disease-related complications (Committee on Infectious Diseases, 1997). Children in daycare, attending special developmental programs, or receiving care in residential centers are exposed to other children who also may not be immunized and are therefore at increased risk for developing pertussis. In such difficult situations, consultation with the child's neurosurgeon or neurologist may help in assessing the child's seizure potential. If the primary care provider—with parental consent—decides early in infancy that the pertussis immunization will be withheld, diphtheria and tetanus vaccines should be given on schedule.

Measles: Measles vaccine has also been implicated in postvaccination seizures, with a higher incidence in infants and children with a personal history of seizures (Committee on Infectious Diseases, 1997). It is not thought that these postvaccine seizures produce permanent neurologic damage, and the high ongoing risk of natural measles with its high morbidity rate justifies measles immunization in children with a personal history of seizures (Committee on Infectious Diseases, 1997).

***Haemophilus influenzae* type b:** Because of the increased risk of CNS infections in children with shunts, children with shunted hydrocephalus should receive the conjugated vaccine starting at 2 months of age (Committee on Infectious Diseases, 1997). Children who have a history of documented Hib disease before 2 years of age may not produce adequate antibodies to prevent a second infection and should therefore also be immunized. Chemoprophylaxis of household or daycare contacts of children with Hib disease is required, even with adequate immunization (Committee on Infectious Diseases, 1997).

Other immunizations: Vaccination for polio, hepatitis B, varicella, mumps, and rubella should be given as routinely scheduled. There is currently no research on the efficacy of giving pneumococcal or influenza vaccines to these children (Committee on Infectious Diseases, 1997), but the primary care provider may elect to administer these additional vaccines to children with multiple shunt infections or severe motor disabilities.

Screening

Vision: Because of the high incidence of visual defects in children with hydrocephalus, practitioners must pay particular attention to visual screening. The Hirschberg light reflex, cover test, tracking, and funduscopic examinations should be performed at each office visit and the results carefully documented in the record. At approximately 6 months of age, the child should be referred to a pediatric ophthalmologist for a thorough examination. Yearly examinations should be scheduled thereafter. Children with hydrocephalus often need surgery on their eye muscles to correct esotropia or exotropia. Practitioners can be instrumental in completing preoperative examinations and preparing the families for surgery. The primary care provider must remember that alterations in the funduscopic examination, eye muscle control, or visual ability may be associated with shunt malfunction and must be evaluated carefully when shunt malfunction or infection is part of the differential diagnosis. Referral to an ophthalmologist for evaluation of an infant or young child for papilledema or evidence of increased pressure may help to differentiate benign headaches from those due to shunt malfunction.

Hearing: In addition to routine office screening for hearing acuity, an auditory evoked response test should be ordered if an infant has a history of CNS infection or antibiotic treatment with aminoglycocides. Subsequent shunt malfunctions or CNS infections require reassessment of hearing. Periodic evaluation by an audiologist is recommended.

Dental: Routine dental care is recommended. If a child is taking phenytoin (Dilantin) for seizure control, dental care may need to be more frequent because of hyperplasia of the gums. Poor dental hygiene and periodontal infections may produce bacteremia—even without dental procedures (Dajani et al, 1990; Helpin et al, 1998). Because intravascular foreign bodies are susceptible to bacterial colonization, any episode of transient bacteremia places a child with a ventriculoatrial shunt at risk for infection (Helpin et al, 1998). Antibiotic prophylaxis is recommended for children with VA shunts undergoing dental work likely to cause gingival bleeding (including routine cleaning of teeth). The spontaneous shedding of primary teeth or simple adjustment of orthodontic appliances do not require prophylaxis to prevent bacterial endocarditis. The recommended prophylaxis is the same for prevention of bacterial endocarditis in children with congenital heart disease (see Chapter 17). Children with ventriculoperitoneal shunts do not require prophylaxis for routine dental procedures.

Blood pressure: Blood pressure readings should be recorded on each clinic or office visit. Elevations in blood pressure with a widening pulse pressure are a late sign of increased ICP. Having an established baseline reading can help the practitioner assess a child for possible shunt malfunctions or progression of disease process.

Hematocrit: Routine screening is recommended.

Urinalysis: Routine screening is recommended.

Tuberculosis: Routine screening is recommended.

Condition-Specific Screening

Head circumference: Head circumference measurements should be taken at every clinic or office visit until a child's sutures are completely fused (see the discussion of growth and development in this chapter).

Common Illness Management

Differential Diagnosis

Unfortunately, many of the symptoms of shunt malfunction or infection are the same symptoms commonly found with routine childhood illness (Box 25-5). It is important to remember that children with hydrocephalus will develop otitis media, gastrointestinal (GI) illnesses, headaches, and viral infections with fever just like their unaffected peers. Primary care providers must approach these children as they would children without hydrocephalus. A calm manner and a thorough history and examination are reassuring to parents and productive for the primary care provider. The most frequent symptoms of shunt malfunction include irritability, headache, nausea, vomiting, lethargy, and delays or loss of developmental milestones. Other symptoms include personality changes, diplopia, new seizures or a change in seizure pattern, and worsening school performance, as well as—in infants—decreased level of consciousness, loss of upward gaze, nuchal rigidity, sixth nerve palsy, papilledema, and hemiparesis or loss of coordination and balance. With a shunt malfunction, the shunt reservoir may not pump and refill as expected, although the sensitivity and predictive value of a shunt pumping is questionable (Piatt, 1992). If the shunt is infected, additional signs and symptoms may include fever, redness and swelling

---

Box 25-5

Differential Diagnosis

Fever—concern about shunt malfunction
Gastrointestinal symptoms—concern about:
Peritoneal shunt placement and malfunction
Abdominal infection may seed shunt
Brain tumors may metastasize to abdomen via shunt
Constipation may result in peritoneal shunt malfunction
Headaches—concern about increased ICP
Scalp infections—concern about spread of infection to shunt reservoir
Alterations in behavior—concern about shunt malfunction

---

along the shunt tract, abdominal pain, skin breakdown or drainage along incision sites, leakage of CSF from a recent surgical wound, nuchal rigidity, neck or back pain, headache, and photophobia (Drake and Sainte-Rose, 1995; Madikians and Conway, 1997).

Fever: Fevers associated with shunt malfunction or infection can be chronic or acute and mild or severe. The more time that has elapsed since a child's last shunt surgery, the less likely the fever is associated with shunt malfunction or infection. One study found that the presence of fever was negatively associated with shunt malfunction in a cohort of children admitted to the hospital for evaluation (Watkins et al, 1994). Other symptoms, especially a change in sensorium or continued irritability or drowsiness after the fever has been controlled, are the most critical observations when trying to rule out shunt malfunction. During an infant's first year when shunt infections are most common, parents should be encouraged to consult the primary care provider whenever the infant has a temperature above 38.5° C. The practitioner, with the consulting physician, can then evaluate the child early in the course of illness and note progression of symptoms. If a focus of infection other than the shunt is identified, it should be treated appropriately. No studies indicate that frequent antibacterial therapy for illnesses of questionable origin reduces the incidence of shunt malfunction. Children being treated for bacterial infections (e.g., otitis media, pneumonia, or streptococcal sore throat) should be carefully reassessed in the office or clinic 24 to 48 hours after treatment is initiated. Continued or worsening symptoms may indicate progression of the infection into bacteremia or a CNS infection caused by the increased susceptibility resulting from the shunt. The primary care provider should obtain a CBC and blood cultures and then immediately consult the neurosurgeon. If shunt malfunction is suspected, imaging studies should be obtained to evaluate ventricular size and evidence of CNS infection (Madikians and Conway, 1997).

If a child has a mild or moderate fever of unknown origin with other symptoms compatible with a common childhood illness and no obvious signs of shunt malfunction, the primary care provider can assume a wait-and-see attitude. Arrangements for telephone follow-up or a return appointment in 24 hours should be made. The parents must be instructed to report symptoms such as lethargy, confusion, or recurrent vomiting (more than 3 times/24 hours), immediately if they occur.

Children who have very high temperatures (i.e., 40° C) and symptoms of moderate to severe illness must be assumed to have a shunt infection until this is proved otherwise. Consultation with the neurosurgeon or neurologist is advised. Blood cultures for both aerobic and anaerobic organisms should be drawn, although they are not often initially positive. A CBC count is also indicated, but minimal leukocytosis does not rule out shunt infection. CSF can be obtained for culture through the shunt reservoir. Although CSF leukocytosis (i.e., 50 to 200 cells per cm^3) is common with shunt infection, an infection can be present despite normal CSF cell count, protein, and glucose. CSF eosinophilia (i.e., more than 7% of the total CSF white blood cell count) is also indicative of shunt infection (Drake and Sainte-Rose, 1995; Madikians and Conway, 1997). Shunt aspiration should be done with meticulous aseptic technique so as not to contaminate a sterile shunt system or introduce a second organism into an already-infected shunt. A lumbar puncture may be helpful but should not be performed in children with noncommunicating hydrocephalus until shunt malfunction has been ruled out. Withdrawing CSF with a lumbar tap in a child with enlarged ventricles and increased ICP may result in downward brain herniation and death.

A chest radiograph and urine culture are recommended to rule out pneumonia or urinary tract infection, but if the history and physical findings strongly suggest shunt involvement, these may be omitted. The neurosurgeon may prefer that all tests be done at the hospital because hospitalization is often required to complete the evaluation and treatment process.

Gastrointestinal symptoms: Nausea and vomiting are common clinical symptoms during childhood, often accompanying such diverse conditions as influenza, otitis media, and urinary tract infections. Diarrhea and abdominal pain are also frequent complaints in childhood. Children with hydrocephalus can be expected to have these common complaints as often as other children. When a child has mild gastrointestinal symptoms, the practitioner must consider the presence or absence of other symptoms and the history of exposure to gastrointestinal illness. The diagnostic workup should include an evaluation for shunt infection and gastrointestinal disease. The primary care provider must recognize that abdominal symptoms may be the presenting symptom of peritoneal shunt malfunction or an acute condition in the abdomen in children with shunts (Pumberger, Lobl, and Geissler, 1998).

A child with a peritoneal shunt infection may have mild-to-moderate fever, abdominal pain, anorexia, nausea, vomiting, and diarrhea. They may guard their abdomen and be unwilling to ambulate. Swelling, redness, or inflammation along the catheter line or at the incision site is highly suggestive of shunt involvement. Abdominal ultrasound and CSF cultures should help differentiate between an acute condition in the abdomen and a shunt infection. Specific signs of appendicitis can be demonstrated by ultrasonography, but identification of an abdominal pseudocyst is more characteristic of a distal shunt infection (Pumberger, Lobl, and Geissler, 1998). Abdominal pseudocysts may develop around the peritoneal end of the VP shunt and usually result from past or current shunt infection. A history of recent or recurrent shunt revisions also substantially increases the risk for infection. The primary care practitioner may be able to differentiate the symptoms of an acute condition in the abdomen from peritoneal shunt malfunction. Consultation with and referral to the attending neurosurgeon are advised.

A chart review reported constipation as the apparent cause of temporary peritoneal shunt malfunction (Bragg et al, 1994). Many children with hydrocephalus have other neurologic problems that may increase the incidence of constipation. Stool trapped in the colon may put pressure on the peritoneal shunt, resulting in a malfunction. Maintenance of regular stool patterns may prevent unnecessary hospitalization and possible shunt revision. Another abdominal concern for infants with inguinal or umbilical hernias is the potential for CSF or shunt tubing to migrate into the hernia. The hernia becomes enlarged with a collection of CSF; treatment includes repair of the hernia and possible shunt revision.

Metastasis of brain tumor cells from the ventricular cavities into the abdominal cavity is a possible side effect of ventriculoperitoneal shunts (Rickert, 1998). This side effect must be considered when a differential diagnosis is made in children with chronic or recurring abdominal complaints if these children also have a history of a brain tumor. Appropriate referral is required to rule out this possibility after more common reasons for the complaint have been proved negative.

Headaches: Children often complain of headaches, which can also occur in children with a shunt and may have the same origin as in children without hydrocephalus. Children with hydrocephalus are reported to have migrainous headaches twice as often (i.e., 8.5% vs. 4%) and nonmigrainous headaches almost 3 times as often as children without hydrocephalus (Stellman-Ward et al, 1997). The incidence of headaches in these children did not decrease with shunt revision and was not associated with seizures or the underlying condition causing the hydrocephalus. These headaches have been called shunt migraines and occur more often in individuals who have very small ventricles after shunting and are thought to be due to poor brain compliance in response to physiologic variations in ICP. If routine treatment with mild analgesics and rest does not relieve the symptom or if the headaches become frequent, affect school attendance, or are associated with lethargy or irritability, then evaluation by the neurologist and neurosurgeon is required. Repetitive and vigorous investigation of shunt malfunction may not be necessary in the absence of other symptoms (Burton et al, 1997; Stellman-Ward et al, 1997). Shunt malfunction can be partial or variable, depending on cerebral blood flow, CSF production, and a child's activity, and may result in periodic episodes of increased ICP (Drake and Sainte-Rose, 1995).

Children with shunts occasionally experience headaches and vomiting in the early morning after sleeping all night. These symptoms may be caused by temporary partial blockage of the shunt from cellular debris, inactivity, and the horizontal sleeping position, which negates the beneficial effect of gravity for ventricular drainage. These symptoms usually subside after children have been up for a few hours. If these episodes are infrequent and self-limited, they do not require treatment other than acetaminophen for pain. Parents should be instructed to call the primary care provider if these symptoms continue for more than 6 hours or are associated with a decrease in the level of consciousness or loss of motor ability.

Scalp infections: A thin layer of skin covers the shunt reservoir on the scalp. If the skin around the shunt reservoir becomes infected, the integrity of the skin barrier may be broken and infection of the shunt is possible. Primary care providers should manage scalp infections in conjunction with the neurosurgeon.

Alterations in behavior: All children experience mood swings and temporary behavior changes. Parents of children with hydrocephalus may comment on them not being themselves; school performance may falter, normal interest in activities may dwindle; and lethargy or irritability may develop. If these changes persist beyond a few days, a child should be seen by the neurosurgeon for an evaluation. Subtle changes in behavior, cognition, or motor ability may be symptoms of shunt malfunction.

Drug Interactions

No routine medications are prescribed for children with hydrocephalus. (See Chapter 21 for drug interactions with anticonvulsant therapy.)

Developmental Issues

Sleep Patterns

Parents may be concerned about their infant or child sleeping in a position that might adversely affect the shunt. During the immediate period after shunt placement, these children should be positioned off the reservoir site to avoid skin breakdown. Except for during this brief period, parents and caretakers must be reassured that their child can sleep in any comfortable position without fear of affecting the shunt. Infants and young children should be encouraged to assume a normal sleeping pattern at night.

Toileting

Children with neurologic deficits associated with hydrocephalus may have a delayed ability to develop bowel and bladder control. Parents need to be counseled on the possibility of this difficulty, and the methods of toilet training should be reviewed. The neurologist and neurosurgeon following a child's development should be consulted about the child's neurologic capability to attain satisfactory toilet training. If necessary, special bowel training and clean, intermittent catheterization education should be provided and can usually be obtained through referral to a pediatric urologist or rehabilitation specialist (see Chapter 29).

Discipline

Discipline for children with hydrocephalus should be managed as for other children, recognizing the limitations of cognitive and motor development of each child. Some parents may have difficulty understanding the discrepancy between their child's verbal and performance skills and may have expectations that are too high for the child to attain, which may lead to inappropriate discipline. On the other hand, parents may be afraid to discipline their child and must be encouraged to set appropriate limits (Gardner, Tholcken, and Quay, 1991).

Practitioners must always be concerned with the increased possibility of child abuse in children with chronic conditions. Head injuries and abdominal injuries are common in child abuse and may result in further brain injury or shunt malfunction.

Child Care

Most mothers work outside the home. Child care and preschool placement are major issues for all working parents but are even more so when a child has a chronic condition. Fortunately, the current shunt systems are self-maintained and do not require special care (e.g., pumping periodically) throughout the day. There are no special care needs for children with hydrocephalus unless other disabilities (e.g., cerebral palsy, seizures, or mental

retardation) are present. If a child has significant disabilities, child care arrangements must be evaluated for their ability to meet the child's needs. Public Law 101-476, the Individuals with Disabilities Education Act (1990), extended services to children with disabilities from birth to school entry, so federally funded programs are accessible to children with disabilities (see Chapter 5).

Children with hydrocephalus, however, are at greater risk for CNS infections than their peers because of their shunt. Parents must understand that children who attend daycare or preschool are exposed to childhood infections and have illnesses (i.e., usually respiratory or gastrointestinal) more often than those who stay at home (Takala et al, 1995; Thacker et al, 1992). Children up to 2 years of age should receive child care at home or in a small home care program to minimize exposure to common pediatric pathogens.

Schooling

In general, 60% of children with hydrocephalus attend regular school, but many function below their expected grade level (Casey et al, 1997; Hoppe-Hirsch et al, 1997). Primary care providers can help families plan their child's individualized educational program (IEP) to ensure appropriate interventions for the child. Although Public Law 101-476 requires the school district to assess a child's needs, financial constraints of the school district may limit neuropsychologic testing, so any testing done before school may be beneficial and should be forwarded to the school district. Parents may need help obtaining medical records to facilitate formulation of their child's IEP.

Because of physical or intellectual limitations, some children with hydrocephalus qualify for separate special education classes. Other children can be mainstreamed into regular classrooms and receive special services (e.g., adaptive physical education to help with motor control and balance, occupational therapy to assist with kinesthetic-proprioceptive deficits, speech therapy, or psychologic counseling to address emotional issues). As these children reach junior high school and high school, some limitations may be made on competitive, high-impact sports. Tackle football, soccer, and ice hockey have a much higher risk of head and abdominal injury than track, swimming, or tennis. If a child has mild-to-moderate neuromotor deficits, an evaluation by a sports medicine professional may help identify sports activities that the child can successfully perform. Being involved in sports activities is often beneficial to a child's self-esteem and encourages peer relationships, both of which may be problematic areas for children with hydrocephalus.

Children with less severe disabilities may experience psychosocial difficulty because they may have a difficult time fitting in with nondisabled peers but also do not fit in with disabled children (Holmbeck and Faier-Routman, 1995). Their disabilities may not be recognized by teachers and peers unable to understand why these individuals have difficulty in school or sports. Adolescents who are trying not to be different may not disclose their learning or motor deficit but will not be able to successfully compete with unaffected peers. The resulting incongruity between expectations and ability can lead to a sense of failure and lowered self-esteem.

Primary care providers should routinely ask parents and children about school progress. If academic difficulties develop, these children should be referred for repeat neuropsychologic testing to rule out medical reasons for these problems. Shunt malfunction may result in gradual changes in cognition, fine motor abilities, or personality and must be ruled out as a contributing factor. If difficulties are assessed to be more emotional, which often happens during adolescence when children struggle with their body image and identity, children should be referred for counseling. This referral should be made to a professional experienced in working with children with disabilities.

Sexuality

As previously mentioned, delayed or precocious puberty may occur in children with hydrocephalus. Their progression through puberty must be assessed and monitored, and counseling may be indicated to support them during this period. Research indicates that children with precocious puberty may have lowered self-esteem, poor peer relationships, and a higher incidence of sexual abuse than normally developing children (Jackson and Ott, 1990). Sexuality and reproductive issues should be managed the same as with other children. Female adolescents receiving anticonvulsive therapy should be informed of the possible teratogenic effects of the medications they are taking (see Chapter 21).

Adolescents with associated motor disabilities may have additional needs (see Chapter 14).

Transition to Adulthood

Beginning in the 1970s, improvements in shunt techniques and management of shunt complications have resulted in a dramatic increase in the survival of individuals with hydrocephalus. Researchers are following these young people as they make their transition into adulthood (Kokkonen et al, 1994; Simpson and Hemmer, 1993; Villani et al, 1995). These researchers have identified concerns about how these individuals deal with vocational training, career placement, sexuality, and family roles. Their social outcomes are highly influenced by their associated disabilities, especially mental retardation and motor handicaps (Kokkonen et al, 1994). Many adults who were shunted during childhood have achieved full-time employment and successful personal relationships because either their disabilities were minor or they were able to overcome them (Simpson and Hemmer, 1993). Results of studies assessing the employment rate of young adults with hydrocephalus associated with spina bifida have been less promising, with as many as 70% to 80% failing to maintain employment (Tew, Laurence, and Jenkins, 1990). Some of these individuals were described as lacking drive or initiative, but both Tew and associates and Kokkonen and associates cite the lack of an environment that fosters independence as a probable factor. Parents are often overcautious and overprotective and do not discipline appropriately, inadvertently causing children to be socially inappropriate and dependent (Gardner, Tholcken, and Quay, 1991).

A supportive climate that encourages independence, maturity, and responsibility is essential if young adults with hydrocephalus are to complete school, maintain employment, and function as adults. Professional guidance is often necessary to create this environment. Health professionals should emphasize a positive prognosis for young adults with hydrocephalus. Parents must be prepared to face the normal problems of adolescence and let their young children develop independence (Gardner, Tholcken, and Quay, 1991; Kokkonen et al, 1994; Simpson and Hemmer, 1993). The National Information Center For Handicapped Children and Youth (NICHY) can provide information and referrals for social skills programs that may be useful to parents, teachers, and others. At the college level, vocational training and special education resources can help young adults prepare for job placement. Young adults dependent on a shunt should be cautious about living alone because they could become acutely ill, confused, or even comatose during a shunt malfunction. These individuals should form a buddy system to ensure their well-being, thereby minimizing their risk of permanent brain injury from an unrecognized shunt malfunction (Rekate, 1997).

Hydrocephalus alone should not interfere with a woman's ability to conceive, but recent reports suggest that shunt function can be affected by pregnancy (Bradley et al, 1998; Wisoff et al, 1991). Wisoff and associates reported the outcome of 16 pregnancies in women with hydrocephalus. Neurologic complications during pregnancy (i.e., including seizures, headaches, nausea, vomiting, lethargy, ataxia, and gaze paresis) occurred in 75% of the women with preexisting shunts. In most cases, symptoms of increased ICP resolved postpartum, but four women required shunt revision during pregnancy or within 1 year of delivery. Bradley and associates reviewed questionnaires from 37 women with shunts and reported that 84% of the pregnancies in this group of women progressed without shunt malfunction or revisions. Therefore prenatal counseling and assessment should include an evaluation of medications—especially anticonvulsants, genetic counseling, and a review of family history for neural tube defects. A complete assessment of shunt function should be obtained if pregnancy is being considered (Wisoff et al, 1991). In addition, maternal supplementation with folic acid has been found to decrease the incidence of neural tube defects by as much as 50%. Therefore women of child-bearing age should be encouraged to supplement their intake of folic acid before conception (Canadian Task Force, 1994; Rieder, 1994).

Special Family Concerns and Resources

Parents of children with hydrocephalus constantly worry about continued shunt function. With every malfunction there is the need for surgery and the perceived threat of further brain damage. This constant worry and the daily responsibility and stress of caring for a child who may have multiple medical problems are hard on families (Jackson, 1985). The financial strain from numerous medical visits or surgical procedures may deplete a family's financial reserve. Private insurance may not be obtainable unless offered through a large group employment policy. Concern about a child's ability to be self-supporting and independent in the future is also an issue for parents as their child grows into adolescence.

Parent-to-parent support groups can offer parental support by publishing newsletters and even hosting major medical conferences for both health professionals and parents. These organizations also provide a network for children with hydrocephalus, offering them the opportunity to make new friends, develop peer support, and exchange knowledge. Primary care providers should become familiar with the organizations in the community so that appropriate referrals can be made. It is better to make such referrals soon after a child's diagnosis than to wait to see how the parents cope. All parents need support above and beyond what is reasonable for a physician or nurse to provide.

Organizations

National organizations:
HOPE (Hydrocephalus Opens People Eyes)
104-47 120th St
Richmond Hill, NY 11419

Hydrocephalus Association
870 Market St #705
San Francisco, Calif. 94102
(415) 7732-7040; (415) 732-7044
hydroassoc@aol.com

National Hydrocephalus Foundation
12313 Centralia Road
Lakewood, Calif. 90715
(562) 402-3532
hydrobrat@aol.com

National Information Center for Handicapped
Children and Youth (NICHY)
PO Box 1492
Washington, DC 20013

National Organization for Rare Disorders (NORD)
PO Box 8923
New Fairfield, Conn. 06812
(203) 746-6518

Spina Bifida Association of America
4590 MacArthur Blvd NW, Suite 250
Washington, DC 20007-4226

United Cerebral Palsy Association, Inc
330 West 34th St
New York, NY 10001
(212) 947-5770

Summary of Primary Care Needs for the Child with Hydrocephalus

HEALTH CARE MAINTENANCE
Growth and development

Height and weight are usually within normal range unless a child is severely handicapped.

If enlarged head size is diagnosed in infancy and a shunt is placed, head size should follow the normal growth curve.

The head should be measured at each visit until the sutures are fused.

Both precocious puberty and short stature are reported.

Standard infant development tests may indicate delay because of poor head control.

Of all children with hydrocephalus, 75% will have some motor disability.

Verbal skills must be assessed and compared with intellectual ability.

Diet: A normal diet is indicated.

There are concerns about and difficulty in assessing infant vomiting as normal or as a sign of increased ICP.

Safety: The risk of head injury is increased because of poor head control.

A rear-facing car seat should be recommended until a child can sit unsupported.

A helmet should be used for bike and skateboard riding.

Neurologic deficits may make competitive sports difficult and operation of motor vehicles hazardous.

Immunization

Pertussis vaccine may be deferred in infants with seizures.

Measles vaccine may cause seizures in children with seizure disorders but is recommended because of the prevalence of measles.

Haemophilus influenzae type b conjugated vaccine is strongly recommended.

Pneumococcal vaccine and influenza vaccine should be considered for children with multiple shunt infections or significant disabilities.

Screening

Vision: Hirschberg's examination, cover test, ability to track, and funduscopic examination should be done at each visit. Children should be examined by an ophthalmologist at 6 months of age and then yearly thereafter.

Alterations in eye examination may be associated with shunt malfunction.

Hearing: A routine office screening is recommended. An auditory evoked response test should be given to children with a history of CNS infection or who have been treated with aminoglycosides.

Dental: Routine dental care is recommended.

Children on phenytoin therapy require more frequent dental care.

Prophylactic antibiotics are recommended for dental procedures likely to cause bleeding.

Blood pressure: Blood pressure should be recorded at each visit.

Blood pressure increases with increased ICP.

Hematocrit: Routine screening is recommended.

Urinalysis: Routine screening is recommended.

Tuberculosis: Routine screening is recommended.

Condition-specific screening

Head circumference: Head circumference should be measured at each visit until the sutures are completely fused.

Continued

Summary of Primary Care Needs for the Child with Hydrocephalus—cont'd

COMMON ILLNESS MANAGEMENT

Differential diagnosis

Fever: Shunt or CNS infection should be ruled out.

Gastrointestinal symptoms: Increased ICP with nausea and vomiting should be ruled out.

Peritonitis with abdominal pain or acute diarrhea should be ruled out.

Shunt infection caused by abdominal infection should be ruled out.

Constipation should be ruled out as cause of shunt malfunction.

Metastatic abdominal tumor should be ruled out in children with primary brain tumors and ventriculoperitoneal shunts.

Headaches: Shunt malfunction should be ruled out as the cause of acute or chronic headaches.

Scalp infections: Possible infection spread to shunt reservoir should be ruled out.

Alterations in behavior: Alterations in behavior should be ruled out as a symptom of shunt malfunction.

Drug interactions

No routine medications are prescribed.

Developmental issues

Sleep patterns: Standard developmental counseling is advised.

Toileting: Delayed bowel and bladder training may occur because of neurologic deficit.

Constipation may cause peritoneal shunt malfunction.

Discipline: Expectations are normal with recognition of the possible discrepancy between verbal and motor abilities. Physical punishment is a hazard because it may cause head or abdominal injury.

Child care: No special care needs are required except when a child has a severe motor disability or seizures.

Home care or small daycare programs are recommended during a child's first 2 years of life to reduce infections.

Schooling: Associated problems are often covered by Public Law 101-476.

Families should be assisted in IEP hearings.

Children may have possible adjustment problems during adolescence.

Children may need psychometric testing for poor school performance.

Low-impact sports should be selected to prevent head trauma and abdominal injury.

Minor, unseen disabilities should not be overlooked.

Sexuality: Children should be evaluated for delayed or precocious puberty.

Standard developmental counseling is advised unless associated problems warrant additional care.

Transition to adulthood

Research has identified difficulty with vocational training, career, sexuality, and family roles associated with hydrocephalus and mental retardation and motor handicaps.

Independence must be fostered from an early age to prepare young adults for independence.

Shunt-dependent individuals should develop a buddy system to ensure that shunt malfunction leading to acute illness, confusion, or coma does not go unrecognized.

Pregnancy may interfere with peritoneal shunt drainage. Securing independent health and life insurance may be difficult for individuals with hydrocephalus.

Special family concerns

Families are concerned about continued shunt function and the possibility of brain damage caused by shunt failure or infection.

References

Abdel-Rahman AM and Rosenberg AA: Prevention of intraventricular hemorrhage in the premature infant, Clin Perinatol 21(3):505-521, 1994.

Albright L: Hydrocephalus in Children. In Rengachary SS and RH Wilkins, editors: Principles of neurosurgery, London, 1994, Wolfe.

Barkovich AJ: Hydrocephalus. In Barkovich AJ, editor: Pediatric neuroimaging, New York, 1995, Raven Press.

Bier JA et al: Medical and social factors associated with cognitive outcome in individuals with myelomeningocele, Dev Med Child Neurol 39(4):263-266, 1997.

Blum RW and Pfaffinger K: Myelodysplasia in childhood and adolescence, Pediatr Rev 15(12):480-484, 1994.

Bradley NK et al: Maternal shunt dependency: implications for obstetric care and neurosurgical management, and pregnancy outcomes and a review of selected literature, Neurosurg 43(3):448-461, 1998.

Bragg CL et al: Ventriculoperitoneal shunt dysfunction and constipation: a chart review, J Neurosci Nurs 26(5):265-269, 1994.

Brockmeyer D et al: Endoscopic third venticulostomy: an outcome analysis, Pediatr Neurosurg 28:236-240, 1998.

Brookshire et al: Verbal and nonverbal skill discrepancies in children with hydrocephalus: a five-year longitudinal follow up, J Pediatr Psychol 20(6):785-800, 1995.

Burton LJ et al: Headache etiology in a pediatric emergency department, Pediatric Emerg Care 13(1):1-4, 1997.

Buxton N et al: Neuroendoscopy in the premature population, Child's Nervous System 14:649-652, 1998.

Canadian Task Force on the Periodic Health Examination: Periodic health examination, 1994 update: primary and secondary prevention of neural tube defect, CMAJ 151(2):159-166, 1994.

Carey CM, Tullous MW, and Walker ML: Hydrocephalus: etiology, pathologic effects, diagnosis, and natural history. In Check WR, editor: Pediatric neurosurgery: surgery of the developing nervous system, ed 3, Philadelphia, 1994, W.B. Saunders.

Casey ATH et al: The long-term outlook for hydrocephalus in childhood, Pediatr Neurosurg 27:63-70, 1997.

Committee on Infectious Diseases: Report of the committee on infectious diseases, ed 23, Elk Grove Village, Ill., 1997, The American Academy of Pediatrics.

Committee on Sports Medicine and Fitness: Medical conditions affecting sports participation, Pediatrics 94(5):757-760, 1994.

Crombleholme TM: Invasive fetal therapy: current status and future directions, Sem Perinatol 18(4):385-397, 1994.

Dajani AS et al: Prevention of bacterial endocarditis: recommendations by the American Heart Association, JAMA 264(22):2919-2922, 1990.

Dias MS and Li V: Pediatric neurosurgical disease, Pediatr Clin North Am 45(6):1539-1545, 1998

Donders J, Canady AI, and Rourke BP: Psychometric intelligence after infantile hydrocephalus, Child's Nervous System 6:148-154, 1990.

Drake JM et al: Randomized trial of cerebrospinal fluid shunt valve design in pediatric hydrocephalus, Neurosurg 43(2):294-303,1998.

Drake JM and Sainte-Rose C: The shunt book, Cambridge, 1995, Blackwell Science Inc.

Du Plessis A and Volpe JJ: Prognosis for development in the newborn requiring neurosurgical intervention, Neurosurg Clin North Am 9(1):187-197, 1998.

Elias ER and Sadeghi-Nejad A: Precocious puberty in girls with myelodysplasia, Pediatrics 93(3):521-2, 1994.

Epstein FJ: How to get rid of the shunt: a comment, Child's Nervous System 10:342-343, 1994.

Frim DM, Scott RM, and JR Madsen: Surgical management of neonatal hydrocephalus, Neurosurg Clin North Am 9(1):105-110, 1998.

Fudge R: Prenatal onset hydrocephalus, San Francisco, Hydrocephalus Association, in press.

Gardner R, Tholcken MF, and Quay NB: Psychosocial implications. In Leech RW and Brumback RA, editors: Hydrocephalus: current clinical concepts, St Louis, 1991, Mosby.

Gaston H: Ophthalmic complications of spina bifida and hydrocephalus, Eye 5:279-290, 1991.

Graham SM et al: Safety of percutaneous endoscopic gastrostomy in patients with ventriculoperitoneal shunt, Neurosurg 32(6):932-934, 1993.

Hack M and AR Cohen: Acetazolamide plus furosemide for periventricular dilatation: lessons for drug therapy in children, Lancet 352:418-419, 1998.

Haines SJ and Walters BC: Antibiotic prophylaxis for cerebrospinal fluid shunts: a metanalysis, Neurosurg 34:87-92, 1994.

Hendrick EB: Results of treatment in infants and children in hydrocephalus. In Schurr PH and Polkey CE, editors: Hydrocephalus, Oxford, 1993, Oxford University Press.

Helpin ML et al: Antibiotic prophylaxis in dental patients with ventriculop-peritoneal shunts: a pilot study, J Dent Child 65(4):244-7, 1998.

Holmbeck GN and Faier-Routman J: Spinal lesion level, shunt status, family relationships, and psychosocial adjustment in children and adolescents with spina bifida myelomeningocele, J Pediatr Psychol 20(6):817-832, 1995.

Hoppe-Hirsch E et al: Late outcome of the surgical treatment of hydrocephalus, Child's Nervous System 14:97-99, 1998.

Hudgins RJ et al: Treatment of intraventricular hemorrhage in the premature infant with urokinase: a preliminary report, Pediatr Neurosurg 20(3):190-197, 1994.

International PHVD Drug Trial Group: International randomised controlled trial of acetazolamide and furosemide in posthaemorrhagic ventricular dilatation in infancy, Lancet 352:433-440, 1998.

Iskandar BJ et al: Death in shunted hydrocephalic children in the 1990s, Pediatr Neurosurg 28:173-176, 1998.

Iskander BJ et al: Pitfalls in the diagnosis of ventricular shunt dysfunction: radiology reports and ventricular size, Pediatrics 101(6):1031-1036, 1998.

Jackson PL: When the baby isn't perfect, Am J Nurs 85:396-399, 1985.

Jackson PL and Ott MJ: Perceived self-esteem among children diagnosed with precocious puberty, J Pediatr Nurs 5(3):190-203, 1990.

Kast J et al: Time-related patterns of ventricular shunt failure, Child's Nervous System 10:524-528, 1994.

Klauschie J and Rose SR: Incidence of short stature in children with hydrocephalus, J Pediatr Endocrinol Metab 9(2):181-187, 1996.

Kokkonen J et al: Long-term prognosis for children with shunted hydrocephalus, Child's Nervous System 10:384-387, 1994.

Lazareff JA et al: Multiple shunt failures: an analysis of relevant factors, Child's Nervous System 14:271-275, 1998

Lumenta CB and Skotarczak U: Long-term follow-up in 233 patients with congenital hydrocephalus, Child's Nervous System, 11:173-175, 1995.

Madikians A and EE Conway: Cerebrospinal fluid shunt problems in pediatric patients, Pediatr Ann 26:613-620, 1997.

Mancao M et al: Cerebral fluid shunt infections in infants and children in Mobile, Alabama, Acta Paediatr 87:667-70, 1998.

Marlin AE and Gaskill SJ: Cerebrospinal fluid shunts: complications and results. In Cheek WR, editor: Pediatric neurosurgery: surgery of the developing nervous system, ed 3, Philadelphia, 1994, W.B. Saunders.

Marlin AE and Gaskill SJ: The etiology and management of hydrocephalus in the preterm infant. In Scott RM, editor: Hydrocephalus: concepts in neurosurgery, Baltimore, 1994, Williams & Wilkins.

Neville BGR: Clinical features of hydrocephalus in childhood and infancy. In Schurr PH and Polkey CE, editors: Hydrocephalus, Oxford, 1993, Oxford University Press.

Paakko E et al: Information value of magnetic resonance imaging in shunted hydrocephalus, Arch Dis Child 70(6):530-534, 1994.

Paley K et al: Transportation of children with special seating needs, South Med J 86(12):1339-1341, 1993.

Piatt JH: How effective are ventriculopleural shunts, Pediatr Neurosurg 21(1):66-70, 1994.

Piatt JH: Physical examination of patients with cerebrospinal fluid shunts: is there useful information in pumping the shunt?, Pediatrics 89(3):470-473, 1992.

Piatt JH and Carlson CV: A search for determinants of cerebrospinal fluid shunt survival: retrospective analysis of a 14-year institutional experience, Pediatr Neurosurg 19(5):233-241, 1993.

Proos LA et al: Increased perinatal intracranial pressure and prediction of early puberty in girls with myelomeningocele, Arch Dis Child 75(1):42-45, 1996.

Pumberger W, Lobl M, and Geissler W: Appendicitis in children with a ventriculoperitoneal shunt, Pediatr Neurosurg 28:21-26, 1998.

Punt J: Principles of CSF diversion and alternative treatment. In Schurr PH and Polkey CE, editors: Hydrocephalus, Oxford, 1993, Oxford University Press.

Raimondi AJ: Hydrocephalus. In Raimondi AJ, editor: Pediatric neurosurgery: theoretical principles, art of surgical techniques, ed 2, New York, 1998, Springer-Verlag.

Reinprecht A et al: The Medos Hakim programmable valve in the treatment of pediatric hydrocephalus, Child's Nervous System 13:588-594, 1997.

Rekate H: Treatment of hydrocephalus. In Cheek WR, editor: Pediatric neurosurgery: surgery of the developing nervous system, ed 3, Philadelphia, 1994, W.B. Saunders.

Rekate H: Recent advances in the understanding and treatment of hydrocephalus, Sem Pediatr Neurol 4(3):167-178, 1997.

Rekate H, McCormick J, and Yamada K: An analysis of the need for shunting after brain tumor surgery. In Marlin AE, editor: Concepts in pediatric neurosurgery, ed 2, Conn., 1991, S. Karger.

Rickert CH: Abdominal metastases of pediatric brain tumors via ventriculo-peritoneal shunts, Child's Nervous System 14:10-14, 1998.

Rieder MJ: Prevention of neural tube defects with periconceptional folic acid, Clin Perinatol 21(3):483-501, 1994.

Riva D et al: Intelligence outcome in children with shunted hydrocephalus of different etiology, Child's Nervous System 10(1):70-73, 1994.

Rosen S: Educating students who have visual impairments with neurological disabilities. In Sacks SZ and Silberman RK, editors: Educating students who have visual impairments with other disabilities, Baltimore, 1998, Paul H. Brookes.

Rotim K et al: Reducing the incidence of infection in pediatric cerebrospinal fluid shunt operations, Child's Nervous System, 13:584-587, 1997.

Sainte-Rose C and Chumas P: Endoscopic third ventriculostomy, Tech Neurosurg 1:176-184, 1996.

Sheiner M: Day to day management of hydrocephalus, Hydrocephalus Association Newsletter 17(2):6-7, 1996.

Shiminski-Maher T and Disabato J: Current trends in the diagnosis and management of hydrocephalus in children, J Pediatr Nurs 9(2):74-82, 1994.

Simpson D and Hemmer R: Social aspects of hydrocephalus. In Schurr PH and Polkey CE, editors: Hydrocephalus, Oxford, 1993, Oxford University Press.

Stellman-Ward GR et al: The incidence of chronic headache in children with shunted hydrocephalus, Eur J Pediatr Surg 7(suppl 1):12-14, 1997.

Takala AK et al: Risk factors for primary invasive pneumococcal disease among children in Finland, JAMA 273(11):859-864, 1995.

Tew B, Laurence KM, and Jenkins V: Factors affecting employability among young adults with spina bifida and hydrocephalus, Zeitschrift fur Kinderchirurgie, Surgery in Infancy and Childhood 45:34-36, 1990.

Thacker SB et al: Infectious diseases and injuries in child day care, JAMA 268(13):1720-1726, 1992.

Tulipan N and Bruner JP: Myelomeningocele repair in utero: a report of three cases, Pediatr Neurosurg 28:177-180, 1998.

Vernet O, Campiche R, and deTribolet N: Long-term results after ventriculoatrial shunting in children, Child's Nervous System 11:176, 1995.

Villani R et al: Long-term outcome in aqueductal stenosis, Child's Nervous System 11:180-185, 1995.

Warnick RE and Edwards MSB: Pediatric brain tumors, Curr Prob Pediatr 21(4):129-166, 1991.

Watkins L et al: The diagnosis of blocked cerebrospinal fluid shunts: a prospective study of referral to a pediatric neurosurgical unit, Child's Nervous System 10:87-90, 1994.

Wisoff JH et al: Management of hydrocephalic women during pregnancy. In Marlin AE, editor: Concepts in pediatric neurosurgery 3:60-68, 1991.

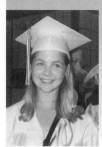

CHAPTER 26

Inflammatory Bowel Disease

Veronica Perrone Pollack and Anne DelSanto Ravenscroft

Etiology

The term inflammatory bowel disease (IBD) encompasses the diagnoses of Crohn's disease (CD) and ulcerative colitis (UC). These two diseases are commonly discussed together because they share many of the same presenting signs and symptoms and approaches to diagnosis and treatment. If they are distinct entities or manifestations of a single disease process is unknown (Hyams, 1996).

CD is a chronic inflammatory disease of the bowel that may occur at any point in the gastrointestinal (GI) tract—from mouth to anus. The inflammation is transmural and may extend from the intestinal mucosal lining through the serosal layer. In this condition, diseased segments of the bowel may border on segments of healthy tissue. The disease commonly affects the terminal ileum and proximal segments of the colon. Ileocecal involvement is present in approximately 80% of children (Kirschner, 1995b). Evidence of gastroduodenal involvement has been reported in 21% to 42% of children in two studies (Mashako et al, 1989; Schmidt-Sommerfeld, Kirschner, and Stephends, 1990). The occurrence rate of perianal disease in children with CD ranges from 14% to 40% (Cohen et al, 1998; Motil et al, 1993). Affected children may have skin tags, fissures, hemorrhoids, and fistulas. Rectal disease, however, is unusual in CD.

UC is an inflammatory disease that affects the colonic and rectal mucosa. In a study of children with UC, 3% had ulcerative proctitis, 19% had disease limited to the proctosigmoid region, 36% had disease affecting the entire descending colon, and 43% had pancolitis at the time of diagnosis (Hyams et al, 1996).

The cause of IBD is a fertile area for research. Environmental, genetic, infectious, and immunologic theories are pursued as potential contributors to the development of both CD and UC. The emphasis of current research for CD and UC is upon

hypothesized abnormalities in the intestinal mucosal immune system (Hyams, 1996; Kirschner, 1996). Current work directed toward a better understanding of the immunologic response of the GI tract, as well as ongoing research elucidating the genetic component of these conditions, is promising.

Incidence

Few epidemiologic studies of IBD directed at the pediatric age group have been conducted. A review of such research shows that most of the published studies have demonstrated incidences of CD and UC in children that mirror those found in adults (Evans, Beattie, and Walker-Smith, 1997). Recent epidemiologic studies of IBD conducted in the United States reported incidences of 7.3 per 100,000 individuals for UC and 7.0 per 100,000 individuals for CD (Loftus et al, 1997).

The incidence of CD increased considerably during the middle of this century. It appears that this overall increase in incidence began to level off in the early 1980s, although there is some controversy over this point. The incidence of CD in children seems to have modestly increased, but this increase may be due to earlier diagnoses rather than a true increase in the occurrence of CD in children (Hyams, 1996; Logan, 1998). An incidence rate for CD recently reported in a U.S. study was 5.8 per every 100,000 individuals per year (Loftus et al, 1997). The incidence of UC is thought to be relatively stable (Kirschner, 1996; Logan, 1998). Incidence figures for UC in children range from 1 to 10 cases per 100,000 individuals (Calkins and Mendeloff, 1995).

The risk for UC and CD is greater for Jewish people of middle European origin living in the United States than for those living in Israel. Blacks are less commonly affected with CD than whites.

Men and women appear to be equally affected (Hyams, 1996).

Clinical Manifestations at Time of Diagnosis

The diagnostic evaluation for IBD most often includes radiographic examination of the GI tract, endoscopy and biopsy, evaluation of growth parameters, and assessment of laboratory values (including stool cultures). Common laboratory findings associated with IBD include increased acute phase reactants (i.e., erythrocyte sedimentation rate [ESR], C-reactive protein, and orosomucoid), thrombocytosis, low serum iron, low hematocrit value, and low hemoglobin level. In CD that affects the small bowel and in severe UC, hypoalbuminemia and a decreased total protein serum value may also be noted.

Serologic assays that are highly specific to UC and CD have been identified. Perinuclear antineu-trophil cytoplasmic antibodies (pANCAs) are highly specific to UC. Anti-*Saccharomyces cerevisiae* antibodies (ASCAs) are highly specific to CD. One study of the use of these assays in the pediatric population showed that "when the results of both tests are taken together . . . a specificity of 95% and a positive predictive value of 96%" were found (Ruemmele et al, 1998).

The symptoms noted depend on the location of the disease. Common presenting symptoms for both CD and UC are abdominal pain, diarrhea, fever, blood in the stool, and weight loss (Table 26-1).

Children with UC typically complain of frequent, watery diarrhea that is grossly bloody. Pus and mucus are often noted, as well. The diarrheal stools may be associated with abdominal cramping and—if rectal disease is present—tenesmus (i.e., cramping pain in the rectum accompanied by urgency that is most commonly noted after a bowel movement is passed). Fever, weight loss, and fatigue may also be seen in children with UC. Growth failure may be seen in 6% to 12% of these children before corticosteroid therapy (Kirschner,

Table 26-1
Comparison of Crohn's Disease and Ulcerative Colitis: Presenting Symptoms

	Crohn's Disease	Ulcerative Colitis
Alteration in bowel pattern	Diarrhea is common; constipation, alternating with diarrhea, may also be seen.	Diarrhea is a hallmark; an increase in frequency of bowel movements with urgency is often a component. Constipation may be seen if the disease is obstructive.
Blood in stool	Grossly bloody stools are occasionally seen, most often when colonic disease is present. Occult blood is not uncommon in Crohn's disease.	It is common to see grossly bloody diarrhea; pus or mucus may also be seen.
Abdominal pain	Abdominal pain is often present in association with meals; pain is often periumbilical.	Abdominal cramping is often present in association with passage of stool. Pain is often noted in the lower part of the abdomen.
Fever	It is not uncommon to have intermittent, usually low-grade fever.	Fever is sometimes seen.
Onset of disease	Classically the signs of Crohn's disease are more subtle than those of ulcerative colitis, though in a smaller percentage onset may be abrupt.	Onset may be insidious or abrupt.
Weight loss/Growth failure	Weight loss is a common feature of Crohn's disease; it may have occurred for many months to years before diagnosis.	Weight loss is not uncommon and is typically more abrupt than in Crohn's disease.
Perianal disease	Perianal disease is common.	Perianal disease is rarely seen.

1995a). The onset of symptoms may be either abrupt or more insidious, occurring over weeks or months. A child may appear essentially well or chronically or acutely ill.

As with UC, the symptoms of CD may manifest in many ways. A child may have an acute, severe attack or—more commonly—the symptoms of the disease are subtle and have been present for months or years before the diagnosis (Colenda and Grand, 1995; Hyams, 1996). Symptoms of CD affecting the small bowel are commonly obstructive. A diffuse abdominal discomfort possibly associated with meals may accompany diarrhea or constipation, and blood may be noted in the stool. Blood is usually occult, although stools may be grossly bloody— particularly in CD of the colon. Fever, anorexia, and weight loss are more commonly seen in these children than in those with UC. Growth failure may precede overt GI symptoms by many months in 20% to 30% of children with CD (Colenda and Grand, 1995; Hyams, 1996; Kanof, Lake, Bayless, 1988) and may have been the original symptom for the GI evaluation to commence.

In children whose disease is limited to the colon, there is a subgroup whose condition cannot be clearly categorized. In their review of the literature, Ruemmele and associates (1998) summarize that individuals with "indeterminate colitis" may compose between 10% to 15% of cases.

IBD may manifest itself as symptoms other than those attributed to the GI tract (Figure 26-1). Children may have or eventually develop extraintestinal symptoms of their disease. Hyams (1994) reports that at least one extraintestinal manifestation is seen in about 25% to 35% of children with IBD. Extraintestinal manifestations of the disease that are not uncommonly seen at diagnosis include aphthous ulcers of the mouth, arthritic inflammation (especially of large joints), anemia, digital clubbing, and growth delay. An unusual but relevant issue to pediatric practitioners is the observation that children's presenting symptoms can sometimes be limited to abnormalities of the anogenital region. Published cases document children with CD being initially referred for evaluation of suspected sexual abuse (Sellman and Hupertz, 1996). Although physical findings consistent with sexual abuse must be appropriately investigated, organic causes of anogenital disease must also be properly evaluated.

The severity of presenting symptoms of IBD may not be indicative of the course that the disease will follow for a child. One of the most frustrating aspects of the diagnosis for children with IBD and their parents is the inability to learn the "anticipated course" of the condition. In one retrospective study of children with UC, 70% were in clinical remission within 3 months of diagnosis. Remission was achieved within 6 months in 80% to 90% of the children studied. The course of the disease beyond 1 year from diagnosis was similar for the children, regardless of the initial degree of severity of their disease. The percentage of children with inactive (absence of GI or extraintestinal symptoms) disease was 55% to 57%. The percentage of children whose disease was moderate to severe ranged from 37% to 39%. The percentage of those who had continuous symptoms (i.e., absence of symptom-free intervals or daily corticosteroid therapy with recurrence of symptoms when corticosteroids are discontinued) ranged from 4% to 8% (Hyams, 1996).

Symptoms seen at diagnosis (e.g., the extraintestinal manifestations previously noted) may remain with a child, reappear with exacerbations of the disease, or never return. New symptoms (i.e., GI or extraintestinal) may also appear with exacerbations. An exacerbation of CD or UC may sometimes be preceded by an intercurrent illness or emotional stress or may occur for no apparent reason. Intercurrent GI infections may also trigger an exacerbation of disease activity, with *Clostridium difficile* and viral infections (e.g., rotovirus and adenovirus) being implicated (Gryboski, 1991; Kirschner, 1996). Exacerbations of symptoms may be seen after dietary indiscretions, but such indiscretions are not considered to be a cause of genuine flare-ups of disease activity because they are not accompanied by changes in histologic, radiographic, or laboratory parameters. Children with IBD often become adept at anticipating which activities are likely to trigger a flare-up of their disease. For example, adolescents with IBD may find that their symptoms worsen during school examinations or near important social events.

Treatment

Treatment of IBD may include pharmacologic (Table 26-2), nutritional, and surgical therapies. The specific treatment plan depends on the location and severity of the disease, the effect of the disease on growth and development, and the degree of de-

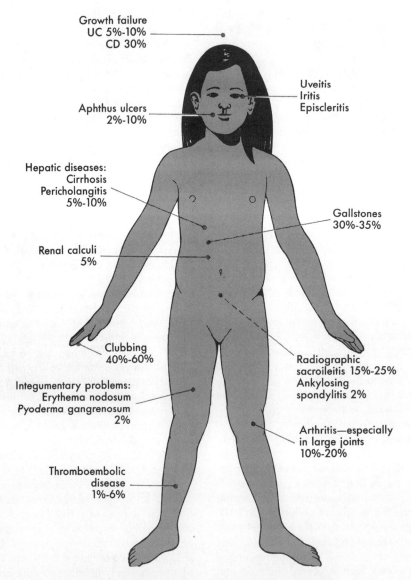

Growth failure
UC 5%-10%
CD 30%

Uveitis
Iritis
Episcleritis

Aphthus ulcers
2%-10%

Hepatic diseases:
Cirrhosis
Pericholangitis
5%-10%

Gallstones
30%-35%

Renal calculi
5%

Clubbing
40%-60%

Radiographic
sacroileitis 15%-25%
Ankylosing
spondylitis 2%

Integumentary problems:
Erythema nodosum
Pyoderma gangrenosum
2%

Arthritis—especially
in large joints
10%-20%

Thromboembolic
disease
1%-6%

Figure 26-1   Extraintestinal manifestations of IBD.

bilitation experienced by the child. When medical therapies do not adequately control symptoms or complications (e.g., toxic megacolon, obstruction, fistulae, or abscesses) do not respond to medical management, surgical intervention is indicated. Children with severe disease who are experiencing debilitating symptoms accompanied by abnormal laboratory values require aggressive medical intervention. These children are generally hospitalized

and placed on restricted diets, as well as receive intravenous corticosteroid therapy and possibly total parenteral nutrition (Box 26-1).

Drug Therapy

The mainstay of treatment and maintenance of remission of IBD are the 5-aminosalicylic acid (5-ASA) preparations and mesalamine (see Table

Box 26-1

Treatment

Drug Therapy

See Table 26-2.

Nutritional Therapy

- An elemental diet is less effective in achieving remission than corticosteroids but can improve nutritional status.
- Total parenteral nutrition is generally reserved for individuals with severe disease who cannot tolerate enteral feedings.

Surgical Intervention

Surgical intervention is indicated when disease activity or complications do not respond to medical management.

- Ulcerative colitis: Colectomy is the procedure of choice. For many individuals the option exists for reanastomosis and surgical construction of a "rectum" or pouch to maintain continence.
- Crohn's disease: Procedures are limited resection of diseased bowel segment or colectomy with permanent ileostomy.

Emotional Support

Stress is a factor in exacerbations. Stress management techniques can be helpful.

26-2). These preparations include the oral agents sulfasalazine, olsalazine (Dipentum), mesalamine (Asacol, Pentasa), as well as mesalamine (Rowasa) in enema and suppository form. For years, sulfasalazine has been the primary drug used to treat UC. Sulfasalazine is a compound that combines 5-aminosalicylic acid with sulfapyridine. Sulfapyridine is primarily used as a delivery agent which—when bound to 5-ASA—prevents its absorption in the proximal GI tract. Unfortunately, 10% to 45% of individuals who take sulfasalazine experience significant side effects, mostly related to the sulfapyridine component (Leichtner, 1995). The most common side effects include headache, malaise, nausea, vomiting, anorexia, heartburn, and diarrhea. Less common but more severe reactions include skin eruptions, hepatitis, pancreatitis, pneumonia, hemolysis or bone marrow toxicity,

and allergic reactions. Sulfasalazine also inhibits folate absorption, which may lead to megaloblastic anemia. This inhibition can be prevented by coadministering 1 mg of folic acid per day (Leichtner, 1995).

When initiating therapy, some clinicians gradually increase a child's dose to the therapeutic range (i.e., 50 to 75 mg/kg/day) in an effort to alleviate or avoid the side effects of sulfasalazine (Kirshner, 1996). During the initiation of therapy, leukopenia and hemolytic anemia should be monitored monthly by a complete blood count (CBC). If either of these occur, the dose should be decreased or stopped until the blood values return to normal. The dose may then be slowly returned to therapeutic range. If this approach is unsuccessful, the drug should be discontinued and therapy with another 5-ASA preparation attempted (Leichtner, 1995).

Newer preparations of 5-ASA have been developed in the past decade. These drugs have the advantage of being more site-specific and having a lower incidence of side effects and are equally as effective in prolonging remission in UC and helpful in treating Crohn's ileitis (Cohen et al, 1998; Hyams, 1996; Sachar, 1995). Olsalazine (Dipentum) is primarily used for UC or Crohn's colitis, and mesalamine (Asacol) is used to treat ileocolonic CD, as well as UC. Mesalamine (Pentasa) releases mesalamine beginning in the duodenum and continuing throughout the intestine, making it well-suited for upper intestinal CD. Griffiths and associates (1993) studied the use of Pentasa in children with small intestine CD and reported improvement in several disease activity scores after treatment.

Adverse effects with the newer 5-ASA preparations occur less frequently than those of sulfasalazine but include nausea, vomiting, dizziness, headache, abdominal pain, diarrhea, rash, and hair loss. Pancreatitis, pericarditis, aplastic anemia, and hypersensitivity reactions are rare but more worrisome (Leichtner, 1995). Although pediatric doses of mesalamine have not been fully established, many authors recommend starting at 30 to 50 mg/kg/day (Hyams, 1996; Leichtner, 1995). Recommended monitoring of toxicity includes monthly complete blood cell (CBC) counts, liver function tests, blood urea nitrogen and creatinine levels, and urinalysis for 3 months, then every 3 to 6 months (Leictner, 1995). Sulfasalazine and Asacol only come in tablet form, which is difficult

Table 26-2
Drugs Used for Treatment of Inflammatory Bowel Disease

Drug/Dosage	Uses in IBD	Side Effects	Special Considerations
Sulfasalazine (Azulfidine) 50-75 mg/kg/day	Treatment of UC and Crohn's colitis	*Common:* headache, malaise GI upset, decreased sperm production *Less common:* skin eruption, hepatitis, pancreatitis, pneumonia, hemolysis, allergic reaction 5-ASA side effects (see below)	Fewer adverse reactions may be noted if the dose is gradually increased to reach the planned therapeutic dosage Enteric coated tablets may alleviate GI upset Monitor WBC count over first 3 months of treatment Impairs folic acid absorption; give folic acid 1 mg/day
Olsalazine (Dipentum) 30-50 mg/kg/day	Treatment of UC and Crohn's colitis	**For all 5-ASAs:** *Common:* GI upset, abdominal pain, dizziness, headache, diarrhea, rash, hair loss *Less common:* pancreatitis, pericarditis, aplastic anemia, allergic reaction	**For all 5-ASAs:** Fewer adverse reactions than sulfasalazine; useful for individuals unable to tolerate sulfasalazine Dipentum and Pentasa capsules may be opened and mixed in food for younger children
Mesalamine (Asacol) 30-50 mg/kg/day	Treatment of UC and ileocolonic CD	5-ASA side effects	5-ASA special considerations
Mesalamine (Pentasa) 30-50 mg/kg/day	Treatment of small intestinal and colonic CD Can be used to treat UC	5-ASA side effects	5-ASA special considerations
Mesalamine (Rowasa Salofalk) enema at hospitalization, suppository twice per day	Topical therapy for distal colitis and rectal disease	5-ASA side effects *Common:* perianal irritation, pruritus *Less common:* pancreatitis, pericarditis	5-ASA special considerations Child should be instructed to try to retain the enema overnight

From Grand, Ramakrishna, and Calenda, 1995; Hyams, 1996; Kirshner, 1995, 1996, 1998; Leichtner, 1995; Podolsky, 1991; Spahn and Kamada, 1995.

for children who cannot swallow tablets; olsalazine (Dipentum) and Pentasa capsules may be opened and mixed in food to ease administration.

Mesalamine (Rowasa) enemas and suppositories are useful in treating distal colonic and rectal disease. These enemas are instilled at bedtime with the goal of retaining the fluid overnight. The suppositories are useful for treating proctitis and are inserted twice a day. Treatment may last from weeks to months. Adverse effects of these topical preparations include perianal irritation and pruritus and, rarely, pancreatitis and pericarditis (Leichtner, 1995).

In moderate to severe disease, as well as during exacerbations, corticosteroids given with an agent containing 5-ASA are effective in achieving remission. Children are first given a dosage ranging from 1 to 2 mg/kg/day, which is maintained until their symptoms diminish and their previous levels of comfort and activity are achieved. The time period often allotted for this is 1 to 2 months (Kirschner, 1996; Hyams, 1996). The dose is then gradually tapered while a child's symptoms and laboratory values—especially ESR, CBC, and albumin—are monitored. The dose continues to be tapered until a child can function normally without it. Side effects of prednisone include Cushingoid features, weight gain, hypertension, hyperglycemia, acne, striae,

Table 26-2
Drugs Used for Treatment of Inflammatory Bowel Disease—cont'd

Drug/Dosage	Uses in IBD	Side Effects	Special Considerations
Corticosteroids (Prednisone, Prednisolone) 1-2 mg/kg/day	Useful in children who do not respond adequately to 5-ASAs Useful in moderate to severe disease Available as foam (Cortifoam) and retention enemas (Cortenema) for rectal disease	*Common:* adrenal suppression, growth retardation, Cushingoid facies, weight gain, striae, mood swings, acne, impaired calcium absorption and osteoporosis, hypertension, hyperglycemia *Less common:* cataracts, aseptic necrosis of the femoral head	Alternate day therapy at lowest possible dose is often used to minimize adverse effects Child should be warned to not discontinue corticosteroid use suddenly; this could result in an adrenal crisis and a flare-up of symptoms Ophthalmic examination, urine dipstick, and blood pressure monitoring should be done at each visit Child should see an ophthalmologist twice a year
Metronidazole (Flagyl) 10-15 mg/kg/day	Effective adjunct treatment for CD Useful in the management of perianal disease, fistulae, and abscesses	*Common:* GI upset, metallic taste in mouth, parasthesias	Assess for parathesias at each office visit; these are usually reversible after discontinuation of the medication Disulfiram-like effect (i.e., vomiting) occurs if taken with alcohol or products containing alcohol
6-Mercaptopurine (6-MP, Purinethol) 1.5 mg/kg/day	Used when 5-ASA therapy and corticosteroids have failed, or when child cannot be weaned from corticosteroids	*Common:* leukopenia, pancreatitis, hepatitis, allergic reactions, increased risk of infection	If fever develops, drug should be discontinued until illness resolves It may take 3 to 4 months to see response
Azathioprine (Imuran) 2.0 mg/kg/day		*Common:* GI upset, leukopenia, hepatitis, pancreatitis, allergy, risk of infection	CBC, transaminases, amylase, and lipase should be monitored during therapy

mood swings, calcium depletion, aseptic necrosis of the hip, immunosuppression, and cataracts (Spahn and Kamada, 1995).

Long-term corticosteroid use also leads to adrenal suppression, which may last 6 months to 1 year after prednisone therapy has stopped. Rapid cessation of prednisone during therapy or any stressful incident (e.g., an accident or surgery) in the year after prednisone therapy may precipitate acute adrenal insufficiency. Symptoms of acute adrenal insufficiency include fever, hypotension, dehydration, electrolyte abnormalities, hypoglycemia, severe abdominal pain, and lethargy. Treatment consists of intravenous hydrocortisone administration until oral therapy can be resumed and, if needed, fluid replacement to treat dehydration.

Children should also be given stress doses of corticosteroids during episodes of significant illness or for scheduled surgical procedures (Spahn and Kamada, 1995) (see Chapter 16). The use of alternate-day corticosteroids has been shown to allow a normal growth rate to occur (Kirshner, 1996; Spahn and Kamada, 1995). Alternative corticosteroid preparations (e.g., retention enemas and foams for rectal instillation) are also available. Rectal administration of the medication allows for local treatment of disease with fewer systemic side effects. Individuals with rectal disease, perianal disease, or disease of the descending colon may benefit from this therapy (Podolsky, 1991).

Metronidazole is effective in the treatment of perianal disease, fistulae, and abscesses, but when its dose is lowered or it is discontinued, perianal disease commonly relapses (Cohen et al, 1998; Grand, Ramakrishna, and Calenda, 1995). The effects of long-term use of metronidazole are not known, but there is concern that it may potentially be carcinogenic or mutagenic because this response has been identified in mice and rats. There have been no cases where either cancer or chromosomal aberrations have been proven to be attributable to metronidazole in humans (Physicians Desk Reference, 1998). The recommended pediatric dosage ranges from 10 to 15 mg/kg/day (Kirschner, 1995a; Markowitz et al, 1991). Side effects of metronidazole include GI upset and a metallic taste. A more worrisome side effect is peripheral neuropathy (Grand, Ramakrishna, and Calenda, 1995). Adolescents should be warned of the disulfiram-like effect if they ingest alcohol while taking metronidazole. Other antibiotics (e.g., ciprofloxacin or clarithromycin) have been useful as an adjunct to other therapies in treating severe colitis, but further research is necessary to document their effectiveness (Grand, Ramakrishhna, and Calenda, 1995; Hanauer, 1996).

6-mercaptopurine (6-MP) and azathioprine are immunosuppressive agents that are widely used to treat IBD in children. They are used as a second-line therapy in children for whom more conservative medical management has failed and for those individuals who have required long-term steroid use to control symptoms (Cohen et al, 1998; Grand, Ramakrishna, and Calenda, 1995; Kirshner, 1996; and Hanauer, 1996). The recommended doses are 1.0 to 1.5 mg/kg/day for 6-MP and 2 mg/kg/day for azathioprine. Response to these agents is not immediate, averaging 3 to 4 months. A new assay test has been developed for use in determining the optimal dose of 6-MP, as well as identifying patients in whom the drug will not be effective or may be severely toxic (Cuffari et al, 1996). The most commonly cited complications of 6-MP and azathioprine are GI upset, leukopenia, hepatitis, and pancreatitis. Other complications include allergy and increased risk of infection (Grand, Ramakrishna, and Calenda, 1995; Kirshner, 1998). Concerns about the possible increased risk of lymphoma for individuals treated with these agents has

been allayed by multiple clinical studies showing their safety for long-term use (Hanauer, 1996; Kirshner, 1998). For the first several months of therapy a CBC count and transaminases, amylase, and lipase levels should be checked every 2 weeks to assess for adverse reactions. These parameters should be checked monthly for several months and then every 3 months thereafter (Kirshner, 1996, 1998). It is recommended that the dose be reduced or therapy terminated if the WBC count falls below normal or the transaminases rise. Therapy may be reattempted after the values return to normal. An elevation in pancreatic function tests necessitates termination of therapy (Hanauer, 1996; Kirshner, 1996). The primary care provider, family, and child must be aware that any febrile illness during therapy with 6-MP or azathioprine is an indication for concern and must be evaluated. Temporary discontinuation of the drug may be necessary until the illness resolves.

Cyclosporine (Sandimmune) is an immunosuppressant therapy for IBD that has an increased acceptance with individuals with refractory UC and—to a lesser extent—CD. This response to cyclosporine therapy has been inconsistent, however, and treated individuals have had a significant incidence of relapse while receiving therapy and recurrence when discontinuing the drug (Kirschner, 1996; Lichtiger et al, 1994; Ramakrisha et al, 1996). Its main use seems to be rapidly inducing remission of disease; although other more effective long-term therapies (e.g., 6-MP, azathioprine, and 5-ASA preparations) are given time to become effective. Once remission has been sustained for several months, individuals can usually be successfully weaned from cyclosporine and corticosteroids and remission can be continued on the other therapies (Grand, Ramakrishna, and Calenda, 1995; Hanauer, 1996; Ramakrishna et al, 1996). Cyclosporine is usually first administered intravenously at 1 to 2 mg/kg/day. Once clinical improvement is seen, children are then changed to the oral form at 4 to 8 mg/kg/day. Because absorption of cyclosporine can be erratic, trough blood levels frequently need to checked and the dosage adjusted to maintain a blood level between 100 to 200 ng/ml (Grand, Ramakrishna, and Calenda, 1995; Ramakrishna et al, 1996). Side effects of cyclosporine include hypertension, tremor, hirsutism, seizures, and the potential for renal insufficiency. Frequent monitoring of vital signs, serum laboratory studies (including blood urea nitrogen and creatinine), and drug levels is mandatory during treatment (Kirshner, 1996; Ramakrishna et al, 1996).

Nutritional Therapy

Nutritional therapy has been used for primary management of disease activity and nutritional replenishment for children with IBD. Children with IBD, particularly with CD, are at significant risk for growth failure. The cause of growth failure is thought to be multifactorial; but the consensus is, however, that inadequate caloric intake is the fundamental cause of growth failure. Children may ingest too few calories because of anorexia associated with the symptoms of disease activity. They may also consciously skip meals to minimize embarrassing symptoms such as diarrhea. Nutritional intervention directed toward achieving adequate caloric intake for growth and development is a crucial goal for treatment of IBD.

The role of nutritional therapy as a primary method of treating IBD is controversial. When elemental nutrition was first proposed as a therapy for IBD, there was optimism that it might offer an acceptable alternative to corticosteroid therapy for treating intractable CD. The initial optimism that nutritional therapy would supplant medical therapy—particularly corticosteroids—in the treatment of CD, however, has not borne out. A recent metaanalysis of enteral therapy for CD found that the results have been disappointing (Tolia, 1997). Findings have consistently shown that enteral therapy with elemental formula is less effective than corticosteroids in achieving remission in active CD. Additional drawbacks of enteral therapy include the difficult choice between the discomfort of daily placement of a nasogastric tube vs. the stigma of being seen in public with a tube in place. Some motivated adolescents, however, can be taught to place the tube themselves and have had success with enteral therapy. Many insurance carriers refuse to cover these costly formulas, and the burden of this expense must be shouldered by the families alone. Some research has supported the position that the composition of the formula used for nutritional replenishment may not be critical. The therapeutic benefit to individuals may result from improvement in nutritional status rather than as a direct result of a benefit from the elemental preparation (Tolia, 1997). The significance

of this is that less expensive, more palatable preparations may be used when indicated.

Enteral nutrition offers important benefits for children experiencing growth failure—particularly when disease affects the small intestine. A suitable management strategy for these children may be to combine use of steroids and nutritional therapy for faster induction and maintain remission by rapidly tapering the steroids to a lower dose (Tolia, 1997).

Total parenteral nutrition (TPN) has shown improvement in disease activity and reversal of growth failure (Seidman et al, 1987). The use of TPN is typically restricted to individuals with fulminant IBD who cannot tolerate enteral feedings.

Surgical Intervention

Indications for surgical intervention for children with UC include intractable disease, refractory growth failure, toxic megacolon, hemorrhage, perforation, and cancer prophylaxis (Kirschner, 1996). Total colectomy with preservation of a rectal stump and creation of a diverting ileostomy is currently the procedure of choice (Cohen et al, 1998; Grand, Ramakrishna, and Calenda, 1995). A second surgery is later performed where the mucosa is peeled away from the muscular layers of the rectal stump, a pouch is formed from the distal ileum, and the pouch is then sutured into the remaining rectal sleeve. A third and final surgery is later performed to close the ileostomy. Benefits of the pouch procedure are resumption of rectal continence and avoidance of a permanent ostomy. Bowel movements initially occur frequently but in time decrease to 4 to 8 times a day (Grand, Ramakrishna, and Calenda, 1995). Although colectomy is curative of the underlying disease in UC, inflammation of the pouch (i.e., pouchitis) may occur but is readily treatable with medical therapy.

Indications for surgery in CD include intractable disease, hemorrhage, toxic megacolon, bowel perforation, stricture with obstruction, and abscesses and fistulae unresponsive to medical management (Cohen et al, 1998; Hyams, 1996). Surgery may also be indicated for prepubertal children or early adolescents who have growth failure and localized, stenotic segments of bowel (Cohen et al, 1998). Recurrence of disease is common in CD after surgery, and 50% of children have a recurrence within 5 years of their first surgery. Because a child with CD may have multiple surgical resections over a lifetime, the goal of surgery should be to relieve symptoms while preserving as much bowel as possible. An isolated, nonprogressive area of bowel may be removed, or strictureplasty, which is aimed at opening a stenotic area while preventing resection of bowel, may be performed. In cases of fulminant colitis, a total proctocolectomy and permanent ileostomy may be necessary. Children with CD are not good candidates for pouch procedures because of the high rate of disease recurrence (Cohen et al, 1998; Grand, Ramakrishna, and Calenda, 1995; Hyams, 1996).

Emotional Support

Because stress has been identified as a factor that may contribute to the exacerbation of IBD symptoms, some children find it helpful to master relaxation and stress management techniques for controlling or preventing flare-ups of their disease, as well as for managing daily stressors. Primary care providers may help families find programs that promote the development of stress management and problem-solving skills.

Recent and Anticipated Advances in Management

Many new therapies for the treatment of IBD have been developed and are undergoing further clinical trials. Much of the data on their effectiveness are from research done with adults; clinical trials are just beginning with children.

A new form of corticosteroid, budesonide, has been widely tested in Europe and Canada (Lofberg et al, 1996; Rutgeerts et al, 1994). This corticosteroid exerts a strong topical antiinflammatory effect in the small intestine or colon but, when absorbed, is rapidly metabolized in the liver and has minimal effect on adrenal suppression. Because of its low bioavailability, the incidence of prednisone-like side effects is much lower. Budesonide has proved almost as effective as prednisone in treating IBD but is unfortunately not yet available in the United States.

Methotrexate (administered in weekly injections) has been studied in both children and adults with CD who have been steroid-dependent (Feagan et al, 1995; Mack et al, 1998). Methotrexate has

been effective in inducing remission and permitting weaning of corticosteroids in children and adults and has generally been well-tolerated. In a recent study of 14 children who were steroid-dependent and had failed treatment with 6-MP or azathioprine (Mack et al, 1998), 64% showed improvement after administration of methotrexate. Methotrexate has also been shown to have a quicker onset of action as compared with 6-MP and azathioprine.

Tacrolimus, or FK-506, is an immunosuppressant agent used to treat cyclosporine-refractory liver rejection in liver transplantation and is the drug of choice for liver-bowel transplants (see Chapter 30). Tacrolimus seems to be more potent than cyclosporine, and the advantage of reliable oral absorption reduces the need for intravenous therapy (Bousvaros et al, 1997; Bousvaros, Wang, and Leichtner, 1996). Ongoing studies of FK-506 in children with fulminant colitis show the effectiveness of this agent in inducing remission while permitting individuals to be weaned from steroids and make a transition to other immunosuppressant medications. The side effects of FK-506 appear to be the same or less than those of cyclosporine.

Remicade (Infliximab), an antibody to tumor necrosis factor alpha, has been approved for adults to treat moderate to severe CD that is unresponsive to other medical therapies. Imfliximab is also effective in treating fistulae (Centocor, 1998; Targan et al, 1997). Given once as an intravenous infusion for active CD or as a series of three infusions for fistula treatment, Infliximab has shown rapid improvement in disease symptoms. Clinical trials in children have not yet been performed.

Associated Problems (Box 26-2)

Growth Failure

Growth failure associated with IBD in childhood affects children with CD more than those with UC. The proposed etiologic theories for growth failure include chronic malnutrition, corticosteroid administration, and the hypothesized growth-retarding effects of chronic inflammation (Hyams, 1996). It is generally believed that inadequate calorie intake resulting from disease related symptoms and anorexia is the primary cause of malnutrition in children with IBD (Kirschner, 1995b; Kirschner, 1996; Hyams, 1996).

Box 26-2

Associated Problems

Growth Failure

Musculoskeletal Problems
Osteoporosis
Peripheral arthritis
Ankylosing spondylitis
Sacroiliitis
Bone demineralization and osteoporosis

Dermatologic Manifestations

Erythema nodosum
Pyoderma gangrenosum

Visual Changes

Iritis
Episcleritis
Uveitis
Conjunctivitis
Cataracts

Hepatobiliary Complications

Primary sclerosing cholangitis
Pericholangitis
Gallstones

Renal Changes

Renal calculi

Perianal Disease

Fistulas, abscesses
Fissures, skin tags

Fulminant Colitis or Toxic Megacolon

Intestinal Malignancy

Lactose Intolerance
Anemia

Vitamin B_{12} deficiency
Iron deficiency due to chronic blood loss

Musculoskeletal Problems

Musculoskeletal problems associated with IBD include peripheral arthritis, ankylosing spondylitis, and sacroiliitis. Peripheral arthritis is seen in approximately 20% of individuals with IBD, usually in association with active intestinal disease (Kirschner, 1995a). Inflammation and discomfort are noted in the large joints, especially those of the hip, knee, and ankle. Inflammation does not occur

symmetrically. Unlike the other musculoskeletal manifestations of IBD, the arthritic symptoms often fluctuate with the activity of the bowel disease and respond to treatment of the disease. Nonsteroidal antiinflammatory agents may be used to treat refractory joint complaints, but due to the possibility of causing a disease exacerbation, their duration is limited (Kirshner, 1996). Ankylosing spondylitis may be seen in up to 11% of individuals with IBD and is more common in individuals with CD (Retsky and Kraft, 1995). Sacroiliitis may be noted on roentgenogram in 4% to 18% of individuals with IBD, with far fewer individuals noting symptoms such as low back pain (Retsky and Kraft, 1995).

Although not manifestations of IBD, osteoporosis and decreased bone mineral density (BMD) can be seen in children with IBD. Reported causes of decreased BMD include malabsorption of calcium and vitamin D, macro- and micronutrient deficiencies, decreased level of physical activity, estrogen deficiency in females, and—importantly—corticosteroid use (Pigot et al, 1992, Semeao et al, 1997). A recent report by Semeao and associates (1997) described five children with CD, all of whom had received significant amounts of corticosteroids, who developed vertebral compression fractures. Examination of BMD by dual energy radiographic absorptiometry (DEXA) showed a BMD more than two standard deviations below the mean. Semeao and associates recommend that all children with CD receive routine DEXA scanning in addition to careful evaluation of back pain complaints. Calcium and vitamin D supplementation may also be considered.

Dermatologic Manifestations

Dermatologic manifestations occur in up to 5% to 15% of individuals with IBD (Retsky and Kraft, 1995). Erythema nodosum is a tender, reddened nodule that commonly appears on the anterior aspect of the lower leg, although it may be seen on the foot, back of the leg, or arm. Erythema nodosum is seen more often with CD (15%) than with UC (10%).

Pyoderma gangrenosum is a more serious dermatologic condition that may be found in 1% to 5% of individuals with UC and 1% to 2% of those with CD and is usually seen in those with active pancolitis. The lesions typically appear on the anterior of the lower leg and have dark red or purple borders surrounding deep skin ulcerations with necrotic centers (Rankin, 1990). Control of the intestinal disease can result in healing of these lesions, but topical or systemic therapy directed at the lesions themselves may also be necessary. Reoccurrence of the pyoderma gangrenosum is common (Hyams, 1994).

Visual Changes

Ocular manifestations of IBD include iritis, episcleritis, uveitis, and conjunctivitis. Children being treated with corticosteroids are also at increased risk for cataracts and elevated intraocular pressure (Kirschner, 1995a).

Hepatobiliary Complications

Other GI manifestations of IBD include hepatobiliary complications, such as pericholangitis, cirrhosis, and primary sclerosing cholangitis. Physical examinations should be closely monitored for hepatic enlargement or signs of portal hypertension. Gallstones are seen more often with CD than with UC and occur in 13% to 34% of individuals with IBD, particularly in those with extensive ileal disease or ileal resection. The occurrence of gallstones seems to be related to the malabsorption of bile salts with concomitant cholesterol precipitation and calculus formation (Retsky and Kraft, 1995).

Renal Changes

Renal calculi may also be seen in individuals with IBD. They have been noted in 8% to 19% of individuals with IBD—the highest incidence occurring in people with CD after small bowel resection or ileostomy. Children with severe ileal disease or resection of the ileum are at risk for formation of calcium oxalate stones (Retsky and Kraft, 1995).

Perianal Disease

Reports of perianal disease in children with CD vary from 14% to 62%. These lesions include fissures, skin tags, fistulae, and abscesses (Cohen et al, 1998). Because of the transmural nature of the inflammation in CD, fistulae and abscesses may form between the bowel and surface of the skin or between the bowel and other orifices. Clinicians

should question children and/or parents about the passage of air or stool through the vagina or the urethra, because this may indicate a rectovaginal or rectourethral fistula. Complaints of pain, fullness, or drainage from the perianal area may alert clinicians to active perianal disease or abscess. Metronidazole has been most useful in treating perianal disease, but other therapies (e.g., corticosteroids, 6-MP, or cyclosporine) may also be used. In cases of refractory perianal disease, surgery may be necessary (Cohen et al, 1998; Markowitz et al, 1995).

Fulminant Colitis or Toxic Megacolon

Fulminant colitis presents with grossly bloody diarrhea, fever, tachycardia, abdominal pain, and abnormal laboratory findings. When these symptoms occur accompanied by a markedly distended colon on radiographs, toxic megacolon is present (Cohen et al, 1998). Although fulminant colitis and toxic megacolon may be managed medically, most individuals eventually receive a colectomy. Both conditions can occur with UC or Crohn's colitis. The incidence of toxic megacolon has decreased over the years due in part to the decreased use of opiates and antispasmodics, as well as the avoidance of tests such as barium enema or colonoscopy during periods of severe colitis—all of which have been known to precipitate toxic megacolon.

Lactose Intolerance

During periods of active disease, some children with IBD may experience symptoms of lactose intolerance including bloating, abdominal cramping, and diarrhea related to the intake of dairy products (Grand, Ramakrishna, and Calenda, 1995). For this reason, some health care providers recommend that children eliminate lactose from their diet during the initial period of diagnosis and recovery to minimize confusion about a child's response to therapy. A breath hydrogen test may be performed to definitively diagnose lactose intolerance if such a clarification is desired. Ultimately, a significant proportion of children with IBD will eventually be able to tolerate some amount of lactose in their diet.

Anemia

As a result of chronic malnutrition, malabsorption, the interference of sulfasalazine in the absorption of folates, and chronic blood loss, children with IBD are at increased risk for vitamin B_{12} deficiency and hypochromic microcytic or iron deficiency anemia. Daily supplementation with folic acid is recommended for children receiving sulfasalazine, and monitoring of the CBC is recommended for all children with IBD. Iron supplementation is recommended for children with iron deficiency anemia.

Prognosis

The overall life expectancy of individuals with IBD is essentially that of the general population (Harper et al, 1987). A significantly greater risk for intestinal malignancies exists among children with IBD than among those who do not have IBD. It seems that the risk of malignancy in UC increases with the extent and duration of the disease, as well as with a younger age at the time of diagnosis (Ekbom et al, 1990). The risk of cancer begins to increase 10 to 15 years after diagnosis (Podolsky, 1991).

Most authors agree that surveillance colonoscopy should be performed on children with UC but disagree on when this should start and how often it should occur. Annual or biannual colonoscopies are recommended when biopsy findings are negative for dysplasia; colonoscopies are recommended every 6 months when biopsies show indeterminate dysplasia; and a colectomy is recommended when a biopsy shows any signs of dysplasia (Cohen et al, 1998). Cohen and associates (1998) also point out that dysplastic lesions and carcinomas may be difficult to detect in early stages, and although frequent biopsy during colonoscopy is recommended, lesions may be missed. Some gastroenterologists recommend prophylactic colectomy for individuals with long-standing UC—especially when diagnosed in childhood (Cohen et al, 1998; Grand, Ramakrishna, and Calenda, 1995). Finally, carcinoma has been detected in ileoanal pouches, which must also be screened for malignancy (Cohen et al, 1998).

Children with CD are also at greater risk for developing an intestinal malignancy in the future. Bernstein and Rogers (1996) reviewed the literature on malignancy in adults with CD and report that the risk of small bowel carcinoma is six times that of the general population. Risk factors include male sex, duration of disease, and associated fistu-las. The risk of colon cancer is debated but may be similar to that of UC. Factors increasing the risk are early age of disease onset, location and extent of the disease, and presence of strictures or fistulae. Recommendations for colon surveillance are the same as for UC.

The information on the long-term effects of IBD on quality of life indicates that a significant percentage of adults with IBD report their overall life satisfaction to be low or negatively affected by their disease. In Gryboski's reviews (1993, 1994) of children with IBD, during the 2 years immediately after diagnosis of UC, 75% of children or their parents felt that the child's quality of life was fair and 25% reported the quality of life as good. Interestingly, after 24 months following diagnosis, these percentages were reversed with 75% of children's quality of life reported to be good. This is in contrast to individuals diagnosed with CD, 70% of whom reported their quality of life to be only fair, with 22% reporting a good quality of life, and 8% reporting an excellent quality of life. Lashner and associates (1993) reported encountering a significant rate of refusal when conducting a peer-nominated control study of teens with IBD. A high portion of teens who refused participation reportedly did so because they were afraid the disease would be disclosed to peers. Social adaptation was not the focus of the research study, but the authors' observation of this phenomenon may indicate the extent to which adolescents with IBD view themselves to be stigmatized by their condition.

PRIMARY CARE MANAGEMENT

Health Care Maintenance

Growth and Development

Children with IBD should have growth parameters measured and graphed on a National Center for Health Statistics chart at each primary care visit. For recently diagnosed children, it is helpful to go back through previous visit records to assess growth in the years before the diagnosis was made. This review will help primary care providers to assess for any deceleration in growth rate. School health or athletic offices may often be of assistance in reconstructing the growth curve. Height and weight for age, Tanner stage, and arm anthropometry are growth parameters of particular importance. Once growth retardation is identified as an actual or potential problem, bone age should be obtained to identify the child's remaining growth potential. Continued careful measurement and graphing of growth parameters are essential. Catch-up growth is considered to be adequate if children return to their preillness growth percentiles.

Cognitive abilities are unimpaired in children with IBD, and development usually progresses normally.

Diet

No specific dietary restrictions have been documented as helpful in controlling symptoms for individuals with IBD. Because some individuals may feel more comfortable when they avoid certain foods, however, the child and family can be helped to identify such foods. Practitioners fear that concerned parents, who feel able to attribute symptoms to multiple foods, may overly restrict the diet. Such overrestriction may result in a diet that is unappealing to the child and too restrictive to provide enough calories for growth and development.

Many centers consider a referral for nutritional consultation to be a standard of care for children and adolescents who have been recently diagnosed with IBD. The dietitian may assess a child's intake and nutritional status and, if necessary, counsel the child and family about how caloric intake may be augmented.

If growth retardation associated with IBD is identified, nutritional supplementation is necessary. It is generally agreed that given adequate calories, children or adolescents (i.e., before epiphyseal closure) may recover lost growth. As nutritional replenishment begins, children or adolescents with IBD may have greater caloric requirements than their unaffected peers. Recommendations for caloric intake range from 75 to 95 kcal/kg/day. It is not routinely necessary for children with IBD to receive more calories than those without IBD (Kirschner, 1995a).

During periods of active disease, many children may feel more comfortable on a low-roughage diet. Children with CD of the small bowel are also more likely to experience some degree of lactose intolerance, which may even persist during periods of re-

mission. During periods of inactive disease, these children may drink Lactaid (Merck) milk or use lactase capsules and tablets, which are readily available. For children who feel especially deprived or set apart from their peers because of their dietary restrictions, such products may be of value. Experience has shown, however, that these products are not helpful for all lactose-intolerant individuals. Children on milk-restricted diets and those taking corticosteroids should receive calcium supplementation because they are at risk for osteoporosis.

Safety

Children with IBD require no special restriction of activities. They should be encouraged to participate in all sports they can enjoy. Vigorous activities (e.g., lacrosse or tackle football) should pose no problem for children in remission. Children with osteoporosis, however, should refrain from such sports. Because—as in many populations with special needs—anxious families may tend to shelter their child from uncomfortable or tense situations, primary care providers can play an integral role in advocating for a normal lifestyle for these children.

Children and adolescents with IBD who plan to travel may need to make some special modifications. Referral or consultation with a tropical medicine or travel clinic may be beneficial when travel abroad is planned. General considerations include the purity of the water supply, ova, parasites, and proper immunization. Children and adolescents who are immunosuppressed should not receive live virus immunizations.

Alcohol consumption by adolescents with IBD who are in remission is of the same concern as alcohol consumption by their unaffected peers. Alcohol ingestion may cause discomfort for some individuals with IBD. If so, these individuals should limit intake. Individuals taking metronidazole should be informed that alcohol intake will induce a disulfiram (Antabuse) type of reaction.

Children who are immunosuppressed should wear a medical alert bracelet or use other easily identifiable methods of communicating this fact to emergency medical personnel. Children who have received steroids in the past year may need a stress dose of corticosteroids at times of serious illness, accident, or surgery (Spahn and Kamada, 1995) (see Chapter 16).

Immunizations

No change from the normal immunization schedule is necessary unless a child receives maintenance therapy of corticosteroids or other immunosuppressive agents (e.g., 6-MP or cyclosporine). These children should not receive live virus immunizations until they have been tapered from these drugs. If this is not feasible or if exposure is of particular concern, a killed virus vaccine or condition-specific immunoglobulin may be given. Children who receive maintenance therapy of immunosuppressive drugs should receive prophylaxis with varicella-zoster immune globulin for varicella exposure. Additionally, children who are immunosuppressed should receive a yearly flu shot, as well (Peter, 1997).

Screening

Vision: Ophthalmic examinations are necessary at each well-child visit because children with IBD are at risk for ocular manifestations of the disease. In the case of iritis, examiners may note redness of the eye, eye pain, photophobia, or blurred vision. In uveitis, abnormal pupillary reaction may also be assessed. A reddened eye may be noted in episcleritis or conjunctivitis. If the child is receiving prolonged corticosteroid therapy, ophthalmologic referral for assessment for cataracts is recommended twice a year (Kirschner, 1996). Any child with an abnormal ophthalmoscopic examination or complaints of the previously mentioned symptoms should be referred to an ophthalmologist, as well as to the gastroenterology team.

Hearing: Routine screening is recommended.

Dental: Children who are being treated with cyclosporine are at risk for gingival hyperplasia. Proper dental hygiene and the need for dental visits twice a year should be reinforced at each well-child visit.

Blood pressure: Children who are taking cyclosporine or corticosteroids are at increased risk for hypertension. Their blood pressures should be measured and graphed at every visit.

Hematocrit: Hemoglobin and hematocrit values should be measured yearly for children who are asymptomatic and have no history of anemia. A CBC count should be checked every 6 months or as needed for children with a history of anemia or those experiencing increased symptoms of their disease.

Urinalysis: No change in the usual protocol for screening is necessary unless the history indicates renal involvement or the child is experiencing symptoms indicative of any of the previously mentioned conditions.

Tuberculosis: Children who are receiving immunosuppressive therapy may not respond to testing. Screening may be withheld until immunosuppressive drugs are discontinued. If exposure is suspected, a control may be placed along with the purified protein derivative of the tuberculosis to assess for anergy. Chest radiography may be necessary to screen for active disease.

Condition-Specific Screening

It is customary for even asymptomatic children and adolescents to be seen on a regular basis by the gastroenterology team. The following condition-specific screening studies are typically obtained at the time of these visits. Primary care practitioners must be aware that these studies should be routinely evaluated. In some circumstances, the primary care setting may be the most convenient or appropriate place to monitor these values.

Erythrocyte sedimentation rate: An ESR should be measured yearly for asymptomatic children. The ESR may be used for some children with IBD as an index of disease activity, which is seen in up to 90% of individuals with CD and over 50% of those with UC (Colenda and Grand, 1995). The ESR should be normal in children with inactive disease. A variation from baseline should be followed with close questioning about current disease activity and onset of new symptoms.

Fecal occult blood test: For asymptomatic children, stool should be monitored yearly with a fecal-occult blood reagent (e.g., Hemocult) for the presence of occult blood. The results should usually be negative in children with inactive disease. Some children with IBD always carry a trace of blood in their stool. Children whose stools are routinely normal but have a positive occult blood result should be assessed more carefully for indications of increased disease activity and anemia.

Chemistries: Children taking cyclosporine, azathioprine, or 6-MP should have renal (i.e., blood urea nitrogen and creatinine levels) and liver function studies (i.e., fractionated bilirubin, aspartate aminotransferase, alanine aminotransferase, and alkaline phosphatase values) monitored at least every 4 months throughout therapy. Liver function studies should be assessed every year in otherwise asymptomatic children with IBD. Children with CD should also have albumin levels checked yearly.

Lactose intolerance: The diagnosis of lactose intolerance may be made empirically by eliminating lactose-containing products from the diet and monitoring for changes in symptoms such as cramping, distention, and diarrhea. The diagnosis may also be made by the breath hydrogen test. Clinicians may also do a cursory screen for lactose intolerance by testing stool for reducing substances or testing the pH of the stool. An acidic pH (i.e., 6.0 or less) could be indicative of lactose intolerance.

Neurologic examination: Children who are being treated with metronidazole should be assessed for peripheral neuropathy at each visit.

Radiologic studies: Children with CD or those treated with long-term corticosteroids, should have their bone mineral density assessed by means of DEXA scanning.

Endoscopy: Endoscopy may be performed during times of disease exacerbation, and routine colonoscopy should be performed in children with UC starting 10 years after diagnosis.

Common Illness Management

Differential Diagnosis (Box 26-3)

The symptoms of IBD and its associated problems vary. Symptoms of common childhood illnesses may be difficult to differentiate from exacerbations of a child's underlying disease process. GI symptoms will most likely concern or alarm the child, family, and primary care provider. An index of disease activity for some—but not all—children is the ESR, which may sometimes help to clarify a child's symptoms. Because this value is a nonspecific indicator of systemic inflammation, however, it is not a specific indicator of IBD activity.

Intercurrent illnesses, such as a viral or bacterial gastroenteritis or another illness that must be

---

Box 26-3

Differential Diagnosis

Diarrhea
Rule out flare-up of disease; obtain cultures

Abdominal Pain
Rule out flare-up of disease, gastritis, fulminant colitis, and obstruction

Vomiting
Rule out flare-up of disease, gastritis; assess for obstruction

Skeletal Complaints
Rule out arthritic manifestations of the disease (i.e., sacroiliitis, ankylosing spondylitis, peripheral arthritis), aseptic necrosis of the femoral head, vertebral compression fractures, and osteoporosis

---

treated with antibiotics, may contribute to flare-ups of a child's IBD. These illnesses may result from the alteration of the normal flora of the bowel (i.e., usually a predominance of *Clostridium difficile*) after antibiotic therapy.

Diarrhea: Children with IBD have bouts of gastroenteritis similar to those of their peers and family members. A child's physical examination and history should include an evaluation of any IBD-like symptoms, including the presence of any blood, pus, or mucus in the stool; cramping or urgency associated with bowel movements; weight loss or anorexia; and any symptoms that might be extraintestinal manifestations of the disease. A child's abdomen should be closely examined for any change. Stool cultures should always be obtained because *Yersinia, Campylobacter,* and *Shigella* organisms, as well as *C. difficile,* may mimic IBD. Children should be treated for any identified pathogen. Any child with prolonged symptoms, significant hematochezia (with no identified pathogen), or weight loss should be referred to the gastroenterology team.

Abdominal pain: Children with abdominal pain should be examined for any changes that might indicate a progression of the disease or fulminant colitis or an obstruction. These children should be questioned about the similarity of their current pain to the pain experienced as a part of the IBD. Similarity to previous episodes, location of known disease, and history of accompanying symptoms that would indicate disease rather than influenza or another acute condition of the abdomen should guide practitioners. Many of the medications used to treat IBD may cause gastritis. Children will often present with epigastric pain or refluxlike symptoms. A child who appears ill with acute pain should be immediately referred to the gastroenterology team; less acute symptoms should be watched carefully, with referral if the symptoms do not abate within 24 to 48 hours.

Vomiting: Vomiting in children with CD could indicate an obstruction. The history and physical examination should elicit information about distention, associated pain and its relation to meals and the nature of the emesis, and accompanying abdominal pain. As always, information about the child's bowel pattern and the nature of the stools should be gathered.

Skeletal complaints: Children who are receiving corticosteroid therapy are at increased risk for osteoporosis, aseptic necrosis of the hip, and spinal fractures. In addition, children with IBD are more likely to have peripheral arthritis, sacroiliitis, and ankylosing spondylitis. Children with IBD who complain of back or hip pain require radiologic examination to adequately assess these symptoms. When children with IBD complain of joint pain, they should be questioned about the presence of erythema or swelling. If joint involvement is a concern, these children should also be assessed for any increased disease activity.

Drug Interactions

Sulfasalazine potentiates the action of both oral-form hypoglycemia agents and may result in blood glucose values that are lower than anticipated. Corticosteroids also diminish the efficacy of oral hypoglycemic agents, resulting in blood glucose levels that are higher than desired (Bradbury and Mehl, 1989). Sulfasalazine potentiates the action of phenytoin (Dilantin), resulting in higher-than-expected blood values of this drug and inhibits absorption of digoxin (Lanoxin), resulting in decreased blood levels of this drug. Metronidazole and corticosteroids potentiate the action of warfarin (Coumadin), but azathioprine (Imuran) may inhibit

its effect. Increased prothrombin time has also been reported in children taking warfarin and olsalazine (Dipentum) simultaneously. Metronidazole has a disulfiram (Antabuse) type of reaction when an individual ingests alcohol or alcohol-containing elixirs during drug therapy. Phenytoin and phenobarbital increase the elimination of metronidazole, but cimetidine decreases its clearance. Individuals taking lithium may experience elevations in lithium levels if they start taking metronidazole. Their lithium levels should be checked carefully to avoid toxicity. Increased bone marrow suppression has been noted in some individuals taking trimethoprim-sulfamethoxazole while on 6-MP therapy (Physicians' Desk Reference, 1998). Corticosteroids also diminish the efficacy of oral hypoglycemic agents, resulting in blood glucose levels that are higher than desired (Bradbury and Mehl, 1989).

Developmental Issues

Sleep Patterns

Children who are taking corticosteroids twice daily may feel agitated or euphoric at bedtime and may have difficulty sleeping. Dosage times may be shifted somewhat to alleviate this problem. Once the dose is decreased, a single dose may be given in the morning. Children experiencing a flare-up of disease or whose disease is under poor control may be troubled by the need to use the bathroom often during the night, which may make it difficult for them to feel well rested and refreshed in the morning.

Toileting

Because most children are diagnosed with IBD after they have usually accomplished toilet training, families of children with IBD do not typically face this issue. For children who are not toilet-trained, however, it is preferable to wait to start toilet training until the disease is quiescent and the character of bowel movements are as close to normal as possible.

Incontinence is experienced by many individuals with IBD; for children who have frequent bowel movements accompanied by urgency, the fear of this occurrence is ever-present. Children and families should be assisted in planning to prevent or handle such eventualities in a low-key way. In the context of an overview of a child's condition and its implications, the possibility of incontinence occurring should be shared with the school nurse and classroom teachers, who may make plans to ensure that incidents will be handled with sensitivity and that the child may retain as much control and dignity as possible. Classroom teachers should be encouraged to move the child's seat closer to the door and to liberalize bathroom privileges so that he or she may leave the room unobtrusively. Primary care providers may suggest that an extra change of clothing be kept in the child's locker or the nurse's office. Reminders to use the bathroom before leaving home and at regular intervals may also help to reduce the occurrence of potentially embarrassing episodes.

Management styles vary among practitioners with respect to the use of antispasmodic agents for the relief of chronic diarrhea in children with mild IBD. Drugs such as loperamide (Imodium) or diphenoxylate with atropine (Di-Atro) may be used cautiously in controlling symptoms during daytime activities (Kirschner, 1996)

Discipline

Behavioral expectations for children with IBD are similar to those for their unaffected peers. One area of concern may be the issue of compliance for children who are responsible or are assuming responsibility for their treatment regimen. Children in whom IBD remains in remission may not perceive the need for their medications because they may essentially be asymptomatic and feeling well. The concept of remission and disease being present but not discernible is difficult for school-aged children or early adolescents to master. Because a large percentage of children diagnosed with IBD are in early to middle adolescence, rebellion and testing are normal developmental issues. For adolescents with IBD, medications and treatment regimens can become a battleground for testing their independence. Primary care providers can help families identify ownership of responsibility for disease management. A particular risk facing children and adolescents with IBD are the hazards of abrupt discontinuation of steroid medications. In addition to a recurrence of IBD related symptoms, children are at risk for adrenal crisis. Adolescents who are responsible for their own medication regimens, as

well as their parents, should be educated about the significant risks associated with abruptly stopping their steroids.

Child Care

Parents of children with IBD should be encouraged to use the same guidelines for choosing child care arrangements as for their well children. Because the onset of IBD most commonly occurs in childhood, the increased risk of diarrheal illness secondary to diaper-changing areas and daycare providers handling food does not often need to be addressed by these families. If a child becomes infected, the illness should be promptly treated and the child monitored for signs of exacerbation of the disease. The overriding philosophy, however, is not to unduly isolate a child from the normal activities of daily living.

Schooling

Children with CD and UC are as able to achieve in the classroom as their unaffected peers. Similar to many children with chronic conditions, children with IBD must juggle treatment schedules and deal with stigma, pain, fatigue, and—occasionally frequent or long school absences. Academic performance may ultimately reflect a child's struggle to overcome these hurdles.

The nature of the disease processes and treatment regimens often set children with IBD apart from their peers in significant ways. These ways include the Cushingoid faces of children receiving corticosteroid therapy, the need for embarrassing treatments such as the instillation of rectal medications, and the use of nocturnal nasogastric feedings or restrictive diets. The isolation felt by children experiencing these treatments may cause them to limit participation in activities that enrich the school experience. Alternatively, these children may choose not to comply with treatment regimens in an effort to "fit in." This behavior may set up a cycle of disease exacerbation and escalation of therapy that may concomitantly affect a child's academic achievement, reinforcing the child's sense of isolation. Sensitivity to these issues, creative problem solving, and anticipatory guidance by the primary care provider support the child and family in achieving as normal a lifestyle as possible. An issue often faced by individuals with IBD is the common misunderstanding by lay people and some of those in the medical community that IBD is a psychologic disease. A primary role of health care providers is to educate school personnel and other significant adults in the child's life (e.g., club leaders, coaches, and daycare providers).

Sexuality

Adolescence is a time when concerns about body image, interpersonal relationships, and plans for the future are paramount. Therefore it is not unusual that adolescents or young adults with IBD are concerned about the effect this diagnosis might have on their appeal as a sexual partner, their ability to perform sexually, and their fertility. The significant changes in appearance that adolescents with IBD must withstand often include the late onset of puberty, weight gain, and acne—all of which contribute to their feelings of self-consciousness and stigmatization. Individuals with CD frequently have stomas or perianal involvement, which is often disfiguring and may also affect their feelings of sexual attractiveness or acceptability to another person. Positive feelings of self-worth and a sense of acceptance must be conveyed to adolescents with IBD. The option of joining a network of other adolescents with common concerns should be offered whenever possible. Formal organizations or casual social gatherings may provide opportunities for teens and families to obtain support and acceptance.

Sulfasalazine has been shown to cause infertility in men, a decrease in sperm count, dysmotility, and malformation. These effects have been shown to be reversible, however, when men stop taking sulfasalazine for 3 months (Physician's Desk Reference, 1998). There have been no reports of infertility in men receiving the newer, oral 5-ASA preparations (Ogorek and Fisher, 1991). Neither UC or CD increases infertility in women with inactive disease. Some studies have indicated that women with CD have higher rates of infertility than control populations. It is believed that the most common cause of infertility in women with CD is the activity of the disease. Other factors include poor nutritional status, rectovaginal fistulas, and fear of becoming pregnant. Pelvic scarring is thought to be the cause of infertility in only a small percentage of individuals (Burakoff, 1995).

The outcome of pregnancy in women with IBD approximates that of the general population, but some researchers have found a somewhat higher incidence of prematurity in infants born to mothers with IBD than in the general population (Burakoff, 1995).

Pregnancy does not increase the likelihood of a relapse of either UC or of CD. In two thirds of all women with active IBD at conception, the disease remains active or worsens during pregnancy.

Surgical resection for CD or UC appears to affect neither fertility nor the outcome of pregnancy. Men who have undergone colectomy with ileostomy or one of the other continent ileostomy procedures have a low risk of impotence as a complication of the surgical procedure (Burakoff, 1995).

Transition to Adulthood

Individuals with IBD do not typically require a specialized environment or assistance with activities of daily living. The embarrassing nature of many of the required medical therapies and symptoms of active disease make private living facilities most desirable for many individuals with IBD. Practitioners may help individuals to secure such accommodations.

There are no reports of specialized programs to transition adolescents with IBD to adult care. Many primary care providers have an informal policy of caring for their adolescent clients with IBD until they have weathered most of the anticipated developmental crises of late adolescence. It is best to wait to make this transition until a time when the individual's disease is quiescent.

Special Family Concerns and Resources

Families of children with IBD, similar to families of children with other chronic conditions, may focus on the child's symptoms and treatment regimen. In the case of the families dealing with IBD, however, this often means disclosing such private and potentially embarrassing issues as toileting and personal hygiene. The invasion of privacy felt by the child may become a source of stress for the entire family. Common concerns shared by children with IBD include personal appearance, physical endurance, and diet and their ability to fit in when sharing a meal or snacks with friends and family.

These issues are magnified as these children enter adolescence and seek increased independence from their families and become increasingly self-conscious and concerned about body image and function. Poor communication and distrust between parent and child about disease activity and compliance with treatment regimens may result. If these children can become relatively independent in disease management before this difficult time, they and their families may develop confidence and trust in one another, perhaps alleviating or avoiding some of these conflicts.

IBD may affect children of many ethnic and religious backgrounds at a wide range of ages and with varied clinical presentations and severity. When cultural or religious practices focus on food and special dietary practices, these children may feel conflicted if disease activity makes some foods difficult to tolerate. Other than during times of disease activity, it is not typically recommended that children limit their diet. Children should be encouraged to maintain a diet as unrestricted and palatable as possible to encourage adequate caloric intake to promote optimal growth and development. Health care team members' sensitivity about dietary issues relating to both everyday life and special celebrations or religious observances is important. Practitioners should work in partnership with the family and child to develop a flexible plan of care that incorporates individual cultural concerns, such as religious feasts or times of fasting.

Organizations

Crohn's and Colitis Foundation of America, Inc
386 Park Ave S, 17th Floor
New York, NY 10016-8804
(800) 932-2423; (212) 685-3440
www.CCFA.org; info@ccfa.org

The Crohn's and Colitis Foundation of America (CCFA) is an organization with many chapters across the country that supports research and provides education and support for its members and for members of the community. Individuals with IBD and their families are encouraged to join and attend meetings and educational offerings. Many chapters have subcommittees that specifically deal with issues related to the needs of children with IBD and their families. The CCFA also publishes educational books, pamphlets, and newsletters written for the lay public. Professional memberships are available.

Summary of Primary Care Needs for the Child with Inflammatory Bowel Disease

HEALTH CARE MAINTENANCE

Growth and development

Growth failure is a common problem for children with IBD but is more commonly seen in CD than UC.

Growth parameters are important to measure and graph at each primary care visit.

Cognitive abilities are unimpaired by IBD.

Diet

No special diet is recommended. Referral to a nutritionist at time of diagnosis is recommended. Some children may be lactose intolerant, particularly when disease is active. Some children during active disease may have less pain on a diet low in roughage. Adequate caloric intake is essential for growth.

If growth retardation has occurred, supplemental diet preparations may be beneficial.

Travel

No special safety recommendations are necessary for a child with inactive disease.

Children with osteoporosis should not participate in contact sports.

Individuals on metronidazole should be cautioned about an Antabuse type of reaction to alcohol.

Children on immunosuppressive therapy should wear medic alert bracelets.

Summary of Primary Care Needs for the Child with Inflammatory Bowel Disease

Immunizations

No change in the normal immunization protocol is indicated unless a child is taking maintenance doses of immunosuppressive agents; in this case, no live vaccines should be administered, but immune globulin may be used with exposures.

Yearly influenza vaccine is recommended for children receiving immunosuppressants.

Take caution with travel, especially to tropical areas. Ova, parasites, and purity of water should be concerns.

Screening

Vision: Ophthalmic examination is necessary at each visit. Twice yearly ophthalmologist visits are recommended for a child taking maintenance doses of corticosteroids.

Hearing: Routine screening is recommended.

Dental: Routine care is adequate, but children taking cyclosporine are at increased risk for gingival hyperplasia.

Blood pressure: Routine screening is recommended; if a child is taking cyclosporine or corticosteroids, blood pressure should be measured at every visit.

Hematocrit: Hematocrit and hemoglobin values should be obtained yearly if a child is asymptomatic and has no history of anemia; otherwise a CBC should be obtained every 6 months or as necessary.

Urinalysis: Routine screening is recommended unless a child has a history of fistulas or abscesses.

Tuberculosis: Routine screening is recommended.

Condition-specific screening

Erythrocyte sedimentation rate: Check annually or as needed if a flare-up of disease is suspected.

Fecal occult blood test: Check stool yearly and with potential disease flare-ups.

Chemistries: Liver function studies should be monitored every year for an otherwise asymptomatic child with IBD. A child taking Dipentum, Asacol, or Pentasa should have renal functions studies monitored at least every 4 months. A child receiving cyclosporine, 6-MP, or azathioprine renal and liver function studies should be monitored every 4 months. A child taking 6-MP should have amylase and lipase levels tested every 4 months.

Lactose intolerance: Check as indicated.

Neurologic examination: Children receiving metronidazole should be assessed for paresthesias at each routine visit.

Bone mineral density: Screening in children with CD is recommended.

Surveillance endoscopy: There are new recommendations for annual or biannual colonoscopies.

COMMON ILLNESS MANAGEMENT

Differential diagnosis

Diarrhea: Rule out flare-up of disease, obtain cultures.

Abdominal pain: Rule out flare-up of disease, gastritis, fulminant colitis, and obstruction.

Vomiting: Rule out flare-up of disease and gastritis; assess for obstruction.

Skeletal complaints: Rule out arthritic manifestations of the disease (i.e., sacroileitis, ankylosing spondylitis, peripheral arthritis), aseptic necrosis of the femoral head, vertebral compression fractures, and osteoporosis.

DEVELOPMENTAL ISSUES

Sleep patterns

Children with IBD generally have no special needs; children receiving an evening dose of corticosteroids may have some difficulty sleeping. These children may also have some nighttime stooling, which interrupts sleep.

Continued

Summary of Primary Care Needs for the Child with Inflammatory Bowel Disease—cont'd

Toileting

Most children with IBD are diagnosed after toilet training has been accomplished. When toilet training is a concern, it may be suggested that toilet training be instituted when the disease activity is quiescent.

For older children with active disease, occasional incontinence may be an issue.

Antispasmodics may be used cautiously for daytime incontinence.

Discipline

Standard developmental counseling is advised; monitor adherence to treatment regimen.

Children and families should be educated on the hazards of discontinuing treatment.

Child care

Standard developmental counseling is advised.

Schooling

Children with IBD are as able to achieve in the classroom as their unaffected peers.

Frequent or prolonged absences may interfere with school performance.

School personnel must be educated about special issues related to IBD; any misunderstandings about a psychologic cause of IBD should be alleviated.

Sexuality

Self-esteem and body image issues are important to adolescents with IBD.

Adolescents may have late onset of puberty due to growth retardation.

Sulfasalazine may cause infertility in men while they are taking the drug.

Pregnancy outcomes are similar to those of the general population.

Transition to adulthood

Self-care responsibilities may be gradually taken on by adolescents. Specialized environments and assistance with activities of daily living are not typically required by young adults with IBD.

The transition to a provider specializing in care of adults is best done during periods of quiescent disease.

Special family concerns

Privacy issues regarding toileting are often difficult for children and families. Because IBD affects individuals of disparate backgrounds and varies in its clinical presentation and severity, care of a child with IBD should be individualized. The practitioner should be sensitive to the needs of children and families whose cultural or religious practices focus on food if dietary restrictions are indicated during periods of active disease.

References

Bernstein D and Rogers A. Malignancy in Crohn's disease, Am J Gastroenterology 91(3): 434-440, 1996.

Bousvaros A et al: Oral tacrolimus treatment of severe colitis in children, platform presentation at the American Gastroenterology Association meeting 1997, Gastroenterology, 112: PA941, 1997.

Bousvaros A, Wang A, and Leichtner A: Tacrolimus (FK-506) treatment of fulminant colitis in a child, J Pediatr Gastroenterol Nutr 23:329-333, 1996.

Bradbury K and Mehl B: Pharmacology focus: drug interactions, Foundation Focus, November 1989.

Burakoff R: Fertility and pregnancy in inflammatory bowel disease. In Kirsner JB and Shorter RC, editor): Inflammatory bowel disease, Baltimore, 1995, Williams & Wilkins.

Calkins BM and Mendeloff AI: The epidemiology of idiopathic inflammatory bowel disease. In Kirsner JB and Shorter RC, editors: Inflammatory bowel disease, Baltimore, 1995, Williams & Wilkins.

Centocor: Prescribing information for Remicade, Website: www.centocor.com, 1998.

Cohen MB et al: Controversies in pediatric inflammatory bowel disease: Inflammatory Bowel Diseases 4:203-227, 1998.

Colenda K and Grand R: Clinical manifestations of pediatric inflammatory bowel disease. In Kirsner JB and Shorter RC, editors: Inflammatory bowel disease, Baltimore, 1995, Williams & Wilkins.

Cuffari C et al: 6-Mercaptopuring metabolism in Crohn's disease: correlation with efficacy and toxicity, Gut 39:401-406, 1996.

Ekbom A et al: Ulcerative colitis and colorectal cancer, New Engl J Med, 323:1228-1233, 1990.

Evans CM, Beattie RM, and Walker-Smith JA: Inflammatory bowel disease in childhood. In Allan et al, editors: Inflammatory bowel diseases, ed 3, New York, 1997, Churchill-Livingstone.

Feagan BG et al: Methotrexate for the treatment of Crohn's disease, New Engl J Med, 332:292-297, 1995.

Grand RJ, Ramakrishna J, and Calenda KA: Inflammatory bowel disease in the pediatric patient, Gastroenterol Clin North Am 24:613-632, 1995.

Griffiths A et al: Slow-release 5-aminosalicylic acid therapy in children with small intestinal Crohn's disease, J Pediatr Gastroenterol Nutr 17:186-192, 1993.

Gryboski JD: Clostridium difficile in inflammatory bowel disease relapse, J Pediatr Gastroenterol Nutr 13:39, 1991.

Hanauer SB: Inflammatory bowel disease, New Engl J Med, 334:841-848, 1996.

Harper RH et al: The long-term outcome in Crohn's disease, Dis Colon Rectum 30:174-179, 1987.

Hyams JS: Extraintestinal manifestations of inflammatory bowel disease in children, J Pediatr Gastroenterol Nutr 19:7-21, 1994.

Hyams JS: Crohn's disease in children, Pediatr Clin North Am 43:255-277, 1996.

Hyams JS et al: Clinical outcome of ulcerative colitis in children, J Pediatr 129:81-88, 1996.

Kanof ME, Lake AM, and Bayless TM: Decreased height velocity in children and adolescents before the diagnosis of Crohn's disease, Gastroenterology 95:1523-1527, 1988.

Kirschner BS: Medical management of inflammatory bowel disease in children. In Kirsner JB and Shorter RC, editors: Inflammatory bowel disease, Baltimore, 1995, Williams & Wilkins.

Kirschner BS: Ulcerative colitis and Crohn's disease in children, Gastroenterol Clin North Am 24:99-117, 1995b.

Kirschner BS: Ulcerative colitis in children, Pediatr Clin North Am 43:235-254, 1996.

Kirschner BS: Safety of Azathioprine and 6-mercaptopuring in pediatric patients with inflammatory bowel disease, Gastroenterology 115:813-821, 1998.

Lashner BA et al: Passive smoking is associated with an increased risk of developing inflammatory bowel disease in children, Am J Gastroenterology 88: 356-359, 1993.

Leichtner AM: Aminosalicylates for the treatment of inflammatory bowel disease, J Pediatr Gastroenterol Nutr 21:245-252, 1995.

Lichtiger S et al: Cyclosporine in severe ulcerative colitis refractory to steroid therapy, New Engl J Med 330:1841-1845, 1994.

Loftberg R et al: Oral budesonide versus prednisolone in patients with active extensive and left-sided ulcerative colitis, Gastroenterology 110:1713-1718, 1996.

Loftus EV et al: Incidence and prevalence of Crohn's disease in Olmsted County Minnesota, 1970-1993, Gastroenterology 112:A1027, 1997 (abstract).

Logan RFA: Inflammatory bowel disease incidence: up, down, or unchanged? Gut 42:309-311, 1998.

Mack DR et al: Methotrexate in patients with Crohn's disease after 6-mercaptopuring, J Pediatr 132:830-835, 1998.

Markowitz J et al: Highly destructive perianal disease in children with Crohn's disease, J Pediatr Gastroenterol Nutr 21:149-153, 1995.

Markowitz J et al: Immunology of inflammatory bowel disease: summary of the proceedings of the subcommittee on immunosuppressive use in IBD, J Pediatr Gastroenterol Nutr 12: 411-423, 1991.

Mashako MNL et al: Crohn's disease lesions in the upper gastrointestinal tract: correlation between clinical, radiological, endoscopic, and histological features in adolescents and children, J Pediatr Gastroenterol Nutr 8:442-446, 1989.

Motil KJ et al: Growth failure in children with inflammatory bowel disease: a prospective study, Gastroenterology 105: 681-691, 1993.

Ogorek CP and Fisher RS: Current therapy for inflammatory bowel disease, Compr Ther 17:31-37, 1991.

Peter G, editor: American Academy of Pediatrics 1997 red book: report of the Committee on Infectious Disease, ed 24, Elk Grove Village, Ill., 1997, The Academy.

Physicians' Desk Reference, Montvale, New Jersey, 1998, Medical Economics Data Production Company.

Pigot F et al: Low bone mineral density in patients with inflammatory bowel disease, Dig Dis Sci 37:1396-1403, 1992.

Podolsky DK: Inflammatory bowel disease, part 2, New Engl J Med 325:1008-1016, 1991

Ramakrishna J et al: Combined use of cyclosporine and azathioprine or 6-mercaptopurine in pediatric inflammatory bowel disease, J Pediatr Gastroenterol Nutr 23(3):296-302, 1996.

Rankin G: Extraintestinal and systemic manifestations of inflammatory bowel disease, Med Clin North Am 74(1):39-50, 1990.

Retsky JD and Kraft SC: The extraintestinal manifestations of inflammatory bowel disease. In Kirsner JB and Shorter RC, editors: Inflammatory bowel disease, Baltimore, 1995, Williams & Wilkins.

Rutgeerts P et al: A comparison of budesonide with prednisolone for active Crohn's disease, New Engl J Med 331:842-845, 1994.

Ruemmele FM et al: Diagnostic accuracy of serological assays in pediatric inflammatory bowel disease, Gastroenterology 115:822-829, 1998.

Sachar DB: Maintenance therapy in ulcerative colitis and Crohn's disease, J Clin Gastroenterol 20:117-122, 1995.

Schmidt-Sommerfeld E, Kirschner, and Stephends: Endoscopic and histologic findings in the upper gastrointestinal tract of children with Crohn's disease, J Pediatr Gastroenterol Nutr 11:448-454, 1994.

Seidman EG et al: Nutritional therapy of Crohn's disease in childhood, Dig Dis Sci 32(suppl):82-88, 1987.

Sellman SPB and Hupertz: Crohn's disease presenting as suspected abuse, Pediatrics 97:272-274, 1996.

Semeao EJ et al: Vertebral compression fractures in pediatric patients with Crohn's disease, Gastroenterology 112:1710-1713, 1997.

Spahn JD and Kamada AK: Special considerations in the use of glucocorticoids in children, Pediatr Rev 16:266-272, 1995.

Targan SR et al: A short term study of chimeric monoclonal antibody cA2 to tumor necrosis factor α for Crohn's disease, New Engl J Med 337:1029-1035, 1997.

Tolia V: Crohn's disease: to feed or not to feed at night is the question, J Pediatr Gastroenterol Nutr 25:246-247, 1997.

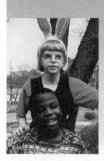

CHAPTER 27

Juvenile Rheumatoid Arthritis*

Gail R. McIlvain-Simpson

Etiology

Juvenile rheumatoid arthritis (JRA) is the official term used in the United States to describe a childhood form of chronic, idiopathic, inflammatory arthritis that differs in many respects from adult rheumatoid arthritis (RA) (Cassidy and Petty, 1995). Diagnostic criteria have been developed and are listed in Box 27-1. Alternative nomenclature, such as juvenile arthritis and juvenile chronic arthritis (preferred in Europe), are used by some researchers but are controversial because of their lack of specificity (Lawrence et al, 1998; Singsen, 1993).

The cause of JRA is unknown. Possible causes include infection, autoimmunity, and genetic predisposition. Although infections are known to cause multiple types of arthritis in children, specific infectious agents that trigger or serve as direct pathogens in JRA have not been isolated. The role of autoimmunity (i.e., immune response toward "self") in the pathogenesis of JRA is suggested by the very high prevalence of autoantibodies, such as antinuclear antibody (ANA) in JRA (Sherry et al, 1998).

JRA is thought to be a complex genetic or polygenic trait (Moroldo et al, 1997; Sherry et al, 1998). Genetics leads to arthritis by defects in immunoregulation. Immunoregulatory imbalances are thought to be important in pathogenesis, but which aberrations are primary and which are secondary is still not clear (Sherry et al, 1998). Studies of histocompatibility antigens have indicated that specific genetic factors exist for JRA

(Cassidy and Petty, 1995; Martin and Woo, 1999; Sherry et al, 1998). Human leukocyte antigen (HLA), the main histocompatibility complex (MHC) in humans, is a chromosomal region containing genes that encode cell surface molecules to facilitate cell-to-cell recognition, which is critical for a regulated immune response. HLA studies have confirmed that the clinical subgroups of JRA are distinct entities (see the discussion of recent and anticipated advances in this chapter) (Moroldo et al, 1997; Prieur et al, 1997). These subgroups can be differentiated on the basis of genetics and are clearly distinguishable from adult RA (Haas et al, 1998).

It is likely that certain genetic types code for surface receptors, which can "handle" foreign or autoantigens in a way that promotes synovial inflammation. The primary lesion in both JRA and RA is synovitis, which is the result of proliferation of synovial cells and bone marrow inflammatory cells (Van Den Berg, 1998). Synovial cells are extremely active immunologically and belong in two macrophage-fibroblast cell lines, which are commonly involved in diseases with an exaggerated immune response.

Trauma and psychosocial factors were thought to play a role in causing arthritis (Cassidy and Petty, 1995), but trauma is now thought to bring attention to—rather than cause—a swollen joint.

Incidence and Prevalence

JRA is the most common chronic rheumatic disease of childhood and also one of the most common chronic illnesses of childhood. The estimates of incidence and prevalence of JRA vary

---

*The authors would like to acknowledge the work done by Patricia M. Reilly on this chapter in the first edition of the book.

Box 27-1

Criteria for the Classification of Juvenile Rheumatoid Arthritis

1. Age at onset <16 years.
2. Arthritis (i.e., swelling or effusion, or presence of two or more of the following signs: limitation of range of motion, tenderness or pain on motion, and increased heat) in one or more joints.
3. Duration of disease ≥6 weeks.
4. Type of onset defined by type of disease in first 6 months:
   a. Polyarthritis: 5 or more inflamed joints.
   b. Oligoarthritis: <5 inflamed joints.
   c. Systemic: arthritis with characteristic fever.
5. Exclusion of other forms of juvenile arthritis.

From Cassidy JT and Petty PE: Textbook of pediatric rheumatology, ed 3, Philadelphia, 1995, W.B. Saunders.

Box 27-2

Clinical Manifestations

Chronic joint inflammation (i.e., swelling, pain, limited range of motion, heat)
Morning stiffness
Fatigue
Limp
Anemia

For specific subtype manifestations see Table 27-1.

because of variations in classification criteria (i.e., American College of Rheumatology [ACR] vs. European League Against Rheumatism [EULAR]) and unrepresentative populations from a variety of areas (i.e., population-based vs. specialty clinic vs. hospital-based). Prevalence is 40/100,000; incidence is 8/100,000 (Petty, 1998). Peterson and associates (1996) reported a cohort spanning 33 years with an incidence of 15/100,000 from 1960 to 1969; 14.1/100,000 from 1970 to 1979; and 7.8/100,000 from 1980 to 1993, with a specific decrease in pauciarticular and systemic subsets (Peterson et al, 1996). An estimated 70,000 children in the United States are currently affected with JRA (Lawrence et al, 1998).

Clinical Manifestations at Time of Diagnosis

JRA is a heterogeneous group of conditions characterized by the presence of chronic synovial inflammation in one or more joints (Figure 27-1 and Box 27-2). Signs of joint inflammation include swelling with heat, pain, and limited range of motion or erythema in one or more joints. Swelling is the result of an intraarticular effusion or hypertrophy of the synovial membrane. Synovitis may develop insidiously and exist for months or years without causing joint destruction, or may damage cartilage, subchondral bone, or other joint structures in a relatively short period of time (Laxer and Schneider, 1998; Prieur, 1998; Sherry et al, 1998). Clinical features range from mild synovitis in one joint with no systemic symptoms to severe disease in many joints with fever, rash, lymphadenopathy, and organomegaly. Common clinical manifestations in addition to the synovial inflammation include morning stiffness, limp, and fatigue. Stiffness in the morning or after rest is a hallmark of inflammatory disease. Children infrequently complain of pain and the manner in which they do so depends on their age and developmental level. Pain can be described during active or passive range of motion. In general, a child's activity may only be slightly limited.

JRA is a diagnosis of exclusion (Laxer and Schneider, 1998; Sherry et al, 1998). There are no pathognomonic signs, symptoms, or laboratory investigations. Manifestations at the time of onset and throughout the first 6 months of the disease determine classification into one of three major subtypes: systemic, polyarticular (i.e., >5 joints), and pauciarticular (i.e., <5 joints). These subtypes are based on the number of joints, variations in patterns and severity of joint disease, extraarticular manifestations, immunogenetic characteristics, age at onset, and sex of the child (Cassidy and Petty, 1995; Laxer and Schneider, 1998; Moroldo et al, 1997; Sherry et al, 1998) (Table 27-1).

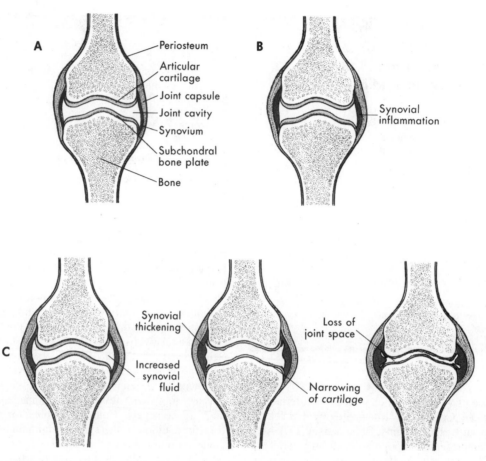

Figure 27-1   **A,** Normal diarthrodial joint. **B,** Early synovitis. **C,** Progressive destruction of an inflamed joint.

In systemic onset disease, systemic toxicity and extraarticular involvement may develop concurrently with arthritis or precede overt arthritis by 3 months, creating a diagnostic challenge. The most characteristic findings are high daily or twice daily spiking fevers (39° C), which return to baseline without intervention. These fevers are accompanied by a discrete, salmon-colored, evanescent, nonpruritic macular rash (3 to 5 mm in diameter with central clearing) that commonly occurs on the trunk and proximal extremities (Laxer and Schneider, 1998). The hallmark of systemic disease is a child who appears toxic during a fever with chills and has severe arthralgias and/or myalgias but feels better once the fever has resolved. Laboratory findings are

not diagnostic and show activation of an acute phase response such as an elevated sedimentation rate (i.e., often greater than 100 mm/hr by Westergren method), C-reactive protein and serum ferritin (Laxer and Schneider, 1998). In addition, hematologic abnormalities including thrombocytosis (usually greater than 500,000), neutrophilic leukocytosis (up to 50×10^9), and normochromic, normocytic anemia of chronic disease may occur (Cassidy and Petty, 1995; Laxer and Schneider, 1998). Other laboratory abnormalities may include hypoalbuminemia, elevated liver function studies, and hypergammaglobulinemia.

The onset of polyarticular JRA can be insidious or acute with progressive symmetric joint involve-

Table 27-1
Clinical Manifestations of Juvenile Arthritis

| Mode of Onset Immunogenetics | Incidence | | Sex (M:F) | Findings | | Prognosis |
	Frequency (% of all Cases)	Age		Articular	Extraarticular	
Systemic (variable # of joints) ANA − (+ in 10%) RF− (+ in 5%) HLA − DR4 HLA − DR5	20	**Any age** (no peak), mean age 4-6 (usually below age 5)	M = F (1:1)	**Multiple joint involvement;** knees, wrists, ankles, cervical spine, Hips, TMJ	**High spiking fever, rash,** hepatosplenomegaly, pericarditis pleuritis, abdominal pain, leukocytosis, anemia, thrombocytosis, mildly elevated LFTs, myalgias, Anorexia, uveitis rare	**Moderate to poor;** severe disabling polyarthritis (20%-50%); good (40% remits); all disease mortality in this group (2%-4%)
Polyarticular (≥5 joints) **Rheumatoid factor +** ANA + (75%) RF+ HLA-DR4	30	**Late childhood** (>8 years), predominantly adolescents	M < F (1:6)	**Symmetrical involvement** of large and small joints plus cervical spine. Early onset of erosive synovitis (unremitting).	**Mild fever, mild to moderate** hepatosplenomegaly and lymphadenopathy, other systemic symptoms, generally mild anemia, rheumatoid nodules, uveitis (5%)	**Poor to moderately good;** severe persistent chronic polyarthritis resembling adult RA
Rheumatoid factor − ANA + (25%) RF− HLA-DpW₃, HLA-DR8, HLA-DQW4		**Any age** (peak between 1-3 years of age)	M < F (1:3)	**Symmetrical involvement** of large and small joints	**Low grade fever,** mild or absent systemic symptoms, anemia, uveitis rare	**Severe** polyarthritis (10%)
Early onset Pauciarticular (<5 joints) ANA +(40%-75%) Homogeneous pattern RF− HLA-DR8, HLA-DR4 HLA-DRw6, HLA-DR5, HLA-PZW2	40-50	**Early childhood** (<5 years) (peak 1-2 years)	M < F (1:4)	**Asymmetrical large joint involvement** of knees, ankles, elbows. Hips and shoulder spared	**Chronic anterior uveitis,** systemic symptoms usually not present	**Excellent except for vision impairment,** 80% no functional disability
Late onset ANA− RF− HLA-B27 +		**Late childhood** (>8 years) of age)	M > F (10:1)	**Asymmetrical large joint involvement,** hips and SI joint involvement common later	**Acute uveitis,** occasional fever, anemia Enthesitis	**Up to ⅓ may** develop true ankylosing spondylosis

ANA, antinuclear antibody; *HLA,* human leukocyte antigen; *RF,* rheumatoid factor.

ment. Children with a positive rheumatoid factor (RF) (i.e., 15%) are the subgroup in JRA equivalent to those with classic adult RA. Adolescent females typically experience early onset of severe erosive arthritis, rheumatoid nodules, and a chronic course persisting into adulthood (Cassidy and Petty, 1995; Laxer and Schneider, 1998). Conversely, children with RF negative arthritis, which is much more common, exhibit less aggressive joint destruction but have widespread large and small joint involvement (Prieur, 1998). Laboratory findings include elevated or normal sedimentation rate, leukocyte count, and platelet count.

Arthritis of pauciarticular onset commonly develops in knees, ankles, or elbows, with shoulder and hip involvement being rare. Children with pauciarticular arthritis are not systemically ill, and nonarticular involvement is rare—except for the ANA-positive subgroup that is at high risk for developing chronic uveitis (Sherry et al, 1998).

JRA is a disease characterized by exacerbations and remissions. Exacerbations may occur during episodes of acute illness or stress, with the frequency and duration of flare-ups being unpredictable. It is difficult, particularly in the course of the disease, to predict when and how a child's disease will flare-up, but a pattern usually becomes clearer 1 year into the disease. Short flare-ups do not require a change in the medication regimen, but flare-ups lasting longer than 2 weeks may require adjustment of interventions. Although the criteria for remission vary among pediatric rheumatology centers, remission is commonly defined as no symptoms of active disease for at least 6 months after cessation of all medications.

Treatment (Box 27-3)

Ultimate goals of early diagnosis, therapy, and management are as follows: (1) to relieve joint pain and inflammation; (2) to minimize joint destruction, deformity, and systemic complications; (3) to maintain musculoskeletal function; (4) to promote and maximize growth and development; (5) to support the psychologic well-being of the child and family; and (6) to help the child be as independent as possible in activities of daily living until the disease is quiescent or in spontaneous remission. These goals are best achieved with a coordinated, multidisciplinary team approach, in-

---

Box 27-3

Treatment

Nonsteroid antiinflammatory drugs (NSAIDs)
Glucocorticoids
Immunosuppressives and/or cytotoxics
Intravenous immunoglobulins
Nutrition
Occupational therapy
Orthoses
Physical therapy
Psychologic support
Slow-acting antirheumatic drugs (SAARD) or disease-modifying antirheumatic drugs (DMARD)
Surgery
Unconventional therapies

---

cluding a pediatric rheumatologist, advanced practice nurse, primary care provider, occupational and physical therapists, and social worker. Consultations with an orthopedist, ophthalmologist, psychologist, dietitian, and orthodontist should be sought as indicated. The family and child should be central components of this team.

Medications

The trend of pediatric rheumatology is to treat JRA earlier and more aggressively, thereby limiting the amount of disability a child may carry into adulthood (Lehman, 1993; Levinson and Wallace, 1992; Singsen and Rose, 1995). Specific pharmacologic agents used to treat JRA are identified in Table 27-2. Other nonsteroidal antiinflammatory drugs (NSAIDs) have gradually replaced salicylates as the treatment of choice because NSAIDs have an easier dosing schedule (i.e., two or three times per day vs. four times per day) and have not been associated with Reye syndrome. The predominant adverse reaction is gastrointestinal irritation, so these medications should be taken with food (Taketomo, Hodding, and Kraus, 1996-1997).

The second group of medications has been referred to as both slow-acting antirheumatic drugs (SAARD) or disease-modifying antirheumatic drugs (DMARD). Medications within this group are gold (oral and injectable), hydroxychloroquine,

Table 27-2
Medications Commonly Used in Treatment of Juvenile Rheumatoid Arthritis

Drug	Trade Name	Daily Dose (mg/kg/day)	Side Effects	Suggested Monitored Parameters
Nonsteroidal Antiinflammatory Drugs				
Salicylates:				
Acetylsalicylate acid	Aspirin	75-100 mg/kg/day (qid), maximum 4 gm/day pediatrics	GI irritation (e.g., abdominal pain/anorexia) and blood loss, mild hepatitis, hematuria, proteinuria, salicylism (e.g., tinnitus, hyperpnea, behavioral change), bleeding (e.g., epistaxis and bruising), anemia, oral ulcers, dental caries, allergic reaction, peptic ulcers.	CBC, platelet count, UA, SGOT and SGPT levels 2 and 6 weeks after initiation of treatment and every 2-3 months. Occult blood in stools as needed. Salicylate levels (5-10 days after initiation). Therapeutic range: 20-30 mg/dl 2 hours after dose. Discontinue 3-5 days after exposure to influenza/varicella.
Proprionic acid derivatives:				
Naproxen	Naprosyn	15-20 mg/kg/day (bid)	Side effects common to all nonsalicylate NSAIDs: GI irritation and blood loss, proteinuria, hematuria, anemia, fluid retention, headache, fatigue, dizziness, mild hepatitis, peptic ulcer, skin manifestations (i.e., pseudoporphyria with Naprosyn).	*Initially:* CBC, platelet count, UA, creatinine, BUN, SGOT, SGPT, then yearly.
Ibuprofen	Advil, Motrin, Nuprin	20-30 mg/kg/day bid/tid)		
Pyrrolealkanoic acid derivative:				
Tolmetin sodium	Tolectin	20-35 mg/kg/day (tid), maximum 1800 mg/day	As listed for Proprionic acid; false positive urine test for protein.	As listed for Proprionic acid.
N-Phenylanthranilic acid derivative:				
Diclofenac sodium	Voltaren	2-3 mg/kg/day (bid/tid)	As listed for Proprionic acid.	As listed for Proprionic acid.

Continued

Table 27-2
Medications Commonly Used in Treatment of Juvenile Rheumatoid Arthritis—cont'd

Drug	Trade Name	Daily Dose (mg/kg/day)	Side Effects	Suggested Monitored Parameters
Nonsteroidal Antiinflammatory Drugs—cont'd				
Indoleacetic acid derivative:				
Indomethacin	Indocin	2-4 mg/kg/day (bid/tid) (qhs)	*More severe* headache, dizziness, GI irritation.	As listed for Proprionic acid.
Slow-Acting Antirheumatic Drugs				
Aurolate		0.5-1.0 mg/kg/wk (after initial test dose) injectable maintenance dose for 20 weeks; .5 mg/kg/wk (oral preparation, 6-9 mg/day)	Nitritoid reaction, hematuria, proteinuria, stomatitis, exfoliative dermatitis, bone marrow suppression, photosensitivity, diarrhea.	CBC, platelet count, UA, and liver function tests before initial dose, CBC, platelet count and UA before each injection. Weekly with oral preparation. Initially, then q 2-4 weeks thereafter.
Aurothioglucose	Solganal			
Auranofin	Ridaura			
D-Penicillamine	Cuprimine, Depen	3 mg/kg/day initially (qd-qid); slowly increased to maximum 10 mg/kg/day (750 mg/day)	Dermatitis, proteinuria, rash, thrombocytopenia, lupuslike syndrome, iron deficiency anemia, vitamin B_6 deficiency nausea, vomiting, diarrhea, alteration in taste, headache, dizziness.	CBC, platelet count, UA, LFTs initially, then monthly.
Sulfasalazine	Azulfidine	*Initial therapy:* 40-60mg/kg/day in 3-6 doses, *Maintenance therapy:* 30 mg/kg/day in divided doses	Hypersensitivity reactions, anorexia, headache, nausea, vomiting, oligospermia, photosensitivity, blood dyscrasias, hematuria, crystalluria, folic acid deficiency, orange discoloration of urine and skin.	CBC, UA monthly; SGOT SGPT, BUN, creatinine periodically.
Hydroxychloroquine	Plaquenil	3-7 mg/kg/day (daily or bid)	GI symptoms, rashes, headache, myopathy, decreased concentration, blurred vision, corneal deposits, keratopathy, retinopathy, neuropathy.	Ophthalmologic exam and central field testing exam initially, then every 6 months. CBC every 6 months.

sulfasalazine, d-penicillamine, and methotrexate and are used when the disease is severe, persistent, or progressive, despite the use of NSAIDs. A widely used medication within this category is low-dose methotrexate, which is efficacious and well-tolerated in the treatment of JRA (Giannini et al, 1992; Hunt et al, 1997; Laxer and Schneider, 1998; Singsen and Rose, 1995; Wallace, 1994).

Glucocorticoids (orally or intravenously as a pulse or bolus) are used in one of the following ways: (1) as a therapeutic bridge before disease control is obtained with other medications; (2) as an agent to control serious systemic features; (3) as an intraarticular injection in persistently inflamed joints; and (4) as an antiinflammatory in the case of primary NSAID intolerance (Laxer and Schneider, 1998; Prieur, 1998; Sherry et al, 1998; Singsen and Rose, 1995). Due to many adverse side effects (e.g., striae, Cushingoid features, hirsutism, weight gain, reduced growth velocity, and osteopenia), efforts are made to limit their use to the shortest possible duration. If required for over 3 months, glucocorticoids must be tapered to an alternate-day schedule if possible.

Immunosuppressive and cytotoxic agents are used for severe illness resistant to the aforementioned forms of therapy (Laxer and Schneider, 1998; Singsen and Rose, 1995). These medications include chlorambucil, cyclophosphamide, azathioprine, and cyclosporine A and are associated with significant short-term and long-term complications such as infertility, mutagenesis, and oncogenesis; therefore their use is clinically limited (Laxer and Schneider, 1998; Singsen and Rose, 1995).

Intravenous immunoglobulins have been used in systemic disease in an attempt to reduce the use of steroids, thereby reducing their toxicity (Laxer and Schneider, 1998). A study by the Pediatric Rheumatology Collaborative Study Group shows that individuals receiving intravenous immunoglobulins did not have a statistically significant improvement when compared with a placebo group, but there was a trend toward overall improvement in the individuals treated with them (Silverman et al, 1994).

Therapies

Physical and occupational therapy evaluations are critical to successful management of children with JRA. Goals of therapy include the following: (1) developing an individualized exercise program (to increase range of motion, endurance, decrease pain, and increase strength); (2) teaching principles of joint protection and energy conservation; (3) fabricating splints; (4) recommending modalities and assistive devices; (5) analyzing the effect of limitations on any current function; and (6) suggesting appropriate recreational activities (Laxer and Schneider, 1998; Scull, 1994). Children with arthritis, along with family members and/or caregivers, are then encouraged to implement the recommended program of therapies at home. Although exercise programs carry potential risks for injury or overuse, preliminary evidence suggests that well-designed, individualized conditioning programs may physically and psychologically benefit children with arthritis (Scull and Athreya, 1995; Klepper and Giannini, 1994). These programs have the potential to increase muscular strength, endurance, and stamina for daily activities without aggravating the joint disease (Klepper and Giannini, 1994). Periodic consultations with therapists are arranged as needed for early recognition of potential problems and analyzation of the effect of any current limitation on present function (Scull, 1994). Depending on their level of involvement, children may need formal therapy 2 to 3 times per week.

Orthoses

Orthoses are used with both the upper and lower extremities. Splints can be useful adjuncts to therapy to rest a joint experiencing a disease flare-up, as well as to maintain or regain motion in an involved joints. Three categories of splints are resting splints, corrective splints, and functional splints (Lindsley, 1999). Resting splints are used during active disease. Night resting wrist splints in a cock-up position (i.e., 20 degrees of wrist extension) are the most common. Resting knee splints are used to help reduce knee flexion contractures in children with pauciarticular JRA. Examples of corrective splints include dynamic wrist splints, knee splints that are periodically adjusted, or serial casting. Functional splints include supportive wrist splints that can be worn during the day, ankle-foot orthoses, molded shoe inserts, and heel cups.

Nutrition

Nutrition counseling is particularly recommended for children who are systemically ill or on long-term steroids. Children with JRA who have or are at risk for developing protein-energy malnutrition can benefit from consultation with a dietitian who can instruct the family on nutrient fortification methods to maximize the child's own food intake and by helping direct enteral feeds if needed (Henderson and Lovell, 1991; Lovell and Woo, 1998). Nutrition education and dietary revisions are also important to help minimize the excessive weight gain associated with the initiation and continuation of corticosteroids.

Psychologic Support

The chronicity of JRA and its inherent unpredictability and pain lead to many situations in which a psychologist may be helpful. For families and children, learning to cope with the emotional difficulties and pain involved in rheumatic disease may need to involve resources outside the realm of family members, friends, and peers. In these situations, consultation with a psychologist knowledgeable about children with chronic conditions can be very useful.

Surgery

Orthopedic surgery plays a limited but valuable role in the management of children with JRA. Relieving pain, overcoming loss of motion, and correcting deformities are the main reasons for a child to undergo surgery. Conversely, age and growth potential are the two main factors supporting a conservative approach. Arthroscopy can be used to perform an intraarticular exam, synovial biopsy, or synovectomy (Laxer and Schneider, 1998). For a child with functional impairment or secondary mechanical problems, soft tissue releases, osteotomies, posterior capsulotomy and tendon lengthening may be performed (Laxer and Schneider, 1998; Prieur, 1998). Prophylactic synovectomies are controversial and their long-term benefits are limited but can be effective in selected cases (Sherry et al, 1998). As a child approaches adulthood and reaches bone maturity, reconstructive surgery plays a more vital role. Children with micrognathia may profit from a combined orthodontic and surgical approach to temporomandibular disease. There have been encouraging results in some children undergoing elongation procedures for the

mandible (Peterson et al, 1997). Total joint replacements (i.e., hip and knee) have been of great benefit in young adults with marked disability and pain (Cassidy and Petty, 1995; Drew, Cohen, and Witt, 1999; Swann, 1998). Total hip replacements have shown a major improvement in functional ability (Drew, Cohen, and Witt, 1999). The materials and methods of fixation have greatly improved. In two studies, 25% of the hips were revised after an average follow-up of 11.5 years, and 15% of the femoral components and 35% of acetabular components required revision for loosening after an average of 12 years follow-up (Chmell et al, 1997; Witt et al, 1991).

The anesthesiologist caring for children with JRA undergoing surgery should be aware that intubation may be challenging given potential limitations at the cervical spine and temporomandibular joint (TMJ). Children with atlantoaxial involvement may get cord compression with excessive flexion. The "sniffing position" (i.e., where the head is hyperextended and flexed) for intubation should best be avoided (Matti and Sharrock, 1998). Use of fiberoptic scopes and keeping the neck in a neutral position is recommended.

Children on long-term corticosteroids over 15 mg/day or 7.5 to 15 mg/day for 1 month should receive corticosteroids before surgery or intravenously during surgery for prophylaxis against adrenal insufficiency (Mackenzie and Sharrock, 1998). Prophylactic antibiotic coverage for surgery is also recommended for children with total joint replacements or taking corticosteroids (see Chapter 17 for the prophylactic schedule). Another preoperative consideration is to monitor a child's complete blood count and platelet count if there has been a history of anemia. If significant blood loss is anticipated, nonsteroidal antiinflammatory medications should be discontinued 7 to 10 days before surgery. If there is an arthritis flare-up due to this discontinuation, the child may need a short course of steroids to control the disease.

Unconventional Therapies

As a result of the chronicity, unpredictability, and sometimes relentless progression of the disease despite treatment, approximately 68% of parents with a child with JRA have used an unconventional therapy or unproved remedy (e.g., wearing copper bracelets or using herbal or nutritional supplements) (Tucker et al, 1996). It is important to foster trust and create an accepting environment where frustrations with conventional treatment can be aired and unproved remedies openly discussed. Primary care providers can help families differentiate between harmless and potentially harmful interventions, as well as help them evaluate the claimed efficacy of unconventional remedies (Ramos-Remus and Russell, 1997; Tucker et al, 1996). Only a few controlled clinical trials on a small number of these therapies have been done and most of the experience is from anecdotal experiences and is rarely consistently reproducible (Eisenberg, 1996). The potential risks include immune system suppression, interaction with prescribed medications, financial considerations, and the perceived strain on the provider-patient relationship (Ramos-Remus and Russell, 1997; Tucker, 1996).

Recent and Anticipated Advances in Diagnosis and Treatment

The most recent model of pathogenetic mechanism for JRA involves trimolecular complexes composed of an HLA product in macrophages, a T-cell receptor (TCR) in lymphocytes, and an antigen (Grom, Giannini, and Glass, 1994). The interplay of certain genetically determined elements of the trimolecular complex is thought to trigger the inflammatory process through local release of cytokines (i.e., tumor necrosis factor [TNF]). An interesting insight into the pathology of different subgroups in JRA has been attained by the measurement of serum and synovial fluid cytokines and their agonists and antagonists (Woo, 1997).

At the 1998 National Scientific Meeting of the American College of Rheumatology, preliminary information on a new medication (etanercept [Enbrel]) was released. This medication is a soluble form of tumor necrosis factor (TNF) receptor that can bind specifically to TNF and blocks its interaction with cell surface TNF receptors, thereby inhibiting the inflammatory effects of this cytokine. Preliminary studies are encouraging (Moreland et al, 1997).

Associated Problems (Box 27-4)

Skeletal Abnormalities

In JRA, the growing skeleton undergoes unique deformities due to systemic and local growth disturbances. Studies of the acquisition of peak skeletal mass in children with and without JRA have led to the following tentative conclusions in children with JRA: (1) the appendicular skeleton is predominately affected; (2) a failure to develop adequate bone mineralization characterized by a failure of bone formation is almost universal in children with JRA; and (3) a failure to undergo the normal increase in bone mass during puberty is common in children with JRA, thereby reducing their potential to achieve an adequate peak skeletal mass and the onset of accelerated skeletal maturation with puberty (Cassidy and Hillman, 1997). Disease severity is a crucial factor in the association between bone mineralization in JRA and low bone formation (Pepmueller et al, 1996). Different subgroups of juvenile chronic arthritis were shown to affect

---

Box 27-4

Associated Problems

Skeletal abnormalities
- Joint deformities, overgrowth, or undergrowth
- Cervical spine fusion C2-C3
- Atlantoaxial subluxation or instability
- Loss of extension and rotation
- Scoliosis
- Hip limitations, erosions, or protrusions
- Knee flexion contractures
- Leg-length discrepancies
- Feet: valgus of hindfoot and/or Hallux valgus
- Gait disturbances

Micrognathia (e.g., mandibular undergrowth, dental malocclusion)

Chronic uveitis

Anemia of chronic disease

Problems common with systemic onset
- Hepatosplenomegaly
- Elevated liver enzymes
- Lymphadenopathy
- Pericarditis
- Pleuritis
- Nutritional problems
- Protein-energy malnutrition

growth differently. Those with systemic onset experienced growth failure much more often than those with pauciarticular onset disease (Laxer and Schneider, 1998; Pepmueller et al, 1996).

Chronic hyperemia in an inflamed joint is thought to stimulate accelerated maturation of the epiphyseal plates resulting in skeletal overgrowth of the extremity (Prieur, 1998). This process is characteristically seen in children with early onset pauciarticular disease who have unilateral knee involvement, bony enlargement of the medial femoral condyle, valgus deformity, and increased leg length in the affected knee (Lovell and Woo, 1998; Sherry et al, 1998). Conversely, in children with older onset (i.e., over 9 years of age) of pauciarticular disease, premature epiphyseal closure can result in a shorter leg on the involved side (Lovell and Woo, 1998). Bone and cartilage erosions are late manifestations of polyarticular disease, but there is potential for cartilage regeneration (Prieur, 1998). Characteristic abnormalities of the cervical spine in systemic and/or polyarticular disease include apophyseal joint space narrowing, irregularity and undergrowth of the vertebral bodies, fusion—especially at C2-C3, and atlantoaxial subluxation or instability leading to impingement on the cord and the brainstem (Cassidy and Petty, 1995; Lovell and Woo, 1998; Prieur, 1998). Stiffness and pain of the cervical spine with rapid loss of extension and rotation are common early findings in polyarticular JRA (Laxer and Schneider, 1998). Children with JRA have been found to have structural scoliosis more often than healthy children due to postural curves associated with asymmetrical involvement of the lower limb joints causing pelvic tilting (Swann, 1998).

Hip pathology occurs in 50% of children with JRA, is almost always bilateral, and is usually associated with polyarticular arthritis. These children experience limitation of full flexion, abduction, and rotation as a result of iliopsoas and adductor spasm (Laxer and Schneider, 1998). In time, anatomical changes in the hip due to persistent inflammation may include femoral head overgrowth, decreased development of the femoral neck, and acetabular modifications with erosions or protrusions (Prieur, 1998). A compensatory lumbar lordosis occurs with a hip contracture. Flexion contractures of the knees are common. Children with arthritis of the knee joint can develop valgus of the knee with compensatory valgus deformity of the hindfoot and varus of the forefoot (Prieur, 1998).

In addition to the foot deformities due to hip involvement, the foot itself is a complex joint with many articular surfaces. Subtalar joint involvement often results in a valgus deformity and, rarely, a varus deformity. Disturbances of gait and balance can occur as a result of retarded growth and development of the feet with active persistent inflammatory disease (Lindsley, 1999).

Micrognathia

Arthritis-induced abnormalities of the TMJ result in mandibular undergrowth, micrognathia, and dental malocclusion. Mechanical feeding problems can occur in 18% to 30% of affected children as a result of their TMJ arthritis (Prieur, 1998). The highest percentage of TMJ abnormalities (e.g., pain, tenderness, or crepitus) are found in the polyarticular subgroup. Combined orthodontic and reconstructive surgical procedures may improve function, decrease pain, and improve appearance in children with TMJ disease (Cassidy and Petty, 1995; Laxer and Schneider, 1998).

Uveitis

Uveitis (i.e., iridocyclitis) is a chronic, nongranulomatous inflammation that primarily affects the anterior uveal tract (i.e., iris and ciliary body) (Cassidy and Petty, 1995; Sherry et al, 1998). JRA-associated uveitis occurs in 13% to 34% of all children with JRA and is characterized by an insidious, asymptomatic, typically bilateral onset that infrequently precedes arthritis (Candell-Chalom et al, 1997). The pattern of remissions and exacerbations of this uveitis does not parallel articular disease (Sherry et al, 1998). Risk factors associated with developing uveitis include female gender, young age, antinuclear antibody (ANA) positivity, RF seronegativity, and pauciarticular onset. Slit-lamp examination by a pediatric ophthalmologist is required for early detection. Early and aggressive treatment with topical steroids and nonsteroidal ophthalmic drops (with or without a mydriatic drug), in addition to frequent ophthalmologic follow-up have been effective in preserving the vision of children without advanced disease. Poorly controlled or untreated uveitis results in ocular complications such as glaucoma, cataracts, band keratopathy, posterior synechiae, and loss of vision (Candell-Chalom et al, 1997). A surprising finding in a retrospective analysis of 760 children from four pediatric rheumatology centers revealed that those with uveitis who were ANA negative had complications twice as often as those who were ANA positive (Candell-Chalom et al, 1997).

Anemia

The anemia seen in JRA is called the anemia of chronic disease. Its pathogenesis is unclear, but its severity correlates with underlying disease activity and inflammation. This anemia usually presents with low iron and transferrin, as well as with an elevated serum ferritin, which does not typically respond to iron supplementation (Richardson et al, 1998). Children with poor nutrition or NSAID-induced gastrointestinal blood loss, however, may also develop iron deficiency anemia, resulting in microcytosis and hypochromia (Laxer and Schneider, 1998; Mulberg et al, 1993).

Problems Associated with Systemic Onset or Course

Systemic onset of JRA can be accompanied by significant extraarticular manifestations. Generalized lymphadenopathy and mild elevations in liver function studies occur in most children with active systemic disease. Pericarditis is a common cardiac finding, with its clinical presentation varying from asymptomatic pericarditis with mild pericardial effusion to severe, life-threatening cardiac involvement. Pleuritis may present with an acute flare-up and can occur alone or with pericarditis. In rare instances, two other serious conditions—amyloidosis and disseminated intravascular coagulation—can occur and are associated with significant mortality and morbidity (Laxer and Schneider, 1998). Nutritional problems are common in systemic JRA. Systemic illness with fever leads to decreased appetite and energy and poor nutrient intake (Lovell and Woo, 1998).

Prognosis

The prognosis for children with JRA depends on the type of disease onset and the course (Flato et al, 1998; Singsen and Rose, 1995). Different criteria for classification and remission, in addition to a lack of multidimensional methods to assess outcome, make a comparison of studies difficult. In a recent Norwegian study (Flato et al,1998) of 72 children with JRA and juvenile spondyloarthropathy over 10 years, remission occurred in 43 (i.e., 60%). This study also showed the following: (1) there were 44 (i.e., 60%) children with no disability on the childhood or adult Health Assessment Questionnaire; (2) there were 18 children (i.e., 25%) with joint erosions; (3) DMARDs were used in 49 children (i.e., 68%) after a disease duration of .8 years; and (4) children having active disease 5 years after onset was a predictor of disability (Flato et al, 1998). This study shows a more favorable course than previously reported (Flato et al, 1998). Early aggressive treatment, as well as including individuals with less severe disease, were thought to be partially responsible. Children with pauciarticular arthritis have a good prognosis for articular disease; 80% of these children have no musculoskeletal disability after 15 years of follow-up (Sherry et al, 1998). Their prognosis in regard to uveitis is less favorable, ranging from remission without sequelae to severe visual loss. Children having no or mild uveitis at diagnosis without posterior synechiae do significantly better that those with persistent uveitis and synechiae. Children with a polyarticular course have a poor prognosis for articular disease. Adolescent females presenting with a positive RF follow a course similar to those with adult onset RA having persistent erosive joint disease (Ansell, 1998). Children with systemic disease can have a monocyclic course with remission, a polycyclic course with exacerbations of systemic disease activity, or a course of persistent polyarticular arthritis without systemic features (Laxer and Schneider, 1998). These children are most prone to developing life-threatening complications, such as amyloidosis or acute hepatic failure. Progressive and destructive arthritis occurs in one third of these children, with this subgroup having the worse outcome of all children with JRA (Laxer and Schneider, 1998).

PRIMARY CARE MANAGEMENT

Health Care Maintenance

Growth and Development

Most children with mild JRA do not experience significant growth failure during the course of their disease, although periodic decreased growth velocity has been observed. Therefore monitoring heights and weights via the growth chart is important. In children with systemic or polyarticular JRA, linear growth is retarded during periods of active disease. Catch-up growth usually occurs during remission or with suppression of disease activity by therapy. Height returns to normal within 2 to 3 years if premature epiphyseal fusion has not occurred. A few children can have growth abnormalities that persist into adulthood. Despite good disease control, long-term treatment with cortisone is also associated with height growth delay.

Motor function is important in growth, development, and social interactions (Sherry et al, 1998). Gross motor delays or temporary regressions are not uncommon in children with JRA. For example, a child with JRA in one knee may have difficulty learning to skip. Age-appropriate physical activities for children with JRA are important as for any child and should be based on their capabilities and energy level. Children should be encouraged and allowed to participate in organized or team activities to their tolerance. Children with JRA can fatigue easily. Daily activities and participation in organized sports were significantly lower in children with JRA when compared with a control group of their peers (Henderson et al, 1995). Strategically planning activities to optimize children's participation in key activities that they enjoy is very helpful. For example, planning activities for one evening but leaving the next evening free allows a child to have rest periods. Fine motor skills are less likely to be delayed as long as the child is provided with toys and activities that encourage manipulation.

Limited mobility and decreased opportunities to actively interact with the environment place a child at risk for cognitive and social delays. Children with severe JRA often fall behind in acquiring hygiene, toileting, dressing, and feeding skills. Regression in performance of these skills is common during acute illness and may be sustained during remissions as a result of lowered parental expectations and continued reinforcement of a child's dependent behaviors. Functional limitations in children with arthritis can be assessed by the following different tools: the Childhood Health Assessment Questionnaire (CHAQ), the Juvenile Arthritis Functional Assessment Report (JAFAF), and the Juvenile Arthritis Self-Report Index (JASI) (Howe et al, 1991; Singh et al, 1994; Wright et al, 1994). Standard infant and early childhood assessment tools (e.g., the Bayley Scales and Denver Developmental Screening Test II) are of questionable value in evaluating delay in seriously affected children. An occupational and physical therapy team familiar with the effect of JRA on a child's overall development can be a valuable resource for primary care providers.

Diet

Nutritional problems are common in JRA. Factors contributing to the occurrence of these problems include increased inflammatory activity (i.e., hypercatabolism in systemic subgroup), anorexia, gastrointestinal side effects of medication, physical limitation, depression, poor food choices, and limited movement of the TMJ or upper extremities. In addition, increased weight gain can occur with corticosteroid use due to increased appetite and fluid retention. Of the children with JRA, 10% to 50% can have protein energy malnutrition (Henderson and Lovell, 1991). Hypoplasia of the mandible occurs in 20% to 30% of the children with JRA, resulting in maldevelopment of the teeth and difficulty swallowing. Children with arthritis in the upper extremities may have difficulty preparing meals or using utensils. A well-balanced diet should be encouraged to ensure adequate nutritional intake. Addition of a vitamin supplement may be recommended. Iron is not routinely recommended because the anemia of chronic disease has a multifactorial cause usually related to ongoing inflammation. Calcium intake should be evaluated and supplementation considered if dietary sources are insufficient—especially in the years following puberty (Lloyd et al, 1993). Evaluation by a dietitian will help to identify, treat, and monitor children at risk for dietary problems. The most popular unconventional dietary remedies for arthritis are avoiding nightshade vegetables (e.g., potatoes and eggplant) and acidic foods (e.g., tomatoes), diets with increased fish or fish oil, fasting, herbal remedies, and megavitamin therapy. There have been no specific diets, dietary restrictions, or supplements that have been effectively proven to treat JRA (Tucker et al, 1996). Given the current knowledge of JRA and diet, educating families about proper nutrition for a growing child with a chronic condition and evaluating potentially harmful dietary manipulations—especially those involving nutrient restrictions—are important responsibilities of the primary care provider.

Safety

Medication therapy is essential to the successful management of JRA. Education about medication safety is an important responsibility of the primary care provider. All medications must be kept in childproof containers out of reach of young children, which is especially important when older children assume responsibility for self-care (due to their limited grip strength, special grippers may be used to open containers). Children taking long-term immunosuppressant drugs are encouraged to wear Medic-Alert bracelets or necklaces. Photo-sensitive skin reactions may occur with several JRA medications including naproxen (Naprosyn), methotrexate (Rheumatrex), sulfasalazine (Azulfidine), and hydroxychloroquine (Plaquenil). Hypoallergenic sun block lotion with a minimum sun protection factor (SPF) of 15 should be used on exposed skin.

Orthotic appliances are often recommended to prevent or correct deformities. Important safety issues related to splint wearing include care of the splint to maintain integrity, proper skin care, signs and symptoms of an ill-fitting splint (e.g., potential pressure points), and proper splint application. The splint should be adjusted to maintain correct function and ensure that the child has not outgrown it.

Superficial heat and cold modalities are often recommended to relieve pain and stiffness. Determining the type of applications used by the family and reviewing safety precautions specific to each type of application are important.

Adaptive equipment (e.g., electric devices, lamp switch extenders, and elevated toilet seats) is used by children with JRA to minimize joint stress and increase independence. Safety can often be maximized with such assistive devices. For example, bath safety can be improved by the use of safety strips, rubber mats, wall grab bars, tub chairs, and one-handed hose attachments (Scull, 1994). Adaptive equipment should be evaluated for the safety of all family members. As with all family members, a home fire safety plan should include a specific plan for the child with JRA.

Immunizations

Children with JRA who are not taking immunosuppressive medications or experiencing disease exacerbations can receive all routine immunizations. Children whose immunocompetence is altered by antimetabolites or large doses of corticosteroids (i.e., 2 mg/kg/day or more, or over 20 mg/day) should not receive live vaccines for at least 3 months after cessation of these medications (Committee on Infectious Diseases, 1997). Live vaccinations may be administered to children with JRA whose only exposure to steroids are topically applied ophthalmic medication, local applications (i.e., intraarticular, bursal, or tendon injections), or maintenance and/or physiologic doses (Committee on Infectious Diseases, 1997). The inactivated poliovirus vaccine (IPV) should be administered to these children, as well as to their immunologically normal siblings.

Children receiving long-term salicylate therapy may be at increased risk for developing Reye syndrome in the presence of influenza and varicella infections (Committee on Infectious Diseases, 1997). Yearly immunizations for types A and B influenza are recommended for children treated with aspirin who are over 6 months of age according to the dosage and schedule set out by the American Academy of Pediatrics Committee on Infectious Diseases (1997). These children should receive the varicella immunization if documented disease has not occurred. Aspirin should be temporarily stopped if a child develops chickenpox or influenza.

A widespread concern of many pediatric rheumatologists is the possibility of immunizations leading to a flare-up of the underlying disease or immunologic disorder in JRA. Anecdotal experience views this as a potential problem, but scientific data to support this theory do not exist. These concerns should not discourage primary care providers from immunizing children with JRA after consulting with their pediatric rheumatologist.

Screening

Vision: A thorough funduscopic examination and visual acuity screening should be performed at each routine office visit. At the time of diagnosis, every child must be examined for uveitis by an ophthalmologist. Frequent ophthalmologic examinations are recommended for children at risk for uveitis, glaucoma, and cataracts. Young children with pauciarticular and ANA-positive arthritis are at greatest risk for development of ocular inflammation. The rheumatology section of the American Academy of Pediatrics (1993) has developed an ophthalmologic screening schedule (Box 27-5).

More frequent follow-up is needed for children with active uveitis.

Corticosteroid-induced glaucoma or cataracts can occur at any time during treatment. Children started on topical corticosteroids should receive baseline intraocular pressure measurements on initiation of treatment with frequent reexamination during continued therapy (Tucker et al, 1996).

Children taking hydroxychloroquine should have a baseline and biyearly ophthalmologic examination, which should at minimum include color vision (visual field determinations should be performed yearly) (Graham and Leak, 1998).

Hearing: Routine office screening is recommended. Decreased acuity in children taking salicylates should be promptly investigated when tinnitus is a complaint because it can herald impaired hearing.

Dental: Salicylates dissolved in the mouth erode the occlusal surfaces of the teeth and cause white, mildly inflamed, oral mucosal lesions to erupt (Tucker et al, 1996). Overretention of salicylate preparations in the mouth should be avoided and rinsing after ingestion of medication is recommended. Dental visits every 6 months are recommended unless erosive signs develop, in which case an increased frequency may be appropriate.

Increased incidence of dental caries can potentially occur in children with JRA, possibly because of poor oral hygiene secondary to TMJ or upper extremity limitations. Malocclusions and crowded teeth occur as a result of micrognathia (Jacobs, 1993). Children with JRA should be checked for bleeding gums and poor dental hygiene. Routine dental visits are recommended, and orthodontic referrals are made as needed. Dental work for children taking sulfasalazine (Azulfidine) who develop thrombocytopenia or leukopenia should be postponed until blood counts have returned to normal (US Pharmacopeia, 1995). In these situations, consultation with the pediatric rheumatology team and the dentist is necessary.

Blood pressure: Routine screening is recommended. Mild hypertension may occur in children taking NSAIDs. Steroid-induced hypertension can occur, although it is less frequent with current treatment regimens (Singsen and Rose, 1995).

Anemia: Hematologic testing is performed by the pediatric rheumatology team depending on a child's medication regimen. Therefore routine screening may not be required.

Tuberculosis: Routine screening is recommended.

Common Illness Management

Differential Diagnosis (Box 27-6)

Fever: Children with JRA may have fever as a response to an infectious process or as a result of their chronic condition. The classic systemic JRA fever is characterized by daily or twice daily temperature elevation to at least 39° C or higher (usually in the afternoon or evening) with a rapid return to baseline without intervention. Remittent and low-grade fevers are less frequent patterns. Children often appear toxic during febrile periods and well when afebrile. Fever typically occurs at disease onset and may recur with arthritis flares. Mild or moderate temperature elevations may occur with polyarticular disease. A careful history and complete physical examination usually determine the source of the fever. Because JRA is a diagnosis of exclusion, the differential diagnosis should consider postinfectious, infectious, and inflammatory diseases and malignancies.

Dermatologic symptoms: The classic systemic JRA fever is usually accompanied by a rash of 2 to 6 mm evanescent, salmon pink, generally circumscribed macular lesions. This rash may become confluent with larger lesions developing

---

Box 27-6

Differential Diagnosis

Fever:
  Rule out systemic JRA fever vs. infectious process
Dermatologic/Rash:
  Rule out systemic JRA rash vs. childhood rash vs. photosensitive skin reaction
Otologic:
  Rule out referred TMJ pain
Respiratory:
  Rule out aspirin intolerance vs. cricoarytenoid arthritis vs. pleuritis
Gastrointestinal:
  Rule out NSAID gastropathy vs. drug-induced GI bleeding vs. inflammatory bowel disease
Renal:
  Rule out urinary urgency with aspirin

---

pale centers and pale peripheries and is most commonly seen on the trunk, extremities, and over pressure areas, but the face, palms, and soles may also be involved. The rash is most prominent during fever spikes and may be visible only after the skin is rubbed or scratched. Stress or a hot bath may also induce the rash (Cassidy and Petty, 1995). Other types of rashes are rarely seen as part of the JRA condition and should be assessed and treated as is routinely done for children without JRA. Photosensitive skin reactions may occur with several of the medications used to treat JRA, including naproxen, methotrexate sulfasalazine, and hydroxychloroquine, with the most common rash being pseudoporphyria associated with naproxen (Naprosyn, Anaprox).

Otologic symptoms: TMJ arthritis may cause referred pain to the ear, which should be considered when evaluating children for otitis media.

Respiratory symptoms: Aspirin intolerance, which is characterized by acute bronchospasm, severe rhinitis, or generalized urticaria and/or angioedema occurring within 3 hours after ingestion of aspirin or another NSAID, has been reported. Any child with recurrent rhinitis or asthma must be considered at risk for bronchoconstriction when exposed to aspirin or other NSAIDs (Drug Facts and Comparisons, 1996). Tachypnea occurs with aspirin toxicity. A serum salicylate level should immediately be drawn when a child on aspirin therapy presents with an increased respiratory rate. Salicylates should be withheld pending laboratory results. Cricoarytenoid arthritis (i.e., laryngeal arthritis) can cause stridor, dyspnea, and cyanosis in systemic JRA (Jacobs, 1993).

Gastrointestinal symptoms: Gastrointestinal tract disease is rarely described in children with JRA. Gastrointestinal symptoms may be difficult to evaluate, however, because NSAIDs cause some degree of nausea, dyspepsia, abdominal pain, and diarrhea. A number of adverse reactions are being noted in children (Lindsley, 1999). Inflammatory bowel disease should be ruled out in children experiencing major gastrointestinal problems (Cassidy and Petty, 1995) (see Chapter 26). A careful history and physical examination, as well as consultation with the pediatric rheumatologist as needed, will help the primary care provider to evaluate differential diagnoses. Drug- or stress-induced gastrointestinal bleeding also must be considered in children receiving NSAIDs or steroids—particularly in those complaining of abdominal pain at night (Keenan, Giannini, and Athreya, 1995). Peptic ulcers may present as chronic anemia secondary to occult blood loss or as acute gastrointestinal hemorrhage. The classic symptom of epigastric pain that improves with eating and worsens with an empty stomach is more common in adolescents and is absent in young children.

Renal symptoms: Children taking aspirin may experience increased urinary urgency and frequency, but this problem is generally temporary. Urinary tract infection must be ruled out first.

Drug Interactions

Many potential interactions exist between medications commonly used to treat JRA and over-the-counter and prescription drugs used to manage other common pediatric conditions. Box 27-7 identifies the major interactions primary care providers must know when providing care to these children. Because of the complexity of possible drug interactions, primary care providers should work in conjunction with the rheumatology team when recommending any medications.

Primary care providers should not discontinue a child's condition-specific medications without consulting the pediatric rheumatologist. Conditions warranting possible temporary cessation of medications include the following: (1) exposure to chicken

Box 27-7

Potential Drug Interactions in Children Treated for Juvenile Rheumatoid Arthritis

- Aspirin plus salicylate-containing medications can cause salicylate toxicity.
- Antacids may alter the absorption rate of NSAIDs, glucocorticoids, or penicillamine, resulting in subtherapeutic serum levels.
- Antacids can alter renal excretion of aspirin, leading to higher serum levels of salicylate with antacid withdrawal or subtherapeutic levels with antacid addition.
- Corticosteroids decrease plasma concentration of salicylates.
- Methotrexate concentrations are increased by salicylates and NSAIDs. Salicylates may displace methotrexate from binding sites and decrease renal clearance, leading to toxic methotrexate plasma concentration
- Sulfonamides may displace or be displaced by other highly protein-bound drugs (e.g., NSAIDs, salicylates, and methotrexate). Monitor children for increased effects (i.e., increased hepatotoxicity) of highly bound drugs when sulfonamides

(e.g., trimethoprim/sulfamethoxazole [Bactrim]) are added.
- Concurrent use of NSAIDs, salicylates, and glucocorticoids may increase risk of gastrointestinal side effects (i.e., ulceration and hemorrhage).
- Estrogen-based oral contraceptives may alter metabolism or protein binding, leading to decreased clearance and increased elimination, half-life, and therapeutic or toxic effects of glucocortosteroids.
- NSAIDs plus acetaminophen increase the risk of adverse renal effects.
- NSAIDs displace anticoagulants from protein binding sites.
- Concomitant use of NSAIDs and alcohol may increase the risk of gastrointestinal side effects including ulceration and hemorrhage.

Data from Drug information for health care professions, ed 15, United States Pharmacopeia of Drugs (USPD), Taunton, Mass., 1995, World Color Book Services.

pox by unimmunized children or influenza-like illness; (2) significant bleeding of the nose, gums, or gastrointestinal tract; (3) dehydration as a result of illness (may result in possible salicylate toxicity and/or acute tubular necrosis); and (4) rapid, deep breathing until salicylate toxicity is ruled out.

Developmental Issues

Sleep Patterns

A child fatigues more readily during flare-ups and requires longer periods of rest during the day. Consequently, the severity and duration of morning stiffness increases. Recommendations to alleviate morning stiffness include the use of flannel sheets, thermal underwear, joint comforters, warmed clothing, and a sleeping bag. An electric blanket with a timer set to warm the blanket 1 hour before a child is scheduled to wake can also reduce morning stiffness. Warm waterbeds may be helpful. Finally, administering medications with food (i.e., a snack)

30 to 60 minutes before rising, and exercising in a warm bath before starting daily activities can increase range of motion. Teaching a child to recognize body signals, set limits and priorities, pace activities, and plan ahead will help conserve energy (Raising a Child with Arthritis, 1998).

Toileting

The acquisition of self-care skills may be delayed in children with JRA. Toilet training should be postponed during periods of active disease because a child may lack the motivation and physical capability to perform tasks necessary for successful toileting. Limitations in the upper and lower extremities make it difficult for children to transfer on and off the toilet, manage toilet paper, and dress and undress for toileting. Safety bars and elevated toilet seats are reliable assistive devices for children with lower extremity involvement. For children with upper extremity limitations, effective aids for wiping after toileting can be obtained from occupational therapists. A bidet can be attached to a toilet, thereby circumventing the need for paper. Adaptive clothing and dressing aids can facilitate toileting. Bedpans, urinals, and commodes may also be required at night if pain and stiffness limit mobility. Consideration should be given to toilet hygiene in facilities outside the home where assistive devices may not be available.

Discipline

Parents of children with JRA may have difficulty with discipline but should continue to use appropriate discipline, as well as establish firm rules at home and enforce them (Raising a Child with Arthritis, 1998; Tucker et al, 1996). Overly protective parents impose unnecessary limitations on activities or enforce excessive safety precautions. Feelings of guilt and sorrow for a child in pain or fear that stress will trigger a flare-up causes some parents to adopt an overly permissive discipline style. In addition, overindulgence during periods of active disease alternating with normalization of discipline practices during remissions fosters inconsistent limit setting. Parent education about every child's need for clear, reasonable, and consistent limits should include a review of alternatives to physical punishment. Guidance about age-specific developmental tasks and the effect of JRA on the acquisition and performance of self-care, language, motor, and social skills offers parents a framework for making decisions about discipline.

Child Care

Parents of children receiving medications may have difficulty locating child care providers who are willing to administer medications. For caregivers who accept this responsibility, parents should prepare a list that includes the name, dose, time, and method of administration, as well as the side effects of each medication. The name and telephone number of the person to contact for questions or problems should be provided. It is important for caregivers to understand that exacerbations and remissions characterize the JRA disease pattern and that a child's functional capacity, energy level, and developmental progress may fluctuate. Education about JRA and about a child's actual or anticipated limitations is likely to decrease anxiety among daycare staff and promote appropriate interactions between caregivers and children with JRA.

Schooling

Children with JRA can attend regular school. Many children have special needs that must be communicated to the school. Discrepancies may exist between what teachers, parents, and students perceive as obstacles. Parents and teachers more often identify limitations in activities of daily living and physical health as primary difficulties. Affected children focus on self-concept and peer relations and prefer to solve peer issues by themselves (Taylor, Passo, and Champion, 1987). Educating school personnel about morning stiffness and variability of clinical manifestations is very important. Certain minor accommodations (e.g., a second set of books, elevator pass, clustering of classes or additional time between classes, and use of a computer or tape recorder) make a large difference in a child's ability to participate in ordinary school activities (Cassidy and Lindsley, 1996). Disease flare-ups or surgery may necessitate temporary home tutoring and should be planned for in a child's individualized education plan (IEP) (see Chapter 5).

Children with JRA face many potential difficulties in school. Inattention and distractibility are most highly related to school performance (Stoff, Bacon, and White, 1989). Primary care providers should periodically question children and parents about school-related problems such as fatigue, distractibility, limited mobility, absences, and medications, as well as work with the family, school staff, and pediatric rheumatology team to identify and remedy problems before—or when—they occur. A student with JRA can participate in modified school athletic programs. It is important to individualize appropriate amounts and forms of exercise depending on the number, type, and severity of joints involved.

Sexuality

Sexual maturation may be delayed in adolescents with JRA—especially in those with systemic disease. Menarche has been shown to occur later in girls with JRA (e.g., mean age = 13.2 years) than in unaffected controls (mean age = 12.5 years) due to active inflammatory disease (Petty, 1998). Contraceptive advice should include discussion of interactions among arthritis medications and various oral contraceptives, as well as any effects of arthritis medications on fertility and fetal development.

If mechanical methods of birth control are difficult for adolescents with hand or hip involvement to use, a review of alternative birth control methods and consultation with the occupational therapist on the pediatric rheumatology team are indicated. Specific issues of sexuality and arthritis are addressed in the pamphlet "Living and Loving: Information about Sex," which is published and distributed by the Arthritis Foundation and in an article by Selekman and McIlvain-Simpson (1991). Obstetrical management of women with JRA who are thinking about getting pregnant or are pregnant is best managed with a team effort between an obstetrician and rheumatologist (Johnson, 1997). In a retrospective study of 76 pregnancies in 51 women with JRA, the following two conclusions were reached: (1) pregnancy had no adverse effects on the signs and symptoms of JRA, and (2) maternal and fetal outcome of pregnancy were good (Ostensen, 1991).

Transition to Adulthood

When preparing for the future, parents and children have questions about what to realistically expect. In the past JRA was stated to be a benign condition because it was thought that approximately 75% of children enter adulthood free of inflammation (Peterson et al, 1997). A controlled, population-based outcome study by Peterson and associates (1997) describes the functional and socioeconomic outcomes in adults who had JRA as children. This study showed that adults who were diagnosed with JRA as children had statistically significant differences in functional outcomes when compared with matched controls (Peterson et al, 1997). Cohorts with JRA were reported to have the following: (1) perceptions of poorer health, less energy, and more fatigue; (2) increased bodily pain; (3) greater limitations in physical functioning with more physical disability; (4) lower employment rates; and (5) lower exercise tolerance than the controls (Peterson et al, 1997). Limitations of this study are its modest sample size and ability to only be generalized for white Americans. These adults who had JRA experienced important physical and social disabilities throughout their lives. Therefore some thoughtful planning for transition is necessary and useful.

Providing a viable medical transition solution for children with JRA can be difficult because of the individual issues of adolescents and their families (i.e., delayed maturity, dependency, and overprotectiveness), the limited number of pediatric rheumatology programs associated with adult tertiary centers, the health insurance restrictions and/or lack of health insurance, as well as the lack of adult practitioners knowledgeable and willing to accept older adolescents as adults.

Another issue for young people with arthritis involves the change from secondary school to higher education or the work environment. Two agencies that work together to help adolescents make a successful transition from students to independent adults are the Department of Education and Vocational Rehabilitation (VR). Students and their parents need to explore transition program options with their school counselor and local VR center (White and Shear, 1992). The Arthritis Foundation provides a pamphlet that outlines many of these services. Adolescents attending college can often access the Office of Students with Disabilities to obtain services such as special scheduling, priority housing, class modifications, and handicapped parking. Outlining needs before searching for a college can be helpful and prevent problems for students in their freshman year. HEATH, which is a national clearinghouse on postsecondary education for individuals with handicaps, and the National Center for Youth with Disabilities (NCYD), which is an informational and resource center focusing on adolescents with chronic illness and their disabilities, are both excellent resources for these young adults and their families.

Special Family Concerns and Resources

Raising a child with JRA is difficult. Families naturally have initial feelings of guilt but must be reminded that they could have done nothing to prevent the JRA from occurring. JRA has an erratic disease course with unpredictable and unpreventable remissions and exacerbations. For many parents, the most difficult burden of this chronic disease is coping with this uncertainty. Families must also learn how to explain a disease that is commonly thought to occur in the elderly to family and friends. After hearing about the diagnosis, well-meaning family and friends sometimes tend to overwhelm the family of a child with JRA (e.g., with speculation about the diagnosis and "cures" of which they have heard or read). Children with JRA often appear healthy, which makes it difficult to explain their need for modifications at school. Children with JRA have concerns about school attendance, sports participation, growth, and any limitations or modifications that make them appear different.

Children with severe disease—especially systemic or polyarticular disease—may require some home modifications depending on the style of the home and the location of the bed and bathroom. Parents have concerns about long-term side effects of medications (i.e., fertility), whereas children are more concerned about the short-term effects (e.g., Cushingoid facies with corticosteroids).

Miller (1993) reviewed studies on the psychosocial factors related to rheumatic diseases in childhood. The consensus was that most children with a rheumatic disease survive the stress of the disease with good psychosocial adjustment, using denial as a necessary coping mechanism. Demographic factors and stresses related to poor maternal function and depression were viewed as major risk factors (Miller, 1993). A mother's sense of mastery was seen as a beneficial factor (Miller, 1993). Psychosocial interventions targeting high-risk families and encouraging families to be self-advocates will provide for good use of resources.

Community Resources

American Juvenile Arthritis Organization (AJAO)
Arthritis Foundation National Office
1330 West Peachtree Street NW
Atlanta, Ga. 30309
(404) 872-7100 (x6277); 1-800-283-7800
www.arthritis.org

The AJAO is a national membership association of the Arthritis Foundation that serves the special needs of young people with arthritis or rheumatic diseases and their families. Videotapes, quarterly newsletters, educational materials for children, parents, and health professionals, as well as information about summer camps, pen pal clubs, and family support groups are available through the national office of AJAO or through local chapters of the Arthritis Foundation. Joining AJAO includes a subscription to *Arthritis Today,* quarterly newsletters, and information on many local and national events.

Key Resources

Arthritis Foundation:
Education material listing—http:\\www.arthritis.org

Raising a Child with Arthritis—A Parents Guide (available from the Arthritis Foundation)

School—Educational Rights for Children with Arthritis: A Manual for Parents (available from the Arthritis Foundation)

General information (key pamphlets)—"Basic Facts," "Arthritis in Children," "Aspirin and Other Non-Steroidal Anti-Inflammatory Medications," and "When your Student Has Arthritis"

Other sources:
Arthritis Foundation: Understanding juvenile rheumatoid arthritis: a health professional's guide to teaching children and parents, Atlanta, 1987, The Foundation.

Tucker LB et al: Your child with arthritis—a family guide for caregiving, Baltimore, 1996, Johns Hopkins University Press.

Transition:
HEATH American Council on Education,
Department 36
Washington DC 20055-0036
(202) 939-9320; (800)544-3284

National Center for Youth with Disabilities
University of Minnesota, Box 721—UMHC
420 Delaware Street
Minneapolis, Minn. 55455
(612) 626-2825
ncyd@gold.tc.umn.edu

Summary of Primary Care Needs for the Child with Juvenile Rheumatoid Arthritis

HEALTH CARE MAINTENANCE

Growth and development

Linear growth may be retarded during active systemic disease.

Catch-up growth occurs with suppression of disease activity or during remission.

Corticosteroids may suppress growth.

Poor weight gain may be a result of systemic disease.

Excessive weight gain may occur as a result of inactivity, depression, poor nutrition, or corticosteroid usage.

Gross motor delays and temporary regressions are not uncommon.

Fine motor skills are less likely to be affected.

Standard infant development screening tests may be of questionable value in evaluating severely affected children.

Age-appropriate physical activities are important and should be based on a child's capabilities and energy level. Children should be allowed to participate in physical activities up to their tolerance.

Diet

The risk of protein-caloric malnutrition is increased.

Increased inflammatory activity, anorexia gastrointestinal side effects of medication, physical limitations, depression, corticosteroid usage, poor food choices, and limited movement of TMJ or upper extremities may contribute to nutritional problems.

A daily vitamin should be added.

"Arthritis diets" should be evaluated for nutritional adequacy, and families should be educated about proper nutrition for a growing child with a chronic disease.

Safety

Childproof containers should be used for medications.

Children taking immunosuppressive agents should wear a Medic-Alert bracelet or necklace.

Safety issues related to splint wearing, heat and cold applications, and adaptive equipment should be reviewed.

Sunblock should be used on exposed skin due to photosensitive skin reactions occurring with some medications.

Immunizations

Children who are not taking immunosuppressive drugs or experiencing systemic disease symptoms should be routinely immunized.

In the absence of neurologic symptoms, a child with classic, intermittent JRA fever can be immunized during febrile episodes.

No live viruses should be given to children receiving antimetabolites or large doses of corticosteroids.

Yearly immunizations for types A and B influenza are recommended for children over 6 months of age who are being treated with aspirin.

Children in whom documented disease has not occurred should receive varicella immunizations.

Immunosuppressed children, as well as immunologically competent siblings, should receive IPV.

Screening

Vision: A funduscopic examination and acuity screening should be performed at each visit.

Children should be examined by an ophthalmologist for uveitis. Children on topical or systemic steroids require close ophthalmologic follow-up.

Hearing: Routine visits (including assessment for tinnitus) are recommended.

Dental: Children taking salicylates should have dental visits every 6 months or more often if erosive signs develop. Children with micrognathia should have frequent dental visits. Prophylactic antibiotics should be used for dental work in children with total joint replacements or those on steroids.

Summary of Primary Care Needs for the Child with Juvenile Rheumatoid Arthritis—Cont'd

Screening—cont'd

Blood pressure: Routine screening is recommended.

Hematocrit: Frequent screening is often performed by rheumatology team to rule out anemia, primarily in those with polyarticular or systemic disease.

Tuberculosis: Routine screening is recommended.

Condition-specific screening:

CBC, differential, ESR, platelet count, and liver function tests are routinely drawn to monitor disease activity, response to therapy, drug toxicity, and review for anemia of chronic disease and are reviewed by pediatric rheumatology staff.

COMMON ILLNESS MANAGEMENT

Differential diagnosis

Fever: Classic, intermittent JRA fever should be differentiated from fevers of infectious origin.

Dermatologic symptoms: Rheumatoid rash should be ruled out in systemic JRA. Drug-related photosensitivity reactions should be ruled out.

Otologic symptoms: TMJ arthritis with referred ear pain should be differentiated from otitis media.

Respiratory symptoms: Salicylate-induced tachypnea or bronchospasm should be ruled out. A cold should be differentiated from influenza symptoms, and all type A influenza should be treated with amantadine. Colds and flu may cause arthritis flare-ups, necessitating increased doses of antiinflammatory medications.

Gastrointestinal symptoms: Rule out drug-induced peptic ulcer and drug-related gastrointestinal symptoms.

Rule out inflammatory bowel disease.

Renal symptoms:

Increased urinary urgency or frequency in a child on aspirin therapy may be temporary drug side effects, but UTI must first be ruled out.

DEVELOPMENTAL ISSUES

Sleep patterns

Recommendations to alleviate morning stiffness (e.g., use of electric blanket with timer) should be discussed with the family.

Toileting

Training should be postponed during periods of active disease.

Assistive devices should be used to compensate for upper and lower extremity limitations.

Situations in public facilities where assistive devices are not available should be anticipated.

Bedpans and urinals may be necessary if pain and stiffness limit mobility at night.

Discipline

Overprotection, overindulgence, and inconsistent limit setting should be identified.

Parents should be guided about the effect of JRA on age-specific developmental tasks to have a framework for decision making about discipline.

Child care

Caregivers must be capable of giving medications, using assistive devices, and applying splints.

Parents should provide caregivers with information about child's medications.

Caregivers should be educated on the effect of JRA on a child's functional capacity, energy level, and developmental progress.

Home-based, single provider daycare setting rather than group child care is recommended for children on steroids or immunosuppressants.

Most infants and young children with JRA are eligible for Public Laws 99-457 and 101-476 educational programs.

Continued

Summary of Primary Care Needs for the Child with Juvenile Rheumatoid Arthritis—Cont'd

Schooling

Public Law 101-476 entitles most students with JRA to occupational therapy, physical therapy, adaptive physical education, and transportation between school, home, and facilities where services are provided.

Most students with JRA can participate in modified school athletic programs.

Disease flare-ups or surgery may necessitate home tutoring.

Sexuality

Pubarche may be delayed in children with JRA.

Adolescents should be referred to physical and occupational therapists on the pediatric rheumatology team for difficulties with sexual postures or problems related to the use of mechanical birth control devices.

Medication modifications must be made prior to planning a pregnancy.

Transition to adulthood

Adolescents should be advised of transitional programs and vocational rehabilitation opportunities.

Special family concerns

The unpredictability of the condition and the family's inability to predict or control flares should be established.

Divergent views regarding perceptions and impact of JRA may exist.

Home remodeling may be necessary.

Parents may be concerned about medication side effects, as well as about the child's inability to attend school, participate in sports activities, and/or participate in social activities.

References

Ansell BM: Juvenile rheumatoid arthritis (rheumatoid factor positive polyarthritis) In Maddison PJ et al, editors: Oxford text of pediatric rheumatology, New York, 1998, Oxford University Press.

American Academy of Pediatrics: Guidelines for ophthalmic examinations in children with juvenile rheumatoid arthritis, Pediatrics 92:295-296, 1993.

Candell-Chalom E et al: Prevalence and outcome of uveitis in a regional cohort of patients with juvenile rheumatoid arthritis, J Rheumatol 24(10):1861-2060, 1997.

Cassidy JT and Hillman LS: Abnormalities in skeletal growth in children with juvenile rheumatoid arthritis, Rheum Dis Clin North Am 23(3):499-522, 1997.

Cassidy JT and Lindsley CB: Legal rights of children with musculoskeletal disabilities, Bull Rheum Dis 45(7):1-5, 1996.

Cassidy JT and Petty RE: Textbook of pediatric rheumatology, ed 3, Philadelphia, 1995, W.B. Saunders.

Chmell MJ et al: Total hip arthroplasty with cement for juvenile rheumatoid arthritis: results at a minimum of ten years in patients less than thirty years old, J Bone Joint Surg 79:44-52, 1997.

Committee on Infectious Diseases: 1997 Red book: report of the Committee on Infectious Diseases, ed 24, Elk Grove Village, Ill., 1997, American Academy of Pediatrics.

Drew SJ, Cohen B, and Witt JD: Surgical management of adolescents with rheumatic diseases. In Isenberg DA and Miller JJ, editors: Adolescent Rheumatology, Malden, Mass., 1999, Blackwell Science Inc.

Drug Facts and Comparisons: 1996 edition, St Louis, 1996, Wolters Kluwer.

Eisenberg D: Alternative medical therapies for rheumatologic disorders, Arthrit Care Res 9:1-6, 1996.

Flato B et al: Outcome and predictive factors in juvenile rheumatoid arthritis and juvenile spondyloarthropathy, J Rheumatol 25(2):366-375, 1998.

Giannini EH et al: Methotrexate in resistant juvenile rheumatoid arthritis—results of the USA-USSR double-blind, placebo-controlled trial, New Engl J Med 326:1043-1049, 1992.

Graham TB and Leak AM: The eye. In Maddison PJ et al, editors: Oxford textbook of rheumatology, ed 2, Oxford, 1998, Oxford University Press.

Grom AA, Giannini EH, and Glass DN: Juvenile rheumatoid arthritis and the trimolecular complex (HLA, T-cell receptor, and antigen), Arthritis Rheum 37:601-607, 1994.

Guidelines for ophthalmologic examinations in children with juvenile rheumatoid arthritis, Pediatrics 92:295-296, 1993.

Haas JP et al: Inversion of MHC-Class II transcription levels in joints of children with EOPA-JCA, Arthritis Rheum(suppl) 41(9):583, 1998 (abstract).

Henderson CJ and Lovell DJ: Nutritional aspects of juvenile rheumatoid arthritis, Rheum Dis Clin North Am 17:403-413, 1991.

Henderson CJ et al: Physical activity in children with juvenile rheumatoid arthritis: quantification and evaluation, Arthritis Care Res 8(2):114-119, 1995.

Howe S et al: Development of a disability measurement tool for juvenile rheumatoid arthritis: the juvenile arthritis functional assessment report for children and their parents, Arthritis Rheum 34:873-880, 1991.

Hunt P et al: The effects of daily intake of folic acid on the efficacy of methotrexate therapy in children with juvenile rheumatoid arthritis: a controlled study, J Rheumatol 24(11):2230-2232, 1997.

Jacobs JC: Pediatric rheumatology for the practitioner, New York, 1993, Springer-Verlag.

Johnson MJ: Obstetric complications and rheumatic disease, Rheum Dis Clin North Am 23(1):169-187, 1997.

Keenan GF, Giannini EH, and Athreya BH: Clinically significant gastropathy associated with nonsteroidal and inflammatory drug use in children with juvenile rheumatoid arthritis, J Rheumatol 22:1149-1151, 1995.

Klepper SE and Giannini MJ: Physical conditioning in children with arthritis, Arthritis Care Res 7:226-236, 1994.

Lawrence RC et al: Estimates of the prevalence of arthritis and selected musculoskeletal disorders in the United States, Arthritis Rheum 41(5):778-799, 1998.

Laxer RM and Schneider R: Systemic-onset juvenile chronic arthritis. In Maddison PJ et al, editors: Oxford textbook of rheumatology, ed 2, Oxford, 1998, Oxford University Press.

Lehman T: Aggressive therapy for childhood rheumatic diseases, Arthritis Rheum 36(1):71-74, 1993

Levinson JE and Wallace CA: Dismantling the pyramid, J Rheumatol 19(suppl 33):6-10, 1992.

Lindsley CB: Rehabilitation and recreation. In Isenberg DA and Miller JJ, editors: Adolescent rheumatology, Malden, Mass., 1999, Blackwell Science Inc.

Lloyd T et al: Calcium supplementation and bone mineral density in adolescent girls, JAMA 270:841-844, 1993.

Lovell DJ and Woo P: Growth and skeletal maturation. In Maddison PJ et al, editors: Oxford textbook of rheumatology, ed 2, Oxford, 1998, Oxford University Press.

MacKenzie CR and Sharrock N: Preoperative medical considerations in patients with rheumatoid arthritis, Rheum Dis Clin North Am 24(1):1-18, 1998.

Martin K and Woo P: Juvenile idiopathic arthritides. In Isenberg D and Miller J III, editors: Adolescent rheumatology, Malden, Mass., 1999, Blackwell Science Inc.

Matti MV and Sharrock NE: Anesthesia on the rheumatoid patient, Rheum Dis Clin North Am 24(1):19-34, 1998.

Miller JJ: Psychosocial factors related to rheumatic diseases in childhood, J Rheumatol 20A(suppl 38):1-11, 1993.

Moreland LW et al: Treatment of rheumatoid arthritis with a recombinant human tumor necrosis factor receptor (p 75)-Fc fusion protein, New Engl J Med 337:141-147, 1997.

Moroldo M et al: Juvenile rheumatoid arthritis in affected sibpairs, Arthritis Rheum 40(11):1962-1966, 1997.

Mulberg AE et al: Clinical and laboratory observations—identification of nonsteroidal antiinflammatory drug-induced gastroduodenal injury in children with juvenile rheumatoid arthritis, J Pediatr 122:647-649, 1993.

Ostensen M: Pregnancy in parents with a history of juvenile rheumatoid arthritis, Arthritis Rheum 34:881-887, 1991.

Pepmueller PH et al: Bone mineralization and bone mineral metabolism in children with juvenile rheumatoid arthritis, Arthritis Rheum 39(5):746-757, 1996.

Peterson LS et al: Juvenile rheumatoid arthritis in Rochester, Minnesota 1960-1993; is the epidemiology changing?, Arthritis Rheum 39:1385-1390, 1996.

Peterson LS et al: Psychosocial outcomes and health status of adults who have had juvenile rheumatoid arthritis, Arthritis Rheum 40(12):2235-2240, 1997.

Petty RE: Clinical presentation in different age groups. In Maddison PJ et al, editors: Oxford text of rheumatology, ed 2, New York, 1998, Oxford University Press.

Prieur AM: Rheumatoid factor negative polyarthritis in children (seronegative polyarthritis). In Maddison PJ et al, editors: Oxford textbook of rheumatology, ed 2, New York, 1998, Oxford University Press.

Prieur A et al: Juvenile chronic arthritis (JCA): 12th International Histocompatibility Workshop study. In Chanon D, editor: Proceedings of the Twelfth International Histocompatibility Workshop and Conference, Paris, 1997, EDK.

Raising a child with arthritis: a parents guide, Atlanta, 1998, Arthritis Foundation.

Ramos-Remus C and Russell A: Alternative therapies medicine, magic or quakery: who is winning the battle?, J Rheumatol 24(12):2276-2278, 1997.

Richardson et al: Haematology. In Maddison PJ et al, editors: Oxford textbook of rheumatology, ed 2, New York, 1998, Oxford University Press.

Scull SA and Athreya BH: Childhood arthritis. In Goldberg B, editor: Sports and exercise for children with chronic health conditions, Champaign, Ill., 1995, Human Kinetics Publishers Inc.

Scull SA: Juvenile rheumatoid arthritis. In Campebell SK, editor: Physical therapy for children, Philadelphia, 1994, W.B. Saunders.

Selekman J and McIlvain-Simpson GR: Sex and sexuality for the adolescent with a chronic condition 17(6):535-538, 1991.

Sherry DD et al: Pauciarticular-onset juvenile chronic arthritis. In Maddison PJ et al, editors: Oxford textbook of rheumatology, ed 2, Oxford, 1998, Oxford University Press.

Silverman ED et al: Intravenous immunoglobulin in treatment of systemic juvenile rheumatoid arthritis: a randomized placebo controlled trial, J Rheumatol 21:2353-2358, 1994.

Singh G et al: Measurement of health status in children with juvenile rheumatoid arthritis, Arthritis Rheum 37:1761-1769, 1994.

Singsen BH and Rose CD: Juvenile rheumatoid arthritis and the pediatric spondyloarthropathies. In Weissan MH and Weinblatt ME, editors: Treatment of the rheumatic diseases: companion to the textbook of rheumatology, Philadelphia, 1995, W.B. Saunders.

Singsen BH: Juvenile rheumatoid arthritis. In Schumacher HR, Klippel JH, and Koopman WS, editors: Primer on the rheumatic diseases, ed 10, Atlanta, 1993, Arthritis Foundation.

Stoff E, Bacon MC, and White PH: The effects of fatigue, distractibility and absenteeism on school achievement in children with rheumatic disease, Arthritis Care Res 2:49-53, 1989.

Swann M: Surgery in children. In Maddison PJ et al, editors: Oxford text of rheumatology, New York, 1998, Oxford University Press.

Taketomo CK, Hodding JH, and Kraus DM: Pediatric dosage handbook, ed 3, Hudson, Ohio, 1996-1997, Lexi-Camp Inc.

Taylor I, Passo MH, and Champion VL: School problems and teacher responsibilities in juvenile rheumatoid arthritis, J Sch Health 57:186-190, 1987.

Tucker LB et al: Your child with arthritis—a family guide for caregiving, Baltimore, 1996, Johns Hopkins University Press.

United States Pharmacopeia of Drug Information: Drug information for the health care professional, ed 15, Taunton, Mass., 1995, World Color Book Services.

Van Den Berg WB: Animal models of arthritis. In Maddison PJ et al, editors: Oxford text of rheumatology, ed 2, New York, 1998, Oxford University Press.

Wallace CA: New uses of methotrexate, Contemp Pediatr 11:43-53, 1994.

White PH and Shear ES. Transition/job readiness for adolescents with juvenile arthritis and other chronic illness, J Rheumatol 19(suppl 33):23-27, 1992.

Witt JD, Swann M, and Ansell BM: Total hip replacement for juvenile chronic arthritis, J Bone Joint Surg 73:770-773, 1991.

Woo P: The cytokine network in juvenile chronic arthritis, Rheum Dis Clin North Am 23(3):491-498, 1997.

Wright VF et al: Development of a self-report functional status index for juvenile rheumatoid arthritis, J Rheumatol 21:536-544, 1994.

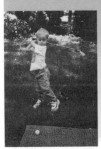

CHAPTER *28*

Learning Disabilities and/or Attention Deficit Hyperactivity Disorder

Janice Selekman and Marybeth Snyder

Etiology

Great confusion exists in the scientific literature about learning disabilities (LDs) and attention deficit hyperactivity disorder (ADHD) because the two conditions were not well differentiated by cause, symptoms, or interventions until the mid-1980s. Although the conditions are distinct, there are areas where they overlap (Figure 28-1). The current diagnoses of LD and ADHD were preceded by many other labels, which sometimes inadvertently combined the two conditions, including brain damaged, minimal brain dysfunction, hyperactive child syndrome, hyperkinetic reaction of childhood, and attention deficit disorder with and without hyperactivity (Barkley, 1998a).

The term *learning disability* was introduced in 1963 and revised in 1994 to refer to a heterogeneous group of disorders manifested by significant difficulties in the acquisition and use of listening, speaking, reading, writing, reasoning, or mathematical skills (National Joint Committee on Learning Disabilities, 1994). The use of this definition, however, differs from state to state (Lester and Kelman, 1997; MacMillan, Gresham, and Bocian, 1998).

The definition of ADHD also continues to change; it is currently defined by the *Diagnostic and Statistical Manual of Mental Disorders IV* (DSM) as a "persistent pattern of inattention and/or hyperactivity-impulsivity that is more frequent and severe than is typically observed in individuals at a comparable level of development" (American Psychiatric Association [APA], 1994).

Both of these disorders are intrinsic to an individual and presumed to be the result of central nervous system (CNS) dysfunction. Even though ADHD or an LD may occur with other handicapping conditions (e.g., sensory impairment, mental retardation, or serious psychosocial and emotional disturbances) or extrinsic influences (e.g., cultural differences or insufficient or inappropriate instruction), LDs and ADHD are not the direct result of those conditions or influences (Accardo, 1996; National Joint Committee on Learning Disabilities, 1994).

The causes and the exact mechanisms involved remain unknown, although multiple areas are being explored. The primary contributors to both LDs and ADHD appear to be genetic and neurologic (Barkley, 1998a; Zametkin and Liotta, 1998). Although the idea of genetic predisposition is supported for both LDs and ADHD in a significant number of cases, most of the work has been in the area of ADHD. Genetic studies with both twins and adopted children have suggested an autosomal gene transmission, although many researchers believe that the condition is polygenic (Barkley, 1998b). There is a 55% to 92% chance that an identical twin of a child with ADHD will develop the condition, which is 11 to 18 times greater than the chance for a child who is not a twin. The risk for developing the condition is approximately 30% for siblings of a child with ADHD (Barkley, 1997). "Siblings of children with ADHD are between five and seven times more likely to develop the syndrome than children from unaffected families. . . and the children of a parent who has ADHD have up to a 50 percent chance of experiencing some difficulties" (Barkley, 1998b).

Although CNS dysfunction is often cited as the general cause for both conditions, most of the cur-

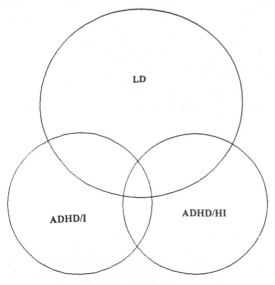

LD - **Learning Disability**

ADHD/I - **Attention Deficit**
        Hyperactivity Disorder-Inattention

ADHD/HI - **Attention Deficit**
        Hyperactivity Disorder-
        Hyperactivity/Impulsivity

Figure 28-1.   Relationship of diagnostic classifications.

rent research is with ADHD. The two most promising areas have been those of neurobiologic and neuroanatomic causes. The neurobiologic hypotheses focus on cerebral glucose metabolism, noradrenergic mechanisms and neurotransmitters—especially catecholamines. Although a decrease in cerebral glucose metabolism in adults with ADHD compared with controls was initially found, studies are now demonstrating inconsistent findings in adolescents (Barkley, 1997; Ernst et al, 1997; Zametkin and Liotta, 1998).

Because most of the medications with proven efficacy for ADHD stimulate alpha-2 adrenergic receptors to increase dopamine release and inhibit reuptake of neurotransmitters, deficits in this system seem to be one of the primary causes of ADHD (Barkley, 1998b). Neurons, especially those related to movement and emotion, secrete dopamine to inhibit or modulate the neuronal activity. The genes that are responsible for dopamine receptors and transporters are very active in the prefrontal cortex

and basal ganglia. Therefore research is now being done to examine the dopamine transporter gene, the dopamine receptor gene, and the dopamine pathways that direct neural activity in the frontal basal ganglia (Barkley, 1998b; Swanson et al, 1998).

The neuroanatomic hypothesis attempts to identify structural anomalies of or damage to the brains of children with LDs and ADHD. Research is now concentrated on frontal lobe anatomy and orbital-limbic pathways (Barkley, 1998a). Most of the positive findings related to ADHD have involved the basal ganglia and its possible asymmetry (Zametkin and Liotta, 1998). In some studies, it appears that the right prefrontal cortex and parts of the cerebellum may be smaller in children with ADHD than in those without the disorder. The right prefrontal cortex is "involved in editing one's behavior, resisting distractions and developing an awareness of self and time" (Barkley, 1998b). The identified areas of the cerebellum are responsible for allowing the cortex time to process stimuli and coordinate input among the regions of the cortex; however, "the structural studies for ADHD . . . have failed to find differences between ADHD and normal populations that would allow for diagnostic utility" (Zametkin and Liotta, 1998).

Barkley (1997) has proposed that ADHD is not a disorder of attention but rather a defect and/or delay in response inhibition that results in difficulty "self-regulating" one's impulsive motor behavior. Consequently, one becomes hyperesponsive to stimuli, and hyperactivity results. This neurologic defect in inhibition and self-control leads to alterations in an individual's ability to carry out executive functions (e.g., deflecting distractions, recalling goals by using hindsight, and taking steps to reach them by using forethought). It also includes changes in the ability to follow rules, control emotions and behaviors, and exhibit flexibility (Barkley, 1997).

Brain damage with resulting LDs or ADHD occurs as a result of brain infections, hypoxic and/or anoxic episodes, or trauma—especially to the prefrontal cortex (Gerring et al, 1998). LDs have been associated with the late effects of cancer treatment from cranial irradiation and intrathecal chemotherapy, although signs are not evidenced until years after the treatment (Foley, Fochtman, and Mooney, 1993). Premature birth—especially for infants weighing 750 to 999 g at birth—and maternal alcohol and tobacco use during pregnancy have also been correlated to the development of LDs and ADHD (Cherkes-Julkowski, 1998; Farel et al 1998; Olson et al, 1997; Resnick et al, 1998). Together, these causes account for less than 30% of cases (Barkley, 1997). LDs may be multifactorial rather than the result of a single etiologic determinant.

There is no empiric support for chemicals and allergies as causes for LDs or ADHD, excluding the permanent damage done by chemicals such as lead. Diets high in sucrose or aspartame and poor child rearing have also been ruled out as causes of LDs or ADHD (Barkley, 1998a).

Incidence

Between 5% and 20% of school-aged children have been identified as having a LD, but there are probably many more still unidentified. In addition to the fact that many cases have not yet been diagnosed, the criteria for the diagnosis differ between states and over time (Lester and Kelman, 1997; MacMillan et al, 1998; Silver, 1997). Half of all children enrolled in federally supported special education programs receive services for LDs (Accardo, 1996). Therefore children with LDs make up more than half of the school age population with disabilities (US Department of Education, 1994). Estimates of the number of children with LDs who also have ADHD range from 20% to 40% (Block, 1998; Silver, 1997).

ADHD has been diagnosed in 3% to 5% of school-age children with a range of 1.3% to 13.3%, although prevalence decreases somewhat with age after elementary school (American Academy of Child and Adolescent Psychiatry [AACAP], 1997; Barkley, 1998a; NIH Consensus Statement, 1998) and is seen in every culture. Of the children with ADHD, 8% to 39% have at least one type of LD, depending on how the definition of LD is used (Barkley, 1998a; Block, 1998). Therefore approximately 4 to 10 million children in the United States have an LD and/or ADHD.

More boys than girls have been diagnosed with these conditions. Although the ratios differ by the setting, the general ratio of male to female with LDs and ADHD is 3:1, with ratios ranging from 9:1 in clinical settings for elementary-age children to 2:1 for the predominantly inattentive type of ADHD (AACAP, 1997). This range may be because those who display aggressive behavior are more likely to be referred to a clinic. Block (1998) found that girls with ADHD usually had the inattentive form.

Clinical Manifestations at Time of Diagnosis (Box 28-1)

Learning Disability

There are two frameworks used to identify LDs. The first is the DSM-IV (APA, 1994), which refers to LDs as learning disorders (formerly called academic skills disorders) and identifies them as "disorders . . . characterized by academic functioning that is substantially below that expected given the person's chronological age, measured intelligence, and age-appropriate education." These disorders are subdivided into reading disorder, mathematics disorder, disorder of written expression, and a learning disorder not otherwise specified. Unfortunately, this format only views learning as academic-related and does not incorporate its effect on a child's life.

Diagnosis is multidimensional and includes standardized testing results and academic achievement that are significantly below those expected given the person's chronologic age, measured intelligence, and age-appropriate education (APA, 1994). There is usually a significant gap of 1.0 to 2.0 standard deviations between a child's achievement on individually administered standardized tests of reading, math, written expression, and intelligence (Lester and Kelman, 1997; MacMillan et al, 1998). This gap significantly affects the number of children diagnosed with a LD and results in different standards between states. Handicapping conditions that may result in LDs (e.g., vision and hearing deficits, mental retardation, psychosocial problems, and environmental conditions) must be ruled out. It should be noted that some schools are identifying children with intelligence quotients (IQs) as low as 58 as learning disabled rather than mildly mentally retarded because it is considered by some to be more socially acceptable to both parents and children (Gresham, MacMillan, and Bocian, 1996; MacMillan et al, 1998). LDs may be diagnosed at any age (APA, 1994).

Reading disorders include deficits in reading accuracy, speed, or comprehension. Mathematics disorders involve a child's ability in mathematic calculations and reasoning. Disorders of written

<table>
<tr><td>

Box 28-1

Clinical Manifestations

Learning Disability
Reduced academic achievement
- 1.5 to 2.0 standard deviations below that projected for age, intelligence, and education in reading, math, and written expression

Alterations in sensory-receptive processing
Visual perceptual deficits
- Decoding language
- Visual memory
- Perception of symbols, depth, distance

Auditory perceptual deficits
- Phonetics
- Directions
- Tone of voice
- Discrimination of sounds

Tactile perceptual deficits
- Kinesthetic

Alterations in integrative processing
- Multitask coordination
- Memory problems

Alterations in motor-expressive performance
- Clumsy, uncoordinated
- Speech disorders
- Fine motor skill delays

Diffuse alterations
- Heterogenous manifestations

Attention Deficit Hyperactivity Disorder
Predominately inattentive
Predominantly hyperactive-impulsive
Combined
(See Box 28-2 for DSM-IV criteria.)

</td></tr>
</table>

expressive output, and diffuse abilities (Selekman, 1997; Silver, 1997).

Alterations in Sensory-Receptive Input

Alterations in sensory-receptive intake involve deficiencies in using and processing information received via the senses, including visual perceptual, auditory perceptual, and sensation-related deficits.

Visual perceptual deficits involve difficulty in decoding and/or comprehending written language because of reversals of letters or words (i.e., dyslexia), difficulty in visual memory and perception of symbols (e.g., musical notes), or misperception of distance and depth. The problem is not with vision, but rather with how the brain interprets the information it "sees." Children with these problems may have difficulty copying and identifying letters or shapes, differentiating right from left, and drawing a clock. The eyes of children with dyslexia may not be able to move evenly across a printed line but instead jump from line to line, causing these children to lose their place. These children may also have difficulty with figure-ground visual perception (i.e., difficulty differentiating an object from its background). They may also have difficulty perceiving speed and distance, leading to an increase in automobile accidents during adolescence (Selekman, 1997; Silver, 1997).

Children with an auditory perceptual deficit have difficulty with phonetics, recitation from memory (e.g., the alphabet), understanding and following directions—especially multi-step instructions, interpreting tone of voice and differentiating auditory "figure-ground noise," making it hard to differentiate background noise (e.g., television, radio, or noise in the hall) from someone speaking to them. Because of these deficits, a child may be erroneously judged to be emotionally disturbed, retarded, noncompliant, or a "problem child," who does not do as told. This deficit also presents as an inability to differentiate similar-sounding words (e.g., pit and pet) (Selekman, 1997; Silver, 1997) and is not due to a hearing problem but rather to how the brain interprets what it "hears."

Children who have difficulty perceiving tactile or body sensations may be unable to read their own body cues. Sensations such as the need to toilet or the onset of menses may be missed or misread, leading to difficulty in toilet training, resolving enuresis or encopresis, and establishing self-care

expression involve writing skills. No differentiating features exist, however, for the category identified as "learning disorder not otherwise specified."

Although these learning disorders are based on academic tasks and test results, the basic problem for children with an LD is processing information—especially if this involves more than one process. A second, more conceptual approach, is to view alterations in the areas of sensory-receptive input, integrative processing and/or memory, motor-behaviors. These children may dislike or misperceive how they are being touched or be supersensitive to the tags on shirts or certain types of fabrics. Such sensations can distract them from the task at hand. Kinesthetic misperception can result in difficulty understanding the body language and facial expressions of others as well as awareness of their own body movements (Silver, 1993).

Alterations in Integrative Processing

Children with an alteration in integrative processing can receive stimuli adequately but have difficulty retrieving and using this information accurately. This manifests itself in several ways, including difficulty sequencing data or parts of a story; difficulty understanding the concepts of time and space, parts and whole, and cause and effect; difficulty with mathematics and the concept of zero; disorganization of thought and planning; slowness in processing problem solving; and difficulty with analysis and abstract thinking. These children may become lost easily and have difficulty reading maps. Children with this condition are limited in the amount of general knowledge they can process from their environment (e.g., knowing the number or sequence of the days in a week) and have difficulty with short-term memory (e.g., memorizing multiplication tables) (Selekman, 1997; Silver, 1997).

Older school-age children with integrative difficulties often find it difficult to process multiple intake stimuli at the same time. To listen to a lecture, observe visual aids, and take notes simultaneously may be confusing because these children may be easily distracted and have difficulty identifying the important points. Organization—whether in plans or on paper—may be a problem. In addition, these children may find it difficult to understand humor, clichés, and puns because they interpret language literally. Their limited understanding of concepts may result in their perception of a problem being worse than in reality (Selekman, 1997).

Alterations in Motor-Expressive Performance

Alteration in the motor-expressive aspects of developmental tasks is a third classification of LDs and ranges from (1) difficulty in performing gross and/or fine motor tasks, resulting in the labels of "clumsy," "uncoordinated," or "accident-prone" to (2) speech disorders, including dysphasia, stuttering, and poor articulation to (3) difficulties in skills such as handwriting, spelling, arithmetic, drawing, and sports activities. These children may try to avoid hobbies and extracurricular activities that require physical activity (Silver, 1993).

Diffuse Alterations

The final category is diffuse alterations, which is a combination of the other three categories. This heterogeneous form is more commonly seen in girls. This diagnosis is often delayed because dyslexia is more common in boys and LDs are rarely considered as a differential diagnosis for girls. Overlap occurs in this category with the signs and symptoms of ADHD-inattention. Children with LDs, as well as those with inattentive ADHD, may appear to be daydreaming or drift off in the middle of an activity.

Additional Findings

One controversial set of findings is that of "soft neurologic signs." These individual minor abnormalities are identified during neurologic assessment and history taking and consist of motor findings (e.g., clumsiness, posturing, repetitive finger tapping), mirror movements, poor directionality—especially left-right orientation, and poor gross motor skills. The incidence of soft signs in children who appear otherwise normal is so high that they have very limited use in diagnosing LDs or ADHD (AACAP, 1997). If a child has soft signs and is happy and doing well, it is recommended that no further intervention be made besides routine follow-up. If a diagnosis of an LD has already been made, the presence or absence of soft signs has not been noted to alter the prognosis.

ADHD

The past emphasis on hyperactivity as the primary component of ADHD has changed because impulsivity and inattention are now given equal importance. These manifestations occur in all facets of a child's life and often become worse in situations requiring sustained attention. The subtypes of

ADHD are the predominantly inattentive type, the predominantly hyperactive-impulsive type, (ADHD-H/I), and the combined type (APA, 1994). The inattentive category appears to have the highest prevalence, but the combined type has the highest incidence of comorbid conditions (Faraone et al, 1998).

To be labeled ADHD predominantly inatten-tive, at least six of the nine symptoms must have persisted for at least 6 months (Box 28-2). For ADHD predominantly hyperactive-impulsive, at least six of the nine characteristics in that category must have persisted for at least 6 months. A diagnosis of the combined type requires at least six symptoms from each of the sets of categories. Regardless of the type of ADHD, some symptoms must

---

Box 28-2

Diagnostic Criteria for Attention Deficit Hyperactivity Disorder

A. Either (1) OR (2):
   (1) Six (or more) of the following symptoms of inattention have persisted for at least 6 months to a degree that is maladaptive and inconsistent with developmental level:
   Inattention
   a. Often fails to give close attention to de-tails or makes careless mistakes in school-work, work, or other activities
   b. Often has difficulty sustaining attention in tasks or play activities
   c. Often does not seem to listen when spo-ken to directly
   d. Often does not follow through on instruc-tions and fails to finish schoolwork, chores, or duties in the workplace (not due to oppositional behavior or failure to understand instructions)
   e. Often has difficulty organizing tasks and activities
   f. Often avoids, dislikes, or is reluctant to engage in tasks that require sustained mental effort (e.g., schoolwork or home-work)
   g. Often loses things necessary for tasks or activities (e.g., toys, school assignments, pencils, books, or tools)
   h. Is often easily distracted by extraneous stimuli
   i. Is often forgetful in daily activities
   (2) Six (or more) of the following symptoms of hy-peractivity-impulsivity have persisted for at least 6 months to a degree that is maladap-tive and inconsistent with developmental level
   Hyperactivity:
   a. Often fidgets with hands or feet or squirms in seat

   b. Often leaves seat in classroom or in other situations in which remaining seated is expected
   c. Often runs about or climbs excessively in situations in which it is inappropriate (in adolescents or adults, may be limited to subjective feelings of restlessness)
   d. Often has difficulty playing or engaging in leisure activities quietly
   e. Is often "on the go" or often acts "as if driven by a motor"
   f. Often talks excessively
   Impulsivity:
   g. Often blurts out answers before questions have been completed
   h. Often has difficulty awaiting turn
   i. Often interrupts or intrudes on others (e.g., butts into conversations or games)
B. Some hyperactive-impulsive or inattentive symp-toms that caused impairment present before age 7 years
C. Some impairment from the symptoms present in two or more settings (e.g., at school or work and at home)
D. Clear evidence of clinically significant impair-ment in social, academic, or occupational func-tioning
E. Symptoms do not occur exclusively during the course of a pervasive developmental disorder, schizophrenia, or other psychotic disorder and are not better accounted for by another mental disorder (e.g., mood disorder, anxiety disorder, dissociative disorder, or a personality disorder)

Data from American Psychiatric Association: Diagnostic and statistical manual of mental disorders, ed 4, Washing-ton, DC, 1994, The Association.

have been present prior to the age of 7 years. The criteria have been found to be valid for children as young as age 4 years (Lahey et al, 1998).

Although symptoms are often identified in early childhood, they may be missed until after a child enters a structured school environment. The DSM-IV (APA, 1994) begins to address symptoms that may help diagnose an adolescent or adult with ADHD. Some controversy has been raised regarding the DSM-IV age-of-onset criterion of 7 years for ADHD, particularly in light of the increasing interest in diagnosis of adolescents and adults with ADHD. Other issues include the following: (1) the validity of historical recollection and self-report of symptoms; (2) the later awareness of impairment, especially with the predominantly inattentive subtype of ADHD; (3) the problem of separating out symptoms of frequent comorbid disorders in adolescents and adults with ADHD; (4) the coupling of a diagnosis of ADHD with eligibility for federally mandated disability services; and (5) the fact that the age of 7 years was selected without empirical field trials (Barkley and Biederman, 1997; Greenhill, 1998; Spencer et al, 1998; Tosyali and Greenhill, 1998).

Although all researchers have acknowledged that many children with ADHD have the disorder into adulthood, it has been implied that there are many adults with ADHD who were never identified as having the disorder as children. Older adolescents and adults suspected of having ADHD exhibit symptoms slightly different than those in the DSM-IV. These symptoms include poor social interaction with possible antisocial behavior; substance and/or alcohol use disorders; high levels of school failure; anxiety disorders; poor work histories; and low self-esteem. These adults are often undereducated and assume lower occupational levels (Spencer et al, 1998).

Diagnostic Measures

Because no "gold standard" exists, no one test or tool can diagnose a child as having an LD or ADHD. Multiple data sources are used over time to make the diagnosis. These sources include the following: (1) family history, (2) perinatal history, (3) developmental history with current developmental assessment, (4) assessment of past and current temperament of the child, (5) health history, (6) assessment of academic performance, (7) com-

prehensive age-appropriate psychologic and intelligence testing, and (8) comprehensive physical assessment with an emphasis on neurologic and motor abilities. Although it is helpful for a clinician to observe a child's performance and behavior in structured and unstructured activities, it is usually not realistic.

A variety of behavior rating scales can be used by parents and teachers for providing supplemental, standardized data when screening for ADHD and assessing treatment efficacy (AACAP, 1997; Reiff, 1998). A teacher's ability to objectively and critically evaluate a child's behavior in comparison with the parent, however, is especially valuable (Block, 1998). Although hyperactivity can be rated as a physical measurement, inattention cannot be measured directly; it must be "inferred" by the rater (Greenhill, 1998). Scales should not be used as the sole diagnostic measure for ADHD (Goldman et al, 1998; Greenhill, 1998). Table 28-1 includes a list of selected behavior rating scales for screening and assessing treatment in ADHD.

LDs are often identified by administering a full psychologic battery of tests (including standardized intelligence tests) and noting discrepancies between IQ and academic achievement (i.e., when the IQ is greater than the achievement) (Vincent, 1996). Gross inconsistencies between verbal and performance scores and among the various components of the testing are also indicative of LDs (MacMillan et al, 1998); gifted students who perform adequately on some sections but are significantly above average in others may be missed. Diagnosing a child with an LD may depend on whether the state uses 1.5 or 2.0 standard deviations below the predicted IQ score as the marker for indicating LDs. "When more liberal criteria are applied, 40% to 60% of ADHD children are identified with a learning disorder, but using more rigid standards, about 20% to 30% of ADHD children will be learning disabled in the area of reading, spelling, or arithmetic" (Pliszka, 1998a).

Primary care providers are responsible for initiating the diagnostic process and obtaining the history and physical and developmental assessments for a child identified as being at risk. Psychologic testing may have to be referred to specially trained individuals. The diagnostic period is difficult for the parents, and guidance and support by the primary care provider is especially helpful. The child should be reevaluated on the same parameters

Table 28-1
Selected Behavior Rating Scales for Screening and Assessing Treatment Efficacy in ADHD

Scales	Source	Age	Method	Comments
Achenbach's Child Behavior Check List (CBCL)	Center for Children, Youth, and Families University of Vermont 1 S. Prospect St. Burlington, VT 05401	4-18 yrs	Observation Interview	Screening provides overview of child's behavior
Teachers Report Form of the CBCL	Same as above	Same	Same	Same
Conners Parent and Teacher Rating Scale	Multi-Health Systems 908 Niagra Falls Blvd. N. Tonawanda, NY 14120	3-14 yrs (long version) 3-17 yrs (short version)	Observation	Screening
Conners Abbreviated Teacher andParent Rating Scale	Same	Same	Observation	For less extensive evaluation
ACTeRS	Meritech, Inc. 111 N. Market St. Champaign, IL 61820	5-13 yrs	Teacher observation	Screening
Barkley Home Situations Questionnaire and School Situation Questionnaire	In Barkley RA: Attention deficit hyperactivity disorder: a clinical workbook, New York, 1990, Guilford Press.		Parent/teacher observation	Screening

(Conners, 1998; Marvin and Vessey, 1997; Miller and Catellanos, 1998; Reiff, 1998).

every 2 to 3 years to identify changes and new areas for needed intervention.

Diagnosis of a child with hyperactive-impulsive ADHD occurs more often during the preschool years (Faraone et al, 1998), whereas diagnoses of LDs and inattentive ADHD do not often occur until a child is in elementary school, usually around the age of 9 years. Increased motor activity—including alterations in sleeping and eating routines, however, has been identified by parents in children as young as 10 to 18 months (Greenhill, 1998). Children with a history of prematurity—especially those who experienced chronic lung disease—should be screened for LDs because they are more at risk for language and memory deficits, lower abstract and/or visual reasoning, and lower achievement in reading and math skills (Cherkes-Julkowski, 1998; Farel et al, 1998). Various behaviors are tolerated and evaluated differently, however, by different cultural groups (Gingerich et al, 1998).

Comorbidity

ADHD commonly occurs in conjunction with other chronic conditions, thus increasing the morbidity that results (Jensen, Martin, and Cantwell, 1997). The most common conditions seen with ADHD include oppositional defiant disorder (ODD), conduct disorder (CD), and LDs. Up to 35% of children with ADHD have ODD (Kuhne et al, 1997), although 62% of males and 71% of females in the ADHD-combined group also meet the criteria for ODD (Carlson, Tamm, and Gaub, 1997). This combination results in increased social isolation. A more serious combination, however, is ADHD with conduct disorder. From 30% to 50% of children with ADHD—most of whom are males—have CD. These children have high levels of aggression, increased anxiety, decreased self-esteem, and increased maternal pathology (Kuhne et al, 1997). Comorbidity rates are much higher in clinic populations than in community samples. Children with

ADHD and ODD generally have better academic achievement and a better prognosis than those with ADHD and CD (Kuhne et al, 1997). Satterfield and Schell (1997) found that hyperactive boys who also had CD were at increased risk for later criminality (i.e., arrest and incarceration), which was not true for those who only had ADHD-H/I. Comorbidity of ADHD with ODD or CD increases the negative outcomes over those of having ADHD alone.

Children with ADHD can also have LDs with the percent involved ranging from 10% to 92% (Jensen et al, 1997). On average, 20% to 40% of children with ADHD also have an LD (Greenhill, 1998; Pliszka, 1998a). Children with LDs have a fourfold increased risk for social, emotional, and behavioral problems compared with children without LDs (Rock, Fessler, and Church, 1997).

Jensen and associates (1997) indicate that internalizing disorders (e.g., anxiety, separation anxiety, and major depressive disorders) occur in between 13% and 50% of those with ADHD. "In both childhood and adulthood, females with ADHD have been found to have higher rates of depression and anxiety than controls" (Gingerich et al, 1998). Tourette's syndrome is a neurologic condition that is also often associated with ADHD.

Treatment

There is no gold standard for therapy for LDs or ADHD. Cognitive, behavioral, and psychosocial strategies are used to treat both conditions. Pharmacologic intervention may also be helpful in treating children with ADHD. No one approach works for all children. Working with the child and family requires an interdisciplinary team approach. This team may include some or all of the following individuals: (1) the primary care provider, (2) the psychologist, (3) occupational and physical therapists, (4) specialists in vision, hearing, and speech and language, (5) educators, and (6) the child and parents. Different strategies may be needed at different ages. Parents and the team should identify the child's strengths and how and when the child learns best and use this modality and timing as the initial approach at home and in school to meet the specific needs of the child (Box 28-3).

For children with a visual perceptual deficit, presenting material verbally in addition to using hands-on experiences is important. A child with an auditory perceptual deficit needs materials presented in writing and pictorially, as well as tactilely. For these children, a short list of directions should be provided with either pictures of a procedure or demonstration on a model (Selekman, 1997). Children with integrative deficits need multisensory approaches. Directions can be written down and explained with the child watching; charts can be used if a child can read. Feedback should constantly be elicited from children to check their understanding. Calendars and lists can be used to help children organize specific tasks or daily health-related activities. These children need shorter learning periods and more time for repetition before mastering a task. Interventions for children with motor deficits are similar to those for children with cerebral palsy (see Chapter 14). Steps of a particular skill need to be broken down to component parts and verbally described so that a child can master one step at a time. These children need extra time to perform or verbalize.

Pharmacologic management is effective for approximately 70% to 75% of children with ADHD (Findling and Dogin, 1998). When prescribing medications for the pediatric population, providers

---

Box 28-3

Treatment

LD

Multiple modalities are needed to counter the area of deficit.

Pharmacologic treatment is not generally used for LD, unless associated psychiatric problems coexist.

ADHD

Pharmacologic intervention is used for ADHD.

Treatment is determined by type of ADHD, age of child, and severity of symptoms.

(See Tables 28-2 and 28-3 for pharmacologic management of ADHD.)

Both

A multidisciplinary approach is most effective.

Interventions are needed for both the child and family members.

Cognitive, behavioral, and psychosocial strategies are used.

should be mindful of the following factors: (1) as children grow, changes in the ratio of body fat to muscle affect the bioavailability of lipid-soluble drugs; (2) as a child's age increases, the metabolism of medications decreases; and (3) gender differences in body fat percentage are generally seen at puberty, with females having more fat than males (Tosyali and Greenhill, 1998). "Only children whose symptoms significantly interfere in at least one area of functioning—socially, academically, or behaviorally—warrant therapy" (Block, 1998). Children with ADHD need supervision in their medication administration to ensure therapeutic adherence because memory problems and distractibility can negatively affect self-administration.

Medications currently used for ADHD include psychostimulants, alpha-2 noradrenergic agonists, and antidepressants. The drugs of choice for treatment of ADHD are the psychostimulants methylphenidate (Ritalin), dextroamphetamine (Dexedrine), mixed salts of a single entity amphetamine product (Adderall), and methamphetamine (Desoxyn) (Table 28-2). Some stimulants come in both short-acting and long-acting preparations, but others are only available in the long-acting form. The effectiveness of stimulants is measured by behavioral changes (e.g., decreased motor activity and increased attention span and concentration). Behavioral changes can be identified 30 to 90 minutes after ingestion. Administering the stimulants with food or shortly after eating enhances their absorption and minimizes anorexia (Kaplan et al, 1998). The mechanism of action for these drugs occurs at the transmitter level of the CNS by increasing the availability of dopamine and norepinephrine at the neural synapse (Findling and Dogin, 1998; Greenhill, 1995; Kaplan et al, 1998). Stimulants can increase attention span and short-term memory, reduce distractibility and motor activity, and improve cognition. These effects can be seen in individuals with ADHD, as well as in unaffected individuals, and are therefore not specific or diagnostic for ADHD (Kaplan et al, 1998). If a child does not respond to one stimulant, others should be tried before moving on to second-line drugs because efficacy may occur with one stimulant but not another (AACAP, 1997). These medications do not alter LDs—if present—but do allow a child with ADHD to be more cognitively available for learning.

Children vary widely both in their response to dose and across domains of behavior and learning. The actual dose for each child should be individually titrated for optimal effects using side effects and therapeutic responses as guides (AACAP, 1997; McEvoy, 1995). The use of stimulants in children with tic disorders is controversial because some children experience a worsening of tic problems. "Behavioral rebound" may occur at the wearing off of some short-acting stimulants, as evidenced by a worsening of behavior beyond baseline for about a half hour. Use of a longer-acting preparation or adjustments in the timing of doses to overlap can prevent this response (Cantwell, 1996). Emotional lability and a dazed, glassy-eyed appearance indicate that a dose is too high. See Table 28-2 for treatment guidelines for specific stimulants.

Methylphenidate (Ritalin) has been the predominantly prescribed stimulant for ADHD, although use of the other stimulants is increasing. A long-acting form of this drug (i.e., Ritalin-SR) is available, but its onset, response, and duration are variable (Findling and Dogin, 1998). The Ritalin-SR 20 tablet must be swallowed—not chewed—or erratic absorption may occur. The long-acting Ritalin preparation is available in only one strength, thus limiting its dosing possibilities (AACAP, 1997).

Dextroamphetamine doses are generally half those of Ritalin (Miller and Castellanos, 1998). D-amphetamine is available as a time-release capsule in 5-, 10-, and 15-mg strengths. The increased duration of action of Dexedrine over Ritalin is an advantage in dosing options.

Adderall, which is a combination of mixed salts of dextroamphetamine and levamphetamine, has recently been remarketed for ADHD treatment, having previously been used as Obetrol for obesity management (Findling and Dogin, 1998). Although less empiric study is available with this drug than with other stimulants, reports of efficacy in treatment are becoming available (Pliszka, 1998b; Swanson et al, 1998). Adderall is available in multiple strengths (i.e., 5-, 10-, 20-, and 30-mg tablets) and can be split to fine-tune dosage further.

Treatment with pemoline (Cylert), which is another long-acting stimulant, has declined following reported problems with liver toxicity, including liver failure (Pliszka, 1998b; Rosh, 1998). Studies now show prompt relief of ADHD symptoms with

Table 28-2
Psychostimulants Used for ADHD

Drug	Dosage (individualized)	Maximum	Onset	Duration	Dosing Schedule
Methylphenidate (Ritalin)	Start with 5 mg bid (2.5 mg for preschoolers; 10 mg for child > 30 kg) with breakfast and lunch; increase by 5 mg/week; a third dose may be required with dinner. *Usual:* 0.6 to 1.0 mg/kg/day	Rarely need >60 mg/day	30 to 60 min	3 to 6 hr	2 to 3 times/day
Dextroamphetamine (Dexedrine)	Start with 2.5 mg (5 mg for child >30 kg) with breakfast and lunch; increase by same increments/week; third dose may be needed with dinner. *Usual:* 0.15 to 0.5 mg/kg/dose	Rarely need >40 mg/day	30 to 60 min	3 to 6 hr	2 to 3 times/day
Pemoline (Cylert)	Start at 18.75 mg (37.5 mg for large child); increase dose/week to 0.5 to 3.0 mg/kg/day	112.5 mg	Gradual	8 to 9 hr	Daily in AM
Mixed salts of Dextro and Levo Amphetamine					
Mixed ampetamine salts (Adderall)	Start with 2.5 mg/day (preschoolers); 5 mg 1 to 2 times/day (≥6 years old)	Rarely need >40 mg/day	Gradual	3 to 6 hr	1 to 2 times/day
Methamphetamine (Desoxyn)	Start with 2.5 to 5 mg each morning; raise by 5-mg increments/week. *Usual:* 20 to 25 mg/day 1 to 2 times/day (≥ 6 years old)		Gradual	8 to 10.5 hr twice daily	1 to 2 times/day

From Findling and Dogin, 1998; Kaplan et al, 1998; Ludwikowski and DeValk, 1998; and McEvoy, 1995.)

pemoline in school-aged children at a starting dose of 37.5 mg (56.25 mg in teens). Pemoline should only be used as a second-line drug choice and only with concurrent monitoring of liver enzymes every 6 months (Kaplan et al, 1998; Pliszka, 1998b; Popper, 1997).

Methamphetamine (Desoxyn) is a long-acting stimulant with a duration of action of 8 to 12 hours and 5-, 10-, and 15-mg formulations. Sources identify Gradumet tablets as effective for once-daily dosing, which is a plus for students who do not want to take medicine at school. There are very few studies of its use in children, and Desoxyn does not seem to be the therapy of choice because of the stigma related to its potential for substance abuse (Popper, 1997).

Stimulant use in preschool children appears more variable with more adverse reactions (Miller and Castellanos, 1998). More research is becoming available on its safety and efficacy (Musten et al, 1997). Children are not usually given medication until after 6 years of age. Psychostimulant use in this age group should be reserved for severe cases or for when parent training and behavioral programs have been ineffective (Block, 1998; Kaplan et al, 1998).

Antidepressants—including the tricyclic antidepressants (TCAs)—are considered second-line drugs for treating children with ADHD, although they are not approved by the FDA for this purpose (Miller and Castellanos, 1998). Antidepressants seem effective in reducing symptoms of ADHD but appear to have fewer positive effects on cognition with stimulants (Biederman, 1998; McEvoy, 1995)

(Table 28-3). For children who fail to respond to stimulants, develop depression, or have adverse effects, TCAs may offer longer duration of action, less behavioral rebound and insomnia, and no risk of abuse (Kaplan et al, 1998). In treating ADHD,

Table 28-3
Nonstimulant Medications for Treating ADHD

Drug	Dosage*	Maximum	Side Effects
Antidepressants			
Imipramine (Tofranil)	Start 10 to 25 mg/day (1.5-5.0 mg/kg/day)	2.0 to 5.0 mg/kg/day	*Common:* cardiac conduction slowing, mild tachycardia, anticholinergic effects
Desipramine (Norpramin)	Start 10 to 15 mg/day (2.5-5.0 mg/kg/day)	2.0 to 5.0 mg/kg/day	*Uncommon but serious:* Heart block or arrhythmias, induction of psychosis, confusion, seizures, hypertension
Amitriptyline (Elavil)	Start 10 to 25 mg/day (Average: 20-150 mg/day	2.0 to 5.0 mg/kg/day	*Occasional:* rash, tics, photosensitization,) gynecomastia
Nortriptyline (Pamelor)	10 to 25 mg/day	1.0 to 3.0 mg/kg/day	May worsen tics and lower seizure threshold
Clomipramine (Anafranil)	Starts 25 mg/day (Average: 85 mg/day)	200 mg or 3.0 mg/kg/day, whichever is less	
Bupropion (Wellbutrin)	3 mg/kg in divided doses	6 mg/kg/day or 450 mg/day	
Alpha Adrenergic Agonists			
Clonidine (Catapres) Adolescents:	8 to 12 yrs: 0.25-0.3 mg/day 0.3 to 0.4 mg/day, give tid with meals and at HS	Rarely .0.5 mg/day	*Common:* sedation, hypotension (usually not clinically significant), headache and dizziness, stomach ache, nausea, and vomiting
Clonidine Transdermal patches	5-day application		*Uncommon but serious:* rebound hypertension, depression
Guanfacine (Tenex)	Start 0.5 mg/day	3 mg	*Occasional:* enhances sedation and hypotension (but less than appetite, Raynaud's with Clonidine)

*Schedule of dosing: consider dividing dose into 2 to 3 doses to minimize adverse effects; otherwise may use daily dosing; initiating at bedtime can reduce sedative effects. Onset of effect is 4 days. (Block, 1998; Kaplan et al, 1998; McEvoy, 1995; Scahill and Lynch, 1994)

desipramine (Norpramin), imipramine (Tofranil), amitriptyline (Elavil), nortriptyline (Pamelor), and clomipramine (Anafranil) are all effective; desipramine and imipramine, however, have been studied more. TCA use in children came under scrutiny after reports of sudden death as a result of cardiac arrest arose in four children being treated with desipramine (Biederman, 1998). Conduction slowing with arrhythmia potentiation is suspected; therefore ECG monitoring after establishing a baseline is recommended for children treated with TCAs. A baseline ECG is rechecked several days after acquiring a dose of 2.5 mg/kg/day (1.0 mg/kg/day with nortriptyline) and after each increase in dose of 50 mg/day to 100 mg/day. After the maintenance dose is reached, ECGs can be twice a year. Nortriptyline or imipramine is favored over desipramine (AACAP, 1997).

The doses for TCA use in ADHD are lower than those for depression, and the onset of response may be more rapid (Popper, 1997) (see Table 28-3). TCA use is effective in reducing hyperactivity, improving mood, and enhancing sleep but does not seem to positively affect concentration (Biederman, 1998; Kaplan et al, 1998). Antidepressants can be used in children with both ADHD and Tourette's syndrome without risk of tic exacerbation (Popper, 1997). Recommendations for starting doses are presented in Table 28-3. Dosing should begin at a low, subtherapeutic dose and be titrated up until the maximum dose, total serum drug or metabolite levels, or untoward effects are observed. The recommendation that TCAs be administered in two or three doses to minimize untoward effects seems prudent. Drugs should be tapered over 2 to 3 weeks when they are being discontinued to prevent withdrawal effects (e.g., nausea, vomiting, fatigue, abdominal pain) (AACAP, 1997).

Bupropion (Wellbutrin), which is a heterocyclic antidepressant, has been suggested as a second-line drug for treating ADHD. Several well-conducted studies have found bupropion to be similar in efficacy to methylphenidate (AACAP, 1997; Popper, 1997). Problems that can occur with its administration include exacerbation of tic disorders, development of a rash, and lowering of the seizure threshold (Miller and Castellanos, 1998).

Clonidine (Catapres), which is an alpha-adrenergic antagonist, has been widely used in the treatment of ADHD, especially for beneficial effects in individuals with a comorbid tic disorder.

The availability of transdermal patches (applied every 5 days) is an advantage, and clonidine can be useful in improving a child's ability to fall asleep. Although not approved by the FDA for these indications, clonidine has been prescribed both alone and in combination with stimulants, reportedly increasing frustration tolerance and cooperation while decreasing distractibility in children with ADHD (AACAP, 1997). Combined pharmacotherapy for ADHD may be useful for the 30% to 40% of children who do not respond to a single agent (Wilens et al, 1995). There are no published studies of the efficacy or safety of the use of a stimulant in combination with clonidine (AACAP, 1997). Practice parameters established by the AACP caution combining clonidine with other medications because four children who had reportedly been taking both clonidine and methylphenidate died. Although the evidence was sparse in linking the medication with the fatalities, a careful cardiovascular history and an electrocardiogram (ECG) should precede onset of clonidine treatment until the details are clarified. Guanfacine (Tenex), which is a longer-acting, less-sedating, more receptor-specific alpha-adrenergic agonist than clonidine, has also been reported to be effective in ADHD treatment (AACAP, 1997; Hunt, Arnsten, and Asbell, 1995).

Despite the fact that ADHD is a chronic condition, controversy exists over what hours to cover with medication. Some children are maintained on medication for attention only during school hours. Not all learning takes place in the classroom, so many children benefit from continual medication. The use of medication during weekends, holidays, and vacations can help a child handle situations that tend to be less structured and are therefore usually more difficult for children with ADHD (Cantwell, 1996).

The effectiveness of stimulant medication should be evaluated periodically and may involve prescribing "drug holidays," during which time no medications are taken. Although the beginning and end of the school year have been proposed as evaluation times, school activities at these times are either new or less predictable and thus more difficult for children with ADHD to manage (Miller and Castellanos, 1998). Therefore evaluations to determine if the medication is still needed should essentially occur at a "neutral" time of the school year. Summer drug holidays give children a break from dependency on drugs that affect their behavior and may allow for catch-up growth in children for whom appetite suppression is a significant adverse effect. Some researchers, however, question the efficacy of removing children from their medications (Cantwell, 1996). These researchers believe that because learning does not stop outside the classroom, children who need pharmacologic support need it continuously. Children who continue taking medication during vacations may have fewer accidents and improved social-emotional growth. Drug holidays occasionally occur accidentally when there has been a failure to take the prescribed medications; these holidays provide excellent opportunities for evaluating the child.

Although pharmacotherapy can significantly improve the behavior of the child with ADHD, education of the child, parents, and teachers is a key component of treatment (AACAP, 1997; Shealy, 1994). Academic and social adjustments are most difficult for these children because of deficient behavioral and cognitive skills. Behavioral interventions are helpful adjuncts to pharmacotherapy, and this combination can offer synergistic and cost-effective benefits (Steinmiller and O'Sullivan, 1997). Health care professionals, educators, and parents must help these children set appropriate goals and then guide them to organize and prioritize strategies to obtain them.

Multimodal, multidisciplinary approaches have traditionally been proposed as most effective in meeting the needs of children with ADHD and LDs (AACAP, 1997), although few controlled studies have evaluated the efficacy of multimodal "packaged" therapy. The support of professionals for child-parent training is important in helping a family and child effectively cope with a chronic, difficult situation.

Controversial Therapies

Numerous alternative therapies have been recommended to correct LDs and hyperactive behavior, but none has been empirically supported by controlled clinical studies or supported by the American Academy of Pediatrics (AAP) as treatment. The different controversial approaches for school-age children include cognitive-behavioristic approaches, neurophysiologic retraining (i.e., patterning, optometric visual training, and applied kinesiology), megavitamins, allergen avoidance, and diet modification—including the Feingold diet or elimination of sorbitol, caffeine, or refined sug-

ars (Barkley, 1998a). The AAP has warned that large amounts of fat-soluble vitamins and vitamin B_6 may result in damage to the nervous system (Silver, 1993). The AAP (1998) has also stated that visual problems are rarely responsible for learning difficulties and that there is no scientific evidence to support the view that correction of subtle visual defects with eye exercises or special lenses can alter the brain's processing of visual stimuli.

Recent and Anticipated Advances in Diagnosis and Management

Research to delineate the various etiologic factors of LDs and ADHD will help in the determination of prevention strategies and tools for early detection. With increased technologic ability to study the genetic, neurobiologic, and neuroanatomic basis for LDs and ADHD, potential new avenues of treatment should emerge. Recognition of the effect of lifespan on LDs and ADHD, coupled with federal support for individuals with disabilities, should broaden treatment options and opportunities for children diagnosed as hyperactive and learning impaired who have "grown up." In addition, expanding the diagnostic criteria to be more applicable to adults will help in diagnosing older teens and adults who were neither diagnosed nor provided educational services during their childhood.

Associated Problems (Box 28-4)

Psychologic Sequelae

Children who are misdiagnosed or not diagnosed in grade school may experience many years of academic failure. The psychologic sequelae of multiple failures can result in poor self-esteem. Chronic school pressures and failure can result in frustration, anxiety, depression, an inner sense of restlessness, psychosomatic complaints, and school absenteeism or resignation (Greenhill, 1998; Silver, 1997). Teachers may misinterpret their behaviors and label these children as lazy or insensitive or dismiss them from the classroom. On average, children with ADHD are rated by their teachers as less popular, less assertive, and less cooperative than their classmates (Lahey et al, 1998).

A number of children with LDs or ADHD have difficulty with peer relationships. This difficulty is especially true for those who have significant psychomotor dysfunction and/or a restricted use of language, or those who are in special education classes or singled out and labeled as "different" in a regular classroom. A similar number of children who are learning disabled, however, are quite popular. Some of the social behavior problems may be the result of the child's impulsivity and difficulty in reading nonverbal social cues, resulting in misjudgment of acceptance or rejection by or increased aggression to peers (Barkley, 1998a). Family relationships are also affected.

One of the problems in identifying children as having an LD or ADHD is the effect of labeling. The label allows the child to receive services to compensate for deficits and adjust to the consequences but may also result in a self-fulfilling prophecy. Educators must be careful not to use the label to separate or identify children in a mainstreamed classroom.

Pharmacologic Sequelae

All medications have side-effects and possible adverse sequelae; those used in the treatment of ADHD are no exception (see Table 28-3). Because medications are the mainstay of therapy for ADHD, providers must have a thorough understanding of their benefits and potential risks and monitor children closely. Children rarely report their side-effects from medications, so direct questioning about potential effects is advised (Tosyali and Greenhill, 1998). If a child has side-effects, the

practitioner may choose to change to another drug in the same class before switching to another category of medication (AACAP, 1997).

Prognosis

A significant number of children diagnosed as learning disabled are affected into adulthood. Most children with LDs continue to be affected throughout life. Those who do not learn to compensate have poorer educational and employment outcomes. Many of these individuals have difficulty succeeding in professions or choosing occupations or professions that match their strengths and are more likely to be underemployed and undereducated, even though their intelligence is at least average. Others have learned to compensate for their areas of weakness and build upon their strengths.

Up to 80% of children with ADHD manifest symptoms as adolescents (AACAP, 1997), and 30% to 65% still meet all or part of the criteria into adulthood (AACAP, 1997; Gingerich et al, 1998). Adults report increased interpersonal problems, increased job terminations (especially in jobs requiring adult problem-solving, prioritizing, and self-control), increased sexual problems, and restlessness (Gingerich et al, 1998; Greenhill, 1998). The rate of ADHD does appear to decline in adulthood "by 50% approximately every 5 years, leading to the estimates of adult ADHD as 0.8% at age 20 and 0.005% at age 40" (Greenhill, 1998). The AACAP (1997), however, indicates that the frequency in adults is from 2% to 7%.

Studies of long-term outcomes in ADHD demonstrate considerable variation in results. This variation is especially true for those with combined ADHD and CD because many of them go on to develop antisocial personality disorder in adulthood (Greenhill et al, 1998). Positive or negative outcomes appear to be mediated by factors such as age at diagnosis, individualized treatment measures instituted, coping mechanisms, mental health of family members, intelligence, cultural expectations, comorbidity of other conditions, and persistence of symptoms (Gingerich et al, 1998). "Comorbid conditions have proven to be the most consistent predictors of later developmental risks and negative outcomes" (Barkley, 1997).

Many children with LDs and ADHD, however, grow up to become successful adults and have learned to compensate for their disability. A number of them have become members of the health care team by entering fields such as dentistry, psychology, medicine, and nursing. Because section 504 of the Rehabilitation Act (1973) indicates that "if otherwise qualified" these individuals must be provided entrance to jobs and continuing education, their potential is limitless.

PRIMARY CARE MANAGEMENT

Health Care Maintenance

Growth and Development

Careful attention must be given to routinely (i.e., about every 6 months) measuring weight and physical growth parameters if a child is taking stimulant medication for hyperactivity. The effect of stimulant medication on growth appears to be temporary and minimal, with no significant differences seen by adolescence (Barkley, 1998a). The side-effect of anorexia, resulting in weight loss of 0.5 kg to 2.25 kg, can be controlled by the timing of the administration of stimulant medications. In many children, this side effect abates after 6 months (Block, 1998). Sleep problems and difficulty with toilet training are also areas that may need attention.

LDs and ADHD are not routinely diagnosed until a child begins school. IDEA requires that children at risk for developing LDs or ADHD be assessed in the first 3 years of life if signs and symptoms are evident (see Chapter 2). This places more responsibility on health care providers to develop and use tools that can measure cognitive abilities and hyperactivity at an earlier age. Because children learn to compensate for their disability, and in some cases the nature of their disability changes as they grow and develop, it is important to reevaluate a child's cognitive, motor, and psychosocial level of development every few years.

Diet

There are no dietary restrictions. Children on stimulant medication may have a decreased appetite, and their increased activity level may warrant an increased caloric intake. These children may be easily distracted from the meal and leave the table before they are finished eating. Therefore meals and snacks that are high in protein and calories and easy to eat should be encouraged to enhance their nutritional status. Establishing a mealtime routine may also be beneficial

Safety

There are a number of safety issues for children and adolescents with LDs and ADHD. Because some children have an increase in impulsive behavior and altered judgment, they are at higher risk for acting without thinking and engaging in unsafe activities. These children are more likely to sustain injuries, especially closed-head injuries, due to behavioral inattentiveness and impulsivity (Gerring et al, 1998). Children with ADHD were reported to have more injuries and more severe injuries related to means of transportation (i.e., motor vehicle, pedestrian, bicycle, motorcycle, all-terrain vehicles and/or recreational vehicles) than children with no preexisting condition, and pedestrian injuries were noted as the major cause of hospital admission for trauma in the ADHD population (DiScala et al, 1998). Children with LDs may get lost more often because of problems in processing information about their environment. Children who have difficulty understanding directions may be unable to safely complete tasks or take appropriate action in an emergency.

Primary care providers may need to help families and older children develop plans to structure their environment and their activities. Breaking down activities into component parts and using checklists may help children be more aware of their behavior. Parents should be advised that normal activities may take more time and they should keep the child's schedule simple to prevent it from becoming overloaded.

A significant number of adolescents with LDs and ADHD have decreased judgment of speed, space, and distance. These deficits, plus a decreased ability to pay attention to things such as conditions of the road and driving speed, result in an increase in motor vehicle accidents in this population (Barkley, 1998a). Driving is an activity that requires multiple tasks and decision-making simultaneously. Adolescents who have difficulty in these areas are advised to delay driving for a few years.

Although no data support abuse of stimulant medications, medication safety should always be a consideration in teaching. Using containers that mark the pills for each day of the week may be helpful for children who are self-administering their medications. Standard precautions for keeping medications safely secured should be followed not only for the child with ADHD but also for siblings and classmates because many of the medications can be easily sold on the street.

Immunizations

No changes in the routine schedule of immunizations are needed.

Screening

Vision: Comprehensive vision testing should be performed at diagnosis, especially if a child is suspected to have a visual-perceptual deficit. Routine screening at recommended intervals should then occur. A child who has a problem with letter reversals may have difficulty when being tested on the Snellen E chart, in which the direction of the letter *E* has to be determined. A short reading test (if age-appropriate) is also helpful in assessing reading comprehension and the ability to read across a line without skipping words or losing place.

Hearing: Comprehensive audiometric testing should be performed at diagnosis, especially if a child is suspected to have an auditory-perceptual deficit. Routine screening at recommended intervals should then occur.

Speech and language: Speech and language assessments should be initiated for children demonstrating receptive or expressive language disorders.

Dental: Routine screening is recommended.

Blood pressure: Routine screening is recommended except for children receiving stimulants, tricyclics, clonidine, or guanfacine. Blood pressure alterations may also occur as a result of the medications used to treat ADHD, thus blood pressure should be monitored every few months—especially in black adolescents, who are more at risk for developing an increase in their diastolic blood pressure (Barkley, 1998a).

Hematocrit: Routine screening is recommended.

Urinalysis: Routine screening is recommended.

Tuberculosis: Routine screening is recommended.

Condition-Specific Screening

Liver function: Children taking pemoline need liver function tests every few months.

Thyroid function: A rare genetic resistance to thyroid hormone has been linked to ADHD. Thyroid function should be checked if a child has any symptoms or a family history of hypo- or hyperthyroid function (AACAP, 1997).

Cardiac function: Children taking TCAs and clonidine will need baseline ECGs repeated with dose increments (AACAP, 1997). Tachycardia, with an increase of 6 to 15 beats per minute over a child's normal baseline has often been reported but does not result in ECG irregularities and is dose-related (Barkley, 1998a).

Common Illness Management

Differential Diagnosis (Box 28-5)

Effects of stimulant therapy: It is important to differentiate the clinical manifestations of LD and ADHD from other problems of childhood (e.g., the irritability and inability to attend to a task) that are common when a child is ill or suffering from emotional trauma. Side-effects of stimulant medications or the characteristics of the conditions themselves (e.g., anorexia, weight loss, stomachache, headache, and insomnia) may mask the symptoms of physical and psychologic illness (Findling and Dogin, 1998).

Developmental and/or behavioral deviations: Numerous developmental deviations (e.g., adjustment disorders, cognitive delay, visual and auditory problems, inadequate sleep, lack of breakfast, and global delays) may be mistaken for ADHD. Absence seizures can be mistaken as inattentive ADHD or LDs. Children must be evaluated carefully to rule out these conditions.

Psychologic conditions such as chronic anxiety, fear of failure, and those that develop from family stress (i.e., divorce, illness and death in the family, teen pregnancy, poverty, and malnutrition) may result in difficulty attending to academic tasks but should not be confused with a worsening of the disability. Adolescents who are found to have depression may have their diagnosis of ADHD delayed because the learning and behavior problems displayed may be classified as secondary to the depression (Biederman et al, 1998).

Characteristics of ADHD and/or LD that Affect Differential Diagnosis

Effects of Stimulant Therapy
Anorexia or weight loss
Insomnia
Headache
Stomachache

Developmental and/or Behavioral Deviations
Adjustment problems
Cognitive delay
Learning disorders
Emotional disorders
Visual and auditory problems
Dysfunctional family

Increased Injuries
Physical and psychological abuse

Comorbidity
Conduct disorder
Depression
Anxiety disorders
Oppositional Defiant Disorder

Increased injuries: Children with ADHD or LDs who are often seen for mild trauma care and are thought to have possibly experienced abuse must be reassessed from the perspective of their LD or ADHD. Children with difficulty following safety directions or who lack hand-eye coordination may be more prone to environmental injury.

Drug Interactions

Medications used to treat ADHD have a number of interactive effects when given with other drugs (Table 28-4). Psychostimulants, the most common medications used to treat ADHD, fortunately have few clinically significant drug-to-drug interactions (Ten Eick, Nakamura, and Reed, 1998). When administered simultaneously with sympathomimetic medications used for cold and allergy symptoms (ephedrine and pseudoephedrine) or other stimulants, stimulants can result in a dangerously heightened stimulant effect (Deglin and Vallerand, 1999). In addition, monoamine oxidase inhibitors (MAOIs)

retard the metabolism of psychostimulants, which can lead to toxic effects, and the coadministration of MAOIs and stimulants can lead to a potentially lethal hypertensive crisis. Stimulant coadministration can decrease neuroleptic drug effects and increase TCA and selective serotonin reuptake inhibitor (SSRI) activity (Tan Eick et al, 1998). Amphetamines can impair the hypotensive effects of guanethidine (Ismelin), possibly resulting in arrhythmias. Clearance of amphetamines is enhanced by urinary acidifiers, resulting in lower levels of the amphetamine; alkalinizers result in impaired renal tubular clearance. Insulin requirements may be decreased in children with diabetes because appetite can be suppressed (Deglin and Vallerand, 1999; McEvoy, 1995).

Some of the psychostimulants have specific precautions that need to be addressed. Methylphenidate may elevate levels of TCAs and warfarin. Dextroamphetamine may increase the risk of cardiovascular effects with beta blockers, and phenothiazines may decrease the effect of dextroamphetamine (Dexedrine). Pemoline may decrease the seizure threshold in children taking anticonvulsants (Deglin and Vallerand, 1999).

Tricyclic antidepressants can cause increased effects with stimulants, CNS depressants (e.g., MAOIs, sympathomimetics, alcohol, or other substance-abuse medications), anticholinergics, thyroid preparations, and seizure-potentiating medications. Tricyclic antidepressants can decrease the effects of clonidine. The effects of the tricyclics are increased by phenothiazine, cimetidine, and oral contraceptives (McEvoy, 1995). The effects of the tricyclics are decreased by barbiturates and smoking.

Clinically important drug-to-drug interactions with TCAs include reactions with carbamazepine, phenobarbital, valproic acid, clonidine, guanfacine, MAOIs, anticholinergics, and sympathomimetics. TCA action is suppressed when carbamazepine or phenobarbital is administered concurrently. TCA toxicity may occur when valproic acid is also being used. Medications frequently used to treat upper respiratory infections and allergies that have anticholinergic and sympathomimetic properties could result in heightened anticholinergic and sympathomimetic effects in children concurrently taking TCAs (Tan Eick et al, 1998). TCAs should not be used with MAOIs to prevent severe hypertension, hyperpyrexia, seizures, and death. MAOIs must be discontinued 2 weeks before TCA therapy is initiated (Deglin and Vallerund, 1999). Increased CNS

Table 28-4
Drug Interactions Relevant in Treating ADHD

Drug A	Combined with Drug B	Interaction
Stimulants	Sympathomimetics, other stimulants	Significantly increased stimulant effect
	MAOIs	Toxic stimulant effect; hypertensive crisis; may be lethal
	Neuroleptics	Decreased seizure threshold
	TCAs	Increased TCA effect
	SSRIs	Increased SSRI effect
	Insulin	Decreased requirements of insulin if eating less
Amphetamines	Urinary acidifiers	Amphetamine effect
	Urinary alkalinizer	Amphetamine effect
	Guanethidine	Guanethidine effect (arrhythmias)
Methylphenidate	Warfarin	Anticoagulant level
	TCA	TCA levels
Dextroamphetamine	Beta blockers	Beta blocker action
	Phenothiazine	Action of both drugs
Pemoline	Antiepileptic medications	Seizure threshold
TCAs	Stimulants	Effects of stimulants
	CNS depressants (MAOI, alcohol sympathomimetics)	CNS depressant effect
	Anticholinergics	Effect of anticholinergics
	Thyroid preparations	Thyroid activity
	Seizure potentiating medications	Seizure potentiation
	Carbamazepine	Decreased TCA action
	Valproic Acid	Increased TCA effect
	Clonidine or guanfacine	Effect of clonidine, guanfacine
	Phenothiazines	TCA effect
	Oral contraceptives	TCA effect
	Barbiturates	TCA effect
	Smoking	TCA effect
Clonidine	CNS depressants	Drug B
	Anticholinergic preparations	Drug B
	Beta-adrenergic blockers	Drug B effect
	Fenfluramine	Clonidine effect
	Thiazide diuretics	Clonidine effect
	Antihypertensive agents	Clonidine effect
	CNS depressants	Sedative effect of clonidine
	TCAs	Hypotensive effect of clonidine
	NSAIDS	Hypotensive effect of clonidine
	Sympathomimetic drugs	Hypotensive effects of clonidine
Bupropion	MAOIs, levodopa	Increased adverse effects

depression is noted with concurrent use of clonidine or guanfacine with TCAs, and the antihypertensive effect of clonidine may be antagonized with TCA use.

There is an increased risk of adverse reactions if bupropion is used simultaneously with levodopa or MAOIs (Deglin and Vallerand, 1999). Clonidine increases the effects of CNS depressants and anticholinergic preparations, although usually less in children than adults. Clonidine decreases the effects of beta-adrenergic blockers, which heightens the rebound hypertension that can occur when it is discontinued. The effect of clonidine is enhanced with fenfluramine, thiazide diuretics, and other antihypertensive agents. The sedative effect of clonidine is increased with use of other CNS depressants. The hypotensive effects of clonidine are impaired with tricyclic antidepressants, sympathomimetic drugs, and nonsteroidal antiinflammatory agents (McEvoy, 1995).

Developmental Issues

Sleep Patterns

LDs have no effect on sleep unless emotional problems are present. In children with ADHD, medication timing or inability to settle down may affect falling asleep. Sleep problems—especially in the time it takes to fall asleep—have been identified by parents as a chronic problem in children with ADHD. These problems are not always related to use of stimulant medications but do result in fewer total sleep hours (Barkley, 1998a). The drug administration schedule should be assessed. Insomnia is a common side-effect of stimulant medication and often resolves as a child develops a tolerance to the medication. If insomnia does not resolve, however, decreasing the doses or scheduling administration earlier in the day may help. Medication rebound, resounding as overactivity and irritability, may necessitate the addition of a small bedtime dose of stimulant (Block, 1998). Practitioners should be alerted to the fact that extreme sleepiness may be a sign of overmedication.

Toileting

Unless a child experiences sensory or tactile deficits, there is no effect on toileting. If a child does experience such deficits, he or she must be walked through the sensations involved in toileting. Routine toilet breaks should be a part of the daily schedule. Elementary schools should also be sensitive to this need and incorporate toileting into a day's activities. Delayed toilet training and the possibility of later enuresis and/or encopresis may occur (Barkley, 1998a).

Discipline

All children act out and misbehave at various intervals in the developmental process. As with other children, discipline should fit the seriousness of the misbehavior. Children with an LD or ADHD, however, do not learn well from past experiences and may not be able to understand cause and effect or verbal sequences of directions. Even after these children have done something wrong, they may not relate their activity to the punishment and will need frequent clarification from adults. Frequent feedback related to progress is important.

Behavior-modification techniques over a prolonged period of time may help a child develop self-control. If time-outs are used, children must be told when the period of restriction has ended. They need to be reminded of the reasons for the punishment and consistently helped to differentiate between "the act being wrong or bad" and "the child being bad." Although behavior modification helps to improve targeted behaviors and skills, it does not reduce inattention, hyperactivity, or impulsivity (AACAP, 1997). Identification of and rewards for good behavior are effective. For hyperactive children, parents need help determining to what degree their child's normal behavior requires discipline. Parenting classes may help them to make this differentiation and provide clear instructions with positive reinforcement.

Discipline should be part of the daily routine for these children and must be consistent. Limit-setting is an important component of the day. Structuring the daily routine of the home environment helps these children establish acceptable patterns of behavior. Parents should be reminded to also teach the recommended behavioral approaches to a child's significant others (e.g., grandparents and babysitters).

Child Care

If daycare is a component of child care, a program that has a small class size, a structured and safe environment, constant adult supervision, and an opportunity to engage in gross motor play outdoors should be selected. Predictability of schedule is reassuring to children with ADHD or an LD because they often do not handle surprises or changes well.

Schooling

LDs and ADHD have a major effect on the education of children and adolescents. Children should be evaluated for school readiness prior to kindergarten. A number of children with LDs spend 2 years in kindergarten or first grade to give them time to develop the psychosocial and cognitive skills necessary for success. Children should also be assessed for prerequisite deficits in knowledge or skills, and remediation should be planned for such deficits. Primary care providers may play a key role in emotionally supporting parents through the difficult decision of holding back their child. Focusing on the long-term gains will help diminish the parents' initial disappointment and grief. Making children feel special and giving attention to their accomplishments is beneficial to these children.

Children who are not yet diagnosed when they enter school may experience a series of barriers. Teachers are not permitted to identify a child as hyperactive, lest they be making a diagnosis. Some districts discourage staff from recommending testing to parents because it is then the district's responsibility to pay for the testing (Bender, 1997). Practitioners should be familiar with the internal policies of the school districts in which they practice and support parents in their requests for testing and evaluation through special education if a child's history and physical findings are consistent with LD or ADHD. There is no benefit in waiting to see if a child "outgrows" the learning difficulty if school failure is already occurring.

Children with LDs and ADHD may be educated in regular classrooms, use the resource room, attend special-education classes, be tutored, or use a combination thereof. The goal is inclusion into normal classrooms, but special-education classrooms and resource rooms are also very acceptable therapies. In resource rooms (supplementary help) and special-education (self-contained) classrooms, teachers can limit the number of students in the classroom, decrease the amount of distraction, and provide specific interventions based on a child's needs (Box 28-6).

According to IDEA, every child with an LD should have an individualized education plan (IEP) developed specifically for them. Children with ADHD are covered under Section 504 of the Rehabilitation Act, thus guaranteeing them reasonable accommodations and the development of an accommodation plan. Children who are severely affected with ADHD may also qualify for an IEP (see Chapter 5).

Children who continue to have academic difficulty resulting in failure need counseling support and assistance in dealing with related stress. By high school, the inattention of ADHD may be manifested as chronic academic underachievement and motivation problems (Reiff, 1998). Children with LDs and ADHD need to understand that even though they failed a course (or examination), they are not failures. It is not appropriate to tell children to "try harder." A child's decreased performance is not often because of a lack of effort or anyone's fault. These children need to be reassured that they are not stupid and that requests for repetition of directions and clarification of content are not a nuisance.

A significant part of the educational plan is to help children learn to compensate for their particular disability. Children need to understand which learning modalities work best for them and have material presented (or available) to them in that modality. For children with visual-perceptual deficits, material can be presented orally, with demonstration or simple pictures; tape recording class lectures may be more helpful than manual note-taking. Written directions should be explained, written test delivery may need to be modified, and a ruler may help a child keep the lines in focus.

It may be more helpful to present material in writing, pictorially, or with hands-on demonstration for children with an auditory perceptual deficit. Short lists of directions or check-off sheets also help with organization. Preventive measures of using a calendar to predict oncoming menses and planning frequent toilet breaks may be helpful for children with tactile deficits.

Children with integrative deficits may benefit from multisensory approaches. Constant feedback to ensure their understanding is essential. These children should be given extra time to answer questions; races to come up with answers may be extremely stressful. It may be helpful to highlight texts to help them find the important information. Calen-

---

Box 28-6

Educational and Environmental Strategies for the Child with LD and/or ADHD

- Identify the child's strengths and build on them.
- Provide positive reinforcement for effort and achievement.
- Implement rules and consequences consistently.
- Pace the student.
- Provide learning activities when medication is at its peak.

Learning Environment:
   Muted wall colors
   Decreased clutter (desks, worksheets, classroom)
   Seat child in front of room, away from doors, windows, and distractions
   Seat child near on-task peer
   Structured environment preferred over open, unstructured environment

- Use calendars, assignment books, structured schedule, untimed and oral testing and/or testing in separate quiet room.
- Give extra time to answer questions.
- Use technologic assistive devices (e.g., tape recorders, word processors).

- Give verbal and written instructions.
- Remind the child of critical behavior before an activity.
- Use physical activities (e.g., role-playing) for instruction.
- Use a notebook for daily homework assignments.
- Institute classroom rules that no laughing is allowed when someone makes a mistake.
- Provide positive reinforcement for effort and achievement.
- Give immediate positive feedback on behavior.
- Help the child to develop a relationship with an adult (e.g., college student, Big Brother) to promote social interaction and supervised learning experiences.
- Divide large projects into smaller parts.
- Keep a second set of books at home.
- Post a daily schedule and make to-do lists.
- Decrease the length of tasks; plan frequent breaks.
- Do not let the child get overloaded.
- Build the child's self-esteem and self-confidence at every opportunity.

---

dars and lists will assist in their organization. Children with altered coordination and difficulty in motor skills may shy away from participation in age-appropriate activities. Being involved in noncompetitive sports, being given a different role in a group activity so as to continue being a member of the group, and finding alternative motor activities (e.g., using a computer rather than being required to use script) will enhance the self-concept of these children and make them less fearful of participation.

Administration of medication during school hours has presented some problems for children. Some children forget to get their lunchtime dose because they often have to leave their friends to go to the infirmary or office, are involved in group activities, or may feel guilty or self-conscious about having to take pills—especially if "Drug-Free Schools" information is being promoted. In addition, state and local policies on administration of medication in schools must be considered when prescribing medicines (see Chapter 5).

Sexuality

Providing sex education for children and adolescents is an important role for the primary care provider. Sex education must be individualized to a child's specific learning abilities using the learning techniques previously identified. Role-playing can be helpful because problem-solving is often difficult for these children.

Transition to Adulthood

The transition of older adolescents into adulthood is a critical point for families of children with ADHDs and LDs. The underlying condition and its associated risks do not go away, so adolescents working on the developmental tasks of separation from parents and family, establishing a sense of identity, and formulating personal and occupational goals often require professional help. Youth with LDs and ADHD often have unresolved issues from earlier developmental phases, less developed executive functioning skills and problem-solving skills, and less confidence, and may have limited awareness of the ramifications of their disability.

Special Family Concerns and Resources

Parents and siblings of a child with LD or ADHD must learn strategies to facilitate their abilities. Children with an LD or ADHD and their families will need to readjust to the child's condition at every new developmental stage. The psychologic effect of LDs or ADHD results in specific psychosocial needs. Building a child's self-esteem and self-confidence, as well as an accurate self-perception, becomes even more important when the child is experiencing chronic academic difficulty.

Environmental control in the home is similar to that discussed for the classroom. Decreasing clutter, developing routines, scheduling ample time for activities, and providing clear directions in the format that best meets the child's needs may be beneficial. Parents typically give more commands, directions, and supervision to these children than to a "normal" child. Parents are concerned about the child's potential for schooling and vocational choices, as well as the child's ability to assume an independent lifestyle. This concern results in increased parental stress, depression, and marital discord. Parents, as well as their children, need coping strategies and consistent support.

Books on LDs and ADHD for Parents and Teachers

Barkley RA: Taking charge of ADHD: the complete authoritative guide for parents, New York, 1995, Guilford Press.

Bender W: Understanding ADHD: a practical guide for teachers and parents, Upper Saddle River, NJ, 1997, Prentice-Hall.

Cooper P and Ideus K: Attention deficit/hyperactivity disorder: a practical guide for teachers, London, 1996, David Fulton Publishers.

Fowler M: Maybe you know my kid: a parent's guide to identifying, understanding and helping your child with ADHD, New York, 1990, Birch Lane Press.

Hallowell EM and Ratey JJ: Driven to distraction: recognizing and coping with attention deficit disorder from childhood through adulthood, Newark, NJ, 1994, Simon & Schuster.

Ingersoll BD and Goldstein S: Attention deficit disorder and learning disabilities: realities, myths and controversial treatments, New York, NY, 1993, Doubleday.

McEwan E: The principal's guide to attention deficit hyperactivity disorder, Thousand Oaks, Calif., 1998, Corwin Press

Reif S: How to reach and teach ADD/ADHD students: practical techniques, strategies, and interventions for helping children with attention problems and hyperactivity, West Nyack, NY, 1993, Center for Applied Research in Education.

Silver L: The misunderstood child: a guide for parents of children with learning disabilities, Blue Ridge Summit, Pa., 1992, TAB Books.

Silver L: Dr. Larry Silver's advice to parents on attention-deficit hyperactivity disorder, Washington, DC, 1993, American Psychiatric Press.

Smith C and Strick L: Learning disabilities: A to Z: a parent's complete guide to learning disabilities from preschool to adulthood, New York, NY, 1997, The Free Press.

Books on LDs and ADHD for Children

Gehret J: Eagle eyes, Fairport, NY, 1991, Verbal Images Press.

Gordon M: Jumpin' Johnny: get back to work: a child's guide to ADHD/Hyperactivity, DeWitt, NY, 1991, GSI Publications.

Mosa D: Shelly, the hyperactive turtle, Bethesda, Md., 1989, Woodbine House.

Quinn P and Stern J: Putting on the brakes: young people's guide to understanding attention deficit hyperactivity disorder, New York, 1991, Magination Press.

Organizations

Attention Deficit Disorder Association (ADDA)
9930 Jonnycake Ridge Road
Mentor, Ohio 44060
(216) 350-9595, (800) 487-2282
http://www.add.org

Children and Adults with Attention Deficit
   Disorders (CHADD)
8181 Professional Place, Suite 201
Landover, Md. 20785
(800) 233-4050
http://www.chadd.org

Council for Exceptional Children, Division of
   Learning Disabilities
1920 Association Drive

Reston, Va. 22091-1589
(703) 620-3660, (800) 328-0272
http://www.bgsu.edu/colleges/edhd/programs/
   DLD

Council for Learning Disabilities
PO Box 40303
Overland Park, Kan. 66204
(913) 492-8755
http://www.iser.com/CLD.html

Heath Resource Center (National Clearinghouse
   for Postsecondary Education for People with
   Disabilities)
1 DuPont Circle NW, Suite 800
Washington DC 20036-1193
http://www.acenet.edu/Programs/heath/home.html

International Dyslexia Association (IDA)
Chester Building
8600 La Salle Road, Suite 382
Baltimore, Md. 21204
(800) 222-03123
http://www.interdys.org

LD Online Home Page
(Learning Disabilities Project at WETA, Washington, DC)
http://www.ldonline.org

Learning Disabilities Association of America
4156 Library Road
Pittsburgh, Pa. 15234
(412) 341-1515
http://www.ldanatl.org

National Center for Learning Disabilities (NCLD)
381 Park Ave S, Suite 1401
New York, NY 10016
(212) 545-7510
http://www.ncld.org

National Information Center for Children and
   Youth with Disabilities (NICHCY)
PO Box 1492
Washington, DC 20013-1492
(800) 695-0285
http://www.nichcy.org

Summary of Primary Care Needs for the Child with Learning Disabilities or Attention Deficit Hyperactivity Disorder

HEALTH CARE MAINTENANCE

Growth and development

Medications for hyperactivity cause appetite suppression; assess height and weight every 6 months.

Manifestations of an LD or ADHD vary with development.

Early identification is beneficial and supported under IDEA.

Diet

Children may be poor eaters. Decreased appetite may occur if they are taking stimulant medication. A nutritious diet with adequate protein and calories for growth is important.

Safety

There is a risk of injury because of impulsive behaviors. Pedestrian, bike, and automobile accidents may occur more often because of spatial-perceptual difficulties.

Medication should be safely kept out of reach of young children.

Immunizations

Routine schedule is recommended.

Screening

Vision: Comprehensive visual testing is done to identify acuity problems and rule out other causes of a visual perceptual deficit.

Children may have difficulty using standard E chart.

Hearing: Comprehensive audiometric testing is done to identify hearing loss and rule out other causes of an auditory perceptual deficit.

Children may have difficulty with audiometric testing because of directionality problems.

Speech and language: Specialized testing is done if a problem is observed.

Dental: Routine screening is recommended.

Summary of Primary Care Needs for the Child with Learning Disabilities or Attention Deficit Hyperactivity Disorder—cont'd

Blood pressure: Routine screening is recommended. If a child is taking medication for ADHD, screening must be done more often because of possible hypo- or hypertension.

Hematocrit: Routine screening is recommended.

Urinalysis: Routine screening is recommended.

Tuberculosis: Routine screening is recommended.

Condition-specific screening: Liver function tests are necessary for children taking pemoline.

Thyroid function may need to be tested.

ECG monitoring is necessary for children on tricyclic antidepressants and clonidine.

COMMON ILLNESS MANAGEMENT

Differential diagnosis

Irritability, anorexia, weight loss, and insomnia are side effects of stimulants.

Illness or need for a change in dose or dosing schedule for medications must be ruled out.

Comorbidity is common in developmental and/or behavioral deviations and must be evaluated.

Change in inattention pattern may require ruling out seizure disorder.

Change in mood may suggest referral for anxiety, depression, and decreased self-esteem.

Injury pattern may be associated with possible abuse or need for greater supervision and/or safety practices.

Drug interactions

See Table 28-4.

Stimulant medications inhibit liver metabolism of other drugs.

Developmental issues

Sleep patterns: Children with ADHD on stimulant medication may have insomnia if it is given late in the day or in large doses.

Toileting: There is no effect on toileting unless a child has sensory tactile deficits.

Discipline: Children may have difficulty responding to directions and may not understand discipline or learn from past experiences. Consistency in expectations is important.

Behavior modification may be effective. A bad deed must be differentiated from a bad child.

Child care: Children perform better in a small, structured safe environment with constant adult supervision.

Schooling: Education strategies to decrease distraction in a regular classroom, in addition to creative teaching modalities appropriate to the specific learning needs of the child, should be implemented. Building a child's self-esteem and confidence are essential. Children should be helped to learn to compensate for their disability. Development of the individualized education plan (IEP) or accommodation plan is a team effort (see Table 28-6).

Sexuality: Learning techniques individualized for particular adolescents must be used when teaching sexuality and birth control material.

Transition to Adulthood

Professional help may be necessary to facilitate the transition to more autonomous living and work situations.

Career development counseling may be helpful in identifying an appropriate vocation based on a child's strengths and weaknesses

Special Family Concerns and Resources

The child and the family need to readjust to this disability at every new developmental stage. Family counseling can provide information and emotional support. An LD is a living disability.

References

Accardo P: The invisible disability: understanding learning disabilities in the context of health and education, Washington, DC, 1996, National Health and Education Consortium.

American Academy of Child and Adolescent Psychiatry: Practice parameters for the assessment and treatment of children, adolescents, and adults with attention-deficit/hyperactivity disorder, 36(10):85S-112S, 1997.

American Academy of Pediatrics: Learning disabilities, dyslexia, and vision: a subject review, Pediatrics 102(5):1217-1219, 1998.

American Psychiatric Association: Diagnostic and statistical manual of mental disorders, ed 4, Washington, DC, 1994, The Association.

Barkley R: Attention deficit hyperactivity disorder and the nature of self control, New York, 1997, The Guilford Press.

Barkley R. Attention-deficit hyperactivity disorder: a handbook for diagnosis and treatment, New York, 1998a, The Guilford Press.

Barkley R: Attention-deficit hyperactivity disorder, Scientific American, September 1998b, Website: http://www.sciam.com/1998/0998issuebarkley.html

Barkley R and Biederman J: Toward a broader definition of the age-of-onset criterion for attention-deficit hyperactivity disorder, J Am Acad Child Adolesc Psychiatry 36(9):1204-1210, 1997.

Bender W: Understanding ADHD: a practical guide for teachers and parents, Upper Saddle River, NJ, 1997, Prentice-Hall.

Biederman J: Attention-deficit/hyperactivity disorder: a life-span perspective, J Clin Psychol 59(Suppl 7): 4-16, 1998.

Biederman J et al: Diagnostic continuity between child and adolescent ADHD: findings from a longitudinal clinical sample, J Am Acad Child Adolesc Psychiatry 37(3):305-313, 1998

Block S: Attention-deficit disorder: a paradigm for psychotropic medication intervention in pediatrics, Pediatr Clin North Am 45(5):1053-1083, 1998.

Cantwell D: Attention deficit disorder: a review of the past 10 years, J Am Acad Child Adolesc Psychiatry 35(8):978-987, 1996

Carlson C, Tamm L, and Gaub M: Gender differences in children with ADHD, ODD, and co-occurring ADHD/ODD identified in a school population, J Am Acad Child Adolesc Psychiatry 36(12):1706-1714, 1997.

Cherkes-Julkowski M: Learning disability, attention-deficit disorder, and language impairment as outcomes of prematurity: a longitudinal descriptive study, J Learning Disabilities 31(3):294-306, 1998

Conners CK: Rating scales in attention-deficit/hyperactivity disorder: use in assessment and treatment monitoring, J Clin Psychiatry 59(suppl 7):24-30, 1998

Daly J and Wilens T: The use of tricyclic antidepressants in children and adolescents, Psychiatric Clin North Am 45(5):1123-1136, 1998.

Deglin J and Vallerand A: Davis's drug guide for nurses, Philadelphia, 1999, FA Davis Company.

DiScala C et al: Injuries to children with attention deficit hyperactivity disorder, Pediatrics 102(6):1415-1421, 1998.

Ernst M et al:. Cerebral glucose metabolism in adolescent girls with attention-deficit/hyperactivity disorder, J Am Acad Psychiatry 36(10):1399-1406, 1997.

Faraone S et al: Psychiatric, neuropsychological, and psychosocial features of DSM-IV subtypes of attention-deficit/hyperactivity disorder: results from a clinical referred sample, J Am Acad Child Adolesc Psychiatry 37(2):185-193, 1998.

Farel A et al: Very-low-birthweight infants at seven years: an assessment of the health and neurodevelopmental risk conveyed by chronic lung disease, J Learning Disabilities 31(2):118-126, 1998

Findling R and Dogin J: Psychopharmacology of ADHD: children and adolescents J Clin Psychiatry 59(7):42-49, 1998

Foley GV, Fochtman D, and Mooney KH: Nursing care of the child with cancer, Philadelphia, 1993, W.B. Saunders.

Gerring J et al: Premorbid prevalence of ADHD and development of secondary ADHD after closed head injury, J Am Acad Child Adolesc Psychiatry 37(6):647-654, 1998.

Gingerich K et al: Diversity and attention-deficit hyperactivity disorder, J Clin Psychology 54(4):415-426, 1998

Goldman L et al: Diagnosis and treatment of attention deficit/hyperactivity disorder in children and adolescents, JAMA 279(14):1100-1107, 1998.

Greenhill L: Attention-deficit hyperactivity disorder, Child Adolesc Clin North Am 4(1):123-168, 1995

Greenhill L: Diagnosing attention-deficit hyperactivity disorder in children, J Clin Psychiatry 59(suppl 7):31-41, 1998

Gresham F, MacMillan D, and Bocian K: Learning disabilities, low achievement, and mild mental retardation: more alike than different?, J Learning Disabilities 29(6):570-581, 1996.

Hunt R, Arnsten A, and Asbell M: An open trial of guanfacine in the treatment of attention-deficithyperactivity disorder, J Am Acad Child Adolesc Psychiatry 34(1):50-54, 1995

Jensen P et al: Comorbidity in ADHD: implications for research, practice, and DSM-V, J Am Acad Child Adolesc Psychiatry 36(8):1065-1079, 1997.

Kaplan D, Grados M, and Reiss A: Attention deficit and developmental disorders. In Enna S and Coyle J, editors: Pharmacological management of neurological psychiatric disorders, New York, 1998, McGraw-Hill

Kuhne M et al: Impact of comorbid oppositional or conduct problems on attention-deficit hyperactivity disorder, J Am Acad Child Adolesc Psychiatry 36(12):1715-1725, 1997

Lahey B et al: Validity of DSM-IV attention-deficit/hyperactivity disorder for younger children, J Am Acad Child Adolesc Psychiatry 37(7):695-702, 1998

Lester G and Kelman M: State disparities in the diagnosis and placement of pupils with learning disabilities, J Learning Disabilities 30(6):599-607, 1997.

MacMillan D et al: Discrepancy between definitions of learning disabilities and school practices: an empirical investigation, J Learning Disabilities 31(4):314-326, 1998.

Marvin S and Vessey J: Diagnosing learning disorders and/or ADHD. In Vessey J, editor: The child with a learning disorder or ADHD: a manual for school nurses, Scarborough, Ma., 1997, National Association of School Nurses, Inc.

McEvoy GK, editor: American hospital formulary service drug information, Bethesda, Md., 1995, American Society of Health-System Pharmacists Inc.

Miller K and Castellanos F: Attention deficit/hyperactivity disorders, Pediatr Rev 19(11):373-384, 1998.

Musten L et al: Effects of methylphenidate on preschool children with ADHD: cognitive and behavioral functions, J Acad Child Adolesc Psychiatry 36(10):1407-1415, 1997

National Institute of Health Consensus Statement, November 16-18 1998. Diagnosis and treatment of Attention Deficit Hyperactivity Disorder.

National Joint Committee on Learning Disabilities: Collected perspectives on issues affecting learning disabilities: position papers and statements, Austin Tx., 1994, Pro-Ed.

Olson H et al: Association of prenatal alcohol exposure with behavioral and learning problems in early adolescence, J Am Acad Child Adolesc Psychiatry 36(9):1187-1194, 1997

Pliszka S: Comorbidity of attention-deficit/hyperactivity disorder with psychiatric disorders: an overview, J Clin Psychiatry 59(Suppl 7):50-58, 1998a.

Pliszka S: The use of psychostimulants in the pediatric patient, Psychiatric Clin North Am 45(5):1085-1098, 1998b.

Popper C: Antidepressants in the treatment of attention-deficit/hyperactivity disorder, J Clin Psychiatry 58(Suppl 14):14-29, 1997.

Reiff M: Adolescent school failure: failure to thrive in adolescence, Pediatr Rev 19(6):199-207, 1998.

Resnick M et al: Educational disabilities of neonatal intensive care graduates, Pediatrics 102(2):308-314, 1998.

Rock E, Fessler M, and Church R: The concomitance of learning disabilities and emotional/behavioral disorders: a conceptual model, J Learning Disabilities 30(3):245-263, 1997.

Rosh J et al: Four cases of severe hepatotoxicity associated with pemoline: possible autoimmune pathogenesis, Pediatrics 101(5):921-923, 1998.

Satterfield J and Schell A: A prospective study of hyperactive boys with conduct problems and normal boys: adolescent and adult criminality, J Am Acad Child Adolesc Psychiatry 36(12):1726-1735, 1997.

Scahill L and Lynch K: The use of methylphenidate in children with attention-deficit hyperactivity disorder, J Child Adolesc Psychiatr Nurs 7(4):44-47, 1994.

Selekman J: Learning disorders and ADHD: an overview. In Vessey J, editor: The child with a learning disorder or ADHD: a manual for school nurses, Scarborough, Ma., 1997, National Association of School Nurses, Inc.

Shealy A: Attention deficit hyperactivity disorder: etiology, diagnosis, and management, J Child Adolesc Psychiatr Nurs 7(2):24-36, 1994.

Silver L: The controversial therapies for treating learning disabilities, Child Adolesc Psychiatr Clin North Am 2(2):339-350, 1993.

Silver L: ADHD: attention deficit-hyperactivity disorder and learning disabilities, booklet for the classroom teacher, Summit, NJ, 1997, Novartis.

Spencer T et al: Adults with attention-deficit/hyperactivity disorder: a controversial diagnosis, J Clin Psychiatr 59(Suppl 7):59-68, 1998.

Steinmiller G and O'Sullivan P: Education and behavioral interventions. In Vessey J, editor: The child with a learning disorder or ADHD: a manual for school nurses, Scarborough, Ma., 1997, National Association of School Nurses, Inc.

Swanson J et al: Attention-deficit hyperactivity disorder and hyperkinetic disorder, The Lancet 351: 429-433, 1998.

Ten Eick A et al: Drug-drug interactions in pediatric pharmacology, Psychiatr Clin North Am 45(5):1233-1264, 1998

Tosyali M and Greenhill L: Child and adolescent psychopharmacology: important developmental issues, Psychiatr Clin North Am 45(5):1021-1035, 1998

United States Department of Education: Sixteenth annual report to Congress,1994.

Vincent L: Neuropsychological assessment of developmental learning disabilities in adults, Sem Speech Lang 17(3):183-200, 1996

Wilens TE et al: Combined pharmacotherapy: an emerging trend in pediatric psychopharmacology, J Am Acad Child Adolesc Psychiatr 34(1):110-112, 1995.

Zametkin A and Liotta W: The neurobiology of attention-deficit/hyperactivity disorder, J Clin Psychiatr 59(Supp. 7):17-23, 1998.

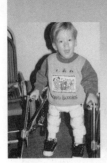

CHAPTER 29

Myelodysplasia

Judith A. Farley and Mary Jo Dunleavy

Etiology

Neural tube defects involve the malformation of the central nervous system (CNS) during embryonic development. The embryologic development of the CNS begins early in the third week of gestation. During this time the neural plate invaginates and folds together, forming the neural tube. The process of neurulation produces the functional nervous system (i.e., the future brain and spinal cord). If the neural tube fails to close the process of neurulation is interrupted, which results in the imperfect formation of the brain and spinal cord at a focal point (Elias and Hobbs, 1998; McComb, 1998).

Myelodysplasia is one form of a neural tube defect, which refers to the defective formation and subsequent development and function of the spinal cord. This defect can occur at any level of the spinal cord; the extent of nerve tissue and spinal cord involvement varies. The malformation results in altered body function at and below the level of the defect (see Table 29-1).

The cause of neural tube defects is unknown. Many potential causes or factors have been considered, but none has been confirmed as an isolated cause. There are insufficient data in the literature to link a specific drug exposure with the development of neural tube defects (McComb, 1998).

Incidence

The incidence of neural tube defects in the United States is approximately 0.7 to 1.0 for every 1000 live births each year. A higher incidence of neural tube defects exists in affected families, as well as an overall increased risk of birth defects with poor prenatal care and maternal nutritional deficiencies. The strong association of fetal demise with neural tube defects reduces the actual prevalence of neural tube defects at birth (McComb, 1998; Shaw et al, 1994).

Clinical Manifestations at Time of Diagnosis

Clinical presentation at the time of diagnosis varies depending on the extent of involvement of the spinal cord and surrounding structures of nerve, bone, muscle, and skin (Box 29-1). Myelodysplasia is classified based on the pathophysiology of the lesion or defect (Figure 29-1).

Spina bifida occulta is the failed fusion of the vertebral arches that surround and protect the spinal cord and may involve a small portion of one vertebra or the complete absence of bone. Absence of the vertebral arches is commonly associated with cutaneous abnormalities such as tufts of hair, hemangiomas, and dermoid cysts located on the surface at the area of the defect. Usually no neurologic deficits are present at the time of birth; but a child with such a defect may develop bowel, bladder, and musculoskeletal difficulties later in life (American Association of Neuroscience Nurses [AAAN], 1996; Gregerson, 1997).

Another example of myelodysplasia is the meningocele, in which the neural tube fails to close, resulting in a cystic dilatation of meninges through the vertebral defect and around the malformed tube. This defect does not involve the spinal cord, and the condition of hydrocephalus can be associated with this diagnosis (AANN, 1996). At birth the infant has a protruding sac on the back at the level of the defect. The sac may be covered by a thin layer of muscle and skin and usually appears as raw, fluid-filled tissue. The child may have abnormal neurologic findings at birth. Manipulation of the sac, surgical closure, and infection may

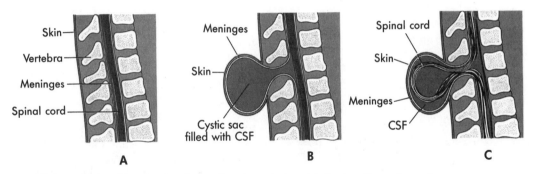

Figure 29-1 Diagram showing section through, **A,** normal spine; **B,** meningocele; **C,** myelomeningocele.

lead to neurologic changes. Functional implications depend on the level and severity of the defect (see Table 29-1).

Myelomeningocele is a particular type of meningocele in which the spinal cord protrudes through the vertebral defect (AANN, 1996). Hydrocephalus is present in virtually all children afflicted with this condition (AANN, 1996). Approximately 85% will require an internal shunt system to control the hydrocephalus (Dias and McClone, 1993) (see Chapter 25). The actual involvement of the spinal cord has greater implications for overall function throughout growth and development (see Table 29-1).

Treatment

Initial treatment for meningocele and myelomeningocele is early surgical closure of the defect (Elias and Hobbs, 1998; McClone, 1998) (Box 29-2). Specific tissue malformation and involvement and the presence of hydrocephalus can only be determined through further diagnostic tests (e.g., ul-

Table 29-1
Functional Alterations in Myelodysplasia Related to Level of Lesion

Level of Lesion	Functional Implications
Thoracic	Flaccid paralysis of lower extremities
	Variable weakness in abdominal trunk musculature
	High thoracic level may have respiratory compromise
	Absence of bowel and bladder control
High lumbar	Voluntary hip flexion and adduction
	Flaccid paralysis of knees, ankles, feet
	May walk with extensive braces and crutches
	Absence of bowel and bladder control
Midlumbar	Strong hip flexion and adduction
	Fair knee extension
	Flaccid paralysis of ankles and feet
	Absence of bowel and bladder control
Low lumbar	Strong hip flexion, extension and adduction, knee extension
	Weak ankle and toe mobility
	May have limited bowel and bladder function
Sacral	"Normal" function of lower extremities
	"Normal" bowel and bladder function

Box 29-2

Treatment

Assess level of involvement:
Ultrasonography
CT scan
MRI scan
Surgical closure of deformity

---

trasonography, computerized tomography [CT] scan, and magnetic resonance imaging [MRI]). Careful assessment of the infant before and during the surgical closure often aids in determination of the depth and extent of involvement. This information is important for habilitative planning and outcome.

The multisystem involvement of this diagnosis requires a comprehensive multidisciplinary team approach to treatment. This team may include nurses, neurosurgeons, urologists, orthopedists, pediatricians, physical therapists, occupational therapists, and social workers.

Recent and Anticipated Advances in Diagnosis and Management

Because the pathophysiology of myelodysplasia is determined early in gestation, prenatal diagnosis is possible. The presence of a neural tube defect may result in an elevation in the maternal serum alpha-fetoprotein (AFP) levels. It is important to note that a closed neural tube defect may not alter the AFP levels. When maternal serum AFP levels are elevated, further testing is indicated. The amniotic fluid can be obtained for evaluation through amniocentesis. Additionally, high-resolution ultrasonography is a noninvasive study to evaluate pregnancies at risk or suspect for neural tube defects (Babcook, 1995; Budorick, Pretorius, and Nelson, 1995).

The purpose of prenatal diagnosis is twofold. First it offers the parents the option to terminate the pregnancy. If the parents choose to continue the pregnancy, prenatal diagnosis provides the family and health-care team the opportunity to physically and emotionally prepare for the birth of the child. Delivery by cesarean section may limit trauma to

the open myelomeningocele (Luthy et al, 1991). Genetic counseling should be offered at this time, as well.

Recent studies indicate that ingestion of multivitamins with folic acid before conception or early in the pregnancy may offer protection against the occurrence of neural tube defects (Daly and Scott, 1998; Elias and Hobbs, 1998; Locksmith and Duff, 1998). Repeated studies demonstrate a 60% to 86% reduction of risks for neural tube defects with the periconceptional ingestion of vitamins containing the U.S. recommended daily allowance of 0.4 mg to 0.8 mg folic acid. All women of childbearing age should take a multivitamin containing 0.4 mg of folic acid (Daly and Scott, 1998).

The Centers for Disease Control and Prevention (CDC) has determined that women who have had a pregnancy resulting in a neural tube defect are at increased risk for recurrence. These women should be counseled and advised that folic acid supplements may substantially reduce this risk. The US Public Health Service, American College of Obstetrics and Gynecology, and the US Preventive Services Task Force recommend that these women take 4 mg of folic acid daily periconceptionally (Daly and Scott, 1998).

Associated Problems (Box 29-3)

Arnold Chiari II Malformation

One associated problem of myelodysplasia is the Chiari II malformation. This deformity involves the downward displacement of the cerebellum, brain stem, and fourth ventricle (Figure 29-2). The exact pathogenesis of the malformation is not known (Madsen and Scott, 1993). The area of the brain involved is the posterior fossa region, which is primarily responsible for vital functions including respirations and protective reflexes directed by the twelve cranial nerves. The downward displacement of this area results in compression and elongation of nerves and tissue, restricting neuronal performance to varying degrees (Madsen and Scott, 1993).

Skin Integrity

Newborns are at great risk for developing infection secondary to the altered skin integrity over the mal-

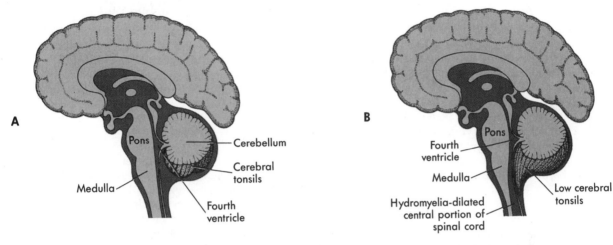

Figure 29-2   Diagram showing, **A,** normal brain; and, **B,** brain with Chiari malformation.

Box 29-3
Associated Problems

Arnold Chiari II malformation
Maintaining skin integrity
Hydrocephalus
Seizures
Visual and perceptual problems
Cognitive deficit
Altered motor and sensory function
Musculoskeletal deformities
Urinary dysfunction
Latex allergic reactions

---

formed spine, which is a possible complication until the lesion has completely healed. The risk of skin breakdown continues throughout a child's life span as a result of altered sensory function below the level of the lesion.

Hydrocephalus and Seizures

Hydrocephalus occurs in approximately 85% of children with myelodysplasia (Dias and McClone, 1993). Seizures occur in approximately 30% of these children (Reigel, 1993). See Chapters 21 and 25 for additional information.

Visual and Perceptual Problems

Visual and perceptual problems including ocular palsies, astigmatism, and visual perceptual deficits are common (Lollar, 1993b). Pressure on cranial nerves that control eye movements—CN III (oculomotor), CN IV (trochlear), and CN VI (abducens)—may result in a mild disconjugate gaze or esotropia.

Cognitive Deficit

Children born with myelodysplasia have mean intellectual quotients (IQs) in the average range (Lollar, 1993b). Children who are shunted as a result of the associated diagnosis of hydrocephalus have been reported to have IQs in the range of low-average or below (Lollar, 1993b). High-resolution prenatal ultrasounds can predict early cognitive development (Coniglio, Anderson, Ferguson, 1997). Hydrocephalus, especially complicated by frequent shunt revisions, malfunctions, or infections, may limit intellectual function (Lollar, 1993b). (Refer to Chapter 25.) These children often exhibit strength in verbal skills; however, limited cognitive skills (e.g., memory, speed of response, acquired knowledge, integrated functioning, and coordination) are common and must be considered in the intellectual assessment of these children (Lollar, 1993b).

Altered Motor and Sensory Function

Motor and sensory functions below the level of the lesions are invariably altered. This dysfunction may include paralysis, weakness, spasticity of lower extremities, and sensory loss. Altered motor and sensory function may also impair peristalsis leading to constipation, impaction, and fecal incontinence. These associated problems may worsen as a child grows and the cord ascends within the vertebral canal, pulling primary scar tissue and tethering the spinal cord. As a result, tethering of spinal cord is present in virtually all cases.

Musculoskeletal Deformities

Musculoskeletal deformities related to myelomeningocele may include club feet, dislocated hips, and improper musculoskeletal alignment from altered embryonic development. Spinal deformities (e.g., scoliosis, kyphosis, and gibbus) are also common. Muscle group imbalance occurs with growth and development and may cause further deformities over time (Karol, 1995; Ryan, Ploski, and Emans, 1992).

Urinary Dysfunction

Depending on the level of the defect, neurogenic bladder may occur. Other potential complications of the urinary system include dyssynergy, hydronephrosis, incomplete emptying of the bladder, urinary reflux, urinary tract infections, and incontinence. Presentation of any of these findings may indicate deterioration of urinary function and could lead to renal damage (Edelstein et al, 1995; Kreder, 1992).

Latex Allergic Reactions

Approximately 18% to 40% of individuals with myelodysplasia have a sensitivity to latex. These individuals are at risk for anaphylaxis during operations and procedures where latex is used (Nieto et al, 1996; Shah et al, 1998; Slater, 1994). Therefore, the primary care provider must inform and educate the parents and individual of this potential sensitivity, observe for signs, and document the allergy. Examples of products that may contain latex are surgical gloves, balloons, catheters, and bandages. (An updated list of such products and alternatives

for use is available from the Spina Bifida Association of America.) Individuals with latex sensitivity should carry an epi-pen, a letter documenting the allergy, and nonlatex gloves, as well as wear a Medic-Alert bracelet indicating the allergy.

Prognosis

Myelodysplasia is a chronic condition. The prognosis depends on the success of prophylactic and acute treatment for potential and actual complications that affect each body system. Children with myelodysplasia are at risk for sudden death as a result of a shunt malfunction or problems related to the Chiari II malformation (Madsen and Scott, 1993; Waters et al, 1998). Improved ventricular shunt systems have helped to minimize infections that may lead to CNS damage. The advent of new urologic interventions (e.g., early urodynamic assessment and intermittent catheterization) also greatly reduces the risk of renal damage (Bauer, 1994; Wu, Baskin, and Kogan, 1997). Further treatments and interventions will be necessary throughout the child's life span. Procedures are individualized to the child's needs and rendered when indicated by the clinical presentation, assessment, and evaluation.

PRIMARY CARE MANAGEMENT
Health Care Maintenance
Growth and Development

The deformity, degree of motor impairment, cognitive function, and personal motivation influence the growth and development of each child (Ryan, Ploski, and Emans, 1992). As with all children, monitoring growth and development by obtaining routine heights and weights and plotting them on a standardized growth chart is crucial. During infancy, problems related to Chiari II malformation may cause feeding problems affecting growth. Growth hormone deficiency may also occur; therefore referral to an endocrinologist may be indicated (Elias and Hobbs, 1998; Rotenstein and Breen, 1996; Rotenstein and Reigal, 1996). Obesity is a common problem in older children with myelodysplasia as a result of decreased levels of activity. Because obesity may lead to problems with skin breakdown, brace fittings, and the ability to ambulate, education for parents and children is essential (Ryan, Ploski, and Emans, 1992). Obesity may also interfere with development of a positive self-image.

Obtaining heights may be difficult, depending on the child's ability to stand. If necessary, the primary care provider should measure the full body length with the child supine or by using arm span. Because of shortening of the spine or muscle atrophy, these children often fall below the 10th percentile in height.

Head circumference should be monitored closely by the primary care provider during infancy and early childhood. If a progressive enlargement in size is noted, referral to a neurosurgeon should be made (see Chapter 25).

Motor development may be affected and is directly related to the level of the lesion (see Table 29-1). The degree of weakness, paralysis, and decreased sensation vary. Early orthopedic and physical therapy assessment and intervention are extremely important to prevent contractures, minimize deformities, and monitor muscle strength and flexibility. This assessment aids in planning for the child's future mobility and independence (Karol, 1995; Ryan, Ploski, and Emans, 1992).

The rate at which cognitive and intellectual skills are acquired depends on a child's interaction with the environment and the severity of the defect. The orthopedist and physical therapist can assist the child by ensuring that the physical developmental sequence proceeds normally. For instance, if a child cannot stand by age 10 to 18 months, the use a standing frame or a parapodium allows the child to accomplish various developmental tasks and stand with his or her hands free for play (Ryan, Ploski, and Emans, 1992).

As the child grows and develops, other adaptive equipment (i.e., braces, wheelchairs) is used to increase mobility and independence. Each child's treatment program varies because of differences in motivation and variability of social resources. Age-related goals are most important (Ryan, Ploski, and Emans, 1992).

Surgical intervention is often recommended and sometimes required to achieve proper muscle balance and body alignment for problems common to this population (e.g., dislocated hips, scoliosis, kyphosis, and club feet) that would limit the child's potential.

Precocious puberty has been noted in a number of children with myelodysplasia and hydrocephalus. The cause is not known but may be related to early pituitary gonadotropin secretion activated by the hydrocephalic brain (Elias and Hobbs, 1998; Elias and Sadeghi-Nejad, 1994; Rotenstein and Breen, 1996; Rotenstein and Reigal, 1996).

Diet

Infancy is an excellent time to guide and educate parents on nutritional needs. It is important to teach parents early about the dangers of overfeeding—especially in children who are less mobile and therefore have fewer caloric needs. Preventing obesity and avoiding the pattern of using food as a reward are primary goals in the nutritional management of these children.

The child's diet should include plenty of fluids to lessen the chance of constipation and the incidence of urinary tract infections. Dietary management is important in controlling the consistency of stools and in avoiding constipation. A diet high in fiber and low in constipating foods is usually recommended. Early nutritional assessment and guidance are essential parts of the care of children with myelodysplasia.

Poor feeding, prolonged feeding time, and poor weight gain are common symptoms of the Chiari II malformation in affected children (Elias and Hobbs, 1998; Madsen and Scott, 1993). In children with severe symptomatology, a gastrostomy tube may be required to avoid malnutrition and aspiration.

Safety

Safety issues particular to infants and children with myelodysplasia are numerous. Because the neurologic system is the primary system involved, parents must be educated on the changes that may occur and threaten their child's safety. The potential for limited cognitive ability and altered judgment exists in these children. An awareness of limitations is essential to help these children with issues such as independence, decision making, self-care, and sexuality. Instructions on the proper use of equipment for mobility (e.g., wheelchairs, braces, and crutches) should be appropriate to the child's developmental and cognitive abilities.

The congenital defect affects nerve function at and below the level of the defect on the spine, thus altering mobility and sensation of bone, muscle, and skin tissue below the level of the defect. This decreased sensation puts a child at greater risk for injuries such as burns, fractures, and skin breakdown. With proper body positioning, frequent position changes, and assurance that adaptive equipment fits properly and is used correctly, this risk can be minimized. Tepid water should be used for bathing to prevent burns. The condition of the child's skin should be checked at least twice a day for redness and irritation. As soon as children are competent to assume this responsibility, they should be taught how to perform a thorough skin check.

Parents of children with seizures should be instructed on how to intervene safely and appropriately during a seizure (refer to Chapter 21).

Immunizations

The recommended schedule for routine immunizations is suggested, although it may be altered as a result of frequent hospitalizations (Hoeman, 1997). The primary care provider should attempt to keep the child up to date with the routine immunizations. Alterations in the immunization schedule for children with hydrocephalus and seizures are addressed in Chapters 21 and 25.

Screening

Vision: Routine screening is recommended. Because of the high incidence of visual and perceptual deficits, ocular palsies, and astigmatism in children with myelodysplasia, practitioners should consider these during routine screening. Referral to an ophthalmologist is indicated for any positive visual findings.

Hearing: Routine screening is recommended. Children with myelodysplasia who are shunted for hydrocephalus are hypersensitive to loud noises. Awareness of this finding may alleviate parental concern. Use of aminoglycocides may cause hearing deficits.

Dental: Routine dental screening and care are recommended. Dentists should be notified of the increased risk of latex allergy. (Information should be given for safe, alternative nonlatex products.)

Children with shunted hydrocephalus should receive prophylactic antibiotics before any dental care that may result in bleeding (see Chapter 17).

Hematocrit: Routine screening is recommended.

Tuberculosis: Routine screening is recommended.

Blood pressure: Routine screening is recommended. Children with known renal problems such as urinary reflux or a history of hypertension should have more frequent assessment. Persistent elevated readings should be communicated to the child's urologist.

Urinalysis: Baseline urinalysis and urine cultures are obtained in newborns. After this time, routine cultures should be obtained every 4 to 6 months. If a urinary tract infection is suspected, a urine culture and sensitivity should be obtained by catheterization (bag specimens have been noted to have a higher chance of contamination). A positive urine culture should be reported to the child's urologist.

Condition-Specific Screening
(Box 29-4)

Complete blood count: If an individual is on long-term antibiotic therapy (e.g., sulfonamides) for prevention of urinary tract infections complete blood counts should be checked approximately every 6 months to monitor changes.

Serum creatinine: This should be checked routinely in newborns as a baseline study for renal function and should be repeated yearly.

Scoliosis: Screening for scoliosis in children with myelodysplasia should begin during the first year of life and continue throughout adolescence. Spine radiographs should be obtained yearly or as indicated.

Box 29-4

Condition-Specific Screening

Complete blood count
Serum creatinine
Scoliosis
Latex allergy

Latex Allergy: Careful history should be elicited regarding signs and symptoms of latex allergy. There are three types of reactions that may occur:

1. Irritant contact dermatitis: dry, itchy, irritated areas, usually on the hands, caused from using gloves—not a true allergy;
2. Allergic contact dermatitis (Type IV): delayed hypersensitivity, may include symptoms such as watery eyes, eczematous skin eruptions or dermatitis;
3. Immediate allergic reaction (Type I) (NIOSH, 1997).

Type I reaction is an immediate hypersensitivity to exposure and may include symptoms such as rhinitis, conjunctivitis, wheezing, bronchospasm, facial swelling, tachycardia, laryngeal edema, and hypotension. Individuals with Type I reaction to latex are at extreme risk for developing anaphylaxis. Those who experience Type IV are at lower risk for developing anaphylaxis, but constant sensitization may predispose them to anaphylaxis. Avoidance of latex products is extremely important in preventing allergic reactions. Refer individuals to an allergist if latex allergy is suspected.

Common Illness Management

Differential Diagnosis (Box 29-5)

Chiari II: Chiari II is a serious, potentially life-threatening malformation that invariably occurs with myelodysplasia. The Chiari II malformation may be a clinically silent phenomenon or cause catastrophic events (e.g., cardiac or respiratory arrest).

Box 29-5

Differential Diagnosis

Chiari II malformation
Tethering of the spinal cord
Hydrocephalus
Urinary tract infections
Fevers
Gastrointestinal symptoms

The malformation compresses and essentially stretches the posterior region of the cerebellum and brain stem downward through the foramen of magnum into the cervical space. Children with Chiari II seldom show immediate signs at birth but more often become symptomatic during the first days to weeks of life. Otherwise, manifestations of the condition may not become obvious until 4 to 5 years of age or older (Elias and Hobbs, 1998; Madsen and Scott, 1993).

The brain stem houses the 12 cranial nerves (CNs) (see Table 29-2). Pressure on this region results in altered function of these vital nerves or actual palsies. Dysfunction of the lower CNs is common. The infant's symptoms may include apnea, respiratory difficulties, stridor, and the classic barking cough of croup. Primary care providers must be cautious not to dismiss these findings as a simple upper respiratory infection but must consider the possibility that these symptoms result from pressure on CN IX (glossopharyngeal), CN X (vagus), and CN XII (hypoglossal). A depressed or absent gag may be present, leading to possible aspiration pneumonia. Feeding difficulties, poor weight gain, and symptoms of failure to thrive may also be present.

Pressure on the CNs that control eye movements—CN III (oculomotor), CN IV (trochlear), CN VI (abducens)—may result in a mild disconjugate gaze or esotropia.

Subtle complaints and changes in hand function or strength, increased upper-extremity spasticity, neck pain, or behavior changes (e.g., irritability) necessitate immediate consultation with the neurosurgeon to rule out shunt malfunction. Treatment is focused on the symptomatic relief of the presenting problems (i.e., gastrostomy tube and tracheostomy may be placed for absent gag and cough). Surgical decompression of the cervical region is controversial and has not yet been proven a reliable solution (Elias and Hobbs, 1998; Madsen and Scott, 1993; Waters et al, 1998).

Tethering of the spinal cord: Tethering of the spinal cord develops with growth. Symptoms related to this problem may include scoliosis, altered gait pattern, changes in muscle strength and tone at or below the lesion, disturbance in urinary and bowel patterns, and back pain. Primary care providers should be alert to these findings and refer the child to the neurosurgeon for further evaluation, which may include urodynamic studies and

Table 29-2
Implications of Cranial Nerve Dysfunction in Myelodysplasia

Cranial Nerve	Functional Implications
I olfactory	Sense of smell
II optic	Visual acuity, visual fields
III oculomotor	Raises eyelids; constricts pupils; moves eyes up, down, and medially
IV trochlear	Moves eyes down
V trigeminal	Sensory innervation to face, tongue; opens and closes jaw
VI abducens	Moves eyes laterally (out)
VII facial	Closes eyelids; motor and sensory for facial muscles; secretion of lacrimal and salivary glands
VIII acoustic	Hearing; equilibrium
IX glossopharyngeal	Gag, swallow; taste
X vagus	Muscles of larynx, pharynx, soft palate; parasympathetic innervation
XI spinal accessory	Shoulder shrug
XII hypoglossal	Moves tongue

MRI. Surgical release may be indicated based on evaluation and symptoms.

Hydrocephalus: Most individuals have an internal shunt system to treat hydrocephalus. The differential diagnosis of shunt malfunction and infection must be considered in the presence of lethargy, fever, gastrointestinal distress, and headache (refer to Chapter 25).

Urinary tract infections: Urinary tract infections (UTIs) are common among children with myelodysplasia. Fever associated with UTIs may be mild or severe. Other symptoms may include abdominal pain; vomiting; cloudy, malodorous urine; and increased wetting. Frequency and burning may be masked because of decreased sensation. These symptoms should alert the primary care provider to obtain a urine specimen by catheterization for culture. A positive culture should be reported to the child's urologist, especially in cases with urinary reflux. Treatment of positive cultures may vary depending on the individual's urologist but is usually only initiated in the presence of

symptoms or urinary reflux (Bauer, 1994). Most children who are on clean intermittent catheterization are chronically colonized with bacteria. Treatment is usually based on the presence of urinary reflux or severe symptoms (e.g., fever, back pain, and/or vomiting) (Elias and Hobbs, 1998). Recommendations for treatment may include a short course of appropriate antibiotics and instillation of an antibiotic solution into the bladder via catheterization. Children with urinary reflux need continuous antibiotic coverage and frequent urine cultures. Repeat cultures should be obtained once during the course of treatment and again approximately 1 week after treatment.

Fevers: Fever is a symptom found in many common childhood illnesses. Causes of fever may include shunt infection and malfunction, UTI, skin breakdown, and cellulitis. Particular consideration must be given to the presence of a fever because it may lower the seizure threshold in these children.

Fever of unknown origin may be the result of an undetected fracture of an insensiate extremity. Osteoporosis associated with paralysis, decreased weight bearing, and inactivity, especially after immobilization in a cast, may contribute to the occurrence of fractures (Ryan, Ploski, and Emans, 1992). An undetected burn of insensiate areas may also result in fever. Careful examination of the area for swelling, redness, or abrasions should be undertaken by the practitioner. Obtaining a complete history from the individual and the parents may assist in determining if there has been recent trauma.

Gastrointestinal symptoms: Nausea, vomiting, and diarrhea are all common symptoms in children. In children with myelodysplasia, however, a heightened concern and consideration to the cause should be given. Nausea and vomiting may be symptomatic of shunt malfunction. UTIs may be the cause of gastrointestinal distress. Children who have had a bladder augmentation and also have referred pain to the shoulder should seek immediate medical attention because this could indicate a urinary leak into the peritoneum. A child with a neurogenic bowel may become impacted with stool, leading to gastrointestinal distress. The presence of diarrhea may be misleading because liquid stool passes around the impacted stool. A KUB may help differentiate diarrhea vs. impaction.

In children with a high lesion, practitioners should consider the possibility of appendicitis as a cause of nausea or vomiting. The classic symptom of pain may be altered as a result of the decreased sensation.

Drug Interactions

Many children with myelodysplasia are on routine medication therapy. Potential interactions among these and other medications must be carefully considered when additional pharmotherapeutics are prescribed. Commonly used drug categories are as follows:

1. Antibiotics for treatment of UTIs or prophylaxis, including amoxicillin (Amoxil), trimethoprim and sulfamethoxazole (Bactrim), sulfisoxazole (Gantrisin), and nitrofurantoin (Furadantin). If a child requires other antibiotic therapy for common childhood illness such as ear infections, the antibiotic for the UTI is discontinued during the needed course of treatment. Bladder irrigations containing antibiotics may also be used.
2. Anticholinergics to assist in urinary continence and reduce high bladder pressure, including oxybutynin chloride (Ditropan) and propantheline bromide (Pro-Banthine) (Levsin and Detrol). Oxybutynin chloride can cause heat prostration in the presence of high environmental temperatures. Installing this medication (i.e., in pill form, crushed and dissolved in normal saline) into the bladder is a new treatment option with fewer side effects. Anticholinergics may delay absorption of other medications given concomitantly in these children (Physician's Desk Reference [PDR], 1998).
3. Sympathomimetics to increase urethral resistance, including ephedrine (Gluco-Fedrin), pseudoephedrine hydrochloride (Sudafed), and phenylpropanolamine. Practitioners should determine if the child is taking any of these drugs before treating cold symptoms.
4. Stool softeners, stimulants, and bulk formers to aid in evacuation of stool. Many products are used for this purpose, and most are over-the-counter drugs. None of these should be administered in the presence of abdominal pain, nausea, vomiting, or diarrhea.

5. Anticonvulsants to control seizure activity, including phenobarbital, phenytoid sodium (Dilantin), and carbamazepine (Tegretol). Concomitant administration of carbamazepine with erythromycin may result in toxicity (PDR, 1998) (see Chapter 21).

Developmental Issues

Sleep Patterns

Individuals with Chiari II malformation may experience sleep apnea, increased stridor, and snoring with sleep. These children are at increased risk for sudden respiratory arrest. Sleep studies are helpful in determining the severity of sleep disorder and the need for bilevel positive airway pressure (BiPAP) (Waters et al, 1998). Therefore children with such symptoms should wear a cardiac/apnea monitor during sleep. Parents must also be able to perform cardiopulmonary resuscitation in the event of an arrest.

Alteration in the child's normal sleep pattern (e.g., longer naps, increased frequency of naps) may indicate increased intracranial pressure from a shunt malfunction (see Chapter 25 on hydrocephalus).

In addition, sleep may be interrupted if a child needs to be repositioned during the night to prevent pressure sores and skin breakdown from developing.

Toileting

Mastery of bowel and bladder continence is crucial to optimal functioning and is of major importance for social acceptance (King, Currie, and Wright, 1994; Sloan, 1993; Younoszai, 1992). A child's physical abilities and psychologic readiness for toileting should be assessed. Children who are unable to sit without adaptive devices or unable to master self-dressing skills need special consideration when toileting is introduced. A physical or occupational therapist should be consulted about the use of bars, adaptive seats, etc. Special clothing or underwear may be helpful to make access to the perineum easier.

It is desirable for children to master self-care methods of toileting before entering school. Urinary and fecal incontinence may partly explain the poor social adjustment experienced by many children with myelodysplasia. Bowel management should be monitored from birth to avoid constipation and impaction. At age 2 to 3 years the concept of toileting should be introduced to children. The goals of bowel management are to maintain soft-formed stools and develop a regular schedule of evacuation on the toilet every 1 to 2 days to avoid impaction or soiling in between bowel movements. These goals can be accomplished by having the child sit on the toilet at regular times, take advantage of the gastrocolic reflex by toileting after meals, and increase abdominal pressure by blowing bubbles, by tickling the child to make him or her laugh, or by placing the child's legs on a stool to increase pressure by hip flexion.

Stool consistency is crucial to developing a good bowel program. Bulking agents (e.g., psyllium) taken with increased fluids are a key factor in avoiding constipation and eventual impaction. Children should assume responsibility for timed evacuation and good perineal care as physical and cognitive development allows. Some children will not be able to assume toileting responsibilities and will require continued assistance by parents or caretakers (Edwards-Beckett and King, 1996).

The use of medicinal aids may also be necessary to control the consistency or to aid in evacuation. A number of agents are available, including stimulants, softeners, and lubricants. Biofeedback, behavior-modification techniques, and the use of an enema continent catheter have also been used with some success in this population to treat fecal incontinence (Blair et al, 1992; Liptak and Revell, 1992; Younoszai, 1992). The antegrade continence enema (ACE) is an increasingly popular way to administer a large-volume enema through a surgically created catheterizable stoma. The goal is to administer the antegrade washout for colonic emptying and to prevent soiling. Electrostimulation for improving fecal continence is also used in some centers (Balcom et al, 1997; Malone, Ransley, and Kiely, 1990; Palmer, Richards, and Kaplan, 1997).

It is important to remember that each program of management varies from child-to-child. A sympathetic manner in working with a child helps to avoid feelings of guilt and blame for unavoidable accidents. Accidents can be avoided with careful attention to diet and timed defecation. Despite a successful continence program, some individuals may need to wear a diaper during sleep.

Clean intermittent catheterization is the most commonly used method to help achieve urinary continence. If catheterization has not been started for other reasons, it may be started in children who are 2 to 3 years of age in an attempt to get them out of diapers when most other children have achieved this milestone (Vereecken, 1992; Wu, Baskin, and Kogan, 1997). If a child has been catheterized from birth, the concept of using the toilet for the procedure should be introduced at this time. The procedure is ideally taught to the parents and other individuals involved in the child's direct care. Instituting this procedure often causes a resurfacing of emotions in parents related to the child's disabilities. Fear of injuring the child, difficulties with genital touching, and frustration with the mechanics of the procedure are common. Psychologic and emotional concerns are usual and must be addressed before parents can be expected to understand and comply with the recommendations.

Self-catheterization is a realistic goal for most children with myelodysplasia. An individualized approach accounting for the child's readiness is of great benefit in achieving this goal. Providing young children with an anatomically correct doll and catheter often helps them master the skill. The goal is to have this task accomplished by early school age. In children with limited cognitive abilities and poor manual dexterity, continued assistance may be necessary. Noncompliance with self-catheterization may become an issue in adolescence when catheterization is used as a focus in the fight for independence.

If continence is not attained by catheterization alone, medications such as anticholinergics and sympathomimetics may be used in conjunction with the procedure. Continence may also successfully be achieved through use of bladder stimulation and surgical interventions (e.g., artificial urinary sphincter, bladder neck reconstruction, bladder augmentation, and creation of continent stomas) (Aprikian et al, 1992; Balcom et al, 1997; Bauer, 1994; Selzman, Elder, and Mapstone, 1993).

Discipline

Children with such a complex chronic condition are at increased risk for experiencing psychosocial adjustment problems, which may affect the parents' and family members' response to discipline. The need for discipline, direction, and encouragement of independence should be addressed early in a child's life (Lollar, 1993b). Referral for parent counseling may be necessary to assist with the particular needs and challenges that may arise (Elias and Hobbs, 1998).

Child Care

Primary care providers should be familiar with resources available for referral because early intervention programs for infants vary from state to state. Preschoolers are eligible for placement in public programs that meet their physical and educational needs. It is important that the daycare or educational setting be notified in advance about a prospective student so that the daycare staff can be educated and a smooth transition can be facilitated (see Chapter 5).

Children with myelodysplasia and a ventriculoperitoneal shunt may exhibit signs of shunt malfunction while in the care of someone besides a parent. That individual should be aware of the signs and alert the parent or guardian. Additional concerns related to the issue of hydrocephalus can be found in Chapter 25.

Knowledge of a child's specific bladder and bowel program should be communicated. Any procedures necessary to carry out the particular program must be taught to the care provider. This instruction is not usually necessary in the birth to 3-year programs unless the child is also in daycare. If so, a trained person should perform the procedure. Care providers should be informed of all medications the child requires and of latex sensitivity.

Many children with myelodysplasia have adaptive equipment to aid in mobilization, maintain appropriate body alignment, prevent further deformity, and increase independence. Primary care providers should be aware of proper application and fit of the equipment. It is also important to communicate the child's actual motor and sensory capacity to prevent injury.

A list of emergency telephone numbers must accompany these children. If possible, primary care providers should be available to answer questions and concerns from child care staff.

Schooling

Learning disabilities are common in children with myelodysplasia. Problems may occur in perceptual motor performance, comprehension, attention, activity, memory, organization, sequencing, and rea-

soning. These areas must be assessed early in the educational process so particular needs may be met and adaptations made to minimize educational problems and frustrations for the child, family, and educators. Neuropsychologic testing is recommended to support this process (Burke and Meeropol, 1994; Elias and Hobbs, 1998; Lollar, 1993a). School performance is further compromised by frequent absences as a result of illness or medical treatment.

Federal laws protect the rights of children with disabilities to have access to an appropriate education (see Chapter 5). Individualized education plans (IEPs) must be formulated to take care of each child's specific needs, including educational and physical requirements. The primary care provider, the child, and the family must actively collaborate with the school in this planning process. Each child's particular needs must be addressed in the IEP, including the need for catheterization, timed toileting, administration of medication(s), physical, occupational and speech therapy, and individual counseling. These particular needs may occasionally require assistance from an aide.

Adaptive equipment may be necessary and depends on a child's degree of disability. School personnel should be aware of what adaptive equipment the child has, how it functions, and what to monitor with regard to fit, skin irritation, etc. (Ryan, Ploski, and Emans, 1992). Elevators may help a child to get to classes in a timely manner and minimize fatigue.

As children age, they may choose to use a wheelchair for mobilization in the school building, which should be viewed as an increase instead of a decrease in independence. Ideally, the school should be free of structural barriers to enable the child to move freely and participate in all activities. Special provisions must be made for safe departure from the building in the event of an emergency, as well as transportation to and from home (i.e., wheelchair van or bus). Individuals with a known latex allergy will need to have adaptations made in all aspects of the school setting to avoid exposure. Common sources of latex in the school environment include art supplies, pencil erasers, and gym mats or floors. Clinical personnel or allergists are possible resources to assist in this adaptation process.

Children with chronic conditions and physical disabilities are at risk for experiencing adjustment problems (Lollar, 1993a). Children with myelodysplasia often have low self-concepts, low levels of general happiness, and high levels of anxiety. Awareness of these potential problems is helpful for those working with children with myelodysplasia. Emotional independence is the foundation that supports the successful development of physical independence. Appropriate referrals for further psychologic intervention and support may be advised. Primary care providers should encourage these children to be involved in extracurricular activities such as clubs, scouting, and sporting activities to enhance peer relationships, self-esteem, and independence (Loller, 1993b).

Academic planning and career counseling must take into consideration an individual's physical— as well as cognitive—abilities. Education and vocational training should prepare individuals to be successful in employment, independent living, and in social relationships (Edwards et al, 1994).

Sexuality

The issue of sexuality is a major area of concern for children with myelodysplasia and their parents. Education, information, and an opportunity to address concerns about sexuality and reproductive function should be discussed early in a child's life (Joyner, McLorie, and Khoury, 1998; Sloan, 1993). Urodynamic studies in the newborn period may help to determine prognosis regarding sexual function (Bauer, 1989). Maximizing urinary and fecal continence, fostering self-esteem, and promoting self-care are all beneficial to children in developing a sexual identity (Sloan, 1993).

The usual sources of sexual information available to adolescents may be difficult to access by individuals with myelodysplasia because of limited mobility and poor peer relationships (Joyner, McLorie, Khoury, 1998; Sloan, 1993). Practitioners should provide anticipatory guidance during routine health maintenance visits and assess for signs of early sexual development associated with precocious puberty (Elias and Sadeghi-Nejad, 1994). If a primary care provider does not feel skilled in gynecologic care, the child should be referred to a sensitive specialist with experience examining individuals with disabilities.

Women with myelodysplasia are capable of normal fertility. Birth control methods must be carefully evaluated on an individual basis. The risk of blood clots and pelvic inflammatory disease make oral contraceptives and intrauterine devices more hazardous (Sloan, 1993). The high incidence of latex allergies in this population prohibits the use of latex condoms and diaphragms. Nonlatex condoms are available but do not provide protection from AIDS or other sexually transmitted diseases. Because of increased risk for UTI with intercourse, women not on routine antibiotics should take prophylactic antibiotics before and after intercourse.

Although individuals with myelodysplasia have normal sex drives, unless sensation exists in the bulbourethral, bulbocavernosus, and perineal muscles of both sexes, orgasm is not likely (Sloan, 1993). Women may benefit from use of additional lubricating gels when attempting intercourse because vaginal lubrication in response to sexual arousal does not occur with lower spinal cord injury.

Severe spinal deformities or complex urologic problems may increase the risk for complications during pregnancy. Women with these problems are also at risk for having a child with a neural tube defect. Genetic counseling should be available to these women and encouraged by their primary care provider (Elias and Hobbs, 1998; Sloan, 1993). The American College of Obstetrics and Gynecology has guidelines on pregnancy and delivery for women with myelodysplasia.

In men with myelodysplasia, the level of spinal lesion will predict their capacity for erection and ejaculation. Because this functional ability varies among individuals, the reproductive potential is much less predictable than in women. Past erections and ejaculations are an important part of the sexual history in males. Penile implants or collection of sperm by electric stimulation may be indicated for this population (Joyner, McLorie, and Khoury, 1998; Sloan, 1993). Technologic advances may offer more possibilities in the future.

Transition to Adulthood

Transition planning is a process mandated by law (Section 204 of the Carl D. Perkins Act) that must begin by age 14 years (Rowley-Kelly, 1993). Amendments under the Individuals with Disabilities Education Act (PL 101-476) require that goals and objectives related to employment and postsecondary education, independent living, and community participation be included in IEPs no later than age 16 years (Burke and Meeropol, 1994).

Of utmost importance for parents and school personnel is to begin as early as possible to work together in fostering necessary skills and traits in adolescents for successful transition from high school to college or to the workplace (Edwards et al, 1994; Rowley-Kelly, 1993).

The survival rate of individuals with myelodysplasia has increased with medical advances, so a new population of adults with myelodysplasia has emerged (Rauen and Aubert, 1992). These young adults often find themselves at a loss for accessing appropriate health care (Schidlow and Fiel, 1990). Depression, chemical addiction, obesity, contractures, decreased ambulation, pressure ulcers, osteoporosis, joint pain, and hydronephrosis are some of the common secondary disabilities seen in this population (Kaufman et al, 1994; Rauen and Aubert, 1992). As in the pediatric multidisciplinary care model, coordinated care is of utmost importance in adults. In a recent symposium on preventing secondary conditions associated with spina bifida, the recommendation made to health care professionals was to "provide a single point entry to a system that coordinates the needed care" (Marge, 1994). Primary health care should be directed by providers interested in and committed to working with this high-risk population. This necessary transition of care has been met with reluctance by many adult health care providers for a number of reasons, including lack of familiarity of the complex needs of individuals with myelodysplasia. Providers may perceive this population as having a negative economic effect on their practice.

Coordinated multidisciplinary care, education of health care providers and clients, costs, and promotion of client-directed care are issues that need to be addressed. A few adult programs have been developed in various parts of the country. Further information can be obtained from the Spina Bifida Association of America.

Special Family Concerns and Resources

Families of children with myelodysplasia suffer chronic grief for the "loss of the normal" child at birth. This grief is expressed repeatedly as the child fails to achieve developmental milestones.

The risk for sudden death as a result of a shunt malfunction or complications related to the Chiari II malformation is a chronic and intense stress on the family system. This stress, in addition to the other complex needs of these children, often results in families becoming overprotective (Lollar, 1993b). Families may be hesitant or fearful of allowing others to care for their child because of the child's special needs. Parents should be encouraged to meet their own individual needs and, as a couple, to participate in activities outside the home independent of the child, as well as to seek respite care if other caretakers are not available (Pavin et al, 1994; Samuelson, Foltz, and Foxall, 1992).

The multisystem involvement of this condition requires frequent hospitalizations, surgeries, outpatient services, and multidisciplinary care. These factors, in addition to items such as special equipment or medications that may be needed by these children, place a tremendous financial burden on parents. Many children with myelodysplasia are eligible for social security benefits. Social service involvement with these families is crucial in providing guidance and support (Elias and Hobbs, 1998).

The health care system recognizes the multitude of needs for children with myelodysplasia and their families and offers physical, emotional, spiritual, and social care. Nevertheless, no individual understands or feels the problems these children and families face in their day-to-day lives as well as another child or family with the same disorder. Therefore support groups and opportunities available to provide this network of support within the community are not only necessary but also have proven to be a major factor in coping and adaptation for these families. The following are a few of the support systems available to families. Each region has its own community-based network or local chapter. It is important that the primary care provider be aware of available local resources.

Spina Bifida Association of America
4590 MacArthur Blvd NW, Suite 250
Washington DC 20007-4226
(202)944-3285 or (800)621-3141
sbaa@sbaa.org

Northeast Myelodysplasia Association
c/o New England Regional Genetics Group
Joseph Robinson, coordinator
P.O. Box 670
Mt. Desert, ME 04660
(207)288-2705

Arnold-Chiari Family Network
c/o Kevin and Maureen Walsh
67 Spring St
Weymouth, MA 02188

Summary of Special Primary Care Needs for the Child with Myelodysplasia

HEALTH CARE MAINTENANCE

Growth and development

Growth hormone deficiency may occur.

Obesity is common in these children.

Head size may be enlarged if diagnosed with hydrocephalus; measure head each visit.

Motor delays are common.

Both precocious puberty and short stature are reported.

Diet

Regurgitation, vomiting, and difficulties with gag reflex need to be evaluated for increased intracranial pressure and Chiari II malformation.

Caloric intake should be monitored to minimize potential for obesity.

Diet should include increased fluids to lessen chance of constipation and urinary tract infections.

Safety

Education on emergency care of seizures is recommended.

Increased risk of injuries as a result of decreased sensation and mobility is possible.

Proper body positioning, frequent position changes, and proper fit of adaptive equipment are recommended.

Increased risk for latex allergy is possible.

Immunizations

Pertussis vaccine may be deferred in infants with seizures.

Measles vaccine may cause seizures in children with seizure disorder but is recommended because of prevalence of disease.

Screening

Vision: Routine screening is recommended.

These children have a high incidence of visual deficits such as ocular palsies, astigmatism, and visual perceptual deficits.

Hearing: Routine screening is recommended. Children may have hypersensitivity to loud noises if shunted.

If children are exposed to aminoglycocides, hearing should be evaluated by an audiologist.

Dental: Routine care is recommended. Latex allergy should be considered before dental work. If a child is shunted for hydrocephalus, he or she will need antibiotic prophylaxis before dental work that may result in bleeding.

Hematocrit: Routine screening is recommended.

Tuberculosis: Routine screening is recommended.

Blood pressure: Routine monitoring is recommended. Children with renal problems may develop hypertension and should have more frequent monitoring.

Urinalysis: Baseline urinalysis and cultures should be obtained in the newborn period.

Bladder catheterization is recommended for obtaining urine for cultures.

Condition-specific screening

Blood tests: CBCs should be obtained frequently on children treated with sulfonamides. Serum creatinine should be done on newborns and then yearly to monitor renal function.

Scoliosis: Screening for scoliosis should be done yearly from birth through adolescence.

Latex allergies: Monitor for signs and symptoms.

Patient, family, and other care providers should be educated.

COMMON ILLNESS MANAGEMENT

Differential diagnosis

If the child presents with:

• Respiratory difficulties, stridor, croupy cough: rule out Chiari II malformation.

Summary of Special Primary Care Needs for the Child with Myelodysplasia—cont'd

- Scoliosis, altered gait pattern, changes in muscle strength and tone, disturbance in urinary and bowel patterns and back pain: rule out tethered cord.
- Headaches: rule out shunt malfunction.
- Fevers: rule out shunt or CNS infection; urinary tract infection; fracture or injury of insensate area.
- Gastrointestinal symptoms: rule out increased intracranial pressure with nausea and vomiting; urinary tract infection; fecal impaction.

Drug interactions

No routine drug therapy exists, therefore any interactions are specific to the individual and any medications they must be taking.

DEVELOPMENTAL ISSUES

Sleep patterns

Apnea, increased stridor, and snoring may occur in children with symptomatic Chiari II malformation. Sleep studies may be indicated.

Lethargy may indicate increased intracranial pressure.

Toileting

Delayed bowel and bladder training may occur as a result of neurologic deficit.

Independence should be encouraged when developmentally and physically appropriate.

Bowel regimens will vary. Antigrade continence enemas are being used. Electrostimulation for fecal control is also used.

Intermittent catheterization is common, and compliance may be an issue during adolescence.

Discipline

These children are at an increased risk of psychosocial adjustment problems.

They have a need for discipline and encouragement toward independence.

Child care

Special medical needs may be necessary with severe physical involvement.

Early intervention programs are ideal for infants and toddlers.

Schooling

Federal laws protect children with disabilities.

Families need assistance in IEP hearings.

Children may have possible adjustment problems.

Neuropsychologic testing is recommended.

Special provisions may be necessary for adaptive equipment, transportation, and accessibility.

Special physical needs must be tended to during school hours.

Sexuality

Precocious puberty may occur.

Sexual functioning may be altered.

Genetic counseling may be necessary.

In choosing birth control, individuals must consider risks of latex allergy and blood clots associated with OCS.

Transition to adulthood

Issue dependent on severity of associated problems: primary health care, independent living, vocational training, socialization.

SPECIAL FAMILY CONCERNS

Parents suffer chronic grief for loss of "normal" child.

Stress is related to frequent hospitalizations, surgeries, and need for multidisciplinary care.

Caring for these children can be a financial burden on families.

References

American Association of Neuroscience Nurses: Core curriculum for neuroscience nursing ed 3, Park Ridge, Ill., 1996, AANN.

Aprikian A et al: Experience with the AS-800 artificial urinary sphincter in myelodysplastic children, Can J Surg 35(4):396-400, 1992.

Babcook CJ: Ultrasound evaluation of prenatal and neonatal spina bifida, Neurosurg Clin N Am 6(2):203-218, 1995.

Balcom AH et al: Initial experience with home therapeutic electrostimulation for continence in the myelomeningocele population, J Urol 158(3):1272-1276, 1997.

Bauer SB: Urologic care of the child with spina bifida, Spina Bifida Spotlight, Washington, DC, 1994, Spina Bifida Association of America.

Blair GK et al: The bowel management tube: an effective means for controlling fecal incontinence, J Pediatr Surg 27(10):1269-1272, 1992.

Budorick NE, Pretorius DH, and Nelson TR: Sonography of the fetal spine: technique, imaging findings, and clinical implications, American Journal of Roentgenology, 164(2):41-428, 1995.

Burke M and Meeropol E: The student with myelodysplasia. In Schwab N, editor: Guidelines for the management of students with genetic disorders: a manual for school nurses, ed 2, Mt Desert, ME, 1994, New England Regional Genetics Group.

Coniglio SJ, Anderson SM, and Ferguson JE: Developmental outcomes of children with myelomeningocele: prenatal predictors, Am J Obstet Gynecol 177(2):319-324, 1997.

Daly S and Scott JM: The prevention of neural tube defects, Curr Opin Obstet Gynecol 10(2):85-89, 1998.

Dias MS and McClone DG: Hydrocephalus in the child with dysraphism, Neurosurg Clin North Am 4(4):715-726, 1993.

Edelstein RA et al: The long term urological response of neonates with myelodysplasia treated proactively with intermittent catharizations and anticholinergic therapy: J Urol 154(4):1500-1504, 1995.

Edwards G et al: Recommendations for vocational and educational professionals. In Lollar DJ, editor: Preventing secondary conditions associated with spina bifida or cerebral palsy; proceedings and recommendations of a symposium, Washington, DC, 1994, Spina Bifida Association of America.

Edwards-Beckett J and King H: The impact of spinal pathology on bowel control in children, Rehabilitation Nursing, 21(6):292-296, 1996.

Elias ER and Hobbs N: Spina Bifida: sorting out the complexities of care, Contemporary Pediatrics, 15(4):156-171, 1998.

Elias ER and Sadeghi-Nejad A: Precocious puberty in girls with myelodysplasia, Pediatrics 93(3):521-522, 1994.

Gregerson DM: Clinical consequences of spina bifida occulta, Journal of Manipulative & Physiological Therapeutics, 20(8):546-550, 1997.

Hoeman SP: Primary care of the child with spina bifida, Nurse Pract 22(9):65-72, 1997.

Joyner BD, McLorie GA, and Khoury AE: Sexuality and reproductive issues in children with myelomeningocele, Eur J Pediat Surg 8(1):29-34, 1998.

Karol LA: Orthopedic management in myelomeningocele, Neurosurg Clin N Am 6(2):259-268, 1995.

Kaufman B et al: Disbanding a multidisciplinary clinic: effects on the health care of myelomeningocele patients, Pediatr Neurosurg 21:36-44, 1994.

King JC, Currie DM, and Wright E: Bowel training in spina bifida: importance of education, patient compliance, age, and reflexes, Arch Phys Ther Rehabil 75(3):243-247, 1994.

Kreder K: Anomalies associated with myelodysplasia, Pediatr Urol 39(3):248-250, 1992.

Liptak GS and Revell G: Management of bowel dysfunction in children with spinal cord disease or injury by means of the enema continence catheter, J Pediatr Surg 120(2):190-194, 1992.

Locksmith GJ, and Duff P: Preventing neural tube defects: the importance of periconceptional folic acid supplements, Obstet Gynecol 91(6):1027-1034, 1998.

Lollar DJ: Educational issues among children with spina bifida, Spina bifida spotlight, Washington, DC, 1993a, Spina Bifida Association of America.

Lollar DJ: Learning among children with spina bifida, Spina Bifida Spotlight, Washington, DC, 1993b, Spina Bifida Association of America.

Luthy DA et al: Cesarean section before the onset of labor and subsequent motor function in infants with myelomeningocele diagnosed internally, New Engl J Med 324(10):662-666, 1991.

Madsen JR, Scott RM: Chiari malformation, syringomyelia, and intramedullary spinal cord tumors, Curr Opin Neurol Neurosurg 6:559-563, 1993.

Malone PS, Ransley PG, and Kiely EM: Preliminary report: the antegrade continence enema, Lancet, 336:1217-1218, 1990.

Marge M: Toward a state of well-being: promoting healthy behaviors to prevent secondary conditions. In Lollar DJ, editor: Preventing secondary conditions associated with spina bifida or cerebral palsy: proceedings and recommendations of a symposium, Washington, DC, 1994, Spina Bifida Association of America.

McClone DG: Care of the neonate with myelomeningocele, Neurosurg Clin N Am 9(1):111-120, 1998.

McComb JG: Spinal and cranial neural tube defects, Seminars in Pediatric Neurology, 4(3):156-166, 1998.

National Institute for Occupational Health Alert: Preventing allergic reactions to natural rubber latex in the workplace, NIOSH No. 97-135. June 1997.

Nieto A et al: Allergy to latex in spina bifida: a multivariate study of associated factors in 100 consecutive patients, J Allergy Clin Immunol 98(3):501-507, 1996.

Palmer LS, Richards I, and Kaplan WE: Transrectal electrostimulation therapy for neuropathic bowel dysfunction in children with myelomeningocele. J Urol 157(4):1449-1452, 1997.

Pavin M et al: Recommendations for parents and families. In Lollar DJ, editor: Preventing secondary conditions associated with spina bifida or cerebral palsy: proceedings and recommendations of a symposium, Washington, DC, 1994, Spina Bifida Association of America.

Physician's Desk Reference, ed 52, Montvale, NJ, 1998, Medical Economics.

Rauen K and Aubert E: A brighter future for adults who have myelomeningocele—one form of spina bifida, Orthop Nurs 11(3):16-26, 1992.

Reigel DH: Infancy through the school years. In Rowley-Kelly F and Reigel DH, editors: Teaching the student with spina bifida, Baltimore, 1993, Brookes.

Rotenstein D, and Breen TJ: Growth hormone treatment of children with myelomeningocele, Journal of Pediatrics, 128(5):S28-31, 1996.

Rotenstein D, and Reigal DH: Growth hormone treatment in children with neural tube defects: results from 6 months to 6 years, J Pediatr 128(2):184-189, 1996.

Rowley-Kelly F: Transition planning to adulthood. In Rowley-Kelly F and Reigel DH, editors: Teaching the student with spina bifida, Baltimore, 1993, Brookes.

Ryan KD, Ploski C, and Emans JB: Myelodysplasia—the musculoskeletal problem: habilation from infancy to adulthood, Phys Ther 71(12):935-946, 1992.

Samuelson JJ, Foltz J, and Foxall MJ: Stress and coping in families of children with myelomeningocele, Arch Psychiatr Nurs 1(5):287-295, 1992.

Schidlow DV and Fiel SB: Life beyond pediatrics, Med Clin North Am 75(5):1113-1120, 1990.

Selzman AA, Elder JS, and Mapstone TB: Urologic consequences of myelodysplasia and other congenital abnormalities of the spinal cord (review), Urol Clin North Am 20(3):485-504, 1993.

Shah S et al: Latex allergy and latex sensitization in children and adolescents with meningomyelocele, J Allergy Clin Immunol 101(6):741-746, 1998.

Shaw GM et al: Epidemiologic characteristics of phenotypically distinct neural tube defects among 0.7 million California births, 1983-1987, Teratology 49:143-149, 1994.

Slater JE: Latex allergy, J Allergy Clin Immunol 94(2 pt1):139-149; quiz 150, Aug 1994.

Sloan SL: Sexuality issues in spina bifida, Spina bifida spotlight, Washington, DC, 1993, Spina Bifida Association of America.

Vereecken RL: Bladder pressure and kidney function in children with myelomeningocele: review article, Paraplegia 30(3):153-159, 1992.

Waters KA et al: Sleep-disordered breathing in children with myelomeningocele, J Pediatr 132(4):672-681, 1998.

Wu HY, Baskin LS, and Kogan BA: Neurogenic bladder dysfunction due to myelomeningocele: neonatal versus childhood treatment, J Urol 157(6):2295-2297, 1997.

Younoszai MK: Stooling problems in patients with myelomeningocele (review), South Med J 85(7):718-724, 1992.

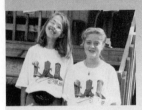

CHAPTER **30**

Organ Transplantation

Beverly Kosmach, Beverly Corbo-Richert, and Nancy Pike

Etiology

Transplantation is an effective treatment for a variety of end-stage organ diseases. This complex procedure is followed by a phase of intensive surgical and medical management—particularly in the early postoperative period. The liver, kidney, and heart are the most commonly transplanted solid organs in the pediatric population; however, heart-lung and intestine transplants in children are increasing.

As transplantation has become a more viable treatment for certain end-stage diseases, the indications for transplantation of the kidney, liver, and heart continue to increase (Table 30-1). The most common indications for renal transplantation in infants and young children are congenital or hereditary disorders, including renal hypoplasia or dysplasia, obstructive uropathy (usually posterior urethral valves), reflux nephropathy, or agenesis of the abdominal musculature (i.e., prune belly syndrome). In contrast, older children or adolescents tend to have glomerulonephritis as the cause of end-stage renal disease (ESRD) (Ellis et al, 1997).

Liver transplantation is a treatment therapy for a variety of end-stage liver diseases (ESLDs) that can generally be categorized as cholestatic disease, metabolic disease, fulminant liver failure, and chronic active hepatitis with cirrhosis (McDiarmid et al, 1998). Biliary atresia, which is an obstructive biliary tract disease, accounts for 50% to 75% of pediatric liver transplants in most centers (Ryckman et al, 1998). A Kasai portoenterostomy may result in improved bile drainage if performed within an infant's first 60 days of life. About 75% of children, however, will eventually require liver transplantation due to jaundice, recurrent cholangitis, portal hypertension, ascites, growth failure, and decreased synthetic function (McDiarmid et al, 1998). The most common metabolic disease requiring transplantation is alpha-1-antitrypsin deficiency.

Cardiomyopathy and congenital heart disease (CHD) are the leading indications for heart or heart-lung transplantation in children, with nearly half of those referred for transplant having CHD (Hosenpud, Novick, and Bennett, 1996). The most common indication for heart-lung transplantation is either surgically corrected or uncorrected CHD, which is associated with end-stage pulmonary vascular disease, primary pulmonary hypertension, and cystic fibrosis (Hosenpud et al, 1998). Fewer children now require heart-lung transplantation as a result of advancements in single or double lung transplants and congenital heart surgery (Hosenpud et al, 1998).

Recipient and graft survival have improved significantly over the past 3 decades due to advances in immunosuppression, surgical techniques, organ preservation, and monitoring for infections, as well as a better understanding of postoperative management and intensive care medicine. Immunosuppressive protocols vary by institution and the organ transplanted. Cyclosporine (CSA) (Sandimmune) has been the mainstay of solid organ transplantation since its introduction in 1983. Used in conjunction with steroids and azathioprine (Imuran), this immunosuppressant revolutionized transplantation and resulted in dramatically improved survival rates. Tacrolimus (Prograf) has been introduced as a primary immunosuppressant and has been shown to be significantly more effective in preventing acute rejection episodes and treating rejection that is refractory to corticosteroids (Pirsch et al, 1997; Reyes et al, 1998b; US Multicenter FK 506 Study Group, 1994; Webber 1997).

Incidence

Renal Transplantation

The first successful clinical trials in renal transplantation were conducted in 1962 at the University of Colorado (Starzl and Demetris, 1997). Prior

Table 30-1
Comparative Indications for Transplantation in Children by Organ*

Renal	Liver	Heart	Dual Transplants
Congenital disease	**Cholestatic disease**	**Cardiomyopathy**	**Heart and liver**
Renal hypoplasia	Biliary atresia	Dilated	Familial hypercholester-
Renal dysplasia	Familial cholestasis	Hypertrophic	olemia with ischemic
Prune belly syndrome	Alagille's syndrome	Restrictive	cardiomyopathy
Congenital nephrotic syn-	Byler's syndrome	**Congenital heart**	Intrahepatic biliary
drome	**Parenchymal disease**	**defects** (select	atresia and dilated
Wilms' tumor	Budd-Chiari syndrome	lesions)	cardiomyopathy
Obstructive uropathy	Congenital hepatic fibrosis		**Liver and kidney**
Acquired disease	Cystic fibrosis		Cystinosis
Glomerulonephritis	Neonatal hepatitis		Oxalosis
Lupus nephritis	Acute fulminant hepatic		**Heart and lung**
Membranous glomeru-	failure		Primary pulmonary hy-
lonephritis	Hepatitis B		pertension
Focal segmental glomerular	Hepatitis C		Congenital heart defects
sclerosis	**Metabolic disorders**		with elevated pul-
IgA nephropathy/	α_1-antitrypsin deficiency		monary vascular re-
Henoch-Schönlein	Wilson's disease		sistance
purpura	Glycogen storage disease,		Cystic fibrosis
Hemolytic uremic syndrome	type IV		
Chronic pyelonephritis	Tyrosinemia		
Renal infarct	**Hepatomas**		
Sickle cell nephropathy			
Hereditary disease			
Alport's syndrome			
Juvenile nephrophthisis			
Polycystic kidney disease			
Metabolic disorders			
Cystinosis			
Oxalosis			

*These are a few of the more common conditions leading to end-stage organ failure; the list is not all-inclusive.

to that series, a few isolated cases of renal transplantation between fraternal and identical twins were reported. Renal transplantation has evolved as the treatment choice for ESRD. Transplantation is a desirable goal early in the disease process so that a child does not have to experience the complications of progressive disease and medical therapies, as well as the emotional stressors of dialysis and chronic illness issues (Ellis et al, 1997).

Renal transplantation from living-related donors reveals a significant graft survival advantage over cadaveric transplants in all age groups, with the best results in infants and toddlers. In this age group, there is a 66% survival rate with cadaveric donors and an 84% survival rate with living-related donors (Cecka, Gjertson, and Terasaki,

1997). There were 636 pediatric renal transplants performed in 1997 (United Network for Organ Sharing, [UNOS], Scientific Registry Data, 1998).

Liver Transplantation

Dr. Thomas Starzl pioneered pediatric liver transplantation, with the first surgery being performed in 1963 (Starzl et al, 1982). Survival in this early period was less than 50% but has greatly improved over the last 30 years. The United Network for Organ Sharing (UNOS) reports an 80% survival at 1 year and a 76% survival at 5 years (UNOS Scientific Registry Data, 1998). In 1997, 552 pediatric liver transplants were performed (UNOS Scientific Registry Data, 1998).

With the demand for donor livers far exceeding the supply, split liver transplantation and living-related liver transplantation (LRLT) have been developed as strategies to increase the donor pool (Reichert et al, 1998). The split liver procedure involves dividing the liver into its left and right lobes and transplanting the lobes into two different recipients, usually an adult and child. LRLT usually involves liver donation between a child with ESLD and an ABO compatible biologic parent. Although the timing of living, related transplantation is advantageous, these recipients endure similar complications (e.g., hepatic artery thrombosis and rejection) to those of individuals receiving cadaveric livers (Heffron, 1993). LRLT also poses the ethical dilemma of placing a healthy donor at risk in order to save the life of a child. The evaluation for LRLT demands a full assessment of the risk-benefit ratio for the child, parent, and family.

Heart Transplantation

Heart transplantation in humans also began in the 1960s. The development of successful orthotopic surgical techniques involving the removal of the recipient's ventricles, leaving the posterior atrial walls and the ridge of the interatrial septum intact was a significant breakthrough (Lower and Shumway, 1960). The first pediatric heart transplant was performed on an 18-day-old infant with Ebstein's anomaly; but this child died 6 hours later from complications (Kantrowitz et al, 1968).

About 25,000 to 30,000 children are born with a congenital heart defect per year in the United States (American Heart Association, 1997). Most of these children can be helped surgically, yet an estimated 10% who have complex, incorrectable CHD require heart or heart-lung transplantation. In 1985, neonatal transplantation was introduced as a treatment option for infants with hypoplastic left heart syndrome. Without surgical intervention, this condition is usually fatal within the first few months of life (Morrow et al, 1997). The number of cardiac transplants in infants has decreased due to the limited supply of donors and the advancement in surgical palliation for congenital heart defects.

The incidence of cardiomyopathy in children is not well documented and varies according to primary (i.e., congenital, acquired) or secondary causes (e.g., infection, systemic disease, toxic ex-

posure, and malnutrition). The most common cardiomyopathy in children is of the dilated type. About 1 in 20 cases of dilated myocardiopathy is idiopathic, which means that there is a positive family history indicating a genetic predisposition to develop the cardiovascular changes (Stockwell, Tobias, and Greely, 1995).

There were 275 pediatric heart transplants performed in 1997 (UNOS Scientific Registry Data, 1998). The 1-year survival rate for heart transplant recipients has remained consistent at nearly 80% over the past 10 years compared with 72% prior to 1988 (Hosenpud et al, 1998).

Small Bowel and Multivisceral Transplantation

Small bowel transplantation has become an increasingly effective treatment for children with end-stage short gut syndrome over the last 10 years. The overall survival rate for these children is approximately 70% (Abu-Elmagd, Reyes, and Todol, 1998). Although the use of total parenteral nutrition (TPN) has extended the lives of children with end-stage short gut syndrome, associated morbidities are common. These morbidities include TPN-related liver failure; venous access complications related to thrombosis, multiple line insertions, and sepsis; and ultimately a lack of venous access. The financial burden of daily TPN and associated care, as well as the psychosocial impact of a permanent indwelling line and connection to an infusion pump, are also stressors for these children and their families.

Multivisceral or composite transplantation involves the replacement of two or more organs in a variety of combinations, depending upon the cause of the disease and/or the complications of treatment of the end-stage disease. This surgery may include combinations of heart-liver, heart-lung, liver-kidney, small bowel-liver, or heart-lung-liver. In rare cases, such as chronic intestinal pseudoobstruction or volvulus with cholestasis, a child may receive an "en-bloc" transplant including the stomach, liver, pancreas, and small bowel. Survival varies, depending upon the number of organs transplanted, the medical status of the child prior to transplantation, and the posttransplant complications, as well as the experience of the transplant center. Actuarial survival rates at 1, 3, and 5 years after multivisceral transplantation involving transplantation of the lungs or intestine in combination with the heart, liver, or kidney are reported to be 57%, 43%, and 43%, respectively (Reyes et al, 1998a). The 1-year survival rate for heart-lung transplants has remained consistent at 60% over the past 10 years as compared with 56% prior to 1988 (Hosenpud et al, 1998).

Clinical Manifestations at Time of Diagnosis

The presenting symptoms and severity of illness of children with end-stage organ disease varies according to the specific disease and affected organ, as well as the length of illness, age of the child, and effectiveness of treatment. Table 30-2 presents the clinical manifestations of end-stage organ disease in children.

Renal Disease

Children with ESRD typically exhibit symptoms related to fluid and electrolyte imbalances, hypertension, and hyperglycemia. Early signs and symptoms may include pallor and fatigue on exertion. Children with renal disease may also present with anorexia, recurrent emesis, edema, anemia, and rickets (Ellis et al, 1997). These children also often exhibit growth failure as a long-term effect of chronic renal disease (Fine, 1997b). A complete

discussion of the manifestations of chronic renal failure is presented in Chapter 34.

Liver Disease

Children with liver disease may have an acute or chronic course of illness. Depending upon the cause of their liver disease, some children may remain stable for several years prior to transplantation with appropriate medical management, but others may have a moderate to rapid decline in hepatic function with serious sequelae. Symptoms of liver dysfunction, such as those seen with biliary atresia, may include jaundice, hepatomegaly, splenomegaly, ascites, pruritus, xanthomas, and variceal bleeding. Hepatic enzymes, bilirubin, gamma GTP, and ammonia levels are elevated. Children who have had a Kasai portoenterostomy are also at risk for cholangitis. Other symptoms associated with liver failure may include delayed growth, malnutrition, rickets, osteomalacia with fractures, increased synthetic function, and encephalopathy.

Acute end-stage liver disease secondary to fulminant hepatic failure may have an insidious onset with rapid clinical deterioration over a few days, characterized by encephalopathy and coagulopathy. With progression of the disease, cerebral edema increases, causing neurologic deterioration—often with intracranial hemorrhage, which is an emergent situation requiring liver transplantation before the child deteriorates to the point of being ineligible for transplantation.

Table 30-2
Comparative Clinical Manifestations of End-Stage Renal, Liver, and Heart Disease in Children

Renal	Liver	Heart
Electrolyte abnormalities	Jaundice	Respiratory distress
Sodium retention	Ascites	Tachypnea
Hyperkalemia	Hepatomegaly	Congestive heart failure
Hypokalemia	Splenomegaly	Cardiomegaly
Metabolic acidosis	Portal hypertension	ST- and T-wave abnormalities
Hyperglycemia	Hypercholesterolemia	Cardiac murmurs
Hyperlipidemia	Hyperammonemia	Growth retardation
Anemia	Hypoalbuminemia	Arrhythmias
Congestive heart failure or pericarditis	Hypoglycemia	
Peripheral neuropathy	Prolonged prothrombin time	
Renal osteodystrophy	Hormone imbalance	
Growth retardation	Encephalopathy	

Heart Disease

Complex CHD and cardiomyopathies requiring transplantation may have similar presenting symptoms (see Chapter 17 for a review of CHD). Symptoms of cardiomyopathy vary depending upon the child's age at presentation of illness and the type of cardiomyopathy. The clinical manifestations of dilated cardiomyopathy include symptoms of congestive heart failure as a result of decreasing myocardial contractility. Other common clinical signs include an enlarged heart by chest radiography, nonspecific ST-T wave changes and sinus tachycardia on electrocardiography, and a gallop rhythm on auscultation. Nonspecific symptoms may include fever, vomiting, weight loss, or failure to thrive.

Most children discovered to have hypertropic cardiomyopathy do not have prominent cardiac symptoms because thickening of the left ventricular wall may remain stable or progress slowly. There is usually a positive family history in 30% to 60% of affected individuals (Park, 1996). Children and young adults are at risk for episodes of syncope and sudden death during exercise when the left ventricular demand increases and obstruction to the outflow tract occurs. This diagnosis is sometimes first made on autopsy. The annual incidence of sudden death is 4% to 6% per year in children and adolescents with hypertrophic cardiomyopathy (Park, 1996).

Treatment

Pretransplant Management

Renal Disease

Conservative therapy consists of managing fluid, electrolyte, and metabolic imbalances, as well as hypertension and anemia (see Chapter 34). When conservative treatment for chronic renal failure is no longer effective, ESRD care consists of hemodialysis and/or peritoneal dialysis or renal transplantation (Fine, 1997b). Recent data, however, support preemptive renal transplantation (i.e., transplantation prior to dialysis) over the use of pretransplant dialysis (Mahmoud et al, 1997). Because this goal is not always immediately attainable, dialysis may need to be initiated. Successful transplantation is the optimum treatment choice for children with ESRD to improve overall health and quality of life (Cecka et al, 1997; Ellis et al, 1997).

Liver Disease

Children with chronic liver disease may be followed on an outpatient basis with medical management designed to optimize and stabilize hepatic function. To meet nutritional requirements, these children may require enteral supplementation, administration of fat-soluble vitamins, and/or TPN. Synthetic function of the liver, coagulation times, and ammonia level, as well as electrolytes, fluid balance, and renal function must be frequently monitored.

Medications may also provide symptomatic relief to stabilize hepatic function. Ursodiol and phenobarbital may be used to decrease cholestasis. Severe pruritus may be treated with ursodiol or diphenhydramine. Hyperammonemia is treated with lactulose. Recurrent cholangitis due to biliary stasis and bacterial contamination in children who have had a Kasai procedure is common. Symptoms may include a fever of greater than 38° C, an elevated white blood cell count, and an increase in serum bilirubin concentration. Positive blood cultures provide a definitive diagnosis. These children are initially treated with an appropriately sensitive intravenous antibiotic followed by long-term prophylaxis with trimethoprim-sulfamethoxazole, metronidazole, or ciprofloxacin hydrochloride.

Bleeding episodes due to esophageal and gastric varices from portal hypertension can be temporized during the waiting period by sclerotherapy and band variceal ligation. Peritoneal-venous shunt surgery may also be performed to decrease ascites, and the splenic artery may be embolized to mediate thrombocytopenia. In the event of massive bleeding refractory to sclerotherapy, transcutaneous intrahepatic portosystemic shunting (TIPS) may be required (Reyes et al, 1999). The TIPS procedure can help stabilize a candidate for pediatric liver transplant, although complications with bleeding due to perforation or extrahepatic portal vein puncture, peritonitis, or hepatic or biliary injury are seen (Reyes et al, 1999).

Heart Disease

Children with cardiomyopathy may be managed on oral medications if symptoms of heart failure are controlled. Medical management of dilated cardiomyopathy consists of maximizing cardiac output and controlling symptoms of heart failure with digoxin, diuretics, and afterload reduction.

Angiotensin-converting enzyme inhibitors (i.e, captopril or enalapril) for afterload reduction have been beneficial in optimizing cardiac function and decreasing the workload of the heart. Antiarrhythmics may be needed in some children. Anticoagulation therapy may help to prevent thrombus formation in a dilated and poorly contracting heart.

Children with CHD who develop ventricular dysfunction, lethal arrhythmias, and/or irreversible pulmonary hypertension are also managed medically until transplantation. Management is similar to dilated cardiomyopathy but may vary slightly depending on the type of CHD and previous operative or palliative procedures. Some children and adolescents with cyanotic heart defects may have additional management issues related to polycythemia, hypoxemia, and CNS sequelae (see Chapter 17).

In contrast, medical management for hypertrophic cardiomyopathy consists of maintaining a normal preload and afterload while reducing ventricular contractility, which is usually accomplished with calcium channel blockers, as well as beta blockers to decrease the septal muscle from obstructing the left ventricular outflow tract. Antiarrhythmics may also be needed for ventricular arrhythmias but have not been shown to prevent sudden death. Surgical intervention can be attempted to remove muscle bundles in the left ventricular outflow tract to relieve obstruction. Surgical intervention is not recommended until medical management has failed because of the possibility of recurrent obstruction.

Additionally, children who have an increased pulmonary vascular resistance (PVR) unresponsive to pulmonary vasodilators will require a heart-lung transplant instead of an isolated heart transplant (Wong and Starnes, 1998). Heart transplantation is the alternative to failed medical and surgical management. Due to the shortage of pediatric donors, however, children at the maximum limits of medical management may not survive until transplantation. A 20% mortality rate for pediatric candidates for cardiac transplants has been reported (Webber, 1997).

Evaluation for Transplantation

Evaluation for organ transplantation is an exhaustive process that includes medical, surgical, nutritional, and psychosocial assessments with multiple diagnostic tests, laboratory data, radiologic testing, and consultant evaluations. Although the evaluation process varies by institution and organ, a multidisciplinary approach is commonly used. The health care team includes the transplant surgery staff: specialty medical services (e.g., nephrology, gastroenterology, anesthesiology, or cardiology) and infectious disease specialists; nursing services with transplant coordinators, clinical nurse specialists or nurse practitioners; psychosocial services through social work and psychiatry; behavioral medicine involving developmental and child life specialists; and physical and occupational therapists. Evaluations are usually scheduled on an outpatient basis in specialty clinics, with individuals having routine outpatient follow-up facilitated by the transplant coordinator during the waiting period. Children with more advanced disease, however, are hospitalized when evaluated and may require continued hospitalization until an organ is available.

Pretransplant surgical procedures may be necessary in some cases to provide corrective or palliative repairs to prepare or stabilize a child for transplantation. For example, a child with urethral valve anomalies in addition to ESRD may benefit from ureteral reimplantation prior to transplantation.

Laboratory data commonly obtained for all organs include a complete blood count and platelet count; a full chemistry profile to assess electrolytes, renal function, and nutritional status; and prothrombin and partial thromboplastin times. Serologic testing is also completed to diagnose previous infections with hepatitis A, B, and C, cytomegalovirus (CMV), Epstein-Barr virus (EBV), human immunodeficiency virus (HIV), herpes, and varicella zoster. A child's immunization record is also reviewed.

Blood typing to achieve ABO-matched organs is required for heart, kidney, and liver transplantation. Additionally, human leukocyte antigen (HLA) matching is necessary in renal transplantation. Cytotoxic antibody cross-match compatibility, percent panel reactive antibody (PRA), and HLA tissue typing are also completed.

Although most children with end-stage organ disease are suitable candidates for transplantation, there are some exclusion criteria. These criteria have decreased significantly over the past several years due to innovations in care and advances in surgical techniques. Exclusion criteria vary by institution, but most centers agree that children with systemic sepsis, multi-organ failure, and metastatic disease are not appropriate candidates. HIV positivity, which was once considered an absolute contraindication, is now under debate (McDiarmid et al, 1998). A history of medical noncompliance and a poor social support system should also be considered as relative contraindications. In the pediatric population, referral to Child and Family Services for foster care when a family is unable or unwilling to care for the child may be indicated.

Once accepted as a transplant candidate, a child is listed with UNOS and the wait begins for the child and family. While waiting at home or in a community hospital for transplantation, the child is medically managed by the primary care provider, who must provide regular updates to the transplant center and inform the center of any deterioration or complications in the child's medical status. Because the primary care provider may also have developed a supportive relationship with the child and family during the diagnosis of the illness and pretransplant care, this caregiver may be best able to assess the child and family's coping abilities, responses to stress, level of understanding, and adaptability. This assessment should be communicated to the transplant team to help them build on the family's strengths as the family learns to cope with and adapt to the various stressors of the transplant process. The waiting period is variable, lasting from a few days to months—and occasionally years. It is a highly stressful time for the family as they hope for an organ before their child's condition deteriorates.

Recent and Anticipated Advances in Diagnosis and Management

Over the past 30 years, transplantation has evolved into an accepted treatment for certain end-stage organ diseases. Pediatric recipients have benefited from advances in surgical techniques, organ preservation, and immunosuppressive protocols. New approaches to standard immunosuppressive protocols that result in optimum graft function with minimal side effects are being explored. Ongoing research is focused on immunosuppressive medications that more specifically inhibit the immune system and decrease the incidence of rejection, subsequently

placing a child at less risk for long-term infection and nephrotoxicity.

Medications

Sirolimus (Rapamycin) is a new immunosuppressive agent that has structural similarities to tacrolimus. This macrolide antibiotic inhibits T- and B-cell activity by blocking the signaling from cytokine and growth factor cell surface receptors to the nucleus (Groth et al, 1998). Sirolimus has synergistic effects with CSA and tacrolimus, and nephrotoxic side effects may be minimized when it is used as an adjunctive immunosuppressant with lower doses of CSA or tacrolimus (Zimmerman and Kahan, 1997). Human studies are currently limited to phase I and II trials in renal transplantation. The International Multicenter Study includes 146 recipients of renal transplant under triple drug therapy with CSA, prednisone (Deltasone), and sirolimus. Observations from this trial show that adding sirolimus to a CSA protocol resulted in a decreased incidence of rejection and that sirolimus as a base therapy prevented acute rejection as competently as CSA. The side effects of sirolimus were quite different than those of CSA and included thrombocytopenia, leukocytopenia, and hypercholesterolemia. Of importance was a normal serum creatinine as compared with those treated with CSA. Although the rate of rejection was lower in the group treated with sirolimus, the 1-year graft survival rates were similar (Groth et al, 1998).

Mycophenolate mofetil (MMF) was approved by the US Food and Drug Administration in 1995 for prevention of acute rejection in renal transplantation. In a trial of nearly 500 recipients of cadaveric renal transplants, MMF was shown to significantly reduce the rate of rejection during the first 6 months after transplantation. The most frequent side effects were gastrointestinal problems, leukopenia, and opportunistic infections (Hausen and Morris, 1997).

Daclizumab (Zenapax) is used for the prophylaxis of acute organ rejection and is a monoclonal antibody that works by directly inhibiting interleukin-2 (IL-2) (Roche product monograph, 1997). Daclizumab is used in combination with CSA or tacrolimus and steroids and can also be used with azathioprine and MMF. A total of five doses are administered, with the first dose being given within 24 hours before the transplant and subsequent doses given every 14 days. Studies of adult renal transplant recipients reported a decreased incidence of rejection in individuals receiving daclizumab prophylaxis. Pediatric studies are limited at this time (n = 25), and the most common side effects in this group were hypertension, pain, diarrhea, and vomiting. In the adult population, the addition of daclizumab did not increase the incidence of lymphoproliferative disorders, and the overall incidence of infection was not higher when compared with those treated with placebos (Roche product monograph, 1997).

Chimerism and Tolerance

Following transplantation, donor cells migrate throughout the recipient's body with an exchange of leukocytes from the donor organ into recipient tissue and a replacement of the same type of leukocytes from the recipient into the donor tissue. Chimerism, which is the coexistence of donor and recipient cells, depends upon effective immunosuppression and is thought to be necessary for the body to accept the transplanted organ (Starzl et al, 1993a). It is theorized that if chimerism can be maintained, chronic rejection may be avoided and less immunosuppression will be required long-term (Starzl et al, 1993a).

Achieving a chimeric state is thought to lead to the development of tolerance. Although it is presumed that transplant recipients will require lifelong immunosuppression, some individuals can achieve tolerance of the transplanted organ after they have been successfully weaned of maintenance immunosuppression. In a study of 95 liver transplant recipients at least 5 years after transplant and over 2 years from a rejection with the goal of immunosuppressive withdrawal (Mazariegos et al, 1997), 18 (i.e., 19%) of these individuals have been drug free for nearly 5 years. Acute rejection occurred in 26% of transplant recipients, but no grafts have been lost and chronic rejection has not developed. Those treated for rejection during the weaning process required less immunosuppression than when they entered the study (Mazariegos et al, 1997).

Due to early observations indicating that bone marrow cells were the most effective antigen-presenting cells to produce the donor-specific effect (Padbury, Toogood, and McMaster, 1998), donor bone marrow infusion at the time of solid organ transplantation is being used to augment the process of chimerism and possibly increase the incidence of immunosuppressive withdrawal in recipients of liver transplants. In transplant recipients receiving immunosuppressive therapy of tacrolimus and prednisone, 138 received bone marrow infusions and were compared with 92 who did not (Zeevi et al, 1997). Chimerism was seen in 90% of the recipients receiving bone marrow infusions and in 52% of those who did not receive bone marrow. Donor-specific immunomodulation was reported in 48% of the bone-marrow recipients as compared with 30% of those not treated with bone marrow. It remains to be seen if bone marrow-augmented transplantation will result in withdrawal of immunosuppression in this population (Zeevi et al, 1997).

Xenotransplantation

Organ donation is unable to meet the demands of the increasing numbers of individuals requiring organ transplantation for end-stage disease. Dialysis and cardiac assist devices may prolong life as candidates wait for an organ, but no such device is currently available for liver transplant candidates. Reduced-size, living related, and split liver techniques have been of some use in increasing the donor pool for liver transplantation, but other strategies are being explored to meet the increasing demand of donor organs. Xenotransplantation, the cross-species transplantation of organs, has been done experimentally in a few cases between pigs and baboons since 1968 (Harland and Platt, 1996). There have been three reported cases of xenotransplantation of the liver in humans. A heterotopic auxiliary transplant of a pig liver into an individual with fulminant hepatic failure was performed in 1993 as a bridge in waiting for a human liver. The pig liver functioned for about 24 hours as evidenced by lactate clearance, bile production, and improved renal function. A rise in anti-pig antibodies was observed, however, and thought to be the cause for graft failure. The individual expired from cerebral edema before a human liver was available (Makowka, Cramer, and Hoffman, 1993; Makowka et al, 1994).

Two xenotransplants of the liver from baboon donors to human recipients were performed at the University of Pittsburgh Medical Center, with one person surviving 70 days posttransplant. Death was due to a subarachnoid hemorrhage secondary to invasive aspergillosis. The immunosuppressive regimen included tacrolimus, cyclophosphamide, prostaglandin E, and steroids. Although liver function was normal for nearly 2 months, an autopsy revealed biliary statis with damage of the intrahepatic ducts and infection (Starzl et al, 1993b).

Further research to understand the immunological barriers to cross-species transplantation is progressing. Because of the liver's relative resistance to hyperacute rejection, as well as the often immediate need for transplantation in end-stage liver disease, xenotransplantation of the liver may be seen before that of other organs (Harland and Platt, 1996). Research has also begun to evaluate the pig heart as an animal source for cardiac transplantation. With the increased need for donor hearts, xenotransplantation and mechanical circulatory support devices for children will continue to be a focus of research to improve survival to transplantation (Morrow et al, 1997; Platt, 1997).

Mechanical Assist Devices

Circulatory support: Mechanical circulatory support as a temporary "bridge" to transplantation is an option for the failing heart. There are a variety of mechanical devices available for adults, but few are designed for long-term pediatric support. If only ventricular support is required, the most common mechanical circulatory support used while an individual is awaiting transplantation is the ventricular assist device. Extracorporeal membrane oxygenation (ECMO) is also used for infants and children requiring both cardiac and pulmonary support. A right and/or left ventricular assist device can be used, depending on the child's need.

Ventricular assist devices have been well-documented as a bridge to transplantation in adults, with 60% of the individuals supported going on to transplantation and 89% discharged from the hospital (Hunt and Frazier, 1998). The better outcomes from the ventricular assist devices can be attributed to improving kidney, liver, and pulmonary function due to improved organ perfusion if no sequelae occur while an individual is being supported by the device. Some ventricular assist devices allow a child to ambulate, which provides physical rehabilitation and places the child in optimal condition prior to transplantation. There are risks associated with any mechanical circulatory device. The most frequent complications are bleeding, infection,

thromboembolism, hemolysis, technical problems, and neurologic dysfunction (Hunt and Frazier, 1998). The ideal long-term mechanical circulatory support device for children has not yet evolved, and current devices on the market are being adapted for pediatric use.

Extracorporeal liver assistance: Because the function of the liver is primarily metabolic, the challenge is to develop a device that could duplicate these complex chemical reactions. One type of hepatic-assist device under development consists of growing hepatocytes in the extracapillary spaces of a hollow fiber cartridge. An individual's blood is pumped through this cartridge as a continuous rather than an intermittent process, and the hepatocytes function as if they were in an intact liver (Sussman and Kelly, 1995). Clinical trials are underway for a limited number of cases of fulminant hepatic failure, and preliminary findings are encouraging. This type of "liver dialysis" could be helpful in sustaining liver function until the liver recovers and begins a regenerative process after injury due to trauma or disease (Sussman and Kelly, 1995). The hepatic assist device may also help maintain a child with end-stage liver disease awaiting transplantation.

Associated Problems after Transplantation (Box 30-1)

Immunosuppression

Immunosuppressive regimens vary according to the organ transplanted and the specific protocols of the institution where the transplant is performed. The most common immunosuppressive medications used alone or in combination therapy to prevent rejection are CSA, tacrolimus, azathioprine, and prednisone. CSA has been the mainstay of immunosuppressive management since 1983 and has resulted in dramatically improved survival rates. Tacrolimus, formerly known as FK-506, has recently been shown to be significantly more effective in preventing acute, corticosteroid-resistant, and refractory rejection (Pirsch et al, 1997; Reyes et al, 1998b; The US Multicenter FK506 Liver Study Group 1994; Webber 1997).

CSA interferes with the production and release of IL-2, which is an essential cytokine in the immune process, by helper T-cells. CSA also inter-

Box 30-1

Associated Problems

Immunosuppression
Side effects of medications
Potential for infection
Nephrotoxicity
Lymphoproliferative disease

Rejection
Acute—first 6 months posttransplant
Reversible
Chronic—slower process lasting months to years; leading cause of late graft loss

Infection
Bacterial
Viral
Fungal
Protozoan
Symptoms of infection masked by immunosuppressive therapy

Table 30-3
Toxicity of Cyclosporine and Tacrolimus

Adverse Effect	Cyclosporine	Tacrolimus
Neurotoxicity	+	++
Nephrotoxicity	++	++
Hyperkalemia	++	+++
Hypertension	+++	+
Diabetogenicity	+	+
Hypercholesterolemia	++	+
Increased low-density lipoprotein levels	++	+
Hyperuricemia	+	+
Gingival hyperplasia	++	−
Hirsutism	++	−
Alopecia	+	++
Anemia	+	++
Hand tremors	+	+

+ to +++ indicate increasing frequency and/or severity of each adverse effect; − indicates adverse effect not observed.
From Jain A and Fung J: Cyclosporin and tacrolimus in clinical transplantation: a comparative review, Clin Immunotherapy 5:365, 1996.

feres with the precursor cytotoxic cell response to IL-2. It is through these mechanisms that CSA can inhibit T-cell–mediated acute rejection (Jain and Fung, 1996). Absorption of CSA is bile-dependent because it is excreted and reabsorbed from bile through enterohepatic circulation (Crandall, 1990). Therefore therapeutic drug levels may be difficult to maintain in liver transplant recipients, other organ recipients who may also have hepatic dysfunction with cholestasis, and children with external bile drainage. A microemulsion formulation of CSA that is absorbed independently of bile is currently available (Trull et al, 1993).

Although nephrotoxicity is the most significant side effect of CSA, it is dosage-dependent and usually reversible (Jain and Fung, 1996) (Table 30-3). Nephrotoxicity may present with hyperkalemia, hypomagnesemia, hyperchloremic metabolic acidosis, hyperuricemia, and transient elevations in blood urea nitrogen (BUN) and creatinine. Acute microvascular disease, chronic progressive interstitial fibrosis, and a decreased glomerular filtration rate of nearly 30% may also be seen (Jordan, Rosenthal, Makowka; 1993; US Multicenter FK506 Liver Study Group, 1994). Hypertension is quite common—especially when CSA is given in combination with high-dose corticosteroids—but is usually responsive to antihypertensive therapy with calcium channel blockers (e.g., nifedipine, verapamil) or beta-adrenergic blockers (e.g., atenolol, propranolol, labetalol). Although nephrotoxicity is a concern in all transplant recipients, it may be more critical in those with renal transplants because renal dysfunction may reflect not only CSA toxicity but also rejection and acute tubular necrosis.

Neurotoxicities are also commonly seen with CSA but are usually level-dependent and reversible. Neurotoxic side effects may include tremor, headache, dizziness, insomnia, photophobia, paraesthesia, and seizures (European FK506 Multicenter Liver Study Group, 1994; The US Multicenter FK506 Liver Study Group, 1994). Other side effects of CSA therapy include gingival hyperplasia, hirsutism, gastrointestinal (GI) disorders, and an increased risk for infection and malignancy. A lower CSA trough level may often decrease the severity or presence of these side effects.

Tacrolimus is a macrolide compound that differs chemically from CSA but has a similar mechanism of action. It is up to 100 times more potent in inhibiting the production of cytotoxic T-lymphocytes and IL-2 and gamma-interferon production than CSA in vitro (Goto et al, 1987). Tacrolimus was initially used in individuals with refractory rejection as a "rescue" therapy for those who failed to respond to conventional immunosuppression, high-dose steroids, antilymphocyte globulin, or azathioprine. Clinical trials followed as a result of favorable outcomes, and tacrolimus was subsequently approved by the US Food and Drug Administration (USFDA) in 1994. Tacrolimus has now replaced CSA as the primary immunosuppressive agent in some centers (McDiarmid et al, 1995a; Shapiro et al, 1996; Webber, 1997). Additionally, tacrolimus does not depend upon bile for absorption, so more stable levels may be seen in recipients with cholestasis or external bile drainage (Jain et al, 1991).

The side effects of tacrolimus are similar to those of CSA including nephrotoxicity, neurotoxicity, hypertension, infection, and gastrointestinal disturbances. As with CSA, the severity of these side effects may be decreased or eliminated after transplantation as levels are decreased over time. Hirsutism and gingival hyperplasia are not reported with tacrolimus therapy.

The ability to wean and withdraw steroids from transplant recipients receiving tacrolimus is of great benefit both medically and psychosocially. Corticosteroid withdrawal has been achieved in most pediatric recipients, resulting in monotherapy with tacrolimus (Reyes et al, 1998b; Shapiro et al, 1998; Webber 1997). With steroid withdrawal, side effects from long-term high-dose steroids (e.g., Cushingoid facies, growth failure, osteoporosis, cataract formation, hypertension, diabetes, and an increased risk of infection) can be avoided.

The goal of any immunosuppressive protocol is to maintain the lowest acceptable level of drug that results in stable and adequate functioning of the transplanted organ without drug toxicity (Kosmach, Webber, and Reyes, 1998). CSA and tacrolimus are usually administered orally every 12 hours. Trough levels are obtained to guide dosing because many factors can affect absorption and metabolism. Children usually require twice the adult dose based on body weight because they metabolize both CSA and tacrolimus faster, resulting in a shorter half-life of the drug and more rapid clearance (Jain and Fung 1996; Jain et al, 1991). Therapeutic levels vary according to the organ transplanted, the length of time posttransplant, and

the presence of infection or rejection (Kosmach et al, 1998) (Table 30-4).

Rejection

Rejection is an inflammatory response of the immune system in which the transplanted tissue is recognized as foreign. Acute cellular rejection most commonly occurs during the first 6 months after transplantation. This type of rejection is a T-cell mediated event and is usually reversible. Chronic rejection develops over a longer period of time and is a combination of cellular and humoral immune responses. Increased immunosuppressive therapies may not resolve chronic rejection, and the graft may be lost. Tacrolimus may be helpful as rescue therapy in some cases if the primary immunosuppressive therapeutic agent is CSA.

Rejection in the pediatric recipient of a liver transplant presents with fever, elevated liver function tests, abdominal tenderness, irritability, and fatigue (Table 30-5). If rejection is not treated at this early stage, symptoms progress to include ascites, jaundice, acholic stools, bile-stained urine, pruritus, and renal dysfunction. A percutaneous liver biopsy may be performed to definitively diagnose rejection because elevated enzymes and fever may also be seen with infectious processes, biliary tract complications, or hepatic artery thrombosis. Chronic rejection is defined by the progressive disappearance of bile ducts with subsequent cholestasis and liver failure (i.e., vanishing bile duct syndrome). Although occurring in only 5% to 10% of recipients, graft loss may result (McDiarmid, 1996a). With the introduction of tacrolimus as rescue therapy, however, chronic rejection was reversed in about 50% of cases (McDiarmid et al, 1995b).

Symptoms of rejection in individuals with a renal transplant include fever, irritability, and malaise. These children also present with oliguria, increased BUN and creatinine levels, weight gain due to fluid retention, swelling and tenderness at the graft site, edema of the lower extremities, and anorexia. A definitive diagnosis to enact treatment is confirmed through a percutaneous renal biopsy, renal flow scan, and clinical assessment.

Unlike rejection of the liver or kidney, rejection in pediatric recipients of a heart transplant does not present with symptoms until the rejection is severe. Symptoms of severe rejection result in graft dys-

Table 30-4
Therapeutic Levels of Cyclosporine and Tacrolimus (ng/ml) following Transplantation

Time	Liver		Kidney		Heart	
	CSA*	Tacrolimus	CSA	Tacrolimus	CSA	Tacrolimus
<1 month	500-800	10-15	500-750	20-25	300-700	15-20
1-3 months	300-500	~10	300-500	10-20	300-500	10-15
Long-term	<200	<10	200-350	5-10	150-300	5-10

Data from the Children's Hospital of Pittsburgh.
From Kosmach B, Webber S, and Reyes J: Care of the pediatric solid organ transplant recipient, Pediatr Clin North Am 45(6):1399, 1998.
*CSA, cyclosporine, measured by monoclonal TDx in whole blood.

Table 30-5
Clinical Signs of Organ Rejection

Liver	Kidney	Heart
Fever	Fever	Heart failure with tachycardia and gallop rhythm
Elevated liver enzymes (ALT, AST, GGTP), bilirubin, and alkaline phosphatase	Elevated BUN and creatinine levels	Cardiomegaly
Lethargy, fatigue, malaise, irritability	Lethargy, fatigue, malaise, irritability	Hepatomegaly
Acholic stools and bile-stained urine	Weight gain	Fever (nonspecific)
Jaundice	Edema (particularly of lower extremities)	Poor feeding and irritability (in infants)
Abdominal tenderness	Tenderness at the graft site	Abdominal pain and vomiting (nonspecific)
Ascites	Anorexia	Sudden increase in blood pressure (diastolic >100)

ALT, alanine aminotransferase; AST, aspartate aminotransferase; GGTP, gamma-glutamyl transpeptidase phosphate.

function, which presents with heart failure including tachycardia, gallop rhythm, hepatomegaly, and cardiomegaly (Kosmach et al, 1998). Other symptoms may include shortness of breath, increased respiratory rate, edema and/or sudden weight gain, and sudden increase in diastolic blood pressure. Other nonspecific findings may include fever, irritability, and poor feeding—particularly in infants. Abdominal pain and vomiting secondary to decreased cardiac output and perfusion to the gastrointestinal tract may also be seen. Rejection is diagnosed through clinical assessment and echocardiography and confirmed by cardiac biopsy. Biopsies are performed more often (i.e., from weekly to every few weeks) in the early postoperative period and then with decreasing frequency as the risk and incidence of rejection wanes (see Table 30-5).

Chronic rejection in pediatric recipients of a heart transplant is a progressive condition that occurs over many years and results in graft loss (Kosmach et al, 1998). Chronic rejection, as evidenced by coronary artery narrowing, is detected by routine arteriography, which is performed every 1 to 2 years. Retransplantation is the only known treatment of chronic rejection, and approximately 3% of recipients require retransplantation (Hosenpud et al, 1998). Syncope or sudden death may be the first clinical signs of chronic rejection.

Most episodes of acute rejection can be reversed with early diagnosis and treatment. Treatment varies based on center-specific immunosuppressive protocols and severity of rejection but usually involves an increased level of baseline immunosuppression, increased corticosteroids, and the possible addition of an adjunctive immunosuppressant (e.g., azathioprine and MMF). Tacrolimus may be used as "rescue" therapy in children receiving CSA, or OKT3, which is a monoclonal antibody, may be administered for refractory rejection. Repeat biopsies may be performed to evaluate the effectiveness of treatment.

Infection

To achieve ideal graft functioning, an adequately suppressed immune system that prevents rejection must be balanced with one that is also competent in resisting infection. This delicate equilibrium can be easily disturbed when immunosuppression is increased to treat or avoid rejection, resulting in infection, which is a significant cause of morbidity and mortality following transplantation (Green and Michaels, 1997; Sager and Ettenger, 1993).

The most significant infections usually occur within the first 6 months posttransplant. During the early period (i.e., the first 30 days posttransplant), bacterial and fungal infections are most common. These infections are usually the result of a preexisting chronic illness or infection, surgical complications, iatrogenic factors, or nosocomial infections (Green and Michaels, 1997).

During the intermediate period (i.e., the next 30 to 180 days), the most common infections are those usually transmitted from the donor, reactivated viruses, or opportunistic infections (e.g., *Pneumocystis carinii* and toxoplasmosis) (Green and Michaels, 1997). CMV- and EBV-associated lymphoproliferative disorders are seen during this time (Cacciarelli et al, 1998; Kontoyiannis and Rubin, 1995).

Long-term infections are difficult to document because most transplant recipients are receiving care through primary settings where data on infections may not be accrued. Reportedly, 80% of recipients of transplants have satisfactory graft functioning and are on maintenance immunosuppression at 6 months posttransplant. Infections in this group are most commonly community-acquired (i.e., influenza, respiratory syncytial virus, and pneumococcal pneumonia) (Kontoyiannis and Rubin, 1995). An additional 10% have chronic viral infections such as CMV, EBV, or the hepatitis viruses that may lead to organ failure or malignancy. The remaining 10% are plagued by acute and chronic rejection and are receiving high-dose immunosuppression. These children are at high risk for opportunistic infections and graft failure (Kontoyiannis and Rubin, 1995).

Cytomegalovirus: CMV is a common viral infection following transplantation with a reported incidence of 13% of recipients with renal transplant (Shapiro et al, 1996), 6% to 8% of those with liver transplant (Podesta, Rosenthal, and Makowka, 1993), and 24% of those with cardiac transplant (Baum et al, 1991). The incidence and severity of this virus has decreased due to prophylaxis and treatment with ganciclovir, acyclovir, and hyperimmunoglobulin (CytoGam) (Green et al, 1997; Sager and Ettenger, 1993; Webber, 1997). CMV usually occurs at 1 to 3 months posttransplant. Children at greatest risk for developing a primary disease are those who are seronegative prior to transplant and receive a seropositive organ. Children who have received antilymphocyte globulins or OKT3, or who have had intensified immunosuppression for rejection episodes are also at increased risk for CMV (Martin, 1994). Presenting symptoms include a prolonged and possibly high fever, malaise, anorexia, myalgias, arthralgias, and hematologic abnormalities including leukopenia, thrombocytopenia, and atypical lymphocytosis (Balfour and Heussner, 1993). Diagnosis is based on clinical presentation, viral cultures, serology, and histopathology.

Recipients of liver and heart transplants who are seropositive before the transplant or who receive seropositive organs receive prophylaxis with ganciclovir (i.e., 5 mg/kg every 12 hours for 14 days). Only seronegative renal transplant recipients receiving seropositive organs, however, are treated. Active CMV disease is treated with the same dose of ganciclovir for 14 to 21 days (Green and Michaels, 1997). Additionally, immunosuppression may be reduced if there is no concurrent rejection.

EBV-associated lymphoproliferative disorders: EBV and associated posttransplant lymphoproliferative disorders (PTLD) may range from a self-limiting mononucleosis to PTLD with polyclonal or monoclonal disease and ultimately lymphoma (Kosmach et al, 1998). Factors influencing the incidence of EBV include the organ transplanted, the time posttransplant, and the immunosuppressive protocols. The incidence of EBV in pediatric recipients is 9% in renal transplantation (Shapiro et al, 1998), 13% in liver transplantation (Cacciarelli et al, 1998), and 8.6% in cardiac transplantation (Webber 1997). Risk factors for EBV include young age, EBV seronegative status pretransplant and receiving an EBV-seropositive organ, and intensified immunosuppression including administration of OKT3 (Katz, 1997; McDiarmid, 1996b). Presenting symptoms may include lymphadenopathy, fever, tonsillitis, upper airway obstruction, rash, or GI disturbances (Cacciarelli et al, 1998). Tumorlike infiltrates, as well as ulcerations of the GI tract with abdominal pain and bleeding, are seen in invasive disease.

Early diagnosis is vital to recovery and is based on clinical presentation, histopathology, laboratory studies, and radiographic findings. A biopsy is often performed on an accessible node, and a computed tomographic (CT) scan is obtained to assess the chest and abdomen for enlarged nodes or disseminated disease. A promising strategy to measure the EBV viral load through serial polymerase chain reactions (EBV-PCR) is being used in some centers to guide management of EBV through initiation of preemptive therapies (Green, Reyes, and Rowe, 1998).

Treatment of EBV and PTLD varies by the institution and the organ transplanted, but the primary strategy is currently to reduce or discontinue immunosuppression. Other treatment protocols include the use of antiviral agents, interferon, radiation, chemotherapy, and tumor resection (Cacciarelli et al, 1998; Green and Michaels, 1997). In a recent study of pediatric liver transplant recipients receiving tacrolimus (n = 282), there was a 13% incidence of PTLD with an overall mortality rate of 22%. Of the survivors, 74% had acute rejection at a median time of 24 days following treatment and two children developed chronic rejection. One child required retransplantation. After resolution of PTLD, 45% of individuals received monotherapy with tacrolimus, and 26% received combination therapy with tacrolimus and prednisone. It is interesting to note that 19% of these children did not require resumption of immunosuppression and developed long-term tolerance after the PTLD resolved (Cacciarelli et al, 1998).

***Pneumocystis carinii* pneumonia:** Recipients of transplants are at risk for *Pneumocystis carinii* pneumonia, which is a rare but serious posttransplant complication. Trimethoprim-sulfamethoxazole (TMP-SMX) is used as prophylactic treatment and is responsible for the low incidence of this infection. Because most transplant recipients are on lifelong immunosuppression, many transplant centers strongly recommend TMP-SMX prophylaxis indefinitely (Olsen et al, 1993). The recommended prophylactic dose of TMP-SMX is 5 mg/kg, three times per week with a maximum daily dose of 80 mg TMP-SMX (McGhee et al, 1998). If a transplant recipient presents with fever and a lower respiratory tract infection and is not receiving prophylaxis, *P. carinii* should always be considered in the differential diagnosis.

Varicella-zoster virus: Varicella zoster can potentially be a severe illness in immunocompromised children. Because many pediatric transplant recipients receive an organ before being naturally exposed to the virus, it is commonly seen posttransplant. Recommended therapy consists of administration of varicella-zoster immune globulin (VZIG) within 72 hours of exposure to help prevent or decrease the severity of the illness. Some transplant centers may hospitalize a child for a few days and administer intravenous acyclovir. Immunosuppression may be decreased for a short period of time with attention to any symptoms of rejection. Varicella-zoster vaccine (Varivax) is not recommended for immunocompromised children because it is a live-attenuated vaccine. Transplant candidates should be vaccinated, however, if they are over 1 year of age and the transplant is not emergent.

Prognosis

Survival Statistics

Nearly 14,000 children have received either a heart, kidney, or liver transplant since 1988 with 1-year survival rates of 76%, 97%, and 81% and 1-year graft survival rates of 75%, 85%, and 68% respectively (UNOS Scientific Registry Data, 1998). According to the UNOS Scientific Registry, approximately 6,000 renal transplants were performed from 1987 to 1996 in recipients up to 21 years of age (Cecka et al, 1997). With survival adjusted for donor source, age, gender, race, disease, year of transplant, HLA mismatch, and transplant center, the 5-year graft survival rates were 60% for children up to age 2 years, 64% for those aged 3 to

12 years, and 57% for those aged 13 to 21 years. An increased graft failure rate is seen long-term in teenagers due to noncompliance and late acute rejection (Cecka et al, 1997).

PRIMARY CARE MAINTENANCE
Growth and Development

The goals of pediatric organ transplantation are for the child to achieve normal growth and development and an improved quality of life. Growth affects the emotional well-being of children and their participation in the routine activities of childhood. Growth retardation has been reported in children both before and after transplantation (Bereket and Fine, 1995; Codonor-Franch, Bernard, and Alvarez, 1994). There have been improvements related to innovative immunosuppressive protocols, weaning or discontinuation of steroids, and optimal nutritional support, however, that have contributed to growth or growth acceleration (Chinnock and Baum, 1998; Kelly, 1997).

Linear growth after liver transplantation has been satisfactory in most cases. About 14% of pediatric recipients exhibit growth failure, however, most likely due to additional requirements for immunosuppressant agents to treat rejection (Podesta, Rosenthal, and Makowka, 1993).

Corticosteroids are also used for immunosuppressant effects and are part of the immunosuppressive regimen at most transplant centers. The mechanism of action is not completely understood, but corticosteroids affect T-lymphocytes and reduce the production of lymphokines (Crandall, 1990). The antiinflammatory effects of steroids may also play a large role in protecting the transplanted organ. Depending on the dose and length of treatment, steroids produce a variety of mild to severe side effects. Stomach irritation, mood swings, acne, swelling and weight gain, hypertension, and insomnia are most commonly seen. Side effects of higher, long-term doses may include cataracts, glaucoma, delayed growth, osteoporosis, and muscular weakness.

Growth after renal transplantation is affected by age at transplant, severity of pretransplant growth suppression, bone age, graft function, and immunosuppressive medications (Fine 1997b). Catch-up growth during the CSA era has been seen mainly in children under 6 years of age at time of transplant. Consequently, normal growth is unlikely to occur in 75% of renal transplant recipients. Improvements in growth velocity have been seen with the use of growth hormone both before and after transplant (Fine, 1997a, b). Another successful strategy that promotes growth in recipients of renal transplants is the ability to wean and eventually withdraw steroids in individuals who receive tacrolimus as the primary immunosuppressant (Shapiro et al, 1998). The majority of pediatric heart transplant recipients demonstrate normal linear growth, neurologic outcome, and development (Baum et al, 1993; Chinnock, 1996; Chinnock and Baum, 1998; Eke et al, 1996).

In following a transplant recipient long-term, the primary care provider has an essential role in monitoring growth and development. Height and weight should be routinely documented along growth curves on standardized growth chartsto evaluate growth and plan for interventions (e.g., increased nutritional support or growth hormone therapy).

Cognitive and emotional functioning: The cognitive and emotional functioning of children after transplantation has been evaluated in several studies with variable findings. This population has been difficult to assess due to the unavailability of baseline data before transplant, the subject variables, the measurement issues, and the impact of medical interventions (Kosmach et al, 1998). In addition, studies with sufficient numbers of subjects that analyze the long-term effects of transplantation on cognitive and emotional functioning are severely lacking. There is a great need for well-designed research studies to examine pediatric transplant recipients in terms of cognitive and emotional functioning.

Of renal transplant recipients who are young, 75% had cognitive functioning at or above the average range (Davis, Chang, and Nevins, 1990; Stewart et al, 1989). Early studies report that most liver transplant recipients are in the appropriate grade for their age or are delayed 1 year, and that most do not have any significant changes in cognitive functioning unless there were cognitive deficits prior to transplantation (Stewart et al, 1989; Zitelli et al, 1988).

After heart or heart-lung transplantation, most children return to school, participate in sports and age-appropriate activities, and are in New York

Heart Association Functional Class I (i.e., no activity limitations) (Conte et al, 1996; Sigfusson et al, 1997). In 85% of cases, individuals who received transplants as infants were in the appropriate grade level at 6 years of age (Chinnock, 1996). Earlier studies, however, reported cognitive and emotional delays that have been associated with frequent hospitalizations, school absences, peer reactions, and the fear of organ rejection and death (Stewart et al, 1994, Wray et al, 1994).

Nutrition

Intensive attention to nutrition for children both before and after transplant surgery is vital to the attainment of normal growth and development through adequate caloric intake. Postoperatively, a child's diet is usually liberalized with few restrictions. Some children, however, may require enteral supplements due to an inability to ingest adequate calories as a result of anatomical space limitations, taste changes, side effects of oral medications, and difficulty in accepting new textures after formula feeds (Kelly, 1997; Wren and Tarbell, 1998). Specifically, children with heart transplants are maintained on a no-added-salt diet. Posttransplant medications may occasionally cause side effects (e.g., hyperkalemia, hypertension, hypomagnesemia, or hyperglycemia) that may warrant a respective dietary restriction or supplement (e.g., a low sodium diet for hypertension) (Guest and Hasse, 1996).

Recipients of transplants whose immunosuppressive management consists of CSA with high-dose steroids may exhibit weight gain and Cushingoid facies. Children who are receiving monotherapy with tacrolimus and are weaned from steroids do not present with these side effects.

Safety

As with all routine pediatric visits, counseling about safety issues (e.g., the proper use of car seats and seat belts, bicycle helmets, and "child proofing" of the home) at a child's age and developmental level is also appropriate in the pediatric transplant population. Because most children have good graft function and are prescribed maintenance doses of immunosuppression within 6 to 12 months after transplant, good handwashing techniques and avoidance of others with obvious infections are sound guidelines to decrease the risk of infection.

Some centers prefer that families notify the transplant center when they plan to travel for an extended period of time or to a foreign country. This notification is particularly important for transplant candidates on the waiting list so that a means of communication is available in case an organ becomes available. Medication doses and schedules should always be maintained while a child is on vacation, and an adequate supply of medication should be taken with them. Medications should be carried on to airplanes rather than being checked with luggage. Parents are encouraged to obtain Medic-Alert bracelets for their child to identify the child as a transplant recipient and provide the name and telephone number of the transplant center in case of an emergency.

In children with a heart or heart-lung transplant, it is important to understand that the incisions in the heart sever the sympathetic and parasympathetic nerves, which ordinarily regulate the heart rate. This lack of neural connections is known as denervation. Without direct control of the CNS, the transplanted heart will beat faster in a resting state (e.g., 90 to 110 bpm). This faster than normal rate is associated with normal cardiac function and the capability of sustaining vigorous physical activity. The transplanted heart depends on circulating adrenalin and related hormones produced by the adrenal gland—instead of a direct impulse from the brain—to change its rate. The transplanted heart may take up to 10 minutes before an increase in heart rate is seen in response to exercise and up to an hour may pass after stopping exercise before a decrease in rate is seen. Another effect of denervation is that chest pain or angina pectoris cannot be perceived if coronary artery disease develops. Thus coronary arteriograms are part of the pediatric transplant annual studies.

Pediatric heart and heart-lung recipients are activity-restricted for the first 6 to 8 weeks after surgery to allow the sternum to heal. Recipients should avoid lifting, pushing, or pulling heavy objects; bike riding; climbing; sit-ups; push-ups; roller skating; and contact sports during this time period. After 8 weeks, all activities, as well as physical education class at school, may be resumed. A physical therapist should instruct children on an exercise program before they leave the hospital. This program consists of a 5-minute warm-up and cool-down period before and after peak physical activity. If a child shows signs of increased shortness of breath or fatigue, then the cool-down period should begin. It is important for physical education teachers to be informed of this information. Exercise should also be decreased during periods of graft rejection.

Children who have received liver or kidney transplants are encouraged to resume previous activities, but there may be limitations. Recipients should avoid heavy lifting for at least 6 months. Push-ups or sit-ups, as well as activities that stretch or put pressure on the abdomen and incision, are to be avoided for 3 to 6 months. Although some centers discourage contact sports, most children can participate in age-appropriate activities as they develop greater endurance and fitness.

Immunizations

Primary care practitioners should follow the guidelines established by the Committee on Infectious Diseases of the American Academy of Pediatrics in immunizing pediatric transplant recipients (Committee on Infectious Diseases, 1997). Live-bacterial and live-virus vaccines are contraindicated in this population and only inactivated vaccines (e.g., the inactivated polio vaccine) should be administered. Siblings of the transplant recipient should also receive the inactivated polio virus to avoid transmitting the disease to the recipient. Unfortunately, no inactivated form of vaccination exists for measles, mumps, and rubella (MMR). Siblings of transplant recipients should receive the MMR. If a child is stable before the transplant and transplantation is not emergent, every effort should be made to maintain the routine pediatric immunization schedule.

Because children are more highly immunosuppressed for the first 3 months after transplantation, no immunizations should be given during this period. If a child is receiving maintenance immunosuppression after this early period, the immunization schedule for immunosuppressed children may be resumed.

In addition, the influenza vaccine should be administered yearly to all transplant recipients if they are at least 3 months posttransplant. All family members living within the household should also receive the vaccine. Although the varicella vaccine (Varivax) is currently available, it is contraindicated in this population because it is a live virus.

The varicella vaccine, however, is recommended for siblings.

Hepatitis B is an infrequent but significant cause of decreased graft survival, morbidity, and mortality. Transplant candidates—particularly renal candidates on dialysis—should be vaccinated against hepatitis B because it can be acquired through contact with blood products. Transplant recipients may receive the hepatitis B vaccine at 3 months after the transplant. This vaccine is also recommended for siblings, caretakers, and household contacts.

Immunization policies vary by transplant center, so the primary care provider should contact the transplant center to determine the desired immunizations for the child, as well as family members or household contacts, after transplantation.

Screening

Vision: Ophthalmologic evaluations are important screening tests for children and should be completed for the pediatric transplant recipient on the same schedule used for well child visits. Cataracts, glaucoma, and pseudotumor cerebri may be side effects of long-term high-dose steroid use, so ophthalmologic examinations should be conducted yearly for children on such therapy. With current immunosuppressive protocols consisting of lower steroid doses with eventual weaning, however, these complications are infrequent.

Hearing: Children who have received ototoxic drugs routinely before or after the transplant may be at risk for hearing deficits and should be referred to an audiologist. Children should have audiograms as recommended to determine the extent of hearing loss and plan for interventions as needed.

Dental: Biannual dental visits and routine oral hygiene are recommended for children after transplantation, as in the general pediatric population. Children receiving CSA as a primary immunosuppressant may develop gingival hyperplasia. In some cases, gingivectomy may be necessary to reduce gum overgrowth and related swelling, pain, or infection. Antibiotic prophylaxis per standard endocarditis protocols is recommended for invasive dental procedures but is not needed for routine cleaning (Kosmach et al, 1998) (see Chapter 17).

Blood pressure: Blood pressure measurement should be a part of all discharge teaching plans because hypertension may be a side effect of immunosuppressive medications. If antihypertensive medications are prescribed, parents should take the child's blood pressure before administering the medication and follow administration guidelines based on blood pressure parameters. A record of blood pressure readings and administered antihypertensive medications should be evaluated by the primary care provider and specialist at each visit. Children can often be weaned from antihypertensives over time as immunosuppressive levels are decreased.

Hematocrit: The hematocrit is obtained with routine laboratory tests as recommended by the transplant center during the early postoperative period and through the primary care provider when the child is discharged from the transplant area. Laboratory tests are obtained more frequently in the first 3 months after the transplant and then with decreasing frequency over time unless there are complications.

It is important for practitioners to assess for anemia because it has been reported under immunosuppression with tacrolimus and cyclosporin. In a study of 49 pediatric heart transplant recipients receiving tacrolimus, severe anemia developed in 16% and moderate anemia in 43% (Asante-Korang et al, 1996). Hemolytic uremic syndrome has also been reported in children receiving cyclosporine (Morris-Stiff et al, 1998).

Urinalysis: In liver and heart transplant recipients, these tests are obtained only when the child is symptomatic or as part of an evaluation for fever, when multiple cultures are drawn. Renal transplant recipients routinely have urinalysis and urine cultures performed as a part of posttransplant management. Because fever can be a symptom of a urinary tract infection, as well as rejection, careful evaluation and analysis of any febrile episode is required.

Tuberculosis: Some transplant centers may recommend a Mantoux-purified protein derivative (PPD) with an anergy panel in addition to chest radiography to evaluate a child for exposure to tuberculosis (TB) prior to transplantation. Risk factors for developing TB after the transplant include a prior exposure to the disease, living in an area endemic for TB, and having a high level of immunosuppression and/or a concurrent HIV infection (Green and Michaels, 1997). Treatment is with isoniazid, which is administered for 6 to 12 months posttransplant, although it is recommended as

maintenance therapy by some experts (Green and Michaels, 1997).

Condition-Specific Screening

Blood work: Laboratory blood testing is usually obtained with every clinic visit (i.e., weekly or biweekly) after the transplant while the child is residing in the area of the transplant center. Laboratory tests vary depending on the organ transplanted, the length of time after the transplant, the current complications, and the center-specific protocols. Trough levels of CSA or tacrolimus are obtained with routine blood work and are obtained more often during times of rejection or infection. In addition to CSA and tacrolimus trough levels, the most commonly obtained laboratory tests include a complete blood cell count with differential, platelets, a full chemistry profile, glucose, BUN, creatinine, uric acid, aspartate aminotransferase (AST), alanine aminotransferase (ALT), gamma-glutamyl transpeptidase phosphate (GGTP), lactic dehydrogenase (LDH), creatine phosphokinase (CPK), CO_2, magnesium, and phosphorus.

For most children, laboratory testing is required less frequently over time if there are no complications. Most transplant recipients have blood testing done every month, but some require laboratory tests to be obtained every 2 months.

After the transplant, as the child's medical status stabilizes and discharge to the home community occurs, the primary care provider is responsible for obtaining laboratory specimens via the transplant center guidelines. Results are usually faxed to the transplant center as soon as they are available. Unless the family resides in an area close to another major transplant center, however, blood samples obtained for CSA and tacrolimus trough levels are mailed to the transplant center for processing. All changes in immunosuppression are made by the transplant center.

Graft evaluation: Most transplant centers prefer that pediatric transplant recipients return to the transplant center for an annual evaluation of the graft. Blood work and organ-specific testing (e.g., an abdominal ultrasound to assess the liver vasculature, an echocardiogram, renal flow scan, or biopsy of the transplanted organ) are completed as indicated. Although a yearly graft evaluation can usually be accomplished on an outpatient basis over 1 to 2 days, a child may need to be briefly admitted for observation after an invasive procedure (e.g., cardiac catheterization, biopsy).

Common Illness Management

Differential Diagnosis (Box 30-2)

Fever: Children are more highly immunosuppressed for the first 3 months after transplantation and consequently are at greater risk for infections. As discussed previously, bacterial infections are most commonly seen in the early period related to the preexisting chronic condition, surgical complications, or nosocomial infections. Viruses and opportunistic infections are more common in the intermediate and late periods after the transplant. Fevers—especially in the first 3 months following transplantation—must be thoroughly assessed with the differential diagnoses usually being rejection vs. infection (e.g., UTI) (see Table 30-6). The primary care provider must work in conjunction with the transplant specialist to evaluate and manage febrile episodes.

Abdominal symptoms: Abdominal pain in liver transplant recipients during the early postoperative period may indicate rejection or a surgical complication. Although uncommon, late acute rejection can occur. Late hepatic artery thrombosis within the context of biliary strictures must also be ruled out. Obstruction of the common bile duct can also occur. As with the general pediatric population, the differential diagnoses that depend upon clinical presentation, laboratory tests, and radiologic testing may include intestinal obstruction, peptic ulcer disease, appendicitis, or viral or bacterial gastroenteritis. In renal transplant recipients, abdominal pain, as well as tenderness in the kidney area, may be a symptom of UTI or acute pyelonephritis in addition to rejection.

Abdominal pain and vomiting in heart transplant recipients warrants an echocardiogram to evaluate for the possibility of rejection secondary to decreased cardiac output and decreased perfusion to the gastrointestinal tract vs. a viral illness.

Vomiting and diarrhea: Prolonged vomiting or diarrhea caused by a community-acquired virus may result in poor absorption of tacrolimus or CSA, leading to nontherapeutic blood levels and subsequently placing a child at risk for rejection. Parents should contact the transplant center for immunosuppressive management and the primary care provider to facilitate the recommendations for immunosuppression and supervise medical management of fluid balance. A protracted course of vomiting or diarrhea may result in a brief hospitalization for intravenous administration of fluids and CSA or tacrolimus until the virus resolves and the child can tolerate an oral diet and retain medications.

Metabolic abnormalities: When stable graft functioning is achieved with maintenance immunosuppression, pediatric transplant recipients usually do not experience metabolic abnormalities. During the early postoperative period as levels of CSA and tacrolimus are being adjusted, children may experience hyperkalemia, hypomagnesemia, or metabolic acidosis.

Drug Interactions

CSA and tacrolimus are metabolized in the liver by the cytochrome P450 III system (Green, Carcillo, and Reyes, 1998). Metabolism of CSA or tacrolimus depends on liver function and other agents that induce or inhibit this enzyme system, subsequently affecting blood levels. Because primary care providers often prescribe medications for a variety of acute and chronic childhood illness, it is important that the family or health care provider contact the transplant center to discuss possible drug interactions. Drugs that interact with CSA or tacrolimus disrupt an otherwise stable level and can predispose a child to drug-related neurotoxicities and nephrotoxicities, as well as to in-

---

Box 30-2

Differential Diagnosis

Fever—Common childhood conditions vs. rejection

Abdominal symptoms—Common childhood conditions vs. obstruction in common bile duct, ulcers, small bowel obstruction, peritonitis, or rejection; vomiting and diarrhea may result in poor absorption of medications

Metabolic abnormalities—Hyperkalemia, hyperglycemia, and low CO_2 levels may be related to immunosuppressant medications

Table 30-6
Drug interactions with Cyclosporine and Tacrolimus

Drug	Cyclosporine Increase	Cyclosporine Decrease	Tacrolimus Increase	Tacrolimus Decrease
Calcium Channel Blockers				
diltiazem	X	X		
nicardipine	X	X		
nifedipine		X		
verapamil	X	X		
Antifungals				
clotrimazole		X		
fluconazole	X	X		
itraconazole	X	X		
ketoconazole	X	X		
Antibiotics				
clarithromycin	X		X	
erythromycin	X		X	
troleandomycin			X	
rifabutin				X
rifampin		X		X
nafcillin		X		
GI Prokinetic Agents				
cisapride			X	
metoclopramide	X		X	
Anticonvulsants				
carbamazepine		X		X
phenobarbitol		X		X
phenytoin		X		X
Others				
octrocotide		X		
ticlopidine		X		
allopurinol	X			
bromocriptine	X		X	
cimetidine			X	
cyclosporine			X	
danazol	X		X	
protease inhibitors			X	

From Cyclosporine Drug Monograph, Sandoz Pharmaceuticals Corp., 1997.
Fujisawa Drug Monograph, Fujisawa, USA, Inc., 1997.

creased risk of infection and rejection (Table 30-6). Acetaminophen should be used for fever or mild management of pain instead of aspirin or ibuprofen.

Developmental Issues

Sleep Patterns

Sleep disturbances in children with end-stage organ disease are common and may be caused by the existing chronic condition, as well as by symptoms of organ deterioration (e.g., severe pruritus from liver disease). Insomnia or sleep disturbances are also seen in children before and after the transplant due to the effects of extended hospitalization. Sleep patterns may also be affected by medications; both tacrolimus and CSA are reported to cause insomnia. During periods of rejection when the child is treated with increased tacrolimus or CSA levels in addition to high-dose oral steroids or intravenous methylprednisolone, sleep patterns may be significantly altered and insomnia and irritability are common.

Parents may find it helpful to maintain familiar home routines and rituals to the fullest extent possible while the child is hospitalized. It may also be helpful to reestablish these patterns once the child is discharged to home. In some cases, professional counseling may help the child and family.

Toileting

Regression in toileting may be expected in toddlers and preschool-age children during and after hospitalization. Care providers must be understanding of this temporary regression and support children in regaining their toileting skills. Pediatric renal transplant recipients may have specific concerns and issues related to toileting and the establishment or reestablishment of urinary flow and continence. Although the initiation of urine flow for a child following renal transplantation is often a time of great excitement for the child and family, the child may require some time to learn to identify the body cues that signal the need to urinate and to control the urine flow.

Some heart transplant recipients may require diuretic medications, which may contribute to increased incontinence and difficulty with training.

Careful timing of these medications is important to promote less insomnia and incontinence at night due to increased urination. Children will benefit from emotional support and understanding throughout this process because episodes of incontinence and enuresis are common.

Discipline

A child's chronic illness affects the entire family, its system of functioning, and the roles within it. As a child with end-stage organ disease improves significantly after transplantation, former coping mechanisms used by the family, as well as parental roles and family dynamics, may no longer be successful. It is often difficult for families to make the transition from parenting a sick child to parenting a healthy one. Many parents continue to overprotect their child but with new concerns of infection and rejection. Parents may have difficulty encouraging children to develop independence, peer relationships, and integrate themselves into the community and community activities. In contrast, other parents may have trouble setting limits on inappropriate behavior and may overindulge the child.

The primary care provider plays an essential role in evaluating family dynamics and the parents' ability to appropriately discipline and nurture a child after the transplant. The caregiver can help parents achieve a balance between establishing age-appropriate and consistent limits and allowing the child some control over decision making. Encouraging independence helps promote confidence and positive self-esteem. Family counseling can be a highly effective method to help families cope with the ongoing stressors of the transplant process.

Child Care

Attendance at daycare centers for the first 3 months following transplantation is generally not recommended by most transplant centers because these children are usually more highly immunosuppressed during that time and therefore at a higher risk for infection. As immunosuppressive levels are decreased, children are at less risk for infection, and routine social contact or participation in small group or home daycare programs may be resumed. Community-acquired viruses are usually tolerated well by children who are receiving lower-dose maintenance immunosuppression. Parents should be informed by the primary care provider or daycare staff of any outbreaks of varicella or measles in the community or daycare center, however, because these viruses could be potentially serious for the transplant recipient.

School

Children are encouraged to return to school as soon as possible after transplantation to resume a normal routine, continue classes, and interact with peers. Although most children can return to the classroom within 2 to 3 months after transplantation, some children may adapt better by attending school for a few hours daily and then increasing this to a full schedule as tolerated over time. Short-term tutoring in the home may be appropriate in some cases when children have missed extensive content.

Parents are often hesitant to return their child to school because they are concerned about exposure to infections, increased demands on the child, and peer influences and teasing, as well as feel that their child is "fragile" after transplantation (Kosmach et al, 1998). In addition, a high immunosuppressant level may also cause mild to moderate hand tremors that may be distracting when the child attempts to perform fine motor activities, such as writing or working on craft activities. It is not surprising that some adolescent organ recipients infrequently engage in dating and display a cautious attitude toward sexuality. Primary care providers should encourage the resumption of routine childhood activities and school and emphasize the benefits of developmentally appropriate play, social interaction, and instruction.

The child's medication schedule should be organized to accommodate the school day with minimal interruptions. Medications prescribed on a once- or twice-daily schedule are easily adaptable to the daily routine. Frequent visits to the health office for medications or having a parent visit daily to administer medications is disruptive to the child's school routine and may emphasize the different needs of the transplant recipient. Children may be particularly sensitive to these intrusions during adolescence.

The transplant center team works with school nurses to educate them on aspects of care after transplantation. School nurses can also be helpful in reintegrating a child into the classroom with age-appropriate discussions of transplantation to increase classmates' understanding and support.

Sexuality

Following transplantation, older school-age children and adolescents are very aware of dramatic physical changes. Most physical alterations, such as increased energy and strength, resolution of jaundice or cyanosis resulting in a natural skin color, resolution of ascites or peripheral edema, increased growth and maturation, or removal of appliances (i.e., Broviac lines, gastrostomy tubes, oxygen cannulas, or dialysis catheters) are very positive. There are, however, alterations to body image due to multiple incisions with scarring. Professional counseling and support groups are encouraged for this population. Physical appearance may also be altered by medications. The physical stigmata of immunosuppressive therapy with CSA and steroids include hirsutism, Cushingoid facies, gingival hyperplasia, obesity, and short stature. Steroids may also intensify outbreaks of acne in adolescents, as well as cause mood changes. Obvious changes in physical appearance are rare with tacrolimus therapy, although a small percentage of children experience alopecia, which usually resolves over time.

Sexual activity can usually resume at 6 to 8 weeks after transplantation. Birth control methods should be discussed as a part of discharge teaching and follow-up care. A referral to a gynecology practitioner for routine gynecologic examination and birth control counseling is necessary.

With an increased survival and a significantly improved physical status, pregnancy is now a more frequent occurrence for female transplant recipients. Female transplant recipients who are interested in becoming pregnant are usually recommended to wait until graft function is stable and immunosuppression is at a maintenance level. Close monitoring of the graft and immunosuppressive levels and routine prenatal care are also required during pregnancy because alterations of CSA or tacrolimus levels may occur due to the physiologic changes of pregnancy (Armenti et al, 1996).

In a review of 25 pregnancies in 22 female renal recipients on CSA immunosuppression, pregnancy-induced hypertension was observed in

24% of women and preeclamptic toxemia in 20% of cases. Infections (i.e., most commonly monilial vulvovaginitis and asymptomatic UTIs) were reported in 44% of women. The incidence of rejection during pregnancy was 9%, which did not differ from the rate of acute rejection in nonpregnant transplant recipients. Infant outcomes included 3 stillbirths (i.e., 12%) due to placental insufficiency. All live births had satisfactory Apgar scores, nearly 90% at the appropriate weight for gestational age, and none had gross abnormalities.

Childbearing was discouraged in the past for women with heart transplants because of concerns about maternal graft function and survival. Although heart transplant recipients often have successful pregnancies, there is a high incidence of prematurity (i.e., <37 weeks) and a low birth weight (Branch et al, 1998). No structural malformations, however, were found in these infants. In another study of pregnancies after heart transplantation, it was reported that a transplanted denervated heart may tolerate the normal rise of 40% in maternal blood volume. The primary complication of these pregnancies was hypertension related to the use of CSA and high-dose steroids (Delforge et al, 1997). No congenital or chromosomal abnormalities were reported, and the most common complications in infants were prematurity and low birth weight (Delforge, 1997).

Pregnancy following liver transplantation now occurs more often. In an analysis of 48 pregnancies in 34 women with liver transplants, the incidence of low birth weight (i.e., <2500 grams) infants was 31% and the incidence of prematurity (i.e., <37 weeks) was 39% (Radomski et al, 1995). The most common complications were hypertension (46%), preeclampsia (21%), infection (26%), and Caesarian section (47%). No birth defects were reported. The liver graft appears to tolerate pregnancy well with only six episodes of rejection reported in this series—all of which responded to treatment (Radomski et al, 1997). In another series involving 27 pregnancies by 21 women on tacrolimus therapy, there was a similar occurrence of preterm births and low birth weight, but the incidences of hypertension and preeclampsia were lower than previously reported. Two significantly premature infants (i.e., at 23 and 24 weeks gestation) died shortly after birth, but the remaining 25 children have had satisfactory growth and development (Jain et al, 1997).

Successful pregnancies in recipients of solid organ transplants are possible—but are not without certain risks and complications. The pregnancy should be carefully monitored with close assessment of graft function and fetal development. Hypertension and preeclampsia are the most common complications of the mother, and the incidence of rejection is similar to that in the nonpregnant population. The most common complications for the infant are low birth weight and prematurity.

Transition to Adulthood

Adolescents with a transplant struggle with the same issues of separation and developing independence and identity but within the context of adapting to the chronicity of transplantation. As a result of immunosuppression, the transplant recipient is at an increased risk for developing sexually transmitted diseases if safe sex practices are not followed. Drugs, alcohol, and cigarette smoking affect the transplanted organs and may possibly interfere with the metabolism of immunosuppressive medications. Tattoos and body piercings, which are popular with this age group, also place transplant recipients at risk for infection. Noncompliance with medication and care routines can result in rejection and ultimately graft loss and death.

Supporting adolescents in this transition may be difficult for parents as they try to give them a greater responsibility in routine care. During this difficult period, effective parenting and supportive peers can contribute to an adolescent's achievement of developmental tasks. Individual and family counseling is recommended and encouraged. Continued follow-up with the transplant center also helps to provide parents with advice about ongoing transplant issues that are additionally affecting an adolescent.

As adolescents complete high school and enter college or the work force, employability and insurability are concerns. Having a preexisting condition, as well as an employer's concerns of possible physical limitations are common issues. Financial aspects of care related to medication coverage, routine lab tests and check-ups, and repeat hospitalizations may arise because young adults have difficulty obtaining health care insurance when childhood health care coverage is discontinued. Counseling through the financial department at the transplant center or with the transplant social worker may be helpful. Support groups and some pharmaceutical companies (often with information available on the Internet) may also be of assistance.

Noncompliance: Noncompliance is a major cause of late rejection in adolescents with heart transplants with a mortality rate of 30% (Douglas et al, 1993). There is a 50% incidence of noncompliance in recipients with renal transplants, with a 71% incidence of rejection and a graft loss of 13% (Ettenger et al, 1991). Similarly, repeated episodes of noncompliance with a 14% graft loss have been seen in adolescents with liver transplants (Molmenti et al, 1999).

During episodes of rejection—particularly if occurring long-term after transplantation, noncompliance should always be considered in the differential diagnosis. Factors or symptoms suggestive of noncompliance may include unexpectedly low trough levels or erratic levels indicating missed doses or drug loading, inconsistencies between the dose and trough level, poor follow-up with the transplant center or community physician, behavior changes, lack of support, dysfunctional family or parental functioning, or decreased socialization (Kosmach et al, 1998).

Special Family Concerns and Resources

In accepting transplantation, the family and child have exchanged end-stage organ disease for the chronic condition of transplantation. Although most families and recipients believe this is an acceptable "trade-off," anxiety and apprehensions about the future may be ongoing. Long-term survival, the fear of rejection, late infections, possible retransplantation, and the child's future employment and quality of life are paramount concerns.

The financial impact of transplantation is another major issue for families. The transplant surgery and initial hospitalization, possible repeat admissions, an array of medications, living expenses while at the transplant center, and ongoing expenses at home amass an enormous financial burden for many families. Financial support can come from third-party health insurance payers, community fund raising, state funding, or the family's own resources.

Families are in need of information and emotional support from the transplant team and primary care providers to help them cope with fears and apprehensions about their child's future and the financial aspects of transplantation. Successful adaptation to the transplant process contributes to an optimum outcome for the child. Supportive services and ongoing information must be provided to the child and family as they encounter the challenges of transplantation.

Organizations

American Association of Kidney Patients (AAKP)
100 South Ashley Drive, Suite 280
Tampa, Fla. 33260
(800) 749-2257; (813) 223-0001 (fax)
http://www.aakp.org

American Heart Association (AHA)
National Center
7272 Greenville Avenue
Dallas, Tex. 75231-4596
(800) 242-8721
http://www.Americanheart.org

American Organ Transplant Association (AOTA)
PO Box 277
Missouri City, Tex. 77459
(281) 261-2682
http://www.aota.phoenix.net

American Kidney Fund
6110 Executive Blvd, No 1010
Rockville, Md. 20852
(800) 638-8299; (301) 881-0898 (fax)
http://www.arabon.com/kidney

American Liver Foundation
1425 Pompton Ave
Cedar Grove, NJ 07009
(800) 223-0179
http://hepar-sfgh.ucsf.edu

American Lung Association
1740 Broadway
New York, NY 10019
(800) 586-4872 or (800) LUNG-USA
http://www.lungusa.org

Children's Liver Alliance
3835 Richmond Ave, Box 190
Staten Island, NY 10312-3828
(718) 987-6200
http://www.asf.org/balt.html;
Livers4Kids@ earthlink.net

Children's Organ Transplant Association (COTA)
2501 COTA Drive
Bloomington, Ind. 47403
(800) 366-2682; (812)-336-8885 (fax)
http://www.cota.org

Coram Prescription Pharmacy
(800) 950-2840
(Transplant mail order prescription services and information)

Hepatitis Foundation International
(201) 239-1035; (800) 891-0707
http://www.hepfi.org

International Transplant Nurses Society
1739 E. Carson Street, Box 351
Pittsburgh, Pa. 15203
(412) 448-0240; (412) 431-5911 (fax)
ITNS@msn.com; http://www.transweb.org/itns

National Disease Research Interchange
1880 JFK Boulevard, 6th floor
Philadelphia, Pa. 19103
(215) 557-7361

National Heart Assist and Transplant Fund
PO Box 258
Bryn Mawr, Pa. 19010
(800) 642-8399 or (800) NHATF99
http://www.libertynet.org/~txfund

National Kidney Foundation, Inc.
30 East 33rd Street
New York, NY 10016
(800) 622-9010
http://www.kidney.org

National Transplant Assistance Fund (NTAF)
(800) 642-8399; (610) 527-5210 (fax)
http://www.LibertyNet.org/~txFund;
  txFund@LibertyNet.org

Organ Transplant Fund (OTF)
National Office
1102 Brookfield Road, Suite 202
Memphis, Tenn. 38119
(800) 489-3863
http://www.OTF.org

Renal Physicians' Association
1101 Vermont Ave, NW, No 500
Washington, DC 20005-3547
(202) 835-0436

Transplant Learning Center (TLC)
1-888-TLCENTER (852-3683)
(A lifestyle management program)

Transplant Recipients' International Organization (TRIO)
PO Box 71122
Pittsburgh, Pa. 15213
(412) 734-5698, or
1735 I Street NW, Suite 917
Washington, DC 20006
(202) 293-0980 or (800) 874-6386
http://www.primenet.com~trio

United Liver Association
11646 West Pico Boulevard
Los Angeles, Calif. 90064
(310) 445-4204

United Network for Organ Sharing (UNOS)
The National Organ Procurement and Transplantation Network
1100 Boulders Parkway, Suite 500
PO Box 13770
Richmond, Va. 23225-8770
(800) 24-DONOR or (888) 894-6361
http://www.unos.org

Summary of Primary Care Needs for the Child with a Solid Organ Transplant

HEALTH CARE MAINTENANCE

Growth and development

Height and weight should be measured each visit.

Linear growth may be affected by long-term corticosteroid use.

Catch-up growth may be attained after transplantation.

Growth hormone may be advised for children before or after renal transplantation.

Improved physical development after transplantation has a positive effect on psychosocial development.

Cognitive functioning should be monitored.

Nutrition

A regular diet is usually allowed.

Enteral supplements are sometimes needed for adequate caloric intake.

Dietary restrictions are instituted as needed; electrolyte imbalance may occur.

Children with heart transplants are on a no-added-salt diet.

Safety

Precautions with animal feces—especially cat litter boxes—are recommended to prevent transmission of disease to children who are immunosuppressed.

Medic-Alert bracelets are recommended.

The transplant center should be contacted prior to travel outside of the country or for extended time.

Exercise restrictions are necessary for the first 6 to 8 weeks to allow for healing. Activity should be decreased when the child is fatigued or during period of rejection.

Immunizations

All recommended immunizations should be administered before the transplant whenever possible.

Interrupted immunization schedules can usually be resumed 3 months after transplantation.

Live virus vaccines are contraindicated in transplant recipients; immunodeficient children should receive inactivated vaccines when available.

Inactivated polio virus (IPV), MMR, varicella should be given to siblings and other close contacts.

The influenza vaccine should be given to the recipient and family members yearly.

Screening

Vision: Yearly examinations should be conducted for children on high-dose steroids to monitor for vision changes.

Pediatric transplant recipients should be screened according to well-child visit guidelines.

Hearing: Audiograms should be done as needed to evaluate hearing loss in children who received ototoxic drugs.

Dental: Biannual dental visits are recommended.

CSA may cause gingival hyperplasia.

Antibiotic prophylaxis is only needed for invasive dental procedures.

Blood pressure: Blood pressure should be checked at each visit.

If antihypertensive medications are prescribed, blood pressure should be checked and recorded prior to administration.

Hematocrit: Screening should be done per transplant center routine.

Urinalysis: Screening for renal recipients should be routine per transplant center.

Additional routine screening is not necessary unless the child is symptomatic.

Immunosuppression may mask symptoms of UTI.

Tuberculosis: Routine screening is recommended. PPD with anergy panal and chest radiography may be ordered.

Children with positive chest radiograph and PPD should take Isoniazid (INH) for life.

Continued

Summary of Primary Care Needs for the Child with a Solid Organ Transplant—cont'd

Condition-specific screening

Blood work: Multiple laboratory tests are obtained at clinic visits per the transplant center routine.

Drug levels of immunosuppressant medications are also monitored and adjusted per transplant center protocol.

Graft evaluation: Diagnostic testing is done yearly to evaluate graft function.

COMMON ILLNESS MANAGEMENT

Differential diagnosis

Fever: The risks for bacterial and viral infection are increased during the first 3 months after a transplant.

Immunosuppression will mask symptoms, so careful assessment of any fever is very important.

Normal childhood illnesses should be ruled out.

Fever may indicate organ rejection or infection.

Abdominal symptoms: Abdominal pain should be investigated to rule out appendicitis or intestinal obstruction, ulcers, and peritonitis.

Abdominal pain in liver transplant recipients may be a sign of rejection or surgical complications.

Abdominal pain and/or vomiting may be a sign of rejection in heart transplant recipients.

Vomiting and diarrhea may lower therapeutic blood levels of immunosuppressant drugs.

Metabolic abnormalities: Hyperkalemia can result from drug therapy.

Hyperglycemia may result from immunosuppressant medications.

Drug interactions: CSA and tacrolimus absorption is altered by phenytoin, phenobarbital, ketoconazole, fluconazole, erythromycin, diltiazem, and other drugs.

When administered with anticonvulsants, higher doses of CSA may be needed to achieve a therapeutic range.

Acetaminophen should be used instead of aspirin or ibuprofen.

If the child is hypertensive, decongestants should be avoided.

DEVELOPMENTAL ISSUES

Sleep patterns

End-stage organ disease, hospitalization, or drugs may alter sleep patterns.

Familiar routines and rituals should be maintained when possible.

Toileting

Regression in toddlers and preschoolers is to be expected.

Children with renal transplantation may need to relearn body cues to achieve toilet traning.

Children taking diuretics may have difficulty with urinary continence and training.

Emotional support is required as children learn skills.

Discipline

Parental overprotectiveness is likely; parents may need help to promote independence in their children.

Noncompliance with medications may occur with adolescents.

Child care

Children may attend daycare by 3 months after surgery if immunosuppression requirements have been reduced.

Precautions should be taken to limit exposure to communicable diseases.

Schooling

Normal schooling should be resumed 2 to 3 months after transplantation.

Additional academic help may be needed to attain grade level skills due to time lost.

An individual education plan (IEP) should be initiated if school problems develop.

Alterations in body image may negatively affect peer interactions.

Summary of Primary Care Needs for the Child with a Solid Organ Transplant—cont'd

Sexuality

The transplant experience may affect body image and self-esteem.

Barrier methods of birth control are recommended.

Childbearing is possible after transplantation.

Physiologic strain on maternal system must be monitored.

Affects of immunosuppression on fetus must be monitored

Transition to adulthood

Most individuals have difficulty attaining independence.

Body image and intimacy may be negatively affected.

Concerns about employment and health insurance develop.

SPECIAL FAMILY CONCERNS

Special family concerns include the fear of rejection, search for a new organ, organ donor issues, and finances.

References

Abu-Elmagd K, Reyes J, and Todo S: Clinical intestinal transplantation: new perspectives and immunologic considerations, J Am Coll Surg 186(5):512-527, 1998.

American Heart Association: If your child has a congenital heart defect, 1997, Dallas, The Association.

Committee on Infectious Diseases: 1997 Red Book: report of the Committee on Infectious Disease, ed 24, Elk Grove Village, Ill., 1997, American Academy of Pediatrics.

Armenti VT et al: National Transplantation Pregnancy Registry (NTPR): cyclosporine dosing and pregnancy outcome in female renal transplant recipients, Transplantation Proceedings, 28(4): 2111-2112, 1996.

Asante-Korang A et al: Experience of FK506 immune suppression in pediatric heart transplantation: a study of long-term adverse effects, J Heart Lung Transplant 15(4):415-22, 1996.

Balfour H and Heussner R: Cytomegalovirus infections and liver transplantation: an overview, Transplant Proceedings 25(2):2012-2013, 1993.

Baum D et al: Pediatric heart transplantation at Stanford: results of a 15-year experience, Pediatrics 88:203-214, 1991.

Baum M et al: Growth and neurodevelopmental outcome of infants undergoing heart transplantation, J Heart Lung Transplant 12(6 Pt 2):S211-217, 1993.

Bereket G and Fine R: Pediatric renal transplantation, Pediatr Clin North Am 42(6):1603-1628, 1995.

Branel K et al: Risks of subsequent preganancies on mother and newborn in female heart transplant recipients, J Heart Lung Transplant 17:698-702, 1998.

Cacciarelli T et al: Management of posttransplant lymphoproliferative disease in pediatric liver transplant recipients receiving primary tacrolimus therapy, Transplantation 66(8):1047-1052, 1998.

Cecka J et al: Pediatric renal transplantation: a review of the UNOS data, Pediatr Transplant 1:55-64, 1997.

Chinnock R: Pediatric heart transplantation at Loma Linda: 1985-1996, Clin Transplant 145-151, 1996.

Chinnock R and Baum M: Somatic growth in infant heart transplant recipients, Pediatr Transplant 2:30-34, 1998.

Codoner-Franch P, Bernard O, and Alvarez F: Long term follow-up of growth in height after successful liver transplantation, J Pediatr 124(3):368-373, 1994.

Conte J et al: Pediatric heart-lung transplantation: intermediate term results, J Heart Lung Transplant 15: 692-699, 1996.

Crandall B: Immunosuppression. In Sigardson-Poor K and Haggerty L, editors: Nursing care of the transplant recipient, Philadelphia, 1990, W.B. Saunders.

Davis D, Chang P, and Nevins T: Successful renal transplantation accelerated development in young uremic children, Pediatrics 86(4):594-600, 1990.

Delforge C et al: Pregnancy after cardiac transplantation, Transplant Proceed 29:2481-2483, 1997.

Douglas J et al: Late rejection as major indicator of noncompliance in pediatric heart transplant patients. Presented at the Annual Meeting of the American Heart Association, Dallas, November 1993 (abstract).

Eke C et al: Neurologic sequelae of deep hypothermic circulatory arrest in cardiac transplant infants, Ann Thorac Surg 61(3):783-788, 1996.

Ellis D et al: Renal transplantation in infants and children. In Shapiro R, Simmons R, and Starzl T, editors, Renal transplantation, Stamford, Conn., 2997, Appleton & Lang.

Ettenger RB et al. Improved cadaveric renal transplant outcome in children, Pediatric Nephrol 5(1):137-142, 1991.

European FK 506 Multicenter Liver Study Group: Randomized trial comparing tacrolimus (FK506) and cyclosporin in prevention of liver allograft rejection, Lancet 344:423-428, 1994.

Fine R: Growth hormone treatment of children with chronic renal insufficiency, end-stage renal disease and following renal transplantation—update 1997, J Pediatr Endocrinol Metab 10(4):361-70, 1997a.

Fine R: Growth post renal-transplantation in children: lessons from the North American Pediatric Renal Transplant Cooperative Study (NAPRTCS), Pediatr Transplant 1:85-89, 1997b.

Fung J et al: Randomized trial in primary liver transplantation under immunosuppression with FK506 or cyclosporine, Transplant Proceedings 25(1):1130, 1993.

Goto T et al: Discovery of FK506, a novel immunosuppressant isolated from Streptomyces tsukubaensis, Transplant Proceedings 19: 4-8, 1987.

Green J, Carcillo J, and Reyes J: Liver transplantation. In Fuhrman B and Zimmerman J, editors: Pediatric critical care, St Louis, 1998, Mosby.

Green M et al: Comparison of intravenous ganciclovir followed by oral acyclovir with intravenous ganciclovir alone for prevention of cytomegalovirus and Epstein-Barr virus disease after liver transplantation in children, Clin Infect Disease 25:1344-1349, 1997.

Green M and Michaels M: Infections in solid organ transplant recipients. In Long S, Pickery L, and Prober C, editors: Principles and practice of pediatric infectious diseases, New York, 1997, Churchill Livingston.

Green M, Reyes J, and Rowe D: New strategies in the prevention and management of Epstein-Barr virus infection and posttransplant lymphoproliferative disease following solid organ transplantation, Curr Op Organ Transplant 3:143-147, 1998.

Groth C et al: New trials in transplantation: how to exploit the potential of sirolimus in clinical transplantation, Transplant Proceedings 30:4064-4065, 1998.

Guest J and Hasse J: Nutritional aspects of pediatric liver transplantation. In Busutil R and Klintmalm G, editors: Transplantation of the liver, Philadelphia, 1996, W.B. Saunders.

Harland R and Platt J: Prospects for xenotransplantation of the liver, J Hepatol 25:248-258, 1996.

Hausen B and Morris R: Review of immunosuppression for lung transplantation: novel drugs, new uses for conventional immunosuppressants and alternative strategies, Clin Chest Med 18(2):353-359, 1997.

Heffron T: Living related pediatric liver transplantation, Sem Pediatr Surg 2(4):248-253, 1993.

Hosenpud J, Novick R, and Bennett L: The registry of the International Society for Heart and Lung Transplantation: thirteenth official report—1996, 15:655-674, 1996.

Hosenpud J et al: The registry of the international society for heart and lung transplantation: fifteenth official report, J Heart Lung Transplant 17:656-668, 1998.

Hunt S and Frazier O: Mechanical circulatory support and cardiac transplantation, Circulation 97:2079-2090, 1998.

Jain A and Fung J: Cyclosporin and tacrolimus in clinical transplantation: a comparative review, Clin Immunother 5(5):352-372, 1996.

Jain A et al: Comparative study of cyclosporine and FK506 dosage requirement in adults and pediatric orthotopic liver transplantation, Transplant Proceedings 23(6):2763-2766, 1991.

Jordan S, Rosenthal P, and Makowka L: Immunosuppression in organ transplantation, Sem Pediatr Surg 2(4):206-217, 1993.

Kantrowitz A et al: Transplantation of the heart in an infant and an adult, Am J Cardiol 22:782-790, 1968.

Katz B: Epstein-Barr virus (mononucleosis and lymphoproliferative disorders). In Long S, Pickery L, and Prober C, editors: Principles and practice of pediatric infectious diseases, New York, 1997, Churchill Livingstone.

Kelly D: Nutritional factors affecting growth before and after liver transplantation, Pediatr Transplant 1:80-83, 1997.

Kontoyiannis D and Rubin R: Infection in the organ transplant recipient: an overview, Infectious Dis Clin North Am 9(4):811-822;1995.

Kosmach B et al: Care of the pediatric solid organ transplant recipient: the primary care perspective, Pediatr Clin North Am 45(6):1395-1418, 1998.

Lower RR and Shumway NE: Studies on orthotopic transplantation of the canine heart, Surg Forum 11:18-19, 1960.

Mahmoud A et al: Outcome of preemptive renal transplantation and pretransplantation dialysis in children, Pediatr Nephrol 11(5):537-541, 1997.

Makowka L, Cramer D, and Hoffman A: Pig liver xenografts as a temporary bridge for human allografting, Xenotransplantation I:27-29, 1993.

Makowka L et al: Immunohistopathologic lesions associated with the rejection of a pig-to-human liver xenograft, Transplant Proc 26:1074-1075, 1994.

Martin M: Combination antiviral strategies in managing cytomegalovirus infection, Transplant Proc 26(5):28-30, 1994.

Mazariegos G et al: Weaning of immunosuppression in liver transplant recipients, Transplantation 63:243-249, 1997.

McDiarmid S: Risk factors and outcomes after pediatric liver transplantation, Liver Transplant Surg 2(5):44-56, 1996a.

McDiarmid S: Special considerations for pediatric immunosuppression after liver transplantation. In Busutil R and Klintmalm G, editors: Transplantation of the liver, Philadelphia, 1996b, W.B. Saunders.

McDiarmid S et al: FK-506 (tacrolimus) compared with cyclosporine for primary immunosuppression after pediatric liver transplantation; results from the US Multicenter Trial, Transplantation 59:530-536, 1995a.

McDiarmid S et al: Indications for pediatric liver transplantation, Pediatr Transplant 2:106-116, 1998.

McDiarmid S et al: The treatment of intractable rejection with FK506 in pediatric liver transplant recipients, J Pediatr Gastroenterol Nutr 20:291-299, 1995b.

McGhee B et al, editors: Pediatric Drug therapy handbook and formulary, Pittsburgh, Pa., 1998, Department of Pharmacy.

Molmenti E et al: Noncompliance after pediatric liver transplantation, Transplant Proceed 31(1-2):408, 1999.

Morris-Stiff G et al: Conversion of renal transplant recipients from cyclosporin (neoral) to tacrolimus (Prograf) for haemolytic uraemic syndrome, Transplant Int 11(Suppl 1):S98-S99, 1998.

Morrow W et al: Outcome of listing for heart transplantation in infants younger than six months: predictors of death and interval to transplantation, J Heart Lung Transpl 16:1255-1266, 1997.

Olsen S et al: Prevention of *Pneumocystis carinii* pneumonia in cardiac transplant recipients by trimethoprim-sulfamethozazole, Transplant 56(2):359-362, 1993.

Padbury RT, Toogood GJ, and McMaster P: Withdrawal of immunosuppression in liver allograft recipients: Liver transplantation and surgery 4(3):242-248, 1998.

Park M: Primary myocardial disease. In Pediatric cardiology for practitioners, ed 3, St Louis, 1996, Mosby.

Pirsch J et al: A comparison of tacrolimus and cyclosporine for immunosuppression after cadaveric renal transplantation, Transplant 63(7):977-983, 1997.

Platt J: Approaching clinical application of xenotransplantation, J Card Surg 12:285-293, 1997.

Podesta L, Rosenthal P, and Makowka L: Pediatric liver transplantation, Sem Pediatr Surg 2(4):265-278, 1993.

Radomski JS et al: National transplantation pregnancy registry: analysis of pregnancy outcomes in female liver transplant recipients, Liver Transplant Surg 1(5):281-284, 1995.

Reichert P et al: Biliary complications of reduced-organ liver transplantation, Liver Transplant Surg 4(5):343-349, 1998.

Reyes J et al: Current status of intestinal transplantation in children, J PediatrSurg 33(2):243-254, 1998a.

Reyes J et al: Primary liver transplantation in children under tacrolimus: three to eight years' follow-up (abstract 347). In Program and Abstracts of the 17th Annual Meeting of the American Society of Transplant Physicians, Chicago, 1998b, The Society.

Reyes J et al: The role of portosystemic shunting in children in the transplant era, J Pediatr Surg 34(1):117-123, 1999.

Roche product monograph, Roche Pharmaceuticals, Nutley, NJ, December 1997.

Ryckman F et al: Biliary atresia—surgical management and treatment options as they relate to outcome, Liver Transplant Surg 4(5):S24-S33, 1998 (supplement).

Sager S and Ettenger R: Kidney transplantation in children, Sem Pediatr Surg 2(4):235-247, 1993.

Shapiro R et al: Tacrolimus in pediatric renal transplantation, Transplant 62(12):1752-1758, 1996.

Shapiro R et al: Pediatric renal transplantation under tacrolimus-based immunosuppression (abstract 21). In Programs and Abstracts of the 24th Annual Scientific Meeting of the American Society of Transplant Surgeons, Chicago, A-21, 1998, The Society.

Starzl T et al: Evolution of liver transplantation, Hepatology 2:614-636, 1982.

Starzl T et al: The role of cell migration and chimerism in organ transplant acceptance and tolerance induction, Transplant Sci 3(1):47-50, 1993a.

Starzl T et al: Baboon-to-human liver transplantation, Lancet 341:65-71, 1993b.

Starzl T and Demetris A: History of renal transplantation. In Shapiro R, Simmons R, and Starzl T, editors: Renal transplantation, Stamford, Conn., 1997, Appleton & Lang.

Stewart S et al: Cognitive function in children who receive organ transplantation, Health Psychol 13(1):3-13, 1994.

Stewart S et al: Mental and motor development, social competence, and growth one year after successful pediatric liver transplantation, J Pediatr 4(1):574-581, 1989.

Stockwell J, Tobias J, and Greeley W: Noninflammatory, noninfiltrative cardiomyopathy. In Nichols D et al, editors: Critical heart disease in infants and children, St Louis, 1995, Mosby.

Sussman N and Kelly J: The artificial liver, Scientific American 5:63-77, 1995.

Trull A et al: Cyclosporin absorption from microemulsion formulation in liver transplant recipients, Lancet 341:433, 1993.

United Network for Organ Sharing (UNOS): Scientific Registry, 1998.

US Multicenter FK-506 Liver Study Group: A comparison of tacrolimus (FK-506) and cyclosporine for immunosuppression in liver transplantation, New Engl J Med 331(17):1110-1115, 1994.

Webber S: 15 years of pediatric heart transplantation at the University of Pittsburgh: lessons learned and future prospects, Pediatr Transplant 1:8-21, 1997.

Wong P and Starnes V: Pediatric heart and lung transplantation. In Chang A et al, editors: Pediatric cardiac intensive care, Baltimore, Md., 1998, Williams & Wilkins.

Wray J et al: Cognitive function and behavioral status in pediatric heart and heart lung transplant recipients: the Harefield experience, Br Med J 309(6958):837-841, 1994.

Wren F and Tarbell S: Feeding and growth disorders. In Ammerman R and Campo J, editors: Handbook of pediatric psychology and psychiatry: disease, injury, and illness, vol II, Boston, 1998, Allyn & Bacon.

Zeevi A et al: Three years of follow-up of bone marrow augmented organ transplant recipients: the impact on donor-specific immune modulation, Transplant Proceed 29:1205-1206, 1997.

Zimmerman J and Kahan B: Pharmacokinetics of sirolimus in stable renal transplant patients after multiple oral dose administration, J Clin Pharm 37:405-415, 1997.

Zitelli B et al: Changes in lifestyle after liver transplantation, Pediatr 82:173-180, 1988.

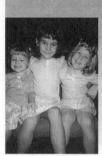

CHAPTER **31**

Phenylketonuria

Kathleen Schmidt Yule

Etiology

Phenylketonuria (PKU) is an autosomal recessive inherited metabolic disorder that causes plasma phenylalanine (phe) levels to rise to more than 1000 μM (16.5 mg/dL).[1] PKU is caused by a mutation of the phenylalanine hydroxylase (PAH) gene and exposure to elevated blood phe. Clinically less harmful than PKU, mild hyperphenylalaninemia (HPA) is a related disorder in which phe levels are greater than 120 μM but less than 1000 μM. PKU is clinically distinguished from non-PKU HPA by a lower tolerance for dietary phe (<500 mg/day). Mild HPA can have the same effects as PKU in some cases (Scriver et al, 1995).

The metabolic pathway for phe is in the liver. PAH, an enzyme, converts phe by hydroxylation to tyrosine (tyr) in the hepatocyte for use in the biosynthesis of (1) protein, (2) melanin, (3) thyroxine, and (4) the catecholamines in the brain and adrenal medulla. Loss of PAH activity causes an accumulation of normal phe metabolites, phenylpyruvic acid, and derivatives (phenylketones), which the kidney has a finite capacity to excrete when plasma phe reaches 1000 μM. There are no abnormal metabolites in PKU, only normal metabolites in abnormal amounts. A high level of phe inhibits the entry of large neutral amino acids into the brain; the essential cellular processes of myelination and protein synthesis in the brain are disrupted, causing a deficient neurotransmitter supply to the brain and the neuropathology of PKU (Cockburn et al, 1996; Hommes, 1991; Kaufman, 1989; Scriver et al, 1995).

In a growing child the recommended dietary allowance (RDA) for phe is used by the body in two major ways: (1) up to 60% is used for new tissue protein synthesis, decreasing with age, and (2) 40% is hydroxylated to form tyr. Homeostasis of phe in the body reflects the interaction among (1) a dietary intake of phe; (2) turnover of the body's tissue protein; and (3) outflow by means of hydroxylation (to form tyr), transamination (to form pheynlypyruvic acid and derivatives), and conversion to other minor metabolites under the control of multiple independent genes and the PAH gene (Scriver et al, 1995; Treacy et al, 1994).

The phe hydroxylation system is a complex biochemical reaction that requires the presence of tetrahydrobiopterin (BH_4), oxygen, and phe. Three enzymes responsible for the synthesis and regeneration of BH_4 are also necessary for the hydroxylation of phe (Figure 31-1). A deficiency of any one of these enzymes causes a deficiency of BH_4 and HPA. Characterized by progressive neurologic deterioration, BH_4 deficiency disorders are phenotypically and genotypically distinct from PKU, require different modes of therapy, and have a different prognosis (Blau et al, 1993; Blau et al, 1995; Leonard, 1998).

Because both PKU and the BH_4 deficiency disorders present with neonatal HPA, screening for BH_4 deficiency should be done in all newborns with HPA. Older children with microcephaly, mental retardation, convulsions (grand mal or myoclonic), disturbances of tone and posture, abnormal movements, drowsiness, diurnal fluctuation of alertness, irritability, hypersalivation, swallowing difficulties, or recurrent hyperthermia without infection should also be tested for HPA and the BH_4-deficiency disorders (Blau et al, 1993).

PKU is the result of over 400 different mutations in the PAH gene on chromosome 12. Because all cases of true PKU and 95% of all cases of mild HPA are the result of a mutation at the PAH locus, this locus is the PKU locus in humans. A mutation changes the DNA code for PAH protein, creating

---

[1]To convert phe from μM (same as μmol/L) to mg/dL, multiply (x phe μM) by .0165. To convert phe from mg/dl to μM, multiply mg/dl by 60.53.

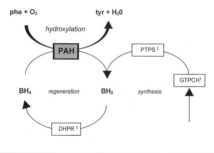

Figure 31-1 The phenylalanine hydroxylation system.

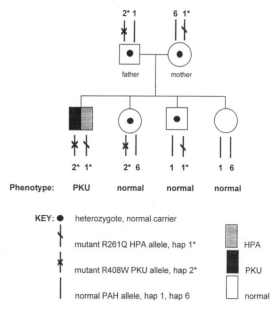

Phenotype: PKU   normal   normal   normal

KEY: ● heterozygote, normal carrier

mutant R261Q HPA allele, hap 1*   HPA

mutant R408W PKU allele, hap 2*   PKU

normal PAH allele, hap 1, hap 6   normal

Figure 31-2 Hypothetical family pedigree showing segregation of mutant PKU and mutant HPA alleles with haplotype.

an unstable enzyme with varying degrees of activity, less than 1% of normal activity for PKU and 2% to 5% for mild HPA (Scriver et al, 1995). This high degree of genetic diversity at the PAH locus partially accounts for the clinical spectrum of HPA observed in PKU and mild HPA.

All individuals inherit two PAH alleles—one from each parent—at the PAH locus. PAH alleles that encode for the abnormal production of little or no functional PAH enzyme are mutant PKU alleles. If both inherited alleles carry identical mutations for PKU, an individual is homozygous for PKU at the locus; if each allele carries a different mutation, an individual is compound heterozygous for PKU at the locus. Mutation analysis of DNA has revealed that approximately 75% of PKU cases are compound heterozygotes for PKU alleles; each parent contributed a different PKU mutation. Alternatively, because PKU alleles and mild HPA alleles are allelic, an individual can inherit them together and be compound heterozygous for both PKU and mild HPA (Figure 31-2). Clinically this explains why individuals with PKU or mild HPA and even affected siblings have different degrees of HPA (Koch et al, 1998a; Weglage et al, 1998).

All individuals have identifiable normal variations in the DNA surrounding the PAH locus on chromosome 12 called *restriction fragment length polymorphisms* (RFLPs). Because eight specific RFLPs segregate with the PKU mutation on the PAH gene, they act as markers for PKU and are called *PKU haplotypes* (haps) (Scriver et al, 1995).

Because PKU and mild HPA follow the Mendelian autosomal recessive pattern of inheritance,

PKU hap analysis can trace the segregation pattern of the PKU alleles in a family at 25% risk for PKU with each offspring without direct mutation analysis (see Figure 31-2). Prenatal diagnosis for PKU is 99% informative when an intragenic polymorphic marker is used together with direct DNA mutation analysis. Direct DNA mutation analysis for PKU is indicated for sperm and ovum donors—with or without phenotypic expression of HPA (Scriver et al, 1995).

Direct DNA analysis in a newborn with PKU is a valuable tool for identifying the specific mutation and further defining the severity of PKU; therapy can be optimized and long-term prognosis anticipated and enhanced. The HPA phenotype, however, is more complex than that predicted by Mendelian inheritance of alleles at the PAH; there are inconsistencies between different individuals with similar PAH genotypes (Enns et al, 1997; Kayaalp et al, 1997). In 112 Midwestern children, a mutation analysis of 12 haps characterized 56.5% of the PKU alleles. In 35% of the children, both PKU alleles were identified and 9.4% of the children were homozygous for the R408W mutation. The rest of the children were compound heterozygous for this specific mutation with another PKU mutation (Kaul et al, 1994).

Incidence

PKU is prevalent in many populations. The incidence of PKU ranges from 5 to 385 cases per 1 million live births (Table 31-1). The worldwide incidence of PKU in white populations is 1:10,000. Based on this incidence, 1 out of 50 whites carries the PKU gene and the PKU gene frequency in whites is 1%, the same as in the Chinese. Carriers, or gene frequency in populations, remain constant from generation to generation despite availability of carrier testing and prenatal diagnosis. The incidence of PKU in the black population in the United States is 1:50,000 (Hofman et al, 1991).

Both PKU and mild HPA are currently screened for using nonselective newborn screening (NBS) in all states, the District of Columbia, Puerto Rico, and U.S. Virgin Islands, and in more than 30 other countries. There will continue to be individuals of all ages who may or may not know whether they were previously screened, diagnosed, and treated for PKU or even that they have mild HPA. It is estimated that at least 10% of individuals with untreated PKU may have near normal intelligence quotients (IQs).

Women with PKU are a clinically significant group because their offspring are at risk for maternal PKU (MPKU) syndrome. Over 50% of all births in North America and Europe are to women unscreened for PKU. Women with mild HPA can produce offspring with severe MPKU embryopathy. Mothers of newborns with transient HPA, as well as mothers who have delivered infants with any of the features of MPKU syndrome, should be tested for PKU (Hanley, 1994).

Case findings for PKU, mild HPA, and MPKU syndrome should be paramount in the primary care provider's mind when (1) a presumptive positive PKU NBS test result is reported, even if the result is found negative on recall testing (mild HPA); (2) the newborn is premature; (3) a child has unexplained microcephaly, intrauterine (Thibaud et al, 1998) or postnatal growth delay, dysmorphic facial features, or congenital anomalies—particularly a congenital heart defect or harsh systolic murmur (MPKU syndrome); (4) an infant has unexplained developmental delay or a child has any degree of

Table 31-1
Incidences of Hyperphenylalaninemia Variants by Phenotype, Region, and Ethnic Group

Variant	Geographic Region or Ethnic Group	Incidence (per 10^6 Births)
PKU	Turkey	385
	Yemenite Jews	190
	Scotland	190
	Eire	190
	Czech and Slovak Republics	150
	Poland	130
	Hungary	90
	France	75
	Denmark	85
	Norway	70
	Sweden	25
	Finland	5
	England	70
	Italy	60
	China	60
	Canada	45
	Japan	7
	Ashkenazi Jews	5
Non-PKU HPA	All regions except Finland	15-75
BH_4-deficiency HPA	Panethnic and panregional	1-2

Adapted from Scriver CR et al: The hyperphenylalaninemias. In Scriver CR, editors: The Metabolic and Molecular Bases of Inherited Disease, vol I, ed 7, New York, 1995, McGraw-Hill.

mental retardation; (5) the family immigrated to the United States; and (6) the maternal history includes a spontaneous abortion (SAB), stillbirth, rash, seizures, poor coordination of unknown cause, any degree of mental retardation, or a mother who was born before 1967 (Acosta and Wright, 1992).

The greatest source of referral for HPA cases are NBS programs. The primary care provider's role in NBS is critical (Buist and Tuerck, 1992). The lack of universal NBS standards, tests, or legislation, and different technologies available for the testing of phe make uniform recommendations for providers difficult. Knowledge about specific regional NBS program practices (Council of Regional Networks for Genetic Services [CORN], 1994; Kling, 1993) and consultation with the regional NBS coordinator are mandatory for the follow-up protocol of presumptive positive HPA NBS test results. Different conditions, treatments, and other biologic variables at the time of testing can alter the phe level; providers must be alert to the causes of false-negative and false-positive results in the newborn (Schmidt, 1989). Early discharge of newborns from the hospital can affect NBS testing for HPA. Follow-up varies depending on the methodology employed by the regional NBS program (Cunningham et al, 1996; Jew et al, 1994; Jew, Kamjou, and McElroy, 1998; Lorey and Cunningham, 1994; Wallman, 1998).

Clinical Manifestations at Time of Diagnosis (Box 31-1)

The NBS test alone does not establish the diagnosis of PKU: a positive PKU test result does not constitute the diagnosis of PKU, nor does a negative PKU test result dismiss the possibility of PKU. Further investigation for PKU is warranted in a child with manifestations of untreated PKU. Berg (1984) states:

> Affected infants usually appear normal at birth, but within several months become irritable and may have recurring vomiting. Though milestones may be reached at a normal time, they are usually delayed in both motor and intellectual skills. Acquisition of speech and language is delayed. Seizures occur in at least 25% of untreated PKU patients and in early life are typically infantile spasms. As the patients become older, the convulsions assume other forms of generalized epilepsies. Microcephaly is common and increased muscle tone with hyperreflexia is generally present. Patients often assume an unusual seated position, "schneidersitz" (tailor's position) and many children have a fine, rapid and irregular tremor at rest as well as with outstretched arms. The plantar responses are variable. Electroencephalograms are usually abnormal and hypsarrhythmia is commonly found, sometimes when no clinical convulsive activity has been noted.

If untreated, the toxic effects of phe in a child with PKU cause a drop in developmental quotient to 50 points by 1 year of age and to 30 points by 3 years

Box 31-1

Clinical Manifestations

Normal appearance at birth
Fair pigmentation
Irritability
Neonatal vomiting
Infantile spasms
Generalized epilepsy
Microcephaly
Atopic dermatitis
Mousey odor of urine and sweat
Increased deep tendon reflexes
Plantar responses variable
Tailor's sitting position
Fine rapid irregular tremor
Parkinson's-like movements
Bony changes in growth plate
Decreased height in males
Increased weight in females
Delayed motor skills
Delayed intellectual skills
Delayed speech and language skills
Decreased IQ
Hyperphenylalaninemia

of age (Koch and Wenz, 1987). Since the advent of NBS and earlier diagnosis and treatment, it has been demonstrated that an average of 10 IQ points are lost if phe homeostasis is not achieved during the first month of life and an additional 10 points are lost if it is not achieved by the second month (Fishler et al, 1987; Smith, Beasley, and Ades, 1990).

Boys with untreated PKU have measurements for height that are consistently 2 standard deviations (SDs) below the mean when compared with boys without PKU. In contrast, mean height and weight measurements for girls with untreated PKU are consistently 2 SDs above the mean when compared with girls without PKU (Fisch, Gravem, and Feinberg, 1966). Mesodermal changes in the growth plate of long bones of intrauterine origin are characteristic in neonates and children with PKU—both untreated and early treated (Fisch et al, 1991a).

Of the children with untreated PKU, 20% to 40% have eczema (i.e., an atopic dermatitis with predilection for flexural creases on the arms and legs) indistinguishable from that in children who do not have PKU (Irons and Levy, 1986). A lingering musty odor sometimes described as mousey, barn-like, or old urine is commonly present and is secondary to the urinary excretion of phenylacetic acid, which accumulates over the first month of life. Children with PKU typically have a fairer complexion than the composite coloring of other family members. This complexion is related to inhibitions of tyr metabolism and reduced melanin production. In ethnic backgrounds where black hair is expected, this feature will be expressed as hair that is brown or even reddish. Whites typically have blonde hair and blue eyes. Because these manifestations are not pronounced at birth, their expression may not be evident until irreversible brain damage has already occurred.

The results of complete blood cell (CBC) count, routine urinalysis, and liver, renal, and endocrine function tests are normal in children with untreated PKU (Koch and Wenz, 1987). The concurrence of PKU with other genetic disorders is relatively uncommon, although it can occur (e.g., with Down syndrome [author's experience] and Goldenhar syndrome) (Tokatli et al, 1994). The concurrence of PKU with multifactorial disorders (e.g., diabetes) is the same as for a child without PKU.

Treatment

Treatment for PKU is simple in theory but difficult in practice (Box 31-2). It involves restricting phe in the diet to maintain a nontoxic level of plasma phe between 120 μM and 360 μM while allowing optimum growth and brain development by supplementing the diet with adequate sources of energy, protein, and other nutrients. Tyrosine is supplemented when plasma tyr levels are less than 20 μM. Optimal management is a phe-restricted diet initiated within the first 2 weeks of life and continued throughout childhood, adolescence, and adulthood, especially before conception and throughout pregnancy for the benefit of the offspring.

Clinical tolerance of phe distinguishes PKU from mild HPA. The phe requirement for infants and young children with PKU is between 250 and 500 mg/day and is not more than 1.5 times greater than this level in the older child. Children with PKU have a narrower tolerance between the lower and upper limits of required phe than individuals with greater PAH activity. An individual with HPA

Box 31-2

Treatment

Phe-restricted diet
Supplement tyr if low
Provide nutrients to support normal growth and development

---

requiring dietary restriction of phe to maintain a plasma phe level of less than 600 μM needs treatment regardless of the distinction made between PKU and mild HPA. Tolerance of phe is observed over time and can change within weeks, months, or even years. Rarely, PKU and mild HPA can be transient, and a child's tolerance for phe can increase to normal levels because of either a regulatory defect affecting PAH activity or a transient disorder of biopterin metabolism. Careful and continuous monitoring of individuals whose phe intake is restricted is necessary to avoid phe deficiency when tolerance changes in these rare cases or because of changes related to growth rate.

Dietary restriction of phe is accomplished by the use of commercially available elemental medical foods (EMFs). These products are modified protein hydrolysates in which phe is removed or are mixtures of free amino acids that do not contain phe. EMFs provide the essential amino acids in suitable proportions for the given age of the individual. Because natural protein contains 2.4% to 9% of phe by weight, adequate protein cannot be obtained from natural foods without ingesting excess phe. Therefore phe-restricted diets are usually designed so that EMF products provide the majority of the essential nutrients with the exception of the caloric requirement, which is derived from no- or low-protein, high-calorie natural sources. Nutrient intakes must be sufficient to meet the anabolic requirements of the individual and maintain essential conversion reactions (Acosta and Yannicelli, 1997).

Phenylalanine-restricted diets are prescribed by the medical genetics PKU treatment center team who continually monitors a child's phe tolerance. An individual's phe requirements depend on PAH activity, age, growth rate, adequacy of energy and protein intakes, and state of health (Table 31-2).

Table 31-2
Recommended Daily Nutrient Intakes (Ranges) for Infants, Children, and Adults with PKU

Age	Nutrient				
	PHE[1] (mg/kg)	TYR[1] (mg/kg)	Protein (g/kg)	Energy (kcal/kg)	Fluid[2] (ml/kg)
Infants					
0 to <3 mo	25-70	300-350	3.50-3.00	120 (145-95)	160-135
3 to <6 mo	20-45	300-350	3.50-3.00	120 (145-95)	160-130
6 to <9 mo	15-35	250-300	3.00-2.50	110 (135-80)	145-125
9 to <12 mo	10-35	250-300	3.00-2.50	105 (135-80)	135-120
	(mg/day)	(g/day)	(g/day)	(kcal/day)	(ml/day)
Girls and Boys					
1 to <4 yr	200-400	1.72-3.00	30	1300 (900-1800)	900-1800
4 to <7 yr	210-450	2.25-3.50	35	1700 (1300-2300)	1300-2300
7 to <11 yr	220-500	2.55-4.00	40	2400 (1650-3300)	1650-3300
Women					
11 to <15 yr	250-750	3.45-5.00	50	2200 (1500-3000)	1500-3000
15 to <19 yr	230-700	3.45-5.00	50	2100 (1200-3000)	1200-3000
≥19 yr	220-700	3.75-5.00	50	2100 (1400-2500)	2100-2500
Men					
11 to <15 yr	225-900	3.38-5.50	55	2700 (2000-3700)	2000-3700
15 to <19 yr	295-1100	4.42-6.50	65	2800 (2100-3900)	2100-3900
≥19 yr	290-1200	4.35-6.50	65	2900 (2000-3300)	2000-3300

From Acosta PB and Yannicelli S: The Ross metabolic formula system nutrition support protocols, Columbus, Ohio, 1993, Abbott Laboratories, USA.
[1]Modify prescription based on frequently obtained blood and/or plasma values and growth in infants and children and frequently obtained plasma values and weight maintenance in adults.
[2]Under normal circumstances offer minimum of 1.5 mL fluid to neonates for each Kcal ingested.

The greatest benefits of continuing the diet are in the areas of cognitive functioning measured by IQ tests and by the reading and spelling subtests of the "Wide Range Achievement Test" (WRAT). There is a strong relationship between the IQ of a child and the age at which dietary control is lost (blood phe level consistently more than 900 μM (Table 31-3). The best predictor of IQ in a child with PKU and of the deficit in IQ between the child and unaffected siblings or parents is the age when dietary control is lost. The IQ deficit is greatest when phe control is lost before 6 years of age. If phe control continues past 8 years of age to at least 12 years of age, IQ remains at the national average; there is virtually no change in IQ between 6 and 12 years of age (Azen et al, 1991; Fishler et al, 1987; Koch, 1993).

Children with late-diagnosed PKU should also be placed on the phe-restricted diet no matter how late they are identified as having PKU (de Koning et al, 1998). Improvements in behavior and cognitive functioning have been seen in individuals with severe retardation who had untreated PKU (Clarke et al, 1987; Koch and Wenz, 1987; Koch et al, 1998b).

Recent and Anticipated Advances in Diagnosis and Management

The correlation of the clinical phenotype of individuals with PKU with their genotype continues in populations worldwide with hopes of improving

Table 31-3
Mean 12-Year WISC-R, WRAT, and Parent WAIS IQ Scores* for PKU Collaborative Study
Children** Grouped by Age at Loss of Dietary Control

Loss of Dietary Control, Age in Years:	<6	6 to 10	>10	ANOVA P
WISC-R[1] IQ scores	n = 23	n = 47	n = 25	
Verbal	85 ± 15	95 ± 14	101 ± 11	.0004
Performance	92 ± 15	95 ± 14	101 ± 11	.0499
Full scale	87 ± 14	96 ± 14	101 ± 11	.0028
WRAT[2] standard scores	n = 22	n = 46	n = 20	
Reading	92 ± 13	97 ± 11	105 ± 12	.0029
Spelling	87 ± 17	92 ± 13	98 ± 17	.0452
Arithmetic	80 ± 11	82 ± 11	84 ± 10	.6033
Parent WAIS IQ[3] scores	n = 23	n = 43	n = 25	
Full scale	104 ± 10	109 ± 9	108 ± 14	.1905

Adapted from Azen CG, Koch R, Friedman EG et al: *Am J Dis Child,* 145:35-39, 1991.
*Values are means ± SDs.
**The PKU Collaborative Study supported by grant 4-RO1-HD-09543 and contract N01-HD-4-3807 from NICHHD, NIH.
[1]Weschler Intelligence Scale for Children-Revised
[2]Wide Range Achievement Test
[3]Weschler Adult Intelligence Scale

the clinical outcome of PKU (Scriver, 1998). Other modes of therapy for PKU continue to be investigated. New protein sources, phe-free genetically modified human therapeutic proteins, are being developed to enhance the diet until there is a cure for PKU (Schuett, 1999). Based on research of the depletion of dopamine in the prefrontal cortex, supplementation of the large neutral amino acids could offset the effects on the brain of persisting phe levels of 120 to 360 μM (Diamond, 1993; Diamond, 1998). Pioneers in hepatic gene therapy are aiming to restore enough PAH enzyme activity to make phe restriction unnecessary; the PAH gene has successfully been delivered to the hepatocyte of the PKU mouse model (Sarkissian, Boulais, and Scriver, 1998). Microencapsulation of recombinant phenylalanine ammonia lyase (PAL), an enzyme capable of being delivered to the gastrointestinal tract by oral ingestion, degrades phenylalanine to a harmless metabolite; work is progressing in the PKU mouse model. If successful, PAL would make the PKU diet less restrictive for humans (Sarkissian et al, 1999). Phenylalanine tolerance was restored to a 10-year-old boy with PKU who received a liver transplant for concurrent active cirrhosis (Vajro et al, 1993). Liver transplantation may potentially benefit the BH_4-deficiency disorders, but because early lifelong dietary restriction of phe improves the prognosis of PKU, it is not warranted.

Associated Problems (Box 31-3)

Neurologic Changes

Parents and children must be apprised of the lifelong vulnerability of the nervous system to HPA. Abnormal findings in cerebral white matter are common on cranial magnetic resonance imaging (MRI) of children treated early or late for PKU; abnormalities in the periventricular and subcortical white matter have been seen in children with PKU aged 7 years and older. Clinically, there was no evidence of neurologic deterioration of the 25 early treated children with PKU studied by MRI, although 40% showed brisk lower-limb reflexes. In anticipation of psychopathology, the use of DNA mutation analysis assists in making decisions about dietary quality and duration. On diet, psychiatric disturbances of anxiety, depression and hysteria are alleviated. Attention deficit and hyperactivity disorder (ADHD) and attention deficit disorder (ADD) are often diagnosed in children even if their phe levels are consistently less than 600 μM and the IQs are in normal range. A characteristic of both PKU and ADHD is a "negative task orientation," but not an increase in "negative social behavior" typical of ADHD. Specific deficits in selective and sustained attention are correlated with elevated phe levels at time of testing phe (Schuett, 1999b).

The extent of changes in the brain as measured by MRI, Visual Evoked Potentials (VEPs), and Brainstem Auditory Evoked Potentials (BAEPs) does not correlate with the start, duration, or quality of dietary treatment, as much as the degree of HPA at the time of the studies and the number of years since the phe-restricted diet was stopped. Normalized MRI scans are found in children whose phe levels are consistently below 360 μM (Schuett, 1997a; Schuett, 1999b; Thompson et al, 1993). Immature myelin, demyelinization, and edema respond within a few weeks or months of re-instituting phe restriction. In young children still receiving a well-controlled, phe-restricted diet, the clinical risk appears to be predominately of impairment of intellectual function, whereas in older individuals with PKU on relaxed or normal diets, the risk is progressive damage to the white matter. The risk of myelin damage increases the longer the individual is exposed to unrestricted amounts of phe. Demyelinization is the extreme manifestation of

more generalized myelin changes and could explain irreversible neurologic deterioration (Cockburn et al, 1996).

Cognitive Deficits

Deficits in cognitive function relative to mathematic conceptualizations are a troubling finding in children with PKU who have maintained good phe control since birth. When tested at 12 years of age, children with well-controlled PKU scored 17 points lower on the WRAT for arithmetic than previous baseline levels. This scoring does not indicate gross deficits in the intellectual status of treated children with PKU but is evidence of subtle deficits that become more pronounced over time (Table 31-3).

Children with PKU who have maintained good phe control often have difficulty with visual perception and linquistic development (Brunner, Berch, and Berry, 1987). Neither the age at which treatment was initiated nor the phe level during the early years of life correlate with a discrepancy in skills of children with PKU compared with their siblings at 5 years of age on tests of visual perception and at 7 years of age on tests of psycholinguistic abilities (Fishler et al, 1987). In a study of 16 young adults ages 13 to 20 years old with PKU, whose phe level ranged between 300 to 500 μM, their mutation genotype correlated with MRI findings of frontal white matter changes and with deficits in visuospatial learning and memory and visuomotor functioning, suggesting that there are limitations to the effect of dietary treatment in HPA (Cockburn et al, 1996; Lou et al, 1992, 1994). In another study (Craft et al, 1992), boys treated early for PKU (mean age 9.76 ± 2.97 years) exhibited right visual field impairment in disengaging attention, indicative of left hemisphere dysfunction, and overall slowed reaction times. The lifelong outcome for children with well-treated PKU is yet to be observed because the history of early-treated PKU is relatively short.

Gammaglobulinemia

Environmental factors and genetic factors affect IgE synthesis in children with PKU. PKU appears to be a metabolic disorder with particular immunologic features (e.g., low IgG levels and high IgE levels), but, when treated with diet therapy, the high rate of allergic pathology—specifically asthma—does not occur. Elevated IgE levels in children with PKU must be considered a gammaglobulinemic disorder, similar to some inherited primary immunodeficiencies in which asthma is exceptional, despite high IgE levels (e.g., common variable immune deficiency, Job syndrome, and Wiskott-Aldrich syndrome). Allergic sensitizations are more frequent in children with PKU (Riva et al, 1994).

Pyloric Stenosis

Pyloric stenosis has been observed more often in males with PKU than in the general male newborn population (male-female ratio is 5:1). Children of either sex identified with pyloric stenosis should be retested for PKU (Koch and Wenz, 1987).

Peptic Ulcer

Peptic ulcer, with the uncommon complication of bleeding or perforation, has been documented in both sexes of individuals (11 to 25 years of age) with PKU. The relationship of peptic ulcer to PKU is not clear. Elevated blood phe concentrations secondary to PAH deficiency may lead to increased gastric secretion, which in some individuals results in peptic ulceration; vomiting, which was formerly a common presenting symptom in untreated children with PKU, could possibly be explained by this same mechanism (Scriver et al, 1995). Peptic ulcer could be related to the dietary treatment; L-amino acid supplements can stimulate gastric acid secretion (Greeves, Carson, and Dodge, 1988).

Prognosis

Three major factors affect the prognosis for PKU: (1) age at time of diagnosis and phe restriction, (2) quality and length of dietary control, and (3) socioeconomic status (Koch et al, 1998). The values of blood phe concentration at the first screening test and before treatment are not predictive of the PKU phenotype or IQ (Enns et al, 1998; Spada et al, 1997). The phenotypic expression of PKU represents the degree of homeostasis achieved given the variables at the PKU locus and in the environment, as well as the variable of the collective genotype at other loci that can neutralize the PKU allele at the

PKU locus. "The most relevant environmental variable for PKU is food intake, which can be influenced by culture, income, and family structure. If the family environment does not support compliance to a special diet, the outcome of a normally predictable course can drastically change" (Valle and Mitchell, 1994, pp 4-5). Imperfections in the dietary treatment of PKU as it is currently known and delays in treatment are all factors evidenced by neuropsychologic and cognitive functions that are slightly less than average in treated individuals with PKU.

PRIMARY CARE MANAGEMENT

Health Care Maintenance

Growth and Development

Growth and development are normal for children with PKU on a controlled, phe-restricted diet. Head circumference, weight, and length are measured at scheduled monthly intervals for the first year, then every 3 months until after the prepubertal growth spurt, and every 6 months throughout adolescence to monitor adequacy of diet. There is a tendency toward obesity in children with PKU (McBurnie et al, 1991) that is related to the high caloric density of natural food sources necessary to meet the child's RDA for calories, the free sugar in the EMF product, and the free foods high in carbohydrates.

Children with PKU are at risk for having low self-esteem. Because they require a special diet and they are different from others are obvious causes. The possible consequences of being taken off the diet and the effect that high blood phe levels have on their behavior contribute to this risk. Children with PKU who are older than age 4 years are at risk for having immature social interaction and interpersonal skills (Kazak, Reber, and Snitzer, 1988). Continuing the phe-restricted diet, becoming involved in PKU peer-support groups, promoting self-control of the diet at an early age, and deemphasizing that children with PKU are "different" are easier said than done. Art therapy with younger children and role-playing for older children are only some of the creative ways to elicit a child's attitudes about having PKU. As children approach school age, parents must be encouraged to enhance their child's social development by allowing them to spend increasing amounts of time outside the immediate family.

Affective disorders and acting out behaviors are not the norm for well-managed children with PKU; the psychologist on the medical genetics PKU treatment team is a resource for dealing with these issues and knowing when professional intervention is required.

Diet

Dietary support at all developmental stages of the individual with PKU is an important component of therapy. Monitoring of phe concentrations with weight and diet changes needs to occur throughout an individual's life. It is important to initiate self-management of the phe-restricted diet early in childhood (Trahms, 1992a,b,c). Some reasons for failure to achieve long-term adherence to the phe-restricted diet include poor family coping skills, increasing independence of children, limited food choices, and unpalatable EMF products.

In infants, protein is initially prescribed in an amount greater than the RDA. When the EMF is the primary source of protein, the requirement for protein increases because of rapid absorption, early and high peak of plasma amino acids, and rapid catabolism of amino acids. Mature human breast milk (>15 days' lactation) is an ideal source of whole protein for the infant with PKU (Greve et al, 1994). Breast milk, compared with cow's milk, contains an amino acid composition that supports adequate growth at a lower protein intake (0.9 to 1.0 vs. 3.3 g/dl) and enhances bioavailability of minerals and trace elements (especially zinc) because of the greater percentage of protein (70% vs. 20%) from the predominant whey fraction. Breast milk, if fed for 4 or more months, supplies docosahexaenoic acid (DHA) and its essential fatty acid precursor, a-linolenic acid (AA), in which bottle-fed infants and—especially—infants fed low-phe formula are deficient. Treated children with PKU have significant deficits in the DHA content of their erythrocyte phospholipid membranes. The phospholipid membranes of their nervous systems may be deficient as well, which would explain some of the neurologic findings on MRIs and VEPs and learning difficulties in even early and well-treated

children (Cockburn et al, 1996). Breast milk has a lower phe content per ounce compared with other formulas.*

Infants with PKU should be given a variety of foods at the appropriate ages so that these foods become part of their diet later in life. It is recommended to ingest one third of the total amount of EMF with main meals to optimize utilization of total protein intake by the body. A system of food exchanges in which phe content is used as the basis for providing specific amounts of foods by food group is employed. Foods of similar phe content are grouped together and are exchanged, one for another, within the list to give variety to the diet (Acosta and Yannicelli, 1997).

EMF products are sensitive to heat and a prolonged shelf life. These products should not be heated beyond 54.5°C because of the Maillard reaction; amino acids, peptides, and proteins condense with sugars, forming bonds for which no digestive enzymes are available. The reaction is initially characterized by a light brown color, followed by buff yellow and then dark brown; caramel-like and roasted aromas develop. Any amino-acid preparation should be inspected for these changes, and the expiration date checked before use. The shelf life for EMF products is generally 2 years. The vitamin C content diminishes initially, followed by the vitamin A and D content, which can decrease to as much as 30% below labeled values after the expiration date. In addition, the fats in EMF products become rancid after the expiration date. Products containing L-amino acids taste best when served cold (i.e., frozen to a slush) to disguise the sulfurous bitter taste. There is no contraindication for freezing EMF products or warming them to under 54.5°C. Terminal sterilization of an infant's EMF formula is contraindicated (Acosta and Yannicelli, 1997).

Activities besides those revolving around food can be promoted with peers. Quality peer relationships are important, not those in which an individual has to eat the same things to be accepted. Food is a social instrument for children of any age, and every effort should be made to use the available

---

*Breast milk = 12.3 mg of phe/oz; Enfamil = 17 mg of phe/oz; Similac[20] = 22 mg of phe/oz; SMA = 24 mg of phe/oz; Isomil and Prosobee = 29 mg of phe/oz; and cow's milk = 104 mg of phe/oz.

tips from an experienced nutritionist to approximate the visual, textural, and taste appeal of the unrestricted diet.

Safety

Children with PKU are not at an increased risk of acute safety hazards. Chronic ingestion of excess dietary phe is more deleterious to the health of a child than the accidental intake of a product containing aspartame. A Medic-Alert bracelet or necklace that indicates "special PKU diet" is added assurance that a child with PKU will receive proper care in case of an emergency.

Because chronic ingestion of EMF products can lead to nutritional deficiencies, these products are contraindicated for individuals not diagnosed as needing a phe-restricted diet.

Pigmented lesions (i.e., melanin spots that are light brown to black) occur in individuals with PKU. The oculocutaneous pigmentary dilution observed even in children with PKU who adhere to a phe-restricted diet is a systemic mechanism related to the disturbed phe-tyr ratio in the circulation. The pigmentary activity of the epidermal melanocytes is unimpaired in individuals with PKU and is normal at the skin level peripherally. Erythema response and ability to tan after exposure to artificial or natural light for individuals with PKU have been demonstrated to be no different than for individuals without PKU who are blonde (Bolognia and Pawelek, 1988; Hassel and Brunsting, 1959). Limiting exposure to the sun and using sunblocks are recommended for children with PKU as they are for any child.

Immunizations

The immunization schedule for children with PKU is the same as it is for any child. Children with PKU must be closely observed for a reaction to the immunization. A febrile reaction can lead to a catabolic state, increasing plasma phe levels. Any illness should be supported with adequate hydration and calories.

Screening

Vision: Routine screening is recommended.

Hearing: Routine screening is recommended.

Dental: The diet for PKU contains sufficient carbohydrate to present more than the usual potential for dental decay. The phe-restricted diet relies on frequent intake of carbohydrates to meet the daily requirement for calories. Explanations to parents about the role that frequency of carbohydrate consumption has and the effects of extremes (e.g., nursing bottle caries or uncontrolled access to candy) helps focus their efforts. Practical goals include weaning children with PKU to a glass as soon as possible, starting with sips at 6 months of age; following retentive foods with fibrous ones to affect food removal; using liquid forms of carbohydrate when possible to promote oral clearance; offering free foods such as fruits in place of more retentive forms of refined sugars; and initiating dental hygiene and screening at the eruption of the first tooth with close follow-up thereafter (Casamassimo et al, 1984).

Blood pressure: Routine screening is recommended.

Hematocrit: Iron status is monitored by plasma ferritin levels at 6, 9, and 12 months of age and then every 6 months thereafter. Hemoglobin and hematocrit values are evaluated at 6 and 12 months of age and annually thereafter. Children with anemia will have a falsely low phe level, and newborns with polycythemia can have a falsely high phe level.

Breast-fed infants with PKU have exaggerated physiologic anemia of infancy, requiring iron supplementation when the hematocrit value approaches 30%.

Urinalysis: Routine screening is recommended.

Tuberculosis: Routine screening is recommended.

Condition-Specific Screening (Box 31-4)

Urine screening for biopterin: The analysis of pterins in urine is done in all newborns with HPA to differentiate PKU and mild HPA from the BH_4-deficiency disorders. This selective screening test is best collected by the primary care provider taking caution not to expose the clean-catch urine to light and delivering by next-day courier at room temperature to the metabolic genetics laboratory designated by the medical genetics PKU treatment center.

Box 31-4

Condition-Specific Screening

Urine biopterin (BH$_2$/BH$_4$) screening
Erythrocyte DHPR screening
Blood phe monitoring
Nutritional indices screening
Auscultation for dysrhythmias
DNA analysis

The qualitative urine test for PKU (ferric chloride reaction or Phenistix) measures phenylpyruvic acid, which is not excreted in the urine until blood phe levels reach 1000 μM. Care must be taken in the interpretation of a ferric chloride reaction because of false-positive and false-negative test results caused by instability of urine specimens and interfering metabolites (Nystaform-HC ointment or iodochlorhydroxyquin, salicylates, phenothiazine derivatives, isoniazid, and L-dopa metabolites). Phenistix is not a substitute for either newborn screening or monitoring of phe levels because blood levels of phe should not be as high as 1000 μM.

Erythrocyte DHPR screening: Dried blood spots collected by heelstick and sent to the designated genetics laboratory for enzymology screen children with HPA for the cofactor variant DHPR.

Blood phe monitoring: The blood test for phe (newborn, child, and adult), whether for screening or diet monitoring, is a capillary blood sample obtained from a free-flowing puncture wound 2 to 4 hours postprandially. Only a blood specimen is reliable in detecting quantitative or semiquantitative levels of phe; phe content can be measured by different laboratory techniques. A fluorometric assay of blood spotted directly onto filter paper yields a mean phe level higher than a spot applied from a capillary tube or dorsal vein, 160 μM, 150 μM and 140 μM, respectively. Using a collection technique other than a heelstick for the collection of a phe level puts a newborn at risk for a false-negative result (Jew et al, 1994; Lorey and Cunningham, 1994).

Immediately after birth (up to 2 hours) the mean phe value in newborns without PKU is 167 μM. This value quickly rises to a peak of 185 μM at 7 to 9 hours of age, and slowly tapers off to 165 μM at 24 hours; after 24 hours of age the mean phe value is 161 μM by fluorometric assay. For infants the upper limit of normal phe is <120 μM, for children 62 ± 18 μM, for teenagers 60 ± 13 μM and for adults 58 ± 15 μM (Scriver et al, 1995).

Plasma phe and tyr levels are evaluated twice weekly by quantitative methods in newborns with PKU until concentrations are stabilized and approximate dietary phe and tyr requirements are known. Thereafter, blood phe is evaluated twice weekly with dietary changes or weekly without dietary changes in both infants and children. The plasma phe and tyr levels are evaluated by the medical genetics PKU treatment center team.

Nutritional indices screening: Nutrient intake is recorded on provided forms for 3 days before each blood phe test and evaluated for phe, tyr, protein, and energy intake by the nutritionist on the PKU treatment team. Protein status is evaluated by plasma albumin or prealbumin levels or both every 3 months in infants and every 6 months in children and adolescents. Individuals on semisynthetic diets are at high risk for deficiencies in the trace elements. Insufficient intake of iron, zinc, and selenium and the interaction of iron with copper and zinc at the intestinal level can cause deficiencies. Safe ranges of fluoride, selenium, and molybdenum are also monitored by the medical genetics PKU treatment team. Overall balance of nutrients is critical in the child with PKU.

Auscultation: Regular auscultation of heart sounds of children with PKU on a phe-restricted diet is advisable for detection of a dysrhythmia. Selenium deficiency related to a low-protein diet and altered bioavailability can cause ventricular tachycardia that is corrected by selenium supplementation (Greeves et al, 1990).

DNA analysis: Nucleic acid analysis can be done from blood spotted onto filter paper as described above. Caution should be taken in prepping the skin with alcohol—not betadine, and blood should not be collected in heparinized (lithium) tubing and transferred to the filter paper. The filter paper should be properly identified and mailed to the DNA lab specified by the medical genetics PKU treatment center team.

Phenylalanine tolerance testing: The practice of phe challenges is no longer warranted with the advent of DNA mutation analysis.

Common Illness Management

Differential Diagnosis (Box 31-5)

Management during illness and surgery: If a child with PKU has a negative nitrogen balance for any reason, the blood phe content can be elevated because body-tissue protein catabolism occurs, releasing phe. The paradox of phe-restricted diets is in the transient elevations of plasma phe when phe is overrestricted; protein synthesis is blocked by nutrient deficiency (negative nitrogen balance), resulting in impaired flow of phe to anabolic nitrogen pools. An elevated temperature is just one of many reasons for a negative nitrogen balance. An accurate history of a child's illness and dietary intake before the illness may help distinguish the cause of a catabolic reaction.

During common childhood illnesses the blood phe level is not tested until the child is well, as long as the illness is less than 3 weeks in duration. During the illness, supportive measures should be undertaken to limit protein catabolism. In infants or adolescents, energy intake should be enhanced by allowing (1) as much fruit juice as tolerated; (2) liquid-flavored gelatin stabilized by carageenan; (3) polycose glucose polymers (liquid or powder) added to the fruit juices; (4) caffeine-free, nondiet soft drinks; and (5) electrolyte formulas (e.g., Pedialyte) without NutraSweet. With close consultation with the medical genetics PKU treatment team, children with PKU are returned to the EMF and preillness diet plan as rapidly as tolerated; usually the EMF product is initiated at one-half original strength, then full strength as tolerated (Acosta and Yannicelli, 1997).

Minor uncomplicated surgery (e.g., tonsillectomy, hernia repair, cytoscopy) with the child under general anesthesia does not cause major alteration in the blood phe level. The highest blood phe levels (1029 μM) occur approximately on the second postoperative day and decline on the fourth postoperative day (605 μM). Because the elevation in phe level is transient, no special dietary measures are needed (Fiedler et al, 1982).

Skin lesions: Localized or generalized eczema and peeling of the soles of the feet and the palms of the hands occur after a long-term catabolic state. Skin lesions related to an amino acid imbalance and disturbed phe-tyr ratio must be distinguished from other rashes by accurate history of the lesion and diet. Establishing phe homeostasis will resolve

eczema and peeling that are not responsive to topical medications.

Children with skin lesions suggestive of scleroderma, severe localized induration of the skin, subcutaneous tissue, and muscle should be tested for PKU. Scleroderma, a rare, often familial, connective tissue disorder and untreated PKU both have a common secondary biochemical deficiency of tryptophan. Tryptophan is an immediate precursor of serotonin and the catecholamines in the tyrosine metabolic pathway. An increased concentration of phe decreases availability of tyr and tryptophan. The scleroderma-like changes observed in PKU appear earlier (first year of life), and have a different distribution and histologic pattern in children in contrast to true scleroderma but become indistinguishable with age (Irons and Levy, 1986; Nova, Kaufman, and Halperin, 1992).

Drug Interactions

Aspartame: Aspartame (APM) is contraindicated in individuals with PKU, and care must be taken to read content labels of food, beverages, vitamins, and medicines for its presence. Marketed under the brand name NutraSweet, the high-intensity artificial sweetener is no longer solely distributed by NutraSweet Company; the familiar NutraSweet swirl logo alerting individuals with PKU to APM in the product may not be displayed on the packaging. The FDA requires the statement "PHENYLKETONURICS: CONTAINS PHENYLALANINE" on the label of all products containing the white, odorless, crystalline powder consisting of two amino acids: L-phenylalanine and L-aspartic acid.

For children with PKU, ingesting 34 mg of APM per kg of body weight will elevate the plasma phe level to approximately 850 $\mu M;$ a quart of APM-sweetened Kool Aid contains 280 mg of phe, which is approximately half the child's daily allowance of phe (Scriver et al, 1995). For individuals with mild HPA who tolerate 50 to 100 mg of phe/kg, APM is not recommended; the acceptable daily intake of APM for individuals without PKU or mild HPA is 40 mg/kg. Individuals who carry the PKU gene and ingest APM have safe levels of phe that persist longer in their bodies than in individuals who are not carriers (Curtius, Endres, and Blau, 1994). During pregnancy, the use of APM by women with PKU is not recommended because of a 1:2 concentration gradient for phe between the maternal and fetal blood (Scriver et al, 1995).

Before prescribing medications for a child with PKU, check the *Physicians' Desk Reference* (PDR), *Drug Facts and Comparisons,* and *Table of Drug Products Containing Phenylalanine* (Arnold, 1998) for the ingredient phenylalanine or L-aspartyl-L-phenylalanine methyl ester (APM). Parents should be cautioned about APM in over-the-counter medications or vitamins or any product labeled "sugar-free." The exact amount of phe in medications must be calculated as part of a child's daily phe intake.

Any drug that affects the neurotransmitters in the CNS should be thoroughly investigated before it is prescribed for children or young adults with PKU. For example, the Daraprim tablet, pyrimethamine, is listed in the PDR as causing HPA and is contraindicated in individuals with PKU. Great care must be taken when individuals with PKU are on any medication, especially when blood phe levels change and when medication is withdrawn (Dolan et al, 1998).

Psychotropic medications: Elevated blood phe and low tyr blood levels affect neurotransmission in the CNS. High blood phe levels decrease the production of serotonin, a neurotransmitter for mood maintenance. Phe/tyr homeostasis should first be achieved in children or young adults experiencing any of the mood disorders previously described. Psychotropic drugs should be used with caution and only as a last resort with the metabolic treatment team's consultation. Neurotoxicity of phenylethylamine is a concern with the use of MAO inhibitors. Use of the serotonin inhibitors for depression in an individual with PKU is yet to be described (Dolan et al, 1998; Kaufman, 1989; Schuett, 1999a).

Oral contraceptives: Fluctuations can occur in plasma amino acids during the menstrual cycle. Plasma phe and tyr levels should be monitored when women with PKU are using oral contraceptives.

Developmental Issues

Sleep Patterns

There are diurnal variations of phe and tyr levels in children who have and do not have PKU. The difference in children with PKU is an elevation of the tyr level in the evening, similar to children without PKU, but a decrease in the phe level at night, unlike unaffected children. The implications of this variation in the phe/tyr ratio are in the relationship to tryptophan, the precursor of serotonin. In the presence of low phe levels, the tryptophan level is elevated. Elevation of tryptophan markedly reduces the total time in rapid eye movement (REM) sleep to 3% (normal REM time in children is 29.5% $\pm$ 4.8%). During lower levels of tryptophan, REM sleep is increased to 8% to 11%. Changes in blood phe levels are related to the timing of EMF (or protein substitute) intake. The greater the quantity of EMF consumed by late afternoon (4 PM), the greater the decrease in phe levels during the day. The less EMF taken before this time, the greater the increase in phe levels. Children with PKU are more susceptible to sleep disturbances, which can be expressed as insomnia or hyperactivity at night. Children who have elevated levels of phe can often have disturbed sleep patterns with nightmares. Any alteration in the ratios of phe, tyr, and tryptophan can cause sleep disturbances; a phe-restricted diet balanced throughout the 24-hour time period optimizes sleep patterns in children with PKU (Herrero et al, 1983; MacDonald et al, 1999).

Toileting

Infants with PKU who are prone to eczema may experience more problems with diaper dermatitis. Careful, explicit instructions on standard management techniques should be given and follow-up appointments made for evaluation of treatment success. Toileting habits become an issue when phe control is lost. When the blood phe level is elevated for any reason, phenylketones are present in the urine and sweat, causing the characteristic musty odor of PKU. Attention to and training of children in their hygiene needs at all ages will avoid unnecessary embarrassment.

Discipline

Consistent discipline for children with PKU is as—if not more—important as it is for any child. Food is a very major social component in any child's life, and how it is managed from the very beginning by parents can determine the success of the only current therapy for PKU, dietary restriction of phe. A major pitfall in disciplining children with PKU is to use food as a reward system and the need for blood tests as punishment. Strategies to help children to adhere to special diets are available.

Child Care

More than one individual in the child's home environment should be knowledgable about the phe-restricted diet and the preparation of EMF products. Materials about PKU written specifically for baby-sitters, grandparents, and teachers, as well as creative ideas on how to deal with these issues, can be found in *National PKU News*.

Schooling

Children with treated PKU experience difficulties in school more often than unaffected children; 33% of children with PKU are 1 or more years below grade level compared with 14% of children in the general white population. For grades 1 through 4, 38% of girls with PKU are 1 or more years below compared with 29% of boys with PKU (Fishler et al, 1987).

Children with PKU need comprehensive integrated psychodiagnostic and neuropsychologic assessments. Developmental testing is ideally performed at the medical genetics PKU treatment center at scheduled intervals starting at 6 months of age and every 6 months until 2 years of age, then annually thereafter. For optimal performance, it is important that the child's blood phe level be in maintenance range on the day of testing.

Anticipatory guidance in the development of visual-spatial skills may be required. Computer games and software programs that train and stimu-

late the development of visual-spatial skills and hand-eye coordination are ideal. Attention to proper lighting is important so that contrasts are clear; black on a white background is perceived better than grey or a monotone by children with PKU (Diamond, unpublished work). Special education in math and language acquisition may also be necessary. Teacher involvement at all stages of the child's schooling is important.

Sexuality

Sexual development and curiosity are no different for children with PKU than for any other child. Genetic counseling specifically for children with PKU is individualized to a child's understanding of PKU and to assessment of a child's readiness. The medical genetics PKU treatment team works closely with families on this issue, and often PKU peer support groups and videos specific to the developmental stage of the child or adolescent with PKU are beneficial.

For the female adolescents with PKU, the onset of menses can cause fluctuations in the plasma amino acid pattern, specifically the tyr level. Monitoring the quantitative plasma amino acid levels is important to ensure that excesses or deficiencies can be alleviated by dietary intervention. Discussions of contraception and the implications of being a woman with PKU should be individualized and approached with sensitivity. PKU peer support groups and written materials and videos designed specifically for female adolescents with PKU are available.

Transition to Adulthood

Individuals with PKU can successfully adjust to society. Worldwide, few adults with PKU are on a phe-restricted diet. It has only been since the 1990s that a *lifelong* diet has been advocated through the developmental stages of adulthood. The first successful pregnancy outcomes from MPKU surveillance were being realized in 1990, when the children enrolled in the PKU Collaborative Study reached 12 years of age, demonstrating that the best performance profiles were by children with PKU who adhered to phe restriction the longest and maintained phe levels (<363 μM) more closely approximating phe homeostasis. These results show the protective benefits of long-term dietary therapy.

To realize optimal psychologic and behavior benefits, adults with PKU should not completely stop the diet but can liberalize phe intake (Koch et al, 1998; Pietz et al, 1993). There is roughly a 30% reduction of serum phe levels with advancing age (Pitt and Danks, 1994).

Although some of the effects of PKU are directly related to phe levels, others seem to be unaffected by institution or reinstitution of phe restriction. A study (Ris et al, 1994) of the late effects of PKU demonstrated that although IQs were normal in adults (>18 years) who benefited from early treatment in childhood, their IQs and performance on measures of attention and complex visuoconstructional ability were lower than their unaffected siblings. Both the age at which blood phe levels rose >1200 μM and the age the EMF was discontinued correlated with intellectual and—to a lesser extent—neuropsychologic variables. This study validates previous observations by others that concurrent elevation of blood phe levels are strongly correlated with lowered, reversible neuropsychologic measures indicative of selective impairment of executive functions: set maintenance, planning, impulse control, organized search, and flexibility of thought and action.

The hazards of losses experienced off dietary control are observed from both the chronic and acute effects of PKU. The natural history of untreated PKU in individuals ages 28 to 72 years (Pitt and Danks, 1994) suggests that PKU does not generally cause a progressive loss of abilities in adult life beyond the irreversible effects sustained in childhood. General health problems, other than those previously associated with untreated PKU in childhood, are not remarkable in adults with PKU; their causes of death are the same as for individuals without PKU and not related to PKU. A vigilant study (Dolan et al, 1998) of untreated older adults with PKU who were started very slowly on a personalized lowering of dietary phe, showed a reduction of behavioral manifestations that previously interfered with abilities, as well as an enhancement of social skills.

Young adults with PKU—especially women—are at risk for depression, anxiety, and agoraphobia that lessen with reinstitution of phe restriction (Waisbren et al, 1997). Emotional effects can persist despite reductions in phe levels. Women with PKU who are treated early in childhood and later go off the diet tend to seek professional help or be on medications for emotional problems that begin in the teens. The biochemical difficulties in PKU, rather than the fact of having a chronic medical problem, are related to personality psychopathology. Although all individuals treated early for PKU function normally within a social context, those who continue or reinstitute phe homeostasis—especially women—benefit in measurable and immeasurable ways. Participation in a Maternal PKU Camp or program is a supportive activity for women with PKU.

Maternal PKU: The first generation of identified and treated infants with PKU are now of childbearing age. The incidence of undiagnosed MPKU is about 1 in 30,000. Sexual activity among adolescents and young women with HPA is no different than it is for their peers without PKU. The success of dietary therapy in arresting the neurologic deficits caused by HPA has inadvertently produced an increasing number of non-HPA mentally retarded offspring with MPKU syndrome; the possibility exists that in one generation the incidence of PKU-related mental retardation could return to the level it was before NBS and treatment were available.

A minimal teratogenic effect of HPA occurs when maternal blood phe levels are maintained between 120 and 360 μM. Women with PKU who do not maintain blood phe control before and throughout an entire pregnancy may have infants without PKU but with other birth defects (Levy et al, 1996). The fetus is at great risk for the teratologic effects of phe exposure because of a positive transplacental gradient of phe approximately 1.13 to 2.19 times higher than the maternal blood phe level. The results of high maternal blood phe levels (>360 μM) in the fetus, especially in the first trimester, are mental retardation, microcephaly, intrauterine and postnatal growth delay, left-outflow-tract cardiac defects, and a constellation of facial dysmorphic features (MPKU syndrome) (Figure 31-3). Compared with those born to women who do not have PKU, 24% of the offspring born to mothers with PKU had abnormal head circumferences (HCs). At levels of 120 to 360 μM, 6% of infants had microcephaly, 4% had postnatal growth retardation, and none had intrauterine growth retardation, in contrast to 85%, 51%, and 26%, respectively, with phe >900 μM. Deceleration of head growth after birth is evident in the first year of life, even if an infant is not microcephalic at birth, in offspring of women with

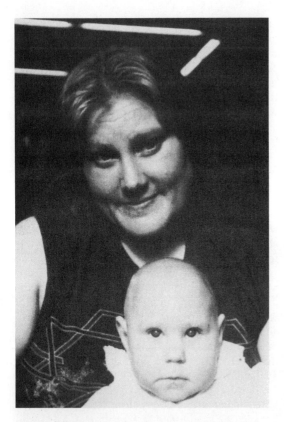

Figure 31-3 Mother with 8-month-old daughter with MPKU syndrome.

PKU who maintained phe levels <600 μ*M*. Women with mild HPA who maintained blood phe levels <360 μ*M* without phe restriction throughout pregnancy had offspring with HCs in the 43rd percentile (Matalon et al, 1994; Rouse et al, 1997). Dose-related effects of phe on pregnancy are evident.

Of women with PKU whose phe levels were >1211 μ*M* throughout pregnancy, 90% had offspring who were microcephalic and whose weight, length, and HC were all below the 3rd percentile; 97% of their offspring had at least one dysmorphic feature. All offspring of women with PKU had at least one dysmorphic feature regardless of how well phe restriction was controlled; facial appearance included epicanthal folds, prominent ears, long philtrum, upturned nose, micrognathia, and wide, depressed nasal bridge. None of the mothers with PKU who maintained their phe level <360 μ*M* had children with the cardiac defects

that were found in the offspring of the mothers with higher phe levels. Defects included ventricular septal defect, hypoplastic left ventricle, coarctation of the aorta, and tetrology of Fallot. The risk of cardiac defects in children born to mothers with PKU whose phe levels are not in control by 8 weeks' gestation is 14% compared with 0.5% to 1.0% risk for the general population (Rouse B et al, 1997).

Pregnancy in women with PKU is a medical challenge. The goals of diet are similar to those for pregnant teenagers without PKU with respect to normal and appropriate weight gain based on height, prepregnancy weight, and gestational age, with indices of nutritional status in the normal range. Concentration of blood phe should be between 121 and 242 μ*M*, and tyr concentration should be 100 μ*M*. The phe requirements vary in the same woman throughout pregnancy depending on age, weight gain, trimester of pregnancy, adequacy of energy and protein intakes, and state of maternal health. At 20 weeks' gestation the phe requirements increase dramatically. Magnesium, copper, and cholesterol levels are significantly lower in MPKU (Acosta and Yannicelli, 1997), and special EMF products have been developed to meet these needs.

Paternal PKU: Historically, few males with PKU have been followed to age 18; therefore primary care providers must educate them on the importance of remaining on diet for the benefits of lessening depression, agitation, and aggressiveness, and improving attention span and concentration. Fertility does not appear to be affected in men with PKU. An inverse correlation between plasma phe level and semen volume and between plasma phe level and sperm count has been observed, however, indicating another benefit of achieving phe homeostasis (Fisch, et al, 1991b).

Special Family Concerns and Resources

PKU is prevalent in all populations. Because PKU is a universal disorder, the cultural and ethnic implications are just as diverse. Cultural and ethnic preferences need to be considered when planning the diet, providing genetic counseling, and discussing family planning options. Maternal PKU is one example of how two different cultures perceive PKU. In a study comparing attitudes of women with PKU in the United States with those in Israel, Israeli women perceived PKU more negatively and had less knowledge about MPKU than women in the United States. Because Israeli women shun premarital sex and use oral contraception more frequently, however, the number of MPKU pregnancies treated before conception in Israel is proportionately greater than those treated in the United States (Shiloh et al, 1993).

Mutation analysis has provided insights into the population genetics of PKU. A founder effect, genetic drift, and heterozygote advantage in the origins and distribution of mutant PAH alleles in the human population have all been proposed (Eisensmith et al, 1995; Scriver et al, 1995). Significant correlations exist between some RFLP haps and HPA phenotypes within specific populations (Scriver et al, 1995). Haps 1 through 6 together account for over 80% of all mutant chromosomes in many European populations; however, it is not an exclusive relationship. Haps 1 and 4 are common among chromosomes in both normal individuals and those with PKU, as is the case with hap 4 which is exclusively found in the Asian population. Most individuals with PKU in northern European populations who have any combination of mutant PAH alleles on hap 2 or 3 exhibit a severe form of PKU, whereas if they have mutant PAH alleles on hap 1 or 4 they display a wide range of HPA phenotypes (Scriver et al, 1995). Genotype-phenotype correlations are less well characterized in the United States and cannot be inferred (Enns, 1997).

The degree of HPA in PKU cannot currently be predicted from hap and DNA mutation analysis. Parents must live with the knowledge that their child's intellectual development depends on how well the diet is managed. Outcome is directly related to the effectiveness of dietary control and genetic potential inherited from the parents. Families with children who have PKU perceive themselves to be less adaptable and cohesive than other families. Mothers of children with PKU particularly feel separated rather than connected within the family structure and feel rigid rather than structured. More rigid family systems may be an adaptive response to children whose daily routine is less flexible than most children. Helping the family discover ways in which to provide a flexible, yet structured organization of the child's management of PKU would be supportive, allowing them to let go of their perceived need for rigidity. On other

measures of family stress, parents of children with PKU did not report significantly greater degrees of parental psychologic distress, marital dissatisfaction, or parenting stress than other parents, although the tendency for stress in these areas was present (Fehrenbach and Peterson, 1989; Kazak, Reber, and Snitzer, 1988).

Reproductive patterns in families after birth of a child with PKU are affected by the birth order of that child, the age of the parents at the time of the birth of the child with PKU, and the expressed intentions of the parents whether to have additional children (Burns et al, 1984). Having a child with PKU does not appear to limit parental reproductive plans. Since the advent of prenatal diagnosis for PKU, another factor that contributes to the reproductive decision-making process includes the parents' perception of the progress of the child with PKU. For families with at least one child with PKU who decided not to have more children, family size was the primary limiting factor (35%), followed by concern about PKU (25%), and finances (20%) (Jew, Williams, and Koch, 1988).

The financial burden of PKU is variable for parents of a child with PKU or young adults with PKU living on their own. The annual cost of feeding a 1-to-2-year-old child with PKU is 10% to 20% higher than the cost of feeding an unaffected 1-to-2-year-old ($2273 vs. $874). The annual cost of a PKU diet for a 15-to-19 year-old is 373% higher than the cost for a teenager without PKU (for a male, $7878 vs. $1664; for a female, $7246 vs. $1394) (California Dept. of Health Services, 1997).

The number of states having some legislated provision for PKU formula is growing: 33 states currently do, 18 of which also cover foods, and 7 of which mandate insurance coverage (www.pkunews.org). The primary care provider can intercede on behalf of the parents in negotiating coverage of the expenses of EMF, low-protein medical foods, and blood phe monitoring. A great deal of parental anguish in the first weeks after the diagnosis of PKU in their newborn can be spared the parents at a time that is already emotionally traumatic for families.

Information about nonselective NBS is optimally given to all expectant parents prenatally. Information should be given to the newborn's parents at least before discharge from the birth facility, assuming that the newborn is under 1 week of age. If information about the significance of

NBS for the child's health and the NBS testing process is not sufficient, parents experience more anxiety and depression about their child's health than about the fact that their child needs to be tested again for a presumptive positive NBS test result (Sorenson et al, 1984). If a child is ultimately diagnosed with PKU, the parents experience guilt over their genetic contribution as a carrier to their child with PKU. The stigma of being a carrier is powerful, but the knowledge that everyone carries several recessive genes for disorders, such as PKU, excluding only 0.01% of all couples that do not, may dispel this stigma for future generations (Burns, 1984). A primary care provider who is astute about PKU can greatly alleviate parents' anxieties of being a carrier.

Informational Materials

Internet Resources:

National PKU News Web site (http://www.pkunews.org). The *National PKU News Literature Listing* describes audiovisual and written materials about PKU by age group of individuals with PKU or for professionals. Ordering information and cost is provided. In addition, the *PKU News Home Page* features "PKU General Information," "PKU Dietary Information," "PKU Support Information," "Rights of the People," "Up Close and Personal," and "PKU Related Links," editor Virginia E. Schuett, M.S., R.D..

PKU Chat Group: America Online (aol), second and fourth Monday of every month at 9PM EST. To access, click on *People Connection,* then *Private Room,* then *PKU Chat.*

PKU Internet Listserve Group. To receive the current dialog or make inquiries regarding issues related to PKU online, sign up by sending an e-mail request to magol@gte.net.

Audiovisual Materials:

Ahn S, Velazquez K, Ojeda N and Cunningham GC, producers: PKU and you: young women share their thoughts, Berkeley, CA, 1988, Maternal PKU Project, Genetic Disease Branch, California Department of Health Services. The purpose of this program is to convey the issues that concern young women with PKU. This video, filmed at California's Maternal PKU Camp, shows young women with PKU, 13 years and older, sharing their experiences of growing up with PKU, giving each other support to stay on or return to the diet, and discussing the importance of returning to the diet be-

fore and throughout pregnancy. Running time is 20 minutes. VHS videotape. To order call the Gene-HELP Resource Center at (510)540-2972.

Helmore JD, producer: A message to PKU parents, Berkeley, CA, 1989, Genetic Disease Branch, California Department of Health Services. The purpose of this program is to help parents of children newly diagnosed with PKU understand the condition and to show that children with PKU can grow to healthy adulthood, leading normal lives. Produced in cooperation with Kathleen Jew, RN, MPH and Julian C. Williams, MD, Children's Hospital of Los Angeles. Running time is 21 minutes and 23 seconds. VHS videotape. To order call the Gene-HELP Resource Center at (510)540-2972.

Koch et al: Maternal PKU: a new crisis on the horizon, March 1995. This video explains the history of PKU from its discovery through the creation of the special medical diet, and how the newborn screening process essentially eliminated the mental retardation caused by PKU. This historical perspective leads naturally into the introduction of MPKU and complications for the fetus. The latter half of the program explains how a multidisciplinary medical team participates in the treatment of successful MPKU pregnancies and how the evidence provided by the 10-year collaborative study of MPKU has led to its successful treatment. The audience is health care providers and policymakers, although the tape is informative for the general public. Directed by Sean P. Dunn, contributors are NICHD, with a supplemental grant from Scientific Hospital Supplies. Running time is 28 minutes, 30 seconds. The cost is $50.00 for rental of a VHS videotape (add $9.00 shipping and handling); $145.00 to purchase. Distributed by Fanlight Productions, (617)524-0980, #LL-170 or (888) 937-4113.

Satter E, producer: *Child of mine: feeding with love and good sense,* Bull Publishing Co, PO Box 208, Palo Alto, CA, 1989. A series of four videotapes of real parents, child care providers, and children shows what works and what does not work in helping children to eat well, stay out of struggles with eating, understand feeding, and know when and when not to hold the line. Video is based on the producer's book by the same title. Running time is 15 minutes for individual tape *(The Infant; The Older Baby; The Toddler;* and *The Preschooler);* 60 minutes for set of four on one VHS videotape. The cost of an individual tape is $54.95; the set of four on one tape costs $164.95; the book costs $14.95. To order call (800) 676-2855.

Written materials for adults:

Acosta PB and Yannicelli S: *A guide for the family of the child with phenylketonuria,* Ross Products Division, Abbott Laboratories, Columbus, Ohio, 1994. This comprehensive guide introduces parents to PKU and its management. Provided free by local representative for Ross. Metabolic Formula Systems, 625 Cleveland Ave., Columbus, OH 43215. (800) 551-5838.

Acosta PB and Yannicelli S: *Nutrition support protocol for previously untreated adults with phenylketonuria,* Ross Products Division, Abbott Laboratories, Columbus, OH, 1997. Designed for use by nutritionists and professionals only. Call (800) 227-5767 for a free copy.

Dolan BE et al: *Guidelines for adults with untreated PKU,* 1998. This guide outlines the process for converting and transitioning untreated adults with classical PKU to diet. To obtain a copy of the guidelines contact Barbara Dolan, RN, MSN, Redwood Coast Regional Center, 1116 Airport Park Blvd, Ukiah, CA 95482-3832, call (707) 462-3832, or access the PKU National News Website at www.pkunews.org

GeneHELP Resource Center, Berkeley, CA. The center maintains a database of public education materials produced nationwide and support groups for PKU, maternal PKU, and other genetic disorders across the USA. For information or to order available materials, write the GeneHELP Resource Center, Genetic Disease Branch, State of California Department of Health Services, 2151 Berkeley Way, Annex 4, Berkeley, CA 94704, or call (510)540-2972.

Koch JH: *Robert Guthrie—the PKU story: crusade against mental retardation,* Pasadena, CA, 1997, Hope Publishing House. To order write Hope Publishing House, PO Box 60008, Pasadena, CA 91116, call (800) 326-2671, or e-mail hopepub@loop.com. The book costs $20.00 (add $3.00 shipping and handling).

Mead Johnson: *Living with PKU,* 1995. This booklet includes a discussion of what PKU is, the genetics and management of PKU, interviews with families, and helpful hints from experienced parents. Provided free by a local representative for Mead Johnson Nutritional Group, Medical Affairs, Evansville, IN 47721, Technical Pediatric Product Information (812) 429-5000.

New York State Department of Health: *Neonatal screening blood specimen collection and handling procedure and simple spot check,* 1994. These posters are provided free by Schleicher and Schuell, Inc, 10 Optical Ave, PO Box 2012, Keene, NH 03431-2012, (800) 245-4024.

PHE Forum: *The California maternal PKU program newsletter,* Berkeley, 1989–present. This newsletter is published twice a year and contains articles and dietary tips relevant to the young adult with PKU and information about the California Maternal PKU Camp activities. To order write the Maternal PKU Program Coordinator, Genetic Disease Branch, State of California Department of Health Services, 2151 Berkeley Way, Annex 4, Berkeley, CA 94704, or call (510) 540-3298.

Schuett V: *Low protein cookery for PKU,* 1997. This cookbook contains over 450 recipes, plus helpful hints for managing the PKU diet. The cost of the cookbook is $21.95 plus shipping and handling. To order write Marketing Department, University of Wisconsin Press, 2537 Daniels St., Madison, WI 53718, or call (800) 829-9559 or access order form at www.pkunews.org.

Schuett V: *Low protein food list for PKU,* 1995. This book lists the phenylalanine content of over 3000 natural and brand name specific foods. This is a flexible, well-designed system for calculating phenylalanine, protein, and calories for both weight of food and household measures; easy for children to use. To order write to Dietary Specialties, Inc, PO Box 227, Rochester, NY 14601, or call (800) 544-0099.

Scientific Hospital Supplies, Inc and Schuett V: *International PKU Cookbook,* 1993. This cookbook contains over 100 simple-to-follow recipes from around the world, with complete phenylalanine content listed. Advice on eating out and holiday meals is given. The cost is $23 Canada, $29.00 US. Checks are payable to SHS. To order write SHS, PO Box 117, Gaithersburg, MD 20884, or call (800) 365-7354.

Taylor JF and Latta S: *Why can't I eat that!: Helping kids obey medical diets,* Saratoga, CA, R&E Publishers, 1993. For parents and members of the helping professions, this book details the psychology of getting children to observe any prescribed diet, and is designed to supplement the dietary measures outlined by the physician and dietitian. The book lists over 50 organizations concerned with children's disorders involving dietary considerations and has over 700 indexed entries. To order write ADD Plus, 1095-25th St SE #107, Salem, OR 97301, call (800) 847-1233, or fax (503) 364-7454.

Children's PKU Network Clearinghouse Publication List. Childrens PKU Network, 1520 State St., Ste #240, San Diego, CA 92101. To order call (619) 233-3202, fax (619) 233-0838, or e-mail pkunetwork@aol.com.

Written materials for children: An extensive list of written materials for children, by age group, is available at www.pkunews.org.

Taylor M and Schuett VE: *You and PKU,* ed 2, 1998. This is a 50-page spiral-bound notebook, with appealing illustrations, for children ages 3 to 8 years. Presented in storybook fashion, the notebook contains information about the PKU diet, blood drawing, and clinic visits. Included are suggestions for parents about teaching their child about PKU. To order call Dietary Specialties, Inc. at (800) 554-0099.

Community Resources

Children's PKU Network: This is a national nonprofit organization dedicated to working together for the benefit of all people involved in the treatment of PKU and other metabolic disorders. As a support service organization, activities include an express "care package" of information to new parents of a child with PKU, a crisis-intervention service to children or adults in need, and the sale of dietary gram scales. The Network administers an educational scholarship program and the Regional Coordinator Network Council for PKU parents' groups nationwide.

Children's PKU Network, 1520 State Street, Suite 240

San Diego, CA 92101

(619) 233-3202; (619) 233-0838 (fax)

pkunetwork@aol.com.

National PKU News: This national nonprofit organization publishes a newsletter 3 times a year to promote exchange of information about PKU. Regular columns include: Research Review, Special Features, Food and Nutrition Notes, The Learning Place, Connections, Just for Kids, and Hang in There . . . the teens and young adults column. Edited by Virginia Schuett. Write to National PKU News, 6869 Woodlawn Ave NE #116, Seattle, WA 98115, (206) 525-5023 (fax); (206) 525-8140; www.pkunews.org; schuett@pkunews.org.

Medical Food Products

Applied Nutrition Corp.,
A Division of FoodTek Manufacturing, Inc.
273 Franklin Road
Randolf, NJ 07869
Customer service: (800) 605-0410
www.medicalfood.com

Dietary Specialties, Inc.
PO Box 227
Rochester, NY 14601-0227
Customer service: (800) 544-0099
www.dietspec.com

Ener-G Foods, Inc.
PO Box 84487
Seattle, WA 98124-5787
Customer service: (800) 331-5222
www.ener-g.com

InterNational Foodbank
1030 St Alexandre, Suite 301
Montreal, QC, Canada H2Z 1P3
Customer service: (514) 395-2394
www.international-foodbank.org

Mead Johnson Nutritional Group,
Medical Affairs
2400 W. Lloyd Expressway
Evansville, IN 47721-0001
Customer service: (800) 457-3550
www.meadjohnson.com/mjn/nutrition/special-needs.html

Med Diet Laboratories, Inc.
3600 Holly Lane North #80
Plymouth, MN 55447
Customer service: (800) MED-DIET
www.med-diet.com

Ross Laboratories,
Ross Products Division
625 Cleveland Avenue
Columbus, OH 43215
Metabolic Formula Systems,
Customer service: (800) 551-5838
www.abbott.com

Scientific Hospital Supplies, Inc.
PO Box 117
Gaithersburg, MD 20884-0117
Customer service: (800) 365-7354
www.shsna.com

Summary of Primary Care Needs for the Child with Phenylketonuria

HEALTH CARE MAINTENANCE

Growth and development

Growth and development are normal on a phe-restricted diet.

Caloric intake of high CHO-free foods should be controlled to avoid obesity.

Adequate protein intake is needed to promote greater dietary phe tolerance.

Children with PKU may have underdeveloped social skills.

Diet

Phe-restricted diet is for life.

Blood phe monitoring with weight and diet changes is for life.

Self-management of phe-restricted diet should be initiated early in childhood.

For optimum availability of nutrients, EMF products should be prepared as prescribed and taken with meals.

Sensitivity to the social and cultural importance of food at each developmental stage is needed.

Safety

A Medic-Alert bracelet or necklace specifying phe-restricted diet is advisable.

Only individuals with a diagnosis of PKU should ingest EMF products as prescribed.

Children and teens need sun protection.

Immunizations

Routine immunizations are recommended.

Any catabolic reaction should be supported with hydration and calories.

Screening

Vision: Routine screening is recommended.

Hearing: Routine screening is recommended.

Dental: Screening should be initiated at eruption of the first tooth and closely followed thereafter.

Frequent CHO intake decreases the risk of caries.

Blood pressure: Routine screening is recommended.

Hematocrit: Hematocrit and hemoglobin values are assessed at 6 and 12 months of age and then annually.

Plasma ferritin levels are checked at 6, 9, and 12 months of age and every 6 months thereafter.

Breast-fed infants have exaggerated physiologic anemia of infancy and require iron supplements.

Urinalysis: Routine screening is recommended.

Tuberculosis: Routine screening is recommended.

Condition-specific screening: All children with persistent HPA require a urine pterin screening test.

Blood phe should be monitored with weight and dietary changes for phe tolerance.

Nutritional indices that should be monitored include tyr, vitamins, prealbumin, albumin, essential fatty acids, selenium, and other trace elements and metals.

Regular auscultation of heart sounds is advisable to identify selenium deficiency.

DNA mutation analysis of blood on filter paper is recommended.

COMMON ILLNESS MANAGEMENT

Differential diagnosis

Elevated blood phe caused by illness should be differentiated from that caused by intake of too little or too much dietary phe by an accurate history.

Catabolic state related to common childhood illness should be prevented with adequate hydration and caloric intake.

Minor surgery results in only a transient level of blood phe.

Skin lesions from allergic sensitivities, eczema, and scleroderma should be differentiated related to imbalance of blood phe, tyr, or tryptophan.

Sun exposure should be limited and sun blocks used, as for any child.

Continued

Summary of Primary Care Needs for the Child with Phenylketonuria—cont'd

Drug interactions

Aspartame ingestion is contraindicated.

Care should be taken to read food labels and medication ingredients for aspartame.

Monoamine oxidase inhibitors are contraindicated.

Daraprim (pyrimethamine) is contraindicated.

Caution should be taken in prescribing drugs that alter neurotransmitters.

Plasma tyr levels of women taking oral contraceptives should be monitored.

DEVELOPMENTAL ISSUES

Sleep patterns

Disturbed sleep patterns or nightmares may occur during loss of phe homeostasis.

Toileting

Infants may be more prone to diaper dermatitis.

Daily hygiene is important, especially for musty odor related to loss of phe homeostasis during illnesses and changes in diet and activity levels.

Discipline

Avoid use of food as a reward system and blood tests as punishment.

Expectations are normal based on age and developmental level.

Child care

Providers should be aware of the need for special diet and hydration and calories during illness and trauma.

Schooling

Visual spatial skills should be promoted.

Good lighting and contrasts of dark on light backgrounds (not greys) promote visualization of detailed subject matter (e.g., letters and numbers).

Annual developmental testing is recommended.

Math and language skills may require tutoring.

School personnel may be made aware of a child's special dietary needs at the parents' discretion.

Sexuality

Young women with PKU should be educated about the risks of MPKU.

Fertility is unaffected in men with PKU, although phe homeostasis is recommended.

Genetic counseling should be provided at the time appropriate for each individual with PKU.

Gamete donors should be tested for PKU by DNA analysis.

Transition to adulthood

All individuals should remain on a phe-restricted diet for life.

Phe homeostasis throughout the lifetime improves the neuropsychiatric executive functions.

Participation in PKU support groups and professional counseling as needed are recommended for adults with PKU and their families.

Psychotropic medication should be a last resort in an individual with PKU, after phe homeostasis is achieved.

SPECIAL FAMILY CONCERNS

Special family concerns include delays in diagnosis after an NBS positive result for PKU, the vigilant supervision of the child's 'diet for life,' the parental guilt at having passed a *hidden gene* on to their child, genetic counseling of immediate and extended family members, family planning and prenatal diagnosis options, inability to predict severity of HPA, and financial support of the lifelong need for EMF products and medical care. Cultural and ethnic sensitivity in planning phe-restricted diet and all aspects of medical care foster a positive attitude toward PKU in the child that will last a lifetime.

References

Acosta PB and Wright L: Nurses' role in preventing birth defects in offspring of women with phenylketonuria, [published erratum appears in JOGNN, 21:352, 1992], JOGNN 21:270-276, 1992.

Acosta PB and Yanicelli S: Protocol 1-Phenylketonuria. In Cameron AM, editor: Ross metabolic formula system nutrition support protocols, ed 3, pp 1-31; maternal PKU pp 32-49, Columbus, Ohio, 1997, Division of Abbott Laboratories.

Acosta PB and Yannicelli S: Nutrition support protocol for previously untreated adults with phenylketonuria, Columbus Ohio, 1997, Division of Abbott Laboratories.

American Academy of Pediatrics Committee on Genetics: Newborn screening facts sheets, Pediatrics 98:473-501, 1996.

Arnold LC: Drug products containing phenylalanine (in the form of aspartame), National PKU News web site, 1998.

Arnopp JJ et al: Results of screening for phenylketonuria using a lower cutoff value in early collected specimens, Screening 3:193-199, 1995.

Azen CG et al: Intellectual development in 12-year-old children treated for phenylketonuria, Am J Dis Child 145:35-39, 1991.

Berg BO: Child neurology, Greenbrae, CA, 1984, Jones Medical Publications.

Blau N et al: A missense mutation in a patient with guanosine triphosphate cyclohydrolase I deficiency missed in the newborn screening program, J Peds 126:401-405, 1995.

Blau N et al: Tetrahydrobiopterin deficiency: from phenotype to genotype, Pteridines 4:1-10, 1993.

Bolognia JL, Pawelek JM: Biology of hypopigmentation, J Am Acad Dermatol 19:217-254, 1988.

Brunner RL, Berch DB, and Berry H: Phenylketonuria and complex spatial visualization: an analysis of information processing, Dev Med Child Neurol 29:460-468, 1987.

Buist NR and Tuerck JM: The practitioner's role in newborn screening, Pediatr Clin North Am 39:199-211, 1992.

Burns JK et al: Impact of PKU on the reproductive patterns in collaborative study families, Am J Med Genet 19:515-524, 1984.

California Department of Health Services, Genetic Disease Branch: Cost of availability of dietary treatment of phenylketonuria (PKU): report of a national survey, Berkeley, California, 1997, The Department.

Casamassimo PS et al: Dental health in children with phenylketonuria and other inborn errors of amino acid metabolism managed by diet, Publication No HRS-D-MC 84-1, Rockville, MD, 1984, US Department of Health and Human Services.

Clarke JTR et al: Neuropsychological studies on adolescents with phenylketonuria returned to phenylalanine restricted diets, Am J Ment Retard 92:255-262, 1987.

Cockburn F et al: Fatty acids in the stability of neuronal membrane: relevance to PKU, Int Pediatr 11:56-60, 1996.

Council of Regional Networks for Genetic Services (CORN), Newborn Screening Committee: National Newborn Screening Report-1991, CORN, New York, 1994.

Craft S et al: Lateralized deficits in visual attention in males with developmental dopamine depletion, Neuropsychologia 30:341-351, 1992.

Cunningham GC et al: Early discharge trends and their effect on PKU screening. In Pass KA and Levy HL, editors: Early hospital discharge: impact on newborn screening, Atlanta, 1996, CORN.

Curtius HC, Endres W, and Blau N: Effect of high-protein meal plus aspartame ingestion on plasma phenylalanine concentrations in obligate heterozygotes for phenylketonuria, Metabolism 43:413-416, 1994.

de Koning TJ et al: Missed PKU cases in the Netherlands: neuropsychological follow-up and clinical outcome, In Proceedings of Society for Inherited Metabolic Disorders, Asilomar, Pacific Grove, California, 1998.

Diamond A: Prefontal cortex cognitive deficits in early-treated PKU: results of a longitudinal study in children and of an animal model, Soc for Neuroscience Abstracts 18:1063, 1993.

Diamond A: Dopamine alterations and their effects on neuropsychologic testing. In Proceedings of Annual Meeting, Society for Inherited Metabolic Disorders, Asilomar, Pacific Grove, CA, 1998.

Dolan et al: Diet intervention guidelines for adults with untreated PKU, National PKU News Website, www.pkunews.org, 1998.

Eisensmith RC et al: Recurrence of the R408W mutation in the phenylalanine hydroxylase locus in Europeans, Am J Hum Genet 56:278-286, 1995.

Enns GM et al: Molecular correlations in phenylketonuria: mutation patterns and corresponding biochemical and clinical phenotypes in a heterogeneous California population, Am J Hum Genet 61:A250, 1998 (suppl).

Fehrenbach AM and Peterson L: Parental problem solving skills, stress, and dietary compliance in PKU, J Consult Clin Psychol 57:237-241, 1994.

Fiedler AE et al: Phenylalanine levels in PKU following minor surgery, Am J Med Genet 11:411-414, 1982.

Fisch RO, Gravem HJ, and Feinberg SB: Growth and bone characteristics of phenylketonurics: comparative analysis of treated and untreated phenylketonuric children, Am J Dis Child 112:3-10, 1966.

Fisch RO et al: Bony changes of PKU neonates unrelated to phenylalanine levels, J Inher Metab Dis 14:890-895, 1991a.

Fisch RO et al: Children of fathers with phenylketonuria: an international survey, J Pediatr 118:739-741, 1991b.

Fishler K et al: Psychoeducational findings among children treated for phenylketonuria, Am J Ment Defic 92:65-73, 1987.

Greeves LG, Carson DJ, and Dodge JA: Peptic ulceration and phenylketonuria: a possible link? Gut 29:691-692, 1988.

Greeves LG et al: Potentially life-threatening cardiac dysrhythmia in a child with selenium deficiency and phenylketonuria, Acta Paediatr Scand 79:1259-1262, 1990.

Greve LC et al: Breast feeding in the management of the newborn with phenylketonuria: a practical approach to dietary therapy, J Am Diet Assoc 94:305-309, 1994.

Hanley WB: Prenatal testing for maternal phenylketonuria (MPKU), Int Pediatr 9(suppl 2):33-39, 1994.

Hassel CW and Brunsting LA: Phenylpyruvic oligphrenia: an elevation of the light-sensitive and pigmentary characteristics of seventeen patients, AMA Arch Dermatol 79:458-465, 1959.

Herrero E et al: Inhibition by L-phenylalanine of tryptophan transport by synaptosomal plasma membrane vesicles: implications in the pathogenesis of phenylketonuria, J Inher Metab Dis 6:32-35, 1983.

Hofman KJ et al: Phenylketonuria in US blacks: molecular analysis of the phenylalanine hydroxylase gene, Am J Hum Genet 48:791-798, 1991.

Hommes FA: On the mechanism of permanent brain dysfunction in hyperphenylalaninemia, Biochem Med Metab Bio 46:277-287, 1991.

Irons M, Levy HL: Metabolic syndromes with dermatologic manifestations, Clin Rev Allergy 4:101-124, 1986.

Jew K: PKU—review of clinical developments and newborn screening aspects. In Levy HL and Pass KA, editors: Proceedings from the Early Discharge: Impact on Newborn Screening, 1996, Washington, D.C., grant MCJ131006010 MCH Bureau HRSA; CORN; ASTPHLD; CDC; and NICHHD

Jew K, Williams JC, and Koch R: Reproductive decision making in PKU families. In Proceedings of the 6th National Neonatal Screening Symposium, Portland, OR, 1988.

Jew K et al: Validity of screening early collected newborn specimens for phenylketonuria using a fluorometric method, Screening 3:1-9, 1994.

Jew K, Kamjou C, and McElroy ME: The shift in early screening practice in California. In Proceedings of 13th National Neonatal Screening Symposium, San Diego, 1998.

Kaufman S: An evaluation of the possible neurotoxicity of metabolites of phenylalanine, J Pediatr 114:895-900, 1989.

Kaul R et al: Frequency of 12 mutations in 114 children with phenylketonuria in the midwest region of the USA, J Inher Metab Dis 17:356-358, 1994.

Kayaalp E et al, Human phenylalanine hydroxylase mutations and hyperphenylalanemia phenotypes: a metanalysis of genotype phenotype correlations, Am J Hum Genet 61:1309-1317, 1997.

Kazak AE, Reber M, and Snitzer L: Childhood chronic disease and family functioning: a study of phenylketonuria, Pediatrics 81:224-283, 1988.

Kling S: Newborn screening—an overview of newborn screening programs in the United States and Canada 1993, Illinois Department of Public Health, Springfield, IL, 1993.

Koch R et al: Mild hyperphe and heterozygosity of the phenylalanine hydroxylase gene, Mol Genet Metab 63(2):148-50, 1998a.

Koch R et al: Long term beneficial effects of the phenylalanine restricted diet in late diagnosed individuals with phenylketonuria with regard to genotype of the phenylalanine hydroxylase gene. In Proceedings of 13th National Neonatal Screening Symposium, San Diego, 1998b.

Koch R and Wenz E: Phenylketonuria, Ann Rev Nutr 7:117-135, 1987.

Leonard CO: Atypical phenylketonuria. In Proceedings of Society for Inherited Metabolic Disorders, Asilomav, Pacific Grove, California, 1998.

Levy HL et al: Fetal ultrasonography in maternal PKU, Prenatal Diagn 16:599-604, 1994.

Lorey FW and Cunningham GC: Effect of specimen collection methods on newborn screening for PKU, Screening 3:57-65, 1994.

Lou HC et al: An occipito-temporal syndrome in adolescents with optimally controlled hyperphenylalaninemia, J Inherit Metab Dis 15:687-695, 1992.

Lou HC et al: Brain magnetic resonance imaging in children with optimally controlled hyperphenylalaninemia. In Proceedings of An International Symposium on the Occasion of the 60th Anniversary of Følling's Discovery of Phenylketonuria, Elsinore, Denmark, 1994.

Matalon R et al: Maternal collaborative study: pregnancy outcome and postnatal head growth, J Inher Metab Dis 17:353-355, 1994.

McBurnie MA et al: Physical growth of children treated for phenylketonuria, Annals Human Bio 18:357-368, 1991.

MacDonald G et al: 24 Hour fluctuations in blood phe levels, Natl PKU News 10(3):2-3, 1999.

Nova MP, Kaufman M, and Halperin A: Sclerodermalike indurations in a child with phenylketonuria: a clinicopathologic correlation and review of the literature, J Am Acad Derm 26:329-333, 1992.

Pietz J et al: EEGs in phenylketonuria: I. follow-up to adulthood, II. short-term diet-related changes in EEGs and cognitive function, Dev Med Child Neuro 35:54-64, 1993.

Pitt DB and Danks DM: The natural history of untreated phenylketonuria over 20 years, J Paediatr Child Health 27:189-190, 1994.

Ris MD et al: Early treated phenylketonuria: adult neuropsychologic outcome, J Peds 124:88-392, 1994.

Riva E et al: PKU-related dysgammaglobulinaemia: the effect of diet therapy on IgE and allergic sensitization, J Inher Metab Dis 17:710-717, 1994.

Rouse B et al: Maternal phenylketonuria Collaborative Study (MPKUCS) offspring: facial anomalies, malformation, and early neurological sequelae, Am J Med Genet 69(1):89-95, 1997.

Sarkissian CN, Boulais DM, and Scriver CR: A new heteroallelic mutant mouse; an ortholoque for human hyperphenylalaninemia, Am J Hum Genet 63(suppl):A273, 1998.

Sarkissian CN et al: A different approach to treatment of phenylketonuria: phenylalanine degradation with recombinant phenylalanine ammonia lyase, Proc Natl Acad Sci USA 96:2339-44, 1999.

Schmidt K: Primer to the inborn errors of metabolism for perinatal and neonatal nurses, J Perinat Neonatal Nurs 2:60-71, 1989.

Schuett V: Off-diet young adults with PKU: lives in danger, Natl PKU News 8(3):1-3, 1997a.

Schuett V: PKU: Lives in danger: responses from families and professionals, Natl PKU News 9(1):1-39, 1997b.

Schuett V: A new approach to PKU diet treatment, Natl PKU News 10(3):1-2, 1999a.

Schuett V: Off-diet young adults with PKU: lives in danger; PKU: lives in danger-responses from families and professionals, www.pkunews.org, 1999b.

Scriver CR: An ongoing debate over phenylalanine hydroxylase deficiency in phenylketonuria, J Clin Invest 101(12):2613-4, 1998.

Scriver CR et al: The hyperphenylalaninemias. In Scriver CR et al, editors: The metabolic and molecular bases of inherited disease, New York, 1995, McGraw-Hill, vol I.

Shiloh S et al: Cross-cultural perspectives on coping with the risks of maternal phenylketonuria, Psych Health 8:435-446, 1993.

Smith I, Beasley MG, and Ades AE: Intelligence and quality of dietary treatment in phenylketonuria, Arch Dis Child 65:472-478, 1990.

Sorenson JR et al: Parental response to repeat testing of infants with 'false positive' results in a newborn screening program, Pediatrics 73:183-187, 1984.

Spada M et al: The impact on PKU screening outcome of patient genotype and phenotype, Am J Hum Genet 63(suppl):A274, 1998.

Thibaud D et al: Diagnosis of phenylketonuria in a 35-year-old mother in relation to prenatal diagnosis of intrauterine growth retardation with microcephaly, Arch Pediatr 5:1229-31, 1998.

Thompson AJ et al: Brain MRI changes in phenylketonuria, Brain 116:811-821, 1993.

Tokatli A et al: Classical phenylketonuria associated with Goldenhar's syndrome: a case report, Turk J Peds 36:153-156, 1994.

Trahms CM: Self-management skills: the key to successful PKU treatment, part I. first steps: teaching your young child the basics, National PKU News 3(3):4-5, Winter 1992a.

Trahms CM: Self-management skills: the key to successful PKU treatment, part II. moving ahead and walking strong: promoting self-management for the school-aged child, National PKU News 4(1):4-5, Spring/Summer 1992b.

Trahms CM: Self-management skills: the key to successful PKU treatment, part III. standing on your own two feet: the adolescent years and beyond, National PKU News 4(2):4-5, Fall 1992c.

Treacy E et al: Phenylalanine metabolism in vivo in mild phenylketonuria, the effect of multiple loci, abstract 106, Am J Hum Genet 55 (suppl):A22, 1994.

Vajro P et al: Correction of phenylketonuria after liver transplantation in a child with cirrhosis, NEJM 329:363, 1993.

Valle D and Mitchell G: Introduction to genetic disorders: sources of variability. In Dietary management of persons with metabolic disorders, Evansville, IN, 1994, Mead Johnson and Company.

Waisbren SE et al: Social factors and the meaning of food in adherence to medical diets: results of a maternal phenoketonuria camp, J Inherit Metab Dis 20:21-7, 1997.

Wallman CM: Newborn genetic screening, Neonatal Network 17:55-60, 1998.

Weglage J et al: Pathogenesis of different clinical outcomes in spite of identical genotypes and comparable blood phenylalanine concentrations in phenylketonurics, J Inherit Metab Dis 21:181-2, 1998.

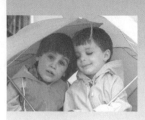

CHAPTER 32

Prematurity

Toshiko Hirata, Elena Bosque, Diane J. Goldman, and Steven L. Goldman

Etiology

Premature, low birth weight (LBW) infants are a heterogeneous group. At one end of the spectrum are infants who spend their first weeks of life critically ill and, if they survive, require life-long chronic care. At the other end are infants who have little or no problems during the perinatal period and require no special long-term care.

Premature, or preterm, refers to infants born before 37 completed weeks of gestation (Committee on Fetus and Newborn, 1967; Sohl and Moore, 1998; World Health Organization, 1969). LBW refers to infants whose birth weight is under 2500 g, *very* low birth weight (VLBW) refers to infants weighing under 1500 g, and *extremely* low birth weight (ELBW) refers to infants weighing under 1000 g. Historically the term *low birth weight* has been used almost synonymously with the term *premature,* but this usage can be misleading. For example, some term infants have birth weights under 2500 g (these infants are small for gestational age [SGA]), and some premature infants have birth weights of over 2500 g (most of these are normal premature infants with longer gestational ages, but some may be large for gestational age [LGA]). Appropriate for gestational age (AGA) infants have a birth weight within the normal range for their gestational age (Sohl and Moore, 1998).

The causes of prematurity are varied, and many are interrelated. There are two main reasons for preterm births: the infant may need to be delivered prematurely because of maternal or fetal problems (indicated births) or is born spontaneously because of spontaneous preterm labor or preterm rupture of fetal membranes (Iams et al, 1998; Meis et al, 1998). Some of the known causes or risk factors are listed in Box 32-1 (Creasy and Iams, 1999). Assisted reproductive technology is associated with an increased incidence of preterm births when compared with either singleton or multiple spontaneous pregnancies. In many other cases a specific cause or risk factor cannot be identified (Creasy and Iams, 1999).

Incidence

Birth certificate gestational data reveal a prematurity rate of 11% in 1995 (Centers for Disease Control and Prevention [CDC], 1997). In 1997 the incidence of LBW among infants in the United States was 7.4%; VLBW infants composed 1.4% of births. A racial disparity in birth weight continues: the incidence of LBW among black infants is approximately 2.1 times that among white infants, which is primarily attributed to a preterm birth rate of 17.4% in black infants compared with 9.8% in white infants (Guyer et al, 1998). The LBW rate in Hispanic infants is 6.3% (CDC, 1997).

Clinical Manifestations

Prematurity is definitively diagnosed at the time of birth (Box 32-2). The degree of prematurity is most accurately assessed using reliable maternal history. When the date of the last menstrual period is uncertain, the gestational age can be estimated using measurements obtained at early ultrasound examinations. In the absence of reliable dates or conflicting data, the physical and neurologic findings in the neonate can be used to estimate gestational age to within 2 weeks (Ballard et al, 1991; Dubowitz, Dubowitz, and Goldberg, 1970).

Instruments that have been developed for the clinical assessment of gestational age take advantage of the profound physical and neurologic changes that occur in the fetus during the last trimester. For example, an infant of 24 weeks' gestation is extremely hypotonic, with fragile, thin,

Treatment

Prevention

The most desirable treatment for prematurity is prevention. To this end, the National Institute of Child Health and Development (NICHD) Preterm Prediction Study is collecting data in a prospective, population-based study to identify markers that might predict preterm delivery (Creasy and Iams, 1999). Through preterm birth prevention programs, educational materials and technology (e.g., home uterine activity monitors and telemetry) can be used by clinicians and pregnant women so that the signs of preterm labor can be identified and treated early (Creasy and Iams, 1999). New markers for preterm birth (e.g., fetal fibronectin and transvaginal ultrasonography measurements of cervical length) are being tested for identification of early signs of labor. When present in cervicovaginal mucus, fetal fibronectin, which is an extracellular matrix protein normally found in fetal membranes and decidua, has been shown to be a good predictor of spontaneous preterm delivery within 7 days of presentation (Iams et al, 1995). In very early gestations where preterm delivery cannot be entirely prevented, prolonging the pregnancy and achieving advancement of gestational age may avoid extreme prematurity and its attendant morbidities and may significantly alter perinatal outcome (Creasy and Iams, 1999; Kilpatrick et al, 1997; Piecuch et al, 1997).

Treatment in Utero

If a preterm birth appears inevitable, treatment should begin in utero (Box 32-3). Corticosteroids given to the mother before delivery will accelerate fetal lung maturation and decrease the risk of

gelatinous skin (Siegfried and Esterly, 1998). Because the chest wall is so flexible at this gestational age, respiratory effort results in substernal retractions (Harris and Wood, 1996). As the fetus matures there is a global increase in resting tone, a flexed posture develops, the skin thickens, and the bone and cartilage become firmer (Siegfried and Esterly, 1998).

Box 32-3

Treatment

Prevention of prematurity

- Ensure prenatal care
- Avoid drugs, tobacco, and alcohol
- Prolong gestation (tocolytics)
- Identify early signs of labor

Treatment in utero

- Corticosteroids given to mother to increase fetal lung maturation
- Prevent infection (antenatal antibiotics)
- Birth at a center for high-risk pregnancies

Management of complications of prematurity

- Metabolic
- Infections
- Respiratory
- Neurologic
- Hematologic
- Cardiovascular
- Gastrointestinal
- Nutritional

---

respiratory distress syndrome (RDS), significantly reduce the incidence of intraventricular hemorrhage (IVH), lower the incidence of cerebral palsy (Garland, Buck, and Leviton, 1995; Salokorpi et al, 1997), enhance the effectiveness of surfactant (Jobe et al, 1993; Kari et al, 1994; Rebello et al, 1996), and improve outcome (Long, Zucker, and Kraybill, 1995). If rupture of the membranes occurs or infection is suspected, prenatal administration of antibiotics improves neonatal survival and outcome (Creasy and Iams, 1999). Mortality rate can increase fourfold among VLBW infants whose mothers develop intraamniotic infection (Riggs and Blanco, 1998). If conditions permit, the mother should be transferred to a center with expertise in the management of preterm labor and high-risk deliveries and in caring for high-risk infants.

After the infant is born, treatment is tailored to existing or anticipated problems. Prophylactic treatment modalities are often used in infants at highest risk. Exogenous surfactant can be given initially at birth to prevent or lessen the severity of RDS (Corbet et al, 1995; Kossel and Versmold, 1997). Indomethacin (Indocin) may be given before or soon after signs of patent ductus arteriosus (PDA) are clinically apparent (Clyman, 1996; Tintoc et al, 1994), and respiratory stimulants (e.g., caffeine or theophylline) may be given before apnea occurs.

Recent and Anticipated Advances in Diagnosis and Management

Prematurity itself does not cause long-range problems for affected infants; the complications associated with prematurity actually cause—in some cases—irreparable damage. In general, VLBW and ELBW infants have a higher incidence of long-range problems.

The most important advance in this area would be to decrease the incidence of premature births. Universal provision of prenatal care would have the greatest effect in reducing preterm births. Social interventions to reduce the use of drugs, including tobacco and alcohol, and improve nutrition and other changes in environment and personal behaviors would also contribute to reducing preterm births (Merkatz and Merkatz, 1995). Medical advances in managing the complications associated with premature birth would lessen the incidence of poor outcomes. Improved techniques (e.g., high-frequency ventilation) decrease the lung damage seen with conventional ventilation (Clark et al, 1992; Gerstmann et al, 1996). Research in liquid ventilation is ongoing (Leach et al, 1996; Shaffer, Greenspan, and Wolfson, 1994). Low-dose prophylactic indomethacin may be useful in prevention of IVH (Ment et al, 1994), and closure of a PDA (Tintoc et al, 1994), allowing surgical closure to be avoided. Detection of abnormalities in the cerebral circulation by near infra-red spectroscopy may further decrease the risk of IVH (Volpe, 1998). New blood bank techniques (e.g., dividing blood units into eight aliquots) have been successful in reducing the number of donor exposures per infant (Lee et al, 1995). Likewise, the use of erythropoietin has reduced the total number of transfusions received

(Kumar, Shankaran, and Krishnan, 1998). The addition of the fatty acids docosahexaenoic acid (DHA) and arachidonic acid (AA) to infant formulas is being investigated for safety in premature infants. These nutrients have been added to infant formulas in European and other countries for several years and have been shown to improve cognitive and visual outcomes in premature infants (Horwood and Fergusson, 1998).

Use of tin mesoporphyrin seems promising for prevention of extreme hyperbilirubinemia and its consequences of kernicterus and hearing loss in term and preterm infants (Martinez et al, 1999; Valaes et al, 1994). Laser therapy for prevention of advanced retinopathy of prematurity (ROP) has proved successful in reducing or eliminating blindness.

Associated Problems

The potential clinical problems associated with prematurity are many (Box 32-4). Any, all, or none of these clinical problems, many of which are risk factors for the development of other problems can develop. For example, an infant with severe RDS is more apt to develop IVH than an infant without respiratory disease; an ELBW infant or one with a delayed establishment of enteral feedings because of feeding intolerance or necrotizing enterocolitis (NEC) is more likely to develop osteopenic fractures or rickets (Dabezies and Warren, 1997; Krug-Wispe, 1998). Recognizing that these problems are possible lets clinicians anticipate and possibly prevent their occurrence and long-term implications.

Intraventricular Hemorrhage

IVH often begins with bleeding into the subependymal germinal matrix (a germinal matrix hemorrhage). This bleeding can extend into the ventricular system or the nearby brain parenchyma. According to Papile, Munsick-Bruno, and Schaefer (1983), IVH has been classified into four grades: grade I, subependymal or germinal matrix hemorrhage; grade II, intraventricular hemorrhage; grade III, IVH with ventricular dilation; and grade IV, IVH and parenchymal hemorrhage.

The germinal matrix is a metabolically active, highly vascularized area that persists until term and is predisposed to hemorrhage for several reasons.

Box 32-4

Associated Problems

Intraventricular Hemorrhage
Respiratory Problems
- Lung damage
- Apnea

Nutritional
- Parenteral feeding
- Enteral feeding
- Necrotizing enterocolitis
- Gastroesophageal reflux

Anemia
- Iatrogenic
- Exaggerated physiologic anemia

Retinopathy of Prematurity
Genitourinary Problems
- Reduce renal function
- Inguinal hernias
- Undescended testicles

Because there is poor autoregulation of blood flow to this area in premature infants, the delicate capillaries of the germinal matrix are vulnerable to damage from acute changes in systemic arterial or venous pressure (Duncan and Chiang, 1999; Lou et al, 1979). Perinatal asphyxia and metabolic or respiratory problems can also damage the capillary bed and further predispose individuals to hemorrhage (Goddard-Finegold, Mizrahi and Lee, 1998; Roland and Hill, 1997).

Treatment is supportive, by minimizing risk factors thought to contribute to further hemorrhage. Serial ultrasound examinations are necessary to document the resolution of the hemorrhage and detect the development of hydrocephalus. If hydrocephalus develops, treatment must be instituted to minimize brain damage (see Chapter 25).

Mortality from IVH is related to severity. Although there is no mortality associated with minimal hemorrhage, over 50% of infants with the most extensive hemorrhage do not survive (Volpe, 1997). Of those who do survive, infants with higher grades of IVH, posthemorrhagic hydrocephalus, and periventricular leukomalacia (PVL) have the worst outcome (Duncan and Chiang, 1999; Khalid et al, 1995; Piecuch et al, 1997; Pinto-Martin et al, 1995; Whitaker et al, 1996).

PVL is generally a result of symmetric, non-hemorrhagic, and ischemic injury to the cerebral white matter of preterm infants and is usually—but not always—a neuropathologic accompaniment of IVH (Volpe, 1995). PVL may not be limited to the periventricular area and has a high incidence of neurologic sequelae. Both IVH and PVL are diagnosed by neuroultrasound examination (Paneth et al, 1994; Volpe, 1995).

Respiratory Problems

Lung damage: Respiratory distress occurs in approximately 10% of all live births. Of these, 60% to 70% have only transient respiratory problems. RDS, aspiration (i.e., of meconium, blood, or amniotic fluid), and congenital pneumonia each occur at a rate of about 10%. The smallest and lowest gestational age infants have the highest incidence of RDS (Kopelman and Mathew, 1995; Martin, Fanaroff, and Klaus, 1993).

Most infants require only supplemental oxygen given through a hood or nasal cannula. Others require continuous positive airway pressure (CPAP), and those most severely affected by RDS require mechanical ventilation through an endotracheal tube. Supplemental oxygen and positive pressure, although lifesaving, may damage the lungs and airways (Kossel and Versmold, 1997). This damage must be viewed as a continuum. The extreme example of this is bronchopulmonary dysplasia (BPD) (see Chapter 12). Premature infants who require mechanical ventilation but do not develop BPD and those who have RDS but do not require mechanical ventilation also have evidence of lung and airway damage. The lung damage is demonstrated only with pulmonary function testing and reflected in increased airway reactivity or increased pulmonary infections in the first years of life (Hansen and Corbet, 1998). The use of surfactant and high-frequency ventilation in recent years has decreased the incidence of BPD (Clark et al, 1992; Kossel and Versmold, 1997).

Apnea: Of LBW infants, 25% to 30% have apnea that is mostly attributable to respiratory center immaturity (i.e., apnea of prematurity). The incidence increases with decreasing gestational age. In most cases, apnea resolves by the time an infant reaches 36 to 40 weeks' maturational age (Poets et al, 1991). Apnea of prematurity, however, often persists beyond term gestation in infants ≤28 weeks' gestational age and is usually associated with chronic lung disease (Eichenwald, Aina, and Stark, 1997). For many VLBW infants, persistence or recurrence of apnea at this stage suggests gastroesophageal reflux (GER) (Gibson, 1996; Hansen and Corbet, 1998). Diagnosis and treatment of reflux result in resolution of the apnea.

There is no evidence that apnea of prematurity increases the risk for sudden infant death syndrome (SIDS) (Barrington, Finer, and Li, 1996). LBW infants—particularly VLBW infants, however, are at much higher risk for SIDS (Hodgman, 1998), whereas SIDS rates are declining for all other infants (Bigger et al, 1998). This risk appears to be magnified by other factors such as BPD, maternal drug abuse (especially of nicotine and cocaine), and prone or side-sleeping position (Gibson, 1996; Hodgman, 1998; Milerad et al, 1998; Oyen et al, 1997). Unfortunately, there is no way to predict which infants will develop SIDS. Although many centers perform pneumograms on LBW infants as a diagnostic tool to determine which infants should be sent home with a cardiorespiratory monitor (Gibson, 1996), their usefulness is controversial (Hodgman, 1998). Preterm infants under 50 to 60 weeks postconceptional age are at high risk for postanesthesia apnea and require monitoring for prolonged periods after surgery. They are not candidates for outpatient surgery after discharge (Hansen and Corbet, 1998; Wellborn et al, 1990).

Most neonatologists require a 5 to 10 day apnea-free period after discontinuing caffeine or theophylline for premature infants who continue to have significant apnea near the time of discharge. Darnall and associates (1997) found that for healthy preterm infants, 8 apnea-free days before discharge proved to be a reasonable margin of safety. Darnall's findings also confirmed the current guidelines of observation of infants in the hospital, after cessation of significant apnea for a prescribed length of time.

Nutrition

Nutrition is a major problem for the smallest premature infants. Generally, infants with birth weights above 1250 g and without significant medical problems tolerate enteral feedings easily. For those with acute problems and for smaller infants, however, enteral feedings are often delayed for days or weeks.

Parenteral nutrition: Parenteral nutrition consisting of dextrose, emulsified fat, amino acids, and other micronutrients can provide infants with adequate calories for growth. Physiologic complications of parenteral nutrition include hyperglycemia, protein intolerance reflected by hyperammonemia or acidosis, elevated triglycerides, and platelet dysfunction. Difficulties related to prolonged intravenous access (e.g., infiltrates and infection) also occur (Chathas and Paton, 1997; Heird and Gomez, 1993). These complications may prevent an infant from receiving adequate nutrition for long periods. Late complications of parenteral nutrition include cholestatic jaundice, often with elevated liver enzymes, which may affect up to 50% of infants who weigh under 1000 g and 15% of infants weighing from 1000 g to 2000 g who receive parenteral nutrition for more than 2 weeks (American Society of Parenteral and Enteral Nutrition, 1993; Berseth, 1998). This jaundice may be prolonged—lasting several weeks or more—but eventually resolves. Early small volume feeding enterally (i.e., "gut stimulation") may reduce the risk for cholestasis (Slagle, Bosque, and Cox, 1991).

The process of weaning parenteral nutrition and slowly introducing breast milk or formula can be frustrating. Feedings are often "not tolerated," a catchall phrase that includes vomiting, abdominal distention, and large gastric residuals. Because these nonspecific symptoms may be early signs of NEC, feeding is often temporarily discontinued. This on-again, off-again phase of enteral feeding results in a period of poor nutrition unless adequate calories are maintained by continuing supplementation with parenteral nutrition.

Enteral feeding: Enteral feeding practices have changed over the past decade. Because premature infants have special nutritional needs (i.e., increased need for protein, calcium, phosphate, and sodium) (Krug-Wispe, 1998), formulas have undergone many changes to meet as many of these needs as possible while maintaining an acceptably high caloric density and an acceptably low osmolality and solute load. Preterm mother's milk supplemented with human milk fortifiers has been shown to be highly suited to an infant's nutritional needs (Goldman et al, 1994; Lucas, 1993; Schanler and

Hurst, 1994; Schanler, 1998; Schanler and Abrams, 1995; Schanler et al, 1999). Preterm formulas with a base of protein from cow's milk are available in varying caloric densities for infants for whom mother's milk is not available. Soy–protein-based formulas are not recommended for preterm infants because of concerns of aluminum toxicity and their failure to achieve equivalent growth and bone mineralization when compared with fortified human milk or cow protein formulas (Committee on Nutrition, 1998). Despite the availability of parenteral nutrition, fortified breast milk, and premature formulas, most small premature infants do not receive adequate calcium and phosphorous intake. Therefore the incidence of bone demineralization, fractures, and rickets in VLBW infants is significant (Dabezies and Warren, 1997; Koo and Tsang, 1993).

Necrotizing Enterocolitis

NEC is a condition in premature infants characterized by ischemic damage to the submucosal layer of the bowel. This condition occurs in about 10% of VLBW infants (Hack et al, 1995) and accounts for approximately 2% of all deaths in premature infants. The highest mortality rates are seen in newborns with the lowest birth weights and gestational ages (Ladd et al, 1998), and mortality is higher when other organ systems are involved (Sonntag et al, 1998). NEC probably has many causes. The long list of risk factors includes asphyxia, hypertonic feedings, umbilical vessel catheterization, exchange transfusion, and polycythemia. NEC is more common in infants who have been fed than in those who have not been fed and more common in infants fed formula than in those fed breast milk (Berseth and Abrams, 1998). In severe cases of NEC, intestinal perforation can occur. Most infants with perforation are treated with immediate surgery after stabilization; however, management by peritoneal drainage for VLBW and ELBW infants may result in lower mortality and fewer long-term gastrointestinal complications (e.g., short bowel syndrome) (Ein et al, 1990; Lessin et al, 1998; Morgan, Shochant and Hartman, 1994). Whether or not perforation occurs, stricture and obstruction, along with symptoms of abdominal distention and vomiting, occur weeks later in approximately 15% of affected infants. Infants who require surgical intervention show higher rates of poor growth (Ladd et al, 1998). Life-long problems may develop in infants with postoperative short bowel syndrome (Vanderhoof et al, 1996).

Gastroesophageal Reflux

GER is another fairly common problem of premature infants that is caused by decreased lower esophageal sphincter (LES) tone. Many therapies used in NICUs, such as caffeine therapy, may exaggerate this problem with LES (Berseth and Abrams, 1998). Premature infants may need prolonged treatment for GER. GER has been associated with increased length of hospital stay and time required to achieve full feedings (Frakaloss, Burke and Sanders, 1998). Treatment depends on the clinical findings and degree of severity and may include positioning, monitoring, and thickened feedings, and medications that suppress hydrogen ion secretion in the stomach, as well as drugs that enhance gastric emptying (Trachtenbarg and Golemon, 1998).

Retinopathy of Prematurity

ROP affects the retina of premature infants. Vascularization of the retina may not be complete until after approximately 42 to 44 weeks' postconceptional age. For reasons that are not clear, abnormal vascularization of the retina develops in some premature infants. In most cases the retinopathy resolves with little or no sequelae; but in a few infants a proliferative neovascularization accompanied by fibrosis and retinal detachment can develop. This development leads to total or partial blindness (International Committee for the Classification of the Late Stages of Retinopathy of Prematurity [ICROP], 1987).

The following stages of ROP are described: stage 1, demarcation line between vascularized and avascular retina; stage 2, ridge (i.e., raised demarcation line); stage 3, ridge with extraretinal fibrovascular proliferation; stage 4, partial retinal detachment; and stage 5, total retinal detachment (ICROP, 1987).

The risk factors for development of ROP have been identified (Fielder et al, 1992), but clear cause-and-effect relationships remain to be confirmed. The most important risk factors appear to be prematurity and the length of time supplemental oxygen is used. Other factors that may increase risk are sepsis, apnea, and transfusion with adult blood

(Phelps, 1995). Over the last 15 years there has been a significant decrease in the rate and severity of ROP (Keith and Doyle, 1995; Quinn, 1998).

Treatment of neovascularization with laser photocoagulation has been effective in preventing progression of the retinopathy in most cases. This treatment appears to have fewer side effects than cryotherapy, with less pain and swelling and less likelihood of damage to the eye (Landers et al, 1990; McNamara et al, 1993). Recent data have suggested that laser photocoagulation also results in better visual acuity and less myopia when compared with cryotherapy, which was used in past years (Connolly et al, 1998).

Anemia

LBW infants are born with reduced iron stores and are particularly vulnerable to developing anemia. Because no single, specific definition for anemia exists in this population, the hemoglobin level or hematocrit value must be assessed in light of an infant's age. For example, a hematocrit value of below 40% at term birth is considered anemic; it is normal, however, for the hematocrit value to be below 40% at very early gestation and to rise with advancing gestational age. All hematocrit values then decrease over the weeks after birth, leading to "physiologic" anemia (Stockman et al, 1984). Anemia of prematurity is thus an exaggeration of this process, and the responsible mechanisms remain undefined. Shortened erythrocyte survival, hemodilution from rapidly increasing body mass, and low serum erythropoietin concentrations, despite diminished available oxygen to tissues, may contribute to anemia of prematurity (Ohls, 1998).

Infants found to have anemia at birth should be evaluated for hemolysis, chronic blood loss in utero, or acute perinatal blood loss. Common causes of anemia that develop in premature infants after the immediate perinatal period are iatrogenic blood loss and anemia of prematurity (Mentzer and Glader, 1998). The blood volume of an infant is only 80 to 100 ml/kg. Even with microtechniques, laboratory tests in sick infants can easily deplete this blood volume. Early iatrogenic anemia in very small, very sick premature infants is virtually universal and most of these infants will require at least one blood transfusion.

Tachycardia, tachypnea, poor growth, increased oxygen requirement, and acidosis are nonspecific symptoms of anemia. Presence of any of these symptoms in the face of a low hematocrit value may indicate the need for a transfusion of red blood cells (RBCs) (Sacher, Luban, and Strauss, 1989). Treatment is not without risk, however. Transfusion reactions are rare but can occur in neonates. With improved screening and the advent of DNA- and/or RNA-directed assays of donor blood for virus detection for agents such as human immunodeficiency virus (HIV) (Hewlett and Epstein, 1997), cytomegalovirus (CMV), and hepatitis B and C, infectious complications from transfusions have decreased significantly (see Chapter 24).

In VLBW or very sick premature infants, recombinant human erythropoietin may be used to treat anemia because physiologic erythropoietin levels are anticipated to be low for a prolonged period. Given with oral elemental iron and vitamin E (Kumar, Shankaran, and Krishnan, 1998; Mentzer and Shannon, 1995; Shannon et al, 1995) or in combination with parenteral iron (Ohls et al, 1997), erythropoietin stimulates erythropoiesis and decreases the need for blood transfusions in VLBW infants.

Genitourinary Problems

Preterm infants have reduced renal function when compared with term infants or older children, and extreme care must be given in the administration of fluids and medication to avoid toxic levels of drugs and other chemicals. Some functions may remain immature beyond the first year of life (Guignard, 1998). LBW and premature male infants have a higher rate of undescended testes than full-term newborns. Nearly all infants weighing approximately 900 g exhibit bilateral undescended testes. In most of these tiny infants, the testes descend during the first year of life. Medical and surgical intervention is indicated soon after 1 year of age for children with undescended testes because there is evidence of decreased spermatogonia if the testes remain in the abdomen (Hawtrey, 1990). The incidence of inguinal hernias is higher in LBW infants (i.e., up to 30%) than those born at term (i.e., approximately 1% to 4%); and occurrence is highest in the first year of life, and six times more common in boys (Kapur, Caty, and Glick, 1998). Inguinal hernias occur more often in infants born under 32 weeks' gestation or who weigh under 1250 g; the risk is highest for SGA male infants

born at less than 32 weeks' gestation. Preterm infants with inguinal hernia may have increased risk of bowel incarceration with possible testicular injury from obstruction of blood flow. Surgical repair of hernias should be accomplished as soon as possible by a qualified pediatric surgeon before these infants are discharged (Kapur, Caty and Glick, 1998). Postoperative complications include recurrent apnea as a common anesthesia morbidity, and outpatient surgery is not recommended in the first few months.

Prognosis

The infant mortality rate continues to decrease. In 1997 the infant mortality rate in the United States was a record low of 7.1/1000 live births. Prematurity and LBW and their associated problems are responsible for over 60% of these deaths. Births of LBW infants increased to 7.5% in 1997 for the fifth consecutive year (Guyer, 1998). Black mothers continue to have twice as many LBW infants as white mothers, and black infant mortality is 2.4 times that of whites. The number of multiple births has also increased since the 1980s (adding to the increase in LBW infants), in large part because of increased use of reproductive technology and an increase in the number of older mothers. RDS accounts for 3.5% of infant deaths, and maternal complications (which often lead to prematurity) account for 3.1% of deaths (CDC, 1997; Guyer, 1998). Preterm and LBW infants have a 3 to 7 times greater chance of dying after discharge from the hospital (Hulsey, Hudson, and Pittard, 1994), and the risk is highest for those of lowest gestational age (23 to 25 weeks) (Cooper et al, 1998).

Overall, survival is directly related to gestational age and/or birth weight (Kilpatrick et al, 1997) and has improved over the past 20 years. Approximately 95% of infants with birth weights of 1250 to 1499 g now survive the first year of life (Guyer, 1998). Improved survival in the smaller infants is due in part to the scientific and technologic improvements in many areas of perinatal and neonatal care. The application of available technology to infants previously thought to be nonviable has been an important reason as well. With increasing survival, however, there has not been a proportionate increase in infants with significant morbidity (i.e., the relative percentages of impairment have not increased (Fanaroff et al, 1995; Hack, Friedman and Fanaroff, 1996; O'Shea et al, 1997, 1998).

A body of outcome data now available for preterm infants consistently indicates that the smaller the baby, the lower the survival rate and the higher the morbidity in relation to medical status, cognitive ability, behavior regulation, and social competence. On average, most VLBW infants do well, but a small yet significant proportion of them develop disabilities of varying degrees of severity (Kaplan and Mayes, 1997; McCarton et al, 1996). Socioeconomic status, parental education, rearing environment, or postdischarge medical morbidity contribute to—and may be more predictive of—later outcome than interventions and complications in the NICU (Leonard and Piecuch, 1997; Monset-Couchard, deBethmann, and Kastler, 1996).

PRIMARY CARE MANAGEMENT

Health Care Maintenance

Growth and Development

When plotted by corrected age (i.e., postnatal age less the number of weeks the infant was premature), the growth pattern of preterm AGA infants follows a different pattern from that of full-term infants, but growth velocity is similar for the first 3 years (Casey et al, 1991). Moderately premature infants without serious medical illness exhibit "catch-up" growth earlier than extremely premature infants or those with serious medical problems (Hack and Fanaroff, 1988). VLBW and ELBW infants demonstrate growth patterns in the lowest percentiles during the first 12 months and remain smaller as a group than term children at 3 years of age (Casey et al, 1991; Hirata and Bosque, 1998). These children may catch up to the general population, however, by school age (Hack, Weissman and Borawski-Clark, 1996; Ross, Lipper, and Auld, 1990) and can reach their genetic potential in stature by adolescence (Hirata and Bosque, 1998).

Premature SGA infants tend to have poor neonatal growth, with the period of rapid catch-up growth occurring between 40 weeks' corrected age and 8 months of age. These children generally have lower rates of catch-up growth when compared with AGA preterm infants of the same birth weight (Strauss and Dietz, 1997).

Head circumference of LBW infants must be followed closely. Catch-up growth, which usually occurs in the first 6 weeks after birth and continues until 6 to 8 months, may result in disproportionately high head circumference percentiles, especially in the first 3 months after term. Primary care providers must be aware of infants with intracranial hemorrhage during the neonatal course to differentiate catch-up growth from developing hydrocephalus (see Chapter 25). Early postnatal head growth is an indicator of positive neurodevelopmental outcome. Lack of catch-up growth or initial catch-up growth followed by slow head growth are ominous signs (Hack and Fanaroff, 1988).

The parameters of growth must be followed closely to determine if an infant is thriving. Corrected age should be used for VLBW infants until 3 years of age. Measurements may be plotted on standard growth charts or on "Infant Health and Development Program" premature infant growth charts. These charts are available for infants up to 3 years corrected age and are separated into categories of 1501 to 2500 g and ≤1500 g for birth weight and for boys and girls (Casey et al, 1991; Ross Products Division, 1994). Infants who fail to grow within or drop off their established growth curves should be examined for undetected or inadequately treated conditions.

Development: Infants with birth weights under 1500 g are at greatest risk for developmental morbidity. Outcomes have improved over time for VLBW infants, particularly for ELBW infants, in whom there has been a dramatic increase in survival without an increase in the incidence of disabilities (Hack, Friedman, and Fanaroff, 1996). If adjustments are made for severity of illness, there is also significant improvement in the disability rate (Perlman et al, 1995; Robertson et al, 1992).

Piecuch and associates (1997) reported outcome for 446 ELBW infants born in a 12-year period and found that 64% demonstrated normal-range cognitive development at a mean age of 55 months and that cognitive outcomes improved with the advent of surfactant. In summarizing the recent developmental literature, Bennett and Scott (1997) and Vohr and Msall (1997) report that for infants with birth weights ≤ 1000 g, 75% can be expected to be free of major impairment at 2 years of age; and 85% of children with birth weights between 1000 and 1500 g will be free of major impairments. For infants weighing more than

1500 g, approximately 92% will be developmentally normal.

Major developmental disabilities associated with VLBW infants include cerebral palsy, mental retardation, sensorineural hearing loss, and visual impairment related to ROP. These conditions are two to five times more frequent in LBW infants than in term infants. In addition, low-average intelligence, static motor disorders other than overt cerebral palsy (CP) (i.e., including motor clumsiness and incoordination), seizure disorders, and behavior disorders are prevalent. Educational disabilities, school failure, and speech delay are found in a high percentage of VLBW children (Bennett and Scott, 1997; Leonard and Piecuch, 1997). Many children have multiple problems, with the most pervasive and global disabilities becoming evident early (Desmond et al, 1980; Ross, Lipper and Auld, 1990).

Premature infants are more vulnerable to environmental deprivation, resulting in more abnormal developmental outcomes in infants of lower SES (Engleke et al, 1995; Hille et al, 1994; Hunt, Cooper and Tooley, 1988; Leonard et al, 1990; Msall, 1991) and more severe disabilities than in their more advantaged peers (Leonard et al, 1990). Premature infants show significantly lower scores in social competence and significantly higher rates of behavior problems. Ross, Lipper, and Auld (1990) showed that intelligence quotient (IQ) test scores best explained social competence scores, and family stability and socioeconomic status have explained behavior problem outcomes. Educational and cognitive disabilities of these infants are influenced differently by perinatal and sociodemographic variables. Both of these sets of variables must be considered to ascertain their contributions to the long-term risk of educational disabilities (Leonard and Piecuch, 1997; Resnick, et al, 1998).

Intervention, as early as in the NICU, may maximize the developmental potential of high-risk infants (Als et al, 1994). Education and parental intervention in the first few years of life enhance early development, particularly in preterm children from disadvantaged environments (McCormick et al, 1993; Ramey et al, 1992); this effect attenuates over time, however, if not reinforced (McCarton et al, 1997).

An essential component of primary care of premature infants is developmental assessment and anticipatory guidance concerning developmental expectations. It is often difficult to perform formal testing in an office setting, but the Denver Developmental Screening Test II can help clinicians effectively screen and formulate a clinical impression of an infant's developmental capabilities. For VLBW infants, corrected age should be used for the first year of life and until 3 years of age. Using chronologic age to assess gross motor abilities will lead to overdiagnosis of neurologic abnormality in VLBW preterm infants (Allen and Alexander, 1990). Corrected age should be used when specific and comprehensive developmental tests are used.

Assessment of motor milestones during sequential visits can be a multistep screening process for CP (Allen and Alexander, 1997). Further evaluation is necessary when a delay is evident or parents are extremely worried about their child's mental development. Referrals can be made to high-risk infant follow-up clinics, child development centers, regional developmental services, Easter Seal centers, or developmental pediatricians with training in assessing premature infants.

LBW infants often show signs of neuromuscular abnormalities that resolve during the second year of life and therefore do not carry the same prognostic importance as in the full-term infant. The most common neurologic abnormalities include increased extensor tone of the lower extremities, shoulder retractions caused by hypertonicity of the shoulder girdle and trapezius muscles, mild or transient asymmetry in tone, mild-to-moderate hypotonicity, and hypertonicity of the upper or lower extremities or trunk (Dubowitz, 1988). Primary care providers must perform thorough neurologic assessments during the first 2 years of life to determine the presence and progress of abnormalities. To ensure early identification of CP, careful examination for abnormal motor patterns and motor delay should be noted, but at the same time one must be cautious about labeling a child as having CP before 18 months' corrected age (Allen and Alexander, 1997; Morgan, 1996) (see Chapter 14).

Diet

Breast and bottle feeding: Primary care providers must encourage breast feeding by providing the family information about its advantages (Box 32-5). The use of an electric pump on each breast every 3 hours helps mothers of premature infants maintain an adequate milk supply while their infants are hos-

Box 32-5

Advantages of Mother's Milk

Antiinfective Properties

Antimicrobial factors
- sIgA
- Lactoferrin
- Lysozyme
- B_{12} and folate binding proteins
- Complement
- Antiviral factors

Live cells
- Macrophages
- Polymorphonuclear leukocytes
- T and B lymphocytes

Growth Enhancing Properties

Hormones and hormone releasors
Growth factors
Enzymes
Nucleotides
Docosahexaenoic acid (DHA) (essential fatty acid)
Arachidonic acid
Preterm mother's milk, which has a higher content of protein, Na, Cl, Mg, Fe, Cu, Zn, and IgA, is adapted to preterm infants.

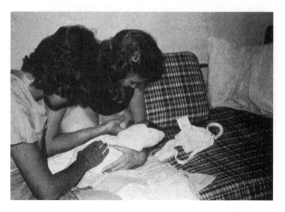

Figure 32-1 Nurse assisting mother with breast feeding her preterm infant.

pitalized and enables transition to breast feeding. Giving premature infants the opportunity to suckle, as early as 32 weeks' gestational age, engenders positive effects for both mother and infant and encourages breast feeding after discharge (Hill et al, 1997). In addition to well-known antiinfective properties and enhanced iron absorption, breast feeding has also been associated with many other benefits including developmental, psychologic, socioeconomic and environmental benefits (Work Group on Breast Feeding, 1997). Statistically significant increases in cognitive outcome at school age were seen in preterm and term infants (Horwood and Fergusson, 1998; Lucas et al, 1992). The presence of DHA and AA in breast milk, which are required for optimal brain and eye development, enhances visual acuity (Birch et al, 1998; Makrides et al, 1995). These findings should encourage health care givers to ensure that parents are given information and support. Anxiety, fatigue, and emotional stress may inhibit lactation, and mothers need support and

guidance while in the hospital, as well as after discharge, to ensure adequate nutritional intake and a healthy feeding environment for the infant-mother dyad (Figure 32-1). Many communities and hospitals have lactation counselors to work with mothers to establish a successful breast feeding regimen.

Certain maternal viral infections may result in transmission of virus to the infant via breast milk feedings, and therefore breast milk is not recommended. Such viruses include human immunodeficiency virus 1 (HIV-1) and human T-cell lymphotrophic virus type 1 (HTLV-1). CMV may be shed intermittently in breast milk, but disease does not usually develop in a term infant, presumably because of passively transferred maternal antibodies. Preterm infants, however, are at a greater potential risk because of low levels of transplacental antibodies, particularly if mothers become CMV-positive during lactation (Ruff, 1994). Preterm infants are at risk for systemic disease and sensorineural hearing loss from CMV infection (Arnold and Radkowski, 1997). Pasteurization of human milk appears to inactivate the CMV virus and allow CMV-positive mothers to provide breast milk for their infant (Committee on Infectious Disease, 1997). There are many preterm infant formulas available for mothers who cannot or choose not to provide breast milk. These formulas are constantly being modified and improved to maintain optimal health status.

Feeding premature infants can be difficult because their mouths are small, oral musculature is weak, and sucking mechanism is disorganized. Premature infants may benefit from any or all of the following interventions: frequent, small-volume feedings; soft bottle nipples; support of head, neck, and hips in slight flexion; minimal talking during eye contact; and a quiet, slightly darkened room (Gorski, 1988). Nonnutritive sucking may have beneficial effects on gastrointestinal function and growth and may facilitate nutritive sucking. Restricted flow devices (i.e., through which milk only flows when the infant sucks) have been shown to facilitate oral feeding in infants of 26 to 29 weeks gestational age (Lau et al, 1997). Prolonged skin-to-skin contact between mother and baby with opportunity for suckling at any time (i.e., kangaroo care) has been used as a means to promote successful breast feeding of hospitalized premature infants. Kangaroo care is physiologically safe for previously ill VLBW and LBW infants and psychologically beneficial for their mothers (Affonso et al, 1993; Bosque et al, 1995).

Abnormal feeding behaviors such as tonic bite reflex, tongue thrust, hyperactive gag reflex, or oral hypersensitivity can be seen. Hypersensitivity secondary to intubation, repeated suctioning, or use of nasogastric or orogastric tubes can make infants resistant to any type of oral stimulation, including nipples, spoons, and cups, and this oral aversion may last months to years after discharge. It is important for primary care providers to continually assess an infant's feeding capabilities and parental concerns about feeding. Referral to an oral-motor therapist (i.e., speech, physical, or occupational) familiar with feeding disorders is warranted when a significant or prolonged problem is recognized.

Maternal breast milk or regular commercial formula (20 kcal/30 ml) is usually nutritionally adequate for larger, healthy preterm infants after discharge (Committee on Nutrition, Nutrition Handbook, 1998). Increased caloric-density feedings are recommended for infants who were VLBW or ELBW, as well as for those who exhibit poor catch-up growth (Lucas et al, 1992). This increased caloric density can be achieved by using commercial formulas of increased caloric density (i.e., 22 kcal/30 ml), which can be purchased without prescription or by adding medium-chain triglycerides, glucose polymers, or milk fortifiers to breast milk. Higher-density formulas of 24 or even 30 kcal/30 ml may be needed for some infants with BPD. The use of additives and very high caloric formulas should be considered after consultation with a neonatologist or pediatric dietitian (Trachtenberg and Golemon, 1998).

A multivitamin supplement should be given until LBW infants are ingesting more than 32 oz of formula per day or until their body weight exceeds 2.5 kg. If breast-fed, an infant should receive a multivitamin supplement until 1 year of age. Infants with poor growth because of recurrent or chronic illness or poor caloric intake should continue to receive a multivitamin supplement until they are consuming a well-balanced diet (Committee on Nutrition, Nutrition Handbook, 1998; Groh-Wargo, 1998). Iron supplementation (2 to 4 mg/kg/day to maximum of 15 mg/day), as either an iron-fortified formula or a ferrous sulfate liquid if breastfeeding, should be given by 2 months' chronologic age and continue for 12 to 15 months until a child is regularly eating iron-rich solid foods (Committee on Nutrition, Nutrition Handbook, 1998; Groh-Wargo, 1998; Trachtenberg and Golemon, 1998). If iron deficiency is anticipated because of the infant's history or VLBW status, iron supplementation can begin by 2 to 3 weeks of age when full oral feedings are established (Ehrenkranz, 1993; Krug-Wispe, 1998). Vitamin E and folic acid supplementation should also continue until an infant is at least 40 weeks' postconceptional age. Multivitamin preparations containing vitamin E should satisfy this requirement. When iron deficiency is proven by laboratory testing, an infant may require increased iron supplementation (i.e., up to 6 mg/kg/day). Increases over this dose may cause hemolytic anemia if an infant is vitamin E deficient, may be poorly tolerated, and do not result in a more rapid response (Ehrenkranz, 1993).

Solid foods can be introduced to premature infants when any one of the following criteria is met: (1) the infant consistently consumes more than 32 oz of formula per day for 1 week, (2) the infant weighs 6 to 7 kg, or (3) the infant's corrected age is 6 months. The American Academy of Pediatrics (AAP) does not recommend feeding solids before 4 months' age. Cow's milk should not be introduced before 12 months past an infant's due date (Committee on Nutrition, 1998).

Safety

Anticipatory guidance about safety must be adjusted to a child's developmental level—not

Box 32-6

Safe Transportation of Premature Infants

- Place the infant in the rear car seat with observation by an adult.
- Infants under 1 year of age or weighing <20 lb must ride facing the rear.
- Infants 1 year of age and >20 lb should ride in rear seats approved for higher weights.
- Blanket rolls should be used inside the car seat for head and lateral trunk control.
- Rolls should be placed between the crotch strap and infant to reduce slouching.
- If the infant's head drops forward, the seat should be tilted back and/or a cloth roll wedged under the safety seat base.
- The seat should be reclined at a 45-degree angle to avoid the head dropping forward.
- Use of convertible car seats with shields, abdominal pads, or arm rests that would contact the infant's face or neck during impact should be avoided.
- The car seat's retainer clip should be positioned on the infant's chest.
- A car seat for young children should never be placed in the front passenger seat of any vehicle with a passenger-side air bag.
- An infant should never be left unattended in a car seat.

Adapted from the Committee on Injury and Poison Prevention and Committee on Fetus and Newborn: Safe transportation of premature and low birth weight infants, Pediatrics 97:758-760, 1996.

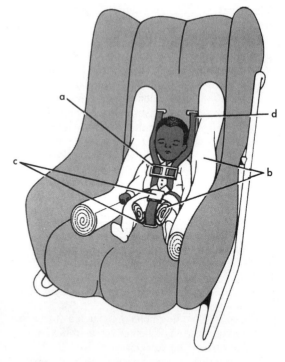

Figure 32-2 Positioning of premature infant in car seat. **A,** Retainer clip positioned on child's chest; **B,** Blanket rolls on both sides of trunk and between crotch strap and infant; **C,** Distance of 5½ inches or less from crotch strap to seat back; **D,** Distance of 10 inches or less from lower harness strap to seat bottom.

chronologic age. Because many parents continue to consider their child weak or vulnerable, they must be encouraged not to restrict activities but to allow exploration and social interaction in a safe setting.

Recommendations for the safe transportation of premature infants are shown in Box 32-6 and Figure 32-2 (Committee on Injury and Poison Prevention and Committee on Fetus and Newborn, 1996).

Safety must be ensured during air travel because of the decreased environmental oxygen concentration in commercial aircraft. Specific recommendations regarding travel for infants at risk for respiratory problems are shown in Box 32-7.

Parents of infants at higher risk for apnea or SIDS should be taught infant cardiopulmonary resuscitation (CPR) before the infant is discharged from the hospital. Home cardiorespiratory monitoring needs to be decided on an individual basis. If parent education and reliable methods of recording events are instituted, home monitoring can reduce hospitalizations for apparent life-threatening events (ALTE) (Gibson, 1996).

Immunizations

The recommendations of the AAP Committee on Infectious Disease (1999) should be used for immunizing preterm infants. Precautions and contraindications for vaccine use designated for term infants also apply to preterm infants (Committee on Infectious Disease, 1999; Khalak, Pichichero, and D'Angio, 1998).

Inactivated polio virus vaccine (IPV) should be given if an infant remains hospitalized. Use of the oral vaccine (live virus) may cause cross-infection in other vulnerable infants. After hospital discharge, standard recommendations for polio vaccination should be followed.

Rotavirus vaccine (RV) (Rotashield) should only be given to preterm infants when final approval is given by the AAP Committee on Infectious Disease. As with OPV, RV is an oral vaccine containing live, attenuated virus and should not be given to hospitalized or immunocompromised infants.

Preterm infants over 6 months of age with long-term pulmonary or cardiac problems should receive the split-virus vaccine yearly. Parents and caretakers of infants under 6 months of age and all preterm infants with pulmonary or cardiac problems should be immunized yearly with influenzae vaccine to decrease the viral exposure to the infant.

Because of the poor transfer of antibodies across the placenta early in pregnancy, all infants born before 28 weeks' gestation (or weighing ≤ 1000 g) who are still hospitalized and exposed to varicella should receive varicella-zoster immune globulin (125 units). The recommendation also applies to premature infants born after 28 weeks' gestation whose mothers have a negative history of infection (Committee on Infectious Disease, 1997).

Screening

Vision: Ophthalmologic problems, as a consequence of ROP—particularly stage 3 or higher—include myopia, amblyopia, and rarely retinal detachment and blindness. Strabismus also occurs with increased frequency among premature infants, particularly the VLBW (Allen, 1998; Phelps, 1992; Quinn, 1998). All oxygen-exposed infants with birth weights under 1500 g (or ≤ 38 weeks of gestation) or those weighing over 1500 g at birth with an unstable clinical course and at high risk for ROP should have an ophthalmologic examination at 4 to 6 weeks after birth, from 31 to 33 weeks postconceptional age, or before discharge to assess for ROP. Those who are still at risk for ROP by virtue of their immature retinae should receive close ophthalmologic follow-up after discharge. The follow-up examinations should occur at 1- to 4-week intervals, depending upon the immaturity of the retinal vessels, until the retina is mature (AAP, American Association for Pediatric Ophthalmology and Strabismus, American Academy of Ophthalmology, 1997).

Eye examinations of LBW infants by the primary care provider should include assessments of vision, the fundus, and the alignment of the eyes. Visual assessment includes the infant's ability to fixate and follow objects. This response should be present by 6 weeks' corrected age (Day, 1988). Continued yearly assessment of visual acuity in these infants is important to identify early myopia and more subtle refractive errors that may affect scholastic achievement. Anisometropia (i.e., unequal refraction) may lead to amblyopia.

Hearing: The incidence of sensorineural hearing loss in preterm infants is reported to be 1% to 3%. Factors associated with prematurity (e.g., hypoxia, mechanical ventilation for 5 days or longer, hyponatremia, metabolic acidosis, hyperbilirubinemia, environmental noise levels, concomitant antibiotic and diuretic therapy, and congenital infections) place LBW infants at particular risk for hearing problems (Borradori et al, 1997; Joint Committee on Infant Hearing, 1995). Significantly better language development was associated with early identification of hearing loss and early intervention (i.e., at under 6 months of age) (Yoshinaga-Itano, 1998).

The AAP Task Force on Newborn and Infant Hearing (1999) recommends implementation of universal newborn hearing screening. VLBW infants or infants with any other risk factors should be screened under the supervision of an audiologist. Screening should optimally be performed before discharge from the newborn nursery—never later than 3 months of age. Initial screening should include auditory brainstem response (ABR) or evoked otoacoustic emissions (EOAE) or both. If the results of an initial screening are equivocal, the infant should be referred for general medical, otologic, and audiologic follow-up, which should include a repeat ABR and a behavioral auditory testing when the child is 4 to 6 months of corrected age. Ongoing testing is necessary when there are conditions that increase the probability of progressive hearing loss, such as family history of delayed onset of hearing loss, degenerative disease, craniofacial anomalies, stigmata associated with hearing loss, meningitis, or intrauterine infections (Task Force on Newborn and Infant Hearing, 1999).

Health care providers should be alerted to children who have delays in speech development, poor attentiveness, and absent or abnormal responses to sound. These findings may indicate hearing loss and necessitate more thorough investigation.

Dental: Prolonged orotracheal intubation affects the palate and possibly the dentition; very high arched palates and deep palatal grooves have been observed. In mild cases, these deformities usually resolve within the first year of life. Abnormally shaped teeth with notching have been observed in some infants. Dental eruption is usually mildly delayed in premature infants (even allowing for corrected age), with greater delays seen in chronically ill infants (Piecuch, 1988). Staining of deciduous teeth as a result of neonatal illness (e.g., hyperbilirubinemia and cholestasis) may be evident (Herbert and Delcambre, 1987). Consultation with a pediatric dentist may be required. Specific guidelines for fluoride use in premature infants do not exist; but routine fluoride supplementation is not recommended for the first 6 months of life (Committee on Nutrition, 1995).

Blood pressure: Premature infants may be particularly at risk for developing hypertension, possibly because of complications of umbilical arterial catheters. Occult renal disease and BPD may also be the cause (Sheftel, Hustead, and Friedman, 1983). Hypertension screening should be done several times in the first year of life and then routinely in childhood. Normal blood pressures, adjusted for height, are within the 90th percentile on the blood pressure tables and graphs produced by the National High Blood Pressure Education Program (NHBPEP, 1996) and should be used for accuracy of diagnosis. Infants with blood pressures above the 95th percentile for age on three separate visits should be considered hypertensive, and the cause should be identified (NHBPEP, 1996). Children with blood pressures between the 90th and 95th percentiles warrant careful follow-up.

Hematocrit: At each visit, hematocrit screening should be tailored to individual preterm infants and the health care provider index of suspicion about the infant's hemoglobin status. History of general nutrition, iron and vitamin intake, and birth weight will help determine the need to check a blood count before the signs and symptoms of anemia (tachycardia, tachypnea, pallor, lethargy, poor feeding, poor weight gain, and apnea with bradycardia) develop. Corrective iron treatment can then be instituted to avoid a transfusion. Routine hematocrit determinations should be performed on infants with hemolytic diseases (e.g., ABO or Rh incompatibility) or those whose vitamin and iron intake is poor. Although hematocrit levels below 25% are not well tolerated, the need for transfusion should be determined by signs and symptoms of anemia rather than a defined hematocrit level (Trachtenberg and Golemon, 1998).

Urinalysis: Routine screening is recommended.

Tuberculosis: Routine screening is recommended.

Condition-Specific Screening

Hernia and testicular screening: At each primary care visit the infant's caretaker must be asked about the presence of inguinal swelling that increases in size with coughing or crying. The inguinal area and canal must be palpated for any swelling or masses. Because of the increased incidence of undescended testicles in premature male infants, a thorough testicular examination is warranted.

Common Illness Management

Differential Diagnosis, Prevention, and Treatment (Box 32-8)

Respiratory infections: Respiratory infections are frequent causes of rehospitalization in premature infants, and viral respiratory disease is particularly dangerous for infants with residual lung disease. These infants must be monitored closely by the primary care provider for signs of respiratory distress (See Chapter 12). The risk of acquiring lower respiratory tract infection is related to an infant's age at acquisition of the primary infection, with highest morbidity in the first year and lower morbidity in the second and third years of life. Because older siblings and adults usually bring viral pathogens into the home, direct contact with the infant by symptomatic individuals should be minimized, especially during the infant's first year of life. Respiratory viruses (e.g., respiratory syncytial virus [RSV], parainfluenza viruses, and influenza viruses) are a major cause of morbidity and late mortality (Committees on Infectious Disease and Fetus and Newborn, 1998). Parents should also be counselled to avoid exposing infants to environmental tobacco smoke, which is known to cause or exacerbate respiratory illness and middle ear effusions in the infant (Committee on Environmental Health, 1997).

Other viral infections: The incubation period for infants with perinatal exposure to herpes simplex virus (HSV) is variable, ranging from 2 days to 6 weeks. Because the attack rate for HSV increases with prematurity and is associated with significant morbidity and mortality, the diagnosis of

---

Box 32-8

Differential Diagnosis

Respiratory Infections

- Increased susceptibility to viral respiratory illnesses, especially RSV
- Increased incidence of wheezing and bronchiolitis
- RSV immune globulin prophylaxis

Other Viral Infections

- Herpes simplex virus type 1 and 2

Bacterial Infections

- Group B *streptococcus, Chlamydia, Staphylococcus aureus,* and *E. coli* require appropriate antibiotics
- Increased risk for *Streptococcus* pneumonial and *Hemophilus influenzae* type b
- Need early identification of possible sepsis

HSV should be considered in high-risk premature infants who have any symptoms compatible with HSV, including lethargy, poor feeding, herpetic (vesicular) lesions, respiratory distress, or seizures (Cole, 1998b). A maternal history of herpes infection or vesicular lesions increases the suspicion. Because the effects of HSV type 1 can be as devastating as HSV type 2, parents must be advised to avoid exposing their infant to individuals with fever blisters, cold sores, or any vesicular lesions suspected to be caused by HSV (Committee on Infectious Disease, 1997). Appropriate cultures should be taken and treatment should be begun with acyclovir when an infant is suspected of being infected with HSV.

Bacterial infections: Organisms such as *Chlamydia,* group B *Streptococcus, Staphylococcus aureus,* or *Escherichia coli* can colonize in an infant during birth or hospitalization and become invasive, causing serious infection characterized by sepsis and/or meningitis after discharge, particularly in the first month of life. In addition, premature infants may be at special risk for organisms such as *Streptococcus pneumoniae* (pneumococcus) and *Hemophilus influenza* type b (Hib). The major sites of infection are the respiratory system, CNS, bones, and joints.

Healthy premature infants who have unexplained fever should be assessed according to their corrected ages. This investigation is similar to that for term infants but with a higher degree of suspicion. In early stages, close follow-up is critical to the evaluation because signs and symptoms may be nonspecific and subtle. Empiric antibiotic therapy must be given immediately after cultures are taken because infection can spread rapidly because of the relative immunodeficiency of preterm infants if the provider awaits culture results. Antibiotic selection must take into account possible neonatal sources of infection (e.g., *S. aureus*), resistant bacteria from the NICU (e.g., *enterococcus* or *enterobacter*), or organisms recovered from or known to inhabit the maternal genital tract (e.g., group B *Streptococcus*) (Cole, 1998). An infant with obtundation, hypothermia, poor color, respiratory distress, seizures, or apnea is a medical emergency, and immediate hospitalization and treatment must be achieved. Parents should be instructed about the possible early signs and symptoms of infection, which may include lethargy, poor feeding, irritability, fever, respiratory distress, skin lesions, and bowel changes. Because some of these symptoms in milder form may be characteristics of a well premature infant's baseline behavior, awareness of changes in this baseline may help to identify illness.

Developmental Issues

Sleep Patterns

The sleep patterns of premature infants may differ from those of full-term infants in the first weeks after hospital discharge. Nutritional needs of premature infants may entail night feedings and establish a pattern of night waking. Some premature infants may be hypersensitive to sights and sounds and, conversely, some have become habituated to the noise and lights of the NICU and have difficulty adjusting to the quiet and dark of the home environment (Gorski, 1988). Premature infants do, however, develop circadian sleep-wake rhythms after exposure to an environment with daily routines and time cues (McMillen et al, 1991) and do not appear to have more sleep problems than term infants beyond the first few months (Wolke et al, 1995). Although an individual infant's ability to sleep through the night is determined by factors

such as age, temperament, and previous sleep patterning, a recent European study showed that night waking is more related to the type of feeding, rather than gestational age. More night waking was seen with breast feeding than with bottle feeding (Wolke et al, 1998), and more support and education by the provider is necessary to prevent early termination of breast feeding.

Toileting

Signs of toileting readiness are more likely to appear at the appropriate corrected—chronologic—age. Abnormal neurologic findings (e.g., increased muscle tone) may have a negative effect on the toilet training process, and training may be effective when muscle tone has decreased.

Discipline

The stress of having an infant in the NICU leaves many parents prone to what Green and Solnit (1964) have called "the vulnerable child syndrome." These attitudes about the child may result in the "compensatory parenting" of overindulgence and overpermissiveness (Miles and Holditch-Davis, 1997). Families often have difficulties setting limits, which can interfere with normal development; these children may exhibit dependent, demanding, or uncontrolled behavior. Guidelines on effective discipline from the AAP Committee on Psychological Aspects of Child and Family Health (1998) are helpful for primary care providers to impart to parents.

Premature infants are often more difficult to care for than full-term infants. Many become agitated or nonresponsive to what is considered average stimulation. These infants are often difficult to soothe, have trouble eating and delayed milestones, and require more care and patience from their parents. Therefore preterm children may be more prone to child abuse than term children.

Child Care

Many studies have shown the increased incidence of infectious diseases (e.g., diarrhea and respiratory illnesses) in infants and children attending daycare centers compared with children cared for in the home (Committee on Infectious Disease, 1997; Hurwitz et al, 1991). Because LBW infants have greater and more prolonged immune deficiencies, the transmission of infectious diseases within day-care centers may affect the morbidity of LBW infants attending these facilities. Based on these considerations, child care at home is preferable to other daycare situations, at least for the infant's first year of life (Committee on Infectious Disease, 1997). Parents must also consider their role in educating daycare providers about the special needs of LBW infants (e.g., nutrition, stimulation, and sleep habits).

Schooling

Many studies have documented an increased frequency of educational problems in premature children. Premature children are more likely to have lower school achievement and greater need for special class placements. These problems are often manifested as subtle visual-motor, perceptual, language, and reading difficulties or hyperactive behavior (Botting et al, 1998; Hack et al, 1994; Leonard and Piecuch, 1997; Resnick et al, 1998). School readiness is often delayed in VLBW infants (particularly in boys), and early school problems may be prevented by starting these children in school a year behind their full-term peers.

The prevalence of learning problems in preterm infants of normal intelligence emphasizes the need for early identification and implementation of individual intervention programs (Committee on Children with Disabilities, 1998; Hille et al, 1994; McCarton et al, 1997; McCormick, Gortmaker and Sobol, 1990). Ideally, these children should be longitudinally followed into their school years in high-risk clinics. If these services are not available, primary care providers should assess the neurodevelopmental progress of a child, including the presence of soft signs, which may indicate poor academic performance (Blondis, Snow, and Accardo, 1990). School performance and progress should be discussed with parents and school personnel; referral for educational testing should be initiated if a problem is suspected.

Sexuality

Preterm children, even ELBW children, do not appear to have problems in becoming parents. Both male and female survivors have had normal progeny (Hirata, 1999). Women who were born SGA have been found to be at increased risk for giving birth to both growth-retarded and preterm infants (Klebanoff, Meirik, and Berendes, 1989). Appropriate counseling and early prenatal referral for parents and adolescents are necessary with regard to these findings.

Transition to Adulthood

Transition to adolescence and adulthood may be more difficult for VLBW premature children, depending on earlier developmental and behavioral problems. Fortunately, most VLBW and ELBW children experience more rapid catch-up growth during adolescence and reach stature closer to their genetic potential. Saigal (1996) found that a majority of ELBW infants 12 to 16 years of age viewed their own health status and quality of life as quite satisfactory, although as a whole this cohort suffered a greater burden of morbidity than the control group. Many VLBW children, however, appear to have lower social competence and more behavior problems in their school years when compared with their peers (Ross, Lipper, and Auld, 1990).

In preterm children, any preexisting developmental or behavioral problems may be exaggerated during the turbulence of adolescence. Feelings of not measuring up to their peers may surface if growth has been poor and health problems have interfered with their quest for independence. Parental overprotection may add to low self-esteem. During adolescence, children are more sensitive about personal appearance, and any cosmetic deformities and scars from their hospital experience (e.g., IV, chest tube, and surgery scars) may cause anguish. Efforts toward cosmetic repair of more pronounced problems should be made.

If a child's concerns during adolescence are addressed with good parental communication, support, and encouragement, the transition to adulthood should be less problematic and more comparable to that of their full-term peers. In some cases, professional psychologic intervention may need to be provided.

Special Family Concerns and Resources

Families with premature infants have multiple issues to address (Able-Boone and Stevens, 1994).

Parents must deal with the grief of delivering a preterm infant while going through the attachment process. The transition from hospital to home is a period of extreme anxiety; parents are faced with caring for their infant without the support of hospital staff. Parents have financial issues, as well as concerns involving the health and developmental outcome of the infant. Families of infants with long hospitalizations reported more problems in family functioning (McCain, 1990). It is often difficult for parents to appreciate the progress of their premature infant while friends, relatives, and strangers continually make comparisons with full-term infants. Education and support from primary care providers may enable parents to create an environment that will encourage infants to attain their full potential. Understanding the preexisting and concurrent personal and family factors that influence the family's experience of having a premature infant may provide opportunities for support and intervention, both during hospitalization and after discharge to home (Miles and Holditch-Davis, 1997).

Today new approaches and programs exist to aid families with high-risk infants after discharge. Anticipatory guidance can help parents deal with premature infants who behave differently from the full-term infants. Parents should be educated about behavioral cues and a developmentally supportive environment, including consistency in caregiving, a structured routine, pacing of caregiving in accordance with the infant's cues for interaction versus rest, and an individualized feeding plan (Berger et al, 1998).

Resources are available for families with premature infants. Many hospitals have parent support groups that work with families during hospitalization and after discharge. Many NICUs have a follow-up clinic that employs an interdisciplinary team for ongoing evaluation of infants considered to be at high risk for physical, developmental, and psychologic problems. Government agencies and regional developmental centers provide funding for evaluation and treatment of the developmental needs of these infants. Ancillary support services such as the La Leche League and the National Center for Learning Disabilities are available and are listed below.

Informational Materials

Klein AH: Caring for your premature baby, 1998, New York, HarperCollins Publishers.

Organizations

The Preemie Store
17195 Newhope, Suite 105
Fountain Valley, Calif. 92708
(800) 676-8469
www.preemie.com

The Federation for Children with Special Needs
1135 Tremont Street, Suite 420
Boston, Mass. 02120
(617) 482-2915
www.fcsn.org

American Speech-Language-Hearing Association
10801 Rockville Pike
Rockville, Md. 20852
(310) 897-5700
www.asha.org

American Foundation for the Blind
11 Penn Plaza, Suite 300
New York, NY 10001
(800) 232-5463
www.afb.org

National Organization of Mothers of Twins Club, Inc.
PO Box 438
Thompson Station, Tenn. 37179-0438
(800) 243-2276
www.nomote.org

Summary of Primary Care Needs for the Premature or Low Birth Weight Infant

HEALTH CARE MAINTENANCE

Growth and development

Use corrected age to plot height, weight, and head circumference.

Preterm infants who are AGA follow growth patterns similar to those of full-term infants.

Infants who are SGA tend to be smaller children.

"Catch-up" growth occurs within the first year to after 3 years of age and may be prolonged to adolescence in ELBW infants.

Head circumference should be monitored for abnormal growth.

VLBW and ELBW infants are at high risk for neurologic, cognitive, or learning abnormalities.

The incidence of abnormal development increases with decreasing birth weight.

Corrected age should be used to assess development.

Transient neuromuscular abnormalities can be present in the first year.

Diet

Breastfeeding is recommended.

There are special concerns regarding viral transmission of HIV, CMV, and Hepatitis B in breast milk.

Feeding problems such as oral hypersensitivity and gastroesophageal reflux are common.

Fortification of breast milk or higher-caloric formula may be needed for ELBW and SGA infants for several weeks after hospital discharge.

Multivitamins should be given for infants who weigh under 2.5 kg or those who have chronic illness or poor growth.

All preterm infants should receive 2 to 4 mg of iron/kg/day for the first year of life.

Safety

Anticipatory guidance is based on developmental age.

Recommendations for car seat use include using blanket rolls for support, observing while driving, and avoiding models with lap pads or shields.

Air travel should be delayed until an infant tolerates lower environmental oxygen concentrations.

Parents should be trained in CPR for infants at high risk for apnea.

Immunizations

All immunizations should be administered at the chronologic ages recommended by the AAP.

Infants should be given IPV while still in hospital.

The effectiveness of the Hepatitis B vaccine is unknown in infants < 2 kg.

Preterm infants with long-term pulmonary or cardiac problems and their caretakers should receive the influenzae vaccine each fall.

Varicella-zoster immune globulin should be given to infants born at <28 weeks who are exposed to varicella while hospitalized.

Breastfeeding infants of mothers who are hepatitis B surface-antigen positive should receive hepatitis B immune globulin.

Screening

Vision: Assessment of fixation following alignment and fundoscopic examination are recommended. Ophthalmologic follow-up is necessary for infants with ROP or positive visual finding.

Hearing: Screening is recommended for all infants—particularly for those with identified risk factors before hospital discharge—and repeated within 3 months of age if abnormal or equivocal.

Dental: Prolonged intubation affects palate and dentition.

Tooth eruptions may be delayed, and teeth may be abnormally shaped or discolored.

Routine fluoride supplementation is recommended after 6 months corrected age.

Continued

Summary of Primary Care Needs for the Premature or Low Birth Weight Infant—cont'd

Blood pressure: Hypertension screenings should be done at 1, 2, 6, 12, and 24 months of age, and then routinely in childhood.

Children with BP > 95% for three screenings should be considered hypertensive and the reason identified.

Hematocrit: Hematocrit values should be checked based on history, nutritional status, and symptoms.

Urinalysis: Routine screening is recommended.

Tuberculosis: Routine screening is recommended.

Condition-specific screening

Hernia and testicular screening: Infants should be screened for inguinal hernia and undescended testicles.

COMMON ILLNESS MANAGEMENT

Differential diagnosis

Risk of infection—particularly respiratory infection—is increased.

RSV, HSV, *Chlamydia,* group B *Streptococcus, Staphylococcus aureus,* and *Escherichia coli* must all be considered possible pathogens.

Risk for *Streptococcus* pneumonia and *Hemophilus influenzae* type b infections must be evaluated.

Possible sepsis must be identified early.

DEVELOPMENTAL ISSUES

Sleep patterns

Children may have disorganized sleep patterns.

Toileting

Toileting readiness is based on developmental age.

Increased muscle tone may impede toilet training.

Discipline

Children should be assessed for vulnerable child syndrome.

Limits should be set as with any other child.

The incidence of child abuse is higher than with other children.

Child care

Home care or small daycare programs are recommended.

Schooling

These children have an increased incidence of educational problems. School readiness should be ascertained before a child enters kindergarten.

Psychometric testing is indicated for poor school performance.

Sexuality

Preterm children have normal offspring.

Standard developmental counseling is advised. There is an increased incidence of SGA and prematurity in the offspring of women who were SGA at birth.

Transition to adulthood

Preexisting developmental or behavior problems may become more exaggerated. Concerns of parental overprotection, adolescent low self-esteem, correction of cosmetic deformities, and parental communications should be addressed.

These children's self-perception of quality of life is good.

SPECIAL FAMILY CONCERNS

Special family concerns include grief, attachment issues as a result of prolonged hospitalization, financial considerations, and concerns about developmental outcomes.

References

Able-Boone H and Stevens E: After the intensive care nursery experience: families' perceptions of their well-being, Child Health Care 23:99-114, 1994.

Affonso D et al: Reconciliation and healing for mothers through skin to skin contact provided in an American tertiary level intensive care nursery, Neonatal Network 12(3):25-32, 1993.

Allen MC: Outcome and follow up of high-risk infants. In Taeusch HW and Ballard RA: Avery's diseases of the newborn, ed 7, Philadelphia, 1998, W.B. Saunders.

Allen MC and Alexander GR: Gross motor milestones in preterm infants: correction for degree of prematurity, Pediatrics 116:955-959, 1990.

Allen MC and Alexander GR: Using motor milestones as a multistep process to screen preterm infants for cerebral palsy, Dev Med Child Neurol 39:12-16, 1997.

Als H et al: Individualized developmental care for the very low birth weight preterm infant, JAMA 272:853-858, 1994.

American Academy of Pediatrics, American Association for Pediatric Ophthalmology and Strabismus, and the American Academy of Ophthalmology: Screening examination of premature infants for retinopathy of prematurity, Pediatrics 100:273, 1997.

American Society of Parenteral and Enteral Nutrition (ASPEN): Section VII: nutrition support for low-birth-weight infants, J PEN 17(4):33S-38SA, 1993.

Arnold JE and Radkowski D: Hearing loss in the newborn infant. In Fanaroff AA and Martin RJ, editors: Neonatal-perinatal medicine: diseases of the fetus and infant, ed 6, St Louis, 1997, Mosby.

Ballard JL et al: New Ballard score, expanded to include extremely premature infants, J Pediatr 119:417-23, 1991.

Barrington KJ, Finer N, and Li D: Predischarge respiratory recordings in very low birth weight newborn infants, J Pediatr 129:934-940, 1996.

Bennett FC and Scott OT: Long term perspective on preterm infant outcome and contemporary intervention issues, Semin Perinatol 21:190-201, 1997.

Berger et al: Caring for the graduate from the neonatal intensive care unit, Ped Clin North Am 45(3):701-712, 1998.

Berseth CL: Disorders of the liver. In Taeusch HW and Ballard RA, editors: Avery's diseases of the newborn, ed 7, Philadelphia, 1998, W.B. Saunders.

Berseth CL and Abrams SA: Special gastrointestinal concerns. In Taeusch HW and Ballard RA, editors: Avery's diseases of the newborn, ed 7, Philadelphia, 1998, W.B. Saunders.

Bigger HR et al: Influence of increased survival in very low birth weight, low birth weight, and normal birth weight infants on the incidence of sudden infant death syndrome in the United States: 1985-1991, J Pediatr 133:73-78, 1998.

Birch EE et al: Visual acuity and the essentiality of docosahexaenoic acid and arachidonic acid in the diet of term infants, Pediatr Res 44(2):201-209, 1998.

Blondis T, Snow J, and Accardo P: Integration of soft signs in academically normal and academically at-risk children, Pediatrics 85(suppl):421-425, 1990.

Borradori C et al: Risk factors of sensorineural hearing loss in preterm infants, Biol Neonate 100:273-278, 1997.

Bosque EM et al: Physiological measures of kangaroo versus incubator care in a tertiary level nursery, JOGNN 24(3):219-226, 1995.

Botting N et al: Cognitive and educational outcome of very-low-birthweight children in early adolescence, Dev Med Child Neurol 40:652-660, 1998.

Casey PH et al: Growth status and growth rates of a varied sample of low birth weight, preterm infants: a longitudinal cohort from birth to three years of age, J Pediatr 119:599-605, 1991.

Centers for Disease Control and Prevention: Births and deaths: United States—1996, MMWR 46(1):1-44, 1997.

Chathas MK and Paton JB: Meeting the special nutritional needs of sick infants with a percutaneous central venous catheter quality assurance program, J Perinat Neonat Nurs 10(4):72-87, 1997.

Clark RH et al: Prospective randomized comparison of high frequency oscillatory and conventional ventilation in respiratory distress syndrome, Pediatrics 89:5-12, 1992.

Clyman R: Recommendations for the postnatal use of indomethacin: an analysis of four separate treatment strategies, J Pediatr 128:601-607, 1996.

Cole FS: Bacterial infections in the newborn. In Taeusch HW and Ballard RA, editors: Avery's diseases of the newborn, ed 7, Philadelphia, 1998a, W.B. Saunders.

Cole FS: Viral infections of the fetus and newborn. In Taeusch HW and Ballard RA, editors: Avery's diseases of the newborn, ed 7, Philadelphia, 1998b, W.B. Saunders.

Committee on Children with Disabilities, American Association for Pediatric Ophthalmology and Strabismus, American Academy of Ophthalmology: Learning disabilities, dyslexia, and vision: subject review, Pediatrics 100:1217-1219, 1998.

Committee on Environmental Health: Environmental tobacco smoke: a hazard to children, Pediatrics 99:639-642, 1997.

Committee on Fetus and Newborn: Nomenclature for duration of gestation, birthweight, and intrauterine growth, Pediatrics 39:935, 1967.

Committee on Infectious Disease: Prevention of rotavirus disease: guidelines for use of rotavirus vaccine, Pediatrics 102:1483-1491, 1998.

Committee on Infectious Disease: Recommended childhood immunization schedule—United States, January-December 1999, Pediatrics 103:182-185, 1999.

Committee on Infectious Disease: Report of the Committee on Infectious Disease, ed 24, Elk Grove Village, Ill., 1997.

Committee on Infectious Disease and Committee on Fetus and Newborn: Prevention of respiratory syncytial virus infections: indications for the use of palivizumab and update on the use of RSV-IVIG, Pediatrics 102:1211-1216, 1998.

Committee on Injury and Poison Prevention and Committee on Fetus and Newborn: Safe transportation of premature and low birth weight infants, Pediatrics 97:758-760, 1996.

Committee on Nutrition: Fluoride supplementation for children: interim policy recommendations, Pediatrics 95:777, 1995.

Committee on Nutrition: Nutritional needs of preterm infants. In Kleinman RE, editor: Pediatric Nutrition Handbook, ed 4, Elk Grove Village, Ill., 1998, The American Academy of Pediatrics.

Committee on Nutrition: Soy protein-based formulas: recommendations for use in infant feedings, Pediatrics 101:148-152, 1998.

Committee on Psychological Aspects of Child and Family Health: Guidance for effective discipline, Pediatrics 101:723-728, 1998.

Connolly BP et al: A comparison of laser photocoagulation with trans-scleral cryotherapy in the treatment of threshold retinopathy of prematurity, Ophthalmology 105:1628-1631, 1998.

Cooper TR et al: Actuarial survival in the premature infant less than 30 weeks' gestation, Pediatrics 100:975-978, 1998.

Corbet A et al: Double-blind, randomized trial of one versus three prophylactic doses of synthetic surfactant in 826 neonates weighing 700 to 1100 grams: effects on mortality rate, J Pediatr 126:969-978, 1995.

Creasy RK and Iams JD: Preterm labor and delivery. In Creasy RK and Resnik R, editors: Maternal-fetal medicine, Philadelphia, 1999, W.B. Saunders.

Dabezies EJ and Warren PD: Fractures in very low birth weight infants with rickets, Clin Orthop 335:233-239, 1997.

Darnall et al: Margin of safety for discharge after apnea in preterm infants, Pediatrics 100:795-801, 1997.

Day S: The eyes of the ICN graduate. In Ballard R, editor: Pediatric care of the ICN graduate, Philadelphia, 1988, W.B. Saunders.

Desmond M et al: The very low birth infant after discharge from intensive care: anticipatory health care and developmental course, Curr Probl Pediatr 10:1-59, 1980.

Dubowitz LMS: Neurologic assessment. In Ballard R, editor: Pediatric care of the ICN graduate, Philadelphia, 1988, W.B. Saunders.

Dubowitz LMS, Dubowitz V, and Goldberg C: Clinical assessment of gestational age in the newborn, J Pediatr 77:1-10, 1970.

Duncan LL and Chiang VL: Intraventricular hemorrhage and posthemorrhagic hydrocephalus. In Albright AL, Pollack IF, and Adelson PD, editors: Principles and practice of pediatric neurosurgery, New York, 1999, Thieme.

Ehrenkranz RA: Iron, folic acid and vitamin B_{12}. In Tsang RC et al, editors: Nutritional needs of the preterm infant: scientific basis and practical guidelines, Baltimore, 1993, Williams & Wilkins.

Eichenwald EC, Aina A, and Stark A: Apnea frequently persists beyond term gestation in infants delivered at 24 to 28 weeks, Pediatrics 100:354-359, 1997.

Ein S et al: A 13-year experience with peritoneal drainage under local anesthesia for necrotizing enterocolitis perforation, J Pediatr Surg 25:1034, 1990.

Engleke et al: Cognitive failure to thrive in high-risk infants: the importance of the psychosocial environment, J Perinatol 15:325-329, 1995.

Fanaroff AA et al: Very-low-birth-weight outcomes of the National Institute of Child Health and Human Development Neonatal Research Network, May 1991 through December 1992, Am J Obstet Gynecol 173:1423-31, 1995.

Fielder AR et al: Light and retinopathy of prematurity: does retinal location offer a clue?, Pediatrics 89:648-653, 1992.

Frakaloss G, Burke G, and Sanders MR: Impact of gastroesophageal reflux on growth and hospital stay in premature infants, J Pediatr Gastroenterol Nutr 26:146-150, 1998.

Garland JS, Buck R, and Leviton A: Effect of maternal glucocorticoid exposure on risk of severe intraventricular hemorrhage in surfactant-treated preterm infants, J Pediatr 126:272-279, 1995.

Gerstmann DR et al: The Provo multicenter early high-frequency oscillatory ventilation trial: improved pulmonary and clinical outcome in respiratory distress syndrome, Pediatrics 98:1044-1057, 1996.

Gibson E: Apnea. In Spitzer AR, editor: Intensive care of the fetus and neonate, St Louis, 1996, Mosby.

Goddard-Finegold J, Mizrahi EM, and Lee RT: The newborn nervous system. In Taeusch HW and Ballard RA, editors: Avery's diseases of the newborn, ed 7, Philadelphia, 1998, W.B. Saunders.

Goldman et al: Immunologic protection of the premature newborn by human milk, Sem Perinatol 18:495-501, 1994.

Gorski PA: Fostering family development after preterm hospitalization. In Ballard R, editor: Pediatric care of the ICN graduate, Philadelphia, 1988, W.B. Saunders.

Green M and Solnit A: Reactions to the threatened loss of a child: a vulnerable child syndrome, Pediatrics 34:58-66, 1964.

Groh-Wargo S: Recommended enteral nutrient intakes. In Groh-Wargo S, Thompson M, and Cox JH: Nutritional care for high-risk newborns, Chicago, 1998, Precept Press.

Guignard JP: Renal morphogenesis and development of renal function. In Taeusch HW and Ballard RA, editors: Avery's diseases of the newborn, ed 7, Philadelphia, 1998, W.B. Saunders.

Guyer B: Annual summary of vital statistics—1997, Pediatrics 102:1333-1349, 1998.

Hack M and Fanaroff A: Growth patterns in the ICN graduate. In Ballard R, editor: Pediatric care of the ICN graduate, Philadelphia, 1988, W.B. Saunders.

Hack M, Friedman H, and Fanaroff AA: Outcomes of extremely low birth weight infants, Pediatrics 98:931-937, 1996.

Hack M, Weissman B, and Borawski-Clark E: Catch-up growth during childhood among very-low-birth-weight children, Arch Pediatr Adolesc Med 150:1122-1129, 1996.

Hack M et al: Very low birth weight outcomes of the NICHD neonatal network, November 1989-October 1990, Am J Ob Gyn 172:457-464, 1995.

Hansen T and Corbet A: Chronic lung disease. In Taeusch HW and Ballard RA, editors: Avery's diseases of the newborn, ed 7, Philadelphia, 1998, W.B. Saunders.

Hansen T and Corbet A: Control of breathing. In Taeusch HW and Ballard RA, editors: Avery's diseases of the newborn, ed 7, Philadelphia, 1998, W.B. Saunders.

Harris TR and Wood BR: Physiologic principles. In Goldsmith JP and Karotkin EH, editors: Assisted ventilation of the neonate, Philadelphia, 1996, W.B. Saunders.

Hawtrey C: Undescended testis and orchiopexy: recent observations, Pediatr Rev 11:305-308, 1990.

Heird C and Gomez MR: Parenteral nutrition. In Tsang RC et al, editors: Nutritional needs of the preterm infant. Scientific basis and practical guidelines, Baltimore, 1993, Williams & Wilkins.

Herbert FL and Delcambre TJ: Unusual case of green teeth resulting from neonatal hyperbilirubinemia, ASDC J Dent Child 54(1):54-6, 1987.

Hewlett IK and Epstein JS: Food and Drug Administration conference on the feasibility of genetic technology to close the HIV window in donor screening, Transfusion 37:346-351, 1997.

Hill PD et al: Breastfeeding patterns of low-birth-weight infants after hospital discharge, JOGNN 26:189-197, 1997.

Hille ETM et al: School performance at nine years of age in very premature and very low birthweight infants: perinatal risk factors and predictors at 5 years of age, J Pediatr 125:426-434, 1994.

Hirata T: Unpublished data, 1999.

Hirata T and Bosque E: When they grow up: the long-term growth of extremely low birth weight infants from birth to adolescence, J Pediatr 132:1033-1035, 1998.

Hodgman J: Apnea of prematurity and risk for SIDS, Pediatrics 102:969-970, 1998.

Horwood JL and Fergusson DM: Breastfeeding and later cognitive and academic outcomes, J Pediatr 101(1):9S 1998 (abstract).

Hulsey TC, Hudson MB, and Pittard III WB: Predictors of hospital postdischarge infant mortality: implications for high risk infant follow-up efforts, J Perinatol 14:219-225, 1994.

Hunt JV, Cooper BAB, and Tooley WH: Very low birth weight infants at 8 and 11 years of age: role of neonatal illness and family status, Pediatrics 82:596-603, 1988.

Hurwitz et al: Risk of respiratory illness associated with daycare attendance: a nationwide study, Pediatrics 87:62-69, 1991.

Iams JD et al: Fetal fibronectin improves the accuracy of diagnosis of preterm labor, Am J Obstet Gynecol 173:141-145, 1995.

Iams JD et al: The preterm prediction study: recurrence risk of spontaneous preterm birth, Am J Obstet Gynecol 178:1035-40, 1998.

International Committee for the Classification of the Late Stages of Retinopathy of Prematurity: An international classification of retinopathy of prematurity II, the classification of retinal detachment, Arch Ophthalmol 105:906-912, 1987.

Jobe AH et al: Beneficial effects of the combined use of prenatal corticosteroids and postnatal surfactant on preterm infants, Am J Obstet Gynecol 168:508-513, 1993.

Joint Committee on Infant Hearing: 1994 position statement, Pediatrics 95:152-156, 1995.

Kaplan MD and Mayes LC, guest editors: Outcomes of low birthweight premature infants, Sem Perinatol 21(3), 1997.

Kapur P, Caty MG, and Glick PL: Pediatric hernias and hydroceles, Ped Clin North Am 45(4):773-789, 1998.

Kari MA et al: Prenatal dexamethasone treatment in conjunction with rescue therapy of human surfactant: a randomized placebo-controlled multicenter study, Pediatrics 93:730-73, 1994.

Keith CG and Doyle LW: Retinopathy of prematurity in extremely low birth weight infants, Pediatrics 95:42-45, 1995.

Khalak R, Pichichero MR, and D'Angio CT: Three-year follow-up of vaccine response in extremely preterm infants, Pediatrics 101:597-603, 1998.

Khalid A et al: Province-based study of neurologic disability of children weighing 500 through 1249 grams at birth in relation to neonatal cerebral ultrasound findings, Pediatrics 95:837-844, 1995.

Kilpatrick et al: Outcome of infants born at 24-26 weeks' gestation: I, survival and cost, Obstet Gynecol 90:803-808, 1997.

Klebanoff M, Meirik O, and Berendes H: Second generation consequences of small-for-dates birth, Pediatrics 84:343-347, 1989.

Koo WWK and Tsang RC: Calcium, magnesium, phosphorus and vitamin D. In Tsang RC et al, editors: Nutritional needs of the preterm infant: scientific basis and practical guidelines, Baltimore, 1993, Williams & Wilkins.

Kopelman AE and Mathew OP: Common respiratory disorders of the newborn, Pediatr Rev 16:209-217, 1995.

Kossel H and Versmold H: 25 years of respiratory support of newborn infants, J Perinat Med 25:421-432, 1997.

Krug-Wispe SK: Osteopenia of prematurity. In Groh-Wargo S, Thompson M, and Cox JH, editors: Nutritional care for high-risk newborns, Chicago, 1998, Precept Press.

Krug-Wispe SK: Vitamins, minerals and trace elements. In Groh-Wargo S, Thompson M, and Cox JH, editors: Nutritional care for high-risk newborns, Chicago, 1998, Precept Press.

Kumar P, Shankaran S, and Krishnan RG: Recombinant human erythropoietin therapy for treatment of anemia of prematurity in very low birth weight infants: a randomized, double-blind, placebo-controlled trial, J Perinatol 18:173-177, 1998.

Ladd AP et al: Long-term follow-up after bowel resection for necrotizing enterocolitis: factors affecting outcome, J Pediatr Surg 33:967-972, 1998.

Landers III MB et al: Argon laser photocoagulation for advanced retinopathy of prematurity, Am J Ophthalmol 110(4):429-431, 1990.

Lau C et al: Oral feeding in low birth weight infants, J Pediatr 130:561-569, 1997.

Leach CL et al: Partial liquid ventilation with perfluoron in premature infants with severe respiratory distress syndrome, N Engl J Med 335:761-767, 1996.

Lee DL et al: Reducing blood donor exposures in low birth weight infants by use of older, unwashed packed red blood cells, J Pediatr 126:280-286, 1995.

Leonard CH and Piecuch RE: School age outcome of low birth weight preterm infants, Sem Perinatol 21(3):240-253, 1997.

Leonard CH et al: Effect of medical and social risk factors on outcome of prematurity and very low birth weight, J Pediatr 116:620-626, 1990.

Lessin MS et al: Peritoneal drainage as definitive treatment for intestinal perforation in infants with extremely low birth weight (less than 750 grams), J Pediatr Surg 33:370-372, 1998.

Long WA, Zucker JA and Kraybill EN, guest editors: Symposium on synthetic surfactant II: health and developmental outcomes at one year, J Pediatr 126 (suppl 5), part 2, 1995.

Lou HC, Lassen NA, and Friss-Hansen B: Impaired autoregulation of cerebral blood flow in the distressed newborn infant, J Pediatr 94:118-121, 1979.

Lucas A: Enteral nutrition. In Tsang RC et al, editors: Nutritional needs of the preterm infant: scientific basis and practical guidelines, Baltimore, 1993, Williams & Wilkins.

Lucas A et al: Breast milk and subsequent intelligence quotient in children born preterm, Lancet 339:261-264, 1992.

Lucas A et al: Randomized trial of nutrition for preterm infants after discharge, Arch Dis Child 67:324-327, 1992.

Makrides M et al: Are long-chain polyunsaturated fatty acids essential nutrients in infancy?, Lancet 345:1463-1468, 1995.

Martin RJ, Fanaroff A, and Klaus M: Respiratory problems. In Klaus M, Fanaroff A, editors: Care of the high-risk neonate, Philadelphia, 1993, W.B. Saunders.

Martinez et al: Control of severe hyperbilirubinemia in full-term newborns with the inhibitor of bilirubin production snmesoporphyrin, Pediatrics 103:1-5, 1999.

McCain GC: Family functioning 2 to 4 years after preterm birth, J Pediatr Nurs 5:97-104, 1990.

McCarton CM et al: Cognitive and neurologic development of the premature SGA infant through age 6, Pediatrics 98:1167-1178, 1996.

McCarton CM et al: Results at age 8 years of early intervention for low-birth-weight premature infants, JAMA 277:126-132, 1997.

McCormick MC, Gortmaker SL, and Sobol AM: Very low birth weight children: behavior problems and school difficulty in a national sample, J Pediatr 117:687-93, 1990.

McCormick MC et al: Early educational intervention for very low birth weight infants: results from the Infant Health and Development Program, J Pediatr 123:527-533, 1993.

McCormick M et al: Hospitalization of very low birth weight children at school age, J Pediatr 122:360-365, 1993.

McMillen K et al: Development of circadian sleep-wake rhythms in preterm and full term infants, Pediatr Res 29:381-384, 1991.

McNamara JA et al: Diode laser photocoagulation for retinopathy of prematurity, Arch Ophthalmol 110(12):1714-1716, 1993.

Meis PJ et al: The preterm prediction study: risk factors for indicated preterm births, Am J Obstet Gynecol 178:562-567, 1998.

Ment LR et al: Low-dose indomethacin and prevention of intraventricular hemorrhage: a multicenter randomized trial, Pediatrics 93:543-550, 1994.

Mentzer WC and Glader BE: Erythrocyte disorders in infancy. In Taeusch HW and Ballard RE, editors: Avery's diseases of the newborn, Philadelphia, 1998, W.B. Saunders.

Mentzer WC and Shannon KM: The use of recombinant human erythropoietin in preterm infants, Int J Pediatr Hematol Oncol 2:97, 1995.

Merkatz IR and Merkatz RB, guest editors: Social interventions in perinatology, Sem Perinatol 19:241-242, 1995.

Milerad J et al: Objective measurements of nicotine exposure in victims of sudden infant death syndrome and in other unexpected child deaths, J Pediatr 133:232-236, 1998.

Miles MS and Holditch-Davis D: Parenting the prematurely born child: pathways of influence, Sem Perinatol 21:254-265, 1997.

Monset-Couchard M, deBethmann O and Kastler B: Mid- and long-term outcome of 89 premature infants weighing less than 1000 g at birth, all appropriate for gestational age, Biol Neonate 70:328-338, 1996.

Morgan AM: Early identification of cerebral palsy using a profile of abnormal motor patterns, Pediatrics 98:692-697, 1996.

Morgan JL, Shochat SJ and Hartman GE: Peritoneal drainage as primary management of perforated NEC in the very low birth weight infant, J Pediatr Surg 29:310-315, 1994.

Msall ME et al: Risk factors for major neurodevelopmental impairments and need for special education resources in extremely premature infants, J Pediatr 119:606-614, 1991.

National High Blood Pressure Education Program: Update on the task force report on high blood pressure in children and adolescents: a working group report from the National High Blood Pressure Education Program, National Institutes of Health Publication No. 96-3790, September 1996, National Heart, Lung and Blood Institute.

Ohls RK: Developmental erythropoiesis. In Polin RA and Fox WW, editors: Fetal and neonatal physiology, Philadelphia, 1998, W.B. Saunders.

Ohls RK et al: The effect of erythropoietin on the transfusion requirements of preterm infants weighing 750 grams or less: A randomized, double-blind, placebo-controlled study, J Pediatr 131:661-665, 1997.

O'Shea TM et al: Survival and developmental disability in infants with birthweights of 501-800 grams, born between 1979 and 1994, Pediatrics 100:982-986, 1997.

O'Shea TM et al: Trends in mortality and cerebral palsy in a geographically based cohort of very low birth weight neonates born between 1982 and 1994, Pediatrics 101:642-647, 1998.

Oyen N et al: Combined effects of sleeping position and perinatal risk factors in sudden infant death syndrome: the Nordic epidemiologic SIDS study, Pediatrics 100:613-621, 1997.

Paneth N et al, editors: Brain damage in the preterm infant, Lavenham Suffolk, 1994, MacKeith Press (Cambridge University Press).

Papile LA, Munsick-Bruno G, and Schaefer A: Relationship of cerebral intraventricular hemorrhage and early childhood neurologic handicaps, J Pediatr 103:273-277, 1983.

Perlman M et al: Secular changes in the outcomes to 18 to 24 months of age of extremely low birth weight infants, with adjustment for changes in risk factors and severity of illness, J Pediatr 126:75-87, 1995.

Phelps DL: Retinopathy of prematurity, Curr Prob Pediatr 22:349-371, 1992.

Phelps DL: Retinopathy of prematurity, Pediatr Rev 16:50-56, 1995.

Piecuch RE et al: Outcome of infants born at 24-26 weeks' gestation: II, Neurodevelopmental outcome, Obstet Gynecol 90:809-814, 1997.

Piecuch R: Cosmetics, skin, scars, and residual traces of the ICN. In Ballard R, editor: Pediatric care of the ICN graduate, Philadelphia, 1988, WB Saunders, pp 50-56.

Piecuch R et al: Outcome of extremely low birth weight infants (500-999 grams) over a 12 year period, Pediatrics 100:633-639, 1997.

Pinto-Martin JA et al: Cranial ultrasound prediction of disabling and non-disabling cerebral palsy at age two in a low birth weight population, Pediatrics 95:249-254, 1995.

Poets CF et al: Oxygen saturation and breathing patterns in infancy, 2: preterm infants at discharge from special care, Arch Dis Child 66:574-578, 1991.

Quinn GE: The eye: retinopathy of prematurity. In Taeusch HW and Ballard RA, editors: Avery's diseases of the newborn, ed 7, Philadelphia, 1998, W.B. Saunders.

Ramey CT et al: Infant health and development program for low birth weight, premature infants: program elements, family participation, and child intelligence, Pediatrics 89:454-465, 1992.

Rebello CM et al: Postnatal lung responses and surfactant function after fetal or maternal corticosteroid treatment, J Appl Physiol 80:1679-1680, 1996.

Resnick MB et al: Educational disabilities of neonatal intensive care graduates, Pediatrics 102:308-314, 1998.

Riggs JW and Blanco JD: Pathophysiology, diagnosis, and management of intraamniotic infection, Sem Perinatol 22:251-259, 1998.

Robertson CMT et al: Population-based study of the incidence, complexity, and severity of neurologic disability among survivors weighing 500 through 1250 g at birth: a comparison of two birth cohorts, Pediatrics 90:750-754, 1992.

Roland EH and Hill A: Intraventricular hemorrhage and post-hemorrhagic hydrocephalus, current and potential future interventions, Clin Perinatol 24(3):589-605, 1997.

Ross G, Lipper EG, and Auld PAM: Growth achievement of very low birth weight premature children at school age, J Pediatr 117:307-309, 1990.

Ross G, Lipper EG, and Auld PAM: Social competence and behavior problems in premature children at school age, Pediatrics 86:391-397, 1990.

Ross Products Division, Abbott Laboratories: IHDP Growth charts for LBW and VLBW boys and girls, 1994, Columbus, Ohio, Abbott Laboratories.

Ruff AJ: Breast milk, breastfeeding and transmission of virus to the neonate, Sem Perinatol 18(6):510-516, 1994.

Sacher RA, Luban NLC, and Strauss RG: Current practice and guidelines for the transfusion of cellular blood components in the newborn, Transfusion Med Rev 3(1):39-54, 1989.

Saigal et al: Self perceived health status and health related quality of life of extremely low-birth-weight infants at adolescence, JAMA 276:453-459, 1996.

Salokorpi et al: Randomized study of the effect of antenatal dexamethasone on growth and development of premature children at the corrected age of 2 years, Acta Pediatr 86:294-298, 1997.

Schanler RJ: The role of human milk fortification for premature infants, Clin Perinatol 25:645-657, 1998.

Schanler RJ and Abrams SA: Postnatal attainment of intrauterine macromineral accretion rates in low birth weight infants fed fortified human milk, J Pediatr 126:441-447, 1995.

Schanler RJ and Hurst NM: Human milk for the hospitalized preterm infant, Sem Perinatol 18:476-484, 1994.

Schanler RJ et al: Feeding strategies for premature infants: randomized trial of gastrointestinal priming and tube-feeding method, Pediatrics 103:434-439, 1999.

Shaffer TH, Greenspan JS, and Wolfson MR: Liquid ventilation. In Boynton BR, Carlo WA, and Jobe AH, editors: New therapies for neonatal respiratory failure, a physiological approach, New York, 1994, Cambridge University Press.

Shannon et al: Recombinant human erythropoietin stimulates erythropoiesis and reduces erythrocyte transfusions in very low birth weight preterm infants, Pediatrics 95:1-8, 1995.

Sheftel D, Hustead V, and Friedman A: Hypertension screening in the follow-up of premature infants, Pediatrics 71:763-766, 1983.

Siegfried EL and Esterly NB: Newborn skin: basic concepts. In Taeusch HW and Ballard RE, editors: Avery's diseases of the newborn, Philadelphia, 1998, W.B. Saunders.

Slagle TA, Bosque E, and Cox KL: Minimal enteral feeding reduces cholestasis in parenterally nourished neonatal rabbits, Pediatr Res 29:304A, 1991.

Sohl B and Moore TR: Abnormalities of fetal growth. In Taeusch HW and Ballard RE, editors: Avery's diseases of the newborn, Philadelphia, 1998, W.B. Saunders.

Sonntag J et al: Multisystem organ failure and capillary leak syndrome in severe necrotizing enterocolitis of very low birth weight infants, J Pediatr Surg 33:481-484, 1998.

Stockman JA et al: Anemia of prematurity: determinants of the erythropoietin response, J Pediatr 105:786-792, 1984.

Strauss RG: Recombinant erythropoietin for the anemia of prematurity: still a promise, not a panacea, J Pediatr 131:653-655, 1997.

Strauss RS and Dietz WH: Effects of intrauterine growth retardation in premature infants on early childhood growth J Pediatr 130:95-102, 1997.

Task Force on Newborn and Infant Hearing: Newborn and infant hearing loss: detection and intervention, Pediatrics 103:527-530, 1999.

Tintoc E et al: Early indomethacin permanently closes the ductus in 88% of infants <1000 grams, Ped Res (abstract) 35:43A, 1994.

Trachtenbarg DE and Golemon TB: Care of the premature infant: part I, monitoring growth and development, Am Fam Physician 57:2383-2390, 1998.

Trachtenbarg DE and Golemon TB: Care of the premature infant: part II, common medical and surgical problems, Am Fam Physician 57:2123-2130, 1998.

Valaes T et al: Control of jaundice in preterm newborns by an inhibitor of bilirubin production: studies with tin-mesoporphyrin, Pediatrics 93:1-11, 1994.

Vanderhoof JA et al: Short bowel syndrome, Clin Perinatol 23(2):377-386, 1996.

Vohr BR and Msall ME: Neuropsychological and functional outcomes of very low birth weight infants, Semin Perinatol 21(3):202-220, 1997.

Volpe JJ: Intracranial hemorrhage: germinal matrix-intraventricular hemorrhage of the premature infant. In Volpe JJ, editor: Neurology of the Newborn, ed 3, Philadelphia, 1995, W.B. Saunders.

Volpe JJ: Brain injury in the premature infant-from pathogenesis to prevention, Brain Dev 19:519-534, 1997.

Volpe JJ: Neurologic outcome of prematurity, Arch Neurol 55:297-300, 1998.

Wellborn et al: Postoperative apnea in former preterm infants: prospective comparison of spinal and general anesthesia, Anesthesiology 72:838-842, 1990.

Whitaker AH et al: Neonatal cranial ultrasound abnormalities in low birth weight infants: relation to cognitive outcomes at six years of age, Pediatrics 98:719-729, 1996.

Wolke et al: An epidemiologic longitudinal study of sleeping problems and feeding experience of preterm and term children in southern Finland: comparison with a southern German population sample, J Pediatr 133:224-231, 1998.

Wolke et al: The incidence of sleeping problems in preterm and term infants discharged from special neonatal care units: an epidemiological longitudinal study, J Child Psychol Psychiatry 36:203-223, 1995.

Work Group on Breastfeeding: Breastfeeding and the use of human milk, Pediatrics 100:1035-1039, 1997.

World Health Organization (WHO): Prevention of perinatal morbidity and mortality, public health papers No. 42, Geneva, 1969, The Organization.

Yoshinaga-Itano C: Language of early- and later-identified children with hearing loss, Pediatrics 102:1161-1171, 1998.

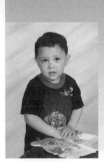

CHAPTER 33

Prenatal Cocaine Exposure

Elizabeth A. Kuehne and Marianne Warguska Reilly

Etiology

Substance abuse during pregnancy is a longstanding problem within our society. It was not until 1973, however, that the term *fetal alcohol syndrome* was first used to describe a distinctive pattern of malformations in infants born to alcoholic mothers (Jones et al, 1973), that these problems began to receive attention from health care professionals and the general public. Since then the effects of alcohol, opiates, marijuana, and other noncocaine substances on the developing fetus have been extensively studied and described (Box 33-1). Since the mid-1980s, cocaine has emerged as a widely used recreational drug and is often used in combination with other substances.

According to the 1997 Household Survey on Drug Abuse, 13.9 million Americans are current users of illicit drugs. Currently, 1.5 million Americans are users of cocaine, and 2.6 million are considered occasional users (Substance Abuse and Mental Health Services Administration [SAMHSA], 1998). With cocaine's rise in popularity among the general public has come a rise in use by women of childbearing age (Azuma and Chasnoff, 1993). Cocaine and marijuana are now the illicit substances most often used by pregnant women and are commonly used in combination with tobacco and alcohol (National Pregnancy and Health Survey [NPHS], 1996).

Cocaine can be administered in a variety of ways: intranasal snorting, intravenous (IV) injection, and smoking (National Institute on Drug Abuse [NIDA], 1998). "Crack" is currently a popular form of cocaine that consists of alkaloid crystals of cocaine that are smoked in a water pipe. Crack became available in the mid-1980s, and its popularity shows no signs of diminishing (SAMHSA, 1998). Crack differs from cocaine hydrochloride (i.e., the preparation used intranasally) in the following three ways: (1) because crack is smoked

and not sniffed, the "high" is reached within 10 seconds and lasts approximately 5 to 15 minutes; (2) crack is absorbed more effectively from the highly vascular surface of the lung, creating a more intense and powerful high; and (3) crack is relatively inexpensive, costing a few dollars per "rock" (Eyler et al, 1998; NIDA, 1998). These factors and elimination of the need for IV injection are believed to contribute to crack's popularity among both young people and women of childbearing age.

Because of crack's dramatic effects on users, a few maternal patterns of abuse have emerged. Many women use crack to abort an unwanted pregnancy or because they think that it will ease their deliveries. Some women use crack to induce labor, thinking that early delivery will prevent further fetal exposure to cocaine. In addition, many women addicted to crack begin prostituting themselves or their children to support their habit. This situation has many grave social and public health implications, including sexually transmitted diseases (STDs), congenital infections, unwanted pregnancies, and the abandonment and/or physical and sexual abuse of children.

Incidence

Each year in the United States, it is estimated that between 212,000 and 956,000 infants are exposed to one or more illicit substances (National Center for Addiction and Substance Abuse at Columbia University, 1996). The National Pregnancy and Health Survey (NPHS, 1996), based on maternal self-report, estimates that 5.5% of all pregnant women use illicit drugs during pregnancy and that 45,000 cocaine-exposed children are born each year. Prevalence reports from around the country vary widely, but documented cocaine use has been reported in 0.5% of all infants born in Georgia during 1994 (Centers for Disease Control and

---

Box 33-1

Effects of Drug Use on Fetal Development

Cocaine

Cocaine causes placental and uterine vasoconstriction, resulting in fetal hypoxia. Associated problems include prematurity, low birth weight, hypertonicity, irritability, tremors, CNS abnormalities, neurodevelopmental problems, and congenital anomalies.

Heroin

Newborns undergo a true withdrawal syndrome that includes irritability, tremors, hypertonicity, and fever. Infants have increased risk for sudden infant death syndrome (SIDS) and are vulnerable to many neonatal infections, including human immunodeficiency virus (HIV).

Alcohol

Infants undergoing withdrawal from alcohol may have tremors, irritability, hypertonicity, muscle twitching, and restlessness. The term *fetal alcohol syndrome* is used to describe a similar pattern of malformations noted in the offspring of alcohol-abusing women. Features of this syndrome include intrauterine growth retardation, slow postnatal growth, microcephaly, mental retardation, and craniofacial abnormalities.

Marijuana

Infants may have tremors, altered visual responses, low birth weight, growth retardation, and neurobehavioral abnormalities. Severity of symptoms is probably related to the amount of the drug used by the mother.

Barbiturates

Severe and prolonged withdrawal syndrome may occur. Symptoms include hyperactivity, restlessness, excessive crying, and hyperreflexia. Sudden withdrawal by the mother or infant can result in seizures.

Tobacco

Smoking in pregnancy is associated with spontaneous abortion, low birth weight, prematurity, and increased perinatal mortality

---

Prevention [CDC], 1996), 5.5% of women giving birth at a Rochester hospital (Ryan et al, 1994), 12% of infants delivered at a Bronx hospital (Wingert et al, 1994), 12.8% of infants delivered at a Manhattan hospital (Bateman et al, 1993), 30.5% of newborns in a Detroit hospital (Ostrea et al, 1997), and 31% of newborns in an inner city hospital in Baltimore (Nair, Rothblum, and Hebel, 1994). The NPHS (1996) found that black women had the highest rates of cocaine (mainly crack) use during pregnancy, whereas white women had the highest rates of alcohol and cigarette use. Use of alcohol and tobacco was strongly linked to use of illicit drugs.

Illicit drug use should be addressed with all pregnant women. Users often deny drug use, so clinicians can accordingly expect an underestimation of drug use when relying entirely on maternal self-report. Other maternal factors that may help clinicians identify children who have been exposed to cocaine in utero are history of drug use, previous birth of a drug-exposed infant, STD, signs of intoxication, lack of prenatal care, physical indications of drug use, and suspicious or erratic behav-

ior. Because of the unreliability of maternal self-report, many hospitals in communities with known drug abuse problems routinely screen all high-risk mothers and their newborns for prenatal drug exposure.

Screening for cocaine and its metabolites using a biologic marker enhances identification of newborns exposed to cocaine in utero. Maternal and infant urine screening has been the marker most widely used. Urine assay can detect benzoylecgonine (i.e., a cocaine metabolite) for 24 to 72 hours after use but cannot detect earlier use or quantify the dose. Because urine toxicologic screening of newborns is only feasible during the immediate postpartum period, primary care providers will find its usefulness limited. Because of the rapid metabolism and excretion of cocaine, it is important to remember that a negative urine assay is *not* conclusive evidence of lack of prenatal exposure.

Meconium has been shown to be a sensitive biologic marker for determining prenatal drug exposure (Ostrea, 1992; Ostrea et al, 1992; Wingert et al, 1994). Drug metabolites are excreted into meconium during the latter part of the pregnancy, so a meconium drug screen will reflect drug use during that time. Studies show that meconium testing can detect significantly more cocaine-exposed infants than urine testing (Ryan et al, 1994). Additionally, meconium may be useful in quantifying drug use during pregnancy and in clarifying issues of dose-response relationship (Delaney-Black et al, 1996). More widespread use of meconium screening will help primary care providers identify children prenatally exposed to drugs.

Other biologic markers under evaluation are hair, amniotic fluid, sweat, and cord blood, but the clinical usefulness of these tests has not been determined. For clinicians working in the newborn nursery, toxicologic screening must be performed within institutional policy and protocol.

Clinical Manifestations at Time of Diagnosis

Pharmacology and Physiologic Effects of Cocaine

Cocaine is benzoylmethylecgonine, which is a local anesthetic and central nervous system (CNS) stimulant prepared from the extract of the leaves of the coca plant (Erythroxylon coca) (Ritchie and Greene, 1980). Cocaine readily crosses from maternal to fetal circulation and, because of metabolic differences, may remain in the fetal system long after it has been excreted by the mother. Cocaine is metabolized by liver and plasma cholinesterases into several major metabolites that are excreted in the urine: benzoylecgonine, ecgonine, and ecgonine methyl ester (Plessinger and Woods, 1998; Wootton and Miller, 1994).

Three additional biologically active cocaine metabolites have been identified: norcocaine, cocaethylene, and methylecgonine (MEG). Norcocaine is water soluble with a high level of CNS penetration. Because of these characteristics, norcocaine does not reenter the maternal circulation, so the fetus may continue to be exposed to this metabolite by ingestion of the amniotic fluid (Wootton and Miller, 1994). Cocaethylene is formed in the liver when cocaine and alcohol are simultaneously ingested. It is a potent stimulant and dopamine uptake blocker that is more car-

diotoxic and longer acting than cocaine alone (Frank et al, 1998; Plessinger and Woods, 1998; Snodgrass, 1994). Methylecgonine (MEG) is a substance formed when cocaine is heated, as with "crack." It has been shown to reach the fetus and is thought to contribute to adverse neonatal outcomes in infants of crack-using mothers (Plessinger and Woods, 1998) (Box 33-2).

Cocaine is a CNS stimulant that can cause feelings of well-being, euphoria, restlessness, and excitement. Overdosage can lead to convulsions, CNS depression, and respiratory failure (Kennedy and Haddox, 1986; Ritchie and Greene, 1980). Cocaine inhibits the reuptake of neurotransmitters at the adrenergic nerve terminals, producing increased levels of norepinephrine, dopamine, and serotonin. These elevated levels of catecholamines result in increased blood pressure, tachycardia, and vasoconstriction. Cocaine also causes elevations in body temperature. Large doses are directly toxic to the myocardium and may result in cardiac failure (Drug facts and comparisons, 1999; Miller, 1991; Wootton and Miller, 1994).

Prenatal Effects of Cocaine

Because cocaine readily crosses the placenta, its physiologic effects (e.g., CNS stimulation, vasoconstriction, tachycardia, and blood pressure elevations) are thought to occur in both the mother and the fetus. In animal studies the fetal complications of cocaine use have included cardiovascular changes and changes in fetal oxygenation resulting

---

Box 33-2

Clinical Manifestations

CNS stimulation
    tremors
    seizures
    hypertonicity
    vasoconstriction
    tachycardia
    blood pressure elevation
Prematurity
Intrauterine growth retardation
Microcephaly
Poor feeding and/or soothing

from reduced uterine blood flow and impaired oxygen transfer (Woods, Plessinger, and Clark, 1987). In addition, the hormonal milieu of pregnancy may increase the hypertensive and cardiovascular effects of cocaine (Plessinger and Woods, 1998). Prenatal manifestations of maternal cocaine use are spontaneous abortion, preterm labor, precipitous labor, fetal distress, meconium staining, in utero intracranial hemorrhage, and abruptio placenta (Cohen et al, 1991; Nair, Rothblum, and Hebel, 1994; Plessinger and Woods, 1998; Robins and Mills, 1993; Sherer et al, 1998; Wootton and Miller, 1994).

Studies in cocaine-exposed rabbits and mice suggest that high levels of neurotransmitters are pooled into the cell spaces of the nervous system, causing the developing brain to undergo permanent changes. When exposed to cocaine, the anterior cingulate cortex, which is involved in attention and learning, develops dendrites that are 30% to 50% longer than normal and formed in a woven configuration. In unexposed brains, dopamine bound to protein receptors inhibits the growth of these neuronal extensions (Vogel, 1997).

Manifestations at Birth

Much literature describes the manifestations of intrauterine cocaine exposure exhibited at birth, including the following: (1) prematurity, intrauterine growth retardation, microcephaly, and low birth weight (Bateman et al, 1993; Chiriboga et al, 1999; Datta-Bhutada, et al, 1998; Eyler, et al, 1998; Richardson, 1998); (2) CNS abnormalities, such as jitteriness, tremors, seizures, electroencephalographic (EEG) abnormalities, hypertonicity, abnormal reflexes, cerebral infarct, and intraventricular hemorrhage (Chasnoff et al, 1986; Chasnoff, MacGregor, and Chisum, 1988; Cohen et al, 1994; Coles et al, 1992; Datta-Bhutada et al, 1998; Doberczak et al, 1988; Kramer et al, 1990; Richardson, 1998; Singer et al, 1994; (3) poor feeding (Barton, 1998); and (4) a higher incidence of necrotizing enterocolitis (NEC) (Czyrko et al, 1991; Porat and Brodsky, 1991). The adverse effects manifested in infants exposed to cocaine are probably not indicative of a true withdrawal syndrome as seen with infants exposed to narcotics. Some believe that these signs of cocaine exposure represent either CNS hyperexcitability as a result of the direct effects of cocaine or indications of CNS damage.

Treatment

Infants who have been exposed to cocaine in utero can be identified based on maternal history, urine or meconium toxicologic screening, and clinical presentation (Box 33-3). Although pharmacologic therapy (including the use of phenobarbital, paregoric, and diazepam) has been advocated for narcotic withdrawal (Committee on Drugs, 1998), infants who have been prenatally exposed only to cocaine do not usually require such therapy. Pacification techniques such as swaddling and decreasing environmental stimuli are used to treat the symptoms of irritability and tremors seen in these infants. Infants exposed to multiple drugs may require treatment if the mother used opiates or methadone in addition to cocaine.

Details of discharge planning for infants with prenatal exposure to cocaine depend on who their caretakers will be after discharge. Planning for discharge is generally done in conjunction with family members and hospital social service staff, as well as child protective workers, in some cases. Once the caretaker has been identified, he or she must be provided with routine discharge information and information on behavioral patterns to expect and pacification techniques to use. A referral to or consultation with a primary care provider familiar with drug misuse and addiction and its associated problems is ideal. The same provider should see these infants often—perhaps monthly—for at least the first year.

Recent and Anticipated Advances in Diagnosis and Management

Over the past decade, the issues surrounding prenatal exposure to cocaine have received attention in both the medical literature and the mass

---

Box 33-3

Treatment

Narcotic withdrawal therapy if indicated
Pacification techniques
Assessment of safety and competence of caretaker

media. Initial media reports described a "lost" generation of children who were "permanently damaged" and would never function well in society. The term "crack baby" was coined, and urban schools braced themselves for classrooms full of disturbed children (Coles, 1993; Zuckerman and Frank, 1992).

Health care providers, particularly those involved in providing obstetric, neonatal, and foster care services, saw increasing numbers of children who were prenatally exposed to cocaine. Without solid research findings, these practitioners had to develop creative ways of providing health care services to these children and their families. Since the mid-1980s, much has been learned about prenatal cocaine exposure, including the following: (1) fetal growth is affected by the continued use of cocaine during pregnancy; (2) most women who use cocaine do so in combination with other drugs, such as alcohol, tobacco, and marijuana; and (3) small differences in IQ scores, behavior and self-regulation problems, and attention difficulties may influence long-term outcomes for these children. This subtle brain damage may eventually lead to a substantial educational burden to society (Lester et al, 1998).

In summary, the verdict is not yet in on children exposed to cocaine in utero. Although health and developmental problems are seen in some of these children, it is difficult to separate the effects of cocaine from those related to a drug-using lifestyle. At this juncture, it seems that cocaine alone may not be responsible for all of the problems reported in exposed children, but conclusive data and studies of long-term outcomes are not available. It is helpful to view maternal cocaine use as a "marker" for other health and developmental risk factors, including inadequate prenatal care, poor nutrition, poly-drug use, poverty, violence, foster-care placement, inadequate parenting, and a chaotic home environment.

Associated Problems (Box 33-4)

Prematurity

Infants exposed to cocaine in utero have an increased risk of preterm birth and consequently require appropriate neonatal intervention and long-term follow-up (see Chapter 32).

Congenital Infections and Infectious Diseases

The general use of illicit drugs is associated with infectious diseases, STDs, and acquired immunodeficiency syndrome (AIDS) (Committee on Infectious Diseases, 1997; Glaser, 1994; Swan, 1997; Wootton and Miller, 1994). Therefore the offspring of women using drugs can be expected to have increased rates of congenitally acquired infections. In particular, congenital syphilis has reached epidemic proportions in many areas (Datta-Bhutada et al, 1998).

Many crack users will exchange sex for drugs; thus frequent sexual activity with multiple partners is believed to be responsible for the recent explosion in the number of syphilis cases. This pattern of behavior also places the mother and infant at increased risk for human immunodeficiency virus (HIV) infection. Many users of crack also inject cocaine or use heroin to bring themselves down from periods of prolonged cocaine use, thus increasing their risk of HIV infection from contaminated needles.

In addition to syphilis and HIV infection, primary care providers must consider infectious diseases such as hepatitis B, hepatitis C, tuberculosis, TORCH (toxoplasmosis, other viruses, rubella, cytomegalovirus, herpes) infections and other STDs (e.g., gonorrhea and chlamydia) when assessing the health status of an infant or child of a cocaine-abusing mother.

Growth Retardation and Microcephaly

Fetal growth, birth weight, and head circumference are affected by continued use of cocaine throughout

---

Box 33-4

Associated Problems

Prematurity
Exposure to congenital infections
Growth retardation
Microcephaly
Congenital anomalies
Sudden Infant Death Syndrome
Neurologic and/or development problems
Feeding difficulties
Continued exposure to drugs
Parental inadequacy

the pregnancy (Coles et al, 1992; Eyler et al, 1998). These effects are thought to be related to chronic uterine and placental hypoxia secondary to cocaine-induced vasoconstriction. Poor maternal nutrition is probably also a factor, especially in light of the anorectic effects of cocaine. A potentially worrisome finding of prenatal cocaine exposure is that of microcephaly. Recent data indicate that the head circumference of cocaine exposed children remains smaller than that of unexposed children for at least 6 years (Chasnoff et al, 1998b).

Congenital Anomalies

Cocaine may be a teratogen. The most common congenital malformations associated with maternal cocaine use are those involving the genitourinary (GU) tract. Other malformations include renal vascular abnormalities, congenital heart disease, skull defects, limb reduction defects, intestinal atresia, and ocular defects—specifically strabismus (Bingol et al, 1987; Block et al, 1997; Chavez, Mulinare, and Cordero, 1989; Hoyme et al, 1990; Lipschultz, Frassica, and Orav, 1991; Ho, Afshani, and Stapleton, 1994). It is thought that vascular compromise or fetal hypoxia resulting from cocaine-induced vasoconstriction may be responsible for the apparently increased rate of congenital malformations in these infants (Bingol et al, 1987; Hoyme et al, 1990).

Sudden Infant Death Syndrome

It is currently not clear whether infants exposed to cocaine prenatally are at an increased risk for sudden infant death syndrome (SIDS). Kandall and associates (1993) reviewed SIDS cases among 1.2 million infants born in New York City between 1979 and 1989. After controlling for high-risk variables such as ethnicity, maternal age, parity, maternal smoking, and low birth weight, the authors found that opiate use was associated with a 2.3 to 3.7-fold increase in SIDS. They also demonstrated a significant yet more modest increase in the rate of SIDS after intrauterine exposure to cocaine. In addition, they noted that cocaine-associated SIDS seems to be increasing, which may be related to the introduction of "crack" in the mid-1980s.

A recent metaanalysis (Fares et al, 1997) of 10 published articles found that an increased risk of SIDS was specific to intrauterine drug exposure, in general. Furthermore, cocaine exposure had a significant effect on risk when exposed infants were compared with drug-free infants, but not when cocaine-exposed infants were compared with poly-drug exposed infants. In contrast, Ostrea and associates (1997) studied mortality rates among 3000 infants in Michigan and found no increased risk for SIDS among infants who were drug-positive. Although no causative relationship between drugs and SIDS has been established, clinicians should be aware that infants of substance-abusing mothers seem to be at an increased risk for SIDS and may have other risk factors (e.g., prematurity and exposure to cigarette smoke).

Neurologic and Developmental Effects

The effects of intrauterine cocaine and/or poly-drug exposure on the developing CNS that have been reported include seizures and perinatal cerebral insults. Neurodevelopmental abnormalities described include irritability, tremulousness, and hypertonicity. The following four common behavioral patterns have been described in cocaine-exposed infants: (1) a deep sleep state, (2) an agitated sleep state, (3) vacillating extremes of state during handling, and (4) a panicked awake state (Schneider, Griffith, and Chasnoff, 1989). These unusual patterns of behavior, combined with inconsolability and irritability, may interfere with appropriate caregiver-infant interactions, potentially hindering the process of bonding and attachment. Delaney-Black and associates (1996) reported significant differences in autonomic stability using the Brazelton Neonatal Behavioral Assessment Scale (BN-BAS) and suggested that a dose-response relationship was evident as measured by cocaine concentration in meconium. Lewkowicz and associates (1998) studied the auditory visual response in 4- and 10-month-old infants who were exposed to cocaine. These infants showed an arousal response difference to "Infant Directed Talk" at 10 months, suggesting a decline in developmental performance beginning at this age.

Motor behavior in these infants is characterized by an increase in extensor tone, which interferes with their ability to explore the environment and their own bodies. When supine, these children often lie in an extended posture and, when held upright, stiffen and extend their ankles, knees, and hips, placing their toes in a weight-bearing position. These children have difficulty bringing their arms to midline and are poorly coordinated. Children with truncal hypertonicity often have difficulty with balance and may not be able to sit. These motor findings are mild or transient in some children and persistent in others. LaGasse and associates (1998) reported a study of infants exposed to cocaine and matched controls reaching for objects in light and dark situations. Infants exposed to cocaine reached for objects less often in the dark using a closed grasp, which may indicate early attentional or motivational deficits.

Chiriboga and associates (1999) studied 104 infants who were exposed to cocaine as documented by maternal hair analysis. Newborns were assessed at ages 1 and 7 days using the Neurological Examination for Children (NEC). When compared with unexposed controls, the newborns exposed to cocaine exhibited higher rates of global hypertonia, coarse tremor, and extensor leg posture. Fetters and associates (1996) studied cocaine-exposed and unexposed infants and evaluated neuromotor development at 1, 4, 7, and 15 months using the Alberta Infant Motor Scale (AIMS), Movement Assessment of Infants (MAI), and the Peabody Developmental Motor Scales (PDMS). They concluded that cocaine exposure was associated with poor motor performance at 4 and 7 months but was no longer evident at 15 months. Belcher and associates (1998) used the BNBAS, AIMS, and the MAI during the newborn period and at 3, 6, and 12 months studying infants with poly-drug exposure. They found numerous early potential and abnormal patterns of tone and movement, which resolved over time. Arendt and associates (1999) used the PDMS to examine 98 toddlers exposed to cocaine. Their findings indicate that abnormalities in fine and gross motor movements may persist at 2 years of age. Children exposed to cocaine had the most difficulty with hand use and eye-hand coordination.

Two recent studies report that behavior problems are evident in preschoolers. Using the Stanford-Binet Intelligence Scales, Richardson (1998) reported decreased attention span, more difficulty focusing, and restlessness during testing in 3-year old children who were prenatally exposed to cocaine. Chasnoff and associates (1998b) studied cocaine and/or poly-drug exposed subjects at 4, 5, and 6 years using the Child Behavior Checklist (CBCL) and concluded that these children had

problems with self-regulation and an inability to manage their behaviors and impulses. Previous studies have suggested early problems with state regulation. In a blinded controlled study, teachers using the Connors Teacher Rating Scale (CTRS) and the Problem Behaviors Scale (PROBS 14) identified significantly more problem behaviors in cocaine-exposed first graders than in the unexposed group (Delaney-Black, 1998).

In terms of cognitive and language development, results from IQ tests are not conclusive at this writing. Hurt (1997) found no differences in cocaine-exposed and matched controls of inner-city children at age 4 years using the Weschler Preschool and Primary Scale of Intelligence-Revised (WPPSI-R). Chasnoff's 4- to 6-year outcome study (1998b) found IQ scores using the WPPSI-R at 4 and 5 years and the Weschler Intelligence Scales for Children-III (WISC-III) at 6 years to be at the low end of the normal range in cocaine- and/or poly-drug–exposed children, but these results were not statistically significant. In Toronto, 23 children who were prenatally exposed to cocaine and then adopted by middle class families were tested using the Bayley Infant Scales of Development, the McCarthy Scales (Koren et al, 1998), and the Reynell Language Test. Findings were statistically significant for language delay. The McCarthy Scales showed a trend toward lower IQ scores, but the results were not statistically significant. This study—unlike others—controlled for maternal IQ and socioeconomic status. Johnson and associates (1997) studied a group of 14- to 15-month-old children prenatally exposed to multiple drugs and cocaine and a matched control group. Results indicated significant differences on the Sequenced Inventory of Communicative Development-Revised (SICD). The researchers concluded that these children were at risk for language delays. Lester and associates (1998) performed a metaanalysis of 101 published studies analyzing the effects of intrauterine cocaine exposure on IQ and reported a statistically significant variation of 3.26 IQ points between the cocaine-exposed and contrast groups. The authors concluded that the prenatal cocaine exposure did not cause devastating brain damage but—rather—subtle damage that may lead to substantial costs in special education.

Studies are needed to examine the intellectual

functioning of cocaine-exposed school-age children who were exposed to cocaine at an age when more complex cognitive skills are necessary for learning. Other problems, such as learning disabilities or attention deficit hyperactivity disorder (ADHD), may be uncovered (see Chapter 28).

Feeding Difficulties

Feeding difficulties and gastrointestinal (GI) symptoms, such as poor suck-swallow response, vomiting, diarrhea, and constipation, have been reported in infants exposed to cocaine in utero (Barton, 1998). These children are also seen to have a voracious appetite from clinical experience. Caretakers will report that an infant will take a full feeding every 2 hours around the clock. These infants are unable to be consoled by anything other than food; they seem genuinely hungry.

Postnatal Exposure to Cocaine and/or Other Drugs

Children of parents who use cocaine can be exposed to cocaine after, as well as before, birth. Cocaine, cocaethylene, and other metabolites are detectable in breast milk, and infants can be exposed to large doses of cocaine by breast feeding. Irritability, tremulousness, and other signs of CNS stimulation are seen in infants who ingest cocaine via breast milk (Bailey, 1998; Chasnoff, Douglas, and Squires, 1987). Children who have been passively exposed to crack smoke have manifested neurologic symptoms such as seizures, drowsiness, and unsteady gait (Bateman and Heagarty, 1989). Lustbader and associates (1998) documented cocaine metabolites in 36.3% of urine samples from infants under 1 year of age brought to Yale-New Haven Hospital's emergency room. Among these infants, upper and lower respiratory symptoms significantly correlated with a positive urine toxicology. Practitioners should consider the possibilities for later cocaine exposure via breast-feeding, passive inhalation, and accidental ingestion when caring for the children of drug-using parents. Because of the known frequency of poly-drug and tobacco use, primary care providers should be mindful of signs and symptoms of exposure to other drugs, including secondhand smoke.

Parenting Issues

Parents dealing with their own addiction may have multiple health and social problems that interfere with their ability to care for their children. They may also have been children of substance-abusing parents (Howard, 1989). Drug-using women have been shown to score higher on measures of potential child abuse and have lower self-esteem than women in a matched control group (Williams-Petersen et al, 1994). These parents, who are often single, may have had few positive parenting experiences in their own lives. If interventions such as preventive social service supports are inadequate, the courts may move to terminate parental rights so that a permanency plan can be made for the young child. Many of these infants are at risk for biologic vulnerability from intrauterine drug exposure exacerbated by inadequate parenting (Chasnoff, 1993).

Prognosis

Conclusive information about the prognosis for children with prenatal exposure to cocaine is unavailable at this time. Two correlates of prenatal drug exposure—HIV infection and preterm birth, however, significantly affect morbidity and mortality and must be considered when determining the prognosis for these children. Ostrea and associates (1997) did not find drug exposure to be associated with an increased risk of mortality within the first 2 years of life. A significantly higher mortality rate, however, was observed among low birth weight infants who were positive for both cocaine and opiates. New York City birth certificate data show that the infant mortality rate for cocaine-exposed infants is about three times that for other infants (Robins and Mills, 1993), but it is currently impossible to separate the direct effect of cocaine exposure from factors related to a family lifestyle of drug use.

PRIMARY CARE MANAGEMENT
Health Care Maintenance

Growth and Development

Primary care providers must closely monitor the physical growth of these infants and young children. Monthly evaluations are prudent during infancy. Accurate measurements for weight, length, and head circumference necessitate use of the same scale and measuring tools at each visit. It is especially important that head size be measured accurately because of the high incidence of microcephaly. Data should be plotted on a standard National Center for Health Statistics growth chart. Data for infants with a history of prematurity should be plotted using the corrected age. Recent data indicate that by the age of 2 years, infants exposed to cocaine "catch up" in height and weight when compared with nondrug-exposed children from a similar background. Children prenatally exposed to cocaine, however, have smaller head circumferences than unexposed children for at least 6 years (Chasnoff, 1998b).

Developmental assessment of infants exposed to cocaine poses a challenge to primary care providers. Routine office screening tools, such as the Denver Developmental Screening Test II, may or may not be helpful. The validity of such tests depends on the stability of the infant's state control during testing. In addition, these infants may exhibit problems with motor development that can affect results.

It is useful to monitor the infant's development at monthly intervals during the first 6 months of life and every 2 months during the second 6 months of life. Frequent assessments by the same provider offer valuable information about the child's developmental progress. Early referrals for a more detailed evaluation by a developmental psychologist may be useful before school entry or if problems are suspected.

For some infants, simultaneous visual and voice stimuli may be too stressful and interfere with parent-infant interaction. Without appropriate guidance, bonding and attachment may be jeopardized. Parents should be advised to make full use of the infant's quiet and alert states and should also be informed that the attainment of developmental milestones can be unpredictable and is generally slower in these fragile infants.

When infants who were exposed to cocaine are evaluated, a complete physical assessment is essential. Abnormal neurologic findings are common in these young children. Examiners should observe for irritability, tremors, extended postures, limb stiffness, hyperreflexia, clonus, persistence of primitive reflexes, subtle signs of infantile spasms, jerky eye movements, and the inability to track visually and respond to sound. Napiorkowski and associates (1996) reported that infants exposed to cocaine showed increased signs of CNS and visual stress using the Neonatal Intensive Care Unit (NICU) network neurobehavioral scale (NNNS). A neurologic consultation is necessary if seizures or other withdrawal symptoms (e.g., persistent hypertonicity, irritability, or disturbance in the sleep-wake state) are noted in newborns. Moreover, early assessment and intervention by a neurodevelopmentally trained physical therapist can provide parents with helpful advice about handling and positioning "stiff" infants.

Diet

Breast feeding is not recommended for women using cocaine because cocaine and cocaethylene are secreted in breast milk (Bailey, 1998). Because cocaine-exposed infants often have low birth weights, careful monitoring of caloric intake and feeding behavior is required. Infants suffering from withdrawal should receive 150 to 250 calories/kg/day; and use of a hypercaloric formula (24 cal/oz) may be necessary (Committee on Drugs, 1998). In addition, caretakers may tend to overfeed or inappropriately feed irritable infants. These infants tend to have poor coordination of sucking and swallowing reflexes, tongue thrusting, and tongue tremors, as well as general oral hypersensitivity (Barton, 1998; Lewis, Bennett, and Schmeder, 1989; Schneider, Griffith, and Chasnoff, 1989).

Parents need continued support in introducing solid foods to infants because their tongue thrust and oral hypersensitivity may persist beyond 6 months. Forced feeding is not appropriate and should be avoided. Primary care providers should encourage parents to give food and fluids that are well-tolerated.

Proper positioning and handling are essential for satisfactory feeding. Parents should have a gentle, calm approach and use a soothing voice while maintaining the infant in a relaxed, flexed posture to assist with feeding. If vomiting or spitting up occurs after feeding, frequent feedings of small amounts may be better tolerated. A side-lying, swaddled position is recommended after feeding.

Safety

Because the chronic use of mind-altering drugs by a parent can interfere with memory, attention, and perception, the safety of children is a major concern for providers. Home visits by health or social service professionals facilitate assessment of the home situation and limit parental supervision for these vulnerable children.

The primary interest of parents who are addicted to drugs—especially those using crack—is often the drug, not their children. When these parents are high, they may be completely unaware of their child's presence. In addition, these children may be living in unstable, dangerous environments with parents who are unable to function as protectors. Therefore it is important to keep children visible in the community. Social service case workers can recommend infant-stimulation programs, daycare programs, and after-school and weekend recreational programs that are appropriate for these children and will allow community workers to regularly assess a child's health and emotional status. All reported and suspected injuries should be assessed to determine if they were unintentional or suspicious of abuse or neglect. When necessary, findings should be reported to Child Protective Services for further evaluation. Substance-abusing parents should also be warned about the danger of their children's passive inhalation or accidental ingestion of the drugs.

Immunizations

No reports have yet been published on the immunization of children who were prenatally exposed to cocaine. Until such recommendations are available, primary care providers must individually assess each child's health status, social situation, and immunization needs. The recommendations published by the American Academy of Pediatrics (AAP) should generally be followed.

Polio vaccine: Children born with prenatal drug exposure are at increased risk for congenital HIV infection, and the AAP guidelines on administration of the live oral polio vaccine should be followed. The inactivated polio virus (IPV) is recommended for children whose HIV status is seronegative or unknown but who are living with an immunocompromised caretaker (Committee on Infectious Diseases, 1997). If there is any question as to the immune status of the parent, the IPV is the prudent choice.

Measles: It is wise to give the measles, mumps, and rubella vaccine at 12 months of age and again before entry to school to children living where measles epidemics are likely to occur (e.g., large urban areas or areas with high concentrations of unimmunized children). Immunogenicity among children immunized at the earlier age has been shown to be adequate (Committee on Infectious Diseases, 1997). During measles epidemics, infants at risk in the community may be immunized at 6 months, again at 12 to 15 months, and again at school entry (Committee on Infectious Diseases, 1997).

Pertussis: Children who have been exposed to cocaine in utero often show CNS manifestations of this exposure, and a small number of these children may have seizures. Infants and children with a history of seizures have an increased risk of seizures after receipt of vaccines containing pertussis (Committee on Infectious Diseases, 1997). Because seizure activity in infants exposed to cocaine is generally limited to the early neonatal period, the pertussis component of the diphtheria, pertussis, tetanus vaccine (DTaP) should be given to all of these infants except those who have persistent, uncontrolled seizures. The AAP recommends that the DTaP be given when children with a history of seizures are vaccinated because it has been shown to be much less likely to precipitate a seizure. Consultation with the child's neurologist is recommended for children exposed to cocaine whose neurologic status is not yet clearly understood.

Hepatitis B: Hepatitis B infection is a common problem among cocaine-using parents. Mothers are generally tested during the prenatal or immediate postpartum period. Doses and timing of these vaccines should be based on the mother's hepatitis B surface antigen (HBSAg) status and AAP recommendations.

Unfortunately, a child's health care maintenance may not be a high priority for drug-using parents. Every effort should be made to encourage these parents to keep their child's immunizations up-to-date, as well as to keep the immunization record intact and in a safe place. Clinicians may choose to administer several immunizations when a child is seen for health care because there may be no guarantee of compliance with follow-up visits. The AAP guidelines should be followed in doing this.

Screening

Vision: The corneal light reflex should be evaluated from birth; the cover test should be performed when a child is able to cooperate. Routine screening for visual acuity is recommended.

Hearing: Routine screening is recommended unless there is a speech delay, in which case a complete audiologic evaluation is warranted.

Dental: Routine screening is recommended.

Blood pressure: Four extremity blood pressures at birth and yearly screenings are recommended as a result of the possibility of renal vascular abnormalities.

Hematocrit: Routine screening is recommended.

Urinalysis: Routine screening is recommended.

Tuberculosis: There is a higher incidence of tuberculosis among people using drugs, especially if infected with HIV. Yearly screening with purified protein derivative (PPD), 0.1 ml intradermally, is recommended starting at age 12 months.

Developmental and/or speech and language: Developmental and/or language delays are often seen. Refer the child for a complete evaluation if a problem is suspected.

Condition-Specific Screening (Box 33-5)

Toxicology screens: If a mother is suspected of substance abuse or has not received prenatal care, the newborn's urine and/or meconium can be screened for drugs.

Congenital infections: Because women who abuse drugs are also at high risk for contracting infectious diseases, it may be wise to obtain TORCH titers to rule out congenital infections, as well as a maternal syphilis serologic test.

Genitourinary abnormalities: The urologist may recommend a renal ultrasonogram or a voiding cystourethrogram to evaluate the urologic system.

Cardiac abnormalities: The cardiologist may recommend an electrocardiogram (ECG) and echocardiogram (ECHO) to evaluate for heart disease.

Neurologic abnormalities: The neurologist may recommend any of the following studies: brainstem auditory evoked response (BAER), magnetic resonance imaging (MRI), EEG, and skull radiographic studies to evaluate the nervous system.

Common Illness Management

Differential Diagnosis (Box 33-6)

Infections: During the first 3 months of life it is often difficult to diagnose illness because of the subtle signs and symptoms newborns exhibit when ill. A change in behavior is often a key factor in the assessment of a child, which complicates diagnosing illness in infants prenatally exposed to cocaine because of the great variability in their sleep-wake state control. Primary care providers should carefully assess irritable or deeply sleeping infants for signs of concomitant illness. Practitioners must be aware of the increased risk of TORCH, HIV, hepatitis B or hepatitis C infections, or sexually transmitted diseases in this population. Accordingly, frequent infections may warrant an immunologic consultation.

Parents should be taught how to take temperatures and encouraged to call the pediatric office or

---

Box 33-5

Condition-Specific Screening

Toxicology screens
Congenital infections
Genitourinary abnormalities
Cardiac abnormalities
Neurologic abnormalities

Box 33-6

Differential Diagnosis

Infections
Gastrointestinal problems
Neurologic symptoms
Potential for child abuse and/or neglect
Continued exposure to drugs

clinic with any concerns. Frequent telephone contact will help parents manage the child at home. If a parent is a poor historian or seems overly concerned on the telephone, the child should be seen in the office or clinic.

Gastrointestinal symptoms: Gastrointestinal symptoms (e.g., poor feeding, vomiting, diarrhea, or constipation) are common in the first 6 to 9 months of life (Barton, 1998; Lewis, Bennett, and Schmeder, 1989). Parents should be advised to report any GI symptoms to their primary care provider. Once serious illness is ruled out, routine advice for handling these problems is helpful.

Neurologic symptoms: Passive exposure to cocaine can cause neurologic symptoms such as seizures, drowsiness, and unsteady gait (Bateman and Heagarty, 1989). Practitioners should include cocaine exposure in the differential diagnosis of children with these symptoms. Seizures may occur in neonates. Parents must be advised of injury prevention when a child is having a seizure, as well as the importance of having the child immediately evaluated by the provider (see Chapter 21). As children enter preschool or school, an evaluation for learning disabilities should be undertaken if there is any indication of difficulty processing information or attending to tasks. These children are considered "at risk" and therefore are eligible for evaluative services under Public Laws 99-457 and 101-476 (see Chapter 5).

Child abuse: These potentially difficult children are at increased risk for child abuse. Providers should be alert to this possibility and take a complete history and thoroughly examine the skin for marks or bruises. Parents who did not have appropriate parenting role models may have difficulty knowing how to care for themselves and may have no understanding of how to care for an irritable infant. In a 1989 fact sheet put out by the National Committee for the Prevention of Child Abuse, it was estimated that 675,000 children are seriously mistreated annually by drug abusing or alcoholic caretakers (Chasnoff, 1998a).

Parental drug use: Providers should also keep in mind that parents who are high on drugs may not follow directions appropriately. Therefore any potentially serious condition warrants an office visit, and children who are ill may need to be hospitalized or placed in temporary foster care to ensure appropriate medical management.

Drug Interactions

If a child is taking anticonvulsants for seizure activity or medications for ADHD, the same precautions outlined in Chapters 21 and 28 should be followed.

Developmental Issues

Sleep Patterns

Because of the variable sleep-wake control state patterns of these infants, establishing regular sleeping patterns is difficult. Techniques that assist parents with sleep problems include swaddling, slow rhythmic rocking, offering a pacifier, and holding the infant in a relaxed, flexed position. Keeping the lights low and reducing environmental noise are also helpful. Fortunately, few sleep problems are reported after the first year. Because drug-exposed infants may have an increased risk of SIDS, they should be placed on their backs or sides for sleep.

Toileting

Persistent motor delays, hyperactivity, and behavioral problems may cause difficulty with toilet training. Parents need a great deal of patience and support for their efforts with the child. Early counseling may help parents avoid potential difficulties. Children with persistent enuresis may require urologic evaluation because of the increased incidence of urinary tract anomalies in cocaine-exposed children.

Discipline

Irritability, excessive crying, and hyperactivity may characterize behavior in these infants and young children. Primary care providers need to assess the parents' ability to parent and their potential for using inappropriate discipline techniques. Suggesting techniques for pacifying these children (e.g., swaddling, offering pacifiers, and decreasing environmental distractions) may be helpful. Older children—especially slow learners—require patient limit-setting, and discipline must be developmentally appropriate. Few resources exist that provide expertise in managing children with difficult behaviors. Primary care providers will need to assess the mental health and developmental services in their communities for appropriate referrals.

Child Care

Parents often place children in daycare and preschool nursery programs. There is currently no clear evidence that children with a history of drug exposure need to be placed in special or therapeutic settings.

Schooling

Children who are prenatally exposed to drugs may be at risk for behavior and/or learning problems. It is wise to make early referrals to Head Start or licensed preschool programs. Head Start programs also have parenting programs to support parents wishing to improve their skills. Enrollment in these programs gives children the added benefit of daily supervision by childcare professionals. Problems such as abuse, neglect, or poor academic performance can be addressed in a timely fashion.

Substance-abusing parents may be unable to assist their children with homework assignments and are sometimes lax about making sure their children attend school regularly. Referrals to after-school and tutorial programs will encourage these children to recognize their strengths, increase their self-esteem, and develop appropriate peer relationships, as well as provide ongoing supervision during the school years.

Any children with behavioral problems or who are performing below grade level should be evaluated for learning disabilities, and a specialized educational program should be developed to meet their needs. Substance-exposed children have difficulty calming themselves, suffer sensory and emotional overload, and are highly sensitive to frustration. Teaching strategies that help children with self-regulation provide a stable structured school environment, predictable day-to-day outcomes, and consistent response to behavior problems (Chasnoff et al, 1998c).

Sexuality

Besides giving routine advice to adolescents, primary care providers must be aware of the potential for desperate drug users to prostitute their children for drugs. In addition, there is the added risk of sex-

ual abuse in these highly dysfunctional families. Providers should be alert to any physical or psychologic indications of sexual abuse and, if suspected, report the situation to the appropriate authorities. Although no published studies describe the sexual behavior of adolescents exposed to cocaine, these teens may be vulnerable to problems such as high-risk sexual activity and teen pregnancy. Social variables, including family structure and parenting practices, are associated with unsafe sexual behaviors (e.g., promiscuity and nonuse of condoms) (Biglan et al, 1990). Teen pregnancy is associated with environmental risks, such as an addicted parent, abuse and/or neglect in childhood, separation from parents by placement in foster care, poor school function, and low self-esteem (Kohlenberg, 1995).

Transition to Adulthood

No data exist to delineate how cocaine-exposed adolescents will handle the transition to adulthood. Unfortunately, these young adults may often encounter substantial problems. Children of substance abusers are three to five times more likely than other children to develop addictions and other problem behaviors (Kemper, 1995). Risk factors for adolescent drug use include parental or sibling alcohol and/or drug use, school failure, low self-esteem, and poor parent-child relationships (Hacker, 1995). School failure is associated with learning disabilities, attentional deficits, temperamental dysfunction, and family dysfunction, which may include substance abuse (Dworkin, 1995). Accordingly, teens exposed to cocaine may be at risk for failure in school. These problems may lead to higher dropout rates, future unemployment, and incarceration. Adolescents in foster care should be encouraged to use "independent living" programs that focus on smoothing the transition between foster care and life on their own. When providing anticipatory guidance for these teens, primary care providers should discuss reducing their health risk, taking responsibility for their own health, and accessing health care. These young adults should also be encouraged to apply for Medicaid or private health insurance before being discharged from foster care, as well as to locate an appropriate primary care provider. Discharge with a medical summary and a current immunization record will promote continuity of care (see Chapter 8).

Children treated for congenital syphilis will continue to have a positive serum treponemal test (i.e., fluorescent treponemal antibody absorption [FTA-ABS] or microhemagglutination assay for *T. pallidium* [MHA-TP]), which is thought to persist into adulthood. Adolescents should be made aware of this fact and have documentation of treatment on their permanent medical record or immunization card.

Special Family Concerns and Resources

The family court system may deem parents to be unfit. In some states, the result of a neonatal drug screen test that is positive for illicit drugs triggers a report to the Child Welfare Administration as evidence of neglect. Neuspiel and associates (1993) found that only 38% of infants exposed to cocaine in one New York City hospital were discharged to their mothers; 28% went to other family members, and 36% entered agency foster care. This situation forces relatives, often elderly grandparents, to assume full responsibility for infants who are drug-addicted and their siblings while parents seek treatment in the limited number of available programs. Few drug treatment programs will accept pregnant women who are addicted to drugs. Low income women and women of color may be more likely to be tested for illicit substances during their pregnancies, but drug use crosses ethnic and socioeconomic boundaries. All women should be treated respectfully, and judgments about their drug use and fitness as a parent should not be based solely on their ethnicity or economic status.

Substance-abusing parents who continue to use illicit drugs must be warned about the possibility of losing custody of their children if they fail to adequately care for them or if they endanger them in any way. Before being placed in either a kinship or temporary foster home, these infants may stay in the hospital for 2 to 4 weeks in the boarder nursery. In other cases, children are quickly moved to preadoptive homes. There is now a growing movement among health and social service professionals to have family assessments done early to improve the potential for family recovery.

Foster and kinship foster parents need respite.

The social service agency responsible for the child should be contacted. Foster parents also need ongoing positive reinforcement. Practitioners must empower them with the strength and resources to cope with these needy children. Professionals also need to examine their own feelings of attachment to children of substance-abusing parents. It may be difficult to maintain empathy and concern for these parents without becoming judgmental. As Weston and associates (1989) have noted, "Stereotypes can blind us to the unique characteristics that both infants and mothers bring to their relationship, despite the impact of drugs."

Despite careful counseling by health care professionals, adoptive parents often have expectations about the infant or child that they accept into their home. Because long-term outcomes are unknown in the cocaine-exposed population, adoptive parents must be advised accordingly. Many of these infants who have had a difficult first few months look "normal" to adoptive parents who so eagerly want a child. It is important for primary care providers to follow a child's progress with adoptive parents while remaining objective and realistic about the outcome.

Across the nation, communities are responding to the devastating problems associated with drug addiction. NAFARE provides research-based information on the effects of substance abuse during pregnancy, treatment options, and long-term prognosis. In addition, many government and private agencies have substance abuse hotlines and Internet websites.

Organizations

National Association for Families and Addiction Research and Education (NAFARE)
122 S. Michigan Ave., Suite 1100
Chicago, IL 60603
(312) 431-0013; (312) 431-8697 (fax)

NAFARE's mission is to develop, synthesize, and disseminate research-based information to professionals working with children and families affected by addiction and to families seeking resources for problems they face.

National Council on Alcoholism and Drug Dependency, Inc.
12 W. 21st St
New York, NY 10010
(212) 206-6770; hopeline: (800) NCA-CALL

National Institute on Drug Abuse (NIDA)
(800) 662-HELP; Infofax: (888) 644-6432 (access science-based facts on drug abuse)
1-800-DRUGHELP, 24-hour confidential information and referral service

Internet Resources:

The National Center on Addiction and Substance Abuse at Columbia University
http://www.casacolumbia.org

National Council on Alcoholism and Drug Dependence, Inc
http://www.ncadd.org

Kuddle Kids Korner
http://www.kuddlekids.com

Information of interest to foster and adoptive families:

National Center for Infants, Toddlers and Families
http://www.zerotothree.org

American Council for Drug Education
1-800-488-DRUG
http://www.acde.org

American Society of Addiction Medicine
http://www.asam.org

Substance Abuse and Mental Health Services Administration
http://www.samhsa.gov

National Clearinghouse on Drug and Alcohol Information (NCADI)
http://www.health.org

National Institute on Drug Abuse
http://www.nida.nih.gov

Web of Addictions
http://www.well.com/user/woa
http://nsawi.health.org

National Substance Abuse Web Index
http://nsawi.health.org

Summary of Primary Care Needs for the Child with Prenatal Cocaine Exposure

HEALTH CARE MAINTENANCE

Growth and Development

Growth parameters, particularly weight and head circumference, should be monitored closely.

Attainment of developmental milestones is unpredictable and generally slower than normal.

Speech and language delays are common.

Motor problems are common in the first year of life.

Behavior problems can occur in the preschool years.

Diet

Breast feeding is not recommended for cocaine-using women because cocaine metabolites are present in breast milk.

Caloric intake and feeding behavior should be monitored.

To enhance feeding, parents should be taught proper positioning and handling techniques.

Safety

Home visits are recommended if parents are suspected substance abusers.

Social service involvement and referrals to after-school and recreational programs are recommended to keep the child visible in the community.

Parents should be warned about the dangers of passive inhalation of crack fumes and the potential for accidental ingestion of drugs by the children.

Injuries should be evaluated for abuse and/or neglect.

Immunizations

Routine immunizations are recommended.

If a child tests HIV seropositive, the guidelines in Chapter 24 should be followed.

Infants with a limited history of seizures in the neonatal period can receive the pertussis vaccine. Infants with persistent seizures require consultation with a pediatric neurologist.

Hepatitis B immune globulin is given if the mother is infected with hepatitis.

If parents who use drugs are not compliant with well-child care visits or if the child has inconsistent health care, the clinician should assess immunization status of each visit and may choose to give several immunizations at one visit.

Screening

Vision: The corneal light reflex should be tested from birth, and the cover test should be administered when the child is able to cooperate. Routine screening for visual acuity is recommended.

Hearing: Routine office screening is recommended unless there is a speech delay, in which case a complete audiologic evaluation is warranted.

Dental: Routine screening is recommended.

Blood pressure: A four-extremity screening is recommended for neonates.

Hematocrit: Routine screening is recommended.

Urinalysis: Routine screening is recommended. The high incidence of urologic abnormalities in these children may require referral to a urologist for testing.

Tuberculosis: Yearly screening with PPD beginning at 12 months is recommended.

Developmental and/or speech and language: Problems are common. Progress should be monitored closely, and the child referred for evaluation if a problem is suspected.

Condition-Specific Screening

Toxicology: Urine toxicologic screening should be done if the mother is a suspected substance abuser or did not receive prenatal care.

Infections: Syphilis serologic testing and TORCH titers should be considered.

Genitourinary screening: Renal ultrasound and/or VCUG may be done in infancy because of a high rate of anomalies.

Cardiac screening: Both ECG and ECHO may be obtained if a heart murmur is detected.

Continued

Summary of Primary Care Needs for the Child with Prenatal Cocaine Exposure—cont'd

---

Neurologic screening: If neurologic problems are suspected, BAER, MRI, EEG, and skull films may be obtained.

COMMON ILLNESS MANAGEMENT
Differential Diagnosis
Infections: Irritable or deeply sleeping infants should be carefully assessed.

Parents should be taught to take temperatures.

An office visit should be scheduled if there are any questions about the child's condition.

These children are at high risk for contracting congenital infections, including HIV, TORCH, and STDs.

Gastrointestinal problems: Gastrointestinal symptoms such as vomiting, diarrhea, and constipation may persist for the first 6 to 9 months. Other illnesses need to be ruled out.

Neurologic problems: The child should be evaluated immediately if a seizure occurs.

These children may experience academic difficulties and school failure.

Child abuse: Behavior should be observed and skin checked closely for signs of abuse.

Parental drug use: If the parents are abusing drugs, the child may need to be hospitalized or placed in temporary foster care during periods of illness to ensure medical management.

Drug Interactions
No routine medications are prescribed. If the child is taking seizure medication or medications for ADHD, see Chapters 21 and 28.

DEVELOPMENTAL ISSUES
Sleep Patterns
Trouble with regulation of the sleep-wake state may occur in the first year of life.

Pacification techniques, low lighting, and a relatively quiet environment are helpful.

Infants should be placed on their back or side to sleep.

Toileting
Persistent motor delays, hyperactivity, and behavior problems may interfere with toilet training.

Children with persistent enuresis may need genitourinary work-up.

Discipline
Parents should be encouraged to be consistent, firm, and patient in their disciplinary efforts.

Child Care
Routine placement is advised and may help improve later school performance.

Early identification of behavior problems and referrals to Head Start or therapeutic programs may be helpful.

Schooling
These children may be at high risk for learning and/or behavior problems.

School attendance and performance should be evaluated.

Referrals for specialized education programs may be necessary.

Sexuality
These children are at high risk for sexual abuse.

Transition to Adulthood
These children are at high risk for substance abuse and school failure.

Teens in foster care should be enrolled in independent living programs.

Access to health care, risk reduction, and health insurance should be discussed.

Treatment for congenital syphilis should be documented on immunization card.

Special Family Concerns
Foster and kinship foster parents need respite.

Adoptive parents require ongoing counseling because long-term outcomes are generally unknown.

Health care providers must try to remain empathic and nonjudgmental.

References

Arendt R et al: Motor development of cocaine-exposed children at age two years, Pediatrics 103:86-92, 1999.

Azuma SD and Chasnoff IJ: Outcome of children prenatally exposed to cocaine and other drugs: a path analysis of 3-year data, Pediatrics 92:396-402, 1993.

Bailey DN: Cocaine and cocaethylene binding to human milk, Am J Clin Pathol 110:491-494, 1998.

Barton SJ: Foster parents of cocaine exposed infants, J Pediatr Nurs 13:104-112, 1998.

Bateman DA and Heagarty MC: Passive freebase cocaine ("crack") inhalation by infants and toddlers, Am J Dis Child 143:25-27, 1989.

Bateman DA et al: The effects of intrauterine cocaine exposure in newborns, AJPH 83:190-193, 1993.

Belcher HME et al: Sequential neuromotor examination of children with intrauterine drug exposure, Annals New York Academy of Sciences 846:362-364, 1998.

Biglan A et al: Social and behavioral factors associated with high-risk sexual behavior among adolescents, J Behav Med 13:245-261, 1990.

Bingol N et al: Teratogenicity of cocaine in humans, J Pediatr 110:93-96, 1987.

Block SS, Moore BD, and Scharre JE: visual anomalies in young children exposed to cocaine Optom Vis Sci 74:28-36, 1997.

Centers for Disease Control and Prevention: Population based prevalence of perinatal exposure to cocaine—Georgia 1994, MMWR 45:887-891, 1996.

Chasnoff IJ: Missing pieces of the puzzle, Neurotoxicol Teratol 15:287-288, 1993.

Chasnoff IJ: Silent violence: is prevention a moral obligation?, Pediatrics 102:145-147, 1998a.

Chasnoff IJ, Douglas EL, and Squires L: Cocaine intoxication in a breast-fed infant, Pediatrics 80:836-838, 1987.

Chasnoff IJ et al: Perinatal cerebral infarction and maternal cocaine use, J Pediatr 108:456-459, 1986.

Chasnoff IJ et al: Prenatal exposure to cocaine and other drugs: outcome at four to six years, Ann NY Acad Sci 846:314-328, 1998b.

Chasnoff IJ, MacGregor S, and Chisum G: Cocaine use during pregnancy: adverse perinatal outcome, Nat Inst Drug Abuse Res Monogr Ser 81:265, 1988.

Chasnoff IJ et al: The drug-exposed child classroom strategies for promoting self-regulation, The Challenge 8:1-4, 1998c.

Chavez GF, Mulinare J, and Cordero JF: Maternal cocaine use during early pregnancy as a risk factor for congenital urogenital anomalies, JAMA 262:795-798, 1989.

Chiriboga CA et al: Dose-response effect of fetal cocaine exposure on newborn neurologic function, Pediatrics 103:79-85, 1999.

Cohen HR et al: Peripartum cocaine use: estimating risk of adverse pregnancy outcome, Int J Gynaecol Obstet 35:51-54, 1991.

Cohen HS et al: Neurosonographic findings in full term infants born to maternal cocaine abusers: visualization of subependymal and periventricular cysts, J Clin Ultrasound 22:327-333, 1994.

Coles CD: Saying "goodbye" to the "crack baby," Neurotoxicol Teratol 15:290-292, 1993.

Coles CD et al: Effects of cocaine and alcohol use in pregnancy on neonatal growth and neurobehavioral status, Neurotoxicol Teratol 14:23-33, 1992.

Committee on Drugs: Neonatal drug withdrawal, Pediatrics 101:1079-1088, 1998.

Committee on Infectious Diseases: Report of the committee on infectious diseases, Evanston, IL, 1997, The American Academy of Pediatrics.

Czyrko C et al: Maternal cocaine abuse and necrotizing enterocolitis: outcome and survival, J Pediatr Surg 26:414-421, 1991.

Datta-Bhutada S et al: Intrauterine cocaine and crack exposure: neonatal outcome, J Perinatol 18:183-188, 1998.

Delaney-Black V et al: Prenatal cocaine exposure and child behavior, Pediatrics 102:945-950, 1998.

Delaney-Black V et al: Prenatal cocaine and neonatal outcome: evaluation of dose-response relationship, Pediatrics 98:735-740, 1996.

Doberczak TM et al: Neonatal neurologic and electroencephalographic effects of intrauterine cocaine exposure, J Pediatr 113:354-358, 1988.

Drug facts and comparisons: Topical local anesthetics, St. Louis, Facts and comparisons, 1999, pp 3194-3195.

Dworkin PH: School failure. In Parker S and Zuckerman B, editors: Behavioral and developmental pediatrics, Boston, 1995, Little, Brown.

Eyler FD et al: Birth outcome from a prospective matched study of prenatal crack/cocaine use: I. Interactive and dose effects on health and growth, Pediatrics 101:229-236, 1998.

Fares I et al: Intrauterine cocaine exposure and the risk for sudden infant death syndrome: a meta analysis, J Perinatol 17:179-182, 1997.

Fetters L et al: Neuromotor development of cocaine-exposed and control infants from birth through 15 months: poor and poorer performance, Pediatrics 98:938-943, 1996.

Frank D et al: Neonatal neurobehavioral and neuroanatomic correlates of prenatal cocaine exposure: problems of dose and confounding, Ann NY Acad Sci 846:40-50, 1998.

Glaser J: Detecting congenital syphilis, Contemp Pediatr 11:57-66, 1994.

Hacker K: Substance abuse in adolescence. In Parker S and Zuckerman B, editors: Behavioral and developmental pediatrics, Boston, 1995, Little, Brown.

Ho J, Afshani E, and Stapleton FB: Renal vascular abnormalities associated with prenatal cocaine exposure, Clin Pediatr 32:155-156, 1994.

Howard J: Long term development of infants exposed prenatally to drugs. In Special currents: cocaine babies, Columbus, Ohio, 1989, Ross Laboratories.

Hoyme HE et al: Prenatal cocaine exposure and fetal vascular disruption, Pediatrics 85:743-747, 1990.

Hurt H et al: Children with in utero exposure do not differ from control subjects on intelligence testing, Arch Pediatr Adolesc Med 151:1237-1241, 1997.

Johnson JM et al: Standardized test performance of children with a history of prenatal exposure to multi drugs/cocaine, J Com Dis 30:45-73, 1997.

Jones KL et al: Pattern of malformation in offspring of chronic alcoholic mothers, Lancet 1:1267-1271, 1973.

Kandall SR et al: Relationship of maternal substance abuse to subsequent sudden infant death syndrome in offspring, J Pediatr 123:120-126, 1993.

Kemper K: Parental drug, alcohol, and cigarette addiction. In Parker S and Zuckerman B, editors: Behavioral and developmental pediatrics, Boston, 1995, Little, Brown.

Kennedy RL and Haddox JD: Local anesthetics. In Craig CR and Stitzel RE, editors: Modern pharmacology, ed 2, Boston, 1986, Little, Brown.

Kohlenberg TM: Teen mothers. In Parker S and Zuckerman B, editors: Behavioral and developmental pediatrics, Boston, 1995, Little, Brown.

Koren G et al: Long-term neurodevelopmental risks in children exposed in utero to cocaine the Toronto adoption study, Ann New York Acad Sci 846:306-312, 1998.

Kramer LD et al: Neonatal cocaine-related seizures, J Child Neurol 5:60-64, 1990.

LaGasse LL et al: Effects of in utero exposure to cocaine and/or opiates on infants reaching behavior, Ann New York Acad Sci 846:405-406, 1998.

Lester BM et al: Cocaine exposure and children: the meaning of subtle effects, Science 282: 633-634, 1998.

Lewis KD, Bennett B, and Schmeder NH: Care of infants menaced by cocaine use, MCN 14:324-329, 1989.

Lewkowicz DJ et al: Effects of prenatal cocaine exposure on responsiveness to multimodal information in infants between 4 and 10 months of age, Ann New York Acad Sci 846:408-411, 1998.

Lipschultz SE, Frassica JJ, Orav EJ: Cardiovascular abnormalities in infants prenatally exposed to cocaine, J Pediatr 118:44-51, 1991.

Lustbader AS et al: Incidence of passive exposure to crack/cocaine and clinical findings in infants seen in an outpatient service, Pediatrics 102:e5, 1998.

Miller NS: Pharmacology of cocaine. In Miller NS: The pharmacology of alcohol and drugs of addiction, New York, 1991, Springer-Verlag.

Nair P, Rothblum S, and Hebel R: Neonatal outcome in infants with evidence of fetal exposure to opiates, cocaine, and cannaboids, Clin Pediatr 33:280-285, 1994.

Napiorkowski B et al: Effects of in utero substance exposure on infant neuro behavior, Pediatrics 98:71-83, 1996.

National Center on Addiction and Substance Abuse at Columbia University: Illicit drug use during pregnancy, substance abuse and the American woman, Website: http://www.casacolumbia.org/pubs/jun96/womc25.html.

National Institute on Drug Abuse: Crack and cocaine: NIDA Infofax, 1998, Website: http://www.nida.nih.gov:80/Infofax/Cocaine.html.

National Pregnancy and Health Survey—Drug use among women delivering livebirths: 1992, HHS, National Institute on Drug Abuse, NIH Publication #96-3819, 1996.

Neuspiel DR et al: Custody of cocaine-exposed newborns: determinants of discharge decisions, Am J Public Health 83:1726-1729, 1993.

Ostrea EM et al: Drug screening of newborns by meconium analysis: a large prospective epidemiologic study, Pediatrics 89:107-113, 1992.

Ostrea EM: Detection of prenatal drug exposure in the pregnant woman and her newborn infant, Nat Inst Drug Abuse Res Monogr Ser 117:61-79, 1992.

Ostrea EM, Ostrea AR, and Simpson PM: Mortality within the first two years in infants exposed to cocaine, opiates, or cannaboid during gestation, Pediatrics 100:79-83, 1997.

Plessinger M and Woods J: Cocaine in pregnancy recent data on maternal and fetal risks, Obstet Gynecol Clin North Am 25:99-118, 1998.

Porat R and Brodsky N: Cocaine: a risk factor for necrotizing enterocolitis, J Perinatol 11:30-32, 1991.

Richardson GA: Prenatal cocaine exposure: a longitudinal study of development, Ann New York Acad Sci 846:144-152, 1998.

Ritchie JM and Greene NM: Local anesthetics. In Gilman AG, Goodman LS, and Gilman A, editors: The pharmacological basis of therapeutics, New York, 1980, MacMillan.

Robins LN and Mills JL, editors: Effects of in utero exposure to street drugs, Am J Public Health Suppl 83:17, 1993.

Ryan RM et al: Meconium analysis for improved identification of infants exposed to cocaine in utero, J Pediatr 125:435-440, 1994.

Schneider JW, Griffith DR, and Chasnoff IJ: Infants exposed to cocaine in utero: implications for developmental assessment and intervention, Infants Young Child 2:25-36, 1989.

Sherer DM et al: Antepartum fetal intracranial hemorrhage, predisposing factors and prenatal sonography: a review, Am J Perinatol 15:431-441, 1998.

Singer LT et al: Increased incidence of intraventricular hemorrhage and developmental delay in cocaine-exposed very low birthweight infants, J Pediatr 124:765-771, 1994.

Snodgrass SR: Cocaine babies: a result of multiple teratogenic influences, J Child Neurol 9:227-233, 1994

Substance Abuse and Mental Health Service Administration, Office of Applied Statistics: Preliminary results from the 1997 National Household survey on drug abuse, Washington, DC, 1998, US Dept. of Health and Human Services, Website: http://www.samhsa.gov/oas/nhsda/nhsda97/htoc.htm.

Swan N: CDC report highlights link between drug use and spread of HIV, NIDA Notes, Website: http://www.nida.nih.gov/NIDA_Notes/ NNVol12N2/CDCReports.html.

Tronick EZ et al: Late dose-response effects of prenatal cocaine exposure on newborn neurobehavioral performance, Pediatrics 98:76-83, 1996.

Vogel G: Cocaine wreaks subtle damage on developing brains, Science 278:38-39, 1997.

Weston DR et al: Drug exposed babies: research and clinical issues, Zero to Three: Bulletin of the National Center for Clinical Infant Programs 9:1-7, 1989.

Williams-Petersen MG et al: Drug-using and nonusing women: potential for child abuse, child-rearing attitudes, social support, and affection for expected baby, Int J Addict 29:1631-1643, 1994.

Wingert WE et al: A comparison of meconium, maternal urine, and neonatal urine for detection of maternal drug use during pregnancy, J Forensic Sci 39:150-158, 1994.

Woods JR, Plessinger MA, and Clark KE: Effect of cocaine on uterine blood flow and fetal oxygenation, JAMA 257:957-961, 1987.

Wootton J and Miller SI: Cocaine: a review, Pediatr Rev 15:89-92, 1994.

Zuckerman B and Frank DA: "Crack kids": not broken, Pediatrics 89:337-339, 1992.

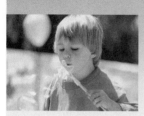

CHAPTER 34

Renal Failure, Chronic

Judy H. Taylor

Etiology

More than 8 million Americans have renal disease, with children representing approximately 10% of this population—a small but significant percentage of the total group. Early recognition and management are essential to minimizing the potentially devastating consequences of renal failure.

Staging of Chronic Renal Failure (CRF)

Assessment of the glomerular filtration rate (GFR) is the most important test for determining kidney function. Because GFR correlates with height and body surface area, estimation of GFR from height and plasma creatinine (calculated using the Schwartz formula) is usually more accurate and reliable in infants and young children than timed urine collections (Chantler, 1997). CRF is a broadly used term relating to GFR and may be described in the following three stages: (1) chronic renal insufficiency (CRI) with a GFR of <75% of normal and associated impairment of excretory and regulatory functions; (2) CRF, with a GFR of 10% to 50% of normal and increasing clinical manifestations of renal failure; and (3) end-stage renal disease (ESRD), with a GFR of <10% of normal and renal replacement therapy (RRT) with dialysis or transplantation necessary to sustain life (Parker, 1998).

Causes of CRF are varied and can be broadly categorized as congenital or hereditary, obstructive uropathy, glomerulopathies, collagen vascular, metabolic or cystic diseases, and malignancies (Table 34-1). Glomerulonephritis accounts for the largest single group of children with ESRD, followed by congenital and other hereditary and/or cystic diseases. Race-related patterns are shown, with hypertension being more common among black children (as in adults) and congenital or hereditary diseases being more common in white

and Native American children (United States Renal Data System [USRDS], 1998).

Children with congenital disorders or whose renal disease begins in infancy are at greatest risk for significant growth failure and progression to ESRD. Children with congenital renal anomalies often have abnormalities of other organ systems, as well, according to the period of embryonic development and gestational stage at which the problem occurred. Genetic counseling is recommended for future family planning. It is important to establish the exact cause of CRF in a child whenever possible, because of the following reasons: (1) disorders may require different treatments and have varying prognoses; (2) genetic counseling and early diagnosis and treatment of similarly affected siblings should be initiated if a hereditary or metabolic disease in involved; and (3) the timing and donor selection for renal transplantation may be altered in diseases with a high incidence of recurrence in renal allografts.

In some cases, early surgical intervention may slow the progression of renal disease. Reimplantation of ureters may prevent further vesicoureteral refluxing and renal scarring from pyelonephritis (Russell, 1998; Walker, 1996). Early ablation of posterior urethral valves, which may be detected prenatally, may delay renal failure and positively affect growth and later sexual development in males (Cendron et al, 1996; Smith and Duckett, 1996). Unfortunately, it is not always possible to determine the cause, especially when a child is already experiencing CRF. A renal biopsy may be indicated for diagnosis and/or prognosis and treatment recommendations.

Incidence and Prevalence

In the most comprehensive collection of data available, the United States Renal Data Service (1998)

Table 34-1

Incidence of Treated ESRD (%) in Pediatric Patients (Age <20), Median Age, Sex, Race[1], and 1-Year Transplant and Death Status by Detailed Primary Disease, 1992-1996

Primary Disease Groups[2]	Total # Patients	Median Age	% Males	% White	% Black	During 1st Year[3] % Tx'ed	During 1st Year[3] % Died
All pediatric ESRD (reference)	**5,155**	**14**	**57.1**	**63.0**	**27.4**	**37.3**	**2.9**
Diabetes	**83**	**16**	**39.8**	**54.2**	**33.7**	**13.3**	**2.4**
Glomerulonephritis (GN)	**1,635**	**16**	**55.0**	**56.9**	**32.8**	**33.3**	**1.6**
• Focal glomerulosclerosis, focal GN	515	16	60.2	44.5	47.0	30.9	1.2
• Membranous nephropathy	23	16	52.2	*	60.9	13.0	4.3
• Membranoproliferative GN	130	15	45.4	68.5	22.3	36.9	0.0
• IgA nephropathy, Berger's disease	66	17	71.2	69.7	*	28.8	0.0
• Rapidly progressive GN	106	14	39.6	69.8	11.3	33.0	0.9
• Goodpastures Syndrome	34	16	47.1	88.2	*	17.6	2.9
• Unspecified GN	683	16	54.8	59.0	30.3	36.5	2.0
• Other proliferative GN	65	16	53.8	66.2	26.2	33.8	3.1
Secondary GN/vasculitis	**470**	**16**	**36.6**	**61.7**	**26.4**	**21.1**	**5.5**
• Lupus erythematosus	257	17	24.5	45.9	40.1	10.1	7.0
• Wegener's granulomatosis	28	17	50.0	85.7	*	17.9	7.1
• Henoch-Schönlein syndrome	50	14	52.0	90.0	*	42.0	2.0
• Hemolytic uremic syndrome	99	9	57.6	83.8	*	34.3	3.0
Interstitial nephritis/pyelonephritis	**558**	**14**	**63.3**	**76.2**	**17.4**	**45.2**	**2.5**
• Chronic pyelonephritis, reflux nephritis	120	16	44.2	80.0	12.5	33.3	0.8
• Nephropathy caused by other agents	71	14	69.0	81.7	*	43.7	2.8
• Nephrolithiasis, obstruction, gout	231	12	76.2	74.9	20.3	49.8	2.2
• Chronic interstitial nephritis	123	15	54.5	73.2	16.3	51.2	4.9
Hypertensive/large vessel disease	**258**	**17**	**57.8**	**38.4**	**52.7**	**25.6**	**4.7**
• Hypertension (no primary renal disease)	237	17	58.6	35.0	56.1	24.9	4.6
• Renal artery stenosis or occlusion	21	9	47.6	76.2	14.3	33.3	4.8
Cystic/hereditary/congenital diseases	**1,259**	**11**	**66.8**	**72.8**	**19.0**	**43.7**	**2.9**
• Polycystic kidneys, adult (dominant)	128	10	44.5	76.6	14.8	46.1	3.1
• Polycystic, infantile (recessive)	31	3	41.9	74.2	*	6.5	9.7
• Medullary cystic, nephronophthisis	40	13	55.0	85.0	*	35.0	0.0
• Alport's other hereditary/familial disease	149	16	85.9	70.5	21.5	40.9	0.7
• Cystinosis	39	12	61.5	92.3	*	61.5	0.0
• Congenital nephrotic syndrome	41	1	39.0	65.9	*	17.1	7.3
• Congenital obstructive uropathy	296	11	80.7	69.6	19.6	50.0	2.4
• Renal hypoplasia, dysplasia	472	8	60.8	72.2	20.3	43.9	3.8
• Prune belly syndrome	42	10	100.0	73.8	*	47.6	0.0
• Other cystic/hereditary/congenital disease	21	37	278.2	292.9	*	104.5	0.0
Neoplasms/tumors	**32**	**6**	**50.0**	**65.6**	*****	**15.6**	**18.8**
• Renal or urological neoplasms	31	6	51.6	64.5	*	16.1	19.4
Miscellaneous conditions	**146**	**13**	**58.2**	**53.4**	**38.4**	**23.3**	**7.5**
• Tubular necrosis (no recovery)	50	10	54.0	70.0	22.0	20.0	6.0
Etiology uncertain	**418**	**15**	**51.7**	**64.6**	**25.8**	**39.5**	**1.9**
Missing	**296**	**13**	**60.5**	**58.8**	**27.7**	**66.9**	**3.4**

Patients in Puerto Rico and U.S. Territories are included. Medicare and Non-Medicare patients are included. Bolded rows represent disease category headings. Percentages are expressed relative to the number of patients in each disease group (row).

*Less than 10 patients per cell.

[1]Percentages for Asian and Native American patients are not shown because of small sample sizes.

[2]Primary diseases with <20 cases total are not listed separately from the corresponding disease group.

[3]1st Year, 1st year of ESRD therapy; Tx'ed, transplanted.

From USRDS 1998 Annual Data Report, US Renal Data System, The National Institutes of Health, National Institute of Diabetes, Digestive, and Kidney Diseases.

identified 73,091 newly diagnosed cases of ESRD in 1996. Children up to 19 years of age beginning treatment for ESRD were 1.5% (i.e., 1129) of this total, at the rate of 13 cases/1 million individuals, which is a slight increase over the past 10 years. Incidence continues to increase with age. Males have a higher incidence and prevalence of CRF than females in all age groups—but especially in the age group of children under 5 years because congenital renal disorders are more common in males (see Table 34-1). By race and/or ethnicity, incidence rates in children per 1 million individuals were 11 for whites, 26 for blacks, 14 for Asian and/or Pacific Islanders, and 21 for Native Americans. In the age group of 15- to 19-year-olds, CRF occurs twice as often in black and Native American adolescents than in white adolescents. Pediatric prevalence counts for 1995 to 1996 show an overall increase (i.e., 67 cases/1 million individuals) from 1993 to 1994 (i.e., 59 cases/1 million individuals), which reflects both the overall higher incidence counts and improved survival in children with CRF. As of December 1998, point prevalence counts listed 283,932 people of all ages with ESRD on Medicare, with children up to 19 years of age representing 1.8% of the total (USRDS, 1998).

Clinical Manifestations at Time of Diagnosis

Symptoms at the time of diagnosis vary depending on the primary renal disease and the amount of residual renal function. Children with CRF may exhibit a few or many common signs and symptoms of renal failure (Box 34-1).

Fluid, Electrolyte, and Acid-Base Abnormalities

As renal function decreases, solute, fluid, and toxins accumulate in the blood (i.e., uremia). Impairment of bicarbonate reabsorption and ammonia excretion causes metabolic acidosis, which is manifested as tachycardia, hyperpnea, hyperkalemia, lethargy, and growth impairment. Hyperkalemia occurs as a result of catabolism, acidosis, and reduced renal excretion and—if untreated—is

---

Box 34-1

Clinical Manifestations

Anemia, pallor
Anorexia, vomiting, weight loss
Metabolic acidosis
Electrolyte imbalance
Renal osteodystrophy, rickets, myopathy
Dry, scaly, itchy skin, poor hair texture
Fluid imbalance, usually overload, edema
Headache, confusion, poor concentration
Fatigue
Growth retardation
Delayed sexual development
Gross and/or fine motor delay
Secondary hyperparathyroidism
Peripheral neuropathy
Congestive heart failure
Pericarditis

---

fatal, causing lethal ventricular fibrillation and cardiac standstill (Lancaster, 1995a). Hypokalemia, although less common, can result from potassium-wasting diuretic therapy or dietary restriction in children with polyuria or tubular disorders (Fine, 1990a).

The ability of the kidneys to conserve sodium and concentrate urine decreases as renal failure progresses. Sodium and water retention, edema, hypertension, pericarditis, and pericardial effusion can occur secondary to impaired sodium excretion (Anderson and Meyer, 1997). Congenital renal abnormalities (e.g., hypoplasia and dysplasia) can produce a "salt-wasting" state, requiring sodium chloride supplementation. In children with salt-losing nephropathy, serum sodium levels may remain within normal limits because of volume contraction. Dietary sodium restrictions may lead to further deterioration in GFR as a result of decreased renal perfusion (Chantler, 1997).

Metabolic Abnormalities

Decreased GFR and tubular defects result in retention of phosphate wastes and impaired vitamin D synthesis. Hyperphosphatemia causes calcium resorption from bone and increased stimulation by the parathyroid gland to secrete more parathormone (PTH) to enhance phosphate excretion. This circular mechanism ultimately results in secondary hyperparathyroidism. As more calcium is removed from bone, it is deposited in soft tissues, joints, and arteries, which causes the following: (1) pain and decreased mobility; (2) dry, itchy, and scaly skin; (3) decreased vascular contractility; and (4) cardiac dysfunction. Disturbance in the calcium-phosphorus-bone metabolism relationship causes renal osteodystrophy, delayed bone growth, renal rickets and other bone deformities, hyperparathyroidism, and metastatic calcifications (Lancaster, 1995a). Hypertriglyceridemia and hypercholesterolemia can occur as CRF worsens.

Decreased Hormone Secretion

Decreased erythropoietin production and a shorter lifespan of red blood cells result in anemia and its manifestations (Wong, 1997a). Decreased renin secretion, coupled with sodium and fluid imbalance, may alter blood pressure control. Hypertension is more common than hypotension in CRF.

Progression of Uremia

Children with CRF may initially exhibit a loss of normal energy and increased fatigue on exertion. Such fatigue often develops gradually and goes unnoticed. These children may prefer sedentary activities over active play. Physical examination may reveal a slightly listless, pale child whose hemoglobin is low. Blood pressure may be high or normal. Secondary amenorrhea is common in adolescent girls. Urine output may decrease or remain normal in volume but with decreased solute clearance.

As renal failure worsens, its manifestations become more pronounced. Children become more fatigued and uninterested in play, have a poor appetite, and are less capable of accomplishing schoolwork as their attention span diminishes and memory becomes erratic from toxin accumulation. Uremic toxicity is characterized by anorexia, nausea, vomiting, malaise, somnolence, and headache (Wong, 1997b). If untreated, a child's symptoms can progress to malnutrition and wasting, gastrointestinal (GI) bleeding, convulsions, and coma. Pericarditis, congestive heart failure, and arrhythmias may develop (Parker, 1998).

Treatment

Treatment goals include restoring and maintaining the child's health and developmental level of function to the highest degree possible. As psychosocial stressors and coping mechanisms affect physical health, the child and family should be included in planning care and treatment to elicit therapeutic adherence (Gilman and Frauman, 1998). Treatment is based on the severity of the clini-cal manifestations of CRF. Approaches include conservative management and—eventually—RRT (Box 34-2).

Conservative Management Therapy

Fluid, electrolyte, and blood pressure control: Early recognition and management of biochemical imbalances may prevent adverse consequences. Fluid overload and hypertension may be controlled by limiting total fluid intake to total output volume plus insensible losses, restricting salt intake, and using diuretic and antihypertensive medications. Loop diuretics help control the volume-dependent hypertension seen in CRF; angiotensin-converting enzyme (ACE) inhibitors reduce glomerular capillary pressure, which may slow the progression of CRF (Giatras et al, 1997). Although beta-adrenergic blockers, alpha-adrenergic antagonists, peripheral vasodilators, calcium channel blockers, and ACE inhibitors are groups of drugs available for CRF-associated hypertension, some of these drugs are not acceptable for use in young children (Chantler, 1997). Hypertension must be controlled primarily by, or in consultation with, a pediatric nephrologist. Less common conditions are hypovolemia and hypotension, which may be seen in some salt-wasting disorders or with overly aggressive fluid restriction (Fine, 1990a).

Hyperkalemia can be controlled through dietary restriction of high potassium foods, use of bicarbonate for intracellular mobilization and acidosis prevention, and use of polystyrene sulfonate (Kayexalate) 1 g/kg once or twice daily to remove potassium from the body (Rastegar and DeFronzo, 1997). Hypokalemia occurs less commonly and is associated with particular renal tubular disorders, prolonged vomiting, or overly aggressive hyperkalemia control. Potassium-restoring medications and dietary supplementation correct the problem. Metabolic acidosis may be controlled

Box 34-2

Treatment of Chronic Renal Failure

Conservative Management
Fluid, electrolyte, and blood pressure control
Anemia management
Hypertension control
Metabolic control and calcium homeostasis
Managing growth retardation

Renal Replacement Therapy
Peritoneal dialysis (CCPD or CAPD)
Hemodialysis
Transplantation

by use of alkalinizing medications (e.g., sodium bicarbonate, sodium or potassium citrate, or Polycitra).

Anemia control: Treatment is aimed at increasing red blood cell (RBC) production and decreasing RBC loss. Oral iron supplementation is prescribed if the serum ferritin is <20 ng/l or the serum iron level is <50 g/dl or both. Blood transfusions carry associated risks of iron overload (i.e., serum ferritin >300 ng/ml), hepatitis-acquired immunodeficiency syndrome, and sensitization to histocompatibility antigens (Cohen and Brattich, 1997; Wong, 1997a). If transfusions are required, filtered and washed leukocyte-poor RBC mass is usually preferred over whole blood.

Administration of synthetic human recombinant erythropoietin (r-HuEPO, epoetin alfa, EPO, Epogen, Procrit) produced by recombinant DNA technology is the gold standard for treatment of anemia associated with CRF. Multicenter studies report variations in frequency (1 to 3 times weekly) and dose (50 to 100 U/kg) according to desired hematocrit (Aufricht et al, 1993; Cohen and Brattich, 1997). The dose must be carefully titrated to prevent a rapid rise in hematocrit and possible hypertensive crisis with seizures (College, 1996; Morris et al, 1993). As the desired erythropoiesis is achieved, iron stores become depleted. Certain foods (e.g., tea, coffee) and medications (e.g., phosphate binders) contribute to iron depletion.

Iron supplementation (oral or intravenous) is usually required (Nissensen, 1998). Reticulocyte count and RBC indices should be monitored. Expected results include an increase in an individual's sense of well-being, energy and endurance levels, exercise tolerance, and appetite, as well as improvement in concentration ability, school performance, and active play (Painter and Carlson, 1994). Significant improvement in cognitive function and intelligence quotient (IQ) testing, in addition to fewer symptoms of anxiety and depression, are also reported (Cohen and Brattich, 1997; Schira, 1994). The present recommendation is toward earlier use of r-HuEPO in children with renal insufficiency before ESRD develops (NAPRTCS, 1998). Refer to the National Kidney Foundation's (NKF) Dialysis Outcome Quality Initiative (DOQI) Guidelines for Anemia Control for further discussion NKF, 1998).

Metabolic control and calcium homeostasis: Control of calcium and phosphate balance prevents renal osteodystrophy and secondary hyperparathyroidism. Dietary phosphate restrictions significantly limit a child's intake of dairy products. Medications used include calcium-based phosphate binders to remove excess phosphate from the blood, calcium supplements, and vitamin D replacement therapy with calcitriol (Rocaltrol) or dihydrotachysterol (DHT) to allow available calcium to be better used (Bruiner, 1994).

Growth retardation is a significant consequence of CRF in children and is the symptom that occasionally leads to the diagnosis of renal disease (Box 34-3). Most children with ESRD are >2 standard deviations (SDs) below the mean height for their age (Stablein, 1992). The younger the age of onset of CRF, the more profound the degree of growth retardation (Fine et al, 1995). Other factors associated with poor growth in CRF include protein and calorie malnutrition, anorexia, electrolyte imbalance, uremic toxicity, and renal osteodystrophy (Fine et al, 1994; Newman, 1998). Dietary manipulations to avoid exacerbation of uremic symptoms (e.g., protein restrictions) can further compromise growth (Fine et al, 1994). Growth retardation continues to be an unresolved consequence of CRF despite optimal clinical management (Chan et al, 1994; Fine, 1996). Recombinant human growth hormone (rhGH) has significant potential for improving the stature of CRF children with growth retardation without advancing bone disease (Daughaday and Harvey, 1994).

Despite its reported safety and the fact that extensive hormonal testing is not necessary prior to initiation, rhGH is underused with children with CRF. Reasons for this include parents or children's lack of interest in performing daily injections and fear of needles and pain, pediatric nephrologists' lack of experience in prescribing and managing the drug, and the prohibitive cost, although financial assistance is available (Greenleaf, 1996; Kohaut and Fine, 1996). The primary care provider and staff can be instrumental in achieving compliance with growth hormone GH therapy through supportive encouragement with injections and assistance in monitoring progress.

Approach to growth retardation: Blood levels of GH are normal to elevated in CRF. Because only a small portion is cleared by the kidney, the half-life of the GH may be slightly elevated. Researchers suggest that it is not the amount—but the action—of the GH that is impaired. Insulin-like growth factors are being studied and may provide a way to evaluate the need for and response to GH (Fine, 1996; Hokken-Koelga et al, 1996). When rhGH is used, response and dosage are reevaluated every 3 months. A normal response includes an increase in height velocity of >2cm/year over the baseline (Kohaut and Fine, 1996). Before starting rhGH, optimal nutritional management and dialysis efficacy should be achieved, the PTH should be normal or reduced if very high, and the baseline parameters should be established for biochemical assays and hip radiographs.

Renal Replacement Therapy

As GFR drops to 5% to 10% of normal, conservative management is no longer adequate and treatment with either dialysis or transplantation is required. As ESRD approaches, it is important to have ongoing discussions about the future and options for dialysis and transplantation with the child (if of suitable age) and parents. Educating the family about the different modalities of therapy, touring the pediatric dialysis center, and introducing the child and parent to one or more well-adjusted families on dialysis or experiencing a transplant are helpful ways to prepare children and families.

Indications for the timing of RRT are individualized, with consideration given to the following factors: (1) the child's age; (2) GFR <10%, or creatinine clearance <10 ml/min/1.73 M^2; (3) primary renal disease and effect of comorbid conditions; (4) eviation from expected growth curve; (5) failure to thrive; (6) developmental delay; (7) inability to function at school; and (8) inadequate control of blood pressure, electrolyte, and metabolic parameters despite aggressive medical management (Evans et al, 1995; Fine, Salusky, and Ettenger, 1987). Absolute indicators include congestive heart failure, uncontrollable hypertension, pericarditis, uremic encephalopathy, and peripheral neuropathy (Fine, 1990a) (Box 34-4).

The many special needs of children help determine the modality of RRT selected. Because of the problems associated with small blood vessels for vascular access, hemodialysis (HD) may not be practical. If a family is supportive and lives a long distance from the pediatric dialysis center, peritoneal dialysis may be preferred, especially for younger children. Middle to older adolescents are more apt to be on HD. Transplantation is by far the preferred modality, however, because it offers greater potential for linear growth than either type of dialysis (NAPRTCS, 1998). From 1992 to 1996, 37% of children starting ESRD therapy were transplanted during the first year (USRDS, 1998). Children may have more live related kidney donors—especially parents—available to them, which may allow for preemptive transplant, foregoing the need for prolonged dialysis. Improved technology and more effective medications promote better survival (i.e., of both patient and graft) with transplantation and offer both the child and family greater potential to live a normal, less restricted life. There are positive and negative aspects for all treatment modalities. The child and family must understand that a kidney transplant is not a cure for CRF but is another treatment and can only be successful through carefully guided immunosuppression management with frequent clinical assessment (see Chapter 30).

The preference among pediatric nephrology practitioners is to initiate RRT early (i.e., before a child is significantly decompensated and susceptible to increased morbidity and mortality) (Tzamaloukas, 1997). Initiation of dialysis or transplantation is traumatic for the child and family, even with pre-ESRD counseling, but is worse if the child is very ill. Denial is a strong coping mechanism, however, and is supported when a child feels "well" despite a significantly elevated creatinine level.

Peritoneal Dialysis

Approximately 60% of children with ESRD are treated by peritoneal dialysis (PD), with 75% using automated cycling PD (NAPRTCS, 1998). The overall survival rates of HD and PD are similar, except that PD is better tolerated in very young and very old individuals (Warady, 1996).

PD incorporates the peritoneum as a filtering membrane to remove renal failure wastes and excess fluid from the vascular system. Silastic peritoneal catheters (curled or straight with one or two polyethylene terephthalate [Dacron] cuffs) are surgically implanted in children (Ash and Daugirdas, 1994; Burrows and Prowant, 1998; Golper et al, 1997). Through the catheter, a sterile solution (dialysate) of electrolytes and glucose is instilled into the peritoneal space. Dialysate volume is calculated at 35 to 50 ml/kg. Waste particles are removed from the blood across the peritoneal membrane by diffusion, and excess water is removed by osmosis. Ultrafiltration is regulated by the amount of glucose in the dialysate in concentrations of 1.5%, 2.5%, and 4.25%. Higher glucose removes more water, which causes increased thirst, fluid intake, and triglycerides and may add 500 to 800 calories/day, which can result in weight gain. The feeling of fullness from dialysate dwelling in the peritoneum may cause decreased appetite, anorexia, and malnutrition (Harum, 1998; Lancaster, 1995b).

Treating a child with home PD offers many psychologic, educational, and emotional advantages, as well as continuous biochemical and fluid control, continued mobility, ease of dietary restrictions, and provision of simple instructions and/or procedures to carry out PD treatments. Continuous ambulatory peritoneal dialysis (CAPD) delivers 4 to 6 dialysate bag exchanges daily into the peritoneum, with dwell times of 3 to 4 hours during the day and a long dwell overnight. CAPD affords greater freedom because no machine is required. Performing 4 to 6 exchanges during the day is time-consuming, however, and inconvenient at work and school (Figure 34-1). Continuous cycling peritoneal dialysis (CCPD) uses a similar concept, but by using an automated cycler, all exchanges can be performed at night while the child and parents sleep, so the daytime is free of exchanges.

With both CAPD and CCPD, meticulous care is crucial to prevent contamination and infection at the catheter exit site and within the peritoneum. Peritonitis, the most common problem associated with PD, is characterized by symptoms of peri-

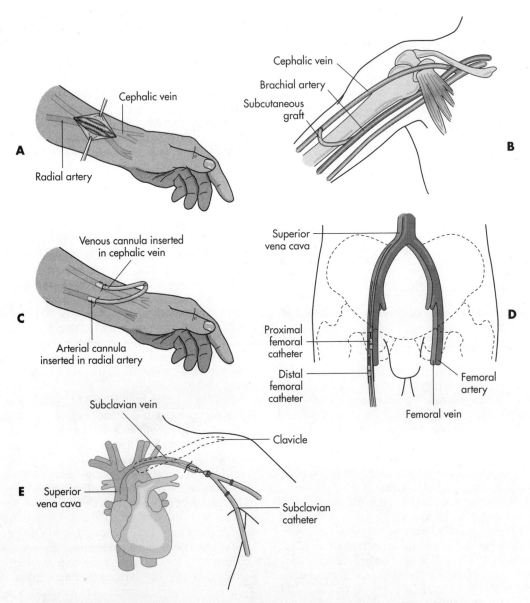

Figure 34-1 Frequently used methods for gaining vascular access for hemodialysis include, **A,** arteriovenous fistula; **B,** arteriovenous graft; **C,** external arteriovenous shunt; **D,** femoral vein catheterization; and **E,** subclavian vein catheterization. (From Phipps WJ et al: Medical-surgical nursing: concepts and clinical practice, ed 6, St Louis, 1999, Mosby.)

toneal inflammation (e.g., pain, fever, cloudy effluent with WBC >100/mm³ and 50% neutrophils, positive Gram stain or positive culture of microorganism) (Burrows and Prowant, 1998). Peritonitis episodes are highest in individuals up to one year of age and decrease in frequency with age (NAPRTCS, 1998). The majority of peritonitis is experienced by a few children who have repeated episodes. Warady (1997) thinks that placement of double-cuffed catheters with a curved tunnel and downward exit site direction helps prevent peritonitis. The most common type of pediatric catheter in use is a Tenckhoff, single-cuffed that is curled with a straight tunnel and a lateral exit site orientation (Burrows and Prowant, 1998; NAPRTCS, 1998). After placement, the catheter should be flushed periodically to maintain patency but not used for full-volume maintenance PD until healing occurs (1 to 2 weeks).

Most peritonitis is caused by Gram-positive organisms, usually *Staphylococcus epidermidis* or *Staphylococcus aureus.* Early use of intraperitoneal antibiotics for suspected peritonitis usually resolves the infection without catheter replacement. Most commonly used antibiotics are the cephalosporins, vancomycin, and aminoglycosides. Many centers find a single daily dose of aminoglycoside and a weekly dose of vancomycin, with a minimum dwell time of 6 hours, to be effective with less risk for ototoxicity (Klaus et al, 1995; Vas et al, 1997). Repeated peritonitis results in loss of membrane permeability by scarring, often requiring a change to HD. Other problems associated with PD include fluid overload or dehydration, membrane failure unrelated to infection, hernia development, bleeding or leaking, catheter exit-site or tunnel infection, catheter obstruction by fibrin or omentum, and catheter perforation (Burrows and Prowant, 1998; Tonshoff and Fine, 1995).

PD has several advantages over HD. It is a simple and safe procedure that can be carried out at home without the psychologic trauma associated with repeated fistula venipunctures. Biochemical and fluid control is maintained at a near-steady state without the nausea, vomiting, and disequilibrium associated with HD. In addition, fewer restrictions are needed with regard to diet, fluid intake, or physical activity. Perhaps the most attractive features of CAPD and CCPD are that they interfere less with normal daily activities and offer more control to the child and family. A child on peritoneal dialysis can attend school every day with little or no interruption, and family vacations are easier to arrange. There is, however, a downside. A common reason for PD failure and change to HD is family "burnout" from the repetitive daily regimen of PD. Providing respite care may provide a solution in some cases. By preventing peritonitis and exit-site infection, as well as promoting good nutrition, PD can be considered a long-term therapy (Oreopolous, 1996).

Hemodialysis

Usually performed three times per week, hemodialysis (HD) has the advantage of more rapid correction of fluid, electrolyte, and metabolic abnormalities over PD. HD requires vascular access, dialyzer and blood lines, an HD delivery system with a blood pump and many monitoring devices, heparin to prevent clotting, and specialized nursing skills. As the blood passes through the filtering membrane, waste particles diffuse across the membrane out of the blood while excess water is ultrafiltrated by negative pressure into the waste dialysate. The 3- to 5-hour process is constantly monitored for pressure changes, air detection or leaks, chemical imbalance, and temperature, in addition to the child's vital signs. Blood flow rates, medications, and fluid volumes are calculated based on the weight of the child (refer to NKF's 1998 DOQI guidelines for HD Adequacy). Risks associated with HD include dialysis disequilibrium, hypotension, accidental blood loss from clotting or dialyzer membrane leak, air embolism, pyrogenic or hemolytic reactions related to dialysate problems, muscle cramps, hypotension, nausea and vomiting, dysrhythmia, hypoxemia, dialysis disequilibrium, seizures, dialyzer membrane reaction, sepsis, hypovolemic shock, cardiopulmonary arrest, and—over time—amyloidosis or acquired cystic disease (Evans et al, 1995; Gilman and Frauman, 1998; Miles and Friedman, 1997; Salai, 1998).

Maintaining a patent and infection-free vascular access is the greatest challenge of HD. An internal or external vascular access is necessary to deliver blood to the extracorporeal dialysis circuit for solute and fluid removal (see Figure 34-1). Internal accesses include the arteriovenous (AV) fistula or synthetic graft (created surgically) and, after a maturation time, are accessed through a special fistula-needle cannulation (Salai,1998). External access devices include central venous catheters (Taylor, 1996). An internal fistula or graft is preferred for larger children (i.e., >12 to 15 kg) because it affords them greater freedom with less risk for infection (Figure 34-2). Access problems account for 30% to 50% of hospitalizations associated with HD (Sands, 1998). One third of vascular accesses initially fail, with 85% due to thrombosis and the remaining 15% from infection (Boag, 1998a). Access sites are at a premium and must be preserved because these children will eventually require multiple vascular accesses. Potential problems warrant early assessment and intervention.

PD is technically easier to perform than HD in infants and small children. In many cases, however, PD may be medically contraindicated. Even very small infants can be successfully hemodialyzed, using central venous, umbilical, or femoral catheters for vascular access and specialized equipment and supplies adaptable to neonatal volume requirements (Knight et al, 1993; Nevins and Maurer, 1986). Infants and small children are hemodynamically more fragile and respond more quickly to sodium and fluid depletion or excess associated with dialysis procedures (Taylor, 1994a). All medications and fluid volumes in pediatric HD are calculated based on a child's weight and medical condition. Pediatric HD should be performed in a pediatric dialysis center. If distance to a pediatric dialysis center is a problem, adolescents may be dialyzed in adult centers but risk the lack of comprehensive assessment and therapies provided by a pediatric center. In such cases, the pediatric primary care provider's role becomes more important in ensuring continuity of care for a child with ESRD. Very stable older children might be considered, on an individual basis, for home HD. HD procedures and access care can be threatening to both the child and family, therefore families should be given as much information as they can handle, and time should be taken to give them basic explanations and elicit their cooperation with procedures (Gilman and Frauman, 1998; Taylor, 1996).

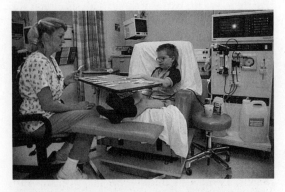

Figure 34-2 Child undergoing hemodialysis. (From Wong DL: Whaley and Wong's Nursing care of infants and children, ed 6, St Louis, 1999, Mosby.)

Renal Transplantation

Renal transplantation is usually preferred for children with ESRD and, with careful planning, may be a primary therapy, bypassing the need for dialysis. Preemptive transplants account for 25% of primary transplants (NAPRTCS, 1998). Children weighing over 5 kg who are over 6 months of age can be transplanted (Matas et al, 1996). Live, related donor sources accounted for 48% of all pediatric transplants reported in the NAPRTCS group (1998). Because transplantation is the preferred option and donor kidneys are scarce, donor eligibility has been expanded to include live, related donors outside the immediate family, as well as live, unrelated donors (Mudge et al, 1998). Transplants across ABO-compatible barriers are being done— mostly in adults—and with higher rates of rejection and failure potential (NAPRTCS, 1998). Adult kidneys may be transplanted into small children with intraabdominal placement (Haggarty and Sigardson-Poor, 1990). The increasing use of laparoscopic nephrectomy can allow live donors to return to work and regular activities sooner and may increase overall use of live donors. Apart from surgical techniques, careful medical management is the key to maintaining a successful kidney transplant (see Chapter 30). With a successful renal transplant, children have a better chance of achieving desired growth and development, attending school regularly, and leading a more normal life.

Recent and Anticipated Advances in Diagnosis and Management

Early Detection and Referral

The primary care provider's early detection of potential renal problems and referral of the child to a pediatric nephrologist can often prevent irreversible renal damage. Earlier and closer monitoring of vesicoureteral reflux, including periodic urine cultures, voiding cystourethrograms to monitor degree of reflux, and renal scans to detect scarring, can sometimes prevent permanent damage. Renal deterioration and failure may be prevented with the use of antibiotic prophylaxis to prevent recurrent urinary tract infections, monitoring for improvement of reflux, and surgical ureteral reimplantation if indicated (Russell, 1998). The condition of posterior urethral valves may be detected by a prenatal sonogram. Placement of stenting, while in-utero, to decrease fetal hydronephrosis and early postnatal urinary diversion until surgical correction of valves can be accomplished and may delay or prevent the renal failure often associated with posterior urethral valves (Cendron et al, 1996; Smith and Duckett, 1996).

Significant technical advances in the treatment of infants and children with CRF have occurred over the past decade. More children are receiving dialysis or transplant for ESRD and surviving longer and living with a higher quality of life. This longevity and improved quality can be credited to some of the following developments: use of recombinant human erythropoietin and GH in children with CRF via subcutaneous, intravenous, and intraperitoneal routes; greater adherence to kinetic modeling calculations, biochemical parameters, and clinical responses to individually tailor the adequacy of dialysis and improve efficiency; early and aggressive correction of electrolyte and metabolic imbalances; and prevention of associated consequences of ESRD.

Because children are such a small percentage of the overall ESRD population, it is not cost-effective for manufacturers to produce dialysis supplies geared to small children. Therefore pediatric supplies are very standardized, costly, and their continued availability is in jeopardy. Pediatric dialysis nurses must be creative and innovative to "rig" adult devices for use with children. Peritoneal dialysis innovations include various disconnect methods and design of smaller and simpler, computer-driven, suitcase-size portable PD cyclers that propose to decrease risk for infection, promote easier PD exchanges, and improve quality of life. HD equipment now has computerization capabilities, allowing for individualization of treatment to be more refined. Some centers use modem connections to connect them with the child's home PD cycler to automatically transmit treatment data and troubleshoot problems (Cresswell and Hicks, 1996). A greater dependence on computerization will guide the future of education, communication, data collection and analysis, and research.

The Internet has opened many doors for both professionals and lay individuals to access education, peer consulting, availability of continuing education for licensure and certification update, and discussion groups. Nutritional information and recipes can be downloaded, and dialysis and transplant medications can be researched. Electronic journals related to nephrology are available for professionals and interested individuals.

Many new medications to treat problems associated with CRF—especially immunosuppressive therapy for transplantation—are being tested, approved, and released for use. Improved immunosuppression may reduce selected side effects of current medications and allow living donors who are related or unrelated to be used with greater success. Experimentation with xenotransplants continues but is still years away from being a practical solution to donor shortages (Boag, 1998b; Caplan, 1998).

Associated Problems (Box 34-5)

Electrolyte Abnormalities

Electrolyte disturbances are probably the most common abnormalities found in renal failure. Hyperkalemia (i.e., potassium > 5.5) is a frequent problem in CRF management, even after initiation of dialysis. Children with ESRD often do not adhere to a low potassium diet. Aggressive infant nutrition to improve brain growth and developmental potential may provide higher dietary potassium

---

Box 34-5

Associated Problems

Electrolyte abnormalities
Anemia
Hypertension
Cardiovascular disorders
Neurologic problems
• Aluminum toxicity
• Uremic neuropathy
• Encephalopathy
Calcium and/or phosphate disorders
• Renal osteodystrophy
Dermatologic manifestations
Gastrointestinal manifestations
Intercurrent illness

than desired. Better overall electrolyte control can be established by CAPD or CCPD because of the continuous steady state of dialysis clearance as opposed to the intermittent clearance of HD.

Anemia

The primary cause of anemia (hematocrit <30) in CRF is decreased red blood cell (RBC) production as a result of decreased production and release of erythropoietin. Other contributing factors include shorter RBC lifespan because of uremic toxins, blood loss as a result of platelet adhesiveness in uremia, retention of uremic toxins and inhibitors, microcytic anemia caused by aluminum toxicity and folate deficiency, and blood loss associated with HD treatments and lab testing (Besarab, 1997; Parker, 1998). Infection, malnutrition, and nephrectomy may further aggravate the decreased erythropoietin production (Roberts, 1998).

Hypertension

The medical management of hypertension associated with CRF depends on the underlying cause (if known), the degree of renal impairment, the relative contributions of extracellular fluid (ECF) volume overload, the renin-angiotensin response, and the severity of the hypertension (Bazilinski and Dunea, 1994; Scribner, 1998).

Managing hypertension in children on dialysis includes restricting fluid and dietary salt and dialytic ultrafiltrating of excess extracellular fluid volume to reach the goal of effective "dry" weight (i.e., the point at which the child is normotensive without use of medications and allows for some intradialytic weight gain without developing hypertension) (Miles and Friedman, 1997). Persistent or uncontrolled hypertension can accelerate the decline in renal function, as well as risk the possibility of hypertensive encephalopathy, seizures, stroke, and death (Anderson and Meyer, 1997). Effective long-term control of hypertension is necessary to prevent cardiac complications.

Cardiovascular Disorders

Abnormal cardiac function associated with CRF can be attributed to hypertension, anemia, and uremia. Congestive heart failure can occur as a result of fluid overload, severe hypertension, or uremic myocardiopathy (Fine, 1990a). The presence of anemia and arteriovenous shunting (from the vascular access) can increase the cardiac workload and contribute to congestive heart failure. As with the general population, cardiovascular disease advances with age, but the risk for cardiovascular disease is 50 times higher for individuals with ESRD than in the general population (Boag, 1998b). Approximately 50% of deaths in individuals with ESRD can be attributed to cardiovascular problems (Foley et al, 1997). Heart murmurs are common in children with CRF as a result of anemia, hypertension, and volume overload. EKG abnormalities include left ventricular hypertrophy, elevated T-waves, and widened QRS complexes (Morris et al, 1994). Uremic pericarditis is a less common manifestation of CRF that is characterized by fever, precordial pain, pericardial friction rub, distended neck veins, hypotension early in HD treatment, a sudden drop in hemoglobin level, cardiomegaly, and cardiac arrhythmias and may lead to cardiac failure (Miles and Friedman, 1997). Treatment of uremic pericarditis may include daily dialysis with ultrafiltration and surgical drainage of the pericardium.

Neurologic Disorders

Neurologic manifestations are attributed to retention of uremic toxins, decreased cerebral blood flow and oxygen use (Parker, 1998). Progressive encephalopathy, developmental delay, microcephaly, electroencephalogram (EEG) and computed tomographic (CT) scan abnormalities have been reported in 80% of children with CRF in infancy (Elzouki et al, 1994). Aluminum toxicity, hyperparathyroidism, undernutrition, and psychosocial problems may be contributing factors in developmental delay. Initiation of chronic dialysis improves many neurologic symptoms of CRF.

Aluminum toxicity: A syndrome of progressive neurologic deterioration in children with CRF has been linked to aluminum toxicity, which depresses bone formation, leading to osteomalacia and bone fractures (Alfrey, 1997; Rotundo et al, 1982; Salusky et al, 1991). When bone does not grow, a child does not grow. Aluminum toxicity is indistinguishable from the dialysis dementia of adults and is characterized by regression of verbal and motor skills, speech disorders, seizures, and dementia and can result in mental retardation or death (Alfrey, 1997). Using calcium-based phosphate binders as a phosphate-binding agent is safer and more effective and will hopefully reduce the incidence of mental retardation and other neurologic dysfunction (Andress and Sherrad, 1997). Aluminum-based antacids are not recommended as phosphate binders for children under the age of 10 years (Salusky et al, 1991). Other agents possibly contributing to aluminum toxicity include total parenteral nutrition (TPN), repeated albumin use (for HD), contamination of intravenous solutions and infant formulas with aluminum salts (Salusky et al, 1990). Deferoxamine (Desferal) is being intravenously administered as a chelating agent without adverse effects in infants and children whose aluminum levels are high despite use of calcium-based phosphate binders (Fraser and Arieff, 1997).

Uremic neuropathy: Uremic neuropathy often affects the lower extremities and involves both motor and sensory function. Signs of neuropathy caused by uremia include muscle weakness; loss of deep tendon reflexes (especially patellar and Achilles); "restless legs" syndrome, including peculiar creeping, crawling, prickly sensations with pruritus; and loss in sensations of pain, light touch, vibration, and pressure (Fraser and Arieff, 1997). Uremic neuropathy may be improved with more efficient or adequate dialysis.

Encephalopathy: Encephalopathy may be seen in advanced renal failure. Children may exhibit early symptoms including headache, fatigue, and listlessness. Memory loss, decreased attention span, drowsiness, and impaired speech appear as deterioration in renal function progresses. Metabolic and biochemical abnormalities associated with CRF may be particularly detrimental to the CNS of the child, which is still developing (Uysal et al, 1990). Rapid reduction of urea from blood through highly efficient HD may cause cerebral edema, which results in the syndrome of dialysis disequilibrium. Symptoms include headache, disorientation, muscle cramps, nausea, and vomiting. If left untreated, seizures, coma, and death may occur (Fraser and Arieff, 1997). When a very high BUN level is present, initial dialysis treatments should be gentle, slow, and moderately efficient for urea clearance to prevent these symptoms from occurring.

Calcium and/or Phosphorus Disorders and Renal Osteodystrophy

Growth retardation and renal osteodystrophy are significant problems for children with ESRD. Loss of renal function has a profound effect on calcium and phosphorus homeostasis and thus on bone integrity (Bruiner, 1994). Bones contain 99% of the body's total calcium. Dietary phosphorus restriction in children with renal problems is difficult because it curtails intake of dairy products and meat. It is especially difficult to provide adequate nutrition to infants with CRF because of this curtailment. Phosphorus restriction and use of calcium-based phosphorus binders, however, help to keep the serum concentration of phosphorus within the normal range to prevent renal osteodystrophy and secondary hyperparathyroidism (Bruiner, 1994).

Renal osteodystrophy is common, occurring in approximately 60% to 80% of children with CRF (Papadopoulou, 1989), and is a significant complication in growing children because of their open epiphyses and rapid bone mineralization and remodeling (Salusky, 1995). There are three types of renal osteodystrophy: osteomalacia, which is attributed to defective bone mineralization through vitamin D deficiency; osteitis fibrosa (i.e., hyperparathyroid or high turnover bone disease), which is the most common bone lesion in renal failure; and osteoporosis, which is a reduction in bone mass (Andress and Sherrard, 1997; Newman, 1998). These children do not usually complain of bone pain but often restrict their physical activity to protect a painful extremity and may develop subtle gait abnormalities. Clinical manifestations include valgus deformities, fractures, rickets, myopathy, growth retardation, bone pain, extra skeletal calcifications in soft tissues and organs, and—in severe bone disease—epiphyseal slipping of the femoral head and metaphyseal fractures (Mehls and Ritz, 1989; Salusky, 1995). Renal osteodystrophy may be improved by early and aggressive calcium and vitamin D therapy with dihydrotachysterol (DHT), 25hydroxy vitamin D, calcitriol or vitamin D_3, 1,25 dihydroxy vitamin D (Rocaltrol), as well as adequate metabolic control by diet, medication, and adequate dialysis (Salusky, 1995). A new drug, paricalcitol injection (Zemplar), has recently been approved for use in adults and older children to reduce the PTH level and renal osteodystrophy (Zemplar, 1998)

Dermatologic Manifestations

Retention of uremic toxins, which are deposited in skin and soft tissue, may contribute to dry, scaly, itchy skin that is characterized by broken skin and scratch marks. Pallor and sallow complexion are improved by anemia control. Capillary fragility contributes to frequent bruising (Parker, 1998).

Gastrointestinal Manifestations

Uremic symptoms of anorexia, nausea, vomiting, stomatitis, and halitosis improve with adequacy of dialysis and control of anemia. Many children gain weight after starting dialysis, and most who are well dialyzed and have normal hemoglobin and hematocrit levels have a good appetite and high energy level.

Intercurrent Illness

The development of intercurrent illnesses in children with CRF must be thoroughly assessed and appropriately managed to prevent further complications and promote optimal health. Infection—especially of the vascular access and peritoneum—is a frequent and common complication. Heart failure, pericarditis, pulmonary edema, and gastrointestinal disease may occur with uremia. Some common childhood viral diseases may be particularly hazardous to children on immunosuppressive therapy because they have received a transplant or have conditions such as lupus or nephrotic syndrome (Gilman and Frauman, 1998).

Prognosis

In infants and younger children, CRF is more likely to be treated by PD than HD, with only 25% of children under 5 years of age and 5% under 1 year on HD (Bunchman, 1996). After 2 years of ESRD treatment, this ratio reverses. Younger children are more likely to receive a transplant and spend less time on dialysis than older children and adults. Of children under 10 years of age, 63% have a functioning transplant graft after 2 years of ESRD therapy, as is true for 67% of children between 10 and 19 years (USRDS, 1998). Medical reasons often dictate the preferred treatment modality. With recent technical advances, small children can be more safely and effectively treated with HD con-

ducted at pediatric dialysis centers. The use of newer medications may delay the onset of CRF in some diseases, more effectively treat problems during HD and PD, and provide better antirejection management for renal transplant patients with fewer adverse reactions or side effects. If a transplant is rejected, children must return to either PD or HD while waiting for another transplant. Unfortunately, many children develop high percentages of reactive antibodies to a large potential donor pool. Therefore the wait for a second or third transplant may be long. This waiting period is when arteriovenous access problems often occur, significantly impairing a child's quality of life. Recent advances in equipment, expendable supplies technology, and medications have improved the potential quality of life for children on HD and PD, allowing them to pursue a more normal lifestyle. The self-esteem of children affects their quality of life and prognosis of morbidity and mortality. Many factors may contribute to poor self-esteem in children with ESRD. Every effort should be made to provide interventions that enhance the self-esteem of children of all ages.

From 1994 to 1996, the mortality rate among children (up to 9 years of age) with ESRD was considerably lower than that among the 20- to 44-year age group. Children on dialysis had a death rate nine times higher than those with transplants, which is partly explained by the fact that the dialysis group included children waiting for transplants and those too ill to receive one. Cardiac problems are the leading cause of death, followed by sepsis (USRDS, 1998). Early recognition and aggressive treatment of uremic symptoms should help reduce morbidity and mortality in children with CRF.

PRIMARY CARE MANAGEMENT

Health Care Maintenance

Growth and Development

Incorporating developmental and behavioral assessments into primary health care evaluations can result in significant advances in early identification and intervention (Finney and Weist, 1992). Children with renal disease may not have any clinical signs besides retarded growth. Many children exhibit growth retardation at the time of referral to the pediatric nephrologist, but inadequate growth remains a problem for many individuals—including those undergoing dialysis. With aggressive nutritional supplementation, infants have achieved better but suboptimal growth (Simonds, 1996). Besides infancy, the next greatest physical growth stage is during puberty. Children with CRF often have delayed linear growth and development of secondary sexual characteristics. Decreased estrogen and testosterone levels may occur.

Accurate growth measurements should be taken at the initial visit and at least every 3 to 6 months thereafter and plotted on appropriate growth charts. Neurologic potential is assessed by following head circumference growth every 3 to 6 months on all children under 3 years of age. The weight-height index provides a measure of a child's weight relative to height, with a low index suggesting malnutrition. Anthropometric measurements of skinfold thickness at the biceps, subscapular, and triceps sites should be obtained every 6 months and with any major change in treatment modality (Papadopoulou, 1989). At the onset of puberty, staging using the Tanner Scale (Hofman and Greydanus, 1989) should be determined every 6 to 12 months for school-aged children until adult staging is reached.

Developmental assessment should be done with the onset of CRF and repeated at 2- to 9-month intervals, depending on a child's age and disease severity. Although the timing may be delayed, children with CRF have the same developmental needs as healthy children and must progress through the same developmental stages. To best help a child attain developmental milestones, the level of development attained must be assessed. Assessment tools (see Chapter 2) are useful in obtaining objective data. The effect of the disease process on the child's psychologic status, school attendance, intellectual performance, and social development should be assessed every 6 to 9 months.

Diet

Although protein restriction may delay progression of CRF, it is not acceptable in children. In addition to growth and developmental delay in children, poor nutrition—especially with low serum albumin levels—is associated with increased morbidity and mortality (Moore, 1991). Nutritional problems are

manifested long before ESRD is reached and continue after RRT is initiated. Based on previous surveys, at least 30% of children with CRF are malnourished, with 6% to 8% being severely malnourished (Kopple, 1997; Roberts, 1998).

Children on PD experience a feeling of fullness soon after eating small amounts because of abdominal distention from the volume of peritoneal fluid, which may be more apparent with CAPD and daytime dwells than with nightly CCPD. In addition with PD, there are obligatory protein losses through the peritoneum because the pore size is easily permeable to albumin transfer (Blake, 1994). Children on PD have increased protein requirements (i.e., 2.5 to 4.0 g/kg in infants, 2.00 to 2.5 g/kg in toddlers and children, and 1.5 g/kg in adolescents).

Energy requirements are also increased, ranging from 98 to 108 kcal/kg in infants to 40 to 50 kcal/kg in adolescents (Rodzilsky and Constantinescu, 1997). Glucose absorption from the dialysate in both HD and PD provides calories, occasionally resulting in obesity. Anemia control via r-HuEPO injections results in increased appetite and energy level and eventual weight gain, which helps reduce the incidence of malnutrition in children with CRF. Intradialytic parental nutrition (IDPN) is provided in some dialysis centers, but reimbursement problems present obstacles to this approach. Lipids increase caloric content significantly but must be monitored closely by lab tests because children on dialysis tend to have higher triglyceride and cholesterol levels (Roberts, 1998; Kopple, 1997).

Parents of infants and small children soon become frustrated with unsuccessful efforts to get children to eat the recommended calories and protein. Children with renal failure are often poor eaters. Supplemental tube feedings by orogastric, nasogastric, or gastrostomy tube or button may be instituted early in renal insufficiency as an important and useful therapy to ensure better nutritional intake with less stress to the family (Brewer, 1990; Gilman and Frauman, 1998). Unpalatable additives of corn or safflower oil and Polycose can easily be instilled by tube along with medications as needed to supplement a child's oral feedings. The formula calculation for supplemental feedings should usually be low in potassium and phosphorus and frequently reevaluated and adjusted for growth and changes in renal function and treatment (Roberts, 1998). The current recommendation is to aggressively treat infants with caloric and protein intake above the recommended daily allowance (RDA) to help improve physical and cognitive growth.

Dietary restrictions change with ESRD modality. In HD, potassium and phosphorus generally govern the dietary prescription. There is greater dietary freedom with PD, and protein may be increased. The posttransplant diet also has restrictions of no added salt, low fat, and low cholesterol to prevent hypertension and obesity. Because eating is a social custom in our society and not just for sustenance, pizza may be the favorite food of a child with CRF, making dietary restrictions difficult. Phosphorus restriction limits dairy products and most children are expected to drink milk. Fluid restriction depends on a child's urinary output volume and is calculated by intake volume allowed being equal to output plus 500 to 600 ml (insensible loss). The primary care provider should obtain the dietary management plan from the nephrology team to reinforce family education.

Safety

Although children with CRF should be encouraged to pursue normal childhood activities, some considerations and limitations must be kept in mind. Delay in cognitive and gross motor development may result in these children being academically and physically slower than classmates, as well as smaller in size. Attempting to keep up with larger and faster children in active play may result in injury to a child with CRF. Children with CRF may become the brunt of jokes and unkind comments. In response to a challenge, these children may retaliate and attempt to accomplish something of which they are not capable, possibly injuring themselves in the process.

Some children require special occupational and physical therapy programs to enhance their physical ability and improve skills and stamina. Bike helmets and knee pads can be used to help prevent easy bruising. Children should be encouraged to wear a Medic-Alert bracelet or necklace to notify other health care providers of their CRF status, medication needs, and other possible complications.

Children on immunosuppressive therapy are more at risk for infections and heal more slowly. Children with an HD internal vascular access (i.e., AV fistula or graft) must be cautioned against allowing blood pressure measurement or venipuncture in their affected arm, wearing restrictive clothing or accessories that can lead to venostasis and clotting, and engaging in activities that may cause bleeding soon after dialysis while they are still heparinized. Children with indwelling central venous catheters should not be allowed to swim to prevent serious infection through the catheter (Berkoben and Schwab, 1995). Swimming with PD catheters is controversial and may require special catheter and exit site care procedures.

Renal osteodystrophy may predispose children to fractures or cause bone pain on exertion. Physical activity, however, should be encouraged to promote physical and mental health. Group aerobic exercise programs, camping, group games at picnics, and other fun outings are excellent ways to promote controlled exercise, encourage independence, and help raise self-esteem.

Immunizations

Routine immunizations should be given to children with CRF except for a few specific disease conditions and therapies. Immunosuppressive therapy is used not only with transplantation but also to treat some renal conditions, including glomerulonephritis, nephrotic syndrome, and lupus nephritis. Immunosuppression is generally an indication for withholding live virus immunizations, including the measles-mumps-rubella (MMR) and varicella vaccines (Committee on Infectious Diseases, 1997). Immunizations should be withheld until a child is in remission and off therapy for 6 months; exceptions are determined by weighing the risks vs. the benefits on an individual basis for children who are steroid-resistant or have frequent relapses. Inactivated polio vaccine (IPV) is preferred for immunosuppressed children (Committee on Infectious Diseases, 1997). Disease-specific immunoglobulins may be given after known exposure. Because the varicella zoster reactions can be severe in children with a transplant (5% to 25% mortality rate with a high potential for graft loss), children without positive antibody titer should be immunized before transplant or immunosuppressive therapy if possible. Seroconversion rates up to 87% have been reported after Varivax (Cohen et al, 1994; Furth et al, 1997). Children should continue to receive varicella zoster virus immunoglobulin (VZIG) after exposure to minimize adverse occurrences (Mudge et al, 1998).

Pneumococcal and influenza vaccines are recommended for children with CRF and active nephrotic syndrome because of their increased susceptibility to infections (Cohen et al, 1994; Sekelman, 1998).

Even though r-HuEPO has decreased the need for blood transfusions in children with ESRD, hepatitis B is still a risk. Hepatitis surface antigen and antibody status should be ascertained before starting dialysis (Parker, 1998). If a child is negative for hepatitis B antigen, the hepatitis vaccine series should be started as soon as possible so it can be completed before transplant. Because the antibody response to the hepatitis B vaccine may be diminished with CRF, these children may require repeated doses until seroconversion is achieved (Committee of Infectious Diseases, 1997). Serum antibody concentrations should be measured every 6 months because antibody protection from the disease may be less complete, which may also be true for responses to other immunizations (e.g., the *Hemophilus Influenza* B virus [HIB] vaccine) (Fivush, 1993). Hepatitis C virus and HIV screening are also recommended in children on dialysis or awaiting transplantation, especially before transplant because these infections are seen more often than in the general population (Chan and Kam, 1997; Shimokura et al, 1998).

Screening

Vision: A yearly eye examination by a pediatric ophthalmologist is recommended. Eyes should be examined for scleral calcification caused by hypercalcemia or uncontrolled hyperphosphatemia. The fundus should be examined for arterial narrowing, hemorrhages, exudates, and papilledema secondary to hypertension. Cataract assessment should be included for any child having been treated with steroid therapy.

Hearing: An annual assessment by an audiologist is recommended. High-frequency sensorineural deafness is characteristic of Alport's syndrome (Gregory and Atkin, 1997). Hearing loss can also result from use of ototoxic drugs (e.g., furosemide and gentamicin).

Dental: Routine dental care (every 6 months) is recommended for children with CRF. Dental procedures may cause breaks in the skin and mucous membranes with bleeding and release of microorganisms into the blood stream, causing infective endocarditis or colonization of the vascular access (Durack and Phil, 1995). A pediatric nephrologist should be consulted to prescribe prophylactic antibiotic coverage for children who are immunosuppressed or have a vascular access prior to dental procedures. See Chapter 17 for prophylaxis protocols.

Children with congenital renal disease often have enamel defects. Poor nutritional intake may lead to poor mineralization of teeth. In an effort to improve nutrition, small children with CRF may be allowed to use a bottle for a longer time, resulting in deformities of the primary teeth. Use of oral iron for anemia may stain teeth; liquid preparations should be placed in the mouth past the teeth.

Drug-induced gingival hyperplasia may occur in children with CRF receiving drugs such as phenytoin (Dilantin) for seizures, calcium channel blockers (e.g., nifedipine [Procardia] or verapamil [Calan]) for hypertension, and cyclosporine (Neoral) or tacrolimus (Prograf, FK506) for immunosuppression in transplant, lupus, and nephrotic syndrome treatment. Good dental and oral hygiene with mechanical stimulation by daily brushing and flossing, gingival massaging, plaque control, and use of folate rinses may aid in prevention. Gingivectomy treatment by surgical excision or laser may be needed periodically (Rossman et al, 1994).

Blood pressure: Blood pressure measurements should be taken at each visit and at periodic intervals, depending on a child's clinical condition. Initiation and follow-up of antihypertensive therapy should be done in consultation with the pediatric nephrologist. The "white coat phenomenon" (i.e., of blood pressure being higher in clinics) is eliminated by use of automated monitoring devices (American College of Physicians, 1993). Small, computerized blood pressure monitors are available to be worn for 24 to 48 hours and can give better insight to the true daily overall blood pressure at rest and during activity and facilitate more ideal medical management (Mensoor and White, 1997).

Hematocrit: Routine screening may be deferred if a recent complete blood cell count (CBC) is included with the other renal function tests. Anemia is a chronic problem that is usually followed by the nephrology team.

Urinalysis: Routine screening is not necessary because of the frequent urinalysis done by the renal team. Some children with CRF have little to no urine output, so urinalysis is not indicated.

Tuberculosis: Yearly screening with PPD testing is recommended.

Condition-Specific Screening

Bloodwork: The nephrology team regularly monitors the CBC, serum ferritin, iron, transferrin, folate, and reticulocyte counts to assess the anemia management. Serum electrolyte, BUN, creatinine, calcium, phosphorus, alkaline phosphatase, protein, albumin, cholesterol, and liver function tests help monitor renal function and treatment efficacy. Metabolic acidosis must be promptly identified and treated to prevent bone demineralization and growth retardation. Parathyroid hormone (PTH) levels should be monitored every 3 to 6 months and correlated with radiological findings for prevention and/or management of renal osteodystrophy. Fasting blood levels are best for monitoring cholesterol and triglycerides, which is difficult in small children or infants. Viral titers for VZV, CMV, HSV, EBV, hepatitis profile (i.e., HAV, HCV, HBV, antibody to HBV), rubella, rubeola, and HIV should initially be monitored as a baseline, then before transplant and periodically as determined by the pediatric nephrologist.

Cardiac screening: A chest radiograph and baseline electrocardiogram and echocardiogram should initially be performed and then again at 6- to 12-month intervals to assess the cardiovascular status of children with CRF.

Radiologic screening: Radiologic bone studies can show evidence of secondary hyperparathyroidism, rickets or osteomalacia, osteosclerosis, and delayed bone age as distinct patterns in children with renal osteodystrophy (Andress and Sherrard, 1997). Examination of the hands and knees should initially be obtained and then again at 6-month intervals to assess for improvement or worsening of renal osteodystrophy and compare bone age with chronologic age to determine growth potential. Bone density studies and bone biopsies are helpful but less commonly used methods of assessing bone mineralization in children.

Common Illness Management

Differential Diagnosis

Infections: Because of a compromised immune system, children with CRF may be at greater risk for routine infections and their sequelae. Primary care providers should evaluate and manage routine pediatric problems (e.g., influenza, urinary tract or gastrointestinal infections, and fever), consulting the pediatric nephrologist about a child's hydration status and residual renal function, as well as antibiotic selection and dose related to a child's renal disease and residual function. Temporary alterations in a child's dialysis program may be necessary during illness. If other common benign causes of fever have been ruled out, fever related to a dialysis access infection or peritonitis should be managed directly by the pediatric nephrologist.

Gastrointestinal symptoms: Nausea and vomiting are common symptoms in childhood. Decreasing renal function must be ruled out in children with mild renal failure, especially in the absence of associated fever.

Headaches: Uncontrolled hypertension should be ruled out in children with CRF complaining of frequent headaches.

Drug interactions: The most important factors to consider in pharmacokinetics are the extent to which the drug is excreted by the kidney, the degree of renal impairment, and the drug's interactions with various other medications needed in the ESRD treatment regimen.

Drug dose regimens are altered with a GFR less than 30 to 40 ml/min (Trompoter, 1987). The initial loading dose of drugs (especially antibiotics) excreted by the kidney, however, is usually the same as it is for children without renal failure. Maintenance doses must be adjusted by either lengthening the interval between doses or reducing individual doses (Swann and Bennett, 1997). CRF may predispose children to bleeding and easy bruising, therefore acetaminophen is preferred over aspirin for pain and fever control.

Anticonvulsants may require dosage adjustments and often interfere with trough drug levels in transplant immunosuppression. Children with anemia and CRF receiving a calcium (not aluminum)-based phosphate binder given with food or within 30 minutes after eating should wait at least 1 hour before taking oral iron because the two medications are antagonistic to each other, compromising the desired effect (Sims et al, 1998). All pediatric medication calculations should be based on the weight—not the age—of a child with CRF. Medications that are removed by dialysis (i.e., vitamins, some antihypertensive medications, and aminoglycoside antibiotics) should be given after dialysis (i.e., at night with CAPD or in the morning with CCPD). The pediatric nephrologist should be consulted for appropriate medication selection and dose adjustment.

Children with CRF may have up to 40 pills to take daily, which requires much determination and perseverance for both them and their parents. Transplant medications can total up to six or seven different medications (and comprise 30 or 40 pills) and are critical to the life of the transplant; even one missed dose can cause a rejection episode. Avenues to promote therapeutic adherence must be explored with the child and family (Wagner, 1997). Refer to "Developmentally Based Teaching Strategies," in Vol. 23, No.6 of *Pediatric Nursing* (November-December 1997) for an excellent reference table for teaching medications.

Developmental Issues

Sleep Patterns

Infants and young children should be encouraged to assume a normal sleep pattern at night. Most children can sleep undisturbed with nocturnal CCPD treatment. An increased need for sleep and lethargy or depression may indicate increasing renal failure and should be reported to the pediatric nephrology team. Restlessness, insomnia, or cramps may indicate the need for more dialysis time or physical activity to promote rest.

Toileting

Children with CRF may be oliguric, anuric, or have normal urine output, as determined largely by the cause of the renal disorder. Some congenital abnormalities require bladder augmentation or creation of a type of urinary diversion with an appliance worn over the stoma (Garvin, 1994). The adolescent with a urinary stoma and appliance may have difficulty emotionally accepting the diversional

system and participating in peer activities. Families and children need instruction in care of the stoma and supportive care as indicated.

Even after corrective urologic surgery, some children may be unable to achieve urinary continence. Toilet training for urinary continence is often deferred until after transplant if a child is capable of urinary continence (DeKernion and Trapasso, 1996). Female children and their parents should be taught to wipe properly to prevent urinary tract infections. Bowel training should be initiated when a toddler is developmentally ready.

Discipline

Parental anxiety, guilt, and despondency over their child's chronic condition may lead to ambivalent feelings toward child rearing or the treatment program, resulting in child behavior problems or nonadherence to the treatment regimen (Grupe, 1986). Parental overprotection of a child with CRF may further reinforce a lack of discipline. Parents need honest answers to questions about their child, as well as encouragement and support in setting and holding limits and behavioral expectations for their child. Children with CRF need the same behavior control and discipline set for their siblings and other healthy children (Gilman and Frauman, 1998).

Children on HD can have difficulty accepting the painful procedure of venipuncture required for each treatment. For pain associated with procedures, management techniques (e.g., play therapy, guided imagery, hypnosis, and progressive muscle relaxation) can be taught to children and their parents. Topical anesthetics (e.g., EMLA cream [Astra Pharmaceutical Company]) are commonly used in many pediatric dialysis centers. Play therapy helps children work through these difficult situations and lets parents or other caregivers know their unexpressed thoughts. A firm but loving disciplinary approach helps to make a positive difference in a child's life (Richardson, 1997).

Children should be encouraged to participate in their care by performing achievable tasks and making decisions. Cooperation can be gained by allowing even 3-year-olds to help select the venipuncture site, remove the tourniquet, rotate the blood tubes, and help place the tape. Singing and other diverting activities also elicit cooperation. Many children on

HD self-cannulate their needles or set up their own dialysis machines for treatment. These children can compete with one another in the dialysis center to complete tasks independently and exercise self-control. Children on CCPD or CAPD can learn to do their own exchanges and care for their exit site. Children may also be taught to subcutaneously self-administer their r-HuEPO or GH (Gilman and Frauman, 1998; Salmon and Broyan, 1991).

Child Care

Children with CRF are not restricted from daycare. Because children receiving corticosteroid therapy are more susceptible to infections, home care or small group child care is recommended. Daycare and preschool settings provide stimulation for learning and sharing with other children and may be a positive situation, especially if classes are small. When child care is used, the caregiver must be taught about the child's dietary restriction, medications, and any special treatment regimen. Specific instructions should be given in writing, with a phone contact in case of questions. The nephrology team should encourage children on CAPD and their parents to arrange the dialysis schedule around the child care hours whenever possible. If a child has a vascular or peritoneal dialysis access, those entrusted as caregivers must be given instructions on potential emergencies and actions to be taken.

Schooling

School-age children must be encouraged to attend school full-time. CAPD exchanges should be scheduled around school activities with the least interference possible, or else nocturnal CCPD might be preferable for school-age children. Changes in schedules to accommodate after-school activities can be discussed with the pediatric nephrology team. Pediatric HD centers should include a school teacher or tutor to help children with missed schoolwork. A dual school-home educational program may be established with both teachers communicating with each other for continuity of the child's learning. Children with renal disease may need a note to be allowed extra trips to the bathroom because of a small bladder capacity or infection, to perform intermittent catheterization, to

drink more or less fluids, or receive assistance with ureterostomy or central venous catheter care. Some children need to be assigned to a school with a nurse in attendance daily, which does not mean that the child needs to be in special education classes. The pediatric nephrology team may need to provide educational materials on specific CRF management and in-service presentations on a child's physical or emotional needs to school personnel, in addition to participating in a child's Individualized Educational Program (IEP) conference. Parents need to be informed about laws protecting their child's education rights (Vessey, 1997).

Poor school performance must be evaluated for contributing factors, including family disharmony. Cognitive deficits have been correlated with more advanced CRF and congenital etiologies (Gilman and Frauman, 1998).

Adolescence can be a time of turbulence that is associated with transition, maturational crises, and adjustment (Wong, 1997b). Table 34-2 highlights some of the differences, problems, and interventions related to cognitive, physical, and psychosocial development in adolescents with ESRD.

Sexuality

Delayed sexual development is common among children with CRF as a result of insufficient production of gonadal steroid and elevated gonadotropin levels (Fine, 1990b). More than half of female adolescents with ESRD have delayed development of secondary sex characteristics and menarche. Although menstrual abnormalities (e.g., amenorrhea, oligomenorrhea, and menorrhagia) and infertility have been described, successful pregnancies in women who were on dialysis have been reported (Scharer, 1990). Adolescent males with ESRD may show delayed development of genitalia, pubic hair, and testicular size, and decreased sperm counts. Impotence may occur in 50% of males on dialysis, but some have still been able to father children (Lewis et al, 1998). Impotence usually improves after transplant. Males have been able to achieve erection through testosterone injections, use of penile injections (Caveject), suppositories (Muse), or Viagra (Lewis et al, 1998; Molzahn, 1998). A successful transplant usually returns hormonal function and fertility capability to normal. These are important issues in adolescent sexuality and preparation for adulthood, as well as for families of small children concerned about the ability of their child to have a normal life.

Adolescents with CRF must be counseled about birth control, sexually transmitted diseases, and acquired immune deficiency syndrome (AIDS). Sexuality is more than just physical intimacy and sexual function. It allows for communication of feelings, provides for physical release and pleasure, and supports feelings of self-worth and identity (Lewis et al, 1998).

Transition to Adulthood

Children with CRF eventually become adults with CRF. The road to independence and career development begins before a child reaches adulthood. Consequences of childhood noncompliance with phosphate binders is evidenced by renal osteodystrophy in adult life. Individuals with short stature from growth retardation or bone disease may require assistive devices to drive. Hypertension, diabetes, and impaired vision may result in other long-term health problems. Individuals must be encouraged to eat a healthy diet and avoid drug, alcohol, and tobacco abuse. Most of all, a successful transition is achieved through a positive mental attitude of overcoming adverse situations into successful lives. The American Association of Kidney Patients (AAKP) can supply dozens of adult role models (see list of resources at end of chapter).

Special Family Concerns

The effect of CRF on a child is felt by the child's entire family. Parents may have to deal with the following: (1) feelings of shock and disbelief, (2) anger, (3) loss, (4) guilt at causing renal failure, (5) depression, (6) fatigue and burnout associated with constant care and appointments, (7) inadequacy at not being able to heal or fix the problem, (8) frustration with the medical establishment for no cure, (9) overprotection vs. being too lenient, (10) marital stress, and (11) financial worries. Frequent trips to the dialysis center or clinic, daily or nightly PD treatments, and additional physical care interfere with family schedules, school, extracurricular activities, and outings.

Family coping and adaptation are improved through maintaining open communication, active participation in care planning and decision making, and the presence of supportive extended family, friends, church members, or renal-focused support or advocacy groups (Travis, Brouhard, and Kalia, 1984). Providing networking sessions is often helpful; new children and families should be grouped with a client who has adjusted well to the dialysis or transplant routine and is willing share information (Gilman and Frauman, 1998). Families should be encouraged to continue normal activities (e.g., family outings, camps for children, and vacations) with previously arranged transient dialysis scheduling at a pediatric dialysis center if necessary.

A family's belief system must be taken into account. Religious practices may prohibit blood transfusions, even in life-threatening situations, or challenge that healing by faith alone is all that is needed. With children who are Jehovah's Witnesses, it may be advisable to start r-HuEPO administration early (before renal failure reaches end-stage), use micro blood tubes for lab tests whenever possible, and use cell-saver reinfusion during surgery. An understanding of the family's background, religious and cultural beliefs and practices, dietary beliefs associated with health care, and identification of the "primary leader" of the family (e.g., a great-grandmother) is valuable to health care professionals when effective interventions require altering a child or family's health care practices (Richie, Mapes, and Dailey, 1995).

Some renal diseases are linked to race and ethnicity. Overall statistics show increased morbidity and mortality in blacks with ESRD and renal transplants, especially in the early post transplant period (Ojo et al, 1994; USRDS, 1998). Some black and Hispanic children wait longer on dialysis for an acceptable transplant match because of ABO compatibility and major histocompatibility complex matching difficulties. The possibility of a better match is secured with a member of the same race for both live related and cadaveric transplantation. Secondly, there are fewer donor organs available from black and Hispanic individuals (Kasiske et al, 1992).

Families need support as they make decisions about their child's care that will have long-range implications. Even the smallest, very ill infant might be treated with life-sustaining dialysis—but at a high cost. Extracorporeal membrane oxygena-

Table 34-2
Characteristics of Adolescents with ESRD by Developmental Domain

Expected Difference from Normal Development	Manifestations or Potential Problems	Prevention and Interventions
Cognitive Aspects: Should move from concrete to abstract thinking at 12-15 years of age. May have excessive school absences for medical reasons and slower or accelerated learning, which must be individualized. Academic achievement is less affected with later CRF onset. RF affects acquisition of new skills, attention, and speed of processing data.	Advanced education requires greater ability to abstract, which is reflected in competency or scholastic testing and academic scores. Concrete thinkers lack ability to apply general principles from one event to another. Academic delay may result in school disinterest and dropout. Hearing and/or vision problems may be CRF-related More difficulty in learning new skills. Attention and responses aided by good biochemical control and worsened by nonadherence.	Concrete thinkers need care plan that realizes immediate goals; abstract thinkers can work with long-range goals. Incorporate results from academic and/or neuropsychomotor skills testing to guide improvement. Encourage school attendance and participation in extracurricular activities. Encourage adherence to care plan. Encourage opportunities for responsible decision making, problem-solving, and development of own beliefs and values. Preparation for transition into adulthood.
Physical Aspects: Linear growth retardation is affected by treatment modality and steroids. Decreased effect and/or production of growth and sex hormones. Delayed puberty onset (refer to Tanner staging, 1962): Girls—10.5-14 years of age, with menarche onset at about 13 years. Boys—12-16.5 years. Delay in development of secondary sexual characteristics and sexually active behavior. Nutritional needs vary with age: Protein—8-1.0 gm/kg needed; Calories—38-60 cal/kg needed. Phosphorus restricted.	Short stature (i.e., 1-3 SD below norm). Does not follow height-weight curve pattern of puberty. Compares size to peers. Girls—delay in breast enlargement, pubic hair, menarche onset (hallmark of womanhood). Boys—delay in testes and/or scrotal growth, pubic hair, penile size and ability to erect and ejaculate, muscle mass increase, voice change to deeper pitch. May be under or overweight. May rebel at ESRD treatment regimen through dietary indiscretions, especially in peer groups. May be nonadherent with medications, especially those causing visible side effects.	Early diagnosis and RRT. Child and family education about normal growth and/or development and expected alterations. Encourage diet and medication adherence, physical activities and exercise, and physical independence. Consider use of growth hormone; teach self-administration. Encourage self-participation in care plan. Provide sexuality education at individual level of understanding. Encourage optimal nutrition to promote best growth potential. Encourage dietary adherence, work with dietitian to include as many favorite foods as possible. Consider meal pattern of school lunches, fast food stops

Anemia present.

May develop ROD with rickets or fractures; hypocalcification by bone radiographs. Fatigue or SOB from anemia.

with peers. Focus on positive—not negative—nutrition. Encourage taking phosphate binders. Consider early use (preRRT) of epoetin alfa; teach self-administration; monitor.

Psychosocial Aspects:
Interruption or inability in mastery of adolescent developmental tasks; dependency vs. independency conflict; identity quest; body image dissatisfaction; peer group identity desired; future planning.
Self-esteem influenced by actual and perceived image and peer response. Risk for lower self-esteem greater with negative body image, poor peer and family relationships, strong family dependence.
Delayed psychosexual development.

Coping behaviors used include denial, regression, projection, displacement, anger, acting out, increased risk taking, disruptive, resentment, argumentative, challenging authority.
Vacillates between child-compliant and rebel-noncompliant. May sublimate poor academic performance with physical prowess. Fears peer rejection, loneliness, depression, and withdrawal despite strong need for friends and social support.
May avoid sexual relationships and activity or experiment to prove sexual worth.

Promote achievement of developmental tasks; foster independence and autonomy. Allow controlled choices. Encourage activities that enhance positive self-esteem and self worth. Encourage healthy group activities in community, school, church, camps, support groups.
Evaluate self-concept through assessment tools
Encourage ventilation of feelings of sexuality and provide education for understanding. Assist in preparation for transition into adulthood.

Adapted from Taylor JH: Enhancing development in the adolescent with ESRD, presentation at ANNA Symposium, Dallas, 1994.
RF, rheumatoid factor; *ROD*, renal osteodystrophy; *SOB*, shortness of breath.

tion (ECMO) with integrated hemofiltration is more widely performed today with positive results. Equipment, supplies, and professional expertise are more costly for infants with ESRD. Many of these infants have other congenital anomalies; morbidity and mortality are high in this early period. Children with mental retardation are being dialyzed and transplanted. Quality of life issues and the rights of parents vs. rights of minor children are being discussed with no black-and-white answers (Currier, 1994). Some infants will not become productive members of society, but others have demonstrated adequate growth and development with early and aggressive RRT and are attending regular school full-time and living fairly normal lives. Children with severe developmental or mental delays require considerable comprehensive and long-term care. Repeated noncompliance of some adolescents to prescribed therapy may result in loss of the transplanted kidney. All of these issues have a significant effect on the families. In addition, families must deal with members of medical and legislative committees who would argue that many children should not receive all ESRD services because of cost containment. Technologic advances in dialysis and transplant have improved the quality of life and increased life expectancy for thousands with ESRD while pacing the resources. For every kidney donor that becomes available, there are four or five individuals waiting. Tighter selection criteria may appear for transplantation. Research continues with porcine xenotransplantation as the logical resource. Both of these options carry strong ethical considerations (Cummings, 1997).

The cost of ESRD treatment is very expensive, ranging from $20,000 to $35,000 or higher per individual per year. On July 1, 1973, the Social Security Act was amended to provide Medicare benefits for persons under 65 years of age who were certified to have chronic kidney failure and require dialysis or transplantation (HR-1, Public Law 92-603, section 2001). The total of all ESRD costs paid by Medicare in 1996 was $10.96 billion for 225,000 individuals with ESRD, compared with $6.03 billion in 1992 (Evans and Kitzman, 1998). Total ESRD costs are much higher because Medicare is considered as secondary payor for the first 30 months of RRT for individuals with private insurance. Because the payment process becomes quite complicated, families should be referred to the nephrology social worker for assistance in accessing available services. Addi-

tional financial assistance information is available through the National Kidney Foundation affiliates, the American Kidney Fund, and the American Association of Kidney Patients.

Resources

American Nephrology Nurses Association (ANNA)
East Holly Drive, Box 56
Pitman, NJ 08071
(609) 256-2320 or (800) 203-5561
(609) 589-7463 (fax)
anna@mail.ajj.com; http://anna.inurse.com

The Pediatric Educational Resource Directory, which is a 5-page listing of available pediatric educational materials, is published in Vol. 24, No. 4 of the ANNA Journal (August 1997).

American Association of Kidney Patients (AAKP)
100 S. Ashley Drive, Suite 250
Tampa, Fla. 33602
(800) 749-AAKP
AAKPnat@aol.com; http://www.aakp.org

Their newsletter and quarterly journal are called, "aakpRENALIFE." Contact the local chapter for educational assistance, summer camps, support groups, and financial information.

National Kidney Foundation (NKF)
30 East 33rd Street
New York, NY 10016
(800) 622-9010
http://www.kidney.org

Contact the local chapter for educational assistance, summer camps, support groups, and financial information.

American Kidney Fund (AKF)
6110 Executive Blvd., Suite 1010
Rockville, Md. 20852
(800) 638-8299
http://www.akfinc.org
Free educational materials are available.
HCFA ESRD Networks

Divided into geographic regions, these networks are assigned to coordinate and review dialysis and transplant facilities to ensure the best possible care for individuals. Call the AAKP or NKF for the location of the network for your state.

Renal Physicians Association (RPA)
1101 Vermont Ave NW, No. 500
Washington, DC 20005-3547
(202) 289-1700

Other online resources:

Medical Matrix—Directory of patient education documents (over 3000) on the Internet: http://www.slackinc.com/matrix/patient.html

United Network of Organ Sharing (UNOS): http://www.unos.org

RENALNET—Comprehensive renal-related site, the Kidney Information Clearinghouse: http://www.renalnet.org

TransWeb—A site for transplant and organ donation information: http://www.transweb.org/tw__contact.html

United States Renal Data Service (USRDS): http://www.med.umich.edu/usrds

Summary of Primary Care Needs for the Child with Chronic Renal Failure

GROWTH AND DEVELOPMENT

Despite advances in medical management, dialysis, and transplant, growth retardation is a major problem in children with CRF (most are at least two SDs below the mean height for their age).

Achievement of developmental milestones (all ages) is delayed; sexual maturation is delayed.

Anthropometric measurements, developmental assessment, and Tanner staging should be monitored.

Aggressive nutrition, adequate dialysis efficiency, and growth hormone injections may improve growth.

DIET

Protein and caloric needs in children with CRF are greater than the normal RDA to enhance growth and development and offset losses (protein in PD). Glucose is absorbed in PD.

Supplemental oral, NG, or G-tube feedings should be considered to improve nutrition.

Dietary restrictions differ with change in ESRD modality.

SAFETY

Children with CRF should be encouraged to live as normal and active lives as possible, with modifications as necessary. Immunosupression and renal osteodystrophy increase risk of infection and fracture.

IMMUNIZATIONS

Routine immunizations are recommended. Live virus vaccines are prohibited in immunosuppressed child.

Influenza, pneumococcal, varicella, and hepatitis vaccines are recommended. Immunoglobulin is given after known exposure to virus (i.e., hepatitis, varicella zoster)

SCREENING

Vision

Routine annual exams by a pediatric ophthalmologist are recommended to assess for calcification, arterial hemorrhages, and cataracts (if child is on steroid therapy), as well as vision testing.

Hearing

Routine annual exams recommended; hearing should be monitored when a child is using ototoxic drugs.

Dental

Routine dental care at 6-month intervals; child with vascular access or immunosuppression is at risk for endocarditis and needs prophylactic antibiotic coverage for dental procedures.

Gingival hyperplasia, enamel defects, and poor mineralization should be monitored.

Blood pressure

Blood pressure should be taken at all medical visits; frequency of measurement depends on BP value. Correctly sized cuff should be used.

Antihypertensive therapy should be managed by the pediatric nephrologist. Goal is normal BP.

Hematocrit

Anemia is a chronic problem. CBCs are monitored by the pediatric nephrology team.

Urinalysis

Routine screening is done by pediatric nephrology team if indicated.

Tuberculosis

Yearly screening by PPD testing is done.

Summary of Primary Care Needs for the Child with Chronic Renal Failure—cont'd

CONDITION-SPECIFIC SCREENING

Bloodwork

CBC and RBC indices and folate studies, electrolytes, BUN, creatinine, calcium, phosphorus, alkaline phosphatase, albumin, ferritin, and iron are monitored monthly. PTH and viral titers periodically.

Cardiac screening

Monitor chest x-ray, EKG, and Echo every 6 months.

Radiologic screening

Monitor bone radiographs for skeletal growth and renal osteodystrophy.

DIFFERENTIAL DIAGNOSIS AND MANAGEMENT OF PEDIATRIC CONDITIONS

Routine pediatric care should be provided by a pediatrician in collaboration with the pediatric nephrologist.

Fever should always be assessed for etiology; fever related to a vascular access or PD catheter infection should be managed by the pediatric nephrologist. GI symptoms should be assessed for decreasing renal function.

Headaches should be assessed for hypertension; BP should be controlled to normal.

DRUG INTERACTIONS AND COMPLIANCE

For all medications in CRF management, the route of excretion, degree of renal impairment, and interaction with other medications in CRF management should be known.

Dosage of all medications should be calculated by weight—not age—of the child.

Renal excreted drugs may require dosage adjustment.

Calcium-based—not aluminum-based— phosphate binders should be used.

Acetaminophen rather than aspirin should be used for pain or fever.

Absolute medication compliance is key to a successful kidney transplant; many graft losses are because of noncompliance, especially in adolescents.

Medication teaching should be related to child's developmental level.

DEVELOPMENTAL ISSUES

Sleep patterns

Increased fatigue and need for sleep may indicate decreasing renal failure.

Toileting

Children with CRF may have normal urine output, oliguria, or anuria. Urinary diversion may present greater difficulty for adolescent.

Not all children can achieve urinary continence.

Bowel training should begin when a child is developmentally ready.

Proper wiping direction should be taught to female children and their parents.

Discipline

Parents' own emotions may interfere with discipline of the child, (e.g., overprotective or too lenient without discipline).

Parents need honest answers and encouragement.

Nonadherence with plan of care is source of conflict.

Children with CRF should learn self-discipline and begin taking responsibility for self-care as possible.

Child care

The child care provider must be taught about diet, medications, special treatment regimen, and emergency measures.

Children may be exposed to more infections in daycare.

School performance

School attendance, when possible, should be encouraged or an alternative (home bound, tutor, teacher in dialysis) provided.

Continued

Summary of Primary Care Needs for the Child with Chronic Renal Failure—cont'd

Teachers should be instructed about child's care plan and needs.

Learning outside the classroom (e.g., in nature) should be encouraged.

Poor school performance should be evaluated for physical vs. psychologic factors contributing to cause.

Adolescence, sexuality, and transition to adulthood

Adolescent characteristics differ between early, middle, and late adolescence, areas of growth, cognition, identity, sexuality, emotionality, family and peer relationships across the age span should be assessed.

Ventilation of emotions; physical activity for emotional health, independence, and support groups should be encouraged.

Counseling on birth control, SDS, HIV exposure should be provided.

Responsibility toward transition to adulthood should be promoted.

SPECIAL FAMILY CONCERNS

CRF affects entire family; the goal is to strengthen the total family unit.

Networking with the other families of children with CRF should be provided.

Religious, ethnic, cultural, and racial factors affect adjustment to CRF and care.

Ethical issues are closely related to economics and highly controversial.

Health care team should practice patient advocacy.

Cost containment has an effect on care.

References

Alfrey A: Phosphate, aluminum and other elements in chronic renal failure. In Schrier RW and Gottschalk CW, editors: Diseases of the kidney, vol. III, ed 6, Boston, 1997, Little Brown.

American College of Physicians: Automated ambulatory blood pressure and self-measured blood pressure monitoring devices: Their role in the diagnosis and management of hypertension, Ann Intern Med 118(11):889-892, 1993.

Anderson S and Meyer TW: Pathophysiology and nephron adaptation in chronic renal failure. In Schrier RW and Gottschalk CW, editors: Diseases of the kidney, vol. III, ed 6, Boston, 1997, Little Brown.

Andress DL and Sherrard DJ: The osteodystrophy of chronic renal failure. In Schrier RW and Gottschalk CW, editors: Diseases of the kidney, vol. III, ed 6, Boston, 1997, Little Brown.

Ash SR and Daugirdas JT: Peritoneal access devices. In Daugirdas JT and Ing RS, editors: Handbook of dialysis ed 2, Boston, 1994, Little, Brown.

Aufricht C et al: Subcutaneous recombinant human erythropoietin in children with renal anemia on continuous ambulatory peritoneal dialysis, Acta Paediatrica 82(11):959-962, 1993.

Bazilinski N and Dunea G: Hypertension. In Daugirdas JT and Ing RS, editors: Handbook of dialysis, ed 2, Boston, 1994, Little, Brown.

Berkoben M and Schwab SN: Maintenance of permanent hemodialysis vascular access patency, American Nephrology Nurses Association Journal 22(1):17-24, 1995.

Besarab A: Anemia in renal disease. In Schrier RW and Gottschalk CW, editors: Diseases of the kidney, vol. III, ed 6, Boston, 1997, Little, Brown.

Blake PG: Malnutrition in peritoneal dialysis—part II, Contemporary Dialysis and Nephrology 15(11):20-21, 1994.

Boag JT: Strategies for influencing outcomes in pre-ESRD and ESRD patients, Part 1, Dialysis and Transplantation 27(9):565-573, 1998.

Boag JT: Strategies for influencing outcomes in pre-ESRD and ESRD patients, Part 1, Dialysis and Transplantation 27(10):656-664, 1998.

Brewer ED: Growth of small children managed with chronic peritoneal dialysis and nasogastric tube feedings: 203-month experience in 14 patients, Adv Perit Dial 6:269-272, 1990.

Bruiner GM: Calcium/phosphorus imbalances, aluminum toxicity, and renal osteodystrophy, American Nephrology Nurses Association Journal 21(4):171-177, 1994.

Bunchman TE: Pediatric hemodialysis: lessons from the past, ideas for the future, Kidney International 49(suppl 53):S64-567, 1996.

Burrows L and Prowant BF: Peritoneal dialysis. In Parker J, editor: Contemporary nephrology nursing ANNA, Pitman, NJ, 1998, AJ Jannetti, Inc.

Caplan AL: . . .And this little pig saved lives!, Dialysis and Transplantation 27(10):618-620, 1998.

Cendron M et al: Perinatal urology. In Gillenwater JY et al, editors: Adult and pediatric urology, vol. 3, ed 3, St Louis, 1996, Mosby.

Chan JC et al: A prospective, double-blind study of growth failure in children with chronic renal insufficiency and the effectiveness of treatment with calcitriol versus dihydrotachysterol: the growth failure in children with renal diseases investigators, J Pediatr 124(4):520-528, 1994.

Chan L and Kam I: Outcomes and complications of transplant. In Schrier RW and Gottschalk CW, editors: Diseases of the kidney, vol. III, ed 6, Boston, 1997, Little Brown.

Chantler C: Kidney disease in children. In Schrier RW and Gottschalk CW, editors: Diseases of the kidney, vol. III, ed 6, Boston, 1997, Little Brown.

Cohen JA and Brattich M: Epoetin alfa: focus on maintaining a higher, stable hematocrit, American Nephrology Nurses Journal 24(5):574-580, 1997.

Cohen J et al: Infectious complications after renal transplant. In Morris PJ: Kidney transplantation: principles and practice, ed 4, Philadelphia, 1994, W.B. Saunders.

College J: Epoetin alfa—focus on nutritional therapy, American Nephrology Nurses Journal 23(4):416-419, 1996.

Committee on Infectious Diseases: Report of the Committee on Infectious Diseases, ed 24, Elk Grove Village, Ill., 1997, The American Academy of Pediatrics.

Cresswell S and Hicks K: A new modem-based communication link for pediatric home peritoneal dialysis patients, Dialysis and Transplantation 25(9):586-590, 1996.

Cummings NB: Ethical and legal considerations in end-stage renal disease. In Schrier RW and Gottschalk CW, editors: Diseases of the kidney, vol. III, ed 6, Boston, 1997, Little Brown.

Currier H: Ethical issues in the neonatal patient with end-stage renal disease, J Perinatal Neonat Nurs 8(1):74-78, 1994.

Daughaday WH and Harvey S: Growth hormone action: clinical significance. In Harvery S, Scanes CG, and Daughaday WH, editors: Growth hormone, Boca Raton, Fla., 1994, CRC Press.

DeKernion JB and Trapasso JG: Urinary diversion and continent reservoir. In Gillenwater et al, editors: Adult and pediatric urology, vol. 3, ed 3, St Louis, 1996, Mosby.

Durack DT and Phil D: Prevention of infective endocarditis, N Engl J Med 332(1):37-44, 1995.

Elzouki A et al: Improved neurological outcome in children with chronic renal disease from infancy, Pediatr Nephrol 8(2):205-210, 1994.

Evans ED et al: Principles of renal replacement therapy in children, Pediatr Clin North Am 42(6):1579-1601, 1995.

Evans RW and Kitzman DJ: An economic analysis of kidney transplantation, Surg Clin North Am 78(1):149-172, 1998.

Fine RN: Recombinant human growth hormone in children with chronic renal insufficiency—clinical update: 1995, Kidney International 49(Suppl 53):S115-118, 1996.

Fine RN: Recent advances in the management of the infant, child, and adolescent with chronic renal failure, Pediatr Rev 11:277-283, 1990.

Fine RN: Recombinant human growth hormone treatment of children with chronic renal failure: update 1990, Acta Paediatr Scand 370:S44-48, 1990.

Fine RN and Ettenger R: Renal transplantation in children. In Morris PF, editor: Kidney transplantation—principles and practice, ed 4, Philadelphia, 1994, W.B. Saunders.

Fine RN et al: Growth after recombinant human growth hormone treatment in children with chronic renal failure: report of a multicenter randomized double-blind placebo-controlled study: Genentech Cooperative Study Group, J Pediatr 124(3):374-382, 1994.

Fine RN, Salusky IB, and Ettenger RB: The therapeutic approach to the infant, child, and adolescent with end-stage renal disease, Pediatr Clin North Am 34:789-801, 1987.

Fine RN et al: Recombinant human growth hormone in infants and young children with chronic renal insufficiency, Pediatr Nephrol 9:451-457, 1995.

Finney JW and Weist MD: Behavioral assessment of children and adolescents, Pediatr Clin North Am 39(3):369-378, 1992.

Fivush BA et al: Defective antibody response to Hemophilus influenza type b immunization in children receiving peritoneal dialysis, Pediatr Nephrol 7(5):548-550, 1993.

Foley RN et al: Cardiovascular complications of ESRD. In Schrier RW and Gottschalk CW, editors: Diseases of the kidney, vol. III, ed 6, Boston, 1997, Little, Brown.

Fraser CL and Arieff AI: Nervous system manifestations of renal failure. In Schrier RW and Gottschalk CW, editors: Diseases of the kidney, vol. III, ed 6, Boston, 1997, Little, Brown.

Furth SL et al: Varicella requiring hospitalization in the first year after renal transplantation: a report to the North American Pediatric Renal Transplant Cooperative Study, Pediatric Transplantation 1(1):37-42, 1997.

Garvin G: Caring for children with ostomies, Nurs Clin North Am 29(4):645-654, 1994.

Giatras I et al: Effects of angiotensin-converting enzyme inhibitors on the progression of nondiabetic renal disease: a meta-analysis of randomized trials, Ann Intern Med 127(5):337-345, 1997.

Gilman C and Frauman AC: The pediatric patient. In Parker J, editor: Contemporary nephrology nursing ANNA, Pitman, NJ, 1998, AJ Jannetti, Inc.

Golper T et al: Peritoneal dialysis. In Schrier RW and Gottschalk CW, editors: Diseases of the kidney, vol. III, ed 6, Boston, 1997, Little, Brown.

Greenleaf K: Barriers to adequate management of growth failure in children with chronic renal insufficiency, guidelines for growth: advocating a standard of care for children with chronic renal insufficiency, Adverceutics 1996.

Gregory MC and Atkin CL: Alport's syndrome, Fabry's disease and Nail-Patella syndome. In Schrier RW and Gottschalk CW, editors: Diseases of the kidney, vol. III, ed 6, Boston, 1997, Little, Brown.

Grupe WE et al: Issues in pediatric dialysis, Am J Kidney Dis 7:324-328, 1986.

Haggerty LM and Sigardson-Poor KM: Kidney transplant. In Sigardson-Poor KM and Haggerty LM, editors: Nursing care of the transplant recipient, Philadelphia, 1990, W.B. Saunders.

Harum P: Protein and your kidneys, aakp RENALIFE 14(2):16-17, 1998.

Hofman A and Greydanus D: Adolescent medicine, ed 2, Norwalk, Conn., 1989, Appleton & Lange.

Hokken-Koelga ACS et al: A placebo-controlled double blind trial of growth hormone treatment in prepubertal children after renal transplant, Kidney International 49(suppl 53):S128-134, 1996.

Kasiske BL et al: The effect of race on access and outcome of transplantation, New Eng J Med 324(5):302-307, 1992.

Klaus G et al: Treatment of peritoneal dialysis-associated peritonitis with continuous versus intermittent vanco/teicoplanin and ceftazidime in children, Adv Periton Dial (11):296-301, 1995.

Knight F et al: Hemodialysis of the infant or small child with chronic renal failure, American Nephrology Nurses Association Journal 20(3):315-323, 1993.

Kohaut EC and Fine RN: Testing for growth hormone release is not necessary prior to treatment of children with chronic renal insufficiency—recombinant human growth hormone, Kidney International 49(suppl 53):S119-122, 1996.

Kopple JD: Dietary considerations in patients with advanced chronic renal failure, acute renal failure, and transplantation. In Schrier RW and Gottschalk CW, editors: Diseases of the kidney, vol. III, ed 6, Boston, 1997, Little, Brown.

Lancaster L: Manifestations of renal failure. In Lancaster LE, editor: Core curriculum for nephrology nursing, ed 3, Pitman, NJ, 1995, AJ Jannetti.

Lancaster L: Peritoneal dialysis. In Lancaster LE, editor: Core curriculum for nephrology nursing, ed 3, Pitman, NJ, 1995, AJ Jannetti.

Lewis S et al: Sexuality, infertility, and impotence—important concerns for dialysis patients, Contemporary Dialysis and Nephrology—For Patients Only: 21-23, May-June 1998.

Matas AJ et al: Recipient evaluation, preparation, and care in pediatric transplant: The University of Minnesota Protocols, Kidney International 49(suppl 53):S99-102, 1996.

Mehls O and Ritz E: Renal osteodystrophy. In Holliday MA, Barratt TM, and Paganini EP, editors: Overview of anemia associated with chronic renal disease: primary and secondary mechanisms, Sem Nephrol 9(suppl 1):3-8, 1989.

Mensoor GA and White WB: Ambulatory blood pressure monitoring is a useful clinical tool in nephrology, Am J Kidney Dis 30(5):591-607, 1997.

Miles AM and Friedman EA: Center and home chronic hemodialysis: outcome and complications. In Schrier RW and Gottschalk CW, editors: Diseases of the kidney, vol. III, ed 6, Boston, 1997, Little, Brown.

Molzahn AE: Psychosocial impact of renal disease. In Parker J, editor: Contemporary nephrology nursing ANNA, Pitman, NJ, 1998, AJ Jannetti, Inc.

Moore LW: Nutrition in end-stage renal disease: a life cycle perspective, Nephrology Nursing Today 1(2):1-8, 1991.

Morris KP et al: Non-cardiac benefits of human recombinant erythropoietin in end stage renal failure and anaemia, Arch Dis Child 69(5):580-586, 1993.

Morris KP et al: Cardiovascular abnormalities in end stage renal failure: the effect of anaemia or uraemia? Arch Dis Child 71(2):119-122, 1994.

Mudge C et al: Transplantation. In Parker J, editor: Contemporary nephrology nursing ANNA, Pitman, NJ, 1998, AJ Jannetti, Inc.

National Kidney Foundation: Dialysis outcome quality initiative (DOQI) guidelines, 1998, NKF Website: http://www.kidney.org/doqi/doqi/exmethodology.html.

Newman M: Growth hormone therapy and chronic renal insufficiency in children, Perspectives on Growth 1(2):1-12, 1998.

Nevins TE and Maurer SM: Infant hemodialysis. In Fine RN and Nissenson AR, editors: Dialysis therapy, Philadelphia, 1986, Harley & Balfur.

Nissensen AR: An update on anemia and iron management in dialysis patients, Contemp Dial Nephrol 19(5):31-34, 1998.

North American Pediatric Renal Transplant Cooperative Study (NAPRTCS): 1998 Annual Report, Potomac, Md., 1998, The Emmes Corp.

Ojo AO et al: Comparative mortality risks of chronic dialysis and cadaveric transplantation in black end-stage renal disease patients, Am J Kidney Dis 24(1):59-64, 1994.

Oreopoulos DG: How can we make peritoneal dialysis a viable long-term therapy?, Nephrology News and Issues 10(6):12-14, 1996.

Painter P and Carlson L: Case study of the anemic patient: Epoetin alfa—focus on exercise, American Nephrology Nurses Association Journal 23(3):304-307, 1994.

Papadopoulou AL: Chronic renal failure. In Barakat AY, editor: Renal disease in children, New York, 1989, Springer-Verlag.

Parker KP: Acute and chronic renal failure. In Parker J, editor: Contemporary nephrology nursing ANNA, Pitman, NJ, 1998, AJ Jannetti, Inc.

Rastegar A and DeFronzo RA: Disorders of potassium and acid-base metabolism in association with renal disease. In Schrier RW and Gottschalk CW, editors: Diseases of the kidney, vol. III, ed 6, Boston, 1997, Little, Brown.

Richardson RC: Discipline and children and chronic illness: strategies to promote positive patient outcomes, American Nephrology Nurses Association (ANNA) Journal 24(1):35-40, 1997.

Richie MF, Mapes D, and Dailey FD: Psychosocial aspects of renal failure and its treatment. In Lancaster LE, editor: Core curriculum for nephrology nursing, ed 3, Pitman, NJ, 1995, AJ Jannetti.

Roberts SD: Nutritional care of renal patients. In Parker J, editor: Contemporary nephrology nursing ANNA, Pitman, NJ, 1998, AJ Jannetti, Inc.

Rodzilsky D and Constantinescu S: Nutritional guidelines for infants and pediatric patients on peritoneal dialysis, Nephrology News and Issues 11(5):22-23, 1997.

Rossmann JA et al: Multimodal treatment of drug-induced gingival hyperplasia in a kidney transplant patient, Compendium 15(10):1266-1274, 1994.

Rotundo A et al: Progressive encephalopathy in children with chronic renal insufficiency in infancy, Kidney Int 21:486-491, 1982.

Russell SS: Conservative management of renal failure. In Parker J, editor: Contemporary nephrology nursing ANNA, Pitman, NJ, 1998, AJ Jannetti, Inc.

Salai PB: Hemodialysis. In Parker J, editor: Contemporary nephrology Nursing ANNA, Pitman, NJ, 1998, AJ Jannetti, Inc.

Salmon K and Broyan P: Epoetin alfa—issues in self-administration, Nephrology Nursing Today 1(5):1-8, 1991.

Salusky IB: Bone and mineral metabolism in childhood end-stage renal disease, Pediatr Clin North Am 42(6):1531-1547, 1995.

Salusky IB et al: Prospective evaluation of aluminum loading from formula in infants with uremia, J Pediatr 116(5):726-729, 1990.

Salusky IB et al: Aluminum accumulation during treatment with aluminum hydroxide and dialysis in children and young adults with chronic renal disease, N Engl J Med 324(8):527-531, 1991.

Sands JJ: A teaching tool for managing hemodialysis access failure, Nephrology News and Issues:25-28, September 1998.

Scharer K: Growth and development of children with chronic renal failure: study group on pubertal development in chronic renal failure, Acta Paediatr Scand 366:S90-92, 1990.

Schira MG: The role of cognitive function in education of patients with ESRD, Nephrology Nursing Today 4(3):1-8, 1994.

Scribner BH: Chronic renal disease and hypertension, Dial Transplant 27(11):702-704, 1998.

Sekelman J: Infectious diseases and immunizations of today and tomorrow, Pediatr Nurs 24(4):309-315, 1998.

Shimokura G et al: Hepatitis C virus in hemodialysis centers, American Nephrology Nurses Association Journal 25(5):541-542, 1998.

Simonds N: Overview of growth failure in children with chronic renal insufficiency, guidelines for growth: advocating a standard of care for children with chronic renal insufficiency, Advolution 7-9, 1996.

Sims TW et al: Pharmacologic agents in renal disease. In Parker J, editor: Contemporary nephrology nursing ANNA, Pitman, NJ, 1998, AJ Jannetti, Inc.

Smith GHH and Duckett JW: Urethral lesions in infants and children. In Gillenwater JY et al, editors: Adult and pediatric urology, vol. 3, ed 3, St Louis, 1996, Mosby.

Stablein DM: Annual report 1992: North American Pediatric Renal Transplant Cooperative Study (NAPRTCS), Potomac, Md., 1992, The EMMES Corporation.

Swann SK and Bennett WM: Use of drugs in patients with renal failure. In Schrier RW and Gottschalk CW, editors: Diseases of the kidney, vol. III, ed 6, Boston, 1997, Little, Brown.

Taylor JH: Care of central venous catheters in children on hemodialysis, aakpRENALIFE 12(1): 8-11, 1996.

Taylor JH: A competency based approach to pediatric hemodialysis, Unpublished lecture presented at ANNA Symposium, Dallas, 1994.

Taylor JH: Enhancing development in the adolescent with ESRD, Unpublished lecture presented at ANNA Symposium, Dallas, 1994.

Tonshoff B and Fine RN: Growth and growth hormone treatment in children with chronic renal insufficiency. In Neissensen AR, Fine RN, and Gentile DE, editors: Clinical dialysis ed 3, E. Norwalk, CT, 1995, Appleton & Lang.

Travis LB, Brouhard BH, and Kalia A: Overview with special emphasis on epidemiologic considerations. In Tune BM and Mendoze SA, editors: Pediatric nephrology: contemporary issues in nephrology, vol. 12, New York, 1984, Churchill Livingstone.

Trompoter RS: A review of drug prescribing in children with end-stage renal failure, Pediatr Nephrol 1:183-194, 1987.

Tzamaloukas AH: Peritoneal dialysis adequacy, Dial Transplant 26(12):834-853, 1997.

US Renal Data System: USRDS 1998 Annual Data Report, The National Institutes of Health, National Institute of Diabetes and Digestive and Kidney Diseases, Bethesda, Md, 1998, Website: http://www.med.umich.edu.usrds/chapters/html.

Uysal S et al: Neurologic complications in chronic renal failure: a retrospective study, Clin Pediatr 29(9):510-514, 1990.

Vas S et al: Treatment in peritoneal dialysis patients of peritonitis caused by gram positive organisms with single daily dose of antibiotics, Perit Dial Int 17(1):91094, 1997.

Vessey JA: School services for children with chronic conditions, Pediatr Nurs 23(5):507-510, 1997.

Walker RD: Vesicoureteral reflux and urinary tract infections in children. In Gillenwater JY et al, editors: Adult and pediatric urology, vol. 3, ed 3, St Louis, 1996, Mosby.

Wagner T: Its up to you: improving medication compliance, Stadtlanders Lifetimes (1):36-37, 1997.

Warady BA: Collaborative efforts enhance peritoneal dialysis prospects for children, Contemp Dial Nephrol 18(2):16-24, 1997.

Warady BA et al: Lessons from the peritoneal dialysis patient database: a report of the NAPRTCS, Kidney International 49(suppl 53):S68-S71, 1996.

Wong DL: The child with hematologic or immunologic dysfunction. In Wong DL, editor: Whaley and Wong's essentials of pediatric nursing, ed 5, St Louis, 1997, Mosby.

Wong DL: The child with genitourinary dysfunction. In Wong DL, editor: Whaley and Wong's essentials of pediatric nursing, ed 5, St Louis, 1997, Mosby.

Zemplar, Paracalcitol, Manufacturer teaching guide, Abbott Park, Ill., 1998, Abbott Labs, Inc.

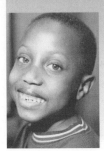

CHAPTER 35

Sickle Cell Disease

Barbara A. Carroll

Etiology

Sickle cell disease (SCD) is a term used to describe several inherited, sickling hemoglobinopathy syndromes, including sickle-β-thalassemia (HgbS-β° thal or HbgSβ+ thal), sickle-C disease (Hgb SC), and—most commonly—sickle cell anemia (Hgb SS). Adult hemoglobin contains two pairs of polypeptide chains, alpha (α) and beta (β). Each of these hemoglobinopathy syndromes involves the mutated sickle hemoglobin (Hgb S), which differs from normal hemoglobin (Hgb A) by the substitution of a single amino acid, valine, for glutamic acid at the sixth position of the β-globin chain.

Red blood cells (RBCs) that contain normal hemoglobin are pliable, biconcave discs with a life span of approximately 120 days. When deoxygenated, RBCs containing predominantly Hgb S polymerize and form microtubules (i.e., rods) that distort the shape of the cell, characteristically to a crescent or sickle shape. In this form the cell is rigid and friable. Hypoxia and acidosis, which may be caused by fever, infection, dehydration, or other factors, are known to induce this change in shape (Figure 35-1). Many times, however, the RBC changes shape without apparent provocation. To a limited degree, this change in shape is reversible, though not indefinitely. These cells eventually become irreversibly sickled cells (ISCs) with a life span of approximately 10 to 20 days. The fragility and shortened life span of these RBCs leads to chronic anemia, which serves as a stimulus for the bone marrow to create new RBCs, resulting in an elevated reticulocyte count.

The sickle "prep" is a solubility test often used to screen infants and children for SCD. This test is inexpensive and rapidly performed but is not very specific. A sickle prep result will be positive for sickle cell trait, sickle cell anemia, and other sickle hemoglobinopathies but will not distinguish one from another. The definitive diagnosis of SCD is made by performing a complete blood count (CBC), peripheral blood smear, and—most importantly—a quantitative hemoglobin electrophoresis. Measurement of hematologic indices are often important in the differential diagnoses of thalassemia syndromes and hemoglobinopathies. It is occasionally helpful to perform hematologic studies on a child's parents to confirm the diagnosis.

SCD has an autosomal recessive inheritance pattern. Both parents must carry some type of abnormal hemoglobin (i.e., one or both of them must carry sickle hemoglobin) for the disease to be manifested in their child. Carriers of SCD are described as having sickle cell trait (Hgb AS). When two individuals, each of whom has sickle cell trait, elect to have a child, there is a 25% chance that they will have a child with sickle cell anemia (Hgb SS). These individuals also have a 50% chance of having a child with sickle cell trait (Hgb AS) and a 25% chance of having a child with entirely normal hemoglobin (Hgb AA) with each pregnancy (Figure 35-2).

In an effort to decrease morbidity and mortality through early identification and prophylactic treatment, most states are now performing routine newborn screening for hemoglobinopathies. These screening methods include electrophoresis or high-performance liquid chromatography (HPLC) and are performed on cord blood or heel-stick blood, usually when blood is obtained for other newborn screening tests (e.g., phenylketonuria, thyroid function).

Fetal hemoglobin (Hbg F) predominates from 10 weeks after conception through the remainder of gestation and normally begins to decline at 34 weeks. Hgb F comprises 60% to 80% of the total hemoglobin at birth and declines to normal adult levels (1% to 2%) by 6 to 9 months of age (Pearson, 1996). In premature infants, however, the

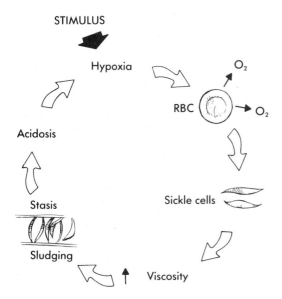

Figure 35-1 Cycle causing vasoocclusive episodes in sickle cell anemia. (From Hockenberry M and Coody D, editors: Pediatric oncology and hematology: perspectives on care, St Louis, 1986, Mosby.)

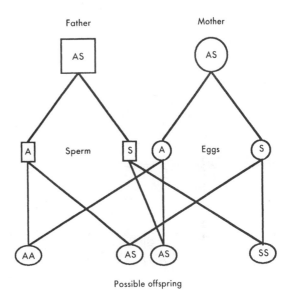

Figure 35-2 Genetics of sickle cell anemia. Both parents possess one gene for normal hemoglobin *(A)* and one for sickle hemoglobin *(S)*. With each pregnancy, there is a 25% statistical chance that the child will have normal hemoglobin *(AA)* and a 25% chance that the child will have sickle cell anemia *(SS)*; 50% of the children will have the sickle cell trait. (From Miller D and Baeher R: Blood diseases of infancy and childhood: in the tradition of CH Smith, ed 6, St Louis, 1990, Mosby.)

falloff in Hgb F is somewhat slower. The remaining 20% to 40% of hemoglobin found at birth has the adult electrophoresis forms, HbA and HbA$_2$ or Hgb S if found to be affected. Hgb F does not sickle, so it is unusual to find clinical manifestations of the disease with significant amounts of Hgb F. Because of this phenomena, manifestations of SCD may not be clinically apparent until 4 to 6 months of age or later.

Incidence

SCD is one of the most common genetic diseases most often seen in individuals of African descent but is also found in other ethnic groups, including those from the Caribbean, Mediterranean, Arabian Peninsula, and India. In the United States, 1 in 12 blacks is a carrier of the sickle cell gene, and 1 in 600 actually manifests the disease (Steinburg and Embury, 1994).

Prenatal diagnosis is available to couples known to be carriers of hemoglobinopathies. Diagnosis may be accomplished via chorionic villi sampling during the first trimester or amniocentesis during the second trimester. The method depends on the risks and benefits of the techniques involved; both are adequate to determine the diagnosis.

Clinical Manifestations at Time of Diagnosis

As a result of current newborn screening programs for hemoglobinopathies, infants are now identified before the onset of acute symptoms (Table 35-1 and Box 35-1). The anemia from which sickle cell anemia derives its name is broadly characterized as an uncompensated hemolytic anemia, in which a markedly shortened overall RBC survival (i.e., an increased rate of RBC destruction) is insuffi-

Table 33-1
Differential Diagnosis of Common Hemoglobinopathies

Diagnosis	Clinical Severity	Hemoglobin (g/dl)	Hematocrit (%)	Mean Corpuscular Volume (MCV) (μ^3)	% of Reticulocytes	RBC Morphology*	Solubility Test	Electrophoresis (%)	Distribution of Hbg F
SS	Moderate-severe	7.5 (6-11)	22 (18-30)	>80	11 (5-20)	Many ISCs, target cells, nucleated RBCs, normochromic H-J bodies	Positive	>90 S <10 F <3.6 A_2	Uneven
SC	Mild-moderate	10 (10-15)	30 (26-40)	75-95	3 (5-10)	Many target cells, aniso/poikilocytosis	Positive	50 S 50 C <5 F	Uneven
S/B° thal	Moderate-severe	8.1 (6-10)	25 (20-36)	<80	8 (5-20)	Marked hypochromia, microcytosis and target cells, variable ISCs	Positive	>80 S <20 F >3.5 A_2	Uneven
S/B + thal	Mild-moderate	11 (9-12)	32 (25-40)	<75	3 (5-10)	Mild microcytosis, hypochromia, rare ISCs	Positive	55-75 S 15-30 A <20 F >3.5 A_2	Uneven
S/HPFH†	Asymptomatic	14 (12-14)	40 (32-48)	<80	1.5 (1-2)	No ISCs, occasional target cells, and mild hypochromia	Positive	<70 S >30 F <2.5 A_2	Even
AS	Asymptomatic	Normal	Normal	Normal	Normal	Normal	Positive	38-45 S 60-55 A 1-3 A_2	Uneven

*ICSs, irreversibly sickled cells.
†S/HPFH, sickle hereditary persistence of fetal hemoglobin.
From Charache, Lubin, and Reid, 1995.

Clinical Manifestations of Sickle Cell Anemia

Neonates

- Normal birth weight
- No evidence of hemolytic anemia
- Hemoglobin electrophoresis shows no evidence of Hgb A production
- Neonatal jaundice (when present) related to ABO hemolytic disease of the newborn, not to SCD

Infants and Toddlers

- Development of anemia
- Coliclike symptoms, often associated with feeding difficulties
- Generalized episodes of bone or abdomen pain preceded by acute, febrile infectious disease
- Hand-foot syndrome associated with heat, pain, swelling, erythema
- Splenic hypofunction marked by presence of Howell-Jolly bodies in the blood smear
- Autosplenectomy preceded by splenomegaly in 73% of infants, followed by decrease in size
- Splenomegaly noted frequently during febrile episodes

Early Childhood

- Generalized vasoocclusive crisis (VOC) of bone or abdomen that may or may not be preceded by acute, febrile infection; seemingly triggered by emotional stress or abrupt weather changes
- Usually nonpalpable spleen but sometimes retained in Hbg SC disease
- Males may develop priapism
- Biliary colic caused by stasis and gallstones
- Development of cerebral vasculopathy with cerebral infarction

Late Childhood

- Gallstones with or without symptoms
- Delayed pubescence
- Females may have increased incidence of VOC with menses, presumably due to hormonal changes
- Males may develop priapism
- Early signs of sickle retinopathy
- Early signs of sickle nephropathy

ciently balanced by the increase in production (i.e., erythropoiesis) to maintain normal levels of total RBC and Hbg concentrations (Bookchin and Virgilio, 1996).

In the first 2 decades of life, sickle cell anemia is marked by periods of clinical quiescence and relative well-being interspersed with episodes of acute illness. These illnesses are treatable by state-of-the-art medical care and are often preventable. The expression of sickle cell anemia is often characterized by septicemia and/or meningitis during infancy, followed by cerebral vasculopathy with cerebral infarction during early childhood. Splenic hypofunction is present in nearly 30% of infants with sickle cell anemia by their first birthday and in 90% by age 6 years. This presence accounts for the high risk of sepsis by polysaccharide-encapsulated organisms (Powars, 1994).

Treatment

There is no cure for SCD short of bone marrow transplantation (BMT). Despite the thorough understanding that exists among researchers and clinicians about the inheritance, diagnosis, and pathophysiology of SCD, treatment is essentially supportive and symptomatic. This therapy is aimed at aggressive treatment of infection and maintenance of optimal hydration and body temperature to prevent hypoxia and acidosis. Standard care implies bed rest, hydration, transfusions, analgesics, oxygen, and folic acid administration to prevent megablastic anemia (Johnston, 1997).

Treatment has recently moved from care during specific crises to the prevention of sickling episodes by inducing production of Hgb F, with hydroxyurea (HU) (Pearson, 1996) (Box 35-2). HU, which is a derivative of urea, has been used for neoplastic diseases. For individuals with SCD, it increases production of Hgb F through mechanisms that remain unclear. Expression of Hgb F, in combination with the native Hgb S, forms a diluted pool of RBCs with HbF and HbS. This combination reduces both the polymerization of the cells and the rate of hemolysis. Six pediatric trials of HU therapy have recently been reported (Vinchinsky, 1997a), indicating significant improvement in Hgb F production, mean corpuscular volume (MCV), and a mild to moderate increase in hemoglobin, which in turn reduces the number of sickle cell crises.

Children are generally started on 15 mg/kg of HU per day, with doses escalating to 5 mg/kg every 8 weeks if no signs or symptoms of toxicity are noted. The maximum dose is usually approximately 35 mg/kg/day (Rogers, 1997).

Charache (1996) suggests that administration of HU should be managed in a research-oriented practice because questions of long-term toxicity, carcinogenesis, growth retardation, and chromosomal damage are unanswered. The future treatment of SCD with HU alone or in combination with other agents (e.g., butyrate, valproic acid, clotrimazole, and erythropoietin) looks promising, and long-term trials are warranted (Vichinsky, 1997a). Although HU has the potential of reducing the incidence of both hemolytic and vasoocclusive manifestation of the disease, it is not an option for treatment of these complications.

From a preventative point of view, providing genetic counseling for those individuals with sickle cell trait, prenatal diagnosis for pregnant women who are at risk for delivering a child with SCD, and education for parents of children newly diagnosed is the standard of care.

Recent and Anticipated Advances in Diagnosis and Management

HU is beneficial in SCD (Charache, 1996; Ohene-Frempong and Smith-Whitley, 1997; Rogers, 1997), and its therapeutic effects may extend beyond its modulating effects on Hgb F. It has been suggested that HU decreases cell density, which indicates a primary membrane effect (Steinburg et al, 1997). Researchers recognize the complex interplay of sickle erythrocytes, leukocytes, vascular endothelium, platelets, plasma clotting factors, and certain mediators of inflammation in producing tissue ischemia and end-organ damage (Adams-Graves et al, 1997). Clinical trials aimed at modulating the effect of these various players are currently being studied.

BMT has effectively cured a small but growing number of individuals with sickle cell anemia. This approach is limited because only 18% of individuals have a matched donor (Mentzer et al, 1994). As with other candidates for BMT, use of umbilical

---

Box 35-2

Treatment

- Genetic counseling for individuals with sickle cell trait
- Prenatal diagnosis
- Parental education
- Aggressive treatment of infection
- Maintenance of optimal hydration
- Maintenance of body temperature
- Transfusion when facing life-threatening events
- Penicillin prophylaxis
- Pneumococcal immunization
- Drug therapy to induce expression of Hgb F
- Bone marrow transplantation in selected subjects

---

cord stem cells is being considered. To date, 200 transplantations have been performed using umbilical cord blood (Kelly et al, 1997). The extent to which human lymphocyte antigen (HLA) incompatibility can be tolerated when cord blood is used has not been determined. These results, however, raise the possibility that umbilical cord blood stem cells could be used in individuals with hemoglobinopathies. There is a dilemma in the selection of candidates for transplant, however, because sickle cell anemia is highly unpredictable in terms of severity and there are no valuable prognostic markers to indicate which individuals will manifest a severe course (Vermylen and Cornu, 1997). In general, children selected for transplant should show a morbid course of disease but not to an extent of irreversible organ damage, which would reduce chances for success.

A further consideration that limits this approach is the morbidity associated with BMT, including risks for death, organ impairment, curtailed sexual functioning, and impaired motor and psychologic functioning (Secundy, 1994). Other considerations include disturbance of family systems, cost-benefit ratios, the rights of siblings, and client compliance (Secundy, 1994). BMT options must be decisions shared by the health care workers and the family; differences in cultural background between the two, however, may impede the ability to negotiate informed consent. External factors (e.g., educational level, economic conditions of the family, and quality of life) are often more critical in minority communities than in other settings (Secundy, 1994).

At a more basic level, recombinant human hemoglobins designed for gene replacement therapy as a cure for SCD are being studied at the biochemical level (McCune et al, 1994). These mutations disrupt the ability of Hgb S to form polymers, suggesting a role for future therapy. Other strategies directed toward the elevation of Hgb F expression through gene therapy manipulation have been suggested. Both constructs may be suitable for future gene therapy for SCD.

The Cooperative Study of Sickle Cell Disease (CSSCD) group has completed two important studies. The Preoperative Transfusion Study group (Vinchinsky et al, 1995) challenged the aggressive practice of transfusing presurgical clients. It is well known that inducing general anesthesia places an individual with SCD at risk for stroke. Standard protocol was to transfuse these individuals to a hemoglobin of 11 g/dl with an Hgb S level of 30%. In the preoperative transfusion study, individuals were transfused to a preoperative level of 10 g/dl with an Hgb S level of 60%. Results suggest that stable individuals with Hgb SS who are undergoing major elective surgery should be transfused to the lower level of 10 g/dl. Transfusion with limited phenotypic units would most likely eliminate the alloimmunization observed from E, K, C, and Fy[a] RBC phenotypes. Definitive data to not recommend preoperative transfusion in SCD are not available. Currently, individuals having tonsillectomies and adenoidectomies should be transfused for surgery (Charache, Lubin, and Reid, 1995).

Because frequent transfusion carries the risk of chronic iron overload, a novel approach is transfusion by erythrocytapheresis (King and Ness, 1996). In this method, sickled cells are selectively removed and replaced with normal red cells via a rapid, continuous flow system that is similar to the production of pheresed units of platelets. Because normal erythrocytes are exchanged for sickled erythrocytes, the net gain of iron is greatly reduced or eliminated. Although this approach has merit, its application is limited to a few sickle cell centers in the United States (Styles and Vinchinsky, 1997).

Another study group of the CSSCD, Stroke Prevention in Sickle Cell Anemia (STOP), looked at genetic markers, laboratory and radiographic indicators, and clinical findings that were predictive of stroke in this population (Adams et al, 1998). Children thought to be at increased risk for stroke were managed more aggressively in hope of preventing serious complications. Recent radiographic developments (e.g., transcranial doppler ultrasound [TCD] and magnetic resonance angiography [MRA]) were used in some centers as a predictors of strokes.

Both techniques reliably demonstrate flow abnormalities consistent with areas of cerebral infarction. In particular, TCD demonstrated that high velocities (i.e., ≥ 200 cm/sec) in either the distal intercerebral or middle cerebral arteries were associated with an increased risk of subsequent stroke (Adams et al, 1997). Sickle cell centers are currently in the process of setting up TCD studies on all children with Hgb SS or Hgb S $\beta°$ thalassemia who have no history of stroke. Children with high velocities are at risk for stroke and offered scheduled transfusions as a means of preventing stroke and its subsequent consequences.

Positive emission tomography (PET) has confirmed areas of irregular brain metabolism in children with SCD. A recent study by Powars and associates (1999) confirms areas of irregular brain metabolism by assessing functional glucose metabolism and microvascular blood flow and confirmed the effectiveness of PET by comparing it with MRI or MRA. Powars and associates concluded the following: (1) the addition of PET to MRI identified a much greater proportion of children with SS neuroimaging abnormalities, particularly in children with no history of overt neurologic events; (2) lesions identified via PET are more extensive (i.e., often bihemispheric) when compared with abnormalities identified via MRI; (3) PET may be useful as a management tool to evaluate metabolic improvement after therapeutic interventions (i.e., chronic transfusions); and (4) the correlation of PET abnormalities to subsequent stroke or progressive neurologic dysfunction necessitates further study.

Associated Problems

Associated problems are primarily caused by the following: (1) blockage of small blood vessels secondary to the clumping of sickled RBCs that cause tissue ischemia, and (2) hemolytic anemia and its sequelae (Figure 35-3 and Box 35-3).

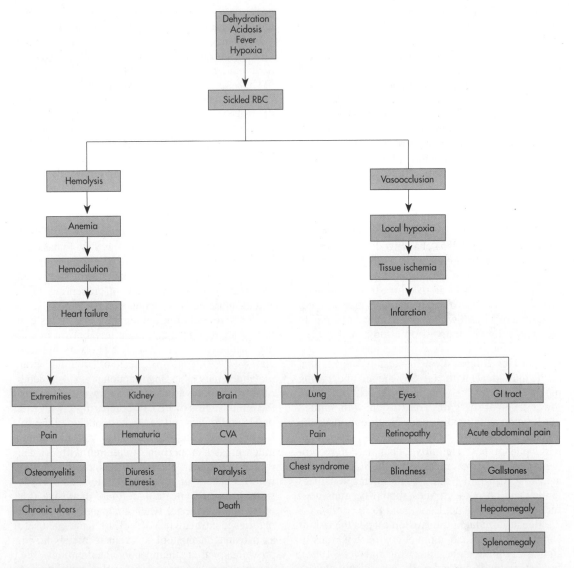

Figure 35-3   Tissue effects of sickle cell anemia. (From Wong D: Nursing care of infants and children, ed 5, St Louis, 1995, Mosby.)

Functional Asplenia

Splenic function is normal at birth, but by 6 months of age a state of splenic dysfunction develops, most likely as a result of massive infarction. Palpation of the spleen on physical examination is no indication of splenic function. A palpable spleen in older children is thought to be the result of fibrosis and is almost exclusively found in individuals with Hgb SC disease. The presence of Howell-Jolley bodies (e.g., "pocked cells") on blood smear confirms the condition of functional asplenia (Pearson, 1996). Functional asplenia occurs when the level of "pocked cells" is greater than 3.5% and the Hgb F level falls below 20%. Without adequate splenic function, children with SCD are at high risk for infection from polysaccharide-encapsulated

---

Box 35-3

Associated Problems

- Functional asplenia
- Splenic sequestration
- Neurologic problems
- Vasoocclusive crisis
- Pulmonary complications
    Acute chest syndrome
    Chronic lung disease
    Hemolysis/anemia
- Aplastic crisis
- Hemolysis
- Renal problems
- Priapism
- Skeletal changes
- Ophthalmologic changes
- Audiologic problems
- Leg ulcers
- Reactions to contrast mediums, anesthesia
- Cardiac problems
- Hepatobiliary problems
- Transfusion complications
    Formation of antibodies
    Iron overload
    Bloodborne pathogens

---

organisms, such as *Streptococcus pneumoniae, Haemophilus influenzae,* and *Neisseria meningitidis.* Less common causes of bacteremia include other streptococci, *Escherichia coli, Staphlococcus aureus,* and Gram-negative bacilli such as *Klebsiella* sp., *Salmonella* sp., and *Pseudomonas aeruginosa* (Committee on Infectious Disease, 1997).

Intervention should be threefold: (1) aggressive management of infectious episodes, (2) timely immunization (including pneumococcal vaccine), and (3) antibiotic prophylaxis. Because current pneumococcal vaccines do not cover all pathogenic strains, antibiotic prophylaxis is the standard of care for all young children with SCD and should be started at the time of diagnosis—preferably by 2 months of age (Committee on Infectious Disease, 1997). The usual doses for penicillin V or G are 125 mg twice daily for children under 3 years of age, and 250 mg twice daily for those over 3 years of age. For children who are not compliant with oral antibiotic therapy at home, .5 to 1.2 million units of a long-acting penicillin may be given intramuscularly each month (Charache, Lubin, and Reid,

1995). If an individual is allergic to penicillin, erythromycin (in appropriate doses) may be substituted. Some experts have recommended amoxicillin (20 mg/kg/day) or trimethoprim-sulfamethoxazole (4 mg/kg/day trimethoprim [TMP] to 20 mg/kg/day sulfamethoxazole [SMX]) for children under 5 years of age (Committee on Infectious Disease, 1997). As with other children taking antibiotics, the potential for monilial infections, gastrointestinal (GI) upset, and allergy exists.

The number of cases of penicillin-resistant invasive pneumococcal infections and the presence of nasopharyngeal carriage on penicillin prophylaxis may no longer be as effective at preventing invasive pneumococcal infections. The age at which prophylaxis should be discontinued is often an empirical decision (Committee on Infectious Disease, 1997). The report of the Prophylactic Penicillin Study II (Falletta et al, 1995) established guidelines for discontinuing prophylaxis at 5 years of age. These guidelines include the following: (1) children receiving regular medical attention, (2) those with no history of prior severe pneumococcal infection, and (3) those without surgical splenectomy. Parents must be counseled to always seek immediate medical assistance with all febrile episodes.

Splenic Sequestration

In this condition, blood flow into the spleen is adequate, but the vascular outflow system from the spleen to the systemic circulation is occluded. This occlusion results in a large collection of blood pooling in the spleen, causing significant enlargement. The systemic circulation may then be deprived of its needed blood volume, causing shock and cardiovascular collapse (Charache, Lubin, and Reid, 1995). The hemoglobin and hematocrit values fall rapidly. Children with Hgb SS are susceptible to this at an early age (i.e., at under 5 years). Those with other variants of the disease may continue to be at risk until their teenage years because they maintain splenic circulation longer than children with Hgb SS. Parents can be taught to palpate and measure their child's spleen using a simple measuring device such as a calibrated tongue blade (Figure 35-4). Knowledge of the child's steady state spleen size is essential in determining appropriate diagnosis and treatment during an acute event.

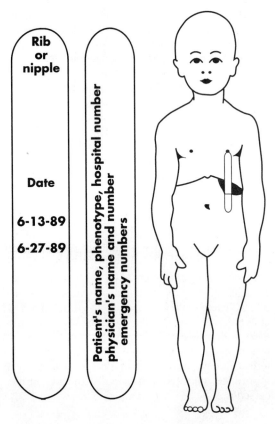

Figure 35-4 Measurement of spleen size with a spleen stick. (From Eckman JR and Platt AF: Problem oriented management of sickle syndromes, Atlanta, 1991, Georgia NIH Sickle Cell Center.)

Management of splenic sequestration necessitates hospitalization with immediate therapy, including transfusion. If shock is present, systemic circulation must be supported with fluids. Once adequate circulation is reestablished, however, the volume of fluid previously sequestered in the spleen is returned to the circulation, and circulatory overload must be avoided. For children who experience recurrent or severe episodes, splenectomy is indicated and curative (Charache, Lubin, and Reid, 1995). Splenectomy, however, places a child at increased risk for infection. It is optimal to splenectomize a child after the age of 2 years and after pneumococcal vaccine has been received. Children under 2 years of age who experience recurrent or severe episodes of splenic sequestration may be

given regular transfusions in an effort to suppress their body's production of Hgb S and prevent further episodes of sequestration until splenectomy can safely be performed. In contrast to the acute episodes, some children develop chronic massive splenomegaly. Splenectomy is indicated in these children when pressure or pain from the enlarged spleen is evident or accompanied by thrombocytopenia, neutropenia, or severe anemia (Charache, Lubin, and Reid, 1995).

Neurologic Problems

The vasculature of the brain is subject to vasoocclusive episodes in children with SCD; by age 14 years the incidence of stroke in children with SCD is 8%, but stroke may occur during infancy (Ferrera et al, 1997). The estimated age of the first cerebrovascular accident (CVA) differs significantly for children with SS and SC. The chances of a child with SS having a first stroke by age 20 years is estimated at 11%, but the estimated risk for a child with SC is 2% (Ohene-Frempong, 1998). Of note, the higher incidence of CVA in the 1- to 9-year age group—as opposed to the 10- to 19-year age group—suggests that a subset of children may have additional risk factors for stroke (Ohene-Frempong, 1998). When a blood vessel is partially occluded by a small embolus or vessel spasm, the manifestations may be focal and last less than 48 hours without residual deficit, which is classified as a transient ischemic attack. When the affected vessel is completely occluded by thrombus or embolus—with or without narrowing of the vessel lining—a CVA occurs. Intracranial hemorrhage is a rare but usually fatal complication that occurs when blood vessel walls are thinned by intravascular sickling and then dilate and rupture (Charache, Lubin, and Reid, 1995). Computerized tomography (CT) and magnetic resonance imaging (MRI) can both show infarcts and areas of hemorrhage. MRI can also show the patchy white matter abnormal signals that are present in individuals with SCD—both with and without neurologic deficits—and are thought to be due to disease in penetrating arterioles (Howlett et al, 1997).

At the time of stroke, most children are at a clinically steady state with no prodrome or symptom warning of any impending neurologic event. Of these children, however, 10% to 30% will experience seizures with stroke (French et al, 1997).

Acute treatment for CVA includes exchange transfusion, stabilization of cardiorespiratory function, and treatment of seizures if present (see Chapter 21). After the acute phase, a lengthy rehabilitation process may be needed. Some children have few or no deficits, but others are neurologically devastated. Strokes usually recur within 3 years if there has been no intervention for the sickle cell condition. Progressive neurologic deterioration occurs with each event.

It is hoped that widespread application of TCD (see the discussion of new therapies later in this chapter) will be effective in prevention because even with proven intervention (i.e., chronic transfusions), some parents and children may refuse this therapy for personal or religious reasons. Reports of recurrence of stroke and silent, undetected central nervous system (CNS) events after cessation of long-term (i.e., 5 to 12 years) transfusion therapy suggest that indefinite transfusions may be required and that—despite compliance with strict criteria—repeated CNS events may occur (Wang et al, 1991).

Vasoocclusive Crisis (VOC)

Painful, vasoocclusive episodes are the most common cause of emergency room visits and hospital admissions for individuals with SCD. Vasoocclusion is a physiologic process, but the resultant pain is a complex biopsychosocial event. Physiologic factors combined with social considerations (e.g., developmental stage, pain history, and family coping skills) contribute to the expression of vasoocclusion. Each child exhibits an individualized pattern of duration, frequency, severity, and location of vasoocclusive crises. The hallmark of these crises is their unpredictability. A few children state that they are always in pain, but approximately one third of children and adolescents rarely seek hospital-based treatment (Charache, Lubin, and Reid, 1995).

Precipitation of painful episodes in SCD has been related to numerous factors, including weather changes (i.e., warm to cold), stress, and menstrual cycles in females (Westerman, 1997). The frequency of painful episodes is indirectly related to the Hgb F level and numerous painful crises are a prognostic sign for further complications as a result of sickling (Embury et al, 1994).

VOCs typically affect the chest, abdomen, and long bones, although any area in the body or organ is subject to sickling episodes. In long bones, infarcts are most common in the shaft and are usually confined to the medulla (Howlett, 1997). Muscular infarcts occasionally occur with secondary hemorrhage and myonecrosis and are clearly seen on CT and MRI scans.

The optimal treatment for VOCs is multimodal and includes treating any antecedent causes, improving circulation, and providing analgesia. Treatment of antecedent causes includes correcting fever, hypoxia, and acidosis, as well as treating infection and dehydration. Primary care providers must be aware that an extraneous illness possibly precipitated a painful episode and the child has two independent problems.

Hydration is an important part of improving circulation to the affected area. Children may be hydrated orally or intravenously with an electrolyte solution. Options for oral hydration include juice, bouillon, water, milk, sports drinks, Pedialyte (Ross), or Infalyte (Mead-Johnson). Fluids given intravenously may include a normal saline bolus with care being taken not to tax the cardiovascular system with too large or rapid of a bolus. Maintenance fluids of 5% dextrose with 0.45% normal saline are then given to replace excess sodium lost in the urine as a result of renal dysfunction in individuals with SCD. Potassium is added as needed after urinary output is established. The rate of fluids given should be approximately 1.5 times the maintenance dosage, or 2500 ml/m^2 daily. Circulation to infarcted areas may also be improved by the local application of heat (e.g., heating pad, warm bath, or whirlpool). Once comfort has been established, passive range of motion and massage may be initiated. These children should be encouraged to be as active as possible.

Analgesia may take several forms, including nonpharmacologic agents, nonsteroidal antiinflammatory drugs (NSAIDs), or oral or parenteral narcotics. Multimodal therapy, which includes several of these approaches, is more effective than single agents because each agent increases analgesia. NSAIDs act on peripheral pain receptors, and narcotics act centrally. This combination therapy may also contravene the "ceiling effect" that occurs with opioids, as well as have a significant narcotic-sparing effect (Martin and Moore, 1997). There are multiple narcotic agents from which to choose, and each child, health care provider, and institution is likely to have a preference. Placebos are never appropriate because they erode the trusting relationship between the health care provider and child. The dose given should begin at a standard therapeutic dose or a dose known to be therapeutic for a given child and then adjusted as needed.

Many narcotics have very brief half-lives, and care must be taken to administer them often enough for analgesic effect. For example, when a medication with a 12-hour half-life is used, dosing should be approximately every 2 hours to maintain consistent pain relief. Early in the course of a vasoocclusive episode, the vascular occlusion is constant—not intermittent. Later in the course, collateral circulation may develop or the occlusion may have decreased, improving circulation to the infarcted area. Therefore early in the course of a painful episode, as needed (i.e., prn) dosing is inappropriate. It is preferable to control a child's pain early in the course of the illness and maintain control. Scheduled doses of narcotics should be given over the first 24 hours after admission for VOC (Charache, Lubin, and Reid, 1995).

It is inappropriate to administer intramuscular injections to children for pain relief because an injection alone can be quite painful unless it is for a single dose and a longer half-life is desired (e.g., for outpatient management) or IV access has not been obtained. Intrathecal catheters have been suggested as a route for analgesic administration for children who are hospitalized with severe, intractable pain (Yaster et al, 1994). This route provides the advantage of pain relief without excessive sedation. Patient-controlled analgesia (PCA) is also recommended if institutions are familiar with its use in children (Martin and Moore, 1997).

Because all pain episodes cannot be prevented, children and their families should be taught to manage mild pain and recognize symptoms that suggest serious problems. For mild pain, nonnarcotic medicines including acetaminophen, aspirin (provided there is no concurrent viral process or other contraindication), ibuprofen, and ketorolac are appropriate and may be given at the standard recommended doses. Caution should be exercised with the use of NSAIDs in children with renal or liver complications. Optimal management requires adequate education of the child, family, and health care providers. Nonpharmacologic forms of pain relief are useful adjuncts to pharmacologic therapy. Self-hypnosis, biofeedback, and distraction are particularly helpful (Charache, Lubin, and Reid, 1995).

When children become significantly uncomfortable, they experience anxiety and, consequently, a heightened perception of pain. They may ultimately develop dysfunctional illness behavior as a result of inadequately treated pain. It is important for the child, family, and health care providers to have realistically attainable goals related to pain control. The goal of pain management should be prompt pain relief. The alleviation of pain provided by narcotics must be balanced against known side effects such as pruritus, nausea, constipation, and respiratory depression.

Shapiro and Ballas (1994) cite several studies that document the low prevalence of drug addiction within this population. Despite these studies, health care providers continue to believe that drug addiction is a major problem among people with SCD, which is unfortunate because this misperception can interfere with the provision of adequate health care. The causes of this misperception are multiple, including—but not limited to—the rampant illicit drug problems in our society; cultural differences between the health care providers, who are often white, and clients, who are often black; and the desire of most individuals with chronic conditions to control some aspects of their treatment.

Pulmonary Complications

Acute chest syndrome (ACS) ranks second as a cause for hospitalization and is responsible for 25% of all deaths from SCD. ACS is most common in younger children (i.e., 2 to 4 years of age) and least frequent in adults (Castro et al, 1994). ACS is a life-threatening complication that results from occlusions in the pulmonary vasculature, resulting in areas of infarcted lung tissue. The occlusion is caused by localized sickling, thromboembolism, or embolism with collections of sickled cells, bone marrow, or marrow fat. The occlusion can also be induced by respiratory depression caused by narcotics. Special instructions for deep-breathing exercises before surgery can prevent certain episodes.

Acute chest pain, a nonproductive cough, leukocytosis, fever, and respiratory distress characterize ACS. Fever, cough, and tachypnea are often the only findings in children (Charache, Lubin, and Reid, 1995). ACS may be difficult to differentiate from, and actually may be concurrent with, pneumonia. Physical examination usually reveals tachypnea, but there may also be evidence of pulmonary consolidation, pleural effusion, a new pulmonary infiltrate, or pleural friction rub. Chest radiographic studies may be normal for the first few days, especially if a child is dehydrated. Lung scans may be useful but are often equivocal because a baseline study is rarely available for comparison.

ACS may be a fulminant process; admission to the intensive care unit may be necessary for close monitoring. Arterial blood gas (ABG) levels should be followed closely; supplemental oxygen and further respiratory support should be provided as needed. Early transfusion may be necessary to prevent progressive problems because hypoxia will induce further sickling; partial or complete exchange transfusion may be needed (Charache, Lubin, and Reid, 1995).

One episode of ACS promotes another with progressive lung scarring and pulmonary hypertension (Castro et al, 1994). Because there are no clear clinical or laboratory parameters that differentiate vasoocclusive disease from pneumonia, primary care providers should empirically use antibiotics directed against *S. pneumonae* and *H. Influenzae,* and other pathogens commonly seen in community-acquired pneumonia (Charache, Lubin, and Reid, 1995).

Aplastic Crisis

Periodically the bone marrow does not respond to a fall in hemoglobin and hematocrit values caused by the rapid turnover of RBCs. The hemoglobin and hematocrit values drop, and there is a lack of compensatory rise in the reticulocyte count, which usually happens during or following a viral infection. Human parvovirus B19 has been implicated in most aplastic crises in this population (Charache, Lubin, and Reid, 1995). Children being cared for during a viral illness should be observed for unusual pallor or prolonged lethargy in the face of improvement of other viral symptoms. Therapy includes slow transfusion to a hemoglobin level slightly above the baseline hemoglobin level. Recovery is indicated by a return of reticulocytosis.

Hemolysis

Hemolysis in SCD is usually of only moderate severity. The symptoms of anemia (e.g., pallor, fatigue, dyspnea) are not the hallmarks of this disease. Hemolysis is generally noted by scleral icterus, tea-colored urine, and elevated bilirubin and urobilinogen levels. One long-term consequence of hemolysis is the high prevalence of gallstones. Increased hemolysis may be triggered by bacterial infections, poisons, or glucose 6-phosphate dehydrogenase (G6PD) deficiency. Hemolysis accompanied by a brisk reticulocytosis requires no treatment (Charache, Lubin, and Reid, 1995).

Renal Problems

The environment within the renal medulla is characterized by low oxygen tension, acidosis, and hypertonicity. Therefore intravascular sickling occurs more rapidly in the kidney than in any other organ (Wong et al, 1996). This leaves the kidney with a relative inability to concentrate urine (i.e., hyposthenuria) or adequately acidify urine, which is an early sign of end-stage renal disease. The relative inability to concentrate urine often leads to enuresis or nocturia and also results in a relative inability to excrete potassium and uric acid. Gross hematuria may occur in children with SCD or sickle trait. Blood loss is usually minimal, resolving within 1 to 3 days with bed rest and hydration and does not require transfusion (Wong et al, 1996). As with all individuals with gross hematuria, diagnoses of glomerulonephritis, tumor, renal stones, urinary tract infection, and bleeding disorders must be excluded. When other diagnoses have been eliminated, hematuria is often attributed to areas of ischemia or necrosis caused by sickled cells (Charache, Lubin, and Reid, 1995). Renal papillary necrosis, renal infarction, and perinephric hematoma (secondary to infarction) are all described. Progressive medullary and cortical infarction leads to the development of chronic renal failure, resulting in death of affected adults over age 40 years (Howlett et al, 1997).

Priapism

Males with sickle cell anemia are subject to episodes of priapism. Priapism occurs when an accumulation of sickled cells obstructs the venous drainage of the corpora cavernosa of the penis, causing a prolonged and exquisitely painful erection of the penis. Priapism is not associated with sexual desire or excitement. In addition, micturition is often difficult, and urinary retention may occur. MRI is useful in demonstrating corporal destruction with development of intracorporal fibrosis and hemosiderin deposition (Howlett, 1997).

Hakim and associates (1994) describe a history of at least one episode of priapism in 42% of males with sickle cell anemia, with a median age of onset of 21 years. Priapism may be seen in boys as young as 7 years. The following four general patterns of priapism are described:

1. Recurrent (i.e., "short stuttering") attacks lasting less than 3 hours several times a week for 4 weeks;
2. Acute (i.e., "major") attacks lasting less than 24 hours, followed by partial or complete impotence;
3. Chronic, persistent, usually painless enlargement or induration that persists weeks to years, which develops after a major episode and is associated with partial or complete impotence; and
4. Acute-on-chronic priapism, which is a chronic induration with a superimposed acute attack that may affect only part of the penile shaft.

Treatment of major episodes begins with conservative measures including hospitalization, hydration, transfusions, and pain management. Surgical intervention is considered if there is no detumescence after 12 to 24 hours of conservative treatment (Charache, Lubin, and Reid, 1995). Surgical measures aim to reestablish adequate venous outflow and circulation of the corporal body via aspiration and—if not successful—placement of a shunt. Prophylactic regimens include the addition of vasodilatory drugs including hydralazine and pentoxifylline, calcium channel blockers (e.g., verapamil), and 6-month transfusion programs, all of which have been clinically efficacious (Hakim, Hashmat, and Macchia, 1994). Despite intervention, impotence is a frequent complication of priapism.

Skeletal Changes

SCD involves both hematologic and osseous abnormalities because it affects the two major functions of bone tissue: hematopoiesis and osteogenesis. Skeletal changes as a result of expansion of the bone marrow and recurrent infarction are often seen in children with SCD. Symptoms of dactylitis

(i.e., hand-foot syndrome) include pain and swelling of the tarsals, metatarsals, carpals, and metacarpals and are often the first symptoms seen in severely affected infants. Because erythropoiesis is critical, the marrow within these small reservoirs is stimulated to produce red cells in these infants. The average age of onset is 9 months, and the risk extends to age 2 years. After this age, red cell production is shifted to the marrow within the long bones and axial skeleton. Dactylitis causes pain and requires frequent hospitalizations for IV administration of fluid. Infants in pain refuse to drink adequate fluids, so hospitalization is necessary to avoid acidosis. These crises do not cause permanent orthopedic problems but are frightening to parents. Back pain is common in older children and is recognized on radiographs by "fish-mouthed" vertebrae, which have decreased vertical height and increased width (Brinker et al, 1998).

Repeated infarction may lead to avascular necrosis. The pathophysiology of bone "erosions" in sickle cell anemia results from necrosis produced by repeated microinfarction (Rothchild et al, 1997). This pathophysiology most commonly involves the head of the femur but may also occur in the head of the humerus or fibula. Treatment initially includes avoidance of weight bearing on or bracing of the joint for up to 6 months. Judicious use of local heat and analgesics for pain relief may be employed. If pain persists along with radiographic progression, treatment consists of surgical core decompression of the femoral head. A newer technique, the injection of acrylic cement, has been used to restore the spherical shape of the femoral head. Both of these procedures are seen as temporary measures to forestall an eventual total hip replacement.

Ophthalmologic Changes

Ophthalmologic complications are a direct result of the vasoocclusive process within the eye. These complications include nonproliferative retinopathy, proliferative retinopathy, or elevated intraocular pressure in the presence of hyphema. Nonproliferative retinopathy may not affect visual acuity. Proliferative sickle retinopathy can cause vitreous hemorrhage and subsequent retinal detachment and blindness. The occurrence of proliferative sickle retinopathy depends on an individual's age and type of hemoglobinopathy, generally beginning in the second decade and progressing. Proliferative sickle retinopathy is more common in people with Hgb SC but also occurs with other forms of SCD. Individuals with sickle hemoglobinopathies who sustain blunt trauma and subsequent hyphema to the eye may quickly develop increased intraocular pressure, which is an ophthalmologic emergency (Charache, Lubin, and Reid, 1995).

Audiologic Problems

Vasoocclusive episodes within the circulation of the inner ear and the administration of ototoxic drugs may cause sensorineural hearing loss. This loss may be unilateral or bilateral but is generally manifested as a high-frequency deficit. Compared with age-matched controls, 22% of children with SCD (compared with 4% of controls) had predominantly high-frequency hearing loss (Adams, 1994). As expected with hearing loss, speech screening should be implemented. A study by Gentry and Dancer (1997) showed 10% of children with SCD as having either an articulation disorder or a fluency disorder. This finding shows a higher speech failure rate than expected.

Leg Ulcers

Leg ulcers are experienced by 25% to 75% of older children and adults with SCD but have also been reported in children as young as 10 years (Cackovic et al, 1998). These ulcers usually begin as a bite or scratch on the lower portion of the leg or the medial or lateral side of the ankle. These ulcers typically form a shallow depression with a smooth and slightly elevated margin and often have a surrounding area of edema. Bacteria are virtually always recovered from the base of an ulcer; although this may represent colonization of devitalized tissue, clinical observation suggests that infection contributes to enlargement and maintenance of ulcers. Ulcers can produce significant pain and limit movement. These ulcers may take 6 weeks to 6 months to heal, and—despite aggressive treatment—a reoccurrence rate of 75.4% in 2 years is reported (Cackovic et al, 1998). Early, prompt treatment includes bed rest, elevation, and wound care with antibiotics for cellulitic areas, but skin grafting and transfusion therapy may also be needed. The specific type of wound care is controversial and should be directed by a competent plastic surgeon.

Preparation for Anesthesia or Contrast Medium

General anesthesia and hyperosmolar contrast medium are both known to induce sickling. If an operative or diagnostic procedure using these agents is anticipated, most hematologists suggest that children with SCD receive transfusion to a hemoglobin of 10 g/dl, giving an Hgb S percentage of less than 40% (Halvorson et al, 1997). All children receiving tonsillectomies and adenoidectomies should be transfused. Additional measures such as warming the operating room, warming the IV fluids, or placing the child on a warming blanket during surgery are warranted. Aggressive hydration of 150% of maintenance fluids given 24 hours before surgery has been recommended (Halvorson et al, 1997).

Cardiac Problems

Over time the cardiovascular system accommodates to chronic anemia with increased cardiac output. This chronic volume overload causes cardiac enlargement. Although dilation and hypertrophy often occur, systolic and diastolic performance of the left ventricle in the resting state are usually preserved (Charache, Lubin, and Reid, 1995). Cardiac enlargement is often apparent on chest radiograph, and a low-grade systolic ejection murmur may be heard in the second and third left intercostal spaces. Cardiomegaly is an adaptation to anemia and alone should not be considered pathologic. Children with sickle cell anemia are subject to the same medical conditions as other children, therefore findings suggestive of congenital, rheumatic, or underlying heart disease should be investigated. In such cases, an echocardiogram and cardiac consultation are recommended. Several studies of children and adolescents document a physical work capacity of 60% to 70% of normal. Electrocardiogram depression in the ST segment occurs during exercise in 15% of children with SCD, suggesting endocardial ischemia (Covitz, 1994).

Hepatobiliary Problems

The ongoing elevated rate of RBC hemolysis generates an increase in serum bilirubin. Likewise, elevations of the serum alkaline phosphatase and lactic dehydrogenase levels as a result of bone metabolism and hemolysis are often seen. Gallstones of bile or calcium bilirubinate are a common finding and easily seen via ultrasound. These gallstones are found in 14% to 30% of children with SCD and are most common in individuals with Hgb SS (Charache, Lubin, and Reid, 1995).

Surgeons should be aware of the finding that concomitant common bile duct (CBD) stones have been reported in individuals with SCD and cholelithiasis. Both laproscopic and open cholecystectomies are approved for individuals with SCD.

A hepatic crisis may be indistinguishable from acute cholecystitis (Chuang et al, 1997). RBC sequestration in the liver causes hepatocellular dysfunction, which decreases bilirubin excretion. Children who have right upper quadrant pain, increased jaundice, and fever need careful evaluation and management. Crisis pain involving the liver is often indistinguishable from acute cholecystitis (Box 35-4). Transfused children are at risk for viral hepatitis and hepatic hemosiderosis, which can result in hepatic injury and fibrosis. Hepatic failure resulting from massive sickling has been reported.

Transfusion Complications

Individuals with SCD may need transfusions emergently, episodically, or chronically. Performing RBC phenotyping before transfusion avoids the problems associated with the development of RBC antibodies. Therefore children requiring RBC transfusions may be administered phenotypically matched units (Vichinsky, 1994). Several centers have been successful in recruiting minority donors for extended matching for RBC antigens. This matching has markedly decreased the occurrence

of alloimmunization and should be the standard for children needing chronic transfusions. The complications of transfusions include possible exposure to blood-borne infectious agents, formation of alloantibodies, and (with chronic or multiple transfusion) iron overload. Individuals with iron overload experience progressive organ dysfunction, leading to iron induced cardiac damage and death. Iron chelation with subcutaneous or intravenous deferoxamine is a difficult but essential treatment. An efficient, easily administered oral chelating agent does not currently exist.

Prognosis

In a classic study done 20 years ago, a group of adults and children was longitudinally followed to determine the natural history of SCD. The disease effects in the adults tended to be chronic and organ related and the problems in the children were acute and often infectious. Overall, there was a 10% expected death rate during the first decade of life and 5% or less during any subsequent decade (Powars, 1975).

It is now known that 20% of all children with Hgb SS will develop the severe form of the disease, which is characterized by frequent pain crises and ultimate end-organ damage; 40% will display moderate symptomatology; and the rest will have a more indolent course. This striking variability between genotypes provides another example of the variable presentation of symptoms and complications that must be considered by the primary care provider. All children with a given genotype (i.e., SS) will not present with either the same symptoms or frequency. Sickle thalassemia is reported to have lower rates of complications and mortality in children who inherit this genetic variant. The β-globin gene cluster haplotypes reported by Powers and associates (1994) further modulate the severity of the disorder.

This information on genotypes assumes urgency in prenatal diagnosis and in making decisions about potentially life-threatening procedures (e.g., BMT) (Serjeant, 1995). In the former case, the decision to continue a pregnancy can rest on the perceived future clinical course of a child. Factors determining the extremely variable clinical course include the following: (1) genetic factors (e.g., α thalassemia, β-globin gene haplotypes, heterocel-

---

Box 35-4

Common Sources of Abdominal Pain in Sickle Cell Anemia

- Gallstones
- Hepatitis
- Biliary sludge
- Small bowel necrosis
- Pancreatic sickling
- Cirrhosis of various causes
- Intrahepatic cholestasis

lular hereditary persistence of Hgb F, and high total hemoglobin) and (2) adherence to suggested clinical guidelines (e.g., penicillin prophylaxis, pneumococcal vaccinations, adequate hydration, and early recognition of life-threatening complications).

Because of penicillin prophylaxis, the mortality rate for children with SCD in the first decade of life has decreased from 10% to 1% (Charache, Lubin, and Reid, 1995). Davis and associates (1997) report that the survival of children with SCD has markedly improved since 1968, but that a substantial number of deaths continue to occur outside the hospital. This finding raises concerns about whether care for acute illness is promptly sought and readily accessible. Compliance with prophylactic recommendations is critical in early years. As early intervention decreases or eliminates deaths from sepsis, ACS, and splenic sequestration, the primary issue will be chronic organ damage—notably renal, neurologic, and pulmonary changes (Davis, 1997).

PRIMARY CARE MANAGEMENT

Health Care Maintenance

Growth and Development

When matched with controls of similar socioeconomic status, children with SCD have comparable physical parameters at birth, including weight, length, and head circumference, as well as similar 1- and 5-minute Apgar scores. Classic studies (Modege and Ifenu, 1993) show that—starting at approximately 6 months of age and being clearly defined by the preschool years—these children demonstrate a pattern of physical growth that is divergent from that of their unaffected peers. That is, these children are shorter, weigh less, and have a smaller percentage of body fat and delayed bone age. Their muscle mass and head circumference, however, are comparable with that of their unaffected peers. Weight is affected more than height, and males are affected more than females.

These changes are coincident with the usual physiologic waning of Hgb F levels. It has also been noted that the growth of children who, for unknown reasons, persist in producing Hgb F is usually not as retarded as that of other children with SCD. Children receiving chronic transfusions, however, show significant growth, which suggests that hemolytic anemia plays a major role in the growth retardation in children with sickle cell anemia. Wang and associates (1993), as part of the CSSCD, concluded that development of children with sickle cell anemia is relatively normal before age 3 years, and that deficits seen in older children may reflect subsequent ischemic events.

As with standard well-child care, physical growth parameters should be measured and plotted on standardized growth charts every 3 to 4 months (Committee on Genetics, 1996). The pattern of growth of an individual child, however, is more important than comparison with unaffected children.

Psychosocial researchers have studied the learning abilities, coping skills, anxieties, and self-concepts of unaffected children and those with SCD. Most studies conclude that children with SCD are well-adjusted but vulnerable to experiencing psychosocial stresses because of the chronicity of their condition. A study comparing the rates of mental illness in children and adolescents with SCD with those of a corresponding control group noted no difference in the risk for clinically significant mental disorders (Cepeda et al, 1997). These findings have been supported by others (Lee et al, 1997).

Beyond the expected significant psychosocial and intellectual deficits experienced by children with a history of stroke, researchers are now focusing on the incidence of subclinical deficits resulting from cerebral microvascular occlusion that are not apparent on routine neurologic examinations. DeBaun and associates (1998) have explored various neurocognitive tests in order to define instruments sensitive and specific for identifying children with silent cerebral infarcts. Selected test results thus far indicate impairment with fine and visual motor tasks, as well as with short-term memory skills.

Standardized tools such as the Denver Developmental Screening Test II are helpful when screening for developmental delay. Children found to be at developmental risk, however, should be referred for a more thorough developmental assessment. The involvement of a consistent caregiver and the caregiver's rapport with a consistent health care provider are invaluable tools for monitoring developmental progress in children with SCD.

Diet

A child's diet should be well-balanced with a generous amount of fluid. Diet during illness or disease exacerbation may include whatever nutritive dense solid foods children desire with oral fluids at one and a half times their usual fluid intake. Maintenance of daily fluid intake is essential in maintaining homeostasis in children with SCD. A fluid sheet, outlining times to increase fluids and amounts of oral fluids to be given, provides a handy reference to parents (Box 35-5).

Because of increased metabolic demands, children with SCD have a relative deficiency of energy, protein, and several micronutrients, so the recommended daily allowances for the normal population may not be applicable (Prasad, 1997). Limited metabolic studies support the hypothesis that chronic hemolysis leads to a state of high protein turnover and increased metabolic requirements. One controlled study measuring energy expenditure in postpubertal males cited reduced physical activity as the compensatory mechanism for low energy intake that is inadequate to meet their higher metabolic demands, which led to a suboptimal nutritional state. Although reduced physical activity may allow the energy balance to be maintained short-term, a persistent energy deficit leads to growth retardation (Singhal et al, 1997).

Folic acid therapy is recommended (Ballas and Saidi, 1997). Usual doses are 0.1 mg/d for children up to 6 months of age; 0.25 mg/d for those between 6 and 12 months of age; 0.5 mg/d for those 1 to 2 years of age; and 1 mg/d for those over 2 years (AAP, 1997). Supplemental iron therapy should not be prescribed unless a child is documented to have reduced iron stores as measured by serum iron, serum ferritin, and iron binding capacity (Charache, Lubin, and Reid, 1995).

Safety

Most children with sickle cell anemia regularly take oral medicines (e.g., folic acid, antibiotics, and narcotics) at home. Ingestion of narcotics beyond the prescribed amount could lead to lethargy and respiratory depression or death. All medicines should be safely stored. Adolescents should be cautioned about driving a car or using machinery while taking narcotics and that substances such as alcohol may potentiate the depressant effects of narcotics. Alcohol should also be avoided because it can cause dehydration and subsequent sickling. Smoking is strongly discouraged because it leads to vasoconstriction and concomitant problems.

Recreational activities that involve prolonged exposure to cold, prolonged exertion, or exposure to high altitudes (i.e., >10,000 feet) in an unpressurized aircraft should be avoided. Sports injuries should not be treated with ice because this can cause localized sickling.

Adolescents with SCD often demonstrate the same limit-testing and risk-taking behaviors as their unaffected peers. Parents must balance their child's need for safety with their child's need to become self-sufficient. An information card or Medic-Alert bracelet is often helpful in emergency situations.

Box 35-5

Children's Center for Cancer and Blood Disorders Sickle Cell Fluid Requirements

A child needs more fluids when:

1. He or she has a *fever*.
2. He or she has *pain*.
3. It's hot *outside*.
4. He or she is very *active*.
5. He or she is *traveling*.

Amount of clear fluids a child needs each day during special times:

Child's weight	Number of 8 oz cups per day
10 lb	2 cups
15 lb	3 cups
20 lb	4 cups
25 lb	5 cups
30 lb	5 to 6 cups
35 lb	6 to 7 cups
40 lb	7 cups
50 lb	8 cups
60 lb	9 cups
Over 60 lb	10 or more cups

Adapted from Earles A et al: A parent's handbook for sickle cell disease (birth to 6 Years), Vienna, Va., 1991, National Maternal and Child Health Clearinghouse.

Immunizations

The conventional schedule may be used for diphtheria-pertussis-tetanus (DaPT) vaccine, inactivated poliomyelitis vaccine (IPV), measles-mumps-rubella (MMR) vaccine, varicella vaccine, and Hepatitis B and Hib vaccines.

The pneumococcal vaccine (Pneumovax) should be given to all children with SCD at 2 years of age. Re-vaccination after 3 to 5 years is recommended for children 10 years of age or younger American Academy of Pediatrics [AAP], 1997), usually when penicillin prophylaxis is discontinued. Only one booster is recommended. It is important to emphasize that even with vigilant immunization and antibiotic prophylaxis, episodes of pneumococcal septicemia have occurred (Vichinsky, 1991). Currently licensed pneumococcal oligo-polysaccharide vaccines are not immunogenic in young children and do not elicit booster responses (Vernocchi et al, 1998). Pneumovax may be given concurrently with the DaPT, IPV, MMR, influenza, and hepatitis B and Hib vaccines. Children with hemoglobinopathies are identified as being at risk for influenza-related complications. Children with SCD are also known to be at high risk for bacterial infection, which could occur associated with concurrent viral infection. Therefore it is recommended that all children with SCD receive influenza vaccine on an annual basis (Committee on Genetics, 1996). Opinions on the use of meningococcal vaccine are divergent. Some centers suggest administering the vaccine to children over 2 years of age, but this is not uniform among all comprehensive care centers. The AAP (Committee on Genetics, 1996) recommends the meningococcal vaccine for all individuals with asplenia.

Screening

Vision: During their first decade of life, children with SCD require routine screening. Thereafter, they need an annual retinal examination by an ophthalmologist to screen for sickle retinopathy and possible intervention. If a child sustains any eye trauma, referral to an ophthalmologist for evaluation of increased intraocular pressure or retinal detachment is necessary.

Hearing: Routine audiologic evaluations are recommended to screen for hearing loss related to vasoocclusion or hyperviscosity in the inner ear.

Sensorineural hearing loss has been well described in this population (Adams, 1994).

Dental: Routine screening is recommended.

Blood pressure: Blood pressure should be measured every year after 2 years of age. Although common in blacks living in the United States, hypertension is uncommon in individuals with SCD. The reason for this is unclear. Most individuals have blood pressures lower than those of their unaffected peers, with differences increasing with age. The risk for occlusive stroke increases with rises in systolic—but not diastolic—pressure. Children with high blood pressure values relative to this population (e.g., 140/90) should be evaluated and considered for treatment (Pegelow, 1997).

Hematocrit: Routine hematocrit testing is deferred because CBC and reticulocyte counts are required every 6 to 12 months (every 6 months for SS and Sβ° thalassemia, and every 12 months for SC and Sβ+ thalassemia).

Urinalysis: Routine urinalysis is deferred because of annual renal function testing.

Tuberculosis: Routine screening is recommended.

Condition-Specific Screening

Hematologic screening: A CBC count with differential, RBC smear, and reticulocyte count is useful in establishing baseline data and ascertaining bone marrow function. Determining the RBC phenotype and alloantibodies of a well child who has not had a transfusion can possibly expedite any future transfusions. Repeat quantitative hemoglobin electrophoresis testing at age 5 to 7 years records nadir levels of Hgb F (Rodgers, 1994). Some comprehensive sickle cell centers test children during this time to correlate Hgb F levels with clinical severity.

Renal function testing: A urinalysis should be done and blood urea nitrogen (BUN) and creatinine levels checked annually after 3 years of age to monitor renal function. An inability to concentrate or acidify urine may be evident in the urinalysis and is commonly seen in children with SCD. Urobilinogen, as a by-product of bilirubin metabolism, is also a frequent finding. Hematuria may be a manifestation of renal dysfunction secondary to SCD or other unrelated pathologic conditions. These children should be referred to a nephrologist for further evaluation and treatment if the hematuria is severe or casts are present in the urine. Proteinuria is the most common clinical manifestation of glomerular injury to the kidney (Wong et al, 1996). Follow-up requires a urine culture and sensitivity, and—if negative—a 24-hour collection of urine for protein quantitation. An elevation requires referral to a nephrologist.

Lead poisoning: Determining erythrocyte protoporphyrin (EP) levels to screen children who may be at high risk for lead intoxication is not valid for children with SCD. Total EP levels may be elevated with iron deficiency, lead intoxication, or reticulocytosis. In a child with SCD, an elevated EP level may reflect the process of accelerated reticulocytosis rather than lead intoxication. Rajkumar and associates (1995) concluded that FEP levels are elevated in children with SCD even in the absence of iron deficiency or lead poisoning. Furthermore, children with Hgb SS have significantly higher FEP levels when compared with children with Hgb SC, suggesting that higher rates of hemolysis may contribute to higher levels of FEP.

Scoliosis: Scoliosis screenings should be done through late adolescence because of the delayed growth spurts of children with SCD.

Cardiac function: Electrocardiography (ECG) and echocardiography (ECHO) should be performed every 1 to 2 years after age 5 to evaluate the impact of chronic anemia on ventricular function. Efforts should be made to establish whether symptoms of chest pain, dyspnea, or decreased exercise tolerance have occurred, and significant symptoms should be evaluated with exercise testing (Covitz, 1994).

Liver function: Yearly liver function studies are helpful to evaluate RBC metabolism and liver function. Bilirubin is often elevated as a consequence of hemolysis, as well as liver disease. Bilirubin levels rise gradually until the third decade of life. Alkaline phosphatase levels fall after periods of most rapid growth in adolescence and reach lower levels in females than in males (Steinburg and Mohandas, 1994).

Common Illness Management

Differential Diagnosis (Box 35-6)

Fever: As a result of functional asplenia, bacterial infection is a significant cause of morbidity and mortality in children with SCD. The incidence of

bacteremia in children with SCD is highest among those under 2 years of age and declines from age 2 to 6 years. The most common pathogen in children under 6 years of age is *Streptococcus pneumoniae.* Antibiotic resistance to *S. pneumoniae* has been reported (Committee on Infectious Disease, 1997). Some children with SCD have cultured *S. pneumoniae* from the tonsillar beds despite appropriate doses of prophylactic penicillin. Therefore caregivers must be alert to these exceptions and closely monitor antibiotic effectiveness and compliance with penicillin prophylaxis. The course of *S. pneumoniae* sepsis is often fulminant, with mortality reaching 24% to 50%. *Escherichia coli* bacteremia is often associated with urinary tract infection and *Salmonella* sp. bacteremia with osteomyelitis (Buchanan, 1994). Capillary blockage by sickle cells causes gut infarction, which—combined with defective function of the liver and spleen—allows for invasion by *Salmonella* sp. This invasion com-

---

Box 35-6

Criteria for In-Patient Management

- "Seriously ill appearance"
- Hypotension
- Severe abdominal pain
- Poor perfusion
- Temperature >40° C
- Hemoglobin <5 g/dl
- Leukocyte count >30,000/mm^3 or <5000/mm^3
- Platelet count <100,000/mm
- Pain crisis that is unrelieved in 48 hours with home pain remedies
- Dehydration by examination or history
- Pulmonary infiltrate
- Prior history of sepsis
- No telephone or immediate access to the hospital
- Poor or no track record with previous prescriptions or appointments
- No prior training on monitoring for early signs of complications

Adapted from Platt OS: The febrile child with sickle cell disease: a pediatricians' quandary, J Pediatr 130:693-694, 1997.

bined with expanded bone marrow and poor blood flow provides an ischemic focus for *Salmonella* sp. localization (Howlett, 1997).

Fever is a common finding during vasoocclusive episodes, as well as during infectious episodes. There is no test or diagnostic tool to differentiate fever of an infectious origin from fever that results from inflammation secondary to infarction. Primary care providers must be aware of the fact that children may have two independent problems (e.g., infection and vasoocclusion), both of which require aggressive treatment and management.

A child under 5 years of age who has a low-grade temperature elevation (i.e., 38.5° C) may be given appropriate antibiotic coverage and treated as an outpatient, provided that a probable cause of temperature elevation can be identified and the child is stable and looks well clinically. There should be careful follow-ups at clinic visits in 24 and 48 hours.

Current treatment consists of prompt assessment of the child, followed by blood and urine cultures and administration of ceftriaxone. Ceftriaxone has a half-life of 6 hours, and effective bactericidal levels persist for 24 hours after a single dose (Buchanan, 1994). Children who appear toxic, have an extremely high fever and/or an unreliable caretaker, or to whom close outpatient follow-up is not possible should be hospitalized (Wilimas et al, 1993).

Fever is usually high with septicemia, but in 20% of the cases studied, the fever was less than 39° C (Buchanan, 1994). All children with SCD should be considered at risk for fatal sepsis regardless of whether they are on penicillin prophylaxis and have received pneumococcal vaccination.

An aggressive search for the cause of the fever should include a CBC count, blood culture, urinalysis, urine culture, chest radiograph, and possibly sinus radiographs. Lumbar puncture should be performed if meningitis is suspected. Clinicians are increasingly aware of the development of penicillin-resistant organisms, which contribute to the difficulty of treating the child with a fever. Bacterial meningitis, suspected or proven to be caused by *S. pneumoniae,* should be treated with combination therapy of vancomycin and cefotaxime or ceftriaxone on all children at least 1 month of age. Based on culture and sensitivity results, penicillin or ceftriaxone should be continued and vancomycin discontinued if not needed. Rifampin is used if found to be sensitive to the offending organism (Committee on Infectious Disease, 1997).

In children over 5 years of age with temperatures above 38.5° C, an aggressive search for the likely cause should be undertaken and antibiotics administered. The location of treatment (i.e., inpatient or outpatient) should depend on the child's clinical condition, anticipated compliance with therapy, and ability to obtain follow-up over the upcoming 24 to 72 hours (Charache, Lubin, and Reid, 1995).

Even common infections such as otitis media or sinusitis may precipitate a vasoocclusive crisis if fluid intake is reduced and dehydration and acidosis result. During periods of illness, a child must be assessed frequently for early signs of crisis. Maintaining fluid intake and controlling fever are critical.

Urinary tract infections: Asymptomatic bacteriuria, symptomatic urinary tract infection, and pyelonephritis occur much more commonly in individuals with SCD than in the general population. A child with a urinary tract infection or pyelonephritis should have a blood culture obtained because bacteremia is present in at least 50% of those with a urinary tract infection. Appropriate antibiotic therapy should be instituted and adequate follow-up—including a repeat culture—arranged. Further diagnostic studies (e.g., renal ultrasound or voiding cystourethrogram) should be done to exclude treatable conditions in children with pyelonephritis or recurrent urinary tract infection.

Orthopedic symptoms: Areas of bone infarction may be easily confused with osteomyelitis or rheumatologic disorders. Even after the diagnosis of SCD is made, it is important to differentiate areas of infarction from areas of infection because children with SCD have an increased incidence of osteomyelitis. With both pathologic processes, a child may have an elevated white blood cell count, fever, and equivocal radiographic findings. Osteomyelitis, however, is more often associated with an increased number of immature granulocytes, bacteremia, and a purulent joint aspirate. Bone scans may be useful in differentiating osteomyelitis from areas of bone infarction. Bone marrow scans have also been used to further discriminate areas of infection from those of infarction, especially when a bone scan is equivocal. Opinions on the use of bone marrow scans are somewhat divergent, however, and largely depend on the level of expertise available at a given facility.

Acute gastroenteritis: Vomiting and diarrhea must be carefully evaluated and managed in children with SCD because these children lack the ability to concentrate urine to compensate for decreased fluid intake or excess losses. Significant dehydration may quickly occur and lead to metabolic acidosis and sickling. If a child's oral fluid intake is less than that needed to maintain hydration, the child must receive IV hydration, often as an inpatient.

Abdominal pain: Episodes of infarction of the abdominal organs (e.g., the liver, spleen, and abdominal lymph nodes) occur and may be quite painful. These abdominal crises should be differentiated from problems that would require surgical intervention (e.g., appendicitis).

Abdominal pain and cramps found commonly in young children are possibly related to mesenteric ischemia (Scott-Conner and Brunson, 1994). Normal bowel sounds and lack of ileus support nonoperative management with adequate pain control. The duration may last days to weeks, with fluctuations in the severity of the pain.

Achord (1994) states that paralytic ileus is common during acute abdominal pain, making the diagnosis problematic. Right upper quadrant pain creates further complications because intrahepatic sickling mimics cholecystitis (Scott-Conner and Brunson, 1994). Neither ultrasound nor laboratory values aid in defining the process. Leukocytosis of 30,000 can be seen with both infarction and infection. Most children find that their sickle cell pain has a unique quality or character and they can often report whether their pain is typical of vasoocclusive pain. Deviation from a characteristic pattern (i.e., lower abdominal pain with persistent local tenderness) with symptoms lasting several hours suggests a surgical problem (Scott-Conner and Brunson, 1994).

Anemia: Virtually all children with SCD are anemic at baseline. A child with SCD may periodically have acute lethargy and pallor. CBC and reticulocyte counts should be obtained. If these reveal a significant drop in the hemoglobin and hematocrit levels, a child is probably experiencing an aplastic crisis or splenic sequestration. A fall in the hemoglobin and hematocrit values is usually a stimulus to the bone marrow, which then produces new RBCs in the form of reticulocytes. If the reticulocyte count is low in the presence of low hemo-

globin and hematocrit levels, a child is experiencing an aplastic crisis (Charache, Lubin, and Reid, 1995). If a child has an enlarged spleen, pallor, lethargy, and an associated drop in hemoglobin, he or she is likely to be experiencing splenic sequestration. Regardless of exact diagnosis, the child will require immediate hospitalization with close observation and transfusion.

Respiratory distress: Increased respiratory rate and effort, chest pain, fever, rales, and dullness to percussion may indicate pneumonia or ACS. Infiltrates on chest radiograph may reflect either process. With ACS the chest radiograph may be clear in the first few days, but a pleural effusion is often seen. These children should receive antibiotics, hydration, analgesics, and oxygen as needed. Transfusion or partial exchange transfusion may be indicated, depending on the degree of respiratory distress. ACS is a medical emergency and necessitates hospitalization.

Neurologic changes: A child who has a seizure, hemiparesis, blurry or double vision, or changes in speech, gait, or level of consciousness should have expedient neurologic and radiologic evaluation for the presence of stroke. These neurologic changes are a medical emergency and require exchange transfusion as soon as possible.

Drug Interactions

Antihistamines and barbiturates given concurrently with narcotics may cause respiratory depression, hypoxia, and further sickling. Diuretics and some bronchodilators, which have a diuretic effect, may cause dehydration and sickling and should be used with caution in children with SCD. Children receiving narcotics for pain control should be given stool softeners and cautioned about the use of alcohol or other sedatives.

Developmental Issues

Sleep Patterns

Because of chronic anemia, some children with SCD may fatigue more easily than their unaffected peers and may desire extra sleep. Parents often report that their child with SCD naps after coming home from school—a routine that can be encouraged.

Toileting

Toilet training should be initiated using the conventional guidelines to assess readiness for training. Bowel training usually progresses without difficulty. Bladder training, however, must take into account the fact that many children with SCD have difficulty concentrating urine and thus produce a large volume of dilute urine. These children may need to be given the opportunity to go to the toilet every 2 to 3 hours during the day. Primary enuresis often occurs in young children and commonly continues into the teenage years. It is especially troublesome when a child requires extra fluids during a vasoocclusive episode. Some children who previously achieve nighttime continence may develop secondary enuresis as subtle insults to the kidney occur. A pattern of enuresis typically emerges as a child begins having more "wet" than "dry" nights. This pattern may reflect the gradual loss of the kidneys' ability to concentrate urine. Daytime continence is unaffected by these renal changes.

Routine counseling regarding enuresis should be offered. Young children may initially use diapers. By the time a child reaches preschool or school age, however, the use of diapers often adversely affects the child's self-esteem and sense of mastery. Many families choose to wake the child once or twice during the night to urinate, but severe restriction of fluids is not wise because hydration needs must be met. Avoidance of caffeine ingestion during the evening hours may help prevent enuresis. Careful questioning by the primary care provider may point to a subclinical infectious process that can be treated.

Discipline

Expectations for the behavior of children with SCD should vary little from those held for their unaffected siblings or peers. These expectations should be as clear and consistent as possible. Likewise, parents should strive to make discipline fair and consistent. Many parents are fearful of disciplining or setting limits for their child with SCD, especially because emotional stress is thought to possibly precipitate a vasoocclusive crisis. Primary care providers can point out to parents that a lack of or inconsistency in setting limits may be more stressful to a child than consistently set limits. Parents should also be encouraged to note which behaviors their child consistently demonstrates when in pain, (e.g., a certain pitch to his or her cry, a change in activity level, or changes in appetite) to help them discriminate episodes of pain from other behavior.

Child Care

Children with SCD can participate in normal daycare centers, although small group or home-centered daycare may be preferable because it provides less exposure to infections. Caregivers must be informed of a child's need for extra fluids and frequent need to void. They may also need to administer medications during daycare hours and must be instructed in this regard. Caregivers must be able to contact a parent or quickly seek medical care for the child in the event of fever, painful vasoocclusive crisis, respiratory distress, or symptoms of stroke, all of which may be life-threatening. Children attending daycare centers are at higher risk for acquiring community-based resistant infections (Armitage et al, 1999), so health care workers must take this into consideration when prescribing antibiotic coverage.

Schooling

Parents are encouraged to meet with school officials before the beginning of each school year to allow them to communicate about the usual symptoms their child has relative to SCD. It further allows for a plan to be developed for absences, make-up work, intermittent home-bound study (if necessary), and transfer of assignments from school to the home.

Many primary care providers play an active role in educating school officials about the needs of children with SCD. Some visit schools and give presentations, and others provide written materials (see the list of resources at the end of this chapter). The needs for adequate hydration, frequent bathroom breaks, rest, physical education, and appropriate dress are all subjects for discussion by the health care team. School officials, in turn, can provide information about learning abilities and behavior. This open exchange of information helps to ensure a successful school year for the student. Knowing whom to call when parents cannot be reached reduces anxiety on the part of school staff (Earles and Dorn, 1994).

Existing studies examining the effect of the disease on academic performance are insufficient (Richard and Burlew, 1997). Children with SCD who have had strokes should be referred for an individualized education program (IEP) (see Chapter 5). Children with splenomegaly should be cautioned about the risks for injury with contact sports. Modified physical education classes should be offered to keep these childen engaged in group activities, which are important to their overall adjustment and well-being. Finally, school personnel should be counseled about the needs of children affected with chronic orthopedic problems (e.g., osteomyelitis or avascular necrosis of the femoral head). These children may need additional time to get to classes, or may need to obtain an elevator key during times of bone healing.

Sexuality

Children with SCD progress through the Tanner stages in an orderly and consistent manner but usually experience puberty several years later than their unaffected peers, which can have significant adverse effects on their self-concepts. Once sexual maturation has occurred, fertility and contraception are important issues that must be addressed by primary care providers. For men, impotence is often a problem after a major episode of priapism. For female adolescents, menarche is often delayed by 2 to 2 and a half years, but fertility is normal. Decisions about contraception must take into account the attitudes, lifestyle, and maturity of the adolescent, as well as the hematologic ramifications of the method chosen.

Various contraceptive choices are available to adolescents with SCD, including all barrier forms of contraception (e.g., condoms for men, and foam and diaphragms for women). Women may also use oral contraceptives, preferably those brands containing low levels of estrogen.

Progesterone-only pills are useful because progestins stabilize the red cell membrane. Medroxyprogesterone (Depo-Provera) has also been used in this population (American College of Obstetricians and Gynecologists, 1995; Hatcher, 1994).

Adolescents with SCD should receive careful, repeated genetic counseling before puberty and during adolescence. They need to understand the pattern of transmission of SCD and the availability of testing for partners before conceiving a child.

Transition to Adulthood

Early vocational counseling should be offered to children and adolescents with SCD. Consideration should be directed toward the child or adolescent's interests and intellectual abilities. Work in a climate-controlled environment is preferred over rigorous, outdoor work, which might trigger a crisis. SCD excludes a person from military service, so technical and academic training is encouraged. Many community-based sickle cell organizations offer scholarships for skilled and academic work. The Sickle Cell Disease Association of America, Inc. can direct families to local resources.

Families should be counseled about the progressive organ damage that develops as a child ages. Continuity of care by a knowledgeable primary care provider will afford the best quality of life and should be encouraged.

Insurance companies may deem individuals with SCD uninsurable, and these individuals may face waiting periods for health insurance. Local Sickle Cell Disease Foundation chapters can provide counseling to such persons about options and resources.

Special Family Concerns and Resources

The families of children with SCD experience the same psychologic ramifications as other families of children with chronic conditions, often in the context of limited resources. These families bear the additional burden of knowing that this disease is genetically transmitted. This knowledge can prompt feelings of overwhelming guilt and responsibility. Exacerbations of the condition often occur without provocation, prompting feelings of helplessness. Many manifestations of the condition are not objectively visible or measurable, therefore children with SCD can appear to be well when they are potentially extremely ill. Many parents are fearful that the therapeutic effects of narcotics and blood transfusions will be outweighed by their potentially deleterious effects. Genetic counseling should be offered to the parents of a child with SCD at the time of the child's diagnosis and when subsequent pregnancies are contemplated. The child's siblings are probably screened at birth to determine their carrier status. Beyond the native black population, permeations of sickle hemoglobinopathies are found in Hispanics, Central Americans, Greeks, Arabs, Asians, and Caribbean natives. Each of these individuals brings his or her own view of health, coping, and wellness. Primary care providers must be mindful of the differences within and between cultures. Emphasis should focus on the different strengths families bring with them. For example, extended family support is a dominant feature in the black community and should play a role during crisis episodes.

Rao and Kramer (1993) show that black families prefer to use their family members as sources of support instead of using formal support groups. Among many blacks, close friends are considered kin and fulfill some functions of extended family members. When working with black families, primary care providers need to explore and understand the effects of ethnicity on the family's daily life. Such understanding seeks out cultural practices (e.g., male and female roles and African-American language, communication styles, and family rituals) (Sterling et al, 1997). Instructions should be delivered to the head of the household. In contrast to the matriarchal leadership found in many black households, Muslim families center their decision-making on the father or male head of the household. Strong church affiliations are often in place and offer consolation and hope leading to greater acceptance and improved quality of life.

Individuals espousing the Jehovah's Witness religion will deny blood transfusions to their children, placing stress on the primary care provider. Sensitive, open communication and vigilant intensive care management may prevent the need for transfusions and thereby support the religious beliefs of the family. In all instances, members of a particular ethnic or minority group should be consulted when actions or choices conflict with those of the medical care team.

Resources

Note that these listings are not all inclusive. Additional material may be available from your own state or local health department, sickle cell agency, or community agency.

A Parents' Handbook for Sickle Cell Disease, Part I: Birth to 6 Years and *Part II: 6 to 18 years.*
Koneksyon Familial: Tras Selil Falsiform

(Family Connection: Sickle Cell Trait) [in Haitian Creole]
Available from National Maternal and Child Health Clearinghouse
8201 Greensboro Dr.
McLean, Va. 22102
(703) 821-8955
www.circsol.com/mch

Sickle Cell Disease—How to Help Your Child to Take It in Stride
A Parent/Teacher Guide
Viewpoints
All available from the National Association for Sickle Cell Disease, Inc
200 Corporate Pointe, Suite 495
Culver City, Calif. 90230-7633
(800) 421-8453
www.sicklecelldisease.org
Also available from this organization are brochures on recent advances; a newsletter on chapter activities; fact sheets; brochures on sickle cell trait, anemia, and other topics; home study kits; games; and a video on parenting.

Thalassemia Information Sheet
Sickle Cell Anemia Public Health Information Sheet
Anemia de células falciformes
Available from the March of Dimes Birth Defects Foundation
1275 Mamaroneck Ave
White Plains, NY 10605
(888) 663-4637
www.modimes.org

Facts about Sickle Cell Anemia
Management and Therapy of Sickle Cell Anemia
Hydroxyurea in Pediatric Patients with Sickle Cell Disease
Available from the NIH/National Heart, Lung and Blood Institute Information Center
PO Box 30105
Bethesda, Md. 20824-0105
(301) 251-1222
www.nhlbi.nih.gov

National Organization for Rare Disorders, Inc. (NORD)
PO Box 8923
New Fairfield, Conn. 06812-8923
(800) 999-6673
www.nord-rdb.com

Summary of Primary Care Needs for the Child with Sickle Cell Disease

HEALTH CARE MAINTENANCE

Growth and development

Children with SCD tend to weigh less and be shorter than their peers. Weight is affected more than height, and males are affected more than females. Weight and height should be checked and plotted every 3 to 4 months.

Puberty is delayed for both sexes.

Developmental impairment varies.

Children with sickle cell anemia are encouraged to participate in physical activities and to set their own limits.

Diet

Diet should be well balanced with a generous amount of fluid; fluid intake should be increased during illness.

Increased metabolic demands require additional protein, micronutrients, and food for energy.

Folic acid supplements are encouraged.

Safety

Ingestion of narcotics could lead to respiratory depression.

Alcohol may dehydrate and potentiate narcotics.

Narcotics may impair driving or safe use of machinery.

Recreational activities that involve prolonged exposure to cold, prolonged exertion, or exposure to high altitudes should be avoided. Ice should not be used to treat injuries.

A Medic-Alert bracelet may be helpful.

Immunizations

Routine standard immunizations are recommended.

The immunogenic response to *Haemophilus influenzae* type b vaccine given at 2, 4, and 6 months of age is not reliable.

The pneumococcal vaccine should be given at 24 months, with a single booster given at 5 years.

An annual influenza vaccine is strongly recommended.

Screening

Vision: Routine screening is recommended until 10 years of age, and then annual retinal examinations are recommended to rule out sickle retinopathy. If a child sustains eye trauma he or she must be referred to an ophthalmologist to rule out increased intraocular pressure or retinal detachment.

Hearing: Routine audiologic examination is recommended.

Dental: Routine screening is recommended.

Blood pressure: Blood pressure should be measured yearly after 2 years of age. Lower pressure readings for age are expected. An increase in systolic pressure increases risk of stroke.

Hematocrit: Hematocrit is deferred because of condition-specific screening.

Urinalysis: Urinalysis is deferred because of condition-specific screening.

Tuberculosis: Routine screening is recommended.

Condition-specific screening

Hematologic screening: A CBC with differential, platelet count, reticulocyte count, and RBC smear should be checked every 6 to 12 months.

Renal function screening: BUN and creatinine levels should be checked and a urinalysis done yearly. A child should be referred to a urologist if severe hematuria or casts are found in urine.

Lead poisoning: Lead screening using the EP level is unreliable; the serum lead level must be determined.

Scoliosis: Screening should be extended to the late teens because of delayed puberty.

Cardiac function: Both ECG and ECHO should be used every 1 to 2 years after age 5 years.

Liver function: Serum liver function tests should be done yearly.

Summary of Primary Care Needs for the Child with Sickle Cell Disease—cont'd

The gallbladder should be assessed via ultrasound every 2 years after age 10 and then as necessary.

Transfused children should be tested for Hepatitis C.

COMMON ILLNESS MANAGEMENT

Differential diagnosis

Fever: *If a child is under age 5 years and has a temperature below 38.5° C,* outpatient management may be considered if the source of the fever can be identified, appropriate antibiotics are given, and follow-up is ensured.

If a child is under 5 years of age and has a temperature above 38.5° C, he or she should be promptly assessed, cultures taken, and Ceftriaxone administered IM or IV, and the child should be reassessed in 24 and 48 hours.

If a child is over 5 years of age, the child's condition, compliance with therapy, and ability to obtain follow-up determine whether or not the child should receive in- or outpatient care.

Urinary tract infections: Asymptomatic bacteriuria, urinary tract infections, and pyelonephritis are more common with SCD.

Blood cultures should be done to rule out bacteremia if a urinary tract infection is diagnosed.

Treatment must cover cultured organisms, and follow-up is essential.

Orthopedic symptoms: It is difficult to differentiate bone infarction from osteomyelitis or rheumatologic disorders.

MRI studies are used to identify bone marrow infarction in adults.

Acute gastroenteritis: Significant dehydration may occur quickly and lead to acidosis and sickling. If oral intake is inadequate, IV hydration is needed.

Abdominal pain: Abdominal pain crises may be differentiated from surgical problems by evaluating fever, hematologic changes, peristalsis, and response to symptomatic, supportive therapy.

Anemia: Hemoglobin and hematocrit levels significantly lower than baseline may reflect aplastic crisis, hyperhemolytic crisis, or splenic sequestration. Splenic sequestration may be life-threatening.

Respiratory distress: It is important that individuals are evaluated for ACS, which may be fulminant and require exchange transfusion.

Neurologic changes: Neurologic changes may indicate stroke. Rapid, thorough evaluation is critical. Exchange transfusion should be performed as quickly as possible if stroke occurs.

Drug interactions: Antihistamines, alcohol, and barbiturates may potentiate sedation with narcotics.

Diuretics and bronchodilators, which may have diuretic effects, may cause dehydration and sickling. Stool softeners are useful while on narcotics.

Developmental issues

Sleep patterns: Routine care is recommended.

Toileting: Enuresis is often a long-term issue because of a large volume of dilute urine.

Nocturia may persist.

Discipline: Expectations should be consistent, fair, and similar to those of unaffected peers and siblings.

Child care: Caregivers must be mindful of fluid requirements and the importance of maintaining normal body temperature and must be able to administer medicines.

Schooling: These children may have frequent, unpredictable absences. While at school, they need access to fluids and liberal bathroom privileges. They may participate in mainstream physical education.

Sexuality: Puberty may be delayed. Women usually have normal fertility but have some special contraceptive concerns. Men are often impotent after an episode of priapism. Genetic counseling is important.

Continued

Summary of Primary Care Needs for the Child with Sickle Cell Disease—cont'd

Transition to adulthood

Early vocational counseling is recommended.
  Insurance problems may be encountered.

SPECIAL FAMILY CONCERNS AND RESOURCES

Because SCD is genetically transmitted, there is a need for genetic counseling, as well as support for feelings of guilt and responsibility.

Support for cultural beliefs and family structure are important components of long-term care.

References

Achord JL: Gastroenterologic and hepatobiliary manifestations. In Embury et al, editors: Sickle cell disease: basic principles and clinical practice, New York, 1994, Raven Press.

Adams RJ: Neurologic complications. In Embury et al: Sickle cell disease: basic principles and clinical practice, New York, 1994, Raven Press.

Adams RJ et al: Long-term stroke risk in children with sickle cell disease screened with transcranial doppler, Ann Neurol 42(5):699-702, 1997.

Adams RJ et al: Prevention of a first stroke by transfusion in children with sickle cell anemia and abnormal results on transcranial doppler, New Engl J Med 33:5-11, 1998.

Adams-Graves P et al: Rheoth Rx (Poloxamer 188) injection for the acute painful episode of sickle cell disease: a pilot study, Blood 90(5):2041-6, 1997.

American Academy of Pediatrics: Red book: report on the committee on infectious disease, Elk Grove Village, Ill., 1997, The Academy.

American College of Obstetrics and Gynecology: Report on hormonal contraception. In American Family Physician, February 1995, 1973-1974, 1976.

Armitage K et al: Respiratory infections: which antibiotics for empiric therapy?, Patient Care for the Nurse Practitioner 2(1):30-46, 1999.

Ballas S and Saidi P: Thrombosis, megaloblastic anaemia and sickle cell disease: a unified hypothesis, Brit J Haemotol 96(4):879-80, 1997.

Bookchin RM and Virgilio LL: Pathophysiology of sickle cell anemia, Hematol/Oncol Clin North Am 10(6):1241-53, 1996.

Brinker MR et al: Bone mineral density of the lumbar spine and proximal femur is decreased in children with sickle cell anemia, Am J Orthoped 43-49, 1998.

Buchanan GR: Infection. In Embury et al, editors: Sickle cell disease: basic principles and clinical practice, 1994, Philadelphia, Raven Press.

Cackovic M et al :Leg ulceration in the sickle cell patient, J Am Coll Surg 187(3):307-309, 1998.

Castro O et al: The cooperative study of sickle cell disease: the acute chest syndrome in sickle cell disease: incidence and risk factors, Blood 84(2):643-649, 1994.

Cepeda ML et al: Mental disorders in children and adolescents with sickle cell disease, South Med J 90(3):284-287, 1997.

Charache S, Lubin B, and Reid CD: Management and therapy of sickle cell disease, NIH Publication no. 95-2117, Washington, DC, 1995, US Government Printing Office.

Charache S: Experimental therapy, Hematol/Oncol Clin North Am 10(6):1373-1382, 1996.

Chuang E et al: Autoimmune liver disease and sickle cell anemia. In Anemia: a report of three cases, J Pediatr Hematol-Oncol 19(2):159-162, 1997.

Committee on Genetics: Health supervision for children with sickle cell disease and their families: Pediatrics 98(3):467-472, 1996.

Committee on Infectious Diseases: Report of the committee on infectious diseases, Evanston, Ill., 1997, The American Academy of Pediatrics.

Covitz W: Cardiac disease. In Embury SH et al: Sickle cell disease: basic principles and clinical practice, New York, Raven Press, 1994.

Davis H et al: National trends in the mortality of children with sickle cell disease, 1968-1992, Am J Pub Health 87(8):1317-22, 1997.

DeBaun MR et al: Cognitive screening examinations for silent cerebral infarcts in sickle cell disease, Neurology 50(6):1678-82, 1998.

Earles A and Dorn L: Nursing considerations. In Embury SH et al, editors: Sickle cell disease: basic principles and clinical practice, New York, 1994, Raven Press.

Eckman JR and Platt AF: Problem oriented management of sickle syndromes, Atlanta, 1991, Georgia NIH Sickle Cell Center.

Embury SH et al, editors: Sickle cell disease: basic principles and clinical practice, New York, 1994, Raven Press.

Falletta JM et al: Discontinuing penicillin prophylaxis in children with sickle cell anemia, J Pediatr 127:685-90, 1995.

Ferrera PC, Curran CB, and Swanson H: Etiology of pediatric ischemic stroke, Am J Emerg Med 15(7):671-79, 1997.

French JA et al: Mechanisms of stroke in sickle cell disease: sickle erythrocytes decrease cerebral blood flow in rats after nitric oxide synthase inhibition, Blood 89(12):4591-4599, 1997.

Gentry B and Dancer J: Screening the speech of young patients with sickle cell disease, Perception and Motor Skills 84:662, 1997.

Groce NE and Zola IK: Multiculturalism, chronic illness, and disability, Pediatrics 91(5 part 2):1048-1055, 1993.

Hakim LS, Hashmat AI, and Macchia RJ: Priapism. In Embury SH et al, et al: Sickle cell disease: basic principles and clinical practice, New York, 1994, Raven Press.

Halvorson DJ et al: Sickle cell disease and tonsillectomy: preoperative management and post-operative complications, Arch Otolaryng Head Neck Surg 123:689, 1997.

Hatcher RA: Contraceptive technology, ed 16, New York, 1994, Irvinton Press.

Hockenberry M and Coody D, editors: Pediatric oncology and hematology: perspectives on care, St Louis, 1986, Mosby.

Howlett C et al: The role of CT and MR in imaging the complications of sickle cell disease, Clin Radiol 52(11):821-9, 1997.

Johnson RB: Folic acid: new dimensions of an old friendship, Adv Pediatr 44:236-238, 1997.

Kelly P et al: Umbilical cord blood stem cells: application for the treatment of patients with hemoglobinopathies, J Pediatr 130(5):695-703, 1997.

King KE and Ness PM: Treating anemia, Hematol/Oncol Clin North Am 10(6):1305-19, 1996.

Lee EJ et al: A comparison study of children with sickle cell disease and their nondiseased siblings on hopelessness, depression and perceived competence, J Adv Nurs 25:79-86, 1997.

Lee SJ, Churchill WH, and Bridges KR: Bone marrow infarcts of severe atypical pain in sickle cell crisis: diagnosis by magnetic resonance imaging and treatment with exchange transfusion. Abstract presented at the 20th Annual Meeting of the National Sickle Cell Disease Program, Boston, March 18-21, 1995.

Martin JJ and Moore GP: Pearls, pitfalls, and updates for pain management, Emerg Clin North Am 15(2):399-415, 1997.

McCune SL et al: Recombinant human hemoglobins designed for gene therapy of sickle cell disease, Proc Nat Acad Sci U S A 91(21):9852-6, 1994.

Mentzer WC et al: Availability of related donors for bone marrow transplantation in sickle cell anemia, Am J Pediatr Hematol Oncol 16(1):27-29, 1994.

Miller DR and Baehner RL, editors: Blood diseases of infancy and childhood, St Louis, 1990, Mosby.

Modege O and Ifenu SA: Growth retardation in homozygous sickle cell disease: role of caloric intake and possible gender related differences, Am J Hematol 44:149-154, 1993.

Ohene-Frempong K and Smith-Whitley K: Use of hydroxyurea in children with sickle cell disease: what comes next?, Sem Hematol 34(suppl. 3):30-41, 1997.

Ohene-Frempong K and Weiner SJ et al: The Co-operative study of sickle cell disease cerebrovascular accidents in sickle cell disease: rate and risk factors, Blood 91(1):288-94, 1998.

Pearson HA: Pharmacologic manipulation of fetal hemoglobin levels in sickle cell diseases and thalassemia: promise and reality, Adv Pediatr 43:309-34, 1996.

Pegelow CH et al: Natural history of blood pressure in sickle cell disease: risks for strokes and death associated with relative hypertension in sickle cell anemia, Am J Med 102(2):171-7, 1997.

Platt OS: The febrile child with sickle cell disease: a pediatricians quandry, J Pediatr 130:693-694, 1997.

Powars DR: Natural history of disease: the first two decades. In Embury SH et al, editors: Sickle cell disease: basic principles and clinical practice, New York, 1994, Raven Press.

Powars DR: Natural history of sickle cell disease—the first 10 years, Sem Hematol 12:267-281, 1975.

Powars DR et al: Beta-S gene cluster haplotype modulate hematologic and hemorrheologic expression in sickle cell anemia: use in predicting clinical severity, Am J Pediatr Hematol Oncol 16(1):55-61, 1994.

Powars D et al: Cerebral vasculopathy in sickle cell anemia: diagnostic contribution of positron emission tomography, Blood 93(1):71-9, 1999.

Prasad AS: Malnutrition in sickle cell disease patients, Am J Clin Nutr 66(2):423-4, 1997.

Rao R and Kramer L: Stress and coping among mothers of infants with a sickle cell condition, Childrens Healthcare 22:169-188, 1993.

Rajkumar K et al: Elevated levels of erythrocyte protoporphyrin (FEP) in children with sickle cell disease in the absence of lead poisoning or iron deficiency. Abstract presented at the 20th Annual Meeting of the National Sickle Cell Disease Program, Boston, March 18-21, 1995.

Richard H and Burlew K: Academic performance among children with sickle cell disease: setting minimum standards for comparison groups, Psychol Rep 81:27-34, 1997.

Rodgers GP: Pharmacologic modulation of fetal hemoglobin. In Embury SH et al, editors: Sickle cell disease: basic principles and clinical practice, New York, 1994, Raven Press.

Rogers ZR: Hydroxyurea therapy for diverse pediatric population with sickle cell disease, Sem Hematol July: 34(suppl 3):22-29, 1997.

Rothschild BM et al: Microfoci or avascular necrosis in sickle cell anemia: pathophysiology of the dot dash pattern, Clin Exp Rheumatol 15:663-666, 1997.

Scott-Conner CEH and Brunson CD: Surgery and anesthesia. In Embury SH et al, editors: Sickle cell disease: basic principles and clinical practice, New York, 1994, Raven Press.

Secundy MG: Psychosocial issues: unanswered questions in the use of bone marrow transplantation for treatment of hemoglobinopathies, Am J Pediatr Hematol Oncol 16(1):76-79, 1994.

Serjeant GR: Natural history and determinants of clinical severity of sickle cell disease, Curr Op Hematol 2:103-108, 1995.

Shapiro B and Ballas SK: The acute painful episode. In Embury SH et al, editors: Sickle cell disease: basic principles and clinical practice, New York, 1994, Raven Press.

Singhal A et al: Is there an energy deficiency in homozygous sickle cell disease?, Am J Clin Nutr 66(2):386-90, 1997.

Steinburg MH, et al: Cellular effects of hydroxyurea in Hbg SC disease, Brit J Haematol 98(4):838-44, 1997.

Steinburg MH and Embury SH: Natural history: overview. In Embury SH et al: Sickle cell disease: basic principles and clinical practice, New York, 1994, Raven Press.

Steinberg MH and Mohandas N: Laboratory values. In Embury SH et al, editor: Sickle cell disease: basic principles and clinical practice, New York, 1994, Raven Press.

Sterling Y et al: American families with chronically ill children: oversights and insights, J Pediatr Nurs 12(5):292-300, 1997.

Styles L and Vinchinsky E: New therapies and approaches to transfusion in sickle cell disease in children, Curr Op Pediatr 9:41-45, 1997.

Vernocchi L et al: Combined schedule of 7-valent pneumococcal conjugate vaccine followed by 23-valent pneumococcal vaccine in children and young adults with sickle cell disease, J Pediatr 133(2):275-278, 1998.

Vermylen C and Cornu G: Hematopoietic stem cell transplantation for sickle cell anemia, Curr Op Hematol 4:377-80, 1997.

Vichinsky EP: Comprehensive care in sickle cell disease: its impact on morbidity and mortality, Sem Hematol 28(3):220-226, 1991.

Vichinsky EP: Transfusion therapy. In Embury SH et al, editors: Sickle cell disease: basic principles and clinical practice, New York, 1994, Raven Press, chap 53.

Vichinsky EP: Hydroxyurea in children: present and future, Sem Hematol 34(suppl 3):22-29, 1997a.

Vinchinsky EP et al: A comparison of conservative and aggressive transfusion regimes in the perioperative management of sickle cell disease, New Eng J Med 333:206-213, 1995.

Wang WC et al: Developmental screening in young children with sickle cell disease. Results of a cooperative study, Am J Pediatr Hematol Oncol 15(1):87-91, 1993.

Wang WC et al: High risk of recurrent stroke after discontinuance of 5 to 12 years of transfusion therapy in patients with sickle cell disease, J Pediatr 118:377-382, 1991.

Westerman MP et al: Assessment of painful episode frequency in sickle cell disease, Am J Hematol 54(3):183-188, 1997.

Wilimas JA et al: A randomized study of outpatient treatment with ceftriazone for selected febrile children with sickle cell disease, New Engl J Med 329:472-476, 1993.

Wong DL: Nursing care of infants and children, ed 5, St Louis, 1995, Mosby.

Wong, W-Y et al: Renal failure in sickle cell anemia, Hematol/Oncol Clin N Am 10(6):1321-31, 1996.

Yaster M et al: Epidural analgesia in the management of severe vasoocclusive sickle cell crisis, Pediatrics 93(2):310-315, 1994.

Photo Credits

The editors wish to thank the numerous contributors who submitted photos for chapter opener photos as well as the following:

Photo Disc: Chapter opener photos for Chapters 5, 11, 18, 21, 24, 30, 32, and 33.

Wong DL et al: Whaley and Wong's Nursing Care of Infants and Children, ed 6, St Louis, 1999, Mosby: Chapter opener photo for Chapter 6.

Ratliffe KT: Clinical Pediatric Physical Therapy, St Louis, 1998, Mosby: Chapter opener photos for Chapters 12, 14, and 20.

Index

A

AAMR Adaptive Behavior Scale, 33-34
Abdominal pain
  in cystic fibrosis, 416
  in hemophilia, 233
  in inflammatory bowel disease, 584,
    598-599
  in sickle cell disease, 828
  in transplant recipient, 694
Absence seizure, 478
Absolute neutrophil count, 282
Acceleration head injury, 514
Acculturation, 69-70
Acesulfame, 434
Acetaminophen
  for cancer pain, 296
  before DTP vaccine, 487
  for joint bleeding-associated pain, 227
Acetazolamide, 565
Acetylsalicylate acid, 611
Achenbach's Child Behavior Check List,
  638
Acid-base abnormalities in chronic renal
  failure, 779
Acquired immunodeficiency syndrome,
  538-559
  bleeding disorders and, 229, 231
  clinical manifestations of, 540-543
  common illness management in, 551-
    553
  developmental issues in, 553-555
  diagnosis and management advances
    in, 544
  diet and, 548
  etiology of, 538-540
  failure to thrive in, 544-545, 546
  fungal infections in, 547
  growth and development and, 547-548
  HIV/AIDS Bureau, 135
  immunizations and, 548-550
  incidence of, 540
  neurologic manifestations of, 545-546
  opportunistic infections in, 546
  pancytopenia in, 546-547
  prenatal and perinatal drug exposure,
    547
  prenatal cocaine exposure and, 762
  primary care needs summary, 556-558
  prognosis in, 547
  pulmonary disease in, 546

Acquired immunodeficiency syndrome—
    cont'd
  safety issues in, 548
  screening and, 550-551
  special family concerns and resources,
    555-556
  treatment, 543-544
ACTeRS, 638
Actinomycin; see Dactinomycin
Activated factor IX complex
    concentrates, 221
Activity
  asthma and, 176
  autism and, 194
  chronic renal failure and, 792
  congenital heart disease and, 392-393
  cystic fibrosis and, 419
  diabetes mellitus and, 438-439
  epilepsy and, 486-487
  hydrocephalus and, 571, 576-577
  inflammatory bowel disease and, 595
  intolerance in bronchopulmonary
    dysplasia, 244
  juvenile rheumatoid arthritis and, 613
Acute adrenal insufficiency, 359, 365
Acute chest syndrome, 818-819, 828
Acute gastroenteritis, 828
Acute lymphoblastic leukemia, 267
  in Down syndrome, 452
  survival rates, 290
Acute megakaryoblastic leukemia, 452
Acute myelogenous leukemia, 267
  alkylating agent-induced, 283
  survival rates, 290
Acyanotic heart disease, 374, 375
Acyclovir, 295
Adaptive behavior screening tools, 33-34
Adaptive equipment
  after head injury, 524
  for cerebral palsied child, 310-311
  in juvenile rheumatoid arthritis, 619
  in myelodysplasia, 663, 669
Adderall, 640, 641
Adolescence, 141-148
  cognitive ability and, 145-146
  developmental parameters in, 143-144
  family factors that moderate transition,
    145
  peer relationships and, 147
  problem solving and autonomy in,
    146-147

Adolescence—cont'd
  self-competence and, 146
  sexuality and, 147-148
Adolescent
  asthma and, 185
  with attention-deficit hyperactivity
    disorder, 645-646
  autistic, 200
  with bronchopulmonary dysplasia, 253
  with chronic renal failure, 796-799
  congenital heart disease and, 394
  developmental tasks of, 23
  diabetes mellitus and, 428-429
  human immunodeficiency virus and,
    539-540
  leading causes of death, 6, 7
  noncompliance in organ transplant
    therapy, 699
  role in treatment decision making,
    109-110, 112
  transition into adulthood, 140-161
    access to health care as adult, 152
    cognitive ability and, 145-146
    coordination of transition planning,
      157-159
    family factors in, 145
    health insurance issues, 152-153
    home to community living in, 156-
      157
    peer relationships and, 147
    planning for health care, 148-152
    problem solving and autonomy in,
      146-147
    school system and, 153-156
    self-competence and, 146
    sexuality and, 147-148
    understanding transition, 142-144
  understanding of medical procedures
    and treatments, 27
Adrenal cortex, 352, 353
Adrenal insufficiency
  in congenital adrenal hyperplasia, 359,
    365
  corticosteroid-related, 589
Adrenal medulla, 352
Adrenalectomy, 359
Adrenocorticotropic hormone
  congenital adrenal hyperplasia and,
    352, 354
  daily blood pressure monitoring during
    therapy, 488
  for infantile spasm, 482, 486